The GALE ENCYCLOPEDIA of GENETIC DISORDERS

SECOND EDITION

The GALE ENCYCLOPEDIA of GENETIC DISORDERS

SECOND EDITION

VOLUME

1

A-L

BRIGHAM NARINS, EDITOR

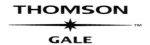

THOMSON

GALE

Detroit • New York • San Francisco • San Diego • New Haven, Conn. • Waterville, Maine • London • Munich

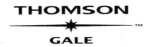

The Gale Encyclopedia of Genetic Disorders, Second Edition

Project Editor
Brigham Narins

Editorial
Erin Watts

Editorial Support Services
Andrea Lopeman

Indexing Services
Synapse

Rights Acquisitions Management
Timothy Sisler, Susan Rudolph

Imaging and Multimedia
Randy Basset, Lezlie Light, Michael Logusz, Dean Dauphinais

Product Design
Michelle DiMercurio, Tracey Rowens

Composition and Electronic Prepress
Evi Seoud, Mary Beth Trimper

Manufacturing
Wendy Blurton, Dorothy Maki

LIBRARY OF CONGRESS CATALOGING-IN-PUBLICATION DATA

The Gale encyclopedia of genetic disorders / Brigham Narins, editor.– 2nd ed.
   p. cm.
   Includes bibliographical references and index.
   ISBN 1-4144-0365-8 (set : hardcover : alk. paper) – ISBN 1-4144-0366-6 (v. 1 : alk. paper) – ISBN 1-4144-0367-4 (v. 2 : alk. paper)
   1. Medical genetics–Encyclopedias. 2. Diseases–Encyclopedias.
   [DNLM: 1. Genetics, Medical–Encyclopedias–English.
2. Genetic Diseases, Inborn–
Encyclopedias–English. 3. Genetic Predisposition to Disease–
Encyclopedias–English.
QZ 13 G515 2005] I. Title: Encyclopedia of genetic disorders. II. Title:
Genetic disorders.
III. Narins, Brigham, 1962-

   RB155.5.G35 2005
   616'.042'03–dc22
                                                    2005007599

This title is also available as an e-book.
ISBN 1-4144-0473-5 (set)
Contact your Gale sales representative for ordering information.
ISBN 1-4144-0365-8 (set)
1-4144-0366-6 (Vol. 1)
1-4144-0367-4 (Vol. 2)
Printed in Canada
10 9 8 7 6 5 4 3 2 1

CONTENTS

LIST OF ENTRIES

A

22q13 deletion syndrome
Aarskog syndrome
Aase syndrome
Abetalipoproteinemia
Acardia
Accutane embryopathy
Achondrogenesis
Achondroplasia
Achoo syndrome
Acrocallosal syndrome
Acromegaly
Adams-Oliver syndrome
Adrenoleukodystrophy
Aicardi syndrome
Alagille syndrome
Albinism
Alcoholism
Alkaptonuria
Alpha-1 antitrypsin
Alpha-thalassemia X-linked mental
   retardation syndrome
Alzheimer disease
Amelia
Amniocentesis
Amyoplasia
Amyotrophic lateral sclerosis
Androgen insensitivity syndrome
Anemia, sideroblastic X-linked
Anencephaly
Angelman syndrome
Ankylosing spondylitis
Apert syndrome
Arginase deficiency
Arnold-Chiari malformation
Arthrogryposis multiplex congenita
Arthropathy-camptodactyly syndrome

Asperger syndrome
Asplenia
Asthma
Ataxia-telangiectasia
Attention deficit hyperactivity disorder
Autism
Azorean disease

B

Bardet-Biedl syndrome
Batten disease
Beals syndrome
Beare-Stevenson cutis gyrata syndrome
Beckwith-Wiedemann syndrome
Beta thalassemia
Bicuspid aortic valve
Biotinidase deficiency
Bipolar disorder
Bloom syndrome
Blue rubber bleb nevus syndrome
Brachydactyly
Branchiootorenal syndrome
Breast cancer
Bruton agammaglobulinemia

C

Cadasil
Campomelic dysplasia
Canavan disease
Cancer
Cardiofaciocutaneous syndrome
Carnitine palmitoyltransferase
   deficiency
Carpenter syndrome

Caudal dysplasia
Celiac disease
Central core disease
Cerebral palsy
Charcot-Marie-Tooth disease
Charge syndrome
Chediak-Higashi syndrome
Chondrodysplasia punctata
Chondrosarcoma
Choroideremia
Chromosomal abnormalities
Chromosome
Cleft lip and palate
Cleidocranial dysplasia
Clubfoot
Cockayne syndrome
Coffin-Lowry syndrome
Coffin-Siris syndrome
Cohen syndrome
Coloboma
Color blindness
Cone-rod dystrophy
Congenital adrenal hyperplasia
Congenital heart disease
Congenital hypothyroid syndrome
Conjoined twins
Corneal dystrophy
Cornelia de Lange syndrome
Corpus callosum agenesis
Costello syndrome
Crane-Heise syndrome
Craniosynostosis
Cri du chat syndrome
Crouzon syndrome
Cystic fibrosis
Cystinosis
Cystinuria

PLEASE READ—IMPORTANT INFORMATION

The *Gale Encyclopedia of Genetic Disorders* is a medical reference product designed to inform and educate readers about a wide variety of disorders, conditions, treatments, and diagnostic tests. Thomson Gale believes the product to be comprehensive, but not necessarily definitive. It is intended to supplement, not replace, consultation with a physician or other health care practitioner. While Thomson Gale has made substantial efforts to provide information that is accurate, comprehensive, and up-to-date, Thomson Gale makes no representations or warranties of any kind, including without limitation, warranties of merchantability or fitness for a particular purpose, nor does it guarantee the accuracy, comprehensiveness, or timeliness of the information contained in this product. Readers should be aware that the universe of medical knowledge is constantly growing and changing, and that differences of medical opinion exist among authorities. They are also advised to seek professional diagnosis and treatment for any medical condition, and to discuss information obtained from this book with their health care provider.

INTRODUCTION

The *Gale Encyclopedia of Genetic Disorders* is a unique and invaluable source for information regarding diseases and conditions of a genetic origin. This collection of over 430 entries provides in-depth coverage of disorders ranging from the exceedingly rare to the very well-known. In addition, several non-disorder entries have been included to facilitate understanding of common genetic concepts and practices such as Chromosomes, Genetic counseling, and Genetic testing.

This encyclopedia avoids medical jargon and uses language that laypersons can understand, while providing the thorough coverage of each disorder that medical professionals will also find beneficial. The *Gale Encyclopedia of Genetic Disorders* fills a gap between basic consumer health resources, such as single-volume family medical guides, and highly technical professional materials.

Each entry discussing a particular disorder follows a standardized format that provides information at a glance. The rubrics used are:

- Definition
- Description
- Genetic profile
- Demographics
- Signs and symptoms
- Diagnosis
- Treatment and management
- Prognosis
- Resources
- Key terms

INCLUSION CRITERIA

A preliminary list of diseases and disorders was compiled from a wide variety of sources, including professional medical guides and textbooks, as well as consumer guides and encyclopedias. The advisory board, made up of seven medical and genetic experts, evaluated the topics and made suggestions for inclusion. Final selection of topics to include was made by the advisory board in conjunction with Thomson Gale editors.

ABOUT THE CONTRIBUTORS

The essays were compiled by experienced medical writers, primarily genetic counselors, physicians, and other health care professionals. The advisors reviewed the completed essays to insure they are appropriate, up-to-date, and medically accurate.

HOW TO USE THIS BOOK

The *Gale Encyclopedia of Genetic Disorders* has been designed with ready reference in mind.

- Straight **alphabetical arrangement** of topics allows users to locate information quickly.
- **Bold-faced terms** direct the reader to related articles.
- **Cross-references** placed throughout the encyclopedia point readers to where information on subjects without entries may be found.
- A list of **key terms** is provided where appropriate to define unfamiliar terms or concepts. Additional terms may be found in the **glossary** at the back of volume 2.
- The **Resources** section directs readers to additional sources of medical information on a topic.
- Valuable **contact information** for organizations and support groups is included with each entry. The appendix contains an extensive list of organizations arranged in alphabetical order.
- A comprehensive **general index** guides readers to all topics and persons mentioned in the text.

GRAPHICS

The *Gale Encyclopedia of Genetic Disorders* contains over 200 full-color illustrations, including photos and pedigree charts. A complete **symbol guide** for the pedigree charts can be found at the beginning of each volume.

ACKNOWLEDGEMENTS

The editor would like to thank the following individuals for their assistance with the *Gale Encyclopedia of Genetic Disorders*: Deepti Babu, MS CGC, Dawn Jacob, MS, and Jennifer Neil, MS CGC, for the creation of the pedigree charts found in entries throughout the main body; K. Lee and Brenda Lerner for their assistance in compiling and reviewing most of the non-disorder entries in this encyclopedia; and to Kyung Kalasky, Beth Kapes, Monique Laberge, PhD, and Lisa Nielsen for their extensive assistance with the final phase of manuscript preparation.

R. Curtis ·Rogers, MD, and William K. Scott, MD, provided invaluable assistance in the preparation of the second edition. Connie Clyde once again contributed outstanding copyediting and good humor during manuscript preparation. And Scott Polzin and Maria Basile both wrote many excellent entries under unique and difficult circumstances—the editor extends special thanks to them and great appreciation to all of the contributors. Finally, Mr. Polzin wishes to dedicate his articles in this and the previous edition to the memory of Betty Wilson, RN.

ADVISORY BOARD

An advisory board comprised of genetic specialists from a variety of backgrounds provided invaluable assistance in the formulation of this encyclopedia. This advisory board performed a myriad of duties, from defining the scope of coverage to reviewing individual entries for accuracy and accessibility. We would therefore like to express our sincere thanks and appreciation for all of their contributions.

CONTRIBUTORS

Christine Adamec
Medical Writer
Palm Bay, FL

Margaret Alic, PhD
Science Writer
Eastsound, WA

Lisa Andres, MS, CGC
Certified Genetic Counselor
Medical Writer
San Jose, CA

Greg Annussek
Medical Writer/Editor
New York, NY

Sharon Aufox, MS, CGC
Genetic Counselor
Rockford Memorial Hospital
Rockford, IL

Deepti Babu, MS, CGC
Genetic Counselor
Edmonton, Alberta, Canada

Kristin Baker Niendorf, MS, CGC
Genetic Counselor
Massachusetts General Hospital
Boston, MA

Maria Basile, PhD
Neuropharmacologist
Newark, NJ

Carin Lea Beltz, MS, CGC
Genetic Counselor and Program Director
The Center for Genetic Counseling
Indianapolis, IN

Abdel Hakim Ben Nasr, PhD
Medical Writer
Dept. of Genetics

Yale University School of
    Medicine
New Haven, CT

Tanya Bivins, BS
Nursing Student
Madonna University
Livonia, MI

Bethanne Black
Medical Writer
Atlanta, GA

Jennifer Bojanowski, MS, CGC
Genetic Counselor
Children's Hospital Oakland
Oakland, CA

Shelly Q. Bosworth, MS, CGC
Genetic Counselor
Eugene, OR

Michelle L. Brandt
Medical Writer
San Francisco, CA

Dawn Cardeiro, MS, CGC
Genetic Counselor
Fairfield, PA

Suzanne M. Carter, MS, CGC
Senior Genetic Counselor
Division of Reproductive Genetics
Montefiore Medical Center
Bronx, NY

Pamela E. Cohen, MS, CGC
Genetic Counselor
San Francisco, CA

Randy Colby, MD
Senior Medical Genetics Fellow
Greenwood Genetic Center
Greenwood, SC

Sonja Eubanks, MS, CGC
Genetic Counselor
Genetic Counseling Program
University of North Carolina at
    Greensboro
Greensboro, NC

David B. Everman, MD
Clinical Geneticist
Greenwood Genetic Center
Greenwood, SC

L. Fleming Fallon, Jr., MD, DrPH
Associate Professor of Public Health
Bowling Green State University
Bowling Green, OH

Antonio Farina, MD, PhD
Medical Writer
Dept. of Embryology
University of Bologna
Italy

Kathleen Fergus, MS, CGC
Genetic Counselor
San Francisco, CA

Lisa Fratt
Medical Writer
Ashland, WI

Sallie B. Freeman, PhD
Assistant Professor
Dept. of Genetics
Emory University
Atlanta, GA

Mary E. Freivogel, MS, CGC
Genetic Counselor
Denver, CO

Rebecca Frey, PhD
Consulting Editor
East Rock Institute
Yale University
New Haven, CT

Sandra Galeotti, MS
Medical Writer
Sau Paulo, Brazil

Avis L. Gibons
Genetic Counseling Intern
UCI Medical Center
Orange, CA

Taria Greenberg, MHS
Medical Writer
Houston, TX

David E. Greenberg, MD
Medicine Resident
Baylor College of Medicine
Houston, TX

Benjamin M. Greenberg
Medical Student
Baylor College of Medicine
Houston, TX

Farris Farid Gulli, MD
Plastic and Reconstructive Surgery
Farmington Hills, MI

Judy C. Hawkins, MS
Certified Genetic Counselor
Department of Pediatrics
University of Texas Medical
    Branch
Galveston, TX

David Helwig
Medical Writer
London, ON, Canada

Edward J. Hollox, PhD
Medical Writer
Institute of Genetics, Queen's
    Medical Center
University of Nottingham
Nottingham, England

Katherine S. Hunt, MS
Genetic Counselor
University of New Mexico Health
    Sciences Center
Albuquerque, NM

Cindy Hunter, MS, CGC
Genetic Counselor
Medical Genetics Department
Indiana University School of
    Medicine
Indianapolis, IN

Kevin Hwang, MD
Medical Writer
Morristown, NJ

Holly A. Ishmael, MS, CGC
Genetic Counselor
The Children's Mercy Hospital
Kansas City, MO

Dawn A. Jacob, MS
Genetic Counselor
Obstetrix Medical Group of Texas
Fort Worth, TX

Paul A. Johnson
Medical Writer
San Diego, CA

Melissa Knopper
Medical Writer
Chicago, IL

Terri A. Knutel, MS, CGC
Genetic Counselor
Chicago, IL

Karen Krajewski, MS, CGC
Genetic Counselor
Assistant Professor of Neurology
Wayne State University
Detroit, MI

Sonya Kunkle
Medical Writer
Baltimore, MD

Dawn Jacob Laney, MS, CGC
Genetic Counselor
Department of Human Genetics
Emory University
Atlanta, GA

Renée Laux, MS
Certified Genetic Counselor
Eastern Virginia Medical School
Norfolk, VA

Marshall Letcher, MA
Science Writer
Vancouver, BC

Christian L. Lorson, PhD
Assistant Professor
Dept. of Biology
Arizona State University
Tempe, AZ

Maureen Mahon, BSc, MFS
Medical Writer
Calgary, AB

Nicole Mallory, MS
Medical Student
Wayne State University
Detroit, MI

Sajid Merchant, BSc, MS, CGC
Genetic Counselor
Department of Medical Genetics
University of Alberta Hospital
Edmonton, Alberta, Canada

Ron C. Michaelis, PhD, FACMG
Research Scientist
Greenwood Genetic Center
Greenwood, SC

Bilal Nasser, MSc
Senior Medical Student
Universidad Iberoamericana
Santo Domingo, Domincan
    Republic

Jennifer E. Neil, MS, CGC
Genetic Counselor
Long Island, NY

Deborah L. Nurmi, MS
Public Health Researcher
Atlanta, GA

Pamela J. Nutting, MS, CGC
Senior Genetic Counselor
Phoenix Genetics Program
University of Arizona
Phoenix, AZ

**Marianne F. O'Connor, MT
    (ASCP), MPH**
Medical Writer
Farmington Hills, MI

Barbara Pettersen, MS, CGC
Genetic Counselor
Genetic Counseling of Central
    Oregon
Bend, OR

Toni Pollin, MS, CGC
Research Analyst
Division of Endocrinology, Diabetes, and Nutrition
University of Maryland School of Medicine
Baltimore, MD

Scott J. Polzin, MS, CGC
Medical Writer
Certified Genetics Counselor
Buffalo Grove, IL

Nada Quercia, Msc, CCGC, CGC
Genetic Counselor
Division of Clinical and Metabolic Genetics
The Hospital for Sick Children
Toronto, ON, Canada

Cristi Radford, BS(s)
Medical Writer
Genetic Counseling Student
University of South Carolina
Columbia, SC

Robert Ramirez, BS
Medical Student
University of Medicine & Dentistry of New Jersey
Stratford, NJ

Julianne Remington
Medical Writer
Portland, OR

Jennifer Roggenbuck, MS, CGC
Genetic Counselor
Hennepin County Medical Center
Minneapolis, MN

Edward R. Rosick, DO, MPH, MS
University Physician/Clinical Assistant Professor
The Pennsylvania State University
University Park, PA

Judyth Sassoon, ARCS, PhD
Medical Writer
Dept. of Chemistry and Biochemistry

University of Bern
Bern, Switzerland

Jason S. Schliesser, DC
Chiropractor
Holland Chiropractic, Inc.
Holland, OH

Charles E. Schwartz, PhD
Director of Center for Molecular Studies
JC Self Research Center
Greenwood Genetic Center
Greenwood, SC

Laurie H. Seaver, MD
Clinical Geneticist
Greenwood Genetic Center
Greenwood, SC

Nina B. Sherak, MS, CHES
Health Educator/Medical Writer
Wilmington, DE

Genevieve Slomski, PhD
Freelance writer/editor
New Britain, CT

Java O. Solis, MS
Medical Writer
Decatur, GA

Amie Stanley, MS
Genetic Counselor
University of Florida
Gainesville, FL

Constance K. Stein, PhD
Director of Cytogenetics
Assistant Director of Molecular Diagnostics
SUNY Upstate Medical University
Syracuse, NY

Kevin M. Sweet, MS, CGC
Cancer Genetic Counselor
James Cancer Hospital
Ohio State University
Columbus, OH

Catherine Tesla, MS, CGC
Senior Associate, Faculty
Dept. of Pediatrics, Division of

Medical Genetics
Emory University School of Medicine
Atlanta, GA

Oren Traub, MD, PhD
Resident Physician
Dept. of Internal Medicine
University of Washington Affiliated Hospitals
Seattle, WA

Amy Vance, MS, CGC
Genetic Counselor
GeneSage, Inc.
San Francisco, CA

Brian Veillette, BS
Medical Writer
Auburn Hills, MI

Chitra Venkatasubramanian, MBBS, MD
Fellow in Stroke/Neurocritical Care
Stanford Stroke Center
Stanford University
Palo Alto, CA

Linnea E. Wahl, MS
Medical Writer
Berkeley, CA

Ken R. Wells
Freelance Writer
Laguna Hills, CA

Jennifer F. Wilson, MS
Science Writer
Haddonfield, NJ

Philip J. Young, PhD
Research Fellow
Dept. of Biology
Arizona State University
Tempe, AZ

Michael V. Zuck, PhD
Medical Writer
Boulder, CO

SYMBOL GUIDE FOR PEDIGREE CHARTS

Pedigree charts are visual tools for documenting biological relationships in families and the presence of disorders. Using these charts, medical professionals such as geneticists and genetic counselors can analyze the genetic risk in a family for a particular trait or condition by tracking which individuals have the disorder and determining how it is inherited.

A standard set of symbols has been established for use in creating pedigree charts. Those found within the body of several entries in the encyclopedia follow the symbol guide explained on the next page. The exact style and amount of information presented on the chart varies for each family and depends on the trait or condition under investigation. Typically, only data that is directly related to the disorder being analyzed will be included. For more information, see the ''Pedigree analysis'' entry in the second volume.

Symbol Guide for Pedigree Charts

☐	Male	△	Miscarriage
○	Female		Pregnancy terminated due to affected condition
■	Affected male		Elective termination of pregnancy
●	Affected female		
☐•	Carrier male	♀	Female with no children by choice
⊙	Carrier female		Female with no children due to medical infertility
▨	Deceased male		Identical twin females
⊘	Deceased female		Fraternal twin females
[☐]	Male adopted into a family	☐═○	Consanguineous relationship
[○]	Female adopted into a family	☐╫○	Relationship no longer exists
◇	Gender not specified	?☐	Unknown family history
◇P	Pregnancy	d.79y	Died at 79 years
☐4	Four males	dx.41y	Diagnosed at 41 years
○3	Three females		Relationship line
			Line of descent
			Sibship line
			Individual line

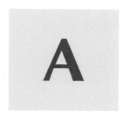

A

22q11 deletion syndrome *see* **Deletion 22q11 syndrome**

22q13 deletion syndrome

Definition

The 22q13 deletion syndrome is a microdeletion syndrome. It results from missing a small segment of genetic material on the end of the long arm (q) of **chromosome** 22. The condition was first described in the literature in the 1980s. Individuals with the condition have a variety of features. The most common features are developmental delay, delayed or absent speech, and weak muscles (also known as hypotonia or low muscle tone).

Description

In 2004, the 22q13 Deletion Syndrome Foundation voted to give the condition a second name. They named it Phelan-McDermid syndrome. Phelan and McDermid are the names of the doctors known for their research on 22q13 deletion syndrome. The condition can be called by either name.

The 22q13 deletion syndrome results from a chromosome difference. People typically have 23 pairs of chromosomes. The first 22 chromosomes are called autosomes and are numbered one to 22. The last pair are the sex chromosomes, identified as X and Y. Each chromosome has a long part (q) and a short part (p). Packed in the chromosomes are genes, which are important because they determine how a person grows, develops, and functions. They also determine physical features of an individual, such as eye color and the shape of a person's face. When a person's genes are missing or not working properly, the result can be health problems, learning difficulties, and/or physical differences.

Individuals with 22q13 deletion syndrome are missing part of a chromosome. The syndrome's name provides the location of the missing part. It is on the long arm of chromosome 22 at the very end (location q13). Since the 22q13 region contains genes, people missing it do not have all the proper instructions for development. As a result, they have similar learning difficulties, physical differences, and behavior problems.

Genetic profile

The 22q13 deletion syndrome is caused by an absence of genetic material on chromosome 22. As of 2005, the specific genes involved in 22q13 deletion syndrome had not been identified. However, several candidate genes had been located to the 22q13 region, including SHANK3, ACR, and RABL2B. Researchers believe an absence of SHANK3 may cause the neurological features of mental retardation and speech delay.

When a person is diagnosed with 22q13 deletion syndrome, it is usually the first time it has been seen in the family. For most parents, the chance of having a second child with the condition is low. In some families, however, an increased risk exists for having a second child with the syndrome. In these families, a parent usually has a balanced translocation, which means that parent has the correct amount of chromosome material, but the material is rearranged. The rearrangement usually does not cause problems in the parent. However, when the parent has a child, the child may receive extra or missing pieces of chromosome material.

If a parent has a balanced translocation involving the 22q13 region, he or she may be at risk of having multiple children with the syndrome. Therefore, parents of a child with 22q13 deletion syndrome should consider testing for balanced translocations. Parents who are found to carry a translocation may decide to pursue prenatal diagnosis for future pregnancies. If an individual with 22q13 deletion syndrome had children, he or she would have a 50% chance of having a child with the condition and a 50% chance of having a child without the condition. As of 2005, there were no known cases of an individual with the condition having children.

Demographics

The 22q13 deletion syndrome affects males, females, and all ethnicities. It is not known how many people have 22q13 deletion syndrome. The syndrome is considered rare and researchers believe it is often underdiagnosed.

Signs and symptoms

Individuals with 22q13 deletion syndrome have a variety of symptoms. In addition, the severity of each feature ranges from mild to severe. Therefore, two people with the syndrome may have very different characteristics. The characteristics most commonly seen are developmental delay, low muscle tone, speech difficulties (lack of speech or absence of speech), and advanced growth. Many individuals also have behavior differences, including autistic-like behavior and/or excessive chewing.

In addition, some children learn a specific skill and lose it. The medical term for the loss of a skill is regression. When children with the condition lose a skill, it is usually in the area of speech. Other characteristics that are not as common in the syndrome, but have been reported include drooping eyelids, large head, webbing between the second and third toes, large hands, lack of sweat, seizures, flaky toenails, and different shaped ears, skull, and/or forehead.

Diagnosis

The diagnosis is made by determining the 22q13 chromosome region is missing. Sometimes the deletion of chromosome 22 can be seen by a routine chromosome analysis. Often, however, the deletion is difficult to see and a special test called **Fluorescence In Situ Hybridization** (FISH) is used. FISH is a molecular cytogenetic technique. It utilizes fluorescent probes to examine the presence or location of specific chromosomes, chromosome regions, or genes. Researchers can determine the presence and location of the probes by looking at them with a microscope. The light causes the fluorescent tag on the probe to glow.

For 22q13 deletion syndrome, a fluorescent probe specific for region 13 on the long arm of chromosome 22 is used. Since people with 22q13 deletion syndrome have one chromosome with the region and one without it, the probe will bind once. Individuals without the syndrome have two copies of the region, so the probes bind twice. As a result, researchers see one fluorescent mark

KEY TERMS

Microdeletion syndrome—A syndrome caused by the deletion of a very small amount of chromosomal material.

Prenatal diagnosis—The use of a medical test to determine if an unborn baby has a genetic condition.

for the 22q13 region in individuals with the syndrome and two fluorescent marks in individuals without the syndrome.

As of 2005, several suggestions regarding testing for the condition were present in the literature. It was suggested that physicians should consider testing babies with an unknown cause of weak muscles at birth. Physicians should also test individuals with severe speech delay and autistic-like behavior or people with developmental delay, absent or delayed speech, and physical differences.

Treatment and management

Treatment for 22q13 varies depending on the presenting symptoms and physical differences. Individuals may see a variety of specialists, including geneticists, psychologists, and neurologists. Most people with the syndrome receive speech, occupational, and/or physical therapy. Each type of therapy helps with specific features of the syndrome. For example, speech therapy can help improve communication, occupational therapy can assist in developing life skills, and physical therapy can help strengthen muscles.

Support groups and resources are available for individuals with 22q13 deletion syndrome and their families. Information can be obtained through the 22q13 Deletion Syndrome Foundation.

Prognosis

In general, most individuals with 22q13 deletion syndrome need help and supervision all of their lives. However, the specific prognosis varies with each person, depending on their characteristics. For example, an individual with mild mental retardation and a few physical differences would be expected to have a better prognosis than a person with severe mental retardation, no speech, and behavior problems. Also, some individuals will have regression or loss of a specific skill, especially in the area of speech. It is not possible to determine which people will lose skills.

Resources

PERIODICALS

Manning, M. A., et al. "Terminal 22q Deletion Syndrome: A Newly Recognized Cause of Speech and Language Disability in the Autism Spectrum." *Pediatrics* 114, no. 2 (August 2004): 451–457.

Phelan, M. C., et al. "22q13 Deletion Syndrome." *American Journal of Medical Genetics* 101 (2001): 91–99.

ORGANIZATIONS

.22q13 Deletion Syndrome Foundation. 250 East Broadway, Maryville, TN 37804. (800) 932-2943. (April 4, 2005.) <http://www.22q13.com>.

Chromosome 22 Central. 237 Kent Avenue, Timmins, ON Canada P4N 3C2. (705) 268-3099. (April 4, 2005.) <http://www.c22c.org>.

Cristi Radford, BS
Gail Stapleton, MS

4p deletion syndrome *see* **Wolf-Hirschhorn syndrome**

5p deletion syndrome *see* **Cri du chat syndrome**

47, XXY syndrome *see* **Klinefelter syndrome**

Aarskog syndrome

Definition

Aarskog syndrome is an inherited disorder that causes a distinctive appearance of the face, skeleton, hands and feet, and genitals. First described in a Norwegian family in 1970 by the pediatrician Dagfinn Aarskog, the disorder has been recognized worldwide in most ethnic and racial groups. Because the responsible **gene** is located on the X **chromosome**, Aarskog syndrome is manifest almost exclusively in males. The prevalence is not known.

Description

Aarskog syndrome is among the **genetic disorders** with distinctive patterns of physical findings and is confused with few others. Manifestations are present at birth allowing for early identification. The facial appearance and findings in the skeletal system and genitals combine to make a recognizable pattern. The diagnosis is almost exclusively based on recognition of these findings. Although the responsible gene has been identified, testing for **gene mutations** is available only in research laboratories. Aarskog syndrome is also called Faciogenital **dysplasia**, Faciogenitodigital syndrome, and Aarskog-Scott syndrome.

Genetic profile

Aarskog syndrome is caused by mutations in the FGD1 gene, located on the short arm of the X chromosome (Xp11.2). In most cases the altered gene in affected males is inherited from a carrier mother. Since males have a single X chromosome, mutations in the FGD1 gene produces full expression in males. Females who carry a mutation of the FGD1 gene on one of their two X chromosomes are usually unaffected, but may have subtle facial differences and less height than other females in the family.

Female carriers have a 50/50 chance of transmitting the altered gene to daughters and each son. Affected males are fully capable of reproduction. They transmit their single X chromosome to all daughters who, therefore, are carriers. Since males do not transmit their single X chromosome to sons, all sons are unaffected.

The gene affected in Aarskog FGD1 codes for a Rho/Rac guanine exchange factor. While the gene product is complex and the details of its function are incompletely understood, it appears responsible for conveying messages within cells that influence their internal architecture and the activity of specific signal pathways. However, the precise way in which mutations in FGD1 produce changes in facial appearance and in the skeletal and genital systems is not yet known.

Demographics

Only males are affected with Aarskog syndrome, although carrier females may have subtle changes of the facial structures and be shorter than noncarrier sisters. There are no high risk racial or ethnic groups.

Signs and symptoms

Manifestations of Aarskog syndrome are present from birth. The facial appearance is distinctive and in most cases is diagnostic. Changes are present in the upper, middle, and lower portion of the face. Increased width of the forehead, growth of scalp hair into the middle of the forehead (widow's peak), increased space between the eyes (ocular hypertelorism), a downward slant to the eye openings, and drooping of the upper eye-

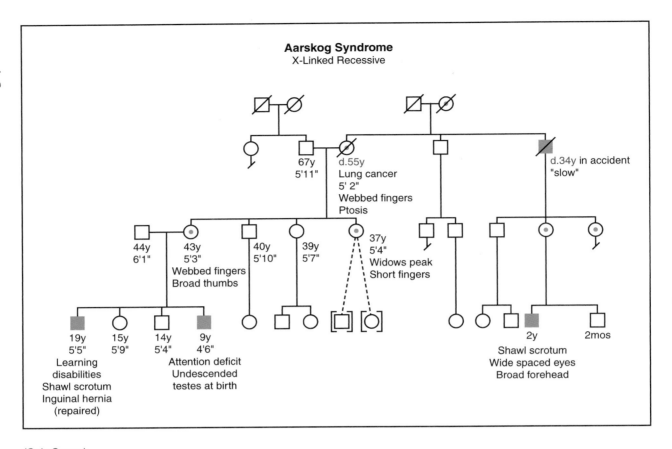

Aarskog Syndrome
X-Linked Recessive

67y
5'11"

d.55y
Lung cancer
5' 2"
Webbed fingers
Ptosis

d.34y in accident
"slow"

44y
6'1"

43y
5'3"
Webbed fingers
Broad thumbs

40y
5'10"

39y
5'7"

37y
5'4"
Widows peak
Short fingers

19y
5'5"
Learning
disabilities
Shawl scrotum
Inguinal hernia
(repaired)

15y
5'9"

14y
5'4"

9y
4'6"
Attention deficit
Undescended
testes at birth

2y
Shawl scrotum
Wide spaced eyes
Broad forehead

2mos

(Gale Group.)

lids (ptosis) are the major features in the upper part of the face. A short nose with forward-directed nostrils and simply formed small ears that may protrude are the major findings in the mid-part of the face. The mouth is wide and the chin small. As the face elongates in adult life, the prominence of the forehead and the increased space between the eyes becomes less apparent. Dental abnormalities include slow eruption, missing teeth and broad upper incisors.

The fingers are often held in a distinctive position with flexion at the joint between the hand and the fingers, over extension at the first joint of the finger and flexion at the second joint. This hand posturing becomes more obvious when there is an attempt to spread the fingers. There may also be some mild webbing between the fingers. The fingers are short and there is often only a single crease across the middle of the palm. The toes are also short and the foot is often bent inward at its middle portion. All of the joints may be unusually loose. Excessive movement of the cervical spine may lead to impingement on the spinal cord. In some cases, the sternum (breastbone) may appear depressed (pectus excavatum).

Changes in the appearance of the genitals may also be helpful in diagnosis. One or both testes may remain in the abdomen, rather than descending into the scrotal sac. The scrotum tends to surround the penis giving a so-called "shawl scrotum" appearance. Hernias may appear in the genital and umbilical regions. Linear growth in childhood and adult height are generally less than in unaffected brothers. The head size is usually normal.

Although most affected males have normal intellectual function, some individuals will have mild impairments. There does not appear to be any particular association with behavioral disturbances. However, attention deficit occurs among some boys with learning difficulties.

Diagnosis

Diagnosis of Aarskog syndrome is made on the basis of clinical findings, primarily analysis of the family history and characteristic facial, skeletal, and genital findings. There are no laboratory or radiographic changes that are specific. Although the diagnosis can be confirmed by finding a mutation in the FGD1 gene, this type of testing is available only in research laboratories.

In families with a prior occurrence of Aarskog syndrome, prenatal diagnosis might be possible through ultrasound examination of the face, hands and feet, or by testing the FGD1 gene. However, this is not generally sought since the condition is not considered medically severe.

Few other conditions are confused with Aarskog syndrome. **Noonan syndrome**, another single gene disorder that has short stature, ocular hypertelorism, downslanting eye openings, and depression of the lower chest, poses the greatest diagnostic confusion. Patients with Noonan syndrome often have wide necks and heart defects, which is helpful in distinguishing them from patients with Aarskog syndrome.

The older patient may pose greater difficulty due to loss of facial findings and obscuring of shawl scrotum by pubic hair.

As in many disorders, there is a range of severity of the clinical appearance even within the same family. In these cases, examination of several affected family members and attention to family history may be helpful.

Treatment and management

Since there are no major malformations or major mental disabilities in Aarskog syndrome, the diagnosis may be reassuring. Developmental milestones and school progress should be monitored, as there may be impairment of intellectual function in some individuals.

The X-linked **inheritance** pattern should be described to the family.

Prognosis

Short-term and long-term prognosis is favorable. Life threatening malformations or other health concerns rarely occur. Special educational attention may be necessary for those with learning difficulties. A minority of affected persons will have spinal cord compression, usually in the neck, causing pain or injury to peripheral nerves. Neurosurgical intervention is necessary in some cases. Hernias in the umbilical and groin areas may be surgically repaired.

Resources

PERIODICALS

Aarskog, D. "A familial syndrome of short stature associated with facial dysplasia and genital anomalies." *Journal of Pediatric Medicine* 77 (1971): 856.

Pasteris, N. G., et al. "Isolated and characterization of the faciogenital dysplasia (Aarskog-Scott syndrome) gene: A putative Rho/Rac guanine nucleotide exchange factor." *Cell* 79 (1994): 669.

ORGANIZATIONS

Alliance of Genetic Support Groups. 4301 Connecticut Ave. NW, Suite 404, Washington, DC 20008. (202) 966-5557. Fax: (202) 966-8553. <http://www.geneticalliance.org>.

National Organization for Rare Disorders (NORD). PO Box 8923, New Fairfield, CT 06812-8923. (203) 746-6518 or (800) 999-6673. Fax: (203) 746-6481. <http://www.rarediseases.org>.

Roger E. Stevenson, MD

Aase syndrome

Definition

Aase syndrome is a rare, autosomal recessive genetic disorder characterized by congenital hypoplastic anemia (CHA) and triphalangeal thumbs (TPT). People with Aase syndrome may have one or more physical abnormalities. Poor growth in childhood is common, but mental retardation and other neurological problems are not associated with Aase syndrome.

Description

Aase syndrome is sometimes also called Aase–Smith syndrome, or Congenital Anemia–Triphalangeal Thumb syndrome. It is a very rare hereditary syndrome involving multiple birth defects. The two symptoms that must be present to consider the diagnosis of Aase syndrome are CHA and TPT. CHA is a significant reduction from birth in the number of red cells in the blood. TPT means that one or both thumbs have three bones (phalanges) rather than the normal two.

Several other physical abnormalities have been described in individuals with Aase syndrome, including narrow shoulders, hypoplastic radius (underdevelopment of one of the bones of the lower arm), heart defect, cleft lip/palate, and late closure of the fontanelles (soft spots on an infant's skull where the bones have not yet fused). The specific cause of Aase syndrome is not known, but recurrence of the condition in siblings implies an abnormal **gene** is responsible.

Genetic profile

The available evidence suggests Aase syndrome is inherited in an autosomal recessive fashion, meaning that an affected person has two copies of the abnormal gene. Parents of an affected individual carry one abnormal copy of that particular gene, but their other gene of the pair is normal. One copy of the normal gene is sufficient for the parent to be unaffected. If both parents are carriers of a gene for the same autosomal recessive condition, there is a one in four chance in each pregnancy that they will both pass on the abnormal gene and have an affected child.

Autosomal recessive **inheritance** is suspected for Aase syndrome based on the pattern seen in the families that have been described. An autosomal recessive pattern requires that only siblings are affected by the condition (parents are unaffected gene carriers), and the disorder occurs equally in males and females. An abnormal gene proven to cause Aase syndrome has not been discovered.

Demographics

Aase syndrome is quite rare, with possibly no more than two dozen cases reported in the medical literature.

Signs and symptoms

CHA and TPT are the two classic signs of Aase syndrome. The anemia may require treatment with steroids, or possibly blood transfusions, but tends to improve over time. TPT may cause a person with Aase syndrome to have difficulty grasping and manipulating objects with their hands. A hypoplastic radius may complicate problems with appearance and movement of the hands and arms. Narrow and sloping shoulders are caused by abnormal development of the bones in that area of the body.

Slow growth in children with Aase syndrome may be partly related to their anemia, but is more likely to be genetically predetermined due to the syndrome. Ventricular septal defect (VSD), a hole between the bottom two chambers of the heart, is the cardiac defect reported most often, and several cases of **cleft lip and palate** have occurred as well.

Diagnosis

The diagnosis of Aase syndrome is made when an infant has CHA and TPT, and one or more of the other symptoms. Children with another more common congenital anemia syndrome, Blackfan–Diamond syndrome (BDS), sometimes have abnormalities of their thumbs. Since the syndromes have overlapping symptoms, there is some question about whether Aase syndrome and BDS are contiguous gene syndromes or even identical conditions. Further genetic research may resolve this issue.

Treatment and management

Anemia associated with Aase syndrome is often helped by the use of a steroid medication. For serious anemia that does not respond to medications, blood transfusions from a matched donor might be necessary. Management of problems related to the skeletal abnormalities should be treated by orthopedic surgery as well as physical and occupational therapy. Heart defects and cleft lip and palate are nearly always correctable, but both require surgery and long–term follow up. A genetic evaluation and counseling should be offered to any individual or couple whose child is suspected of having Aase syndrome.

Prognosis

While major medical procedures such as blood transfusions and corrective surgeries might be needed for a child with Aase syndrome, the long–term prognosis seems to be good. Discovery of the specific genetic defect is not likely to immediately change the prognosis. Development of a reliable genetic test, however, might allow for carrier testing for other family members, and prenatal diagnosis for couples who already have an affected child.

Resources

ORGANIZATIONS

Aicardi Syndrome Awareness and Support Group. 29 Delavan Ave., Toronto, ON M5P 1T2. Canada (416) 481-4095.

March of Dimes Birth Defects Foundation. 1275 Mamaroneck Ave., White Plains, NY 10605. (888) 663-4637. resourcecenter@modimes.org. <http://www.modimes.org>.

National Heart, Lung, and Blood Institute. PO Box 30105, Bethesda, MD 20824-0105. (301) 592-8573. nhlbiinfo@rover.nhlbi.nih.gov. <http://www.nhlbi.nih.gov>.

National Organization for Rare Disorders (NORD). PO Box 8923, New Fairfield, CT 06812-8923. (203) 746-6518 or (800) 999-6673. Fax: (203) 746-6481. <http://www.rarediseases.org>.

National Society of Genetic Counselors. 233 Canterbury Dr., Wallingford, PA 19086-6617. (610) 872-1192. <http://www.nsgc.org/GeneticCounselingYou.asp>.

Scott J. Polzin, MS, CGC

Aase-Smith syndrome *see* **Aase syndrome**

Abetalipoproteinemia

Definition

Abetalipoproteinemia (ABL) is a rare inherited disorder characterized by difficulty in absorbing fat during digestion. The result is absence of betalipoproteins in the blood, abnormally shaped red blood cells, and deficiencies of vitamins A, E, and K. Symptoms include intestinal, neurological, muscular, skeletal, and ocular problems, along with anemia and prolonged bleeding in some cases.

Description

An unusual sign first described in ABL is the presence of star-shaped red blood cells, which were dubbed "acanthocytes" (literally, *thorny cells*). Thus, ABL is also known by the name acanthocytosis. Less commonly, ABL may be referred to as Bassen-Kornzweig syndrome.

The underlying problem in ABL is a difficulty in absorbing fats (lipids) in the intestine. Most people with ABL first develop chronic digestive problems, and then progress to neurological, muscular, skeletal, and ocular disease. Disorders of the blood may also be present. Severe vitamin deficiency causes many of the symptoms in ABL. Treatments include restricting fat intake in the diet and vitamin supplementation. Even with early diagnosis and treatment, though, ABL is progressive and cannot be cured.

Genetic profile

Fats are important components of a normal diet, and their processing, transport, and use by the body are critical to normal functioning. Lipids bind to protein (lipoprotein) so they can be absorbed in the intestine, transferred through the blood, and taken up by cells and tissues throughout the body. There are many different lipoprotein complexes in the body. One group, the betalipoproteins, must combine with another protein, microsomal triglyceride transfer protein (MTP). ABL is caused by abnormalities in the **gene** that codes for MTP. When MTP is nonfunctional or missing, then betalipoproteins will also be decreased or absent. The MTP gene has been localized to **chromosome** 4.

ABL is an autosomal recessive genetic disorder. This means that both copies of the MTP gene are abnormal in a person affected with the disorder. Since all genes are present at conception, a person cannot "acquire" ABL. Each parent of an affected child carries the abnormal MTP gene but also has a normally functioning gene of that pair. Enough functional MTP is produced by the normal gene so that the parent is unaffected (carrier). When both parents are carriers of the same recessive gene, there is a one in four chance in each pregnancy that they will have an affected child.

Demographics

ABL is rare, and the true incidence of the disorder is unknown. Prior to the description of ABL in 1950, it is believed that people with ABL were diagnosed as having either **Friedreich ataxia** (a more common form of hereditary ataxia) or some other neurologic disorder. Misdiagnosis may still occur if all of the symptoms are not present, or if they do not occur in a typical fashion. Most of the reported cases of ABL have been in the Jewish population, but individuals from other ethnic backgrounds have been described as well. As many as one-third of people with ABL have had genetically related (consanguineous) parents. Higher rates of consanguinity are often seen in rare autosomal recessive disorders.

Signs and symptoms

Too much fat left unabsorbed in the intestine results in the symptoms that are often noticed first in ABL, such as chronic diarrhea, loss of appetite, vomiting, and slow weight gain and growth due to reduced uptake of nutrients.

Various lipids, such as cholesterol and its components, are important in the development and normal functioning of nerve and muscle cells. Decreased lipid levels in the bloodstream, and thus elsewhere in the body, are partly responsible for the neuromuscular and ocular problems encountered in ABL. Neurological symptoms include ataxia (poor muscle coordination), loss of deep tendon reflexes, and decreased sensation to touch, pain, and temperature.

Muscular atrophy, the weakening and loss of muscle tissue, is caused by the decreased ability of nerves to control those muscles, as well as lack of nutrients for the muscles themselves. Weakened heart muscle (cardiomyopathy) may occur, and several severe cases have been reported that resulted in early death.

Retinitis pigmentosa is progressive, especially without treatment, and the typical symptoms are loss of night vision and reduced field of vision. Loss of clear vision, nystagmus (involuntary movement of the eyes), and eventual paralysis of the muscles that control the eye may also occur.

Skeletal problems associated with ABL include various types of curvature of the spine and clubfeet. The abnormalities of the spine and feet are thought to result from muscle strength imbalances in those areas during bone growth.

Severe anemia sometimes occurs in ABL, and may be partly due to deficiencies of iron and folic acid (a B vitamin) from poor absorption of nutrients. In addition, because of their abnormal shape, acanthocytes are prematurely destroyed in the blood stream.

Vitamins A, E, and K are fat soluble, meaning they dissolve in lipids in order to be used by the body. Low lipid levels in the blood means that people with ABL have chronic deficiencies of vitamins A, E, and K. Much of the neuromuscular disease seen in ABL is thought to be caused by deficiencies of these vitamins, especially vitamin E.

Approximately one-third of all individuals with ABL develop mental retardation. However, since the proportion of cases involving consanguinity is also reported to be about one-third, it is difficult to determine if mental retardation in individuals with ABL is due to the disease itself or to other effects of consanguinity. Consanguinity may also be responsible for other birth defects seen infrequently in ABL.

Diagnosis

The diagnosis of ABL is suspected from the intestinal, neuromuscular, and ocular symptoms, and is confirmed by laboratory tests showing acanthocytes in the blood and absence of betalipoproteins and chylomicrons in the blood. Other diseases resulting in similar intestinal or neurological symptoms, and those associated with symptoms related to malnutrition and vitamin deficiency must be excluded. There is no direct test of the MTP gene available for routine diagnostic testing. Accurate carrier testing and prenatal diagnosis are therefore not yet available. However, this could change at any time. Any couple whose child is diagnosed with ABL should be referred for **genetic counseling** to obtain the most up-to-date information.

Treatment and management

The recommended treatments for ABL include diet restrictions and vitamin supplementation. Reduced triglyceride content in the diet is suggested if intestinal symptoms require it. Large supplemental doses of vitamin E (tocopherol) have been shown to lessen or even reverse the neurological, muscular, and retinal symptoms in many cases. Supplementation with a water-soluble form of vitamin A is also suggested. Vitamin K therapy should be considered if blood clotting problems occur.

Occupational and physical therapy can assist with any muscular and skeletal problems that arise. Physicians that specialize in orthopedics, digestive disorders, and eye disease should be involved. Support groups and specialty clinics for individuals with multisystem disorders such as ABL are available in nearly all metropolitan areas.

Prognosis

ABL is rare, which means there have been few individuals on which to base prognostic information. The effectiveness of vitamin supplementation and diet restrictions will vary from person to person and family to family. Life span may be near normal with mild to moderate disability in some, but others may have more serious and even life-threatening complications. Arriving at the correct diagnosis as early as possible is important. However, this is often difficult in rare conditions such as ABL. Future therapies, if any, will likely focus on

KEY TERMS

Acanthocytosis—The presence of acanthocytes in the blood. Acanthocytes are red blood cells that have the appearance of thorns on their outer surface.

Ataxia—A deficiency of muscular coordination, especially when voluntary movements are attempted, such as grasping or walking.

Chylomicron—A type of lipoprotein made in the small intestine and used for transporting fats to other tissues in the body. MTP is necessary for the production of chylomicrons.

Clubfoot—Abnormal permanent bending of the ankle and foot. Also called *talipes equinovarus*.

Consanguinity—A mating between two people who are related to one another by blood.

Lipoprotein—A lipid and protein chemically bound together, which aids in transfer of the lipid in and out of cells, across the wall of the intestine, and through the blood stream.

Low density lipoproteins (LDL)—A cholesterol carrying substance that can remain in the blood stream for a long period of time.

Neuromuscular—Involving both the muscles and the nerves that control them.

Ocular—A broad term that refers to structure and function of the eye.

Retinitis pigmentosa—Progressive deterioration of the retina, often leading to vision loss and blindness.

Triglycerides—Certain combinations of fatty acids (types of lipids) and glycerol.

Vitamin deficiency—Abnormally low levels of a vitamin in the body.

improving lipid absorption in the digestive tract. Further study of the MTP gene may lead to the availability of accurate carrier testing and prenatal diagnosis for some families.

Resources

ORGANIZATIONS

March of Dimes Birth Defects Foundation. 1275 Mamaroneck Ave., White Plains, NY 10605. (888) 663-4637. resourcecenter@modimes.org. <http://www.modimes.org>.

National Foundation for Jewish Genetic Diseases, Inc. 250 Park Ave., Suite 1000, New York, NY 10017. (212) 371-1030. <http://www.nfjgd.org>.

National Organization for Rare Disorders (NORD). PO Box 8923, New Fairfield, CT 06812-8923. (203) 746-6518 or (800) 999-6673. Fax: (203) 746-6481. <http://www.rarediseases.org>.

National Society of Genetic Counselors. 233 Canterbury Dr., Wallingford, PA 19086-6617. (610) 872-1192. <http://www.nsgc.org/GeneticCounselingYou.asp>.

National Tay-Sachs and Allied Diseases Association. 2001 Beacon St., Suite 204, Brighton, MA 02135. (800) 906-8723. ntsad-Boston@worldnet.att.net. <http://www.ntsad.org>.

Scott J. Polzin, MS, CGC

Acanthocytosis *see* **Abetalipoproteinemia**

Acardia

Definition

Acardia is a very rare, serious malformation that occurs almost exclusively in monozygous twins (twins developing from a single egg). This condition results from artery to artery connections in the placenta causing a physically normal fetus to circulate blood for both itself and a severely malformed fetus whose heart regresses or is overtaken by the pump twin's heart.

Description

Acardia was first described in the sixteenth century. Early references refer to acardia as chorioangiopagus parasiticus. It is now also called twin reversed arterial perfusion sequence, or TRAP sequence.

Mechanism

Acardia is the most extreme form of twin-twin transfusion syndrome. Twin-twin transfusion syndrome is a pregnancy complication in which twins abnormally share blood flow from the umbilical artery of one twin to the umbilical vein of the other. This abnormal connection can cause serious complications including loss of the pregnancy.

In acardiac twin pregnancies, blood vessels abnormally connect between the twins in the placenta. The

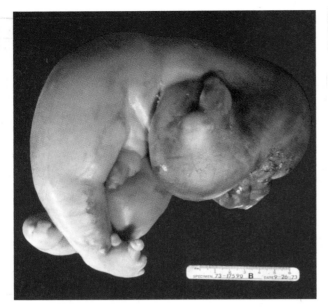

This infant shows partial development of the lower extremities and early development of the head. Acardia almost always occurs in monozygotic twins, with one twin (such as that shown here) unable to fully develop as a result of severe heart complications. *(Greenwood Genetic Center.)*

placenta is the important interface of blood vessels between a mother and baby through which babies receive nutrients and oxygen. This abnormal connection forces the twin with stronger blood flow to pump blood for both, straining the heart of this "pump" twin. This abnormal connection causes the malformed twin to receive blood directly from the pump twin before this blood gathers new oxygen. The poorly deoxygenated blood from the normal twin as well as the pressure deficiency as a result of trying to serve both infants may be the cause of the other twin's malformations.

The acardiac twin

The acardiac twin is severely malformed and may be incorrectly referred to as a tumor. In 1902, a physician named Das established four categories of acardiac twins based on their physical appearance. There is controversy surrounding the use of these traditional four categories because some cases are complex and do not fit neatly into one of Das's four categories. These four traditional categories include acardius acephalus, amorphus, anceps, and acormus.

Acardius acephalus is the most common type of acardiac twin. These twins do not develop a head, but may have an underdeveloped skull base. They have legs, but do not have arms. On autopsy they are generally found to lack chest and upper abdominal organs.

Acardius amorphus appears as a disorganized mass of tissues containing skin, bone, cartilage, muscle, fat, and blood vessels. This type of acardiac twin is not recognizable as a human fetus and contains no recognizable human organs.

Acardius anceps is the most developed form of acardiac twin. This form has arms, legs, and a partially developed head with brain tissues and facial structures. This type of acardiac twin is associated with a high risk for complications in the normal twin.

Acardius acormus is the rarest type of acardiac twin. This type of acardiac twin presents as an isolated head with no body development.

Genetic profile

There is no single known genetic cause for acardia. In most cases, the physically normal twin is genetically identical to the acardiac twin. In these cases, physical differences are believed to be due to abnormal blood circulation.

Aneuploidy, or an abnormal number of chromosomes, has been seen in several acardiac twins, but is rare in the normal twins. Trisomy 2, the presence of three copies of human **chromosome** 2 instead of the normal two copies, has been reported in the abnormal twin of two pregnancies complicated by TRAP sequence in different women. For both of these pregnancies the pump twin had normal chromosome numbers. Since monozygotic twins are formed from a single **zygote**, scientists theorize that an error occurs early in cell division in only one of the two groups of cells formed during this process.

Demographics

TRAP is a rare complication of twinning, occurring only once in about every 35,000 births. Acardia is believed to complicate 1% of monozygotic twin pregnancies. Risks in triplet, quadruplet, and other higher order pregnancies are even higher. Monozygotic twinning in higher order pregnancies are more common in pregnancies conceived with in vitro fertilization (IVF), hence increased risk for TRAP sequence is also associated with IVF.

This condition has been documented over five centuries occurring in many countries and in different races. Specific rates for recurrence are unknown. However, a mother who has had a pregnancy complicated by TRAP sequence is very unlikely to have another pregnancy with the same complication.

Two cases of acardia have been associated with maternal **epilepsy** and the use of anticonvusants. One report, in 1996, describes an acardiac twin pregnancy in an epileptic mother who took primidone, a seizure medication, in the first trimester of her pregnancy. Another report, in 2000, describes an acardiac twin pregnancy in an epileptic mother who took a different seizure medication, oxcarbazepin.

Diagnosis

A mother carrying an acardiac twin pregnancy is not likely to have any unusual symptoms. An acardiac twin is most often found incidentally on **prenatal ultrasound**. No two acardiac twins are formed exactly alike, so they may present differently. During ultrasound, an acardiac twin may appear as tissue mass or it may appear to be a twin who has died in the womb. Acardia is always suspected when, on ultrasound, a twin once considered to be dead begins to move or grow, or there is visible blood flow through that twin's umbilical cord. In 50% of cases the acardiac twin has only two, instead of the normal three, vessels in the umbilical cord. A two vessel umbilical cord may also be found in some normal pregnancies.

Ultrasound diagnostic criteria for the acardiac twin usually include:

- absence of fetal activity
- no heart beat
- continued growth
- increasing soft tissue mass
- undergrowth of the upper torso
- normal growth of the lower trunk

An acardiac fetus may also be missed on prenatal ultrasound. A 1991 report describes an acardiac twin who was missed on ultrasound and only detected at delivery. In rare cases a diagnosis of acardia is not possible until autopsy.

Treatment and management

There is no consensus on which therapy is best for pregnancies complicated by TRAP sequence. No treatment can save the acardiac twin, so the goal of prenatal therapy is to help the normal twin. The normal twin is not always saved by prenatal treatment.

Specialists have used laser and electrical cauterization, electrodes, serial **amniocentesis**, medications, and other treatments successfully. Physicians often recom-

---

> ### KEY TERMS
>
> **Amniocentesis**—A procedure performed at 16-18 weeks of pregnancy in which a needle is inserted through a woman's abdomen into her uterus to draw out a small sample of the amniotic fluid from around the baby. Either the fluid itself or cells from the fluid can be used for a variety of tests to obtain information about genetic disorders and other medical conditions in the fetus.
>
> **Dizygotic**—From two zygotes, as in non-identical, or fraternal twins. The zygote is the first cell formed by the union of sperm and egg.
>
> **Fetus**—The term used to describe a developing human infant from approximately the third month of pregnancy until delivery. The term embryo is used prior to the third month.
>
> **Monozygotic**—From one zygote, as in identical twins. The zygote is the first cell formed by the union of sperm and egg.

---

mend prenatal interruption of the blood vessel connections (thus sacrificing the acardiac twin) before heart failure develops in the pump twin.

Cutting off blood circulation to the acardiac twin can be accomplished by cauterizing or burning the blood vessel connections. In a 1998 study of seven pregnancies treated with laser therapy the rate of death in the normal twin was 13.6%, a vast improvement over the expected 50% death rate. Medications like digoxin may be used to treat congestive heart failure in the normal twin. Current studies examining the success and failure rates of these treatments will be helpful in determining which therapy is the best option.

Fetal echocardiography is recommended to assist with early detection of heart failure in the normal twin. Chromosome studies are recommended for both fetuses in all pregnancies complicated by TRAP sequence.

Prognosis

The acardiac or parasitic twin never survives as it is severely malformed and does not have a functioning heart. Complications associated with having an acardiac twin cause 50-70% of normal twins to die. The normal twin is at risk for heart failure and complications associated with premature birth. Heart failure in the normal twin is common. The normal twin of an acardiac twin pregnancy has about a 10% risk for malformations. Therapy is thought to decrease the normal twin's risk for heart failure and premature birth. Improvement of therapies will undoubtedly lead to a better outlook for pregnancies complicated by TRAP sequence.

Resources

PERIODICALS

Arias, Fernando, et al. "Treatment of acardiac twinning." *Obstetrics & Gynecology* (May 1998): 818-21.

Brassard, Myriam, et al. "Prognostic markers in twin pregnancies with an acardiac fetus." *Obstetrics and Gynecology* (September 1999): 409-14.

Mohanty, C., et al. "Acardiac anomaly spectrum." *Teratology* 62 (2000): 356-359.

Rodeck, C., et al. "Thermocoagulation for the early treatment of pregnancy with an acardiac twin." *New England Journal of Medicine* 339 (1998): 1293-95.

ORGANIZATIONS

Twin Hope, Inc. 2592 West 14th St., Cleveland, OH 44113. (502) 243-2110. <http://www.twinhope.com>.

Judy C. Hawkins, MS

Accutane embryopathy

Definition

Accutane is commonly used to treat severe acne that has not responded to other forms of treatment. Accutane embryopathy refers to the pattern of birth defects that may be caused in an embryo that is exposed to Accutane during pregnancy. Accutane-related birth defects typically include physical abnormalities of the face, ears, heart, and brain.

Description

Accutane is one of several man-made drugs derived from vitamin A. The generic name for Accutane is *isotretinoin*. Accutane and other vitamin A-derivatives are referred to as *retinoids*. Vitamin A is an essential nutrient for normal growth and development. It is found in foods such as green leafy and yellow vegetables, oranges, pineapple, cantaloupe, liver, egg yolks, and butter. It is also available in multivitamins and separately as a daily supplement. Vitamin A is important in a number of biological processes. Included among these is the growth and differentiation of the epithelium, the cells that form the outer layer of skin as well as some of the layers beneath. Deficiency of vitamin A may lead to increased susceptibility to infection and problems with vision and growth of skin cells. The potential risks of supplemental

vitamin A in a person's diet have been a matter of some debate. However, excess vitamin A during pregnancy does not seem to be associated with an increased risk for birth defects.

The same cannot be said for drugs derived from vitamin A. Accutane, like other retinoids, displays some of the same biologic properties as vitamin A, such as its role in stimulating the growth of epithelium. For this reason, it is an effective method of treatment for severe cases of nodular acne, a condition characterized by cystic, painful, scarring lesions. Four to five months of Accutane treatment usually leads to clearing of the acne for one year or more, even after the medicine is stopped. Accutane may also be prescribed for moderate acne that has not responded to other forms of treatment, usually antibiotics taken every day by mouth. Milder cases of acne that produce scarring or other related skin disorders may also be treated with this medication. Often, dermatologists prescribe Accutane only after other methods of treatment have been unsuccessful.

Common side effects of Accutane are chapped lips, dry skin with itching, mild nosebleeds, joint and muscle pain, and temporary thinning of hair. **Depression**, including thoughts of suicide, has been reported more recently as another, much more serious, potential side effect. Severe acne on its own is associated with lower self-esteem. No studies have been published to try to determine if Accutane use somehow makes it more likely for a person to be depressed or to attempt suicide.

The United States Food and Drug Administration (FDA) approved the use of Accutane in September 1982. It had previously been shown to cause birth defects in animals. Consequently, its approval was granted with the provision that the drug label would describe its risk of causing birth defects. The patient information brochure also included information for women taking the medication about avoiding preganancy.

The first report of an infant with Accutane-related birth defects was published in 1983. At least ten additional cases were subsequently reported to the FDA and Centers for Disease Control (CDC). A pattern of birth defects involving the head, ears, face, and heart was identified. In 1985, Dr. Edward Lammer reviewed a total of 154 pregnancies exposed to Accutane. Each of the pregnancies had included use of the drug during the first three months of pregnancy. This period, referred to as the *first trimester*, is a critical and sensitive time during which all of the organs begin to develop. Chemical insults during this part of pregnancy often result in abnormal formation of internal organs with or without external abnormalities.

Each of the 154 pregnancies had been voluntarily reported to either the FDA or CDC. The pregnancy outcomes included 95 elective pregnancy terminations and 59 continuing pregnancies. Of these, twelve (20%) ended in a spontaneous pregnancy loss, or miscarriage. The remaining 47 pregnancies resulted in six stillborn infants with obvious abnormalities, 18 live born infants with abnormalities, and 26 apparently normal babies. The abnormalities observed among the stillborn and living infants were similar, most frequently involving the head, face, heart, and central nervous system. Thus, use of Accutane during the first several months of pregnancy was shown to be associated with an increased risk of pregnancy loss (miscarriage or stillbirth) as well as with a significant risk of birth defects in living children. This pattern of abnormalities has since become known as Accutane embryopathy. The term >retinoic acid embryopathy is also occasionally used to describe the same condition because other retinoids, such as Tegison (etretinate), have been associated with a similar pattern of birth defects. Tegison is commonly used to treat severe psoriasis and can cause birth defects even if stopped years before becoming pregnant.

Genetic profile

Accutane embryopathy (AE) is not an inherited or hereditary type of abnormality. Rather, it is caused by exposure of a developing embryo to the drug, Accutane, during the first trimester of pregnancy. Accutane is a well known, powerful **teratogen**, or agent that causes physical or mental abnormalities in an embryo. Use anytime after the fifteenth day after conception, or approximately four weeks of pregnancy dating from the first day of the mother's last menstrual period, is associated with a significantly increased risk for pregnancy loss or an infant with AE. The dose of Accutane is unimportant. If Accutane is stopped prior to conception, no increased risk for loss or birth defects is expected.

Demographics

The total number of women of reproductive age (15-44 years old) taking Accutane is unknown. However, since the 1990s, the overall number of prescriptions written for Accutane has increased over two hundred percent. Prescriptions are evenly divided between men and women, but women 30 years old or younger account for 80% of the patients among their sex.

A Dermatologic and Ophthalmic Drug Advisory Committee was convened at the FDA in September 2000. Patterns of Accutane use and the outcomes of Accutane-exposed pregnancies were presented at this meeting. Two overlapping sources of pregnancy data exist: one sponsored by the manufacturer of the drug, Roche Laboratories, and a second study maintained by the Slone Epidemiology Unit at the Boston University School of Public Health. Representatives from both institutions reviewed their outcome data up to that time. This data supports previous estimates of the frequency of AE.

A total of 1,995 exposed pregnancies have been reported between the years 1982 and 2000. These pregnancies have been voluntarily reported either directly to the manufacturer or to the Slone Survey. Although doctors have referred some, a majority of participating women obtained the appropriate phone numbers from the insert included with their medication. Elective terminations of pregnancy were performed in 1,214 pregnancies. Spontaneous pregnancy losses were reported in 213 pregnancies and 383 infants were delivered. Of these, 162, or 42%, were born with malformations consistent with AE.

The numbers from the Slone Survey, which began in 1989, represent a large subset of the data reported by Roche. Any woman to whom Accutane is prescribed is invited to contact and participate in the project. As of September 2000, the survey had identified a total of 1,019 pregnancies out of more than 300,000 women enrolled. Some women were already pregnant when they had started Accutane but others conceived while taking the drug. The pregnancy data allows for examination of the risk factors that lead to becoming pregnant as well as the pregnancy outcomes. Among the 1,019 pregnancies that occurred, 681 were electively terminated, 177 resulted in a spontaneous loss, and 117 infants were delivered. Only 60 of these infants were either examined or had medical records available to review. Eight of the 60 (13%) were diagnosed with AE. No information was available on the remaining 57 pregnancies.

Each couple in the general population has a background risk of 34% of having a child with any type of congenital birth defect. The medical literature has suggested a 25–35% risk of AE in infants exposed to Accutane prenatally. The combined Roche and Slone Survey data provided a risk of 42%. Although consistent with the medical literature, this slightly higher number probably reflects some bias in reporting. In other words, some mothers may report their pregnancy only after the birth of a child with AE. Normal births may go unreported. This type of retrospective analysis is not as helpful as prospective reporting in which pregnancies are enrolled before the outcome is known. To ensure objective reporting, the Slone Survey only enrolls their participants prospectively, ideally before the end of the first trimester of pregnancy. Even still, the Slone Survey estimates that it likely only has information on roughly 40% of all Accutane-exposed pregnancies.

Signs and symptoms

AE is characterized by a number of major and minor malformations. Each abnormality is not present in every affected individual.

Craniofacial

• Malformed ears. Abnormalities of the ears, when present, involve both ears but may show different levels of severity ranging from mild external abnormalities to a very small or missing ear.

• Underdevelopment of the skull and facial bones. This leads to a specific facial features including a sharply sloping forehead, small jaw (*micrognathia*), flattened bridge of the nose, and an abnormal size and/or placing of the eye sockets and eyes.

Heart

• Structural defects, most of which require surgery to correct.

Central nervous systerm

• **Hydrocephalus**, or abnormal accumulation of fluid within the brain. This is the most common type of brain abnormality and often is treated by placement of a shunt within the head to drain the fluid.

• Small head size (*microcephaly*)

• Structural or functional brain abnormalities

• Mild to moderate mental retardation or learning disabilities later in life. Either may be present even in the absence of physical abnormalities.

Other

• Abnormal or very small thymus gland

• Cleft palate, or opening in the roof of the mouth

Diagnosis

A diagnosis of AE is based on two pieces of information: (1) report of Accutane use by the mother during the first trimester of pregnancy, and (2) recognition of the physical abnormalities in an exposed infant. The latter is accomplished by a physical examination by a doctor familiar with AE. Special studies of the heart, such as ultrasound, may be required after delivery to determine the specific nature of any structural heart defect.

Prenatal diagnosis is theoretically possible armed with the knowledge of early pregnancy exposure. A **prenatal ultrasound** evaluation may detect abnormalities such as heart defects, hydrocephalus or microcephaly, or some craniofacial abnormalities. However, not all fea-

tures of AE will be apparent even with ultrasound, and a careful examination after delivery is still indicated.

Treatment and management

The care of an infant with AE after delivery is primarily symptomatic. Infants with serious heart abnormalities will need to be evaluated by a heart specialist and may require surgery in order to survive. Infants with brain abnormalities, such as hydrocephalus may require shunt placement soon after birth and monitoring by a brain surgeon on a regular basis. Ear malformations may be associated with hearing loss in affected children. Depending on the severity of the ear abnormality, sign language may be needed for communication. Some infants with very severe internal birth defects, particularly of the heart, may die at a young age.

Based on the features associated with AE and the long-term medical care that may be required, the focus of the manufacturer of Accutane has long been on the prevention of as many pregnancies as possible. Roche Laboratories has made numerous efforts since 1982 to achieve this, including periodic changes in the drug label and attempts to increase doctor and consumer awareness about the teratogenic nature of Accutane during pregnancy.

In 1988, Roche developed the Accutane Pregnancy Prevention Program (PPP). It was fully implemented in mid-1989. The goal of the PPP was to develop educational materials about Accutane for both patients and their doctors. A PPP kit included a consent form and a patient information brochure. Prescribing physicians were encouraged to obtain informed consent from all of their patients after a verbal discussion of the risks and benefits of the drug. Pregnancy tests were strongly encouraged prior to beginning treatment. The patient information brochure included information about, as well as a toll-free phone number for, the patient referral program sponsored by Roche. The program offered to reimburse women for the cost of a visit to their doctor to review effective methods of birth control. Finally, warnings about the risks associated with Accutane were printed directly on the box and the individual drug packages.

An Accutane tracking study was implemented to evaluate how often doctors were using the PPP kit and following other major components of the program. The results of the study revealed that many doctors were inclined to rely only on oral communication about Accutane with their patients rather than using each of the elements of the PPP kit. The patient brochure was frequently used but other components of the kit were considered inconvenient and too time-consuming. Both Roche and the FDA agreed that certain parts of the PPP needed strengthening.

Additional support came in the form of a report published in the CDC-sponsored periodical, *Morbidity and Mortality Weekly Report* (MMWR), in January 2000. A group of 23 women was identified in California, all of whom had taken Accutane while pregnant. During March 1999, a representative from the CDC interviewed a total of 14 of these women in an attempt to learn why pregnancies exposed to Accutane continued to occur despite the efforts of the PPP. Five women had electively terminated their pregnancies and had no information on whether birth defects had been present in the fetus. Four women experienced a spontaneous pregnancy loss, and four infants were born without obvious abnormalities. The last infant was born with features of AE, including a complex heart defect, hydrocephalus, and abnormal facial features. He subsequently died at the age of nine weeks.

Of greater interest to the authors, however, were some of the factors that contributed to the occurrence of these pregnancies in the first place. Some of the women had obtained Accutane from a source other than their doctor, such as in another country or from an associate. Another woman reported using medication left over from a previous prescription. In other cases, the prescription was filled before a pregnancy test was performed (usually the woman was already pregnant) or was started before day two or three of her menstrual period.

In March 1999, Roche submitted plans to the FDA for its revised Targeted Pregnancy Prevention Program. Over the course of the year 2000, the Targeted PPP was put into place, and efforts were resumed to educate doctors and patients alike. In May 2000, the FDA approved a new label for all Accutane packages. The label now includes the following recommendations:

- Two independent pregnancy tests are required, one before treatment begins and the next on the second day of the next normal menstrual period or 11 days after the last unprotected act of sexual intercourse, whichever is later.

- The prescription cannot be filled without a report from a physician documenting a negative pregnancy test result.

- If treatment is started while a woman has her menstrual period, it should be started on the second to third day of her period.

- Only a one-month supply of the drug will be given at a time.

- Two reliable forms of birth control, one primary, another secondary, must be used at the same time before treatment starts, during treatment, and one month after treatment ends. Examples of a primary method of birth control include birth control pills, a history of a sterilization procedure, such as a tubal ligation or vasectomy, or other form of injectable or implantable birth control product. Examples of a secondary form of birth control include use of a diaphragm, condom, or cervical cap, each with spermicide.

- Monthly contraceptive and pregnancy counseling are required as are monthly pregnancy tests.

The FDA's Dermatologic and Ophthalmic Drug Advisory Committee additionally recommended that doctors and their patients participate in a mandatory Accutane registry. Such a registry would be used to track how well prescribers and patients follow the elements of the Targeted PPP, such as pregnancy tests, informed consent, and use of birth control. A similar system has been developed to regulate the use of the drug thalidomide, another powerful human teratogen. Additionally, a centralized database could be maintained to track the outcomes of all Accutane-exposed pregnancies. As of early 2001, such a registry had not yet been established.

The possibility of a registry has met with criticism from professional organizations such as the American Academy of Dermatology (AAD). Critics have charged that a mandatory registry system would restrict access to the drug, particularly for those individuals with severe acne who may live in rural areas or otherwise do not have access to a doctor who is a member of the registry. The AAD agrees that education about Accutane as well as its potential hazards and safe and responsible use of the drug are of utmost importance.

To date, none of the efforts put forth by the drug manufacturer or the medical community has been 100% effective. Pregnancies while women are taking Accutane are still occurring, and infants with AE are still being born. As highlighted by the recent MMWR report, establishment of a registry or other strict methods of control are still unlikely to completely eliminate the birth of children with AE. It is possible in some cases to obtain Accutane without using the services of a knowledgeable physician. Also, many pregnancies are unplanned and unexpected. Since first trimester exposure to Accutane may have serious consequences, time is of the essence in preventing as many prenatal exposures as possible. Doctors and their patients need to be equally attentive to the prevention of pregnancies and, thus, the continuing births of children with AE.

Prognosis

Accutane is a safe and highly effective drug when used properly. However, Accutane embryopathy is a

KEY TERMS

Embryo—The earliest stage of development of a human infant, usually used to refer to the first eight weeks of pregnancy. The term *fetus* is used from roughly the third month of pregnancy until delivery.

Miscarriage—Spontaneous pregnancy loss.

Psoriasis—A common, chronic, scaly skin disease.

Stillbirth—The birth of a baby who has died sometime during the pregnancy or delivery.

Thymus gland—An endocrine gland located in the front of the neck that houses and tranports T cells, which help to fight infection.

serious medical condition that is directly related to a mother's use of Accutane during the first trimester of her pregnancy. Although most individuals with AE will have a normal lifespan, others may die at a young age due to complex internal abnormalities. Mild or moderate mental handicap is common even when there are no obvious physical features of AE.

Resources

BOOKS

"Retinoic acid embryopathy." In *Smith's Recognizable Patterns of Human Malformations,* edited by Kenneth Lyons Jones, W.B. Saunders Company, 1997.

PERIODICALS

"Accutane-exposed pregnancies—California 1999." *Morbidity and Mortality Weekly Report* 49, no. 2 (January 21, 2000): 28-31 <http://www.cdc.gov/epo/mmwr/preview/mmwrhtml/mm4902a2.htm>.

Mechcatie, Elizabeth. "FDA panel backs new pregnancy plan for Accutane." *Family Practice News* 30, no. 2 (November 1, 2000): 20.

ORGANIZATIONS

American Academy of Dermatology. PO Box 4014, 930 N. Meacham Rd., Schaumburg, IL 60168-4014. (847) 330-0230. Fax: (847) 330-0050. <http://www.aad.org>.

Organization of Teratology Services (OTIS). (888) 285-3410. <http://www.otispregnancy.org>.

WEBSITES

"Accutane." *Food and Drug Administration.* <http://www.fda.gov/cder/drug/infopage/accutane/default.htm>.

"Accutane: Complete Product Information." *Roche U.S. Pharmaceuticals.* <http://www.rocheusa.com/products/accutane/pi.html>.

"Accutane and other retinoids." *March of Dimes.* <http://www.modimes.org/HealthLibrary2/factsheets.Accutane.htm>.

Stagg Elliott, Victoria. "More restrictions expected on acne drug." *AMNews.* (October 16, 2000) <http://www.ama-assn.org/sci-pubs/amnews/pick-00/hlsd1016.htm>.

Terri A. Knutel, MS, CGC

Achondrogenesis

Definition

Achondrogenesis is a disorder in which bone growth is severely affected. The condition is usually fatal early in life.

Description

General description

The syndrome achondrogenesis results from abnormal bone growth and cartilage formation. It is considered a lethal form of infantile dwarfism. Dwarfism is a condition that leads to extremely short stature. In achondrogenesis, the abnormalities in cartilage formation lead to abnormalities in bone formation. The lethality of the disorder is thought to result from difficulty breathing, probably due to having a very small chest. Achondrogenesis usually results in a stillborn infant or very early fatality. Achondrogenesis can be subdivided into type 1 and type 2. Type 1 can further be subdivided into type 1A and type 1B. Types 1A and 1B are distinguished by microscopic differences in the cartilage and cartilage-forming cells. Cartilage-forming cells (chondrocytes) are abnormal in type 1A, whereas the cartilage matrix itself is abnormal in type 1B.

Previously, health care professionals had recognized achondrogenesis types 3 and 4, but those classifications have been abandoned. Types 3 and 4 are now considered to be slight variations of type 2 achondrogenesis. Types 1A, 1B, and type 2 all have different genetic causes, and that is one factor supporting the current classification.

Synonyms

Synonyms for achondrogenesis include chondrogenesis imperfecta, **hypochondrogenesis**, lethal neonatal dwarfism, lethal osteochondrodysplasia, and neonatal dwarfism. Achondrogenesis type 1A is also known as Houston-Harris type, achondrogenesis type 1B is also known as Fraccaro type chondrogenesis, and achondrogenesis type 2 is also known as Langer-Saldino type achondrogenesis or type 3 or type 4 achondrogenesis.

Genetic profile

As previously mentioned, achondrogenesis is currently divided into three distinct subtypes: type 1A, type 1B, and type 2. It appears that each subtype is caused by mutations in different genes.

The **gene** for type 1A has not yet been isolated, but it does follow an autosomal recessive pattern of **inheritance**.

Type 1B follows an autosomal recessive pattern of inheritance as well, but the gene has been isolated. It is the **diastrophic dysplasia** sulfate transporter gene (DTDST), which is located on the long arm of **chromosome** 5 (5q32-q33 specifically). Abnormalities in the DTDST gene result in abnormal sulfation of proteins, which is thought to result in disease.

The severity of mutation determines which disorder the patient will have. The most severe of these disorders is type 1B. Since both type 1A and 1B follow autosomal recessive patterns of inheritance, the chance of parents having another child with the disorder after having the first child is 25% for both disorders.

Similar to achondrogenesis type 1B, achondrogenesis type 2 represents the most severe disorder of a group of disorders resulting from the mutation of a single gene—the collagen type 2 gene (COL2A1), located on the long arm of chromosome 12 (12q13.1-q13.3 specifically). In addition to its important role in development and growth, collagen type 2 plays an important structural role in cartilage and in the ability of cartilage to resist compressive forces. Type 2, however, does not follow an autosomal recessive pattern of inheritance. Most of the mutations that cause type 2 are new mutations, meaning they are not passed from parents to children. Also, most of these mutations are considered autosomal dominant. However, some family members of affected children may have the mutant gene without having the disease. This is not a classical pattern of dominance and implies the involvement of other genes in the disease process.

Demographics

Achondrogenesis is equally rare in males and females of all races in the United States. Although the

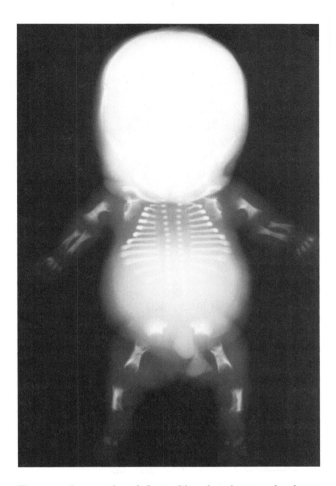

The x-ray image of an infant with achondrogenesis shows the absence of spinal ossification as well as short bone formation throughout the body. *(Greenwood Genetic Center.)*

exact incidence is unknown, one estimate places the incidence at 1 case in every 40,000 births.

Signs and symptoms

Traits found in all subtypes of achondrogenesis

All infants with achondrogenesis share these characteristics: an extremely short neck, underdeveloped lungs, a protuberant abdomen, low birth weight, extremely short limbs (micromelia) and other skeletal abnormalities. The most defining feature of this condition is the extreme shortness of the limbs.

Additionally, fetuses with achondrogenesis may have the condition polyhydramnios, a condition in which there is too much fluid around the fetus in the amniotic sac, and/or fetal hydrops, a condition in which there is too much fluid in the fetal tissues and/or cavities. Infants with achondrogenesis are also often born in the breech position (hindquarters first).

Differences in traits shared by all subtypes of achondrogenesis

Although all the subtypes of achondrogenesis share some characteristics, there are differences in some of these characteristics between subtypes. Type 1 achondrogenesis is generally considered to be more severe than type 2. This is supported by the shorter limbs found in type 1 and the lower average birth weight of type 1 infants compared to type 2 infants. Although any birth weight below 5.5 lbs (2,500 g) is considered to be low, type 1 infants average 2.6 lbs (1,200 g), whereas type 2 infants average 4.6 lbs (2,100 g). Additionally, both groups have a number of subtle skeletal abnormalities in addition to those already discussed.

Traits found in type 1 not shared by type 2 achondrogenesis

Type 1 achondrogenesis has two non-subtle characteristics that type 2 does not. Type 1 is often accompanied by abnormal connections either on the inside of the infant's heart or in the major blood vessels leading to and away from the heart. These defects are formally known as either atrial septal defects, ventral septal defects, or a **patent ductus arteriosus**. These connections allow oxygenated blood and deoxygenated blood to mix. Normally, oxygenated and deoxygenated blood are separated to ensure enough oxygen makes it to important tissues, like the brain. Mixing the blood results in less oxygen being pumped into the body and insufficient oxygenation of tissues around the body.

The other type 1 characteristic is incomplete ossification. Ossification is the process of bone formation. In type 1A, incomplete ossification can be seen in many bones, including the skull. In type 1B, the skull is ossified, but bones other than the skull reveal incomplete ossification. No deficiency in ossification can be seen in type 2 achondrogenesis.

Diagnosis

Prenatal diagnosis of a skeletal disorder may be made by ultrasound. **DNA** testing may be used to determine the type of disorder, or to confirm the presence of a suspected disorder. Otherwise, diagnosis may be made by the physical appearance of the infant at birth, and/or x rays. DNA analysis or a microscopic examination of cartilage tissues may be used to identify the type of disorder.

Treatment and management

There is no treatment for the underlying disorder. Parents should consider mental health and **genetic**

KEY TERMS

Chondrocyte—A specialized type of cell that secretes the material which surrounds the cells in cartilage.

Fetal hydrops—A condition in which there is too much fluid in the fetal tissues and/or cavities.

Micromelia—The state of having extremely short limbs.

Ossification—The process of the formation of bone from its precursor, a cartilage matrix.

Polyhadramnios—A condition in which there is too much fluid around the fetus in the amniotic sac.

---

counseling to deal with the grief of losing a child, and to understand the risks of the disorder recurring in subsequent children. Support groups may be helpful in the pursuit of these goals. It is important for genetic counseling purposes to determine the type of achondrogenesis that affected the child, since different types of achondrogenesis carry very different prognoses for future children.

Prognosis

This disorder is fatal at birth or soon after. Type 1 is considered more severe, partly because infants with type 1 are more likely to be stillborn and generally succumb to the disorder earlier than infants with type 2 achondrogenesis.

Resources

ORGANIZATIONS

International Center for Skeletal Dysplasia. St. Joseph Hospital, 7620 York Road, Towson, MD 21204. (410) 337-1250.

International Skeletal Dysplasia Registry. Cedars-Sinai Medical Center. 444 S. San Vicente Boulevard, Suite 1001, Los Angeles, CA 90048. (310) 855-7488. priore@mailgate.csmc.edu.

Little People of America, Inc. National Headquarters, PO Box 745, Lubbock, TX 79408. (806) 737-8186 or (888) LPA-2001. lpadatabase@juno.com. <http://www.lpaonline.org>.

Parents of Dwarfed Children. 2524 Colt Terrace, Silver Spring, MD 20902. (301) 649-3275.

WEBSITES

"Achdrogenesis." *National Organization of Rare Disorders (NORD).* <http://www.nord.org>.

Lewit, Eugene M., Linda Schuurmann Baker, Hope Corman, and Patricia H. Shiono. "The direct cost of low birth weight." *The Future of Children* 5, no.1 (Spring 1995). <http://www.futureofchildren.org/LBW/04LBWLEW.htm>.

"Polyhydramnios." *Dartmouth-Hitchcock Medical Center—Division of Maternal-Fetal Medicine.* <http://www.dartmouth.edu/~obgyn/mfm/PatientEd/Polyhdramnios.html>.

Schafer, Frank A. MD. "Achdrogenesis" In *Pediatrics/Genetics and Metabolic Disease, e-medicine* <http://www.emedicine.com/ped/topic2.htm>. (April 24, 2001).

Michael V. Zuck, PhD

Achondroplasia

Definition

Achondroplasia is a common form of dwarfism or short stature due to an autosomal dominant mutation (a mutation on one of the first 22 "non-sex" chromosomes) that causes an individual to have short stature with disproportionately short arms and legs, a large head, and distinctive facial features, including a prominent forehead and a flattened midface.

Description

Achondroplasia is a genetic form of dwarfism due to a problem of bone growth and development. There are many causes for dwarfism, including hormone imbalances and metabolic problems. Achondroplasia belongs to a class of dwarfism referred to as a chrondrodystrophy or **skeletal dysplasia**. All skeletal dysplasias are the result of a problem with bone formation or growth. There are over 100 different types of skeletal **dysplasia**. Achondroplasia is the most common and accounts for half of all known skeletal dysplasias.

Achondroplasia is easily recognizable. Affected individuals have disproportionate short stature, large heads with characteristic facial features, and disproportionate shortening of their limbs. Most individuals with achondroplasia have a normal IQ. The motor development of infants is delayed due to hypotonia (low muscle tone) and their physical differences (large heads and small bones). The motor development of children with achondroplasia eventually catches up with that of their peers. Individuals with achondroplasia can have medical complications that range from mild to severe. Because of the differences in their bone structure, these individuals are prone to middle ear infections. They are also at risk for neurologic problems due to spinal cord compression. The spinal canal (which holds the spinal cord) is smaller than normal in achondroplasia. The American Academy of Pediatrics' Committee on Genetics has developed guidelines for the medical management of children with achondroplasia.

The short stature of achondroplasia can be a socially isolating and physically challenging. Most public places are not adapted to individuals of short stature and this can limit their activities. Children and adults with achondroplasia can be socially ostracized due to their physical appearance. Many people erroneously assume that individuals with achondroplasia have limited abilities. It is very important to increase awareness with educational programs and to take proactive steps to foster self-esteem in children with achondroplasia.

Genetic profile

Achondroplasia is caused by a mutation, or change, in the fibroblast growth factor receptor 3 **gene** (FGFR3) located on the short arm of **chromosome** 4.

Genes contain the instructions that tell a body how to form. They are composed of four different chemical bases–adenine (A), thymine (T), cytosine (C), and guanine (G). These bases are arranged like words in a sentence and the specific order of these four bases provide the instructions that a cell needs to form a protein.

FGFR (fibroblast growth factor receptor) genes provide the instruction for the formation of a cell receptor. Every cell in the body has an outer layer called a cell membrane that serves as a filter. Substances are transported into and out of the cells by receptors located on the surface of the cell membrane. Every cell has hundreds of different types of receptors. The fibroblast growth factor receptor transports fibroblast growth factors into a cell. Fibroblast growth factors play a role in the normal growth and development of bones. When the receptors for fibroblast growth factors do not work properly, the cell does not receive enough fibroblast growth factors and results in abnormal growth and development of bones.

Achondroplasia is caused by mutations in the FGFR3 gene. Two specific mutations account for approximately 99% of achondroplasia. The FGFR gene is comprised of 2,520 bases. In a normal (non-mutated) gene, base number 1138 is guanine (G). In most individuals with achondroplasia (98%), this guanine (G) has been replaced with adenine (A). In a small number of individuals with achondroplasia (1%), this guanine (G) has been replaced with cytosine (C). Both of these small substitutions cause a change in the fibroblast growth factor receptor (FGFR) that affects the function of this receptor.

Mutations in the FGFR3 gene are inherited in an autosomal dominant manner. Every individual has two FGFR3 genes—one from their father and one from their mother. In an autosomal dominant disorder, only one gene has to have a mutation for the person to have the disorder. Over 80% of individuals with achondroplasia are born to parents with average stature. Their achondroplasia is the result of a *de novo* or new mutation. No one knows the cause of *de novo* mutations or why they occur so frequently in achondroplasia. For reasons that are not yet understood, most new mutations occur in the FGFR3 gene that is inherited from the average-size father.

An individual with achondroplasia has a 50% chance of passing on their changed (mutated) gene to their children. An achondroplastic couple (both parents have achondroplasia) has a 25% chance that they will have a child with average stature, a 50% chance that they will have a child with one achondroplasia gene (a heterozygote), and a 25% chance that a child will get a two copies of the achondroplasia gene (a homozygote). Babies with homozygous achondroplasia are much more severely affected than babies with a single achondroplasia gene. These infants generally die very shortly after birth because of breathing problems caused by an extremely small chest.

Demographics

Because individuals with other forms of dwarfism are often misdiagnosed with achondroplasia, the exact incidence of achondroplasia is unknown. Estimates of the incidence of achondroplasia vary between 1/10,000 to 1/40,000 births. It is estimated that there are approximately 15,000 individuals with achondroplasia in the United States and 65,000 worldwide. Achondroplasia affects males and females in equal numbers.

Signs and symptoms

Individuals with achondroplasia have disproportionate short stature, large heads with characteristic facial features, and rhizomelic shortening of their limbs. Rhizomelic means "root limb." Rhizomelic shortening of the limbs means that those segments of a limb closest to the body (the root of the limb) are more severely affected. In individuals with achondroplasia, the upper arms are shorter than the forearms and the upper leg (thigh) is shorter than the lower leg.

In addition to shortened limbs, individuals with achondroplasia have other characteristic limb differences. People with achondroplasia have a limited ability to rotate and extend their elbows. They generally develop bowed legs and may have in-turned toes. Their hands and feet are short and broad, as are their fingers and toes. Their hands have been described as having a "trident" configuration. This term is based upon the trident fork used in Greek mythology and describes the unusual separation of their middle fingers. This unusual separation gives their hands a "three-pronged" appearance with the thumb and two small fingers on the side and the index and middle finger in the middle.

Individuals with achondroplasia have similar facial features and a large head (megalencephaly) due to the difference in the growth of the bones of the face and head. The exact reason for the increase in head size is not known, but it reflects increased brain size and can sometimes be due to **hydrocephalus**. People with achondroplasia have a protruding forehead (frontal bossing) and a relatively prominent chin. The prominent appearance of the chin is in part due to the relative flatness of their midface. While people with achondroplasia do resemble one another, they also resemble their family of origin.

Individuals with achondroplasia have shortening of their long bones. Women with achondroplasia have an average adult height of 48 in (122 cm). Men have an average adult height of 52 in (132 cm).

Diagnosis

Achondroplasia is generally diagnosed by physical examination at birth. The characteristic findings of short stature, rhizomelic shortening of the limbs, and specific facial features become more pronounced over time. In addition to being diagnosed by physical examination, individuals with achondroplasia have some specific bone changes that can be seen on an x ray. These include a smaller spinal canal and a small foramen magnum. The foramen magnum is the opening at the base of the skull. The spinal cord runs from the spinal canal through the foramen magnum and connects with the brain.

The diagnosis of achondroplasia can also be made prenatally either by ultrasound (sonogram) or by prenatal **DNA** testing. Sonograms use sound waves to provide an image of a fetus. The physical findings of achondroplasia (shortened long bones, trident hand) can be detected in the third trimester (last three months) of a pregnancy. Prior to the last three months of pregnancy, it is difficult to use a sonogram to diagnose achondroplasia because the physical features may not be obvious. Because of the large number of skeletal dysplasias, it can be very difficult to definitively diagnose achondroplasia by sonogram. Many other dwarfing syndromes can look very similar to achondroplasia on a sonogram.

Prenatal testing can also be done using DNA technology. A sample of tissue from a fetus is obtained by either chorionic villi sampling (CVS) or by **amniocentesis**. Chorionic villi sampling is generally done between 10-12 weeks of pregnancy and amniocentesis is done between 16-18 weeks of pregnancy. Chorionic villi sampling involves removing a small amount of tissue from the developing placenta. The tissue in the placenta contains the same DNA as the fetus. Amniocentesis involves removing a small amount of fluid from around the fetus. This fluid contains some fetal skin cells. DNA can be isolated from these skin cells. The fetal DNA is then tested to determine if it contains either of the two mutations responsible for achondroplasia.

Prenatal DNA testing for achondroplasia is not routinely performed in low-risk pregnancies. This type of testing is generally limited to high-risk pregnancies, such as those in which both parents have achondroplasia. It is particularly helpful in determining if a fetus has received two abnormal genes (homozygous achondroplasia). This occurs when both parents have achondroplasia and each of them passes on their affected gene. The baby gets two copies of the achondroplasia gene. Babies with homozygous achondroplasia are much more severely affected than babies with heterozygous achondroplasia. Infants with homozygous achondroplasia generally die shortly after birth due to breathing problems caused by an extremely small chest.

DNA testing can also be performed on blood samples from children or adults. This is usually done if there is some doubt about the diagnosis of achondroplasia or in atypical cases.

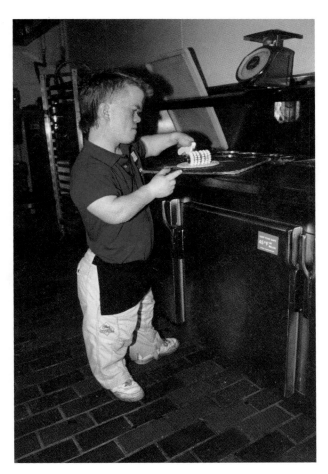

This man has achondroplasia, a disorder characterized by short stature. (Photo Researchers, Inc.)

Treatment and management

There is no cure for achondroplasia. The recommendations for the medical management of individuals with achondroplasia have been outlined by the American Academy of Pediatrics' Committee on Genetics. The potential medical complications of achondroplasia range from mild (ear infections) to severe (spinal cord compression). By being aware of the potential medical complications and catching problems early, it may be possible to avert some of the long-term consequences of these complications. An individual with achondroplasia may have some, all, or none of these complications.

All children with achondroplasia should have their height, weight, and head circumference measured and plotted on growth curves specifically developed for children with achondroplasia. Measurements of head circumference are important to monitor for the development of hydrocephalus—a known but rare (<5%) complication of achondroplasia. Hydrocephalus (or water on the brain) is caused by an enlargement of the fluid-filled cavities of the brain (ventricles) due to a blockage that impedes the movement of the cerebrospinal fluid. Suspected hydrocephalus can be confirmed using imaging techniques such as a CT or MRI scan and can be treated with neurosurgery or shunting (draining) if it causes severe symptoms. Any child displaying neurologic problems such as lethargy, abnormal reflexes, or loss of muscle control should be seen by a neurologist to make sure they are not experiencing compression of their spinal cord. Compression of the spinal cord is common in individuals with achondroplasia because of the abnormal shape and small size of their foramen magnum (opening at the top of the spinal cord).

All children with achondroplasia should be monitored for sleep apnea, which occurs when an individual stops breathing during sleep. This can occur for several

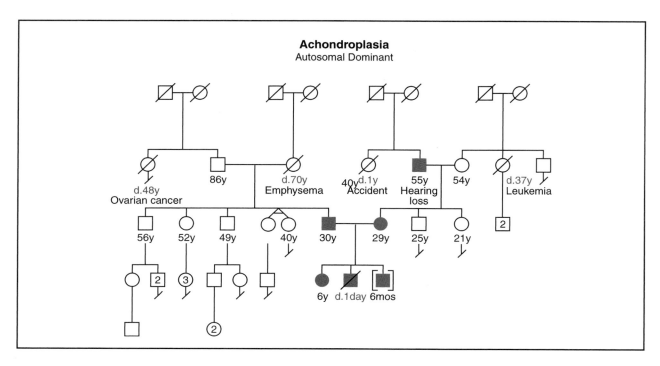

Achondroplasia
Autosomal Dominant

(Gale Group.)

reasons, including obstruction of the throat by the tonsils and adenoids, spinal cord compression and obesity. Individuals with achondroplasia are more prone to sleep apnea due to the changes in their spinal canal, foramen magnum, and because of their short necks. Treatment for sleep apnea depends on its cause. Obstructive sleep apnea is treated by surgically removing the tonsils and adenoids. Neurosurgery may be required to treat sleep apnea due to spinal cord compression. Weight management may also play a role in the treatment of sleep apnea.

Other potential problems in children with achondroplasia include overcrowding of the teeth (dental malocclusion), speech problems (articulation), and frequent ear infections (otitis media). Dental malocclusion (overcrowding of teeth) is treated with orthodontics. All children with achondroplasia should be evaluated by a speech therapist by two years of age because of possible problems with the development of clear speech (articulation). Articulation problems may be caused by orthodontic problems. Due to the abnormal shape of the eustachian tube in an individual with achondroplasia, they are very prone to ear infections (otitis media). Approximately 80% of infants with achondroplasia have an ear infection in the first year of life. About 78% of these infants require ventilation tubes to decrease the frequency of ear infections.

Weight management is extremely important for an individual with achondroplasia. Excess weight can exac-

erbate many of the potential orthopedic problems in an individual with achondroplasia such as bowed legs, curvature of the spine, and joint and lower back pain. Excess weight can also contribute to sleep apnea. Development of good eating habits and appropriate exercise programs should be encouraged in individuals with achondroplasia. These individuals should discuss their exercise programs with their health care provider. Because of the potential for spinal cord compression, care should be used in choosing appropriate forms of exercise.

The social adaptation of children with achondroplasia and their families should be closely monitored. Children with visible physical differences can have difficulties in school and socially. Support groups such as Little People of America can be a source of guidance on how to deal with these issues. It is important that children with achondroplasia not be limited in activities that pose no danger. In addition to monitoring their social adaptation, every effort should be made to physically adapt their surroundings for convenience and to improve independence. Physical adaptations can include stools to increase accessibility and lowering of switches and counters.

Two treatments have been used to try to increase the final adult height of individuals with achondroplasia–limb-lengthening and growth hormone therapy. There are risks and benefits to both treatments and they are still considered experimental.

KEY TERMS

Fibroblast growth factor receptor gene—A type of gene that codes for a cell membrane receptor involved in normal bone growth and development.

Rhizomelic—Disproportionate shortening of the upper part of a limb compared to the lower part of the limb.

Limb-lengthening involves surgically attaching external rods to the long bones in the arms and legs. These rods run parallel to the bone on the outside of the body. Over a period of 18-24 months the tension on these rods is increased, which results in the lengthening of the underlying bone. This procedure is long, costly, and has potential complications such as pain, infections, and nerve problems. Limb-lengthening can increase overall height by 12-14 in (30.5-35.6 cm). It does not change the other physical manifestations of achondroplasia such as the appearance of the hands and face. This is an elective surgery and individuals must decide for themselves if it would be of benefit to them. The optimal age to perform this surgery is not known.

Growth hormone therapy has been used to treat some children with achondroplasia. Originally there was doubt about the effectiveness of this treatment because children with achondroplasia are not growth hormone deficient. However, studies have shown that rate of growth in children with achondroplasia treated with growth hormone does increase during the first two years of treatment. It is too early to say how effective this treatment is because the children involved in this study are still growing and have not reached their final adult height.

Prognosis

The prognosis for most people with achondroplasia is very good. In general, they have minimal medical problems, normal IQ, and most achieve success and have a long life regardless of their stature. The most serious medical barriers to an excellent prognosis are the neurologic complications that can arise in achondroplasia. Spinal cord compression is thought to increase the risk for SIDS to 7.5% in infants with achondroplasia and can lead to life-long complications such as paralysis if untreated. Obesity can increase the risk for heart disease and some studies have revealed an increased risk of unexplained death in the fourth and fifth decade of life.

Successful social adaptation plays an important role in the ultimate success and happiness of an individual with achondroplasia. It is very important that the career and life choices of an individual with achondroplasia not be limited by preconceived ideas about their abilities.

Resources

BOOKS

Ablon, Joan. *Living with Difference: Families with Dwarf Children.* Westport, CT: Praeger Publishing, 1988.

PERIODICALS

American Academy of Pediatrics Committee on Genetics. "Health Supervision for Children With Achondroplasia." *Pediatrics* 95, no 3 (March 1995): 443-51.

ORGANIZATIONS

Little People of America, Inc. National Headquarters, PO Box 745, Lubbock, TX 79408. (806) 737-8186 or (888) LPA-2001. lpadatabase@juno.com. <http://www.lpaonline.org>.

WEBSITES

The Human Growth Foundation <http://www.hgfound.org/>.

Little People of America: An Organization for People of Short Stature. <http://www.lpaonline.org/lpa.html>.

Kathleen Fergus, MS

ACHOO syndrome

Definition

ACHOO syndrome is a generally benign condition characterized by sudden, uncontrollable sneezing after viewing a bright light.

Description

The ACHOO syndrome, standing for autosomal dominant compelling heliopthalmic outburst syndrome, is an inherited condition where a person will involuntarily sneeze after seeing a bright light. A person with this condition will sneeze multiple times, and in rare cases may sneeze 30-40 times. The syndrome is usually more intense if the person with the condition moves suddenly from darkness into an area with bright lights or sunlight.

Genetic profile

The ACHOO syndrome is thought to be inherited in an autosomal dominant pattern. This means that only

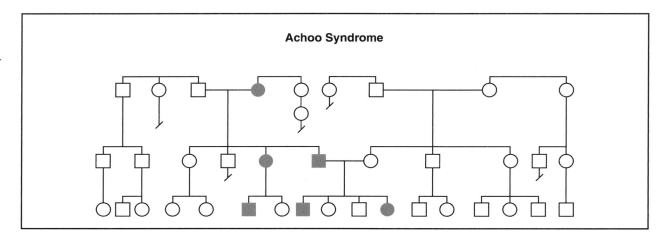

Achoo Syndrome

(Gale Group.)

one copy of the abnormal **gene** needs to be present for the syndrome to occur. If one parent has the condition, their children will have a 50% chance of also having the syndrome. One physician reported the condition in a family, where it was observed in the father and his brother, but not seen in the father's mother or his wife. Both the father and brother would sneeze twice when going from an area of darkness to an area of light. At four weeks of age, the father's daughter also started to sneeze whenever she was moved into bright sunlight.

Because of the relatively benign nature of the condition, there has been no reported scientific work trying to locate the gene responsible for the syndrome.

Demographics

Occurrence of the ACHOO syndrome is widespread in the general population. The few well-documented studies performed report the condition as being present in 23-33% of individuals. Men seem to be affected more than women. Studies on the occurrence of the syndrome in various ethnic groups are very limited. One study showed differences between whites and non-whites, while another study showed no difference.

Signs and symptoms

The prominent symptom of people with the ACHOO syndrome is sudden, involuntary sneezing when they see a bright light or sunlight. The way in which sneezing is triggered is not very well understood, but there are several theories that attempt to explain the syndrome.

One theory is that people who have the ACHOO syndrome have a hypersensitive reaction to light, just like some people have a sensitivity to cat hairs or pollen. When a person with the syndrome is exposed to a bright light, the same mechanism in the body that triggers a sneeze due to an irritant such as pollen somehow confuses light with that irritant and causes a sneeze to occur. Another idea is that the sneeze reflex in people with the ACHOO syndrome is somehow linked to real nasal allergies, although this does not explain the syndrome in people without nasal allergies. A third theory is that people with the ACHOO syndrome are very sensitive to seeing bright light. The sneeze reflex of the syndrome can then be thought of as an involuntary defense reaction against bright light; when the person sneezes, they automatically close their eyes.

Diagnosis

The ACHOO syndrome is diagnosed simply by observing the sneezing pattern of a person, and by looking into the sneezing patterns of the person's close relatives. If the person seems to sneeze every time they are exposed to a bright light, and if their parents and offspring do the same, then the diagnosis of the ACHOO syndrome can be made.

Currently, there are no known blood tests or other medical tests that can help diagnose the syndrome.

Treatment and management

There are no specific treatments for the ACHOO syndrome. Common measures, such as wearing sunglasses, can help people who are severely affected.

There have been reports that people who have nasal allergies have a higher incidence of the ACHOO syndrome. Therefore, it is sometimes assumed that medica-

KEY TERMS

Allergy—Condition in which immune system is hypersensitive to contact with allergens; an abnormal response by the immune system to contact with an allergen; condition in which contact with allergen produces symptoms such as inflammation of tissues and production of excess mucus in respiratory system.

Antibody—A protein produced by the mature B cells of the immune system that attach to invading microorganisms and target them for destruction by other immune system cells.

Antigen—A substance or organism that is foreign to the body and stimulates a response from the immune system.

Hypersensitivity—A process or reaction that occurs at above normal levels; overreaction to a stimulus.

Immune response—Defense mechanism of the body provided by its immune system in response to the presence of an antigen, such as the production of antibodies.

Immune system—A major system of the body that produces specialized cells and substances that interact with and destroy foreign antigens that invade the body.

tions that are used for allergies, such as antihistamines, could perhaps play a beneficial role in the ACHOO syndrome. However, no studies have successfully demonstrated that the syndrome is relieved by this type of medication. Alternative medicine, including homeopathy and herbal medicine, recommend a wide range of remedies for nasal allergies, these may accordingly also be helpful for the ACHOO syndrome.

Prognosis

People with the ACHOO syndrome generally have the condition for life. There is no evidence showing that the ACHOO syndrome in any way affects a person's life span.

Resources

BOOKS

Knight, Jeffrey, and Robert McClenaghan. *Encyclopedia of Genetics.* Pasadena: Salem Press, 1999.

PERIODICALS

Askenasy, J. J. M. "The Photic Sneeze." *Postgraduate Medical Journal* (February 1990): 892-893.

Whitman, B. W., and R. J. Packer. "The Photic Sneeze Reflex." *Neurology* (May 1993): 868-871.

Edward R. Rosick, DO, MPH, MS

Acid maltase deficiency *see* **Pompe disease**

Acrocallosal syndrome

Definition

Acrocallosal syndrome is a rare congenital disorder in which the individual has absence or only partial formation of the corpus callosum. This is accompanied by skull and facial malformations, and some degree of finger or toe malformations. Individuals may display motor and mental retardation. The cause of this genetic disorder is unknown, and the severity of the symptoms vary by individual.

Description

Acrocallosal syndrome was first described by Schinzel in 1979, and also may be referred to as Schinzel acrocallosal syndrome. The term acrocallosal refers to the involvement of the acra (fingers and toes) and the corpus callosum, the thick band of fibers joining the hemispheres of the brain. Reported in both males and females, the cause of the disorder is unknown. The major characteristic of the syndrome is the incomplete formation (hypoplasia) or absence (agenesis) of the corpus callosum. Facial appearance is typically similar among affected people. This includes a prominent forehead, an abnormal increase in the distance between the eyes (hypertelorism), and a large head (macrocephaly). Individuals have a degree of webbing or fusion (syndactyly), or duplication (**polydactyly**) of the fingers and toes. Occasionally, those affected may have a short upper lip, cleft palate, cysts that occur within the cranium (intracranial), hernias, or may develop seizure disorders. Less frequently, affected children have congenital heart defects, internal organ (visceral) or kidney (renal) abnormalities.

Moderate to severe mental retardation is reported with acrocallosal syndrome. Individuals usually display some form of poor muscle tone (hypotonia), and there may be a delay or absence of motor activities, walking, and talking. There is great variation of functioning and symptoms with this disorder, ranging

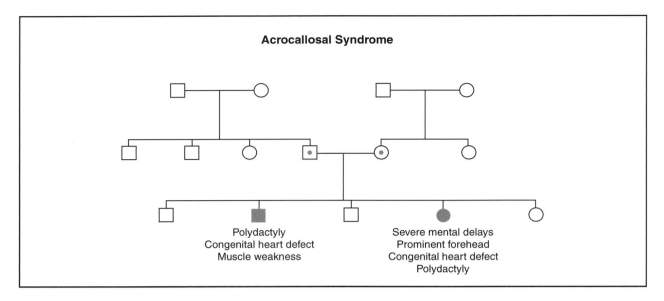

Acrocallosal Syndrome

Polydactyly
Congenital heart defect
Muscle weakness

Severe mental delays
Prominent forehead
Congenital heart defect
Polydactyly

(Gale Group.)

from normal development to severe mental and motor retardation.

Genetic profile

The cause of acrocallosal syndrome is unknown. There are sporadic, or random, cases, and reports of multiple cases within families. Studies involving affected families have suggested an autosomal recessive pattern of **inheritance**. This means that both parents carry the altered form of the **gene**, and the affected child inherited both copies. Following this pattern, each child born will have a 25% risk of being affected.

To help determine which **chromosome** or gene location causes the syndrome, acrocallosal syndrome has been compared with similar disorders. One condition that presents similar symptoms and has a known genetic cause is **Greig cephalopolysyndactyly** syndrome. However, there is no genetic similarity between the two conditions. To date, no specific genetic cause for acrocallosal syndrome is known, and the disorder can only be identified by clinical symptoms.

Demographics

Acrocallosal syndrome is extremely rare. Reports of this disorder may occur within family lines, or randomly. It affects both males and females. There are some reports of webbing of the fingers or toes (syndactyly) and relatedness (consanguinity) of the parents of affected children. However, affected children may also have unrelated, healthy parents and unaffected siblings.

Signs and symptoms

At birth, those with acrocallosal syndrome present the characteristic pattern of facial and limb malformations. Limb appearance ranges from minor webbing between the fingers or toes to near duplication of the hands or feet. Forehead prominence, increased distance between the eyes, and an enlarged head are the main features of facial appearance. X-ray tests will reveal the absence or incomplete formation of the corpus callosum, and the presence of any cysts within the cranium. The infant will usually display reduced muscle tone (hypotonia). This may lead to a drooling condition or feeding difficulties. Hypotonia can also contribute to a delay in growth and motor skills. Severe hypotonia is usually associated with a form of mental retardation.

Progress and functioning during the first year of life is dependent upon the severity of the symptoms. There has been a wide range of individual variation reported, and the degree to which symptoms affect each child may differ. Some children develop normally and will walk and talk within normal age limits, while others may experience a delay or absence of certain motor activities. Mental retardation may be moderate or severe. Some children may develop seizure disorders. The degree and progression of mental retardation also varies by individual.

Diagnosis

The diagnosis of acrocallosal syndrome is based initially on the distinct pattern of facial and limb malforma-

KEY TERMS

Computed tomography (CT) scan—An imaging procedure that produces a three-dimensional picture of organs or structures inside the body, such as the brain.

Consanguinity—A mating between two people who are related to one another by blood.

Corpus callosum—A thick bundle of nerve fibers deep in the center of the forebrain that provides communications between the right and left cerebral hemispheres.

Hypertelorism—A wider-than-normal space between the eyes.

Hypotonia—Reduced or diminished muscle tone.

Polydactyly—The presence of extra fingers or toes.

Syndactyly—Webbing or fusion between the fingers or toes.

tions. Computed tomography (CT), or a similar radiographic procedure, of the head reveals the absence of the corpus callosum. Hand and foot x rays can be taken to confirm finger or toe abnormalities, and will determine the extent of fusion, webbing, or duplication of the fingers or toes.

Prenatal diagnosis may not be possible due to the variability of the condition. However, **prenatal ultrasound** can detect duplication of the digits (polydactyly) and cerebral malformations. This may be especially informative for a woman who already has an affected child and has a 25% risk of having another affected child.

Treatment and management

Beginning in infancy, physical therapy may assist in the development of motor skills and muscle tone. Surgery to remove extra fingers and release fused fingers may improve movement and grasp, though the muscle tone may remain poor. Surgery to separate or remove affected toes may assist in walking and the comfort of footwear. Anti-epileptic therapy should be considered if a seizure disorder develops. Special education may be required, depending on the level of mental impairment.

Prognosis

At present, there are no preventative measures for acrocallosal syndrome, and the severity of symptoms and outcomes varies by individual. It has been found that the lifestyle of an individual with acrocallosal syndrome is dependent upon the degree of mental retardation and reduced muscle tone, rather than the extent of facial and limb malformations.

Resources

PERIODICALS

Bonatz, E., et al. "Acrocallosal Syndrome: A Case Report." *The Journal of Hand Surgery* 22A (1997): 492-494.

Fryns, J. P., et al. "Polysyndactyly and Trignocephaly with Partial Agenesis of the Corpus Callosum: An Example of the Variable Clinical Spectrum of the Acrocallosal Syndrome?" *Clinical Dysmorphology* 6 (1997): 285-286.

Fryns, J. P., et al. "The Variable Clinical Spectrum and Mental Prognosis of the Acrocallosal Syndrome." *Journal of Medical Genetics* 28, no. 23 (March 1991): 214-215.

Hendriks, H.J.E., et al. "Acrocallosal Syndrome." *American Journal of Medical Genetics* 35 (1990): 443-446.

Schinzel, A., and U. Kaufmann. "The Acrocallosal Syndrome in Sisters." *Clinical Genetics* 30 (1986): 339-405.

Thyen, U., et al. "Acrocallosal Syndrome: Association with Cystic Malformation of the Brain and Neurodevelopmental Aspects." *Neuropediatrics* 23 (1992): 292-296.

ORGANIZATIONS

Agenesis of the Corpus Callosum (ACC) Network. Merrill Hall, University of Maine, Room 18, 5749, Orono, ME 04469-5749. (207) 581-3119. um-acc@maine.edu.

WEBSITES

AboutFace U.S.A. <http://www.aboutface2000.org>.

FACES: The National Craniofacial Association. <http://www.faces-cranio.org>.

Maureen Teresa Mahon, BS, MFS

Acrocephalopolysyndactyly type II *see* **Carpenter syndrome**

Acrocephalosyndactyly type I *see* **Apert syndrome**

Acrocephalosyndactyly type III *see* **Saethre-Chotzen syndrome**

Acromatopsia *see* **Color blindness**

Acromegaly

Definition

Acromegaly is a rare condition caused by abnormally high amounts of human growth hormone (HGH). An organ in the brain known as the pituitary gland, normally secretes this growth hormone. Normal amounts of HGH are needed for normal growth and physical maturity in children. However, in acromegaly, there is an increased amount of HGH released, generally by a tumor that forms in the pituitary. Untreated, acromegaly can lead to numerous disabling conditions, as well as a significantly decreased life span.

Description

Acromegaly was first described in scientific detail by the French physician, Pierre Marie. In 1886, Dr. Marie, along with his assistant, Souza-Leite, described in detail 48 patients with acromegaly. These patients all exhibited a rapid growth in their height; significantly enlarged hands and feet; change in appearance of their faces; frequent headaches; and a high incidence of visual problems. Dr. Marie believed all of these problems were due to a defect in the patients' pituitary gland, a small glandular structure located in the middle of the brain.

While Dr. Marie was the first to formally state that a problem in the pituitary gland was responsible for the condition of acromegaly, the link between pituitary defects and acromegaly remained controversial for many years. It was not until 1909, when Dr. Harvey Cushing introduced the concepts of hyperpituitarism in reference to acromegaly, that the association became generally accepted. Dr. Cushing believed acromegaly was due to the pituitary gland, a small structure located deep in the brain and known to be somehow involved in growth, over-secreting some type of substance that caused patients to become "giants." Dr. Cushing also put forth the idea that the over-activity of the pituitary gland was caused by a tumor in the gland, an idea that was proven by autopsies done on patients with acromegaly. At the time, however, it still was not clear how a tumor in the pituitary gland could cause such changes in people afflicted with the tumor.

In the decades after World War II, the structure and function of the pituitary gland was further studied. Dr. Herbert Evans at the University of California at Berkley was the first to isolate many secretions, also known as hormones, which were found to be made in and secreted from the pituitary gland. One of these hormones was found to be human growth hormone, or HGH. It was also discovered that certain tumors can form in the pituitary gland and secrete high levels of HGH, resulting in abnormal growth and, as time progresses, acromegaly.

Acromegaly is a rare condition, with only about 1,000 cases per year in the United States among a total population of 250 million. Its striking consequence of excessive height has caused it to remain a fascinating disease among both scientists, doctors, and the public. Besides causing great height and unusual facial features, it is now known that acromegaly also causes serious conditions that can be life threatening, such as heart disease, respiratory disease, arthritis, neuromuscular problems, and **diabetes**. With early detection and treatment, the consequences of acromegaly can be minimized and patients afflicted with the condition can lead mainly healthy, productive lives.

Genetic profile

The genetics behind the majority of cases of acromegaly is still poorly understood. The most common cause of acromegaly is a benign (non-cancerous) tumor in the pituitary gland that secretes HGH. It is known that the benign tumor arises from cells in the pituitary gland, possibly due to a defect in the pituitary gland itself. The **gene** responsible for this tumor formation is unknown.

Even though the genetics of tumor formation in the pituitary gland leading to most cases of acromegaly is not yet known, there are other conditions that lead to acromegaly in which the genetic causes of the conditions are known. In a very rare condition called familial acromegaly, there is a gene on **chromosome** 11 believed to cause the formation and growth of an HGH-secreting tumor in the pituitary gland. Familial acromegaly is transmitted in an autosomal dominant pattern—which means that it has an equal chance of affecting both boys and girls in a single family. This condition can also cause tumors in other areas of the body besides the pituitary, including the parathyroid gland, which controls the amount of calcium in the bloodstream, and the pancreas, which regulates insulin needed for the body to process sugars.

Another uncommon condition causing HGH-secreting tumors in the pituitary gland is called multiple endocrine neoplasia-1, or MEN-1. This is an autosomal dominant condition characterized by a combination of pituitary, parathyroid, and pancreatic tumors. The gene for this condition has also been found on chromosome 11 and is known as the MEN-1 gene. About half the patients with this abnormal gene will eventually develop acromegaly.

Carney syndrome is a rare autosomal dominant disorder that can cause HGH-secreting pituitary tumors and acromegaly in about 20% of patients who have the syndrome. Carney syndrome is associated with a defective gene on chromosome 2. Besides acromegaly, people with Carney syndrome also frequently have abnormal skin pigmentation, heart tumors, and tumors of the testicles and adrenal glands.

McCune-Albright syndrome is a very rare disorder that can cause acromegaly through HGH-secreting tumors in the pituitary. Other conditions associated with this syndrome are polycystic fibrous **dysplasia** (affecting bone growth, especially in the pelvis and long bones of the arms and legs), abnormal skin pigmentation, early puberty, and thyroid problems. The gene for the syndrome, named GNAS1, is located on chromosome 20.

Demographics

Acromegaly is a very rare condition. It is estimated to occur in about 30-60 individuals per million people. Both males and females seem to be affected equally. There also does not seem to be any difference in secondary complications of acromegaly between males and females. The condition has been recorded at all ages of life, from early childhood into old age. The frequency of chronic complications increases with age in both men and women.

Most cases of acromegaly are detected on an initial visit to a family physician, although some early or mild cases may be missed, causing a delay in the diagnosis. Some patients with acromegaly are initially diagnosed in specialty clinics, such as cardiology clinics and diabetic clinics when they present with secondary problems caused by the condition.

There is very little data on the differences of the occurrence of acromegaly among various ethic and racial lines. The few studies that have been done show no real difference among racial or ethnic groups, with acromegaly showing up equally in Caucasians, African-Americans, and Asian-Americans.

Signs and symptoms

The signs and symptoms of acromegaly can range from striking to almost unseen. The most visible signs of the condition are greatly increased height and coarse facial features. People with acromegaly who have not received treatment early in the course of their condition have grown to be well over seven feet tall. Almost always with this spurt in height there is coarsening of facial features due to abnormal growth of the facial bones. Another very noticeable feature is enlargement of both the hands and feet, which, like the abnormal facial features, is the product of hormones and results in increased bone growth.

Other less visible, yet common, signs of acromegaly are increased sweating, constant and at times debilitating

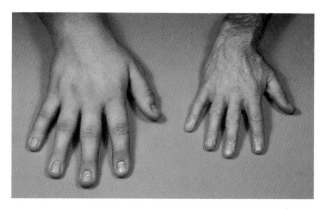

Comparison of hand size between a patient with acromegaly (left) and that of an unaffected adult (right). *(Custom Medical Stock Photo, Inc.)*

headaches, visual disturbances, and increase in hair growth. Loss of sexual desire is often seen in both men and women. Amenorrhea, the cessation of menses (stopping of menstruation), is often a secondary condition associated with acromegaly in women.

There are further secondary complications of acromegaly that are not visible but can be life threatening. People with acromegaly are at greater risk for developing high blood pressure, cardiac disease, high cholesterol levels, arthritis and other degenerative diseases of the joints and spine, and diabetes. Acromegly also increases the risk of other tumors, some of them cancerous, in other areas of the body, especially the breast, colon, and to a lesser degree, prostate.

With adequate treatment, especially early in the course of the condition, many of the secondary symptoms of acromegaly can be halted or even reversed. Less life-threatening complications, such as headaches, visual problems and increased sweating can be almost eliminated after adequate and timely treatment. More serious conditions such as heart disease, high blood pressure, and diabetes can be brought under control with treatment, although many times not totally eliminated.

Diagnosis

For most forms of acromegaly, there are no genetic tests yet available to diagnosis the condition in newborns or before birth. Diagnosis is made by recognizing the clinical signs and symptoms previously described. In certain very rare conditions such as multiple endocrine neoplasia-1 and Carney syndrome, the genetics of the conditions are known and can theoretically be tested for. However, the conditions are so seldom encountered that unless a family member has the condition, **genetic test-**

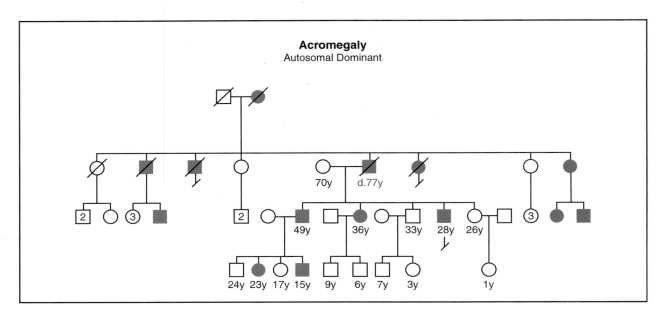

Acromegaly
Autosomal Dominant

(Gale Group.)

ing is usually not done until clinical signs and symptoms are apparent.

Treatment and management

The treatment and management of acromegaly has evolved over the past one hundred years from crude surgery to genetically engineered medications. Today, through precise surgery and medications, a large percentage of patients with acromegaly can have their symptoms brought under control, and in some cases totally cured.

The goal of all therapies, be it surgery or medications, is a reduction in the level of HGH to levels seen in people without acromegaly. This goal can be achieved either through the removal or destruction of the tumor secreting the hormone, inhibition of HGH from the tumor, or blocking the effects of increased HGH on organs and other body systems outside the pituitary.

Surgical removal of the pituitary tumor is still the first treatment of choice for acromegaly. The rate at which a cure is achieved is determined by several factors, including the size of the tumor, whether or not it has spread outside the pituitary, and the level of HGH before the surgery. In patients with small tumors confined to the pituitary and exhibiting only moderately high HGH levels, the cure rate can be as high as 80–90%. In patients with larger tumors, especially those extending out of the pituitary, cure rates with surgery can be reduced to 40–60%.

Radiation therapy is often a second line choice of treatment for acromegaly, especially in patients who have not achieved a cure with surgery. The treatment of acromegaly with radiation was used early on in the history of the condition, with the first report being written in 1909. Careful application of radiation can significantly reduce the size of pituitary tumors, subsequently decreasing high HGH levels. However, this decrease is often very slow, and it can take over ten years for the HGH levels to drop to normal. Treatment with radiation can also have significant side effects, including damage to the pituitary gland itself, visual loss, and brain damage. Some studies have also suggested that treatment with radiation can lead to tumor formation in other areas of the brain.

The use of medications in the treatment of acromegaly has gained importance over the past few decades in the treatment of the condition. Medications available today include Bromocriptine, octreotide and lanreotide, and a genetically engineered HGH receptor antagonist known as Pegvisomant. All of these medications are generally used in combination with surgery or radiation, although there is debate whether or not the medications could or should be used as first-line agents.

Bromocriptine is known as a dopamine agonist, and was one of the first pharmaceutical agents to be used to lower HGH levels in acromegaly. However, bromocriptine is not effective in a majority of cases,

KEY TERMS

Dopamine—A neurochemical made in the brain that is involved in many brain activities, including movement and emotion.

Hormone—A chemical messenger produced by the body that is involved in regulating specific bodily functions such as growth, development, and reproduction.

Somatostatin—A body chemical, known as a cyclic peptide, involved in the release of human growth hormone from the pituitary gland.

and the medications octreotide and lanreotide have supplemented its use. These medications are also known as somatostatin analogues. They decrease both the size of HGH-secreting pituitary tumors and the secretion of HGH itself. In multiple studies, they have been shown to normalize HGH levels in about 50% of cases and show significant tumor shrinkage in 45% of cases. The drawbacks to using both octreotide and lanreotide include multiple weekly dosing over a 12-month period, as well as acute side effects such as nausea, stomach pain, and diarrhea. Also, long term use of these medications results in an increased risk of developing gallstones.

Pegvisomant is a unique, recently developed genetically engineered HGH receptor antagonist. This medication does not decrease the amount of HGH secreted from pituitary tumors; rather, it desensitizes other organs of the body to the effects of the increased HGH circulating in the body. In medical trials, Pegvisomant was well tolerated and resulted in significant symptomatic improvement. It is hoped that with a combination of surgery to decrease the tumor size and the use of a HGH antagonist like Pegvisomant, both the acute and chronic debilitating symptoms of acromegaly can be greatly diminished, if not totally eliminated.

Prognosis

The prognosis for patients with acromegaly who receive prompt treatment is good, although there are still complications. Patients who do not receive treatment, or those who receive it late in the course of the condition, have frequent and debilitating secondary complications as well as a greater chance for early death.

There are only a few reliable studies examining the overall health benefits of treatment versus no treatment for patients with acromegaly. One study showed that those receiving treatment before the age of 40 years had a much better chance of not developing serious complications then those who were treated after 40 years of age. Those receiving earlier treatment had less chance of developing heart disease, high blood pressure, and diabetes, as well as other secondary complications of the condition.

Even with treatment, mortality rates for people with acromegaly are increased when compared to the rest of the population. The principal causes of early death are cardiac disease, strokes, **cancer**, and respiratory failure. The level of HGH after treatment appears to offer the best statistics for predicting early mortality, with higher levels of post-treatment HGH corresponding to a greater, earlier mortality risk.

Resources

BOOKS

Braunwald, Eugene, et al. *Harrison's Principles of Internal Medicine.* 15th ed. New York: McGraw-Hill Publishing, 2001.

Gelehrter, T., F. Collins, and D. Ginsburg. *Principles of Medical Genetics.* Baltimore: Williams and Wilkins, 1998.

PERIODICALS

Stewart, Paul M. "Current Therapy of Acromegaly." *Trends in Endocrinology and Metabolism* 11, no. 4 (May/June 2000): 128–132.

Wass, John A. H. "Acromegaly." *Pituitary* 2, no. 1 (June 1999): 7–91.

WEBSITES

Acromegaly Information Center. <http://www.acromegaly.com>.

Update on Acromegaly. <www.dotpharmacy.com>.

Edward R Rosick, DO, MPH, MS

Adams-Oliver syndrome

Definition

Adams-Oliver syndrome (AOS) is a condition involving the combination of congenital scalp defects (called aplasia cutis congenita) and a specific type of limb defect.

Description

Adams-Oliver syndrome is a genetic condition characterized by aplasia cutis congenita, most commonly of the scalp and skull, and terminal transverse limb defects. **Congenital heart disease** has also been reported in individuals with this condition. The exact cause of the condition is not well-understood. There is extreme variability in the severity of problems between families with AOS.

Genetic profile

There have been both familial and non-familial cases of Adams-Oliver syndrome reported. The majority of genetic cases have been inherited in an autosomal dominant manner, but since autosomal recessive and sporadic **inheritance** have also been reported. A difference in the presentation of AOS in the dominant versus recessive form has not been documented.

Autosomal dominant inheritance means that only one abnormal **gene** copy is required for the disease to occur. For persons with a copy of the gene, the risk of passing it to their offspring is one in two or 50%.

Autosomal recessive inheritance means that two defective gene copies must be inherited, one from each parent, for the disease to manifest itself. Persons with only one gene mutation are carriers for the disorder. Individuals who are carriers for the recessive type of Adams-Oliver syndrome do not have any symptoms (asymptomatic) and do not know they are carriers unless they have had a child with the syndrome. Carrier testing is not available since the gene location is not known at this time. The likelihood that each member of a couple would be a carrier for a mutation in the same gene is higher in people who are related (called consanguineous). When both parents are carriers for the recessive type of Adams-Oliver syndrome, there is a one in four chance (25%) in each pregnancy for a child to have the disease. There is a two in three chance that a healthy sibling of an affected child is a carrier.

Sporadic occurrences of AOS may be caused by a dominant gene with variable expressivity (no one else in the family has symptoms, but some are actually gene carriers), a new (dominant) mutation occurring during the formation of the embryo where neither parent is a carrier, or the existence of both genetic and non-genetic causes for the same syndrome.

Different mechanisms have been postulated to explain how Adams-Oliver syndrome occurs. They include trauma, uterine compression, amniotic band sequence (a condition resulting from strands of the amnion membrane causing amputation of parts of the fetus),

vascular disruption (blockage of blood flow to a developing part or parts of the fetus), and a large blood clot in the placenta which blocks certain important blood vessels and interrupts blood supply to developing structures. Recently, Adams-Oliver syndrome has been hypothesized to occur as a result of abnormalities in small vessel structures that occur very early in embryo formation. The vascular anomaly could be the result of a genetic defect causing decreased stability of embryonic blood vessels in the presence of specific forces.

Demographics

Adams-Oliver syndrome was first described in 1945. There have been over 125 cases reported in the medical literature. There does not appear to be any ethnic difference in prevalence of this condition.

Signs and symptoms

Limb defects are the most common occurrence in Adams-Oliver syndrome, affecting about 84% of patients. The type of limb defect is usually asymmetrical (not the same on both sides), with a tendency to involve both sides of the body (bilateral), more often the lower limbs than the upper limbs. There is a wide range of severity in the limb defects, from something minimal like small or missing finger or toenails (called nail hypoplasia), to the more severe absence of hands, feet, or lower legs. Other more moderate limb defects that have been reported include webbing (syndactyly) of the skin (cutaneous syndactyly) or bones (bony syndactyly) of the fingers or toes, claw-hand malformation (ectrodactly), and **brachydactyly** (shortened fingers or toes). Brachydactyly is the most common limb defect in AOS.

Congenital cutis aplasia is the second most common problem and is present in about 75% of patients with Adams-Oliver syndrome. In 64% of patients with congenital cutis aplasia, there is also an underlying scull defect. More rarely, scull defects can be seen without scalp defects and may be mistaken for an enlarged soft spot (fontanelle).

Congenital heart defects have been reported to occur in between 13%-20% of patients with Adams-Oliver syndrome.

Many different types of vascular (involving the blood vessels) and valvular (with heart valves) problems have been reported in these patients.

Other clinical features seen with AOS, include short stature, kidney (renal) malformations, cleft palate, small eyes (micropthalmia), **spina bifida** occulta, extra (accessory) nipples, undescended testes, skin lesions, and neurological abnormalities. Mental retardation is present in a few cases.

KEY TERMS

Aplasia cutis congenita (ACC)—A group of disorders with different causes whose common characteristic is absence of skin in a defined area.

Congenital—Refers to a disorder which is present at birth.

Genetic heterogeneity—The occurrence of the same or similar disease, caused by different genes among different families.

Incomplete penetrance—Individuals who inherited an abnormal gene for a disorder, but do not exhibit symptoms of that disorder.

Variable expression—Instances in which an identical genetic mutation leads to varying traits from affected individual to affected individual. This variance may occur between members of two separately affected families or it may occur between affected members of the same family.

Diagnosis

Aplasia cutis congenita is a physical finding that has many causes. To determine whether a patient has Adams-Oliver syndrome clinically, all individuals with aplasia cutis congenita should have a complete pregnancy and family history taken, as well as a complete medical evaluation. When possible, relevant family members should be examined for evidence of the condition. When aplasia cutis congenita is discovered at birth, the placenta should be evaluated. Physical exam of the affected infant includes evaluation of other related structures, specifically teeth, hair, and other areas of skin, nails, and central nervous system. Once this evaluation has been completed and a specific diagnosis of Adams-Oliver syndrome has been established or refuted, **genetic counseling** can be provided.

Prenatal diagnosis by ultrasound of the limb defects and possibly some other abnormalities associated with AOS is possible, but clinical confirmation of the diagnosis occurs after birth. Since the gene (or genes) causing AOS have not been isolated, prenatal diagnostic procedures such as **amniocentesis** or chorionic villus sampling are not indicated.

Treatment and management

The treatment for AOS is different for each individual and is tailored to the specific symptoms. If leg-length discrepancy is present, corrective shoes that increase the sole for the unaffected leg to prevent **scoliosis** and ambulation difficulties can be worn. Orthopedic devices such as prostheses are sometimes recommended. Patients should be referred to a physician specializing in treating patients with limb defects early in life. Surgery for congenital defects and skin grafting for scalp defects may be necessary (about 30% of patients required skin grafting in one study).

Special devices for writing or other activities may be necessary if hand malformations are present.

About 30% of patients in one study suffered major hemmorrhage from the scalp defect. Twenty percent of patients had local infection of the scalp defect. Treatment such as transfusion or antibiotic therapy may be required in these cases.

Appropriate special education services are necessary for those with mental retardation. Counseling and support related to limb defeciency issues are essential for coping. Support groups can provide valuable peer referrals and information.

Prognosis

AOS does not usually alter life span, although complications from associated abnormalities such as mental retardation can cause problems. About 5% of the scalp defects that hemorrhaged severely were fatal. Rare cases of meningitis as a result of infection of the scalp defect have been reported. Asymmetry of the limbs can interfere with their proper function and cause pain. Psychological issues relating to disfigurement are possible.

Resources

BOOKS

Sybert, V. P. "Aplasia cutis congenita: A report of 12 new families and review of the literature." *Pediatric Dermatology*, volume 3. Blackwell Scientific Publications, 1985, pps 1-14.

PERIODICALS

Amor, D., R. J. Leventer, S. Hayllar, and A. Bankier. "Polymicrogyria associated with scalp and limb defects: Variant of Adams-Oliver syndrome." *American Journal of Medical Genetics* 93 (2000): 328.

Swartz, E. N., S. Sanatani, G. S. Sandor, and R. A. Schreiber. "Vascular abnormalities in Adams-Oliver syndrome: Cause or effect?" *American Journal of Medical Genetics* 82 (1999): 49.

ORGANIZATIONS

Cherub Association of Families & Friends of Limb Disorder Children. 8401 Powers Rd., Batavia, NY 14020. (716) 762-9997.

REACH—Association for Children with Hand or Arm Deficiency. 12 Wilson Way, Earl's Barton,

Northamptonshire, United Kingdom, NN6 9NZ. 01 604 811041.

WEBSITES

OMIM—Online Mendelian inheritance in Man <http://www.ncbi.nlm.nig.gov>.

Amy Vance, MS, CGC

Addison disease *see* **Adrenoleukodystrophy (ALD)**

Adenomatous polyposis of the colon (APC) *see* **Familial adenomatous polyposis**

▌Adrenoleukodystrophy

Definition

Adrenoleukodystrophy is a progressive condition that affects the adrenal glands, the glands atop the kidneys responsible for the production of adrenalin, and myelin, which insulates the nerves in the brain and spinal cord.

Description

Adrenoleukodystrophy (ALD) was first described in the early 1900s and was originally called Schilder-Addison disease. It is named for the different parts of the body that are affected; "adreno" refers to the adrenal glands, "leuko" is the Greek word for white (myelin is often called the white matter in the brain and spinal cord) and "dystrophy" meaning impaired growth. Therefore, this disease affects the adrenal glands and the growth of the myelin in the brain and spinal cord. There is a wide range in the severity of symptoms. ALD mainly affects males, but occasionally females have mild or moderate symptoms.

Causes and effects

ALD is caused by problems in the peroxisomes. The peroxisomes are tiny structures in cells that help break down large molecules of fats into smaller ones so that they can be used by the body. In ALD the peroxisomes cannot break down a type of fat called very long chain fatty acids (VLCFA). There are two types of problems that occur because the VLCFA are not broken down. First, because the VLCFA cannot be broken down, they accumulate throughout the body, especially in the brain and the adrenal glands. Very high levels of VLCFA are also seen in the blood. The second type of problem occurs because the fats that are usually made when

VLCFA are broken down are not produced. This is in part what happens in the adrenal glands and in the myelin.

The adrenal glands are located on top of each kidney in the abdomen. Part of the job of the adrenal glands is to use cholesterol (a type of fat made in the body when VLCFA are broken down) to make a few different steroids—chemical combinations that form the basis of hormones, body acids, and anabolic agents. The steroids are used to help the body properly use sodium and potassium and to break down proteins, carbohydrates, and other fats. Some of these steroids are also involved with sexual development and function.

The insulation that surrounds the nerves is called myelin and is also affected by the VLCFA not being broken down. Myelin is made up of a number of different proteins and fats. Normally the VLCFA break down and produce fats that make up part of the myelin. When the VLCFA cannot break down, the fats necessary to make the myelin are not made and the myelin is abnormal. In addition, for reasons not well understood, there is also active breakdown of myelin, also known as demyelination.

Genetic profile

ALD is caused by a mutation in a **gene** called the ALD gene. Genes contain the instructions for how the body grows and develops before and after a person is born. The ALD gene makes a protein called ALDP (ALD protein). Different proteins put together make the tissues and organs in the body such as myelin. ALDP is important because it helps VLCFA get into the peroxisomes. When there is a mutation in the ALD gene, the ALDP is abnormal or not present at all. As a result, the VCLFA cannot get into the peroxisomes and the VLCFA accumulate in other places in the body.

Genes are organized on structures called chromosomes. Hundreds to thousands of genes are found on each **chromosome**. There are 46 chromosomes in each cell of the body. These are grouped into 23 pairs. The first 22 pairs are the same in both males and females. The 23rd pair is called the sex chromosomes; having one X chromosome and one Y chromosome causes a person to be male; having two X chromosomes causes a person to be female. People get one member of each pair from the mother's egg and one member from the father's sperm.

The ALD gene is located on the X chromosome. Since males only have one X chromosome, they only have one copy of the ALD gene. Thus, when a male has a mutation in his ALD gene, he will have ALD. However, females have two X chromosomes and therefore have two copies of the ALD gene. If they have a mutation in one copy of their ALD genes, they may only have mild symptoms of ALD or no symptoms at all. This is because their normal copy of the ALD gene does make normal ALD protein. Females who have one copy of the ALD gene with a mutation and one normal copy are called carriers.

Inheritance

ALD is passed on through families by X-linked recessive **inheritance**. This means that affected males are related through females in the family and there are no males in the family that have passed ALD onto their sons. Females pass on one of their X chromosomes to their children—sons or daughters. For a female carrier, if her normal X chromosome is passed on, her son or daughter will be unaffected and cannot pass ALD onto their children. However, if the X chromosome with the ALD mutation is passed on, a daughter will be a carrier and the son would have ALD. Therefore, a female carrier has a 50% or one in two chance of having an unaffected child (son or daughter), a 25%, or one in four, chance of having a carrier daughter, and a 25% or one in four chance of having an affected son.

When males pass on an X chromosome, they have a daughter. When they pass on a Y chromosome, they have a son. Since the ALD mutation is on the X chromosome, an affected male will always pass the ALD mutation on to his daughters. However, when he has a son, he passes on the Y chromosome, and the son is not affected. Therefore, an affected male passes the ALD gene mutation on to all of his daughters, but none of his sons.

Demographics

ALD has been described in people from all different ethnic groups. Approximately one in 20,000 to one in 42,000 people have ALD.

Signs and symptoms

Adrenal insufficiency

Almost all individuals affected with ALD have problems with their adrenal glands not working properly. This is called adrenal insufficiency. These problems include sluggishness, weakness, weight loss, hypoglycemia, nausea, vomiting, darkening of the skin color, and mental changes. Because adrenal insufficiency can cause problems with regulating the balance of sodium and potassium in the body, a person can go into shock and a coma, which can be potentially life threatening. Since this aspect of ALD is readily treatable, it is important to

identify these patients in order to prevent these complications.

Types of ALD

There is a wide range in the severity of symptoms and age of onset of ALD. All different severities have been seen within the same family. Therefore, a family who has many mildly affected members could still have a more severely affected member. ALD is roughly divided into three different types according to severity and age of onset. However, some patients do not fall neatly into one of these categories and instead fall somewhere in between. Each type is given a different name, although all have mutations (changes in the genetic code) in the same gene and the same type of inheritance.

The most severe form of ALD is called childhood ALD. About 35% of people with ALD have this type. These children usually have normal development in the first few years of life. Symptoms typically begin between four and eight years of age. Very rarely is the onset before the age of three or after the age of 15. In some boys, the first symptom may be seizures. In other children, they become hyperactive and have behavioral problems that may initially be diagnosed as attention deficit disorder. Early signs may also include poor school performance due to impaired vision that is not correctable by eyeglasses. Although these symptoms may last for a few months, other more severe problems develop. These include increasing problems with schoolwork and deterioration in handwriting and speech. They usually develop clumsiness, difficulty in reading and comprehension of written material, aggressive or uninhibited behavior, and various personality and behavioral changes. Most of these boys have problems with their adrenal glands by the time their first symptoms are noticed.

A milder form of ALD called adrenomyeloneuropathy (AMN) usually has a symptom onset at the age of 20 or later. Approximately 40–45% of people with ALD have this type. The first symptoms are typically a progressive stiffness and weakness in the legs. Problems with urination and sexual function may also develop. Symptoms slowly progress over many years. Less than 20% of men with AMN will develop significant brain involvement that leads to cognitive and behavioral problems that are severe and may cause a shortened life span. About 70% of men with AMN will have problems with their adrenal glands when other symptoms are first noticed.

A third type of ALD is called Addison disease and affects about 10% of all of those with ALD. In this condition, people do not have the neurologic symptoms associated with ALD and AMN, but do have problems resulting from adrenal insufficiency. Symptoms typically begin between two years of age and adulthood. The first symptoms are often vomiting, weakness or coma. People with Addison disease may or may not have darker skin. Many who are initially diagnosed with Addison disease will later develop symptoms of AMN.

In female carriers, about 20% will develop mild to moderate progressive stiffness and weakness in the legs and sometimes problems with urination. Rarely do they develop adrenal insufficiency. Symptoms in women generally do not begin before middle age.

Diagnosis

When the diagnosis of ALD is suspected, a test called magnetic resonance imaging (MRI) is usually required. In this test, pictures of the brain are taken and the amount of white matter (myelin) in the brain is measured. In people with symptoms of ALD, there are usually characteristic changes in the white matter. An MRI can be helpful in making the diagnosis of ALD, but if changes are seen on MRI, it does not confirm the diagnosis of ALD. Changes in the white matter may only be seen after 1–2 years of age when the brain has matured.

A definitive diagnosis of ALD can be made by measuring the level of the VLCFA in the blood. In 99.9% of males with all types of ALD, the level of the VLCFA in blood is very high. This is diagnostic of ALD.

When ALD is suspected, testing should also be performed to measure the adrenal function. In 90% of boys with symptoms of ALD and 70% of men with AMN, the adrenal glands are affected.

Approximately 85% of female carriers will have higher than normal levels of VLCFA in their blood. However, 15–20% of female carriers will have normal levels of VLCFA in their blood, which gives a "false negative" result. If a woman wants to be certain about her carrier status, **genetic testing** to look for a specific mutation in the ALD gene can be performed. This testing usually involves drawing a small amount of blood. Before a woman could have testing to determine her carrier status, a mutation in the ALD gene must have already been found in an affected member of the family. If a mutation in the ALD gene has already been found in another family member, testing on another child suspected on having ALD would be done to look at the mutation known to cause ALD in the family.

Treatment and management

When the diagnosis of ALD is made, an important first step is to measure the level of adrenal function. If there is adrenal insufficiency, treatment should be given by steroid replacement, which can prove to be life saving. Adrenal function should be tested periodically.

Early on, it was thought that reducing the VLCFA in a person's diet would help reduce the symptoms of ALD. Although some VLCFA does comes from diet, most of it is produced in the body. Therefore, altering the diet alone does not cure ALD.

Lorenzo's oil

In the early 1990s, a film called *Lorenzo's Oil* told an embellished account of a real life family who had a young son with ALD and their search to find a cure for him. A possible treatment was found and was named Lorenzo's oil, after their son, Lorenzo. The Lorenzo's oil therapy worked to reduce the level of VLCFA in the blood. The idea was that if the level of VLCFA could be reduced, perhaps it would cure or help the symptoms. After a number of years of use, Lorenzo's oil unfortunately does not seem to be an effective treatment, at least in those with advanced signs and symptoms. Although it does reduce the level of VLCFA in blood, it does not seem to alter a person's symptoms.

Bone marrow transplant

One promising treatment is bone marrow transplant. However, this is a potentially dangerous procedure that has a 10–20% rate of death. Information is available on a limited number of patients. In the very small number of patients who have had a bone marrow transplant, a few have had their condition stabilize and a few have even made slight improvements. However, all of these people had the bone marrow transplant at an early stage of their disease. This treatment does have drawbacks including the fact that there are limited numbers of donors who are a suitable "match" and a significant chance that complications will develop from the transplant. Early data suggests that bone marrow transplant is most effective when it is performed at an early stage of the disease when abnormalities are first seen through MRI. Additional long term studies are necessary to determine the overall success of these procedures.

Other treatments

Research is being done with other treatments such as lovastatin and 4-phenylbutyrate, both of which may help lower VLCFA levels in cells, but more work is necessary to determine their effectiveness. **Gene therapy**, a possible method of treatment, works by replacing, changing, or supplementing non-working genes. Although different gene therapy methods are being testing on animals, they are not ready for human trials.

KEY TERMS

Adrenal insufficiency—Problems with the adrenal glands that can be life threatening if not treated. Symptoms include sluggishness, weakness, weight loss, vomiting, darkening of the skin and mental changes.

Central nervous system (CNS)—In humans, the central nervous system is composed of the brain, the cranial nerves and the spinal cord. It is responsible for the coordination and control of all body activities.

Leukodystrophy—A disease that affects the white matter called myelin in the CNS.

Myelin—A fatty sheath surrounding nerves in the peripheral nervous system, which helps them conduct impulses more quickly.

Peroxisomes—Tiny structures in the cells that break down fats so that the body can use them.

Very long chain fatty acids (VLCFA)—A type of fat that is normally broken down by the peroxisomes into other fats that can be used by the body.

Other types of therapy and supportive care are of benefit to both affected boys and their families. Physical therapy can help reduce stiffness and occupational therapy can help make the home more accessible. Support from psychologists and other families who have been or are in a similar situation can be invaluable. Many men with AMN lead successful personal and professional lives and can benefit from vocational counseling and physical and occupational therapy.

Prenatal diagnosis

Prenatal testing to determine whether an unborn child is affected is possible if a specific ALD mutation has been identified in a family. This testing can be performed at 10–12 weeks gestation by a procedure called chorionic villus sampling (CVS), which involves removing a tiny piece of the placenta and examining the cells. It can also be done by **amniocentesis** after 14 weeks gestation by removing a small amount of the amniotic fluid surrounding the baby and analyzing the cells in the fluid. Each of these procedures has a small risk of miscarriage associated with it and those who are interested in learning more should check with their doctor or genetic counselor. Couples interested in these options should have **genetic counseling** to carefully explore all of the benefits and limitations of these procedures.

An experimental procedure, called preimplantation diagnosis, allows a couple to have a child that is unaffected with the genetic condition. This procedure is only possible for those families in which a mutation in the ALD gene has been identified. Those interested in learning more about this procedure should check with their doctor or genetic counselor.

Prognosis

The prognosis for people with ALD varies depending on the type of ALD. Those diagnosed with childhood ALD usually have a very rapid course. Symptoms typically progress very fast and these children usually become completely incapacitated and die within three to five years of the onset of symptoms.

The symptoms of AMN progress slowly over decades. Most affected individuals have a normal life span.

Resources

PERIODICALS

Laan, L. A. E. M., et al. "Childhood-onset cerebral X-linked adrenoleukodystrophy." *The Lancet* 356 (November 4, 2000): 1608–1609.

Moser, H. W., L. Bezman, S. E. Lu, and G. V. Raymond. "Therapy of X-linked adrenoleukodystrophy: Prognosis based upon age and MRI abnormality and plans for placebo-controlled trials." *Journal of Inherited Metabolic Disease* 23 (2000): 273–277.

Moser, H. W. "Treatment of X-linked adrenoleukodystrophy with Lorenzo's oil." *Journal of Neurology, Neurosurgery and Psychiatry* 67, no. 3 (September, 1999): 279–280.

Shapiro, E., et al. "Long-term effect of bone-marrow transplantation for childhood-onset cerebral X-linked adrenoleukodystrophy." *The Lancet* 356, no. 9231 (August 26, 2000): 713–718.

Suzuki, Y., et al. "Bone marrow transplantation for the treatment of X-linked adrenoleukodystrophy." *Journal of Inherited Metabolic Disease* 23, no. 5 (July, 2000): 453–458.

Unterrainer, G., B. Molzer, S. Forss-Petter, and J. Berger. "Co-expression of mutated and normal adrenoleukodystrophy protein reduces protein function: Implications for gene therapy of X-linked adrenoleukodystrophy." *Human Molecular Genetics* 9, no. 18 (2000): 2609–2616.

van Geel, B. M., et al, on behalf of the Dutch X-ALD/AMN Study Group. "Progression of abnormalities in adrenomyeloneuropathy and neurologically asymptomatic X-linked adrenoleukodystrophy despite treatment with 'Lorenzo's oil.'" *Journal of Neurology, Neurosurgery and Psychiatry* 67, no. 3 (September, 1999): 290–299.

Verrips, A., M. A. A. P. Willemsen, E. Rubio-Gozalbo, J. De Jong, and J. A. M. Smeitink. "Simvastatin and plasma very long chain fatty acids in X-linked adrenoleukodystrophy." *Annals of Neurology* 47, no. 4 (April, 2000): 552–553.

ORGANIZATIONS

National Organization for Rare Disorders (NORD). PO Box 8923, New Fairfield, CT 06812-8923. (203) 746-6518 or (800) 999-6673. Fax: (203) 746-6481. <http://www.rarediseases.org>.

United Leukodystrophy Foundation. 2304 Highland Dr., Sycamore, IL 60178. (815) 895-3211 or (800) 728-5483. Fax: (815) 895-2432. <http://www. ulf.org>.

WEBSITES

"Entry 300100: Adrenoleukodystrophy, (ALD)." *OMIM— Online Mendelian Inheritance in Man.* <http://www.ncbi.nlm.nih.gov/htbin-post/Omim/dispmim?300100>.

Moser, Hugo W., Anne B. Moser, and Corinne D. Boehm. "X-linked adrenoleukodystrophy." (March 9, 1999). University of Washington, Seattle. *GeneClinics.* <http://www.geneclinics.org/profiles/x-ald/>.

Karen M. Krajewski, MS, CGC

A-gammaglobulinemia tyrosine kinase *see* **Bruton agammaglobulinemia**

Aganglionic megacolon *see* **Hirschsprung disease**

Agenesis of clavicles and cervical vertebral and talipes equinovarus *see* **Crane-Heise syndrome**

Aicardi syndrome

Definition

Aicardi syndrome is a rare genetic disorder that causes defects of the eyes and brain. It is believed to be an X-linked dominant genetic trait. Aicardi syndrome is named after Dr. Jean Aicardi, who first described this syndrome in 1965.

Description

Aicardi syndrome is an X-linked dominant genetic condition primarily found in females because males with the disease do not survive to birth. It is alternately

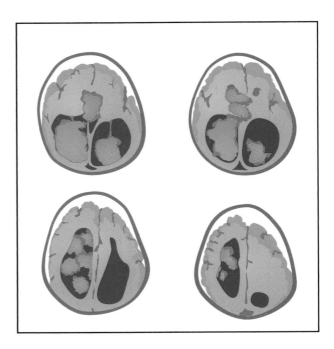

Patients diagnosed with Aicardi syndrome may develop tumors in the tiny blood vessel masses found in the third, lateral, and fourth ventricles of the brain. The tumors, referred to as choroid plexus papillomas, are green in the images above. *(Gale Group.)*

called Agenesis of Corpus Callosum (ACC) with Chorioretinal Abnormality because of the associated abnormal formation of the connection between the right and left hemispheres of the brain (the corpus callosum) and abnormal development of the choroid and retinal sections of the eye.

The eye is composed of three layers: the sclera, the choroid, and the retina. The sclera is the tough white outer coat of the eyeball; it is unaffected in individuals with Aicardi syndrome. The choroid is the middle layer of the eye. It serves to nourish the retina and absorb scattered light. The retina is the inner, light-sensitive, layer of the eye. The retina receives the image produced by the lens and contains the rods and cones that are responsible for color vision. Both the choroid and the retina are abnormally formed in individuals affected with Aicardi syndrome.

Genetic profile

The location of the **gene** mutation responsible for Aicardi syndrome has been localized to Xp22.3. At or near this same locus is the gene responsible for **microphthalmia with linear skin defects (MLS)** and the gene responsible for **Goltz syndrome**. Because only one male has ever been diagnosed with Aicardi syndrome, it is assumed that Aicardi syndrome is dominant and X-linked with near 100% fetal mortality in males. Nearly all of the cases of Aicardi syndrome are believed to result from *de novo* mutations (new mutations that occur after conception) since parents of affected individuals have normal chromosomes.

Demographics

Approximately 300 to 500 individuals, all female except for one, have been diagnosed with Aicardi syndrome worldwide. Aicardi syndrome is not associated with any particular sub-populations. It appears with equal frequency in all races and across all geographies. Because it is an X-linked dominant trait, it is observed almost exclusively in females.

Signs and symptoms

Aicardi syndrome is characterized by abnormalities of the connection between the left and right hemispheres of the brain (the corpus callosum), infantile spasms in affected infants and seizures in older affected individuals, developmental delays, lesions and other abnormalities of the eye, and possible other defects in the brain such as holes where healthy brain tissue should be (brain cysts) and an enlargement of the connecting cavities (ventricles) of the brain. It is these abnormalities of the brain, including the corpus callosum, that lead to the observable symptoms of seizures and developmental delays. Aicardi syndrome may also be complicated by brain tumors, benign tumors of the scalp (lipomas) and **cancer** of the blood vessels (angiosarcoma).

The onset of infantile spasms in individuals with Aicardi syndrome is generally observed between the third and fifth months of life. It is at this time that the final connections (neural synapses) are made in the developing human brain. These infantile spasms are a form of the full seizures that are experienced by older affected individuals. A seizure is the result of sudden abnormal electrical activity in the brain. This electrical activity can result in a wide variety of clinical symptoms including muscle twitches; tongue biting; fixed, staring eyes; a loss of bladder control resulting in involuntary urination; total body shaking (convulsions); and/or loss of consciousness.

There are several types of seizures. Focal, or partial, seizures are characterized by a brief and temporary change in movement, sensation, or nerve function. Examples of this type of seizure include drooling, head turning, eye movements, lip biting, or rhythmic twitching of muscles. Focal seizures usually cause no change in awareness or alertness. An absence seizure is a brief seizure with an accompanying loss of awareness or alertness such as a staring spell. Focal and absence

seizures are types of petit mal seizures. A grand mal seizure is characterized by a loss of consciousness, a loss of bladder control, generalized muscle contractions, and tongue biting. Grand mal seizures are also followed by a period of lethargy, confusion, and deep breathing (post-ictal state) that may last from a few minutes to several hours.

Individuals affected with Aicardi syndrome also have vision problems including blindness. These vision problems are the result of abnormal development of the two inner layers of the eye (the choroid and the retina). The most common type of malformation in the eyes of individuals with Aicardi syndrome is the appearance of small cavities or holes in the retina (retinal lacunae). Instances of small eyes (micropthalmia) and missing structures of the eye (**coloboma**) are also common.

Diagnosis

Aicardi syndrome is generally first diagnosed in affected individuals between the ages of three and five months. It is at this age that the final connections in the brain are completed. Once these connections are completed in an affected individual, this individual will begin to have infantile spasms. These spasms are akin to seizures in older children. Infantile spasms combined with defects of the retina and choroid of one eye or both eyes is sufficient evidence for the diagnosis of Aicardi syndrome. Magnetic resonance imaging (MRI) can confirm the brain malformations including the absence of the corpus callosum. Prenatal diagnosis is not yet available, but connection to the Xp22.3 locus makes **genetic testing** for this dominant trait potentially possible.

Treatment and management

Treatment of an individual with Aicardi syndrome generally consists of seizure management, vision treatment for those individuals born with sight or partial sight, and early and continuing intervention programs for developmental delays. Because of the severe neurological damage, many individuals are unable to chew and swallow and must be fed with pureed food. The most common medications for affected individuals are anti-convulsive drugs such as valproic acid (brand names: Depakene, Valproate, Valrelease); clonazepam (brand names: Klonopin and Rivotril); phenobarbitol (available as a generic drug); and phenytoin (brand name: Dilantin).

Prognosis

Aicardi syndrome is lethal in males prior to birth. The prognosis in females varies on a case-by-case basis. The estimated survival rate is 76% at six years and 40%

KEY TERMS

Absence seizure—A brief seizure with an accompanying loss of awareness or alertness.

Choroid—A vascular membrane that covers the back of the eye between the retina and the sclera and serves to nourish the retina and absorb scattered light.

Corpus callosum—A thick bundle of nerve fibers deep in the center of the forebrain that provides communications between the right and left cerebral hemispheres.

De novo **mutation**—Genetic mutations that are seen for the first time in the affected person, not inherited from the parents.

Focal seizure—A seizure that causes a brief and temporary change in movement, sensation, or nerve function.

Grand mal seizure—A seizure that causes a loss of consciousness, a loss of bladder control, generalized muscle contractions, and tongue biting.

Infantile spasms—The form of grand mal or focal seizures experienced by infants prior to the development of many voluntary muscular controls.

Post-ictal state—A period of lethargy, confusion, and deep breathing following a grand mal seizure that may last from a few minutes to several hours.

Retina—The light-sensitive layer of tissue in the back of the eye that receives and transmits visual signals to the brain through the optic nerve.

Retinal lacunae—Small abnormal cavities or holes in the retina.

at 14 years of age. There has been a report of a surviving individual with Aicardi syndrome in her late forties. Most individuals with Aicardi syndrome are either born blind or will become blind. Developmental delays and mental retardation are seen in all individuals affected with Aicardi syndrome ranging from mild to severe.

Resources

PERIODICALS

Aicardi, J. "Aicardi syndrome: Old and new findings." *International Pediatrics* (March 1999): 5-8.

King, A., S. Buchner, and P. Itin, "Aicardi syndrome." *British Journal of Ophthalmology* (April 1998): 456.

Trifiletti, R. et al. "Aicardi syndrome with multiple tumors: A case report with literature review." *Brain Development* (July-August 1995): 283-5.

ORGANIZATIONS

Aicardi Syndrome Foundation. 450 Winterwood Dr., Roselle, IL 60172. (800) 373-8518. <http://www.aicardi.com>.

WEBSITES

"Entry 304050: Corpus callosum, agenesis of, with chorioretinal abnormality." *OMIM—Online Mendelian Inheritance in Man.* <http://www.ncbi.nlm.nih.gov/htbin-post/Omim/dispmim?304050> (February 9, 2001).

Reader's Digest Health—Focal Dermal Hypoplasia. <http://rdhealth.com/kbase/nord/nord49.htm> (February 9, 2001).

Paul A. Johnson

Alagille syndrome

Definition

Alagille syndrome is a genetic condition characterized by liver disease, typical facial features, heart murmurs or defects, vertebral changes, and eye changes as well as a variety of less frequently noted features. Alagille syndrome is also called arteriohepatic **dysplasia**, cholestasis with peripheral pulmonary stenosis, syndromatic hepatic ductular hypoplasia, and Alagille-Watson syndrome.

Description

Alagille syndrome is a rare condition occurring either sporadically or in an autosomal dominant pattern of **inheritance**. Approximately 70% of cases are caused by changes in the Jagged1 **gene** on **chromosome** 20. However, the diagnosis of Alagille syndrome is based on clinical features and family history. Obtaining medical information about family members can be difficult as some people with Alagille syndrome are so mildly affected or have variable symptoms that the condition may go unrecognized. Prognosis depends on the extent of major organ involvement, especially of the liver, heart, and kidneys. Liver transplantation is needed in some cases. Prenatal testing is available to families in which a genetic change has been identified. The interpretation of this testing is limited by the variability of clinical features, even within the same family. People with the same genetic change can have a wide range of medical problems with varying degrees of severity.

Genetic profile

Alagille syndrome occurs sporadically in 15-56% of cases, but has been noted to follow an autosomal dominant pattern of inheritance in some families. In sporadic cases, the gene change occurred for the first time in the affected individual, and neither parent has the same gene change. In autosomal dominant inheritance, multiple generations of a family are affected with the condition. In either case, people who have the genetic change have a 50% chance to pass the altered gene on to each of their children. Since the gene is dominant, passing on one copy of the gene is enough to cause symptoms. However, the condition exhibits variable expressivity. This means that different people with the condition may experience different features of the disease or levels of severity. One explanation for this is that different changes in the gene may cause different features of the syndrome. However, even in families that all have the same genetic change, different features and degrees of severity can occur. In addition, the condition is not fully penetrant. Some people who have the gene change, due to an affected parent and child, do not show any features of the disease.

Changes in a gene called the Jagged1 (Jag1) gene on the short arm of chromosome 20 have been shown to be the underlying defect in many patients. The Jag1 gene encodes a cell surface protein that plays a role in the regulation of development. The protein is active in many cell types and directs cells to their proper place in the embryo. Seventy to 75% of Alagille syndrome probands have had an identifiable change within this gene. Of that 70%, 6% have been shown to have a small deletion of a piece of the short arm of chromosome 20 (20p), which includes the Jag1 gene, using a laboratory technique called **fluorescent in situ hybridization**. There are a variety of other molecular changes in the gene that have been detected by sequencing the gene. Thirty percent of people with the condition do not have an identifiable change in this gene. It is possible that there are other genes that cause the disease in these families.

Demographics

Alagille syndrome is rare, occurring in one in 70,000-100,000 live births. The condition affects males and females equally. Most patients with Alagille syndrome come to medical attention in the first four months of life with jaundice, an enlarged liver, severe itching of skin, or multiple raised nodular areas on the skin.

Signs and symptoms

Liver manifestations

One of the most common and most serious symptoms of Alagille syndrome is liver disease. Liver disease occurs in 90-100% of patients and often leads to growth delay or failure as a result of malnutrition. Because there is a reduction in the number of bile ducts in the liver, there are elevated bile acids in the blood and an arrest of bile excretion from the body. This results in jaundice, pruritus (severe skin itching), and xanthomas (raised nodules on the skin, especially at skin creases or areas of friction). Some patients have mild or no liver problems, while others have progressive liver failure.

Cardiac manifestations

Heart defects and murmurs have been noted in 85-95% of patients with Alagille syndrome. The most common type of defect is pulmonary artery stenosis, although other types of defects also occur. Many of these defects do not have clinical significance to the patient. However, complex and severe heart defects occur and are one of the more common causes of mortality in patients with Alagille syndrome.

Eye manifestations

An important diagnostic feature of Alagille syndrome is a particular eye finding called posterior embryotoxon. This is an anterior chamber defect of the eye caused by a prominent, centrally positioned Schwalbe ring. This feature can be seen through a split lamp examination and does not affect vision. Since 56-90% of patients have this or other changes in the eye, including retinal pigmentary changes, an eye examination can aid in diagnosis.

Skeletal manifestations

A particular finding called a butterfly vertebra is associated with Alagille syndrome. The term butterfly vertebra refers to the appearance of the space around the vertebrae due to clefting or disruption of formation of a vertebra. There are usually no physical problems associated with this radiological finding. The frequency of butterfly vertebrae in this syndrome is uncertain, with estimates from 33-87% in different studies. Other skeletal malformations are also noted in these patients, such as **spina bifida** occulta and hemivertebrae. Therefore, radiological examination of the spine may aid in diagnosis.

Facial manifestations

The occurrence of particular facial features has been noted in 70-95% of patients with Alagille syndrome. The facial features include a prominent forehead, deep-set and widely spaced eyes, a pointed chin, and a straight nose with a bulbous tip. These features are more subjective, but one of the most consistent features of the diagnosis.

Other manifestations

Problems with the structure and function of kidneys have been noted with an occurrence of 40-70%. Most often symptoms are mild, but renal disease has caused mortality in severe cases. Mild delays in gross motor function have been noted in 16% of children. Most of these children were those with severe organ disease. Intracranial bleeding has also been noted with increased frequency and is associated with mortality in this syndrome.

Diagnosis

The diagnosis of Alagille syndrome is based on clinical features and can be made by the presence of liver disease plus two of the other major features. An ultrasound of the liver can rule out other causes of liver disease and a liver biopsy can determine if there is a reduction in the number of bile ducts. However, this finding occurs in other conditions as well as Alagille syndrome, and the timing of the biopsy is important. Older patients are more likely to have fewer bile ducts than patients under five years of age. An echocardiogram for heart defects, a radiological examination of the spine, blood tests for renal function, an ophthalmologic examination, and an examination of facial features are important diagnostic tools. A careful family history is also important in diagnosis. When a first- or second-degree relative has already been diagnosed with Alagille syndrome, the presence of even one feature of the condition may constitute a diagnosis.

Once a diagnosis has been made in an individual, the parents should undergo an evaluation for subtle features of the condition. If a parent is diagnosed, then evaluation for appropriate extended family members would be offered. A correct diagnosis is important since there are other syndromes that exhibit similar liver disease, heart defects, and eye findings. These syndromes are inherited in different ways, so the recurrence risk for offspring and other family members may be different.

Two different types of testing are used: fluorescence in situ hybridization (FISH), which detects the small percentage of patients who have a deletion of the entire gene; and sequencing, which looks at changes within the gene. Sequencing is not clinically available. New technologies may make gene sequencing for mutations more readily available in the near future. If a genetic change is identified in the family, prenatal testing would be available through chorionic villus sampling or **amniocentesis**. However, the interpretation of this testing is difficult since the presence of a gene change does not allow one to predict the severity of the condition or which medical problems may occur.

Treatment and management

Liver transplantation is needed in 15-20% of patients. Other treatments depend on which of the other features of the condition are present and the degree of severity. Repair of heart defects is another surgical treatment needed in some cases.

Prognosis

Prognosis for Alagille syndrome is quite variable and depends on the degree of liver, heart, and kidney disease and the presence of intracranial bleeding. Overall, survival rates are 72-85%. The survival rate of those undergoing liver transplantation is 60-80%. There is currently no method to determine which patients will reach end-stage liver disease.

Resources

BOOKS

Jones, Kenneth Lyons. *Smith's Recognizable Patterns of Human Malformation.* 5th ed. Philadelphia: W.B. Saunders, 1997.

McKusick, Victor. *Mendelian Inheritance in Man: A Catalog of Human Genes and Genetic Disorders.* 12th ed. Baltimore: The Johns Hopkins University Press, 1998.

Scriver, Charles, et al. *The Metabolic and Molecular Bases of Inherited Disease.* 8th ed. McGraw-Hill, 2001.

PERIODICALS

Emerick, Karan, et al. "Features of Alagille Syndrome in 92 Patients: Frequency and Relation to Prognosis." *Hepatology* (1999): 822-828.

Krantz, Ian, et al. "Alagille Syndrome." *Journal of Medical Genetics* (February 1997): 152-157.

Krantz, Ian, et al. "Clinical and Molecular Genetics of Alagille Syndrome." *Current Opinions in Pediatrics* (December 1999): 558-563.

Quiros-Tejeira, Ruben, et al. "Variable Morbidity in Alagille Syndrome: A Review of 43 Cases." *Journal of Pediatric Gastroenterology and Nutrition* (October 1999): 431-437.

Rand, Elizabeth. "The Genetic Basis of Alagille Syndrome." *Journal of Pediatric Gastroenterology and Nutrition* (February 1998): 234-237.

WEBSITES

Children's Hospital and Regional Medical Center, Seattle, WA. *GeneTests: Genetic Testing Resource.* <http://www.genetests.org/> (February 20, 2001).

Sonja Rene Eubanks

Albinism

Definition

Albinism is an inherited condition that causes a lack of pigment in the hair, skin or eyes.

Description

People with albinism typically have white or pale yellow hair, pale skin and light blue or gray eyes. Since their irises have little pigment, their eyes may appear pink or violet in different types of light. This is because light is being reflected from the reddish part of the retina

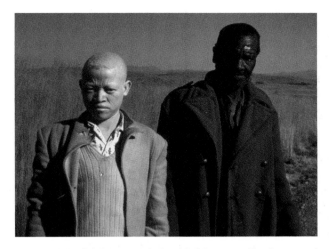

A man with albinism stands beside his normally pigmented father. *(Photo Researchers, Inc.)*

in the back of the eye. Their skin usually does not tan and their eyes are often sensitive to light. Many have trouble with vision. Some children may be born with albinism, but develop some pigmentation as they grow older.

In albinism, the body does not produce enough of a pigment called melanin, which creates hair, skin and eye color. Melanin protects the body by absorbing the sun's ultraviolet light. There are several types of albinism: some affect only the eyes, while others affect the skin and hair or other parts of the body.

Types of albinism

Ocular: A form of albinism that mainly affects the eyes. People with ocular albinism have some pigmentation, but may have lighter skin, hair and eye color than other family members. Scientists have identified five different types of ocular albinism.

X-linked ocular: This type of albinism occurs mostly in males, who inherit the **gene** from their mothers. It causes visual disabilities.

Oculocutaneous: A type of albinism that affects the hair, skin and eyes. Researchers have classified 10 different types of oculocutaneous albinism.

Tyrosinase-negative oculocutaneous: Also known as Type 1A, this is the most severe form of albinism, marked by a total absence of pigment in hair, skin and eyes. People with this type of albinism have vision problems and sensitivity to sunlight. They also are extremely susceptible to sunburn.

Tyrosinase-positive oculocutaneous: People with this type of albinism have light hair, skin and eye coloration and fewer visual impairments.

Hermansky-Pudlak syndrome (HPS): This rare type of albinism is common in the Puerto Rican community. Approximately one person in every 1,800 people in Puerto Rico will be affected by it. The lack of pigmentation can vary widely. People with HPS may have white, pale yellow or brown hair, but it always is lighter than the rest of the population. Their eyes range from blue to brown, and their skin can be creamy white, yellow or brown. HPS also often causes visual changes, along with other physical symptoms.

Chediak-Higashi syndrome: A rare type of albinism that interferes with white blood cells and the body's ability to fight infection.

Black Locks Albinism Deafness syndrome (BADS): Another rare form of albinism identified by a black lock of hair on the forehead. BADS causes deafness from birth.

Piebaldism: Also known as partial albinism, this condition is marked by patches of white hair or lighter skin blotches on the body.

Genetic profile

Children inherit the genes for albinism from their parents. The parents may have normal pigmentation, but if both the mother and father carry a recessive gene, there is a one in four chance their child will have albinism.

A specific genetic abnormality causes tyrosinase-negative oculocutaneous albinism (Type 1A). In this type, also called "ty-neg albinism," the body is unable to convert the amino acid tyrosine into pigment. The genes for producing the enzymes related to ty-neg albinism are located on **chromosome** 11 and chromosome 9.

Similarly, scientists believe the gene that causes Hermansky-Pudlak syndrome is on chromosome 10. They are studying two other genes that appear to be involved in melanin pigment formation: the P gene on chromosome 15 and the ocular albinism gene on the X chromosome.

Women who carry the gene for X-linked ocular albinism may have normal vision, but they have a one in two chance of passing it on to their sons. This type of albinism occurs mainly in males because the gene that causes it is located on the X chromosome. Since males only have one X chromosome, genetic abnormalities on this chromosome will almost always be expressed.

Demographics

Albinism affects one in every 17,000 people. All racial groups, including African-Americans and Latinos are affected by albinism. Asians have the lowest incidence of this condition.

Signs and symptoms

Eye problems

The lack of pigment in albinism causes abnormal development in the eye. For example, the iris (the colored ring around the center of the eye), which normally acts as a filter, may let too much light into the eye. Communication between the retina (the surface inside the eye that absorbs light) and the brain may also be altered in people with albinism, causing a lack of depth perception. These changes can lead to visual impairments, such as sensitivity to sunlight, near-sightedness, far-sightedness, or astigmatism (a curvature in the lens that makes it difficult to focus on objects). Other common affects of albinism on the eyes include nystagmus, a constant, involuntary shifting of the eyes from side to side; and strabismus, a disorder of the muscles in the eyes that causes a wandering eye or crossed eyes. Strabismus can interfere with depth perception.

Skin conditions

People with albinism burn easily in the sun. Since they have no pigmentation, or very little, they typically do not tan. Without adequate protection, they are more likely to develop skin **cancer**. Some people with albinism will have freckles, or large blotches of pigmentation, but they still will not develop a suntan.

Other rare symptoms

People with HPS may experience a variety of health problems related to their unique form of albinism. For example, HPS can cause scarring of the lungs, or fibrosis, which leads to restrictive lung disease and causes fatigue and problems with breathing. Some people with HPS have trouble healing when they cut their skin because the disorder interferes with normal platelet function. Platelets are a component of blood needed for clotting. This complication may cause people with HPS to bruise easily, have frequent nosebleeds or trouble with bleeding gums when brushing their teeth. It also could cause heavy menstrual bleeding and excessive bleeding when a pregnant woman with HPS delivers a child. Intestinal difficulties also are associated with HPS. It can cause a condition called granulomatous colitis, which causes abdominal cramps, intestinal bleeding and diarrhea. People with HPS may also have kidney disease.

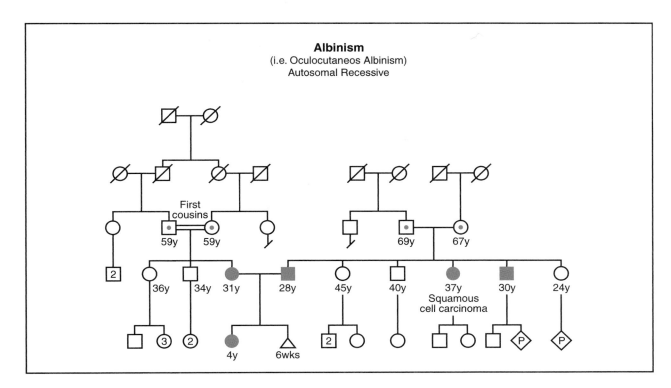

Albinism
(i.e. Oculocutaneos Albinism)
Autosomal Recessive

(Gale Group.)

Other rare forms of albinism may cause deafness or decrease the body's ability to fight infection.

Diagnosis

Physicians are able to diagnose albinism by carefully examining a person's hair, skin, eyes, and family history. Diagnostic testing usually is not necessary, but a genetic test is now available for parents who want to find out if they are carriers of ty-neg albinism. The test also can be performed on an infant by **amniocentesis** at 16 to 18 weeks gestation.

In the past, doctors used to examine a sample of the root of a person's hair, in a procedure known as a hairbulb pigmentation test. They also tested hair for the presence of tyrosine, a substance in the body that produces melanin, to determine the type of albinism a person had. Today, however, most physicians believe these tests are not reliable and they are not often used.

To find out if a person has HPS, physicians can take a sample of their blood and examine the platelets under a microscope to look for a lack of clotting ability.

Eye doctors may be able to identify subtle eye changes in women who carry the gene for X-linked ocular albinism. While their eye color may appear normal, female carriers of this type of albinism often have a slight lack of pigment in their retinas.

Treatment and management

People with albinism must shield their sensitive eyes from the sun with UV protected sunglasses. Some find bifocals and other corrective lenses to be helpful. For those with severe forms of albinism, however, corrective lenses may not be able to overcome problems caused by developmental changes in the retina. Children with albinism may require special accommodations, such as large-print textbooks, for reading in school. If visual impairment is severe, it may affect the individual's ability to drive.

For those with strabismus, surgery can alter their appearance, although the procedure may not significantly improve their vision. Before trying surgery, some doctors have children wear an eye patch in an attempt to strengthen the weaker eye. Eye surgery may also help reduce the involuntary eye movements associated with nystagmus, but vision will not always improve.

To prevent sun-related health problems, people with albinism must cover up with a sunscreen of SPF 20 or higher. Protective clothing, hats or visors are essential.

KEY TERMS

Hermansky-Pudlak syndrome (HPS)—A rare form of albinism, most common in the Puerto Rican community, which can cause pigment changes, lung disease, intestinal disorders, and blood disorders.

Iris—The colored part of the eye, containing pigment and muscle cells that contract and dilate the pupil.

Melanin—Pigments normally produced by the body that give color to the skin and hair.

Nystagmus—Involuntary, rhythmic movement of the eye.

Ocular albinism—A type of albinism that affects the vision.

Oculocutaneous albinism—Inherited loss of pigment in the skin, eyes, and hair.

Platelets—Small disc-shaped structures that circulate in the blood stream and participate in blood clotting.

Retina—The light-sensitive layer of tissue in the back of the eye that receives and transmits visual signals to the brain through the optic nerve.

Strabismus—An improper muscle balance of the ocular musles resulting in crossed or divergent eyes.

Physicians also recommend keeping a careful watch for any changes in birth marks or moles that could become cancerous.

People with HPS should be careful to avoid aspirin, which can reduce clotting, and notify their dentist before having any dental work done. Women with HPS should alert their gynecologist or obstetrician. Some physicians recommend wearing a medical alert bracelet for the bleeding disorder. To avoid exacerbating the lung disease, people with HPS should not smoke.

Children with albinism may need extra support from family or a counselor if they are exposed to teasing or hurtful comments at school. Many families also find support groups to be helpful.

Prognosis

People with albinism can easily adapt to this condition and live healthy, productive lives. Albinism does not affect a person's lifespan, although it may lead to an increased risk of skin cancer if protective measures are not taken.

Resources

BOOKS

Larry. National Association for the Visually Handicapped, New York.

Wiley, Jean. *To Ride the White Rainbow*. National Organization for Albinism and Hypopigmentation (NOAH), 1998.

PERIODICALS

"*NOAH News.*" Newsletter of the National Organization for Albinism and Hypopigmentation, Philadelphia.

Wilson, Tracy. "The paler side of beauty." *Heart and Soul.* Vol. 6, Issue 1 (February, 1999): 30-33.

ORGANIZATIONS

American Academy of Dermatology. PO Box 4014, 930 N. Meacham Rd., Schaumburg, IL 60168-4014. (847) 330-0230. Fax: (847) 330-0050. <http://www.aad.org>.

American Council of the Blind. 1155 15th St. NW, Suite 1004, Washington, DC 20005. (202) 467-5081 or (800) 424-8666. <http://www.acb.org>.

American Nystagmus Network. PO Box 45, Jenison, MI 49429-0045. <http://www.nystagmus.org>.

Hermansky-Pudlak Syndrome Network. 39 Riveria Court, Malverne, NY 11565-1602. (800) 789-9477 or (516) 599-2077. <http://www.medhelp.org/web/hpsn.htm>.

International Albinism Center. University of Minnesota, PO Box 420, Delaware St. SE, Minneapolis, MN 55455. <http://www.cbc.umn.edu/iac>.

National Association for Parents of Children with Visual Impairment (NAPVI). PO Box 317, Watertown, MA 02472. (617) 972-7441 or (800) 562-6265. <http://www.spedex.com/napvi>.

National Organization for Albinism and Hypopigmentation. 1530 Locust St. #29, Philadelphia, PA 19102-4415. (215) 545-2322 or (800) 473-2310. <http://www.albinism.org>.

WEBSITES

"Images of albinism in pop culture." *Lunaeterna.* <http://www.lunaeterna.net/popcult/intro.htm>.

"International Albinism Center fact sheet." *University of Minnesota.* <http://www.cbc.umn.edu/iac/facts.htm>.

"Positive Exposure: Albinism and photography." <http://www.rickguidotti.com>.

OTHER

Albinism: The People, The Challenge. Videotape. Chrysalis Films.

Melissa Knopper

Albright syndrome *see* **McCune-Albright syndrome**

Alcoholism

Definition

Alcoholism is a chronic physical, psychological, and behavioral disorder characterized by excessive use of alcoholic beverages; emotional and physical dependence on them; increased tolerance over time of the effects of alcohol; and withdrawal symptoms if the person stops drinking.

Description

Alcoholism is a complex behavioral as well as medical disorder. It often involves the criminal justice system as well as medicine and other helping professions. Its emergence in an individual's life is affected by a number of variables ranging from age, weight, sex, and ethnic background to his or her family history, peer group, occupation, religious preference, and many other categories. Moreover, persons diagnosed with alcoholism may demonstrate considerable variety in their drinking patterns, age at onset of the disorder, and the speed of its progression.

The *Diagnostic and Statistical Manual of Mental Disorders*, 4th edition (DSM-IV), distinguishes between Alcohol Dependence and Alcohol Abuse largely on the basis of a compulsive element in Alcohol Dependence that is not present in Alcohol Abuse. Some psychiatrists differentiate between so-called primary alcoholism, in which the patient has no other major psychiatric diagnosis; and secondary alcoholism, in which the problem drinking is the patient's preferred way of medicating symptoms of another psychiatric disorder, such as **depression**, **schizophrenia**, post-traumatic stress disorder, or one of the dissociative disorders. Experts in other branches of medicine tend to emphasize patterns of and attitudes toward drinking in order to distinguish between nonproblematic use of alcohol and alcohol abuse or dependence. Classification is typically based on the following five categories:

- Social drinkers. Individuals who use alcohol in minimal to moderate amounts to enhance meals or other social activities. They do not drink alone.

- Situational drinkers. These people rarely or never drink except during periods of stress. They are far more likely to drink alone than social drinkers.

- Problem drinkers. These individuals drink heavily, even when they are not under overwhelming stress. Their drinking causes some problems in their lives (e.g., DUI arrests), but they are capable of responding to warnings or advice from others.

- Binge drinkers. This type of drinker uses alcohol in an out-of-control fashion at regular intervals. The binges may be planned in advance. This pattern is a growing problem on many college campuses.

- Alcoholic drinkers. These are drinkers who have no control of any kind over their intake, and find that their lives are unmanageable.

Other factors have complicated definitions of alcoholism in the United States, including: 1) the increasing tendency to combine alcohol with other drugs of abuse, sometimes called cross-addiction; and 2) the rising rates of alcohol abuse and dependence among children under 12 years of age.

Genetic profile

Alcoholism was one of the first behavioral disorders tackled by genetic research, partly because it is a widespread problem and partly because the cost to society is so high. It has been known since the 1960s that alcoholism has a genetic component. A family history of alcoholism is presently considered the strongest risk factor for developing alcoholism. The risk increases with the number of alcoholic relatives in a person's family, the genetic closeness of the relationships, and the severity of the alcohol problems in the affected relatives. As of 2000, researchers estimate that 40%-60% of a person's vulnerability to alcoholism is genetically based. About 20% of the sons and 5% of the daughters of alcoholic parents develop the disorder, compared to 5% of men and 1% of women in the general North American population.x

Alcoholism is thought to be a polygenic disorder; that is, more than one **gene** appears to be involved in its transmission. The Collaborative Study on the Genetics of Alcoholism (COGA) has pinpointed several areas in the brain that may contain genes for alcoholism. Begun in 1989, COGA has compiled a database from over 300 alcoholic families at six research sites (SUNY-Downstate, University of Connecticut, Indiana University, Washington University, University of Iowa, and University of California at San Diego). The completed mapping of the human genome is also expected to help researchers identify the specific genes that affect an individual's vulnerability to alcohol abuse.

Recent COGA findings suggest that a gene or genes on human **chromosome** 1 may influence vulnerability to affective disorders as well as to alcoholism. The researchers found that first-degree relatives of subjects diagnosed with depression as well as alcoholism had a higher prevalence of both disorders than relatives of subjects diagnosed with alcoholism alone.

Earlier genetic studies

MULTIGENERATIONAL STUDIES The first studies of the genetics of alcoholism were performed in the 1960s. One investigator noted that the brain wave patterns in alcoholics are lower in height (amplitude) than those of normal people and studied children of alcoholics to determine whether this brain wave pattern might be hereditary. He used two groups of boys between the ages of six and 18, one group comprised of sons of alcoholic men. More than 35% of the sons of alcoholics had the brain wave pattern characteristic of alcoholism, whereas fewer than 1% of the boys in the control group had it. Another multigenerational brain wave study involved type 2 alcoholism, a variant of the disorder in which the alcoholic's father is always an alcoholic. This study found that 89% of the sons of type 2 alcoholics had the characteristic brain wave pattern.

Other studies of children of alcoholics have focused on the effects of alcohol on the body. A study published in 1991 reported that the sons of alcoholics perform better on tests of hand-to-eye coordination after drinking a specified amount of alcohol than the sons of nonalcoholics who had consumed the same amount. The researchers hypothesized that low sensitivity to the effects of alcohol may point to higher levels of alcohol consumption in adult life.

TWIN STUDIES Studies of twins performed in Finland and the United States indicate that people with an alcoholic monozygotic (identical) twin have a significantly higher risk of becoming alcoholics than people with alcoholic dizygotic (fraternal) twins.

STUDIES OF ADOPTED CHILDREN A longitudinal Swedish study known as the Stockholm Adoption Study was performed on children of type 2 alcoholics reared by adoptive parents. The researchers reported in the mid-1980s that 34% of these children became alcoholics in adult life, even when they had been reared by adoptive parents who abstained from alcohol.

Another longitudinal study of adopted children done at the University of Kansas Medical School found that sons of alcoholic parents were four times as likely to become alcoholics as sons of nonalcoholics, even if they had been separated from their parents shortly after birth and reared by nonrelatives with no history of problem drinking. On the other hand, the sons of nonalcoholic parents had a low rate of alcoholism in later life even if their adoptive parents were alcoholics. Studies of adopted daughters yielded less clear-cut results.

STUDIES OF GENDER AND ETHNIC VARIABLES It has been known for several decades that different nations and ethnic groups have widely varying rates of alcohol-ism, with Ireland, the countries of the former Soviet Union, and the Baltic countries having relatively high rates. Far Eastern and Mediterranean countries (with the exception of France) have relatively low rates. With regard to Asians, researchers have found that a large proportion of the general population—as high as 50% among the Japanese and Koreans—has an aldehyde dehydrogenase deficiency, related to a variation in a gene known as the ALDH2 gene. People with this deficiency experience a disulfiram-like reaction to small amounts of alcohol, which appears to protect them from becoming alcoholics.

Studies of women indicate that Caucasian women in the United States have a higher rate of aldehyde dehydrogenase deficiency than men. It is not known, however, how important this factor is in explaining the overall lower rate of alcoholism among women. One study of Australian twins found that the variation in the ALDH2 gene that decreases the risk of alcoholism in men does not have this protective effect in women. Race and ethnicity affect both patterns of alcohol consumption in women and physical vulnerability to the effects of alcohol. Although African American women and Caucasian women are equally likely to be heavy drinkers, African American women are more likely than Caucasians to abstain from alcohol (46% versus 34%). Among Hispanic women, American-born Hispanics are more likely to be moderate or heavy drinkers than Hispanic immigrants.

Another important variable in assessing the role of ethnicity in alcohol dependence is educational attainment. According to one 2000 study, low levels of educational attainment are correlated with alcohol dependence among African Americans, while high levels of education are associated with alcohol dependence among Caucasians. Another 2000 study found that dropping out of high school was associated with an increased risk of alcohol abuse among both groups, while entering college without completing the course of studies was associated with a higher rate of alcohol abuse only in Caucasians. The long-term effects of educational level on alcohol dependence in different subcultures, however, require further study.

STUDIES OF BRAIN TISSUE In 1990, researchers at UCLA and the University of Texas studied tissue samples from the brains of 70 deceased persons (men and women from a variety of ethnic groups); half the samples were from known alcoholics. Of the tissue samples from alcoholics, 69% had an abnormal gene for dopamine reception whereas 80% of the nonalcoholics' samples had a normal gene. Dopamine is a neurotransmitter associated with a sense of pleasure; its receptor gene is located on human chromosome 11. The researchers speculated that the atypical form of the gene may direct the formation of defective dopamine receptors in the brain, which in turn may cause the person to crave alcohol and other substances that increase the body's dopamine production.

Newer genetic engineering techniques

The introduction of newer techniques developed in the 1990s has contributed to a greater understanding of the complexity of the genetic transmission of alcoholism in humans.

KNOCKOUT AND TRANSGENIC EXPERIMENTS Newer genetic engineering techniques that were developed in the 1990s allow researchers to deactivate, or knock out, a gene that is thought to be involved in sensitivity to or desire for alcohol. Alternately, researchers can insert a gene into an animal's genetic material, thus producing transgenic offspring. Several knockout experiments have produced strains of mice with a craving for alcohol that can be traced to specific proteins in the brain. Both knockout and transgenic experiments on mice have confirmed the hypothesis that low sensitivity to the effects of alcohol appears to be related to a high preference for consuming alcohol.

MICROARRAYS Microarrays are glass slides or silicon chips with selected genes—as many as 10,000—arranged on them for scanning by an automated system. Because alcoholism is a polygenic disorder, and because genes often change their levels of activity in response to the effects of alcohol, microarrays allow researchers to track the activity levels of a large number of genes simultaneously. As of 2001, it is thought that changes in gene function may be a factor in the human brain's long-term adaptations to heavy drinking.

Demographics

Health professionals estimate that 70% of the adult population of the world's developed countries drink alcohol, with a slightly higher rate (75%) in the United States. Of those who drink, about 10% will become alcoholics. This group of heavy drinkers spends more time in the doctor's office or the ER than most other adults; it is estimated that 20% of hospital inpatients and 15% of outpatients have alcohol problems. There is a definite gender imbalance in alcoholism, with males predominating by a ratio of 4:1 or 3:1. According to a 2000 report from the Centers for Disease Control, 22.3% of men are binge drinkers, compared to 6.7% of women. On the other hand, evidence accumulating in the 1990s suggests that the gender ratio is dropping among younger drinkers. A 1997 U.S. Department of Health and Human Services (DHHS) survey found that the current use of alcohol among women is highest in the 26 to 34 age group, and

that binge and heavy drinking are highest among 18- to 25-year-olds. The smallest sex differences in heavy drinking are for youths aged 12 to 17 (2% of boys and 1% of girls in 1993; 2% of boys and 1.5% of girls younger than 12 in 1999).

Studies of women alcoholics indicate that women are at higher risk than men for serious health problems related to alcoholism. Because women tend to metabolize alcohol more slowly, have a lower percentage of body water and a higher percentage of body fat than men, they develop higher blood alcohol levels than men at a given amount of alcohol per pound of body weight. Thus, even though women typically begin to drink heavily at a later age than men, they often become dependent on alcohol much more rapidly. This relatively speedy progression of alcoholism in women is called telescoping.

At the other end of the age distribution, alcoholism among the elderly appears to be on the increase as well as underdiagnosed. Confusion and other signs of intoxication in an elderly person are often misinterpreted as side effects of the patient's other medications. In addition, many older people turn to alcohol to medicate feelings of depression. It is estimated, as of 1999, that 15% of older women in treatment for depression are alcoholics. The elderly are at higher risk for becoming dependent on alcohol than younger people because their bodies do not absorb alcohol as efficiently; a 90-year-old who drinks the same amount of alcohol as a 20-year-old (of the same sex) will have a blood alcohol level 50% higher.

Signs and symptoms

The symptoms of alcohol intoxication often include talkativeness and a positive mood while the drinker's blood alcohol level is rising, with depression and mental impairment when it is falling. Blood alcohol concentration (BAC) produces the following symptoms of central nervous system (CNS) depression at specific levels:

- 50 mg/dL: feelings of calm or mild drowsiness
- 50-150 mg/dL: loss of physical coordination. The legal BAC for drivers in most states is 100 mg/dL or lower.
- 150-200 mg/dL: loss of mental faculties
- 300-400 mg/dL: unconsciousness
- Over 400 mg/dL: may be fatal.

The symptoms of long-term heavy consumption of alcohol may take a variety of different forms. In spite of a long history of use for "medicinal" purposes, alcohol is increasingly recognized to be toxic to the human body.

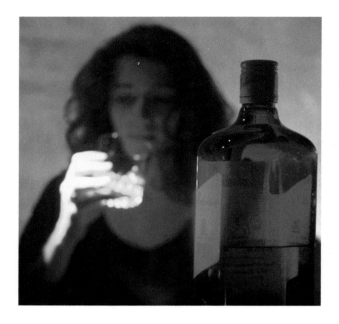

Women are at higher risk for serious alcohol related health problems then men. Because women tend to metabolize alcohol more slowly, have a lower percentage of body water and a higher percentage of body fat than men, they develop higher blood alcohol levels than men at a given amount of alcohol per pound of body weight. *(Custom Medical Stock Photo, Inc.)*

It is basically a CNS depressant that is absorbed into the bloodstream, primarily from the small intestine. Regular consumption of large amounts of alcohol can cause irreversible damage to a number of the body's organ systems, including the cardiovascular system, the digestive tract, the central nervous system, and the peripheral nervous system. Heavy drinkers are at high risk of developing stomach or duodenal ulcers, cirrhosis of the liver, and cancers of the digestive tract. Many alcoholics do not eat properly, and often develop nutritional deficiency diseases as well as organ damage.

In addition to physical symptoms, most alcoholics have a history of psychiatric, occupational, financial, legal, or interpersonal problems as well. Alcohol misuse is the single most important predictor of violence between domestic partners as well as intergenerational violence within families. In 1994 (the latest year for which statistics are available), 79% of drivers over age 25 involved in fatal automobile accidents were intoxicated. In the states that provided data in 1994 for arrests for driving while impaired (DWI) by alcohol, about one-third of the arrested drivers had previous DWI citations. Since the early 1990s, most states have passed stricter laws against alcohol-impaired driving. These laws include such provisions as immediate license suspension for the first DWI arrest and lowering the legal blood alcohol limit to 0.08 g/dL for adults and 0.02 g/dL for

drivers under 21. Penalties for repeated DWI citations include prison sentences; house arrest with electronic monitoring; license plates that identify offending drivers; automobile confiscation; and putting a special ignition interlock on the offender's car.

Diagnosis

The diagnosis of alcoholism is usually based on the patient's drinking history, a thorough physical examination, laboratory findings, and the results of psychodiagnostic assessment.

Patient history and physical examination

A physician who suspects that a patient is abusing or is dependent on alcohol should give him or her a complete physical examination with appropriate laboratory tests, paying particular attention to liver function and the nervous system. Physical findings that suggest alcoholism include head injuries after age 18; broken bones after age 18; other evidence of blackouts, frequent accidents, or falls; puffy eyelids; flushed face; alcohol odor on the breath; shaky hands; slurred speech or tongue tremor; rapid involuntary eye movements (nystagmus); enlargement of the liver (hepatomegaly); hypertension; insomnia; and problems with impotence (in males). Severe memory loss may point to advanced alcoholic damage to the CNS.

Diagnostic questionnaires and checklists

Since some of the physical signs and symptoms of alcoholism can be produced by other drugs or disorders, screening tests can also help to determine the existence of a drinking problem. There are several assessment instruments for alcoholism that can be either self-administered or administered by a clinician. The so-called CAGE test is a brief screener consisting of four questions:

- Have you ever felt the need to *cut down* on drinking?
- Have you ever felt *annoyed* by criticism of your drinking?
- Have you ever felt *guilty* about your drinking?
- Have you ever taken a morning *eye opener*?

One "yes" answer should raise a suspicion of alcohol abuse; two "yes" answers are considered a positive screen.

Other brief screeners include the Alcohol Use Disorder Identification Test, or AUDIT, which also highlights some of the physical symptoms of alcohol abuse that doctors look for during a physical examination of the patient. The Michigan Alcoholism Screening Test, or MAST, is considered the diagnostic standard. It con-

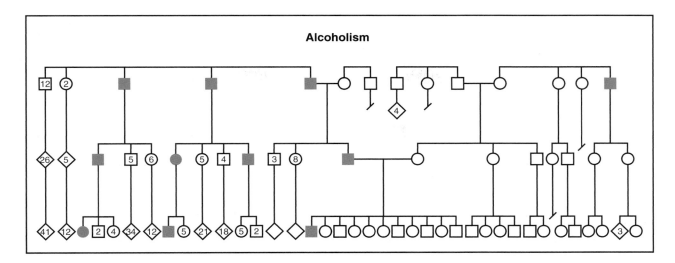

Alcoholism

(Gale Group.)

sists of 25 questions; a score of five or higher is considered to indicate alcohol dependency. A newer screener, the Substance Abuse Subtle Screening Inventory, or SASSI, was introduced in 1988. It can be given in either group or individual settings in a paper-and-pencil or computerized format. The SASSI is available in an adolescent as well as an adult version from the SASSI Institute.x

According to one 1998 study, some brief screeners may be inappropriate for widespread use in some subpopulations because of ethnic and sex bias. The CAGE questionnaire often yielded inaccurate results when administered to African American men and Mexican American women. The AUDIT does not appear to be affected by ethnic or gender biases. Another study of the use of alcohol screening questionnaires in women found that the AUDIT was preferable to the CAGE questionnaire for both African American and Caucasian women.

Laboratory tests

Several laboratory tests can be used to diagnose alcohol abuse and evaluate the presence of medical problems related to drinking. These tests include:

• Full blood cell count. This test indicates the presence of anemia, which is common in alcoholics. In addition, the mean corpuscular volume (MCV) is usually high in heavy drinkers. An MCV higher than 100 fL suggests alcohol abuse.

• Liver function tests. Tests for serum glutamine oxaloacetic transaminase (SGOT) and alkaline phosphatase

can indicate alcohol-related injury to the liver. A high level (>30 units) of gamma-glutamyltransferase (GGT) is a useful marker because it is found in 70% of heavy drinkers.

• Blood alcohol levels.

• Carbohydrate deficient transferrin (CDT) tests. This test should not be used as a screener, but is useful in monitoring alcohol consumption in heavy drinkers (those who consume >60 grams of alcohol per day). When CDT is present, it indicates regular daily consumption of alcohol.

The results of these tests may not be accurate if the patient is abusing or dependent on other substances.

Treatment and management

Because alcoholism is a complex disorder with social and occupational as well as medical implications, treatment plans usually include a mix of several different approaches.

Medications

Most drugs that are now being used to treat alcoholism fall into one of two groups: those that restrain the desire to drink by producing painful physical symptoms if the patient does drink; and those that appear to reduce the craving for alcohol directly. Several medications in the second category were originally developed to treat addiction to opioid substances (e.g., heroin and morphine).

ALCOHOL-SENSITIZING MEDICATIONS The most commonly used alcohol-sensitizing agent is disulfiram (Antabuse), which has been used since the 1950s to deter alcoholics from drinking by the threat of a very unpleasant physical reaction if they do consume alcohol. The severity of the disulfiram/ethanol reaction, or DER, depends on the amount of alcohol and disulfiram in the blood. The symptoms of the reaction include facial flushing, rapid heart beat, palpitations, difficult breathing, lowered blood pressure, headaches, nausea, and vomiting.

A DER results when the drinker consumes alcohol because disulfiram inhibits the functioning of an enzyme called aldehyde dehydrogenase. This enzyme is needed to convert acetaldehyde, which is produced when the body begins to oxidize the alcohol. Without the aldehyde dehydrogenase, the patient's blood level of acetaldehyde rises, causing the symptoms associated with DER.

Another alcohol-sensitizing agent is calcium carbimide, which is marketed in Canada under the brand name Temposil. Temposil has been used clinically although it has not been approved by the FDA for use in the United States as of 2001. Calcium carbimide produces physiological reactions with alcohol similar to those produced by disulfiram, but the onset of action is far more rapid and the duration of action is much shorter.

ANTI-CRAVING MEDICATIONS One medication that has been studied in recent years for the treatment of alcoholism is naltrexone, which appears to reduce the craving for alcohol. In addition, naltrexone, which is sold under the brand names Trexan and ReVia, appears to cause few side effects. One 1992 study suggested that naltrexone-treated alcoholics who did have one or two drinks were less likely to continue drinking. Naltrexone has been the subject of a number of clinical trials in the United States; as of August 2000, 10 out of 30 NIH-sponsored clinical trials were studies of naltrexone. On the other hand, a review of medications presented to the National Institute on Alcohol and Alcohol Abuse (NIAAA) in November 1999 concluded that the effectiveness of naltrexone in the treatment of alcoholism appears to be limited.

An anti-craving drug that is presently approved for use in the European Community, acamprosate (calcium acetyl-homotaurinate), has no psychotropic side effects nor any potential for abuse or dependence. Although acamprosate is being used in clinical trials in the United States as of 2000, its effects are unclear. It appears to reduce the frequency of drinking, but its effects on enhancing abstinence from alcohol are no greater than those of naltrexone. In addition, acamprosate does not appear to enhance the effectiveness of naltrexone if the drugs are given in combination.

KEY TERMS

Acamprosate—An anti-craving medication used in Europe to reduce the craving for alcohol. It is presently undergoing tests for approval in the United States.

Disulfiram—A medication that has been used since the late 1940s as part of a treatment plan for alcohol abuse. Disulfiram, which is sold under the trade name Antabuse, produces changes in the body's metabolism of alcohol that cause headaches, vomiting, and other unpleasant symptoms if the patient drinks even small amounts of alcohol.

Ethanol—The chemical name for beverage alcohol. It is also sometimes called ethyl alcohol or grain alcohol to distinguish it from isopropyl or rubbing alcohol.

Knockout experiment—A type of genetic experiment in which researchers are able to deactivate, or knock out, a gene that may influence a particular trait, such as vulnerability to alcohol.

Longitudinal study—A type of research project in which the same subjects are interviewed repeatedly at intervals over a period of time.

Microarray—An ordered arrangement of many different genes on a glass slide or silicon chip. Microarrays allow researchers to study large numbers of genes simultaneously in determining different levels of gene activity in such complex processes as the body's response to alcohol.

Naltrexone—A medication originally developed to treat addiction to heroin or morphine that is also used to treat alcoholism. It works by reducing the craving for alcohol rather than by producing vomiting or other unpleasant reactions.

Polygenic—A trait, characteristic, condition, etc. that depends on the activity of more than one gene for its emergence or expression.

Telescoping—A term sometimes used to describe the relatively rapid progression of alcoholism in women, even though women usually begin to drink heavily at later ages than men do.

Transgenic experiment—A genetic experiment in which a gene can be added to a laboratory animal's genetic material. The behavior of the altered animal can be compared with the behavior of an unaltered animal to help pinpoint the role of the gene in affecting it.

Psychosocial treatment options

Most alcoholics are treated with a variety of psychosocial approaches, including regular attendance at Alcoholics Anonymous (AA) meetings, group therapy, marital or family therapy, so-called community-based approaches, social skills training, relapse prevention, and stress management techniques. Insight-oriented individual psychotherapy by itself is ineffective with the majority of alcoholics.

The most effective psychosocial treatments of alcohol dependence incorporate a cognitive-behavioral approach. Relapse prevention utilizes cognitive-behavioral approaches to identifying high-risk situations for each patient and restructuring his or her perceptions of the effects of alcohol as well as of the relapse process. Network therapy, which combines individual cognitive-behavioral psychotherapy with the involvement of the patient's family and peers as a group support network, is a newer approach to alcohol dependence. One recent study found that while cognitive-behavioral therapy is effective in treating alcohol dependence, the reasons that are usually offered to explain its effectiveness should be reexamined.

Prognosis

The prognosis for recovery from alcoholism varies widely. The usual course of the disorder is one of episodes of intoxication beginning in adolescence, with full-blown dependence by the mid-20s to mid-30s. The most common pattern is one of periodic attempts at abstinence alternating with relapses into uncontrolled drinking. On the other hand, it is thought that as many as 20% of persons diagnosed as alcohol-dependent achieve long-term sobriety even without medical treatment. It is difficult to compare the outcomes of the various treatment approaches to alcoholism, in part because their definitions of "success" vary. Some researchers count only total abstinence from alcohol as a successful outcome, while others regard curtailed drinking and better social adjustment as indicators of success. The role of genetic factors in the prognosis is still disputed. Available evidence suggests that such factors as the presence of a spouse, partner, or close friend in the alcoholic's life, or religious commitment, can outweigh genetic vulnerability to the disorder.

Resources

BOOKS

"Alcoholism." *The Merck Manual of Diagnosis and Therapy*, edited by Mark H. Beers, MD, and Robert Berkow, MD. Whitehouse Station, NJ: Merck Research Laboratories, 1999.

American Psychiatric Association. *Diagnostic and Statistical Manual of Mental Disorders*, 4th edition. Washington, DC: American Psychiatric Association, 1994.

Batey, Robert G., MD. "Alcohol-Related Problems." In *Conn's Current Therapy*, edited by Robert E. Rakel, MD. Philadelphia: W. B. Saunders Company, 2000.

Gearheart, W. W. "Alcoholism." In *Encyclopedia of Genetics*, vol. I, edited by Jeffrey A. Knight. Pasadena, CA: Salem Press, Inc., 1999.

Goodwin, Donald W. "Alcoholism." In *Encyclopedia of Neuroscience*, vol. I, edited by George Adelman. Boston, Basel, and Stuttgart: Birkhaeuser, 1987.

Hobbs, William R., Theodore W. Rall, and Todd A. Verdoorn. "Hypnotics and Sedatives; Ethanol." Chapter 17. In *Goodman & Gilman's The Pharmacological Basis of Therapeutics*, 9th edition, edited by Joel G. Hardman and Lee E. Limbird. New York: McGraw-Hill, 1995.

Lyon, Jeff, and Peter Gorner. *Altered Fates: Gene Therapy and the Retooling of Human Life*. New York and London: W. W. Norton & Co., Inc., 1996.

O'Brien, Charles P. "Drug Addiction and Drug Abuse." Chapter 24. In *Goodman & Gilman's The Pharmacological Basis of Therapeutics*, 9th edition, edited by Joel G. Hardman and Lee E. Limbird. New York: McGraw-Hill, 1995.

Seixas, Judith S., and Geraldine Youcha. *Children of Alcoholism: A Survivor's Manual*. New York: Harper & Row Publishers, 1985.

PERIODICALS

Anton, R. F., et al. "Posttreatment results of combining naltrexone with cognitive-behavior therapy for the treatment of alcoholism." *Journal of Clinical Psychopharmacology* 21 (February 2001): 72-77.

Bowers, B. J. "Applications of transgenic and knockout mice in alcohol research." *Alcohol in Research and Health* 24 (2000): 175-84.

Bradley, K. A., et al. "Alcohol screening questionnaires in women: A critical review." *Journal of the American Medical Association* 280 (July 8, 1998): 166-71.

Crum, R. M., and J. C. Anthony. "Educational level and risk for alcohol abuse and dependence: Differences by race-ethnicity." *Ethnicity and Disease* 10 (Winter 2000): 39-52.

Cunradi, C. B., et al. "Alcohol-related problems and intimate partner violence among white, black, and Hispanic couples in the U.S." *Alcoholism: Clinical and Experimental Research* 23 (September 1999): 1492-1501.

Enoch, M. A., and D. Goldman. "The genetics of alcoholism and alcohol abuse." *Current Psychiatry Reports* 3 (April 2001): 144-51.

Galanter, M., and D. Brook. "Network therapy for addiction: Bringing family and peer support into office practice."

International Journal of Group Psychotherapy 51 (January 2001): 101-22.

Heath, A. C., et al. "Towards a molecular epidemiology of alcohol dependence: Analyzing the interplay of genetic and environmental risk factors." *British Journal of Psychiatry Supplement* 40 (April 2001): s33-s40.

Holtzman, D., et al. "State- and sex-specific prevalence of selected characteristics—Behavioral Risk Factor Surveillance System, 1996 and 1997." *Morbidity and Mortality Weekly Report* CDC Surveillance (July 2000): 1-39.

Larimer, M. E., et al. "Relapse prevention. An overview of Marlatt's cognitive-behavioral model." *Alcohol Research and Health* 23 (1999): 151-60.

Morgenstern, J., and R. Longabaugh. "Cognitive-behavioral treatment for alcohol dependence: A review of evidence for its hypothesized mechanisms of action." *Addiction* 95 (October 2000): 1475-1490.

Nurnberger, J. I. Jr., et al. "Evidence for a locus in chromosome 1 that influences vulnerability to alcoholism and affective disorder." *American Journal of Psychiatry* 158 (May 2001): 718-24.

Paschall, M. J., et al. "Alcohol misuse in young adulthood: Effects of race, educational attainment, and social context." *Substance Use and Misuse* 35 (September 2000): 1485-1506.

Rodriguez, E., et al. "Family violence, employment status, welfare benefits, and alcohol drinking in the United States: What is the relation?" *Journal of Epidemiology and Community Health* 55 (March 2001): 172-78.

Steinbauer, J. R., et al. "Ethnic and sex bias in primary care screening tests for alcohol use disorders." *Annals of Internal Medicine* 129 (September 1998): 353-62.

Stromberg, M. F., et al. "Effect of acamprosate and naltrexone, alone or in combination, on ethanol consumption." *Alcohol* 23 (February 2001): 109-16.

Wall, T. L., et al. "A genetic association with the development of alcohol and other substance use behavior in Asian Americans." *Journal of Abnormal Psychology* 110 (February 2001): 173-78.

Wall, T. L., et al. "Hangover symptoms in Asian Americans with variations in the aldehyde dehydrogenase (ALDH2) gene." *Journal of Studies on Alcohol* 61 (January 2000): 13-17.

ORGANIZATIONS

Alcoholics Anonymous World Services. PO Box 459, Grand Central Station, New York, NY 10163. (212) 870-3400.

American Psychiatric Association. 1400 K St. NW, Washington, DC 20005. (202) 682-6220.

National Clearinghouse for Alcohol and Drug Information. PO Box 2345, Rockville, MD 20847. (800) 729-6686.

National Council on Alcoholism and Drug Dependence Hopeline. 12 West 21st St., New York, NY 10010. (800) 622-2255.

National Institute on Alcohol Abuse and Alcoholism. 5600 Fishers Lane, Rockville, MD 20852.

WEBSITES

American Psychiatric Association. <http://www.psych.org>.

National Institute of Mental Health. <http://www.nimh.nih.gov>.

National Institute on Alcohol and Alcohol Abuse (NIAAA). <http://www.niaaa.org>.

Rebecca J. Frey, PhD

Aldrich syndrome *see* **Wiskott-Aldrich syndrome**

Alkaptonuria

Definition

Alkaptonuria is a rare, inherited disorder characterized by urine that turns dark when exposed to air, dark pigmentation of the cartilage and other tissues, and arthritis.

Description

Alkaptonuria (AKU) (sometimes spelled alcaptonuria) is a disorder in which a substance called homogentisic acid (HGA) accumulates in cells and connective tissues throughout the body. Large amounts of HGA also are excreted in the urine. In a process known as ochronosis, deposits of HGA form dark pigments in the skin, joints, and other tissues of the body. Over the long term, ochronosis leads to ochronotic arthritis, which is a painful inflammation and stiffening of the joints. AKU is also known as homogentisic acid oxidase deficiency, ochronosis, alkaptonuria ochronosis, or ochronotic arthritis.

History

The black urine that characterizes AKU has been recognized throughout history. It sometimes was considered to be a bad omen. The dark pigmentation of ochronosis has been identified in an Egyptian mummy from 1500 B.C.

AKU was one of the first inherited disorders to be identified as a deficiency in a single enzyme in one pathway of the body's metabolism. In 1902, Sir Archibald Garrod, after consultation with the famous geneticist William Bateson, proposed that the **inheritance** of AKU could best be described by Gregor Mendel's theory of the inheritance of recessive characteristics. These are inherited traits expressed in some of the offspring of parents who both carry the trait. The parents may or may not express the trait. In 1908, Garrod coined the term "inborn error of metabolism" to describe AKU and three other metabolic disorders. Furthermore, he suggested that AKU was due to a deficiency in a specific enzyme, a protein that catalyzes one step of a metabolic pathway.

Homogentisic acid

During normal metabolism, the 20 common amino acids, that are the building blocks of enzymes and other proteins, are broken down into simpler substances. This process provides energy for the body. The amino acids phenylalanine and tyrosine are converted to simpler substances in a series of eight steps. Each step in this pathway occurs through the action of a different enzyme. The first step in the pathway converts phenylalanine to tyrosine. The inherited disorder known as **phenylketonuria** results from a deficiency in the enzyme that carries out this first step.

AKU results from a deficiency in an enzyme called homogentisate 1,2-dioxygenase (HGD). This enzyme also is called homogentisic acid oxidase. It is responsible for the fourth step in the breakdown of phenylalanine and tyrosine, the conversion of HGA to 4-maleylacetoacetic acid. When there is a deficiency in active HGD, as in AKU, HGA cannot be broken down further. It accumulates in cells and tissues throughout the body, and large amounts of HGA are excreted in the urine.

Oxygen causes HGA molecules to combine with each other to form a very large molecule called a polymer. This polymer is a dark pigment similar to melanin, the pigment responsible for skin color. This pigment is formed in the tissues of the body, as well as in urine exposed to the oxygen in air. Oxygen can also convert HGA into a toxic substance called benzoquinone acetic acid.

HGA is excreted very quickly. In general, levels of HGA are kept quite low in individuals with AKU. Nevertheless, over time, large quantities of HGA, either as individual molecules or as a polymer, are deposited in the cartilage (the flexible tissue of the joints and other bony structures) and in other connective tissues of the body.

Granules of HGA pigment collect around collagen. This is the protein that makes up the fibers of connective tissues. Collagen is the most abundant protein in the body. It is a major structural component of cartilage, bone, tendons, ligaments, and blood vessels. Collagen also forms an important structural layer beneath the skin, and it holds together the cells of various tissues. The accumulation of HGA in connective tissues interferes with the body's ability to make new collagen. As a result, collagen fibers throughout the body are weakened. In particular, HGA weakens the collagen fibers in the cartilage of the joints.

Ochronosis

Initially, an ochre or yellowish-colored HGA pigment is deposited in the tissues of individuals with AKU. Over a period of years, the cartilage, bones, and skin begin to turn a slate-blue or blue-black color. This pigmentation, or ochronosis, of the tissues eventually leads to a serious form of arthritis. Furthermore, as the HGA polymer accumulates, inflammation occurs. This causes calcium to be deposited in the joints in a process called calcification.

Genetic profile

AKU is an autosomal recessive disorder. It is autosomal because the **gene** encoding the HGD enzyme is located on **chromosome** 3, rather than on either of the X or Y sex chromosomes. AKU is a recessive trait because it only occurs when an individual has two copies of the defective gene, one inherited from each parent. The two defective HGD genes do not need to carry the same mutations. If the two mutations are identical, the individual is a homozygote. If the two mutations are different, the affected individual is called a compound heterozygote.

In individuals with a single defective HGD gene, at least 50% of the HGD enzyme has normal activity. These individuals have no symptoms of AKU. However, they are carriers of AKU and can pass the gene on to their offspring.

All of the offspring of two parents with AKU will inherit the disorder. All of the offspring of one parent with AKU and one parent with a single defective HGD gene will inherit at least one defective HGD gene. These offspring have a 50% chance of inheriting two defective genes and developing AKU. The offspring of one parent with AKU and one parent with normal HGD genes will inherit a defective gene from the affected parent, but will not develop AKU. The offspring of parents who both carry one defective HGD gene have a 50% chance of inheriting one defective HGD gene. They have an additional 25% chance of inheriting two such genes and developing AKU. Finally, the children of one parent with a single defective HGD gene and one parent with normal HGD genes have a 50% chance of inheriting the defective gene, but will not develop AKU.

A large number of different mutations have been identified in the HGD gene. These changes reduce or destroy the activity of the HGD enzyme. Mutational hot spots have also been identified in the gene. These are regions of the gene in which mutations are particularly likely to occur.

Demographics

As a recessive disorder, AKU requires two copies of the defective gene, one inherited from each parent. Thus, AKU is much more common in the offspring of couples who are related to each other, such as first or second cousins. As an autosomal disorder, AKU occurs equally among males and females. However, in general, the symptoms of arthritis appear at an earlier age in males and tend to be more severe than in females. The reason for this difference is not known.

AKU occurs with equal frequency among various races; however, the frequency varies substantially among different populations. It is most common in geographically isolated populations. The worldwide prevalence of AKU is estimated at between one in 100,000 and one in 250,000 individuals. However, some estimates are as low as one in a million individuals and, in the United States, AKU frequency is estimated to be only one in four million.

AKU occurs with particularly high frequency in the Dominican Republic, Slovakia, and the Czech Republic. The frequency has been reported to be as high as one in 19,000 live births in Slovakia. The frequency of AKU is particularly low in Finland. Certain mutations occur only in HGD genes from Slovakia. Two specific mutations occur in 50% of all Slovakians with AKU. Other mutations in HGD appear to be unique to the Finnish population.

Signs and symptoms

Early symptoms

Often, the first sign of AKU is the dark staining of an infant's diapers from the HGA in the urine. However, a significant number of AKU-affected individuals do not have blackened urine, particularly if their urine is acidic. Other than darkened urine, AKU generally has no symptoms throughout childhood and early adulthood. Nevertheless, pigment is being deposited in the tissues throughout the early years. Occasionally, black ear wax and pigmentation under the arms may develop before the age of 10.

Ochronosis

Ochronosis, the pigmentation of the cartilage, usually does not become apparent until the fourth decade of life. Small rings or patches of slate-blue, gray, or black discoloration of the white, outer membranes of the eyeballs are one of the first visible symptoms. This usually begins when affected individuals are in their 30s. Thickening and discoloration of the cartilage of the ear usually begins in the following decade. This is indicative of the widespread staining of cartilage and other tissues. The ear cartilage may become stiff, irregularly shaped, and calcified (hardened with deposits of calcium).

Discoloration of the skin is due to the depositing of ochronotic pigment granules in the inner layer of the skin and around the sweat glands. The outer ear and nose may darken with a bluish tint. Pigmentation also may be visible on the eyelids, forehead, and armpits. Where the skin is exposed to the sun, and in the regions of the sweat glands, the skin may become speckled with blue-black discoloration. Sweat may stain clothes brown. Fingernails may become bluish.

The ochronotic effects of AKU on the cartilage and tendons are most visible on parts of the body where the connective tissues are closest to the skin. Pigmentation may be visible in the genital regions, the larynx (voice box), and the middle ear. Dark-stained tendons can be seen when the hand is made into a fist.

Arthritis

The symptoms of ochronotic arthritis are similar to those of other types of arthritis. However, the large, weight-bearing joints usually are the most affected in ochronotic arthritis. These include the joints of the hips, knees, and shoulders, and between the vertebrae of the spine. The joints become stiff and difficult to move. This arthritis develops at an unusually early age. In unaffected individuals, similar arthritis usually does not develop before age 55. Men with AKU develop arthritis in their 30s and 40s. Women with AKU usually develop arthritis in their 50s.

AKU can lead to osteoarthrosis, a degenerative joint disease, and ochronotic arthropathy, which is characterized by the swelling and enlargement of the bones. Ankylosis, the adhesion of bones in the joints, also may occur. The pigment deposits may cause the cartilage to become brittle and susceptible to fragmenting. Individuals with AKU may be at risk for bone fractures.

Calcium deposits can lead to painful attacks similar to those of gout. This calcification may occur in the ear cartilage and in the lumbar disks of the lower back. The disks between vertebrae may become narrowed and eventually may collapse.

Organ damage

The coronary artery of the heart can become diseased as a result of AKU. The aortic valve of the heart may harden and narrow from calcification. Similar problems may develop with the mitral or left atrioventricular valve of the heart (mitral valvulitis). Deposits of pigment can lead to the formation of hard spots of cholesterol and fat (atherosclerotic plaques) in the arteries. This can put a person at risk for a heart attack.

Complications from the deficiency of the HGD enzyme arise primarily in the kidneys and the liver. HGD normally is most active in the kidneys, liver, small intestine, colon, and prostate. The calcification of the genital and urinary tract may lead to blockages in as many as 60% of individuals with ochronosis. Kidney stones and other kidney diseases may develop. Stones in the urine may occur in middle to late adulthood. Increasingly though, this condition is seen in children with AKU under the age of 15 and even as young as two. In men, pigment deposits may lead to stones in the prostate.

The teeth, the brain and spinal cord, and the endocrine system that produces hormones also may be affected by ochronosis. Breathing may become restricted due to the effects of ochronosis on the joints where the ribs attach to the spine. Deposits of pigment on the ear bones and on the membrane of the inner ear may lead to tinnitus, or ringing of the ears, and hearing problems.

Diagnosis

Visual diagnosis

AKU is often detected in early childhood because of the characteristic dark-staining of the urine. In adults, diagnosis usually is made on the basis of joint pain and skin discoloration. Most individuals with AKU have pigment visible in the whites of their eyes by their early 40s.

A family history of AKU helps with the diagnosis. Since many individuals with AKU have no symptoms, siblings of affected individuals should be tested for the disorder.

Identification of HGA

An individual with AKU may excrete as much as 4-8 g of HGA per day in the urine. There are several simple methods to test for HGA in the urine: the addition of sodium hydroxide (an alkali) to the urine will turn it dark; urine with HGA turns black when reacted with iron chloride; and alkaline urine containing HGA blackens photographic paper. In the laboratory, HGA can be identified in the urine using a technique called gas chromatography-mass spectroscopy. This technique separates and identifies the components of a mixture.

There are a number of methods for identifying HGA in the blood and tissues. These include procedures for separating HGA from other components of the blood and instruments that can detect the characteristic color of HGA. With AKU, the concentration of HGA in the blood is approximately 40 micromolar, or 40 micromoles of per liter.

Microscopic examination

With AKU, there usually is visible black staining of cartilage in various body regions, particularly the larynx, trachea (windpipe), and cartilage junctions. Heavy deposits of pigment also occur in the bronchi (the air passages to the lungs). Pigment on the inside and outside of the cells of these tissues can be seen with a microscope.

A skin biopsy, the removal of a small piece of skin, may be used to obtain tissue for examination. The tissue is stained with dyes to reveal the yellowish-brown pigment deposits on the outside of skin cells. Pigment deposits also occur in cells of the endothelium (the thin layer of cells that line blood vessels and other tissues), in the sweat glands, and in the membranes below the skin. These pigments will not fade, even after three days in a solution of bleach.

Skeletal x rays

X-ray examination is used to detect calcification of the joints. Since many individuals with AKU do not have dark-staining urine, x-ray evidence of **osteoarthritis** may indicate a need to test for the presence of HGA in the urine. However, osteoarthritis usually affects the smaller joints; whereas ochronosis most often affects the large joints of the hips and shoulders. Spinal x rays may show dense calcification, degeneration, and fusion of the disks of the vertebrae, particularly in the lumbar region of the lower back. Chest x rays are used to assess damage to the valves of the heart.

Other procedures

Physicians may order computerized tomography (CT) scans of the brain and chest or magnetic reso-

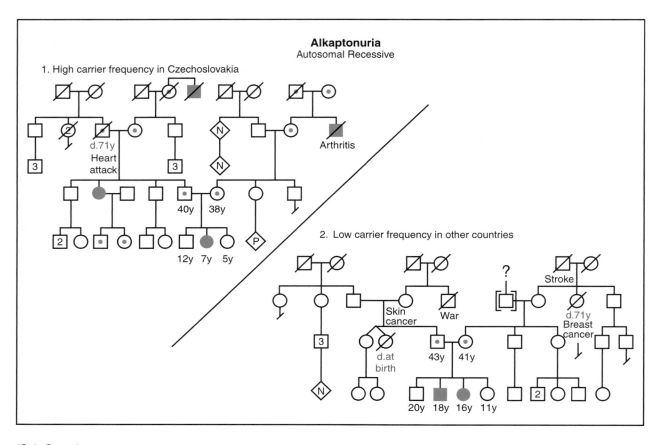

Alkaptonuria
Autosomal Recessive

1. High carrier frequency in Czechoslovakia

2. Low carrier frequency in other countries

(Gale Group.)

nance imaging (MRI) of affected joints. An electrocardiogram (ECG or EKG) may reveal signs of heart complications resulting from AKU. Kidney problems may be diagnosed by ultrasound, the use of sound waves to obtain images of an organ. Lung function tests and hearing tests may be performed to assess additional complications.

Acquired ochronosis

In addition to being a complication of AKU, ochronosis can be acquired. In the past, ochronosis developed from the repeated use of carbolic acid dressings for treating chronic skin ulcers. The prolonged use of the drug quinacrine (atabrine) can cause ochronosis, with pigmentation occurring in many of the same sites as with AKU. Ochronosis can also result from the use of bleaching creams containing hydroquinone. Certain other substances, including phenol, trinitrophenol, quinines, and benzene, can cause ochronosis. However, these forms of ochronosis do not lead to joint disease and, unlike ochronosis from AKU, are reversible.

Treatment and management

The binding of HGA to collagen fibers is irreversible. Treatment of AKU is directed at reducing the deposition of pigment and thereby minimizing arthritis and heart problems in later life.

Vitamin C

Often, high doses (about 1 gm per day) of ascorbic acid (vitamin C) are administered to older children and adults with AKU. Ascorbic acid appears to slow the formation of the HGA polymer and decrease the binding of the polymer to connective tissues. Vitamin C reduces the amount of toxic benzoquinone acetic acid in the urine. However, the amount of HGA in the urine does not decrease. Furthermore, vitamin C does not appear to interrupt the progress of the disease.

Dietary restrictions

Sometimes individuals with AKU are placed on low-protein diets. This limits the intake of phenylalanine and tyrosine from proteins. If the body has lower

KEY TERMS

Alkaline—Having a basic pH; not acidic.

Amino acid—Organic compounds that form the building blocks of protein. There are 20 types of amino acids (eight are "essential amino acids" which the body cannot make and must therefore be obtained from food).

Autosomal recessive—A pattern of genetic inheritance where two abnormal genes are needed to display the trait or disease.

Benzoquinone acetic acid—Toxic compound that is formed when oxygen reacts with homogentisic acid.

Calcification—A process in which tissue becomes hardened due to calcium deposits.

Collagen—The main supportive protein of cartilage, connective tissue, tendon, skin, and bone.

Compound heterozygote—Having two different mutated versions of a gene.

Homogentisate 1,2-dioxygenase (HGD)—Homogentisic acid oxidase, the fourth enzyme in the metabolic pathway for the breakdown of phenylalanine.

Homogentisic acid (HGA)—2,5-Dihydroxyphenylacetic acid, the third intermediate in the metabolic pathway for the breakdown of phenylalanine.

Homozygote—Having two identical copies of a gene or chromosome.

Melanin—Pigments normally produced by the body that give color to the skin and hair.

Mendel, Gregor—Austrian monk who discovered the basic principals of hereditary.

Ochronosis—A condition marked by pigment deposits in cartilage, ligaments, and tendons.

Phenylalanine—An essential amino acid that must be obtained from food since the human body cannot manufacture it.

Polymer—A very large molecule, formed from many smaller, identical molecules.

Tyrosine—An aromatic amino acid that is made from phenylalanine.

amounts of phenylalanine and tyrosine to break down, less HGA will be formed. However, both of these amino acids are necessary for making proteins in the body. Furthermore, phenylalanine is an essential amino acid

that must be obtained from food, since the human body cannot produce it. Adult males require approximately 2 gm per day of phenylalanine. Phenylalanine also is present in some artificial sweeteners.

Restricting protein intake to no more than the daily protein requirement may be beneficial for children with AKU. Such diets appear to substantially reduce the amount of benzoquinone acetic acid in the urine. In children under the age of 12, low-protein diets significantly reduce the amount of HGA in the urine, as well. However, these diets seem to have little effect on older children and young adults with AKU, and low-protein diets are difficult to maintain. When low-protein diets are prescribed, the levels of amino acids in the blood must be monitored, to assure that there is no deficiency in phenylalanine.

Ochronosis

Most treatment of AKU is directed at the diseased joints. The treatment for ochronosis is the same as for other forms of degenerative arthritis. Treatments include painkillers, physical therapy, rehabilitation, orthopedic supports, and rest. Chiropractic manipulations and exercise regimens also are utilized.

Treatment of ochronotic arthritis eventually may require hip and/or knee joint replacements with artificial materials. In older individuals, fusion of the lumbar discs of the lower spine may be necessary. Aortic valve replacement may be necessary to treat heart disease.

Future drug treatment

The National Institutes of Health are undertaking clinical research studies to better understand the clinical, biochemical, and molecular aspects of AKU. These studies are in preparation for clinical trials of a new drug to treat AKU. It is hoped that this drug will block the production and accumulation of HGA.

Prognosis

There is no cure for AKU. Essentially all individuals with AKU eventually experience arthritic symptoms, particularly arthritis of the hips, knees, and spine. The bone and joint disease may become debilitating by the sixth to eighth decades of life. Furthermore, cardiovascular involvement and ochronotic skin abnormalities are to be expected with AKU.

Despite these difficulties, individuals with AKU have normal life expectancies. Although there is an increased risk of heart attack in later life, most individuals with AKU die of causes unrelated to the disorder.

Resources

BOOKS

La Du, B. N. "Alkaptonuria." In *The Metabolic and Molecular Bases of Inherited Disease*, edited by C. R. Scriver, A. L. Beaudet, W. S. Sly, and D. Valle. New York: McGraw Hill, Inc., 1995, pp. 1371-86.

PERIODICALS

Titus, G. P., et al. "Crystal Structure of Human Homogentisate Dioxygenase." *Nature Structural Biology* 7, no. 7 (2000): 542-46.

Zatkova, A., et al. "High Frequency of Alkaptonuria in Slovakia: Evidence for the Appearance of Multiple Mutations in HGO Involving Different Mutational Hot Spots." *American Journal of Human Genetics* 6, no. 5 (November 2000): 1333-39.

ORGANIZATIONS

AKU Hotline. <http://www.goodnet.com/~ee72478/enable/hotline.htm>.

National Heart, Lung, and Blood Institute. PO Box 30105, Bethesda, MD 20824-0105. (301) 592-8573. nhlbiinfo@rover.nhlbi.nih.gov. <http://www.nhlbi.nih.gov>.

National Institute of Child Health and Human Development (NICHD). Patient Recruitment and Public Liaison Office, Building 61, 10 Cloister Court, Bethesda, MD 20892-4754. (800) 411-1222, (301) 594-9774 (TTY), (866) 411-1010 (TTY). prpl@mail.cc.nih.gov. <http://clinicalstudies.info.nih.gov/detail/A_2000-CH-0141.html>.

WEBSITES

"Alkaptonuria." *AKU Database*. <http://www.cib.csic.es/~akudb/alkaptonuria.htm>.

Burkhart, Craig G., and Craig Nathaniel Burkhart. "Ochronosis." *Dermatology/Metabolic Diseases*. 25 July 2000. <http://www.emedicine.com/DERM/topic476.htm>.

"Clinical, Biochemical, and Molecular Investigations into Alkaptonuria." *NIH Clinical Research Studies*. Protocol Number: 00-CH-0141. (March 10, 2001). <http://clinicalstudies.info.nih.gov/detail/A_2000-CH-0141.html>.

Medical College of Wisconsin Physicians and Clinics. "Alkaptonuria and Ochronosis." *HealthLink*. (March 18, 1999). <http://healthlink.mcw.edu/content/article/921733488.html>.

Roth, Karl S. "Alkaptonuria." *Pediatrics/Genetics and Metabolic Disease*. (December 10, 2000). <http://emedicine.com/ped/topic64.htm>.

Margaret Alic, PhD

Alpha-1 antitrypsin

Definition

Alpha-1 antitrypsin is one of the most common inherited diseases in the Caucasian population. The most common symptom is lung disease (emphysema). People with alpha-1 antitrypsin may also develop liver disease and/or liver **cancer**. The disease is caused by a deficiency in the protein alpha-1 antitrypsin, which is why the condition is sometimes called alpha-1 antitrypsin deficiency. Other names include anti-elastase, antitrypsin, and ATT. The development of lung disease is accelerated by harmful environmental exposures, such as smoking tobacco. Alpha-1 antitrypsin is inherited. The age of onset, rate of progression, and type of symptoms vary both between and within families.

Description

The protein alpha-1 antitrypsin is a protease inhibitor, which means that it inactivates other proteins called proteases. This is an important function, as proteases themselves disable proteins. In our bodies the levels of proteases and their inhibitors are balanced so that proteases can perform their functions but not over-perform, which leads to problems.

A protease called *elastase* is the most important target of alpha-1 antitrypsin. Elastase protects the lungs against bacteria and other foreign particles. However, if the action of elastase is not kept in check, elastase destroys lung tissue. Alpha-1 antitrypsin ensures that elastase is not overactive.

Individuals with alpha-1 antitrypsin have inadequate levels of the protein alpha-1 antitrypsin. Thus, certain proteases (especially in the lungs) are overactive, which leads to emphysema and sometimes to liver disease. Alpha-1 antitrypsin is made mostly in the liver.

Some alpha-1 antitrypsin proteins are abnormal in addition to being deficient. These abnormal proteins may not move from the liver to the blood stream correctly. The build-up of the proteins in the liver may lead to liver disease. Also, the abnormal proteins may not neutralize elastase as effectively. Thus, people with alpha-1 antitrypsin have fewer proteins; those they do have do not work as effectively.

Genetic profile

The genetics of alpha-1 antitrypsin are complicated. Scientists have identified many different forms of the **gene** that codes for the alpha-1 antitrypsin protein. This protein is often called Pi and the gene called PI, for protease inhibitor. One form of the gene, which scientists call Z, or *PI Z*, greatly reduced the amount of the active Pi protein. Because every person inherits one of each gene from his or her mother, and another copy of each gene from his or her father, everyone has two copies of every gene. People who have two copies of the PI Z gene have 85% less alpha-1 antitrypsin protein. These people have only 15% of the normal level of protein. The protein that they do have does not function as well as the normal protein. People who have one PI Z gene and one normal PI gene have about 60% of the normal level Pi protein. Other forms of the alpha-1 antitrypsin gene are associated with more or less severe deficiencies in protein.

Two other common forms of the Pi protein are called *S* and *M*. Pi M is the normal protein and PI M is the normal gene. The Pi M protein has many subtypes within the population, designated M1, M2, etc. A few abnormal alpha-1 antitrypsin genes also have unique names. The PI S gene is slightly abnormal, but not as abnormal as PI Z. Individuals with one PI S gene and one PI Z gene have approximately 38% functioning of the Pi protein (Pi SZ).

The **inheritance** of alpha-1 antitrypsin is autosomal recessive. This means that a person with alpha-1 antitrypsin has inherited one abnormal gene from each of his or her parents. The parents are most likely carriers, meaning they each have one normal gene and one abnormal gene. Two carriers have a one in four chance to have an affected child with each pregnancy. However, not all people with alpha-1 antitrypsin develop symptoms. Whether and when a person with two abnormal alpha-1 antitrypsin genes develops symptoms is related to the degree of harmful exposures, such as tobacco smoke. A person who is affected with alpha-1 antitrypsin is only at risk to have an affected child if the child's other parent is a carrier.

Although the inheritance of alpha-1 antitrypsin is autosomal recessive, the activity of the protein is equally determined by the gene inherited from either parent. For example, if a gene inherited from one parent codes for a protein with 100% activity, and the gene inherited from the other parent codes for a protein with 0% activity, the offspring would have 50% protein activity. The physical expression of the genes is autosomal recessive, but each gene has an equal effect on the protein activity—neither gene is dominant over the other gene. The gene for alpha-1 antitrypsin is on **chromosome** 14. More than 90 different forms of the gene have been identified.

Demographics

Alpha-1 antitrypsin is most common in Caucasians, especially those of Northern European descent. Alpha-1 antitrypsin is less common in populations of Asian, African, and American Indian descent. Approximately one in 2,500 Caucasians have two Z genes. These individuals account for 1% of all emphysema patients. Because people with one PI Z gene and one other deleterious PI gene may also have symptoms, the number of people at risk to have alpha-1 antitrypsin associated lung disease is greater than one in 2,500. Approximately one in 20 Caucasians has one Z gene and one normal gene. The number of Caucasians with one S gene and one normal gene is even higher. Approximately one in 1,000 Caucasians of Northern European descent have two S genes (and no normal alpha-1 antitrypsin gene).

Signs and symptoms

The main symptom of alpha-1 antitrypsin is a risk for early-onset, rapidly progressive emphysema. People with alpha-1 antitrypsin who smoke tobacco are at especially high. Emphysema is chronic lung disease that begins with breathlessness during exertion and progresses to shortness of breath at all times, caused by destructive changes in the lung tissue. The risk for liver disease in adults is increased, as is the risk for **hepatocellular carcinoma** (liver cancer). Some children with alpha-1 antitrypsin develop liver disease as well. Individuals with alpha-1 antitrypsin are also at risk for chronic obstructive lung disease and reactive airway disease (**asthma**). Chronic obstructive lung disease is decreased breathing capacity, which may be caused by emphysema but also has other underlying causes.

Lung disease

Approximately 60–70% of the people with two PI Z genes develop chronic lung disease. Shortness of breath with exertion may begin before the age of 40 years and progress rapidly to incapacitating emphysema. Life expectancy may be reduced by 10–15 years and is reduced further if people with two PI Z genes smoke tobacco. A portion of the people with two PI Z genes never develop chronic lung disease.

The age of onset and severity of symptoms associated with alpha-1 antitrypsin are quite variable, even within the same family. Environmental exposures significantly effect whether a person will develop symptoms. Smoking puts individuals with alpha-1 antitrypsin at much greater risk to develop emphysema. The already abnormal and deficient Pi Z protein functions 1,000 times less effectively in smokers. Researcher Ronald Crystal states, "Cigarette smoking renders an already poorly defended lung completely defenseless." People with alpha-1 antitrypsin who are not exposed to harmful environmental factors are less likely to develop emphysema. If people with two PI Z genes stop smoking before they develop lung disease, their life expectancy increases and the risk of lung disease decreases.

Individuals who have one abnormal gene with very little protein function and one gene with somewhat reduced protein function may also at risk for chronic obstructive lung disease. It is possible that people with one Z gene and one normal gene are also at risk to develop chronic lung disease if they are exposed to harmful environmental factors such as tobacco smoke. The age symptoms begin in this group would be later than that seen in people with two abnormal genes. Some researchers disagree, stating that people with PI SZ and PI MZ genes are not at significant risk for lung disease.

Liver disease

The risk of liver disease and liver cancer are increased in individuals with alpha-1 antitrypsin. Babies and children with alpha-1 antitrypsin may have abnormal liver function and inflammation. The abnormal liver function they develop is called cholestasis, which is when the liver stops secreting a digestive fluid called bile. A build-up of bile causes cholestatic jaundice (yellowing of the skin). These abnormalities sometimes progress to liver disease and liver failure, which is fatal without a liver transplant. In other babies and children, liver function returns to normal.

A small number of adults with alpha-1 antitrypsin develop liver disease, and some develop liver cancer. The age at which the liver disease begins, the rate at which it progresses, and the stage at which it is usually diagnosed are quite variable. Adults with alpha-1 antitrypsin who had liver abnormalities as children may be at increased risk to develop liver disease or liver cancer. People with one normal PI gene and one PI Z gene may be at increased risk for liver disease.

The likelihood that a child or adult with alpha-1 antitrypsin will develop liver disease can be predicted to some degree based on which change in the gene (mutation) they have as well as their family history. The risk that a baby with two Z genes will develop significant liver disease is approximately 10%. However if a person has a family history of alpha-1 antitrypsin with liver disease, this risk may be higher. Males (both adult and children) develop liver disease more often than females. Alpha-1 antitrypsin is the most common genetic cause of liver disease in infants and children. Researchers do not know why some people with alpha-1 antitrypsin develop progressive liver disease and many others do not. The liver disease appears to be related to abnormal antitrypsin protein remaining in the liver instead of being secreted.

Diagnosis

Alpha-1 antitrypsin may be suspected in a newborn with cholestatic jaundice, swollen abdomen, and poor feeding. In later childhood or adulthood, fatigue, poor appetite, swelling of the abdomen and legs, or abnormal liver tests may trigger the need for testing. The diagnosis of alpha-1 antitrypsin is based on measurement of antitrypsin (Pi) in the blood. If levels of Pi are deficient, genetic studies may be performed to determine which abnormal forms of the gene are present. The Pi protein can also be studied to determine which type a person has. Prenatal diagnosis is available, however, it is recommended that parental genetic studies precede prenatal testing to ensure accurate interpretation of results.

Levels of antitrypsin protein in the blood may be normal in individuals who have one PI Z gene and one normal gene, and in individuals who have one PI S gene and one PI Z gene. Studying the Pi protein will more accurately diagnose these individuals.

Lung disease in people with alpha-1 antitrypsin is diagnosed by the same methods used to diagnose lung disease in people who do not have alpha-1 antitrypsin. These studies include breathing tests such as total lung capacity and pulmonary function tests. Total lung capacity is measured with a device called a spirometer. Pulmonary function tests measure oxygen/carbon dioxide exchange by determining the amount of air exhaled, the time to exhale, and the efficiency of oxygen transport. X rays and other studies may also be performed.

Liver disease in children and adults with alpha-1 antitrypsin is diagnosed by the same methods used to diagnose liver disease in people who do not have alpha-1 antitrypsin. Liver function studies include tests measuring two liver proteins called serum glutamic oxaloacetic transaminase (SGOT) and serum glutamic pyruvic transaminase (SGPT). SGOT is sometimes called aspartate transaminase (AST), and SGPT is sometimes called alanine aminotransferase (ALT). Studies may also be performed looking for deposits within the cells of the liver called inclusions.

Once the diagnosis of alpha-1 antitrypsin has been made, it is important to share this information with relatives related by blood, especially parents and children. These relatives may also have alpha-1 antitrypsin. If they know that they have it before they develop lung disease, they can take preventative measures such as avoiding exposure to smoke and other lung toxins. Some organizations have recommended that individuals with asthma be tested for alpha-1 antitrypsin.

Treatment and management

Although alpha-1 antitrypsin cannot be prevented, many of the condition's consequences can be prevented. People with alpha-1 antitrypsin should not smoke cigarettes and should not be exposed to smoke or other lung irritants. Respiratory infections should be treated promptly because they increase the level of harmful elastase in the lungs. Some doctors recommend avoiding alcohol and oxidants; keeping hepatitis A and B vaccinations, pneumococcal vaccinations, and influenza shots up-to-date; and preventing hepatitis C exposure.

Protein augmentation

Treatment is available if individuals with alpha-1 antitrypsin develop lung disease. Infusion of alpha-1 antitrypsin protein into the bloodstream may halt or slow progression of respiratory problems. The protein is put into a blood vein weekly, biweekly, or monthly. Treatment with the replacement protein may not be effective if tissue damage to the lungs is severe. This is often called augmentation therapy. This therapy is safe and people who receive it have few adverse reactions. However, some researchers are not convinced that it is an effective treatment.

People with alpha-1 antitrypsin who have diminished lung air capacity but no other symptoms may be given prophylactic replacement antitrypsin infusions. The success of prophylactic treatment has not been confirmed.

Treatments in development

People who have two abnormal PI genes have reason to be hopeful that effective treatments may be available by 2010. The Pi protein may be available in an inhaled form in the first few years of the new millennium. Biotechnology based treatments such as aerosols that deliver the normal gene to lung tissue are being studied. Lung transplant may be an option in the future.

Liver disease treatments

Some doctors advocate regular monitoring of liver function in elderly patients with alpha-1 antitrypsin. In most people with alpha-1 antitrypsin, an initial liver function evaluation will be performed but it will only be repeated if the person has symptoms. Augmentation therapy (replacing the protein in the blood) does not effectively treat the liver disease. **Gene therapy** for liver disease is not possible.

The treatment for children with alpha-1 antitrypsin who develop liver disease is a liver transplant. Alpha-1

antitrypsin is a common reason for liver transplant in the pediatric population. If the new liver is from a donor with normal alpha-1 antitrypsin, the new liver will have normal, functional protein after the transplant.

Prognosis

Individuals with alpha-1 antitrypsin who have never smoked nor been exposed to other respiratory irritants have the best prognosis. They may never develop lung disease. If they do develop lung disease, the age of onset is usually later than that of smokers—10 or more years later. Prognosis is improved if people with alpha-1 antitrypsin stop smoking before the onset of lung disease.

The lung disease people with alpha-1 antitrypsin develop typically progresses rapidly. Affected individuals may progress from decreased respiration during exertion to incapacitation in five years. Smoking cessation and prompt treatment are critical. Prompt treatment with replacement protein improves prognosis. Some scientists recommend delaying treatment until the affected person has quit smoking.

Prognosis of infants with liver disease is poor. If a donor is found and transplant successful, the new liver has the alpha-1 antitrypsin gene of the donor. Therefore, if the liver transplant is successful the prognosis related to alpha-1 antitrypsin is very good.

A great deal of research is done on the prevention and cure of alpha-1 antitrypsin. In 1996, the World Health Organization sponsored a meeting of experts who study the disease. The experts outlined specific topics to be researched, which included studying treatments. In 1997, 12 countries with registries of alpha-1 antitrypsin patients formed an international registry. This will make it easier for researchers to complete studies involving large numbers of patients, which are absolutely necessary to answer research questions (especially treatment questions). Pharmaceutical companies are also studying new treatment options. Researchers are hopeful about new treatments that may become available. Even with new medicines, the most important treatment for alpha-1 antitrypsin will probably be prevention.

Resources

BOOKS

Crystal, Ronald G., ed. *Alpha 1-Antitrypsin Deficiency.* Lung Biology in Health & Disease Series, vol. 88. New York: Marcel Dekker, Inc., 1995

ORGANIZATIONS

Alpha 1 National Association. 8120 Penn Ave. South, Suite 549, Minneapolis, MN 55431. (612) 703-9979 or (800) 521-3025. julie@alpha1.org. <http://www.alpha1.org>.

Alpha One Foundation. 2937 SW 27th Ave., Suite 302, Miami, FL 33133. (305) 567-9888 or (877) 228-7321. mserven@alphaone.org. <http://www.alphaone.org>.

Alpha to Alpha. RR#5 Box 859, Warsaw, MO 65355. (660) 438-3045. <http://www.alpha2alpha.org>.

AlphaNet. (800) 557-2638. <http://www.alphanet.org>.

American Liver Foundation. 75 Maiden Lane, Suite 603, New York, NY 10038. (800) 465-4837 or (888) 443-7222. <http://www.liverfoundation.org>.

American Lung Association. 1740 Broadway, New York, NY 10019-4374. (212) 315-8700 or (800) 586-4872. <http://www.lungusa.org>.

WEBSITES

"A1AD Related Emphysema." Fact sheet. *American Lung Association.* <http://www.lungusa.org/diseases/luna1ad.html>.

"Alpha1-Antitrypsin Deficiency or Inherited Emphysema." Fact sheet. *National Jewish Medical and Research Center.* <http://www.nationaljewish.org/medfacts/alpha1.html>.

Michelle Queneau Bosworth, MS, CGC

Alpha-thalassemia X-linked mental retardation syndrome

Definition

Alpha-thalassemia **X-linked mental retardation** syndrome is a rare, inherited condition characterized by severe mental retardation, characteristic facial features, and mild anemia. Due to the **inheritance** pattern of this disorder, only males are affected.

Description

Alpha-thalassemia X-linked mental retardation syndrome is also known as ATRX syndrome, X-linked mental retardation hypotonic facies syndrome, and alpha-thalassemia/mental retardation, X-linked. This condition is characterized by mental retardation, severe developmental delay, unique craniofacial features, skeletal abnormalities, hypotonia, and genital abnormalities. These patients often have a form of anemia, called alpha **thalassemia**, which results from a defect in the production of hemoglobin. The syndrome has been recognized fairly recently and, thus, information about it is still evolving.

Genetic profile

Alpha-thalassemia X-linked mental retardation syndrome is caused by mutations in the ATRX **gene** that is located on the X **chromosome**. Males only have one X chromosome, which they always inherit from their mother. Thus, males who inherit a mutation in the ATRX gene are affected with the disorder. Females who inherit a mutation in the ATRX gene are carriers of the disorder—this is because they have a second X chromosome with a functional copy of the ATRX gene. This functional copy compensates for the mutated copy. Carrier females rarely show clinical signs of the disorder. Due to the X-linked recessive inheritance pattern, only males can be affected with this condition.

If a male is affected with alpha-thalassemia X-linked mental retardation syndrome, it is impossible for him to reproduce due to the associated genital abnormalities. However, there are implications for other family members. For example, his mother may be a carrier of an ATRX mutation. If this is the case, each subsequent male child will have a 50% to inherit the abnormal ATRX gene. Since there is a 50% chance that a child will be male, this means that any given pregnancy from a carrier mother has a 25% (50% × 50%) chance to be affected with alpha-thalassemia X-linked mental retardation syndrome. It is important to remember that an ATRX mutation may also have implications for the affected individual's maternal aunts and their offspring.

However, it is also possible that the ATRX mutation is a new (*de novo*) mutation in the affected individual, meaning that his mother would not be a carrier. It is unknown how often a *de novo* mutation occurs in ATRX. The possibility of a *de novo* mutation is much less likely if there are two or more affected brothers in the family. If there are no other affected individuals in the family and if the mother's X-inactivation studies are normal, the mother is very unlikely to be a carrier. Thus, it is likely a *de novo* mutation in the affected male and the recurrence risk to siblings is very small.

Another possibility is germline mosaicism. In this case, the ATRX mutation may be present only in the egg cells of the mother. Thus, her blood cells would be normal and, therefore, X-inactivation studies and molecular genetic tests would be normal as well. However, the ATRX mutations present in her egg cells would leave a significant recurrence risk for future pregnancies.

Demographics

The prevalence of alpha-thalassemia X-linked mental retardation syndrome is not currently known. Between 150 and 200 affected patients are known worldwide. There are no reports of the condition being more common in specific ethnic groups or geographical regions.

Signs and symptoms

There are distinctive features that accompany alpha-thalassemia X-linked mental retardation syndrome. The most noticeable clinical sign is the severe developmental delay and mental retardation that is almost always present. From very early in life, affected individuals will be delayed in meeting developmental milestones. Some will fail to walk independently and many will not learn to speak coherently. Poor muscle tone (hypotonia), which is also very common in this condition, plays a role in the developmental delay. More recently, there have been reports of affected individuals with less severe developmental delay and mental retardation, however, it is unclear as to why this is.

There are unique craniofacial features associated with alpha-thalassemia X-linked mental retardation syndrome. Affected individuals often have a small head (microcephaly), widely spaced eyes (telecanthus), flat mid-facial area (mid-face hypoplasia), small and low-set ears, small triangular nose, tented upper lip, and full, everted lower lip with a protruding tongue. About two-thirds of affected individuals have short stature. In some patients, growth retardation is present throughout life and, in other cases, it manifests around puberty. Other minor skeletal abnormalities have been observed as well, such as joint contractures, abnormalities of the fingers

and toes, foot deformations, and **scoliosis**. Additionally, genitalia of affected individuals are often abnormal and underdeveloped. These abnormalities may be minor, such as undescended testes, or major, such as **ambiguous genitalia** that appears female in nature. In many cases, patients do not progress through puberty as expected, probably due to inadequate amounts of the male hormone testosterone.

In addition, patients with alpha-thalassemia X-linked mental retardation syndrome can have abnormal gut function and resulting problems with digestion. Feeding problems are fairly common as well, such as swallowing difficulties, regurgitation of food, and/or vomiting. Constipation becomes an issue in some patients. These difficulties often resolve with age. Seizures occur in approximately one-third of cases. Cleft palate, deafness, cardiac defects, and renal/urinary abnormalities are less common, but have been reported.

About 85% of the time, blood tests in affected individuals show a mild form of anemia, also known as alpha thalassemia. This results from a defect in the production of an important component of hemoglobin. However, this mild anemia does not appear to have any adverse consequences in patients with the disorder.

Diagnosis

Alpha-thalassemia X-linked mental retardation syndrome can be suspected clinically in an individual who has mental retardation, hypotonia, characteristic physical features (i.e., craniofacial, skeletal, genital), and a family history consistent with X-linked recessive inheritance. Usually, the most obvious signs of the disorder are developmental delay and severely impaired cognitive function.

The most ideal way to diagnose this condition is to identify a gene mutation in the affected individual via molecular **genetic testing** of the ATRX gene. Then, the mother can be tested for this mutation to determine her carrier status. This type of analysis will detect mutations in approximately 90% of individuals with alpha-thalassemia X-linked mental retardation syndrome. This testing is done by gene sequence analysis either of the entire ATRX gene or of a portion of the gene that is known to contain 40–50% of ATRX mutations.

If molecular genetic testing is not available or is uninformative in a family, linkage analysis may be helpful. In this genetic test, **DNA** markers that are located very close to the ATRX gene are used to track the damaged copy through a family. This technique is most effective in large families with multiple affected males.

In some cases, blood abnormalities can be detected by various laboratory tests. For example, molecules called hemoglobin H (HbH) inclusions may be seen in the red blood cells of affected individuals. This is a feature of the alpha thalassemia that is associated with this condition. HbH inclusions are less helpful in identifying female carriers and are only seen in approximately 25% of women who carry an ATRX mutation. Additionally, microcytic, hypochromic anemia can be detected by a blood test and may be a sign of alpha thalassemia and, therefore, alpha-thalassemia X-linked mental retardation syndrome. However, the absence of either of these blood abnormalities does not rule out this condition—many affected individuals will not demonstrate these abnormalities.

Another option for detecting female carriers of the ATRX gene is X-chromosome inactivation studies. In a typical female, each cell has two X chromosomes (X1 and X2) and one of them will be inactivated. This inactivation is a random process meaning that, if one were to look at a significant number of cells, X1 would be inactivated in approximately the same number of cells as X2. This process is skewed in females who are carriers of the ATRX gene mutation because the X chromosome that carries the ATRX mutation will be preferentially inactivated. A laboratory test can detect this skewed X inactivation. However, this characteristic is not always present in carriers of ATRX mutations and, also, can be present for other reasons. Thus, it is not diagnostic and must be interpreted in the context of the clinical findings and family history. X-chromosome inactivation studies can be especially useful if molecular testing is not available or is uninformative in a family.

Prenatal testing is available for pregnancies that are at risk for alpha-thalassemia X-linked mental retardation syndrome. For pregnancies in which the mother is a definite carrier of the ATRX mutation, fetal sex is determined via cells obtained from **amniocentesis** or chorionic villus sampling (CVS). If the fetus is male, DNA from the fetal cells can be analyzed for the ATRX mutation that has been found in the family. For pregnancies in which the mother has tested negative for the ATRX mutation but has previously birthed an affected child, prenatal diagnosis should still be offered to all male fetuses. This is due to the possibility of germline mosaicism.

Treatment and management

Very few of the abnormalities that result from alpha-thalassemia X-linked mental retardation syndrome are life-threatening. Thus, treatment and management are often unnecessary. However, some interventions can be helpful depending on the clinical signs and symptoms that are present. For example, feeding problems can be managed with tube feeding in the early months and, in

KEY TERMS

Amniocentesis—A prenatal test in which a hollow needle is inserted through the abdominal wall and into the uterus of a pregnant female in order to obtain amniotic fluid, which contains cells from the fetus. These cells can be examined to determine the sex of the fetus or to look for genetic diseases.

Anemia—A condition in which the blood is deficient in red blood cells and, as a result, tissues and organs do not get a sufficient amount of oxygen.

Chorionic villus sampling (CVS)—Biopsy of the placenta through the abdominal wall or by way of the vagina and uterine cervix to obtain fetal cells for the prenatal diagnosis of a genetic disorder.

Hemoglobin—A component of red blood cells that functions to transport oxygen from the lungs to the tissues of the body.

Microcytic, hypochromic anemia—An anemia marked by deficient hemoglobin and small red blood cells.

rare cases, with a permanent feeding tube passed through the abdominal wall into the stomach (feeding gastrostomy). An operation known as fundoplication may be necessary to correct problems with regurgitation. Additionally, other surgeries may be required for certain clinical manifestations, such as cleft palate, cardiac defects, and abnormal genitalia. Again, the anemia that often accompanies this condition is mild and does not require any treatment.

Prognosis

Alpha-thalassemia X-linked mental retardation syndrome was discovered and characterized fairly recently. Thus, detailed information about prognosis has not been collected. There are reports of adults surviving into their 30s. However, some children will die at an early age. One of the main causes of early death in this condition is pneumonia, which can result from food entering the lungs due to vomiting and regurgitation problems.

Resources

PERIODICALS
Gibbons, R. J., and D. R. Higgs. "Molecular-clinical Spectrum of the ATR-X Syndrome." *American Journal of Medical Genetics* 97 (2000): 204–212.

WEB SITES

"ATRX Syndrome." The Gibbons Laboratory. (April 3, 2005.) <http://www.imm.ox.ac.uk/mhu/Home_Pages/Gibbons/index.html>.

Stevenson, Roger E. "Alpha-thalassemia X-linked mental retardation syndrome." Gene Reviews. (April 3, 2005.) <http://www.genetests.org/servlet/access?db=geneclinics&site=gt&id=8888891&key=FnPPkP-SrKElS&gry=&fcn=y&fw=CjU5&filename=/profiles/xlmr/index.html>.

Mary E. Freivogel, MS, CGC

Alzheimer disease

Definition

Alzheimer disease is a form of **dementia** caused by the destruction of brain cells. Dementia is the loss, usually progressive, of cognitive and intellectual functions. Alzheimer type dementia can be characterized by initial short-term memory loss, which eventually becomes more severe and finally incapacitating.

Diagnosis before death is based upon clinical findings of unexplained slowly progressive dementia and neuroimaging studies that show gross cerebral cortex atrophy (changes in the structure of the brain, usually in the form of shrinkage). Neuroimaging refers to the use of positron emission tomography (PET), magnetic resonance imaging (MRI), or computed topography (CT) scans. These are special types of pictures that allow the brain or other internal body structures to be visualized. Professor Alois Alzheimer of Germany first described the condition is 1907.

Description

Sporadic Alzheimer's accounts for over 75% of cases of Alzheimer disease. Sporadic Alzheimer patients do not have a family history of Alzheimer disease and may develop the disease at any time during their adult life. A family history is positive for Alzheimer's if three or more generations of a family exhibit signs of the disease. Patients are diagnosed with sporadic Alzheimer disease after all other causes of dementia are excluded.

There are five common causes of dementia. If a patient has a history of strokes (blood clot in the brain) and stepwise destruction of mental capacities, multi-infarct vascular (arteries) dementia must be considered. Diffuse white matter disease is another form of vascular dementia that must be excluded as a possible cause of dementia. Diagnosis of diffuse white matter disease is made by MRI, which shows generalized death of large parts of the brain.

Parkinson disease is a brain nerve disease, which causes abnormalities in movement and functioning. Parkinson's can be excluded by clinical presentation because most patients experience tremors and rigidity of arms and legs.

Alcoholism can also lead to dementia because patients who ingest increased quantities of alcohol over many years may have digestive problems that lead to nutritional deficiencies. These patients may experience malnutrition and possible lack of absorption of vitamins such as thiamine (B1), cobalamin (B12) and niacin (nicotinic acid). These vitamins are essential for proper function of the body and brain. Continued use of certain drugs or medications such as tranquilizers, sedatives, and pain relievers can also cause dementia. It is important to note that alcoholism and over use of medications are potentially reversible causes of dementia.

The less common causes of dementia that must be excluded as possible contributors are endocrine abnormalities (abnormalities in the hormones of the body). Thyroid dysfunction is the leading abnormality. The thyroid gland produces hormones that are essential for the basic functions of the body such as growth and metabolism. Abnormalities of the thyroid can be diagnosed by a blood test. Chronic infections, trauma or injury to the brain, tumors of the brain, psychiatric abnormalities such as **depression**, and degenerative disorders should also be ruled out as causes of dementia. (A degenerative disorder is a condition that causes a decrease in mental or physical processes).

Familial Alzheimer disease accounts for approximately twenty-five percent of cases of Alzheimer disease. Familial Alzheimer's is diagnosed if other causes of dementia are ruled out and if there is a family history of the disease. Familial Alzheimer's is further subdivided into early and late onset. Early onset indicates that the patients exhibit unexplained dementia before the age of 65. Late onset refers to the development of unexplained dementia after the age of 65. Late onset is two to four times more prevalent than early onset.

Alzheimer disease associated with **Down syndrome** accounts for the remaining less than one percent of Alzheimer cases. Studies have shown that Down syndrome patients over the age of forty all develop the brain cell changes that are characteristic of Alzheimer disease. Because the function of the brain is already impaired in a

Down syndrome patient it is difficult to determine if changes in outward actions are related to Down syndrome or to the progression of Alzheimer disease.

Genetic profile

The **gene** that causes sporadic Alzheimer disease has not been identified. Currently sporadic Alzheimer's is believed to be the result of a combination of multiple environmental influences and genetic mutations. This view is supported by research involving identical twins. Both twins develop Alzheimer disease only one third of the time. This supports the view that something besides genetic predisposition has an affect on whether sporadic Alzheimer disease develops. Females who have the Apolipoprotein E (ApoE) gene on **chromosome** 19 have been shown in certain cases to have an increased risk for developing sporadic Alzheimer disease. A mutation in the ApoE gene has been shown to cause an increase in the amount of A-beta Amyloid. A-beta Amyloid is a protein that is deposited in increased amounts in the brain of patients with Alzheimer's. Deposits of this protein in the brain are thought to interfere with another protein, which maintains nerve cell shape. A genetic test is available that detects the defect in ApoE.

Familial early onset Alzheimer's has been associated with several genetic mutations. Identification of several genetic mutations has led to the further subdivision of early onset disease into three categories. AD3 refers to a genetic defect in the presenilin 1 (PSEN1) gene located on chromosome 14. AD1 is a genetic defect in the Amyloid precursor protein (APP) gene located on chromosome 21. AD4 is a genetic defect in the presenilin 2 (PSEN2) gene located on chromosome 1. The three genetic mutations account for approximately 50% of early onset familial Alzheimer's. All three of these genetic mutations result in an increased amount of A-beta Amyloid. AD3 has a genetic test currently available that has been shown to detect the AD3 mutation with 20-27% accuracy. Genetic tests for AD1 and AD4 are in the research stage of development. Familial early onset Alzheimer's is most commonly transmitted by autosomal dominant **inheritance**. Autosomal dominant means that either affected parent has a 50% chance of transmitting the disease to their male or female children.

The gene for familial late onset Alzheimer disease (AD2) has not been identified. An association has also been found with mutations in ApoE.

The normal person has two copies (one from each parent) of each of the 22 chromosomes. Down syndrome patients have three copies of chromosome number 21. Brain changes that are similar to those that occur in sporadic and familial Alzheimer's patients are attributed to the gene defect in chromosome 21. Down syndrome patients also experience additional brain related changes that are similar to Alzheimer's patients, but the gene defect for these changes has not been determined.

Demographics

Alzheimer disease is the most common form of dementia in North America and Europe. Alzheimer disease occurs most often in people over age 60 and affects 5% of individuals over the age of 70. It is estimated that four million people in the United States are afflicted with Alzheimer disease and this number is expected to increase as the estimated life expectancy of Americans increases. Females may be at greater risk than males.

Signs and symptoms

Patients with Alzheimer disease progress at different rates. Progression of memory loss will vary from person to person. Impaired memory will eventually begin to interfere with daily activities. Patients may not be aware that they are experiencing failure in memory, a condition referred to as agnosognosia. Other patients are keenly aware of their memory loss and may become anxious and frustrated. Early phase manifestations of Alzheimer's often include anxiety and frustration. Patients may also begin to experience disorientation to place and become confused by changes of environment.

During the middle phase of the disease an individual may not be able to be left unattended. The patient can become easily confused and lost. Difficulty in many aspects of language appears at this time. Patients experience problems with comprehension and remembering the names of things in their environment. Their speech may not flow smoothly when they talk and they may experience difficulties repeating previously explained information. Simple mathematical calculations or performing tasks such as dressing or preparing a meal at the correct time may also become impaired. Because there is individual variation in the progression of the disease, some patients may still be able to continue routine behavior and engage in a generalized type of conversation during this phase of the disease. A small number of patients may experience difficulties seeing. Changes in vision are frequently denied and only confirmed by autopsy results after death that indicate destruction in the areas of the brain, which process visual images.

If a patient remains able to get out of bed in the late phase of Alzheimer disease they may wander aimlessly. Wandering must be monitored at night because

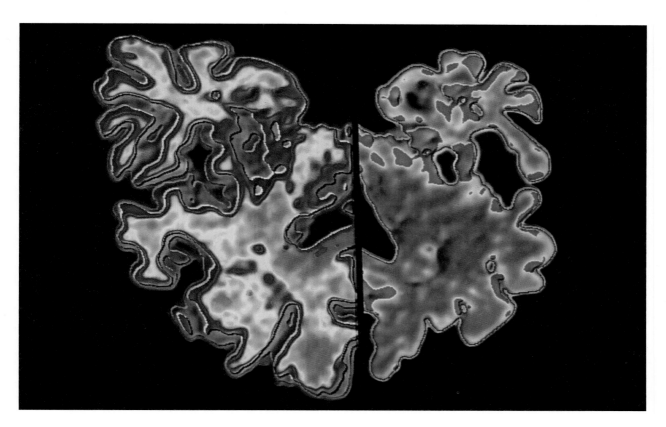

Computer graphic comparing the brain affected by Alzheimer disease (right) to that of a normal brain (left). Due to degeneration and death of nerve cells, the affected brain is considerably smaller. *(Photo Researchers, Inc.)*

sleeping patterns may become altered. Walking may become difficult in the late phase of Alzheimer's because some patients experience stiffening of muscles that causes their movement to be awkward and slow. Patients will require constant supervision. Rationalizing with patients becomes very difficult at this time because they experience severe mental changes. They are often unable to reason or demonstrate appropriate judgment. Patients may become uninhibited and confrontational. They may experience delusions, which are false beliefs despite ample evidence to the contrary. This can be manifested in ways such as not recognizing a family member or accusing a spouse of infidelity. A patient with Alzheimer's may also perceive objects in their environment that do not actually exist.

In the final stage of Alzheimer's, patients may need assistance with the simplest activities of daily living such as feeding ones self and changing clothes. A majority of patients will be bedridden and their muscles will be stiff to the point where they cannot bend. Many are unable to talk and have lost total control of their bowel and urinary functions. Abnormal jerking move-

ments of the body may occur for no reason. Touching a patient or certain noises may precipitate these abnormal body movements. When reflexes such as the knee (tapping of the leg below the knee) are tested, there are frequently exaggerated responses. Some patients additionally experience whole body contractions, known as a generalized seizure.

Diagnosis

Diagnosis is established based upon exclusion of other possible causes for dementia. Obtaining an accurate medical history is essential in this process. An accurate family history including a history of family members who have had Alzheimer disease and age of onset must be obtained.

The earliest changes in the structure of the brain are seen using PET scans. MRI and CT scans are most useful in the early phase of the disease to exclude other brain abnormalities that may be causing dementia. As the disease progresses, use of MRI and CT scans will show changes in the structure of the brain tissue that indicate brain cell death. Studies indicate that MRI is statistically

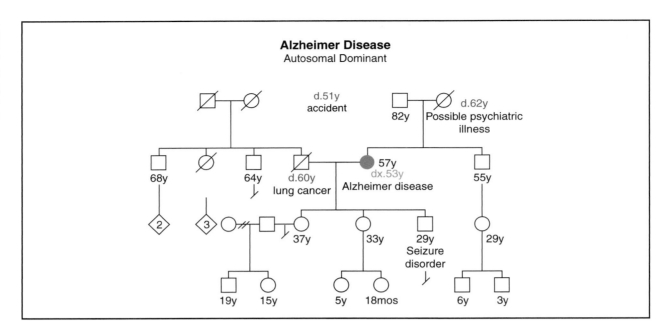

Alzheimer Disease
Autosomal Dominant

(Gale Group.)

accurate in predicting who may or may not develop Alzheimer disease in the future.

Diagnosis is not confirmed unless an autopsy is preformed after death. The brain of a patient with Alzheimer's will have A-beta amyloid neuritic plaques (senile plaques) and intraneuronal neurofibrillary tangles. These are changes in specific proteins and nerve structures of the brain that occur normally as an individual ages but are greatly increased in patients with Alzheimer disease. These brain changes are similar in sporadic, familial early onset, familial late onset, and patients with Down syndrome related Alzheimer disease. It is also noted that the longer the disease process for an individual lasts, the smaller their brain is upon death.

Treatment and management

Because the course of Alzheimer disease has great individual variation, treatment is aimed at being supportive of both patient and caretakers. Neurological and behavioral problems are treated as needed.

Alzheimer disease is associated with decreased levels of specific chemicals called acetylcholine and norepinephrine. Acetylcholine and norepinephrine are chemicals important in many processes in the body including digestion, blood vessel dilation and constriction (usually refers to blood vessel diameter becoming smaller), and regulation of heart beat. Acetylcholinesterase is an enzyme in the body that breaks down acetylcholine. One class of drugs is currently available in the United States that inhibits this process. Use of these medications has been shown to increase levels of acetylcholine in the brain, resulting in improved brain function in patients who are in the early phase of the disease.

Many early phase patients with Alzheimer's experience depression. Antidepressants such as selective serotonin reuptake inhibitors are the most commonly used class of drugs for treatment of depression. This class of drugs helps to stabilize certain chemicals in the brain. Seizures, anxiety, agitation, defiant behavior, inability to sleep, and hallucinations are treated on an as needed basis. Patient and caregiver should establish a relationship with a primary care provider. Nutritional intake needs monitoring since patients will eventually lose capabilities required for maintaining their diet and also because advancing age itself results in decreased appetite. The home environment must be made as safe as possible and the patient should be monitored closely for the point at which they are no longer able to drive safely. Because disorientation is frequently experienced, it is important to maintain the patient within a stable and familiar environment.

Caregivers need to remain calm and offer reassurance. Community organizations that offer help should be sought. Support groups for caretakers offer places to express feeling and help in anticipating future problems.

The patient must be monitored closely during the times when they are unable to determine their own care. Financial assets and plans for the ongoing management of the disease should be addressed before this advanced stage is reached. Nursing home placement is an option for patients with Alzheimer disease without caretakers or for patients who become unmanageable in the home environment.

Individuals who have a history of familial Alzheimer disease in their family should consider **genetic counseling**. Genetic counseling will help to clarify possible risk factors and determine the appropriate usefulness of available genetic tests. The test for the ApoE genetic defect is not considered to be useful for prediction of sporadic Alzheimer disease in patients who do not currently have signs or symptoms of the disease.

Research treatment

Patients with Alzheimer disease have abnormal amounts of A-beta Amyloid deposited in their brain as plaques. Research involving mice in 1999 demonstrated that immunizing the animals with certain protein components of amyloid prevented the development of Alzheimer's related changes, such as plaque formation, in the brains of the mice. Immunization was also shown to slow down the brain changes in older mice. Future benefits for human use are still under investigation.

Several other drugs and combinations of drugs are currently in the beginning and end stage of research studies. Drugs affecting several different chemicals in the brain are being investigated in addition to the use of non-steroidal anti-inflammatory drugs (drugs that reduce inflammation in the body), estrogen, and vitamin E in the prevention and alleviation of Alzheimer disease.

In April of 2001 the first use of human **gene therapy** for the treatment of Alzheimer disease was undertaken. Scientists isolated the gene of a protein found in healthy brains called nerve growth factor. This gene was transplanted into the brain of a woman with early stage Alzheimer disease. Because nerve growth factor has been shown to increase the amounts of acetylcholine in the brain, hope is that this will delay the Alzheimer's process. Further studies in this area are ongoing.

Prognosis

On average, the duration of the disease process associated with Alzheimer disease lasts eight to ten years. Death is most frequently related to malnutrition, secondary infection (infection that is not the initial medical problem) or heart disease. Malnutrition is a state when

not enough calories are taken in to support the normal functions of the human body. An individual is additionally more susceptible to infections when they are malnourished. Having Alzheimer disease does not mean a patient is more likely to have heart disease. The correlation that occurs between heart disease and Alzheimer disease is the fact that both increase in incidence as patients age.

> ## KEY TERMS
>
> **Dementia**—A condition of deteriorated mental ability characterized by a marked decline of intellect and often by emotional apathy.
>
> **Plaques**—Abnormally deposited proteins that interfere with normal cell growth and functioning and usually progresses to cell death.

Resources

BOOKS

Bird, T. D. "Alzheimer's Disease and other Primary Dementias." In *Harrison's Principles of Internal Medicine,* 14th ed., edited by Anthony S. Fauci et. al. McGraw-Hill, 1998, pp. 3248-56.

Wiedemann, H. R., J. Kunze, and F. R. Grosse. "Down Syndrome." In *Clinical Syndromes,* 3rd ed., edited by Gina Almond. Mosby-Wolfe, 1997, pp. 306-7.

PERIODICALS

de la Monte, S. M. "Molecular abnormalities of the brain in Down syndrome: Relevance to Alzheimers neurodegeneration." *Journal of Neural Transmission* Supplementation. 57 (1999): 1-19.

Emilien, G., K. Beyreuther, C. L. Masters, and J. M. Maloteaux. "Prospects for pharmacological intervention in Alzheimer Disease." *Archives of Neurology* 57, no. 4 (April 2000): 454-9.

Killiany, R. J., et al. "Use of structural magnetic resonance imaging to predict who will get Alzheimers Disease." *Annals of Neurology* 47, no. 4 (April 2000): 430-9.

Nochlin, D., G. van Belle, T. D. Bird, and S. M. Sumi. "Comparison of the Severity of Neuropathologic Changes in familial and Sporadic Alzheimer's Disease." *Alzheimer's Disease and Associated Disorders* 7, no. 4 (1993): 212-22.

Schenk, D., and P. Seubert. "Immunization with amyloid-B attenuates Alzhemer-disease-like pathology in the PDAPP mouse." *Nature* 400 (July 1999): 173-77.

ORGANIZATIONS

Alzheimer's Association. 919 North Michigan Ave., Suite 1000, Chicago, IL 60611-1676. (800) 272-3900.

Council of Regional Networks for Genetic Services. Genetic Services Program, Wadsworth Center Labs & Research, PO Box 509, Room E299, Empire State Plaza, Albany, NY 12201-0509. (518) 474-7148. <http://www.cc.emory.edu/PEDIATRICS/corn/corn.htm>.

Laith Farid Gulli, MD
Nicole Mallory, MS

Amelia

Definition

Amelia is an extremely rare birth defect marked by the absence of one or more limbs. The term may be modified to indicate the number of legs or arms missing at birth, such as tetra-amelia for the absence of all four limbs. A related term is meromelia, which is the partial absence of a limb or limbs. Several older terms are no longer in use in international nomenclature because of their imprecision: phocomelia, peromelia, dysmelia, ectromelia, and hemimelia.

Description

The complete absence of an arm or leg in amelia occurs when the limb formation process is either prevented or interrupted very early in the developing embryo: between 24 and 36 days following fertilization. Nearly 25% of all congenital limb defects are amelia. A single limb is involved about 60% of the time and symmetrical amelia is uncommon. The likelihood for upper versus lower limb absence varies with the syndrome.

Amelia may be present as an isolated defect, but more than 50% of the time it is associated with major malformations in other organ systems. The malformations most frequently seen with amelia include cleft lip and/or palate, body wall defects, malformed head, and defects of the neural tube, kidneys and diaphragm. Facial clefts may be accompanied by other facial anomalies such as abnormally small jaw, and missing ears or nose. The body wall defects allow internal organs to protrude through the abdomen. Head malformations may be minor to severe with a near absence of the brain. The diaphragm may be herniated or absent and one or both kidneys may be small or absent.

Other abnormalities associated with amelia include severe defects of the lungs, vertebrae, heart, internal and external genital system, and anus. There is usually a severe growth deficiency, both before and after birth,

and mental retardation may be present in survivors. Benign facial tumors made up of clusters of blood vessels (hemangiomas) may be present.

Amelia was traditionally thought to be a sporadic anomaly with little risk of recurrence, or evidence of genetic origins. However, an estimated 20% of amelia cases can now be traced to probable genetic causes. These genetic conditions may be due to recessive or dominant mutations, or involve chromosomal aberrations where entire sections of chromosomes are deleted, duplicated or exchanged. The best defined of these genetic diseases is known as **Roberts SC phocomelia** or, pseudothalidomide syndrome, caused by an autosomal recessive mutation of unknown location. There is a great variability of expression of the disease, even within families. Classic signs of Roberts SC phocomelia include symmetrical defects of all four limbs including amelia, severe growth deficiency, head and face (craniofacial) abnormalities such as small head and cleft lip or palate, also sparse, silvery blond hair, and facial hemangiomas.

A very small group of genetically based amelia cases is referred to as "autosomal recessive tetra-amelia" which consists of an absence of all four limbs, with small or absent lungs, cleft lip or palate, malformed head and other anomalies. A similar "X-linked tetra-amelia" is highly lethal to the fetus and involves the same set of abnormalities. The abnormal **gene** for X-linked tetra-amelia is assumed to be located on the X **chromosome**. Very few cases have been documented for either of these inherited conditions but the defective gene seems to be more prevalent in Arab populations of the Middle East or in small isolated cultures where consanguineous relationships (intermarriage within extended families) is more common. There is disagreement as to whether these conditions represent new syndromes or are severe cases of Roberts SC phocomelia.

Amelia is associated with various other genetic syndromes. It is seen in the autosomal recessive Baller-Gerold syndrome and **Holt-Oram syndrome**, an autosomal dominant condition that sometimes involves amelia. It has been proposed that many of the new, isolated cases of amelia are due to autosomal dominant mutations where only one copy of an abnormal gene on a non-sex chromosome is powerful enough to cause amelia to be displayed. Absent limbs have also been seen in chromosomal aberrations such as **Trisomy 8** (three copies of chromosome 8) and a deletion of region 7q22 found on the long arm of chromosome 7.

Sporadic amelia may be the end result of various types of disturbances of limb development in the embryo. These disturbances can be vascular, mechanical, due to teratogens (substances that can cause birth defects) or accompany other disease processes such as **diabetes**. An example of vascular disturbance would be hemorrhage in the embryo causing lack of blood and oxygen flow to surrounding tissue. The type and number of resulting defects would depend on the location of the hemorrhage and the point of embryo development when the bleed took place. Defects in limbs and the body wall tend to result from this type of disturbance.

Mechanical disruption can be seen following rupture of the amnion (the thin but tough membrane surrounding the embryo) due to infection, direct trauma such as attempted abortion or removal of IUD, or familial predisposition to rupture. Strands of the collapsed amnion and adhesions (fibrous bands which abnormally connect tissue surfaces) may entangle and amputate developing limbs and cause a variety of other defects including facial clefts.

Various teratogens are well-established causes of amelia. A well-documented historic instance was due to thalidomide use by pregnant women from 1958 to 1963. Thalidomide was used as a sedative and anti-nausea drug but was found to cause a wide array of limb deficiencies, including amelia. It is estimated to have caused 5,800 cases of malformed fetuses, mostly in Europe, but also in North America and wherever it was available worldwide. The mechanism by which thalidomide causes birth defects is still not known but may involve disruption of nerve processes. Although thalidomide is again in use today to treat certain cancers, infections and arthritis, it should not be used by women of childbearing age.

Alcohol (ethanol) consumption by pregnant women, especially in the first trimester, has been documented by several surveys to cause limb deformities. The abnormalities range from frequent, minor defects such as shortened fingers to the much rarer amelia. It is hypothesized that alcohol interrupts the blood supply to the developing limb resulting in malformation or nongrowth. Additional teratogens known to cause amelia include methotrexate, other chemotherapeutic agents and potent vasoconstrictive drugs such as epinephrine and ergotamine.

Maternal diabetes mellitus (non-gestational) has long been associated with congenital anomalies, rarely including amelia. There is a two to threefold risk for congenital abnormalities in children of diabetic mothers and limb defects of various types occur in about one percent of infants of these mothers. It is thought that either abnormal maternal carbohydrate metabolism, or vascular disease resulting in decreased oxygen flow to the fetus, might play a role in causing malformations.

Genetic profile

Amelia is generally considered to be sporadic with scattered cases occurring infrequently. These rare events are presumably influenced by environmental factors, such as teratogenic drugs, maternal factors such as diabetes mellitus, and vascular accidents in the uterus. The role of genetics in causing this condition is still undetermined but two large epidemiological studies estimate that nearly 20% of amelia cases are of genetic origin. Mutations in more than one gene with different modes of transmission can lead to this severe limb deficiency.

Recurrence of amelia within families is the exception. When this occurs, it is most often associated with other malformations in autosomally recessive syndromes such as Roberts SC phocomelia, autosomal recessive amelia and X-linked amelia. Roberts SC phocomelia has a clearly identifiable genetic abnormality that can be seen during chromosome analysis. The abnormality is called either Premature Centromeric Separation (PCS) or Heterochromatin Repulsion (HR). The darkly staining heterochromatin of the chromosome can be seen puffing and splitting. The PCS test is positive in almost 80% of patients with Roberts SC phocomelia.

Demographics

The rarity of amelia makes the study of it on a population level speculative. A few large-scale studies pooling decades of information from malformation registries in several countries do provide preliminary data. Amelia has an incidence of 11-15 cases per million live births and 790 cases per million stillbirths. The condition is probably under reported due to lack of documentation of some miscarriages, stillbirths, and neonatal deaths.

There is no significant difference between number of males and females affected except in the select, extremely rare cases of X-linked amelia, which are all male. Only men would be affected since the abnormal gene is inherited on the X chromosome and men only receive one copy of an X chromosome. Since females inherit two copies of the X chromosome, the normal copy of the gene on the second X chromosome can usually mask the more severe complications that would result if only the abnormal gene was expressed.

The disorder occurs worldwide and there are no geographic clusters except for two. Amelia resulting from the use of thalidomide occurred primarily in Europe and other areas where the drug was available. Autosomal recessive and X-linked amelia has mostly occurred in Arabic and Turkish families. This suggests ethnic differences for an abnormal recessive gene but is based on less than 20 cases. Such a recessive gene is likely to be homozygous (meaning two copies of the abnormal gene need to be inherited for amelia to result), and thus expressed in malformation more often in any culture that tends to be isolated and has more intermarriage from a limited **gene pool**.

Signs and symptoms

Prior to clinical observation of absent limbs, certain signs in the pregnant mother may indicate a greater likelihood of amelia. Abnormal vaginal bleeding, diabetes mellitus, and toxemia (disturbed metabolism during pregnancy characterized by high blood pressure, swelling and protein in the urine) are all associated with amelia in the fetus. Alpha fetoprotein is a protein normally produced by the liver of the fetus which then circulates in the mother's blood. An increased alpha fetoprotein in the maternal blood may indicate **neural tube defects** that can accompany limb defects. Besides seeing missing limbs by ultrasound, signs in the fetus accompanying amelia include breech and other non-cephalic presentations at birth (where the baby is not in the normal head-first, face-down delivery position), an increased frequency of only a single artery in the umbilical cord, low placental weight and extremely low birth weight, not accounted for by the lack of limbs. The average birth weight for an infant with amelia is less than the third percentile for its age.

Diagnosis

Detection of an absent limb is generally simple. Clinical observation of the missing limb is either made at birth or prenatally by ultrasonography. However, more than 50% of amelia cases are accompanied by malformations of other organ systems, and in these cases, determination of a specific syndrome can be difficult. Defects overlap greatly between conditions. A family history including a pedigree chart to map other affected family members can be very helpful in detecting genetic causes. A prenatal history should include determination of maternal exposure to alcohol, thalidomide and other teratogenic drugs. Maternal diabetes mellitus should be considered a risk factor for congenital abnormalities.

Roberts SC phocomelia must be differentiated from other autosomal recessive or X-linked amelias. **Genetic testing** for PCS should be performed on cells from amniotic fluid. Darkly staining heterochromatin of the chromosome puffs out abnormally and splits in a positive test. The PCS test will be positive in nearly 80% of Roberts SC phocomelia cases but negative in the other syndromes. A positive PCS test along with some of the signs listed above, is diagnostic for Roberts SC phocomelia. Further chromosome studies should be done to detect gross chromosomal aberrations such as deletions or Trisomy 8.

Treatment and management

Preventive measures to avoid serious limb defects such as amelia include avoidance of thalidomide and other teratogens in women of childbearing years, avoidance of alcohol during pregnancy and comprehensive management of diabetes mellitus throughout pregnancy. A **prenatal ultrasound** that detects an absence of limbs can be followed by chromosome analysis and **genetic counseling** to make informed decisions regarding termination.

Children with amelia can be fitted with a prosthesis to substitute for the missing limb. Surgery is often performed to repair craniofacial defects. Minimal to full time care may be needed depending on the degree of mental retardation.

Prognosis

When amelia occurs as an isolated abnormality, prognosis is good. However, when amelia is combined with multiple other defects, the prognosis is grim. Abnormalities accompanying amelia may include cleft lip and/or palate, body wall defects, malformed head, and abnormalities of the neural tube, kidneys and diaphragm. Many infants die prior to birth. Sixty percent of newborns die within the first year, with half not surviving the first day. Mild cases of Roberts SC phocomelia are likely to survive past the first few years and reach adulthood. Patients with more severe forms of amelia, such as severe growth deficiency and craniofacial defects, do not live past the first few months.

Resources

BOOKS

Moore, Keith L., and T. V. N. Persaud. "Anomalies of Limbs." In *The Developing Human, Clinically Oriented Embryology,* 6th ed. Philadelphia: W.B. Saunders Company, 1998.

Stevenson, Roger E., and Leslie C. Meyer. "The Limbs" In *Human Malformations and Related Anomalies* Vol. II. edited by Roger E. Stevenson, et al. New York: Oxford University Press, 1993

Watts, Hugh G., and Mary Williams Clark. *Who is Amelia? Caring for children with limb difference.* American Academy of Orthopedic Surgeons, 1998.

PERIODICALS

Froster-Iskenius, Ursula G., and Patricia A. Baird. "Amelia: Incidence and Associated Defects in a Large Population." *Teratology.* 41 (1990): 23-31.

Van Den Berg, David J., and Uta Francke. "Roberts Syndrome: A Review of 100 Cases and a New Rating System for

KEY TERMS

Amnion—Thin, tough membrane surrounding the embryo and containing the amniotic fluid.

Autosomal dominant mutation—An abnormal gene on one of the 22 pairs of non-sex chromosomes that will display the defect when only one copy is inherited.

Autosomal recessive mutation—A pattern of genetic inheritance where two abnormal genes are needed to display the trait or disease.

Consanguineous—Sharing a common bloodline or ancestor.

Craniofacial—Relating to or involving both the head and the face.

Hemangioma—Benign tumor made up of clusters of newly formed blood vessels.

Homeotic genes—Developmental control genes active in the embryo.

Homozygous—Having two identical copies of a gene or chromosome.

Teratogen—Any drug, chemical, maternal disease, or exposure that can cause physical or functional defects in an exposed embryo or fetus.

X-linked mutation—An abnormal gene transmitted on the X chromosome.

Severity." *American Journal of Medical Genetics.* 47 (1993): 1104-1123.

ORGANIZATIONS

National Organization for Rare Disorders (NORD). PO Box 8923, New Fairfield, CT 06812-8923. (203) 746-6518 or (800) 999-6673. Fax: (203) 746-6481. <http://www.rarediseases.org>.

Marianne F. O'Connor, MT (ASCP), MPH

▮ Amniocentesis

Definition

Amniocentesis is an optional procedure offered to women during pregnancy in order to obtain more information about a developing fetus. A doctor uses a thin, hollow needle to remove a small sample of amniotic fluid from around the developing baby. An ultrasound exam is usually performed at the same time to help guide the needle. The fluid sample is used to look for specific types of medical problems in the fetus. Tests done on amniotic fluid obtained by amniocentesis cannot evaluate the fetus for every potential kind of problem. The information it does provide, however, is very accurate. The procedure is associated with a slightly increased chance for pregnancy loss. Women who undergo amniocentesis typically do so either to obtain reassurance about fetal well-being or, if the results are abnormal, to plan for the remainder of their prenatal care.

Description

Amniocentesis is the most common invasive prenatal diagnosis technique offered to pregnant women. A sample of amniotic fluid can be used to detect **chromosomal abnormalities** in a fetus, certain other types of congenital disorders, or other medical indicators. Its safety and accuracy are well-established, and it is generally considered the "gold standard" by which other prenatal diagnosis techniques are measured.

The word amniocentesis is derived from the Greek words, *amnion* and *kentesis*, meaning "lamb" and "puncture," respectively. In order to perform the procedure, a doctor inserts a thin needle into the mother's uterus and the amniotic sac. A continuous ultrasound evaluation is typically used so that the doctor can avoid touching both the baby and the umbilical cord with the needle. The amniotic sac is made up of two membranes: the inner *amnion* and the outer *chorion*. The amnion and chorion both develop from the fertilized egg. They are initially separate but begin to fuse early in pregnancy. This fusion is usually completed by approximately the fourteenth to fifteenth week of pregnancy.

Amniocentesis is usually performed in the second trimester, usually during weeks 16–18 (mid-trimester). The amniotic sac holds the fetus suspended within the amniotic fluid, an almost colorless fluid that protects the fetus from harm, helps maintain a consistent temperature, and prevents the fetus, or parts of it, from becoming attached to the amnion. The amniotic fluid is produced and absorbed by the fetus throughout pregnancy. Fetal cells, primarily derived from the skin, digestive system, and urinary tract, are suspended within the fluid. A smaller number of cells from the amnion and placenta are also present. Finally, the fetus produces a number of different chemical substances that also pass into the amniotic fluid. These substances may be used, in some higher-risk pregnancies, either to assess fetal lung maturity or to determine if the fetus has a viral infection. In the second trimester of pregnancy, one particular protein, called *alpha-fetoprotein*, is commonly used to screen for certain structural birth defects.

It is possible to perform amniocentesis in a twin pregnancy. Amniocentesis in some higher-order pregnancies, such as triplets, has also been reported. In a multiple pregnancy, it is important to ensure that a separate sample of amniotic fluid is obtained from each fetus. To accomplish this, a doctor injects a small amount of harmless blue dye into the amniotic sac of the first baby after a sample has been withdrawn. The dye will temporarily tinge the fluid blue-green. A second needle is inserted into the next amniotic sac with ultrasound guidance. If the fluid withdrawn is pale yellow, a sample from the next fetus has been successfully obtained. In the case of monoamniotic (in one amniotic sac) twins or triplets, the genetic material in each fetus is identical, so only one sample needs to be taken.

Indications for amniocentesis

Amniocentesis has been considered a standard of obstetrical care since the 1970s. It is not, however, offered to all pregnant women. The American College of Obstetricians and Gynecologists (ACOG) recommends that amniocentesis be offered to all expectant mothers age 35 and older. This age cut-off has been selected because advancing maternal age is associated with an increasing risk of having a baby with a numerical **chromosome** abnormality. At age 35, this risk is approximately equivalent to the risk of pregnancy loss associated with amniocentesis.

A person normally has a total of 46 chromosomes in each cell of his or her body, with the exception of sperm or egg cells, which each have only 23. As women get older, there is an increased risk of producing an egg cell with an extra chromosome. This leads to an egg cell with 24 chromosomes rather than the normal 23. Pregnancies with an abnormal number of chromosomes are referred to as aneuploid. Aneuploidy results in a conceptus (product of conception) with either too much or too little genetic material. This, in turn, leads to abnormal development. Common effects of aneuploidy include an increased risk for pregnancy loss or, in live borns, for mental retardation and physical abnormalities.

Down syndrome is the most common form of aneuploidy in live born infants, occurring in approximately 1 in 800 births, regardless of maternal age. In women who are 35 years old, the risk of having a child with Down syndrome is higher, or roughly one in 385 at delivery. It is important to realize that Down syndrome is not the only chromosome abnormality that may occur. Other numerical abnormalities are possible, yielding genetic conditions that may be either more or less severe than Down syndrome. Thus, a woman is often given a risk, based solely on her age, of having a child with *any* type of chromosome abnormality. At age 35, this total

risk is approximately one in 200. By age 40, this risk has increased to one in 65, and, at age 45, this risk is one in 20. These numbers reflect the risk at the time of delivery.

Women younger than 35 years may also have children with chromosomal or other **genetic disorders**. Therefore, other indications for amniocentesis or other forms of prenatal diagnosis include a family history of, or a previous child with a known genetic condition; abnormal prenatal screening results, such as ultrasound or a blood test; or one parent with a previously identified structural chromosome rearrangement. All of the above may make it more likely for a couple to have a child with a genetic condition.

Side effects

Women who have had an amniocentesis often describe it as uncomfortable, involving some mild pressure or pain as the needle is inserted. Fewer women describe it as extremely painful. A local anesthetic may be used to numb the upper layer of the mother's skin prior to testing. This medicine has no effect on the fetus, but may help the mother feel more comfortable during the procedure. An experienced physician can, on average, perform amniocentesis in approximately one to two minutes.

Common complaints after amniocentesis include mild abdominal tenderness at the site of needle insertion or mild cramping. These usually go away within one to two days. More serious complications are significantly less common but include leakage of amniotic fluid, vaginal bleeding, or uterine infection. These complications are estimated to occur in fewer than 1% of pregnancies. In some women, complications after amniocentesis may lead to a miscarriage, or loss of the pregnancy. A woman's background risk of having a miscarriage, without amniocentesis, is approximately 2–3% in her second trimester. When performed by an experienced physician or technician, the risk for an amniocentesis-related pregnancy loss is estimated to be an additional 0.25%–0.50%, or roughly one in every 200–400 pregnancies.

Much attention is often paid to the physical side effects of amniocentesis. However, it is important to also emphasize some of the emotional side effects of amniocentesis. Many of these are applicable to other forms of prenatal diagnosis.

The offer of prenatal testing is associated with increased anxiety. This appears to be true whether a woman knew prenatal testing would be offered to her during the pregnancy or if it comes about unexpectedly, as is usually the case following abnormal screening results. Women to whom genetic amniocentesis is presented must consider the perceived benefits of testing, such as the reassurance that comes when results are normal, and compare them to the possible risks. Potential risks include not only complications after testing but also learning that the child may have a serious disability or chronic medical condition. The nature of the child's possible diagnosis is also important. For example, could it lead to an early death, be more subtle and cause few outward signs of a problem, or be somewhere in between? There are few treatments available to correct the hundreds of genetic disorders so far described. Couples may consider early termination of the pregnancy if a serious abnormality were detected. The definition of "serious" is often a matter of personal opinion. A couple's value system and family history, including that of other pregnancies and their outcomes, all influence their decision regarding amniocentesis. Ideally, a woman and her partner will have discussed at least some of these issues with each other and with either the woman's doctor or a genetic counselor prior to testing. The choice to have amniocentesis depends on many factors and should remain a personal decision.

Results

Genetic testing is available on amniotic fluid obtained by amniocentesis. The most common test result is a complete analysis of the fetal chromosomes. After a sample of amniotic fluid is obtained, the genetic laboratory isolates the cells, referred to as amniocytes, out of the fluid. The cells are placed into two or more containers filled with liquid nutrients, establishing different cultures in which the cells will continue to grow. The cells are cultured anywhere between one to two weeks before the actual analysis begins. This is done in order to synchronize the growth of the cells within a culture. Also, chromosomes are only microscopically visible at a specific point during cell division.

Once there appears to be an adequate number of cells to study, the cultures are harvested. Harvesting prevents additional cell growth and stops the cells at whatever point they were in their division process. A careful study of the total number and structure of the chromosomes within the cells may now be performed. Typically, chromosome results are available within 7–14 days after amniocentesis. Results may be delayed by slow-growing cultures. This rarely reflects an abnormal result but does extend the time until final results are ready.

Many laboratories are beginning to incorporate a special technique called **fluorescence in situ hybridization** (FISH) into their chromosome studies. This adjunct testing provides limited information about certain chromosomes within one to two days after amniocentesis. It does not replace a complete chromosome study using amniocyte cultures. In fact, FISH results are often reported as preliminary, pending confirmation by cul-

tured results. They can, however, be very useful, particularly when there is already a high level of suspicion of a fetal chromosome abnormality.

FISH is performed using a small sample of uncultured amniotic fluid cells. Special molecular tags for particular chromosomes are used. These tags attach themselves to the chromosome. Under specific laboratory conditions, they can be made to "light up" or fluoresce. Their signals can then be counted using a special kind of microscope. FISH is most often used to quickly identify a change in the number of chromosomes from pairs 13, 18, 21, and the two sex chromosomes, X and Y. Abnormalities of these chromosomes account for nearly 95% of all chromosomal abnormalities. Other chromosomal abnormalities will be missed since FISH cannot identify structural rearrangements of the chromosomes or abnormalities involving other pairs. A full chromosome evaluation on cultured cells is a necessary follow-up to interphase FISH results.

A sample of amniotic fluid may be used to measure alpha-fetoprotein (AFP). AFP is a protein made by the fetal liver. It passes out of the fetus and enters both the amniotic fluid and the mother's blood. Screening for open **neural tube defects**, abnormal openings in the fetal head or spinal cord, or ventral wall defects, openings along the belly wall, can be done by measuring AFP during the fifteenth to twentieth weeks of pregnancy. AFP levels normally show a gradual increase during this time. An unusually high level of serum AFP does not necessarily indicate a problem with fetal development, but is cause for some concern. A high AFP level in amniotic fluid will detect up to 98% of all openings on the fetal body that are not covered by skin. Further studies may be suggested if the AFP is high. Most initial AFP results are available within two to three days after amniocentesis.

Finally, amniotic fluid samples obtained by amniocentesis may also be used for more specialized genetic studies, such as biochemical or **DNA** testing. Both often require cell cultures and additional time to complete. These studies are not done on every sample. Rather, they are offered to those couples who, based on their family history or other information, are at increased risk of having a child with a single **gene**, or Mendelian, disorder. Hundreds of such disorders have been described. Examples include **Tay-Sachs disease**, **cystic fibrosis**, and sickle cell anemia. If biochemical or DNA studies are performed, all of the results may not be ready until three to four weeks after testing, although for each patient, the waiting time may be slightly different.

It is important to emphasize that normal results from tests done on amniotic fluid do not necessarily guarantee the birth of a normal infant. Each couple in the general population faces a risk of roughly 3–4% of having a child with any type of congenital birth defect. Many of these will not be detected with tests done on amniotic fluid samples obtained by amniocentesis. Babies with birth defects are often born into families with no history of genetic disorders.

Chorionic villus sampling

Mid-trimester amniocentesis has been available for nearly thirty years. Chorionic villus sampling (CVS) has been available in the United States since the 1980s. CVS is usually performed between ten to twelve weeks of pregnancy. It involves the removal of a small sample of the developing placenta, or chorionic villi. It has been an attractive alternative to amniocentesis, particularly for those women who desire both testing and results earlier in their pregnancies. Some of the benefits of earlier testing include reassurance sooner in pregnancy and fewer physical complications following first trimester pregnancy termination, for those couples who choose this option after testing. CVS is, however, associated with a higher risk of miscarriage than mid-trimester amniocentesis. At experienced centers, this risk is approximately 1% (or, one in 100).

Early amniocentesis

Early amniocentesis is performed before the thirteenth completed week of pregnancy. It has been considered experimental for many years. The results of the largest early amniocentesis trial, published in 1998, have caused physicians worldwide to reconsider the benefit and risks of this procedure.

The Canadian early and mid-trimester amniocentesis trial (CEMAT) is the largest multi-center, randomized clinical trial of early amniocentesis to date. The purpose of the trial was to examine and compare the safety and accuracy of early (EA) versus mid-trimester amniocentesis (MTA). In order to accomplish this, 4,374 pregnant women were identified and enrolled in the study. Ultrasound was performed in the first trimester to confirm the gestational age of all pregnancies. Computer randomization was used to evenly divide the women into either the EA or MTA groups. Ultimately, 1,916 women underwent EA and 1,775 women had MTA. Follow-up was obtained on nearly all pregnancies. Two striking conclusions were reached: EA is associated with an increased incidence of **clubfoot** and an increased risk of procedure-related pregnancy loss.

Clubfoot, also referred to as *talipes equinovarus*, occurs in approximately one in 1,000 live births (0.1%) in the general population. It may involve either one foot (unilateral) or both feet (bilateral). Males are affected slightly more often than females. There are several proposed mechanisms by which clubfoot could occur: due to the interaction of several genes during development, as a direct consequence of environmental factors, such as an abnormal position in the uterus, or as a physical component of a single gene disorder. Any such disorder would be expected to also cause other abnormalities.

Overall, the CEMAT study found an incidence of clubfoot in the EA group of 1.3% (29 infants). None of the affected infants had other abnormalities. This is nearly ten times higher than the risk in the general population. The frequency of clubfoot in the MTA group was the same as in the general population (0.1%). Prior studies of mid-trimester amniocentesis did not reveal an increased frequency of infants with clubfoot or other birth defects.

Clubfoot was more common when testing was performed during the eleventh, rather than the twelfth, week of pregnancy. This suggests that there may be a specific window sometime in the eleventh to twelfth weeks during which the fetus may be particularly vulnerable to developing clubfoot. It is possible that EA causes a temporary, but still significant, loss of amniotic fluid. This loss may go unrecognized. However, it could, in turn, affect the flow of blood to the foot or cause direct pressure on the developing limb, either of which could lead to clubfoot. It is difficult to know which potential mechanism could be correct since the number of affected infants born after EA is relatively small.

Of note, a separate, much smaller, study also demonstrated an increased incidence of clubfoot (1.7%) among the set of women who underwent EA. The study consisted of patients randomized between EA and CVS and examined the risk of miscarriage after EA. Enrollment in the study was stopped once the association between EA and clubfoot was identified. There were no birth defects identified after CVS.

An additional concern recognized from CEMAT was a higher rate of miscarriage after EA. A procedure-related loss was defined as one that occurred either shortly after the testing or before twenty weeks of pregnancy. Fifty-five women (2.5%) experienced a miscarriage after EA. In contrast, miscarriage occurred in seventeen (0.8%) of the MTA patients. An increased rate of loss appeared to more often follow technically challenging procedures. Difficult procedures included those pregnancies in which bleeding occurred prior to amniocentesis or in which uterine fibroids were present. Tenting of the membranes also made early amniocentesis difficult. Tenting occurs when the amnion and chorion are not yet completely fused, as is

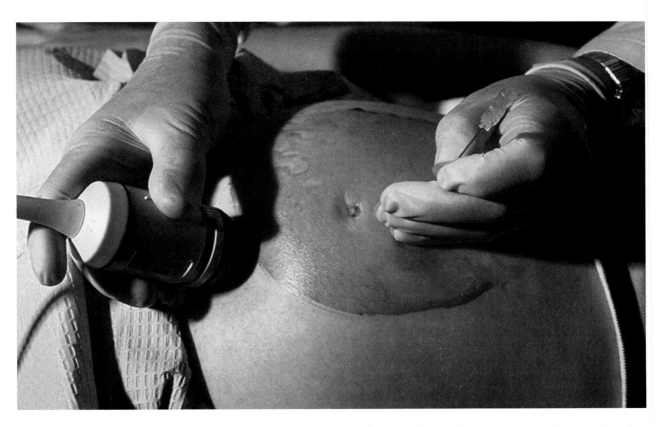

Amniocentesis may be performed to detect several types of genetic disorders. Here, a physician uses an ultrasound monitor (left) to position the needle for insertion into the amnion during the amniocentesis procedure. *(Photo Researchers, Inc.)*

true for the majority of first trimester pregnancies. The separation between the membranes makes insertion of the amniocentesis needle more difficult.

In the absence of a difficult EA procedure, a higher rate of loss was also observed among those pregnancies in which the mother experienced obvious leakage of amniotic fluid or vaginal bleeding after testing. The level of physician experience with EA did not influence the rate of loss.

Finally, EA was also linked to an increased number of laboratory culture failures (no growth of cells and no results) compared to MTA. The total waiting time for results was slightly longer in the EA group. This is not entirely a surprise, since a smaller amount of fluid is obtained when EA is performed. Hence, there are fewer cells, and culturing takes longer.

Demographics

According to the National Center for Health Statistics (NCHS), 112,776 amniocentesis procedures were performed in the United States in 1998, the most recent year for which data is available. The annual birth rate that year was approximately 3.9 million infants. Thus,

approximately 3% of pregnant women in the United States had this procedure performed. It is likely that this is an underestimate, however. The NCHS obtains information from birth certificates registered in each state and the District of Columbia. Although almost all deliveries are registered in the United States, records are still submitted with incomplete information. It is also not possible to know how many amniocentesis procedures were performed for genetic testing, as compared to other indications, as this information is not requested.

Summary

Amniocentesis is a reliable procedure for prenatal diagnosis in the second trimester of pregnancy. It is primarily offered to pregnant women who are at increased risk, based on their age, family history, or other factor, of having a child with a genetic condition. Amniocentesis provides accurate information about fetal chromosomes or the likelihood of certain physical abnormalities. Additional specialized studies may be performed on an as-needed basis. Despite these benefits, amniocentesis is associated with a slightly increased chance of pregnancy loss. Each woman

KEY TERMS

Amnion—Thin, tough membrane surrounding the embryo and containing the amniotic fluid.

Anesthetic—Drug used to temporarily cause loss of sensation in an area of the body. An anesthetic may either be general, associated with a loss of consciousness, or local, affecting one area only without loss of consciousness. Anesthetics are administered either via inhalation or needle injection.

Chorion—The outer membrane of the amniotic sac. Chorionic villi develop from its outer surface early in pregnancy. The villi establish a physical connection with the wall of the uterus and eventually develop into the placenta.

Chromosome—A microscopic thread-like structure found within each cell of the body and consists of a complex of proteins and DNA. Humans have 46 chromosomes arranged into 23 pairs. Changes in either the total number of chromosomes or their shape and size (structure) may lead to physical or mental abnormalities.

Conceptus—The products of conception, or the union of a sperm and egg cell at fertilization.

Cystic fibrosis—A respiratory disease characterized by chronic lung disease, pancreatic insufficiency and an average age of survival of 20 years. Cystic fibrosis is caused by mutations in a gene on chromosome 7 that encode a transmembrane receptor.

Down syndrome—A genetic condition characterized by moderate to severe mental retardation, a characteristic facial appearance, and, in some individuals, abnormalities of some internal organs. Down syndrome is always caused by an extra copy of chromosome 21, or three rather than the normal two. For this reason, Down syndrome is also known as *trisomy 21*.

Fetus—The term used to describe a developing human infant from approximately the third month of pregnancy until delivery. The term embryo is used prior to the third month.

Fibroid—A non-cancerous tumor of connective tissue made of elongated, threadlike structures, or fibers, which usually grow slowly and are contained within an irregular shape. Fibroids are firm in consistency but may become painful if they start to break down or apply pressure to areas within the body. They frequently occur in the uterus and are generally left alone unless growing rapidly or causing other problems. Surgery is needed to remove fibroids.

Sickle cell anemia—A chronic, inherited blood disorder characterized by sickle-shaped red blood cells. It occurs primarily in people of African descent, and produces symptoms including episodic pain in the joints, fever, leg ulcers, and jaundice.

Tay-Sachs disease—An inherited biochemical disease caused by lack of a specific enzyme in the body. In classical Tay-Sachs disease, previously normal children become blind and mentally handicapped, develop seizures, and decline rapidly. Death often occurs between the ages of three to five years. Tay-Sachs disease is common among individuals of eastern European Jewish background but has been reported in other ethnic groups.

Trimester—A three-month period. Human pregnancies are normally divided into three trimesters: first (conception to week 12), second (week 13 to week 24), and third (week 25 until delivery).

Uterus—A muscular, hollow organ of the female reproductive tract. The uterus contains and nourishes the embryo and fetus from the time the fertilized egg is implanted until birth.

should discuss the potential risks and benefits of amniocentesis with a doctor or genetic counselor to make a decision about whether or not she has this testing. Early amniocentesis, or procedures performed before the thirteenth week of pregnancy, has been associated with an increased risk of clubfoot and of procedure-related pregnancy loss.

Resources

BOOKS

"Amniocentesis and chorionic villus sampling (CVS)." In *Medical Tests Sourcebook*. 1st ed. Health Reference Series, edited by Joyce Brennfleck Shannon, Detroit: Omniographics Inc., 1999, pp. 517–522.

Elias, Sherman, Joe Leigh Simpson, and Allan T. Bombard. "Amniocentesis and Fetal Blood Sampling." In *Genetic Disorders and the Fetus: Diagnosis, Prevention, and Treatment*. 4th ed. Edited by Aubrey Milunsky, Baltimore: The Johns Hopkins University Press, 1998, pp. 53–82.

PERIODICALS

The Canadian Early and Mid-trimester Amniocentesis Trial (CEMAT) Group. "Randomized trial to assess the safety and fetal outcome of early and mid-trimester amniocentesis." *Lancet* 351 (January 24, 1998): 242–247.

Farrell, Sandra A., A.M. Summers, Louis Dallaire, Joel Singer, JoAnn M. Johnson, and R. Douglas Wilson, members of CEMAT. "Club foot, an adverse outcome of early amniocentesis: disruption or deformation?" *Journal Medical Genetics* 36, no. 11 (November 1999): 843–846.

ORGANIZATIONS

American College of Obstetricians and Gynecologists. PO Box 96920, 409 12th St. SW, Washington, DC 20090-6920. <http://www.acog.org>.

National Center for Health Statistics. Division of Data Services, 6525 Belcrest Rd., Hyattsville, MD 20782-2003. <http://www.cdc.gov/nchs>.

WEBSITES

"Amniocentesis." <http://www.medicinenet.com/script/main/Art.asp?li=MN1&ArticleKey=268>.

"Amniocentesis." <http://www.modimes.org/HealthLibrary2/factsheets/Amniocentesis.htm>.

"Prenatal diagnosis: Amniocentesis and CVS." <http://www.familydoctor.org/handouts/144.html>.

Terri A. Knutel, MS, CGC

Amyoplasia

Definition

Amyoplasia is a rare congenital disorder characterized by multiple joint contractures of the arms and legs. These contractures result in the wasting of skeletal muscle, which can be replaced by a mixture of dense fat and fibrous tissue. The contractures can be improved with early physical therapy and splinting, however, surgery is often necessary for affected patients.

Description

Amyoplasia, meaning "absent muscle development," is also referred to as amyoplasia congenita. It the most common form of arthrogryposis multiplex congenital (AMC). AMC is a term used to describe a condition where multiple joint contractures are present at birth. Arthrogryposis is derived from the Greek word meaning "with crooking of joints," and AMC can be translated to mean "curved joints, multiple, evident at birth." It occurs in about one out of every 3,000 live births. There are more than 150 types of AMC. Amyoplasia accounts for 40% of AMC cases.

The most striking feature of amyoplasia is the multiple joint contractures, which appear between birth and a few months of age. These joint contractures may affect upper extremities, lower extremities, or both. As a result of these contractures, muscles will often atrophy and become replaced by fat and fibrotic tissue. Additionally, joints can become encased in thickened, fibrotic tissue. More severe cases of amyoplasia may involve other internal organ abnormalities or central nervous system conditions. Individuals affected with amyoplasia are most often of normal intelligence, although they may demonstrate delays in gross and fine motor skills.

Amyoplasia results when a fetus is unable to move sufficiently in the womb. Mothers of children with the disorder often report that their baby was abnormally still during the pregnancy. The lack of movement in utero (also known as fetal akinesia) allows extra connective tissue to form around the joints and, therefore, the joints become fixed. This extra connective tissue replaces muscle tissue, leading to weakness and giving a wasting appearance to the muscles. Additionally, due to the lack of fetal movement, the tendons that connect the muscles to bone are not able to stretch to their normal length and this contributes to the lack of joint mobility as well.

The fetal akinesia in amyoplasia is thought to be caused by various maternal and fetal abnormalities. In some cases, the mother's uterus does not allow for adequate fetal movement because of a lack of amniotic fluid, known as oligohydramnios, or an abnormal shape to the uterus, called a bicornuate uterus. There may also be a myogenic cause to the fetal akinesia, meaning that fetal muscles do not develop properly due to a muscle disease (for example, a congenital **muscular dystrophy**). Similarly, connective tissue (i.e., tendon) and skeletal defects may contribute to the fetal akinesia and be the primary cause of amyoplasia. Additionally, malformations may occur in the central nervous system and/or spinal cord that can lead to a lack of fetal movement in utero. This neurogenic cause is often accompanied by a wide range of other conditions. Other causes of fetal akinesia may include a maternal fever during pregnancy or a virus. There is no single factor that is consistently found in the prenatal history of individuals affected with amyoplasia and, in some cases, there is no known cause of the disorder.

Genetic profile

Amyoplasia is a sporadic condition that occurs due to lack of fetal movement in the womb. There is no specific **gene** that is known to cause the disorder. It is thought to be multifactorial, meaning that numerous genes and environmental factors play a role in its development. The recurrence risk is minimal for siblings or children of affected individuals. There have been no reports of recurrent cases of amyoplasia in a family.

Demographics

Amyoplasia occurs in approximately one in 10,000 live births. There are no reports of the condition being more common in specific ethnic groups or geographical regions.

Signs and symptoms

Delivery of infants with amyoplasia may be difficult and they may deliver in breech presentation. It is possible for limb fractures to occur during a traumatic delivery. However, in general, infants with amyoplasia are most often full term, average weight, and healthy.

Joint contractures will be evident either at the time of birth or in the first few months of life. The primary joints involved are the foot, hip, knee, wrist, elbow, and shoulder. Typically, the contractures will be symmetrical, occurring on both the right and left side of the body. The majority (60–84%) of cases involve all four limbs. Less involve only the lower limbs and even fewer involve only the upper limbs. Often, the involvement of the lower limbs is more extensive than that of the upper limbs. Upper limb involvement may include internal rotation of shoulders, hyperextended elbows, flexed wrists, or "policeman tip" hands (thumb-in-palm). Lower limb involvement may include hip flexion and abduction contractures, dislocated hips, knee flexion or extension contractures, congential dislocation of the knee, and foot deformities (i.e., **clubfoot**). The affected joints will demonstrate limited range of motion. There is diminished muscle mass and limbs may be spindle-shaped (narrower at the ends when compared to the middle). Additionally, there is often a lack of skin creases seen over the affected joints and webbing across the elbow and/or knees may occur. Individuals with amyoplasia have normal sensation, although deep tendon reflexes may be decreased or absent. Cognition and speech are usually normal in individuals with amyoplasia.

Other conditions can be associated with amyoplasia as well. For example, patient often have growth retardation are of small stature compared to the general population. **Scoliosis** is also fairly common and occurs in approximately 30% of affected individuals. Lung hypoplasia is frequently a problem and leads to recurrent respiratory infections in some patients. Facial abnormalities are common, including capillary hemangioma (strawberry birthmark), micrognathia (small jaw), and small, upturned nose. Amyoplasia is occasionally accompanied by genital abnormalities, such as undescended testes, inguinal hernia, and hypoplastic (underdeveloped) external genitalia. Abnormalities in the abdominal wall may be observed as well, for example, **gastroschisis**, a defect of the ventral abdominal wall in which the internal abdominal organs protrude out of the abdomen.

Diagnosis

There are no tests available to definitively diagnose amyoplasia prior to or after birth. The condition may be suspected prenatally if limb deformities are seen on ultrasound (i.e., clubfoot) or if decreased fetal movement is noted. Generally, the diagnosis of amyoplasia is made by ruling out other disorders that cause joint contractures. This is often done via muscle biopsies, blood tests, computed tomography (CT) scans, chromosomal studies, and clinical findings.

Treatment and management

Treatment and management of amyoplasia should involve a multidisciplinary team of health care providers, including pediatrics, neurology, orthopedic surgery, genetics, physical therapy, and occupational therapy. The main goal of treatment is to improve function, not to improve cosmetic appearance.

Generally, it is important to focus on the elbow and wrist in the upper extremity, as contractures in these joints are more problematic than those in the shoulder. Particular attention should be paid to the upper extremity. Due to the emphasis that parents place on encouraging their child to walk, the importance of the function of the arms is often overlooked. For the lower extremity, it is important to pay attention to all joints, however, it is recommended that deformities of the feet are treated first, followed by the knees and then the hips.

Most often, intervention begins immediately after birth with physical therapy and range of motion exercises designed to improve flexibility in muscles and joints. Once the joint is positioned adequately by these exercises, splinting is used to maintain the gains in range of motion. If the joint cannot be positioned adequately with range of motion exercises, casting or soft-tissue release surgery with subsequent casting may be necessary.

In addition to physical therapy, surgery is often necessary for patients with amyoplasia. Muscle transfer is a surgical procedure that involves moving muscles from one location in the body to another location where they might perform better. This is an option for affected patients. However, if muscles are nonfunctional or limited in function as they often are in amyoplasia, this procedure may not be effective. Osteotomy is the surgical cutting of a portion of the bone to correct deformity and may be necessary in some cases of amyoplasia. However, due to the possibility of the recurrence of a bone deformity, this procedure should be postponed until an individual has reached skeletal maturity. Other surgery may be necessary to correct clubfeet, scoliosis, or joint dislocations. Additionally, hernias and other conditions associated with amyoplasia may require surgical intervention.

Prognosis

Amyoplasia is not a progressive disorder and it does not worsen with age. Usually the outlook is very good, especially with early intervention via physical therapy, mobilization, and other treatment. Overall function has been shown to be related to family support, patient personality, education, and early efforts to encourage independence. In rare cases, survival can be poor, particularly if other conditions are associated (i.e., central nervous system disorders). However, most people with amyoplasia are able to lead productive, independent adult lives with minor modifications to daily activities.

Resources

PERIODICALS

Bernstein, Robert M. "Arthrogryposis and Amyoplasia." *Journal of the American Academy of Orthopaedic Surgeons* 10 (November/December 2002): 417–424.

ORGANIZATIONS

Avenues. PO Box 5192, Sonora, CA 95370. (209) 928-3688. (April 3, 2005.) <http://www.sonnet.com/avenues>.

National Organization for Rare Disorders (NORD). 55 Kenosia Avenue, PO Box 1968, Danbury, CT 06813-1968. (800) 999-6673. (April 3, 2005.) <http://www.rarediseases.org/search/rdbdetail_abstract.html?disname=Arthrogryposis%20Multiplex%20Congenita>.

WEB SITES

"Arthrogryposis." *Orthoseek.* (April 3, 2005.) <http://www.orthoseek.com/articles/arthrogryposis.html>.

Stevenson, Roger E. "Alpha-thalassemia X-linked mental retardation syndrome." Gene Reviews. (April 3, 2005.) <http://www.genetests.org/servlet/access?db=geneclinics&site=gt&id=8888891&key=FnPPkP-SrKElS&gry=&fcn=y&fw=CjU5&filename=/profiles/xlmr/index.html>.

"Your child has been diagnosed with arthrogryposis." Shriners Hospital for Children. (April 3, 2005.) <http://www.shrinershq.org/patientedu/arthrogryposis.html>.

Mary E. Freivogel, MS, CGC

Amyotrophic lateral sclerosis

Definition

Amyotrophic lateral sclerosis (ALS) is a fatal disease that affects nerve cells in the brain and spinal cord that are responsible for movement. The motor neurons (nerve cells which send an impulse to illicit muscular contraction or movement) in an ALS patient die as a result of rapid degeneration. Voluntary muscles, controlled by motor neurons, lack proper nourishment and will weaken and atrophy (shrink) as a result. Examples of voluntary movement include stepping off of a curb or reaching for the top shelf. These activities rely on the muscles of the arms and legs. Paralysis sets in at the end-stages of ALS and leaves the patient unable to function physically, despite remaining mentally intact. There are no known causes or cures for amyotrophic lateral sclerosis, and the disease can afflict anyone. The usual cause of death is paralysis of the respiratory muscles which control breathing.

Description

Amyotrophic lateral sclerosis is a progressive disease of the central nervous system. "A" means "no," "myo" implies muscle cells, and "trophic" refers to nourishment. The nerve cells that extend from the brain to the spinal cord (upper motor neurons), and from the spinal cord to the peripheral nerves (lower motor neurons), for unexplained reasons, degenerate and die. "Lateral" refers to the areas of the spinal cord that are affected, and "sclerosis" occurs as hard tissue replaces the previously originally healthy nerve.

The parts of the body that are not affected by ALS are those areas not involved in the use of motor neurons. The mind remains very sharp and in control of sight, hearing, smell, touch and taste. Bowel and bladder functions are generally not affected. Amyotrophic lateral sclerosis rarely causes pain, yet leaves patients dependent on the care of others during advanced stages.

At any given time there are about 30,000 people in the United States with amyotrophic lateral sclerosis, and about 5,000 new cases are reported each year. ALS progresses rapidly and paralyzed patients are usually under the intensive care of nursing facilities or loved ones. This can have a devastating psychological effect on the family members and the patient. In most cases ALS is fatal within two to five years, although approximately 10% live eight years or more.

Amyotrophic lateral sclerosis is not a rare disease. ALS affects approximately seven people out of every 100,000. Most people with ALS are between 40 and 70 years of age. Approximately 5-10% of cases show a heredity pattern.

ALS, or Lou Gehrig's disease, is named after the great New York Yankee's first basemen. Lou Gehrig, known as the "Ironman" of baseball, died two years after he was diagnosed with amyotrophic lateral sclerosis.

Genetic profile

In 1991 a team of ALSA researchers linked familial ALS to **chromosome** 21. In 1993 it was found that there were structural defects in the SOD1 (superoxide dismutase) **gene** on chromosome 21. The SOD1 gene is an enzyme that protects the motor neurons from free radical damage. There is a high incidence of ALS on the island of Guam, in the Western New Guinea and on Kii peninsula of Japan leading some theorists to believe that genetic makeup may be susceptible to an environmental cause, such as the high levels of mercury and lead in these areas.

The **inheritance** pattern is autosomal dominant, which means that children of an affected parent have a 50% chance of inheriting the disorder. The majority of cases are due to a sporadic gene mutation, which means the mutation occurs only in the affected person. It is thought that sporadic mutations result from both biological and environmental causes. In rare cases, a mutation in NFH, the gene encoding for neurofilament (a structure that maintains cell shape) is apparent. Familial amyotrophic lateral sclerosis has been linked to other chromosomal locations but the exact genes involved have not been identified. The Institutional Review Board at Thomas Jefferson University in Philadelphia recently approved the ALS **gene therapy** project. The goal of the project is to inject an adeno-associated virus carrying a normal copy of an EAAT2, into an ALS patient's spinal cord where the motor neurons are dying. The hope is that the cells in that area will not die off.

Demographics

Amyotrophic lateral sclerosis affects anyone and both men and women are at equal risk. ALS may occur at any age and the odds of developing it increase with age. There have been reported cases of teenagers with ALS. A person only needs to inherit a defective gene from one parent to develop the disease.

Signs and symptoms

The disease starts slowly, affecting just one limb, such as the hands or feet, and steadily progresses to more limbs and muscles. When muscles lack the proper nourishment they require, they begin to thin and deteriorate. This condition is the hallmark of amyotrophic lateral sclerosis. Muscle wasting is due to the inability of degenerating motor neurons to elicit a signal to the muscles that allow them to function and grow. Common examples of symptoms for ALS are muscle cramps and twitching, weakness in the hands, feet, or ankles, speech slurring, and swallowing difficulties. Other early symptoms include arm and leg stiffness, foot drop, weight loss, fatigue, and difficulty making facial expressions.

One of the earliest symptoms of ALS is weakness in the bulbar muscles. These muscles in the mouth and throat assist in chewing, swallowing, and speaking. Weakness of these muscle groups usually cause problems such as slurred speech, difficulty with conversation and hoarseness of the voice.

Another symptom of ALS that usually occurs after initial symptoms appear is persistent muscle twitching (fasciculation). Fasciculation is almost never the first sign of ALS.

As the disease progresses the respiratory muscles (breathing muscles) weaken, resulting in increased difficulty with breathing, coughing and possibly inhaling food or saliva. The potential for lung infection increases and can cause death. Many patients find it more comfortable and extend their lives when assisted by ventilators at this stage of the disease. Communication becomes very difficult. One way to accomplish feedback with others is to make use of the eyes. Blinking is one mode that patients of amyotrophic lateral sclerosis will be forced to utilize, in order to continue communication.

As the disease progresses, victims gradually lose the use of their feet, hand, leg, and neck muscles, and paralysis results in affected muscle groups. They are able to speak and swallow only with great struggle. Sexual dysfunction is not affected. Breathing will become increasingly difficult and the patients of ALS may decide to prolong life with the use of assisted ventilation, which may decrease the risks of death from infections such as pneumonia.

Diagnosis

ALS is difficult to diagnose. There is no one set way to test for the disease. A series of diagnostic tests will

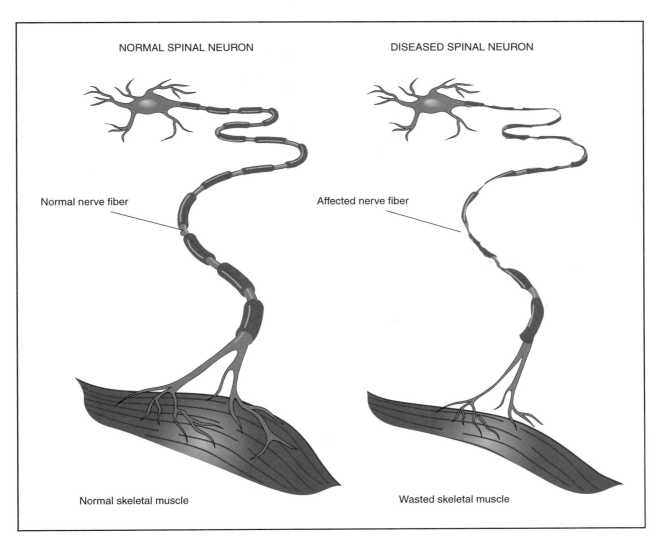

NORMAL SPINAL NEURON DISEASED SPINAL NEURON

Normal nerve fiber Affected nerve fiber

Normal skeletal muscle Wasted skeletal muscle

The degeneration and death of motor neurons in the spinal cord and brain results in amyotrophic lateral sclerosis (ALS). These neurons convey electrical messages from the brain to the muscles to stimulate movement in the arms, legs, trunk, neck, and head. As motor neurons degenerate, the muscles are weakened and cannot move as effectively, leading to muscle wasting. *(Gale Group.)*

rule out and exclude other possible causes and diseases that resemble ALS. Electro diagnostic tests such as electromyography (EMG) and nerve conduction velocity (NCV) are used to help diagnose ALS. Blood and urine tests, spinal taps, x rays, and muscle and/or nerve biopsy are performed, as well as magnetic resonance imaging (MRI), myelograms of the cervical spine and a complete neurological exam.

A second opinion is frequently recommended if ALS is suspected since it is a fatal neurological disease. After a complete medical exam and family history check has been administered, other tests such as a CT (computed tomography) scan may be done to continue ruling out other causes. Many symptoms mimic ALS such as tumors of the skull base or upper cervical spinal cord, spinal arthritis, thyroid disease, lead poisoning, and severe vitamin deficiency. Other possibilities to rule out are **multiple sclerosis**, spinal cord neoplasm, polyarteritis, syringomyelia, **myasthenia gravis**, and **muscular dystrophy**. Amyotrophic lateral sclerosis is hardly ever misdiagnosed after this intensive series of diagnostic tests.

Treatment and management

Currently, there is no treatment for ALS. Management aims to control the symptoms that patients

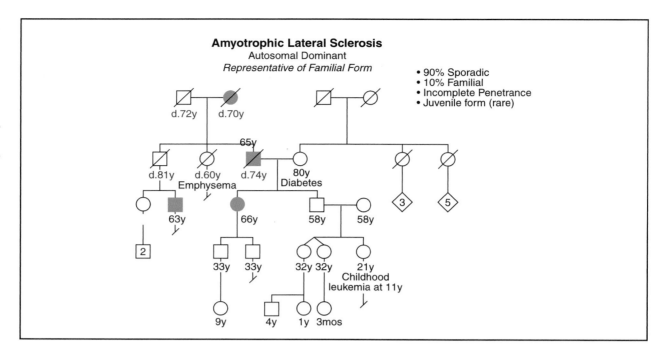

Amyotrophic Lateral Sclerosis
Autosomal Dominant
Representative of Familial Form

- 90% Sporadic
- 10% Familial
- Incomplete Penetrance
- Juvenile form (rare)

(Gale Group.)

experience. Emotional, psychological and physical support, are provided to ease the difficulty associated with this disorder.

Moderate activities are recommended in the early stages of the disease. Physical therapy can help muscles stay active and delay the resulting weakness. ALS patients are encouraged to maintain a healthy diet and exercise regularly for as long as possible. Education of ALS is very important in developing an understanding of the disease, and is vital for family members as well as patients.

Although there are no set treatments for ALS there are still many special considerations that can assist in the quality of lifestyle for the patient. Implementing a physical therapy program, providing a wheelchair or walker, assistance when bathing, and suction machines to help evacuate accumulated secretions all help the ALS patient. Other considerations include providing foods that are soft and easy to swallow, skin maintenance, feeding tubes, ventilation maintenance and emotional support.

Researchers have developed a drug approved by the Food and Drug Administration (FDA) called Rilutek (riluzole). The drug was the first to have a positive effect in that it appears to extend the life of ALS patients by about three months.

Another drug, Myotrophin (somatomedin C), appears to prevent neuron loss and enhance neuron generation in animal studies.

Prognosis

Amyotrophic lateral sclerosis normally progresses rapidly and leads to death from respiratory infection within three to five years. If the person involved is young and the initial symptoms appear in the limbs, the disease tends to develop more slowly. Improved medical care prolongs the lives of ALS patients and shows promise for more effective treatments in the future.

Resources

BOOKS

Adams, Raymond D., Maurice Victor, and Allan H. Ropper. *Adam's & Victor's Principles of Neurology,* 6th ed. New York, McGraw Hill, 1997.

Brown, Robert H. "The motor neuron diseases." In *Harrison's Principles of Internal Medicine, 14th ed.,* edited by Anthony S. Fauci, et al. New York: McGraw-Hill, 1998, pp. 2368-2372.

Feldman, Eva L. "Motor neuron diseases." In *Cecil Textbook of Medicine,* 21st ed., edited by Lee Goldman and J. Claude Bennett. Philadelphia: W.B. Saunders, 2000, pp. 2089-2092.

PERIODICALS

Foubistor, V. "Gene therapy fosters hope." *American Medical News* 43 (March 6, 2000).

ORGANIZATIONS

Association of America (ALSA). 27001 Agoura Rd., Suite150, Calabasas Hills, CA 91301-5104. (818) 800-9006. Fax: (818) 880-9006. <http://www.alsa.org>.

Center for Neurologic Study. 9850 Genesee Ave., Suite 320, Lajolla, CA 92037. (858) 455-5463. Fax: (858) 455-1713. cns@cts.org. <http://www.cnsonline.org>.

Forbes Norris ALS Research Center. Caifornia Pacific Medical Center, 2324 Sacramento St., San Francisco, CA 94115. (415) 923-3604. Fax: (415) 673-5184.

Laith Farid Gulli, MD
Brian Veillette, BS

Androgen insensitivity syndrome

Definition

Androgen insensitivity syndrome is a genetic condition where affected people have male chromosomes and male gonads (testicles). The external genitals, however, have mild to complete feminization.

Description

Normal sexual development

In normal development, the **chromosome** sex determines the gonadal sex, which in turns determines the phenotypic sex. The chromosome sex is determined at conception; a male has the sex chromosome pair XY and a female has the chromosome pair XX. During the first 40 days of gestation, a male and female embryo appear the same and have undifferenti-ated gonads, which have the potential of becoming testes or ovaries. The presence of the Y chromosome in the male directs the undifferentiated gonads to become testicles. If no Y chromosome is present, such as in the female chromosome pair, the undifferentiated gonads become ovaries.

In males, the phenotypic sex, including the internal male structures and the external male genitalia, arises as a result of the hormones secreted from the testicles. The two main hormones secreted by the testicles are testosterone and mullerian duct inhibitor. Testosterone acts directly on the wolffian duct, which give rise to the internal male structures including the epididymides, vasa deferentia, and seminal vesicles. Testosterone is converted into dihydrotestosterone, the hormone responsible for the development of the male urethra and prostate, and the external genitalia of the penis and the scrotum. The mullerian duct inhibitor is the hormone that suppresses the mullerian ducts and prevents the development of fallopian tubes, upper vagina, and uterus in males.

If no testicles are present, as with females, no mullerian duct inhibitor is formed and the mullerian ducts become the fallopian tubes, the upper vagina, and the uterus. The wolffian ducts regress. Due to the lack of dihydrotestosterone, the external genitals are not masculinized and become female. Studies have shown that an ovary is not required for the formation of the internal female structures or the feminization of the genitals. If a testicle is not present, the development of the embryo will default to female development.

In most cases, the chromosomal sex, the gonadal sex, and the phenotypic sex are in agreement. Males have 46,XY chromosomes, testicles, and male internal structures and genitals. Females have 46,XX chromosomes, ovaries, and internal female structures and genitals.

Androgen insensitivity syndrome

Androgen insensitivity syndrome (AIS), also known as testicular feminization, is one of the most common conditions where the chromosome sex and gonadal sex do not agree with the phenotypic sex. Affected people have normal male chromosomes, 46,XY and testicles. The testicles secrete both testosterone and mullerian duct inhibitor as normal and no internal female structures form. However, due to defective androgen receptors, the wolffian ducts and genitals cannot respond to the androgens testosterone and dihydrotestosterone. As a result, no male internal structures are formed from the wolffian ducts and the external genitals are feminized.

The amount of feminization depends on the severity of the androgen receptor defect and is often characterized as complete androgen insensitivity (CAIS), partial androgen insensitivity (PAIS), and mild androgen insensitivity (MAIS). In complete androgen insensitivity, the alteration in the androgen receptor results in complete female external genitals. In partial androgen insensitivity, also called Reifenstein syndrome, partial androgen insensitivity results in female genitalia with some masculinization, **ambiguous genitalia**, or male genitalia with partial feminization. With mild androgen insensitivity, mild androgen resistance results in normal male genitals or a male with mild feminization.

In both CAIS and PAIS, affected individuals are sterile (can not have a child). In MAIS, the affected male may have fertility problems because of oligospermia, low sperm production, or azoospermia, no sperm production. In all types of AIS, secondary sex characteristics such as body and pubic hair can be abnormal. Mental impairment is not found in any of the types of androgen insensitivity syndromes, though poor visual-spatial ability has been observed. People with AIS can also be rather tall, though bone age is usually normal.

Genetic profile

Androgen insensitivity syndrome is a genetic condition that results from mutations (alterations) of the **gene** for the androgen receptor. The androgen receptor is located on the long arm of the X chromosome (Xq11-q12). As women have two X-chromosomes, they also have two androgen receptor genes. Men have only one X chromosome and a Y chromosome; hence they only have one copy of the androgen receptor gene.

When women have one copy of the androgen receptor altered, they are considered carriers of AIS. In most cases, the second, normal copy of the androgen receptor can compensate for the altered copy. However, in approximately 10% of women who are carriers for the altered androgen receptor gene, clinical signs such as sparse pubic hair and armpit hair or a delay to the start of their first menstrual period is observed.

46,XY conceptions that have alterations in the androgen receptor gene do not have a second copy to compensate for the altered copy. Hence, these people will have AIS. If the androgen receptor is severely altered, they will have CAIS. If not severely altered, they will have PAIS or MAIS.

All forms of AIS are inherited in an X-linked recessive pattern. This means women who are carriers have a 25% chance of having an affected child. If a carrier woman has a 46,XY conception, there is a 50% chance the child will have AIS. If a carrier woman has a 46,XX

conception, there will be a 50% chance the daughter will also be a carrier.

When a person has AIS and has no other family history of the condition, approximately 2/3 of the time the affected person inherited the gene alteration from his or her mother. The other 1/3 of the time, the alteration of the androgen receptor was a new event (new mutation) in the affected person and was not inherited.

Cases of both gonadal mosaicism and somatic mosaicism have been reported with AIS. Gonadal mosaicism occurs when the alteration in the androgen receptor occurred not at conception, but in one of the gamete cells (sperm or egg). The rest of the cells of the body do not have the altered androgen receptor. With AIS, this can occur when one of a woman's early gamete cell has the new alteration in the androgen receptor but the rest of the cells in her body do not. All the eggs that come from the early gamete cell will also have the alteration. Her risk for having a child with AIS is increased. Somatic mosaicism occurs when the alteration in the androgen receptor occurs after conception but not in a gamete cell. Some of the person's cells will have the altered androgen receptor and other cells will not. The amount of cells with altered receptors and the location of those cells within the body will determine how severely affected a person will be.

Mutations within the androgen receptor gene are also responsible for the neuromuscular condition spinobulbar muscular atrophy or **Kennedy disease**. See separate entry for more information.

Demographics

Complete androgen insensitivity syndrome occurs in approximately one in 64,000 46,XY births or 2-5 in 100,000 births overall. Partial AIS is at least as common as complete AIS. The incident of mild AIS is unknown, but is estimated to account for approximately 40% of male infertility due to severe oligospermia or azoospermia.

Signs and symptoms

Complete androgen insensitivity

Individuals with CAIS are born looking like normal female babies. Often, the condition is discovered in one of two ways. The child can have an inguinal hernia that upon repair is found to contain testicles. The most common presentation is during puberty with primary amenorrhea, or lack of the onset of the menstrual period. Affected individuals have a short, blind ending vagina and no uterus, cervix, fallopian tubes, or ovaries. During puberty, some girls will have absent or decreased sexual hair. Breasts develop normally and can be large in size

Classification of AIS Phenotypes

Type	External genitalia (synonyms)	Findings
CAIS	Female ("testicular feminization")	Absent or rudimentary wolffian duct derivatives Inguinal or labial testes; short blind-ending vagina Little or no pubic and/or axillary hair
CAIS or PAIS	Predominantly female (incomplete AIS)	Inguinal or labial testes Labial fusion and enlarged clitoris Distinct urethral and vaginal openings or a urogenital sinus
PAIS	Ambiguous	Microphallus (<1 cm) with clitoris-like underdeveloped glans; labia majora-like bifid scrotum Descended or undescended testes Perineoscrotal hypospadias or urogenital sinus Excessive development of the male breasts during puberty
	Predominantly male	Simple (glandular or penile) or severe (perineal) "isolated" hypospadias with a normal-sized penis and descended testes or severe hypospadias with micropenis, bifid scrotum, and either descended or undescended testes Excessive development of the male breasts during puberty
MAIS	Male (undervirilized male syndrome)	Impaired sperm development and/or impaired masculinization Overdevelopment of the male breasts during puberty

with pale and immature nipples and areola. People with CAIS are usually raised as females and have normal female sexual orientation. All women with CAIS are sterile. In families with CAIS, all affected members will have complete androgen insensitivity and similar physical features.

Partial androgen insensitivity syndrome

Children with PAIS usually present at birth due to ambiguous genitalia. The genitalia can look like female genitals with some masculinization, completely ambiguous genitals where the sex of the baby cannot be immediately determined, or male genitals with some feminization. The degree of severity is a direct result of the degree of severity of the genetic alteration in the androgen receptor and resulting amount of functional androgen receptor. The internal structures of PAIS are the same as CAIS, with absent fallopian tubes, cervix, uterus, and ovaries. Testes are present but do not produce sperm. Hence, people with PAIS are also sterile. People with PAIS also have primary amenorrhea, and breast development occurs in puberty. Unlike CAIS, affected individuals in the same family with presumably the same genetic alteration can have varying degrees of masculinization. As a result, some affected people may be raised as females whereas others may be raised as males. Sex assignment is made based upon the structure of the genitals, the surgical correction needed, and the predicted response to androgens during puberty.

Mild androgen insensitivity

Males with mild androgen insensitivity usually have normal male genitals and internal male structures. During puberty, males with MAIS may have breast enlarge-

ment, sparse facial and body hair, and small penis. Some affected males may also have impaired sperm production resulting in oligospermia or azoospermia, decreased or absent sperm. As with CAIS, affected men within the same family usually have similar features.

Diagnosis

Diagnosis is usually made based upon clinical features, chromosome analysis, hormone levels, and analysis of androgen receptor function in skin fibroblasts. Clinical features are listed above for CAIS, PAIS, and MAIS. Chromosome analysis reveals normal male chromosomes. Affected individuals can have elevated luteinizing hormone, normal to slightly elevated testosterone, and high estradiol for men. Follicle stimulating hormone may also be normal to elevated. Reduced androgen receptor function in skin fibroblast cells is also used to aid in a diagnosis.

Direct **genetic testing** for molecular defects in the androgen receptor gene is being done on a research basis only.

Treatment and management

Complete androgen insensitivity

Treatment of CAIS requires the removal of the testicles from the pelvis or inguinal canal to decrease risk of testicular malignancy. Because the overall risk of malignancy is approximately 5% and rarely occurs before age 25, the testicles are usually removed after the development of the secondary sex characteristics, as the testes are needed for estrogen formation. After the removal of the testes, estrogen supplementation is started to aid in the development of secondary sex characteristics and to help prevent **osteoporosis**. Surgery to lengthen the vagina may be necessary.

Partial androgen insensitivity syndrome

For those affected individuals raised as females, treatment is similar to CAIS except the removal of the testicles is done earlier because it may cause enlargement of the clitoris during puberty. Reconstructive surgery of the genitals and lengthening of the vagina may be necessary.

People with PAIS raised as boys may need surgery to improve the appearance of the genitals. Androgen supplementation may be implemented, though long-term affects of androgen therapy are not known. Breast reduction surgery may be necessary after puberty.

Mild androgen insensitivity

Males with MAIS may require no treatment at all or breast reduction surgery after puberty. Males who are infertile may benefit from assisted reproductive technologies.

Prognosis

For CAIS and MAIS, the prognosis is excellent. Generally, gender assignment is not difficult and sexual orientation is female for CAIS and male for MAIS. Treatment usually involves minimal surgery and hormone supplementation. For individuals with PAIS, the prognosis is very dependent upon the severity of the condition. Assignment of gender can be difficult and genital surgery can be more involved. Recently, some individuals with PAIS and other intersex conditions have encouraged the delay of assigning gender until the child is old enough to express a preference. This idea has not been readily embraced in the medical community of the United States.

Resources

BOOKS

Wilson, J. D., and J. E. Griffin. "Disorders of Sexual Differentiation." In *Harrison's Online,* edited by Eugene Braunwald, et al. New York: McGraw-Hill, 2001.

PERIODICALS

Warne, G. L., et al. "Androgen insensitivity syndrome in the era of the molecular genetics and the internet: A point of view." *Journal of Pediatric Endocrinology & Metabolism* 11 (1998): 3-9.

ORGANIZATIONS

AIS Support Group (AISSG). PO Box 269, Banbury, Oxon, OX15 6YT UK <http://www.medhelp.org/www/ais>.

Intersex Society of North America. PO Box 301, Petaluma, CA 94953-0301. <http://www.isna.org>.

WEBSITES

Androgen Receptor Gene Mutations Database. <http://www.mcgill.ca/androgendb>.

Pinsky, L. P. "Androgen Insensitivity Syndrome." *Gene Clinics: Clinical Information Resource* University of Washington, Seattle. <http://www.geneclinics.org/profiles/andrgoen/details.html>. February 6, 2001 (Updated March 23, 1999).

Carin Lea Beltz, MS, CGC

Anemia, sideroblastic X-linked

Definition

X-linked sideroblastic anemia is a hereditary enzyme disorder in which the body has adequate iron but is unable to incorporate it into hemoglobin.

Description

X-linked sideroblastic anemia is the hereditary form of sideroblastic anemia, also known as iron overload anemia or sideroblastosis. Another, more common type of sideroblastic anemia is called acquired sideroblastic anemia.

In sideroblastic anemia, iron enters a developing red blood cell and is not incorporated properly into the hemoglobin molecule (the cell's oxygen carrier). This causes iron to accumulate in the mitochondria and sideroblasts. The defective hemoglobin then transports oxygen poorly, resulting in decreased tissue oxygenation.

This build-up of iron gives the cell nucleus its ringed appearance, called ringed sideroblast, which is the primary sign of sideroblastic anemia.

Sideroblastic anemia is often mistaken for iron deficiency anemia, but tests usually reveal normal or increased levels of iron.

X-linked sideroblastic anemia

The hereditary form of the disorder is rare. The primary type of inherited sideroblastic anemia was first described in 1945 by Thomas Cooley. He identified cases of X-linked sideroblastic anemia in two brothers from a family with a six-generational history of the inherited disease. The genetic abnormality that causes X-linked sideroblastic anemia was identified almost 40 years later. Identification has aided diagnosis of this disorder.

X-linked sideroblastic anemia nearly always manifests in infancy or childhood.

Other inherited forms of sideroblastic anemia

There are other inherited forms of sideroblastic anemia, which are also rare. A rare autosomal recessive form of inherited sideroblastic anemia occurs in both males and females of affected families. Autosomal dominant **inheritance** has also been reported. The abnormalities that cause these anemias are not yet identified. Also, Pearson's syndrome, an inherited disorder caused by abnormal mitochondria, is sometimes called sideroblastic anemia with marrow cell vacuolization and exocrine pancreatic dysfunction.

Acquired sideroblastic anemia

Acquired sideroblastic anemia often results from prolonged exposure to toxins (such as alcohol, lead, or drugs), or nutritional imbalances (such as deficiency in folic acid or copper or excess in zinc). Other causes may be inflammatory disease, cancerous conditions, or kidney, endocrine, or metabolic disorders. Acquired sideroblastic anemia sometimes surfaces in the context of a myelodysplastic syndrome.

Removal of the toxin or treatment of the underlying disease will reverse this type of sideroblastic anemia.

Acquired anemia is usually seen in patients over 65, particularly in those cases associated with myelodysplasia. The disorder can appear as early as the midfifties.

Genetic profile

Hereditary sideroblastic anemia is most commonly inherited as an X-linked recessive trait.

Typical X-linked genetics

The following concepts are important to understanding the inheritance of an X-linked disorder. All humans have two chromosomes that determine their gender: females have XX, males have XY. X-linked recessive, also called sex-linked, inheritance affects the genes located on the X **chromosome**. It occurs when an unaffected mother carries a disease-causing **gene** on at least one of her X chromosomes. Because females have two X chromosomes, they are usually unaffected carriers. The X chromosome that does not have the disease-causing gene compensates for the X chromosome that does. For a woman to show symptoms of the disorder, both X chromosomes would need to have the disease-causing gene. That is why women are less likely to show such symptoms than males.

If a mother has a female child, the child has a 50% chance of inheriting the disease gene and being a carrier who can pass the disease gene on to her sons. On the other hand, if a mother has a male child who inherits the disease-causing gene, he will be affected and has a 100% chance of passing the disease gene on to his children. Since the gene is defective and in the XY state there is no normal gene, the singular flawed gene is expressed.

Genetics of X-linked sideroblastic anemia

The genetic abnormality that causes X-linked sideroblastic anemia is a mutation in the erythroid (red blood cell) specific form of delta-aminolevulinate synthase (ALAS2). ALAS2 is the first enzyme in the heme biosynthetic pathway and the mutation, when present, results in the inability to transport the heme (iron) into the hemoglobin, making it ineffective.

The ability to test for this genetic disorder has improved diagnosis.

Demographics

X-linked sideroblastic anemia occurs in young men. It may be seen in maternal uncles and male cousins of men with the disorder.

Autosomal transmitted forms of the disease may occur in both men and women.

Hereditary sideroblastic anemia generally occurs during the first three decades of life especially during adolescence, but it has been diagnosed in patients over 70 years old.

Signs and symptoms

General weakness, fatigue, dizziness, and difficulty breathing are associated with the disorder. Exertion may cause chest pains similar to angina.

The mucous membranes and skin of hands and arms may be pale, possibly with a lemon-yellow cast. Subcutaneous bleeding may occur, causing a brownish-red effect.

Excess iron accumulation, known as **hemochromatosis**, accumulates over years in the bone marrow, liver, heart, and other tissues. This progressive deposition of toxic iron may result in an enlarged spleen or liver, liver disease, **diabetes**, impotence, arthritic signs, and heart disease, particularly cardiac arrhythmia.

Diagnosis

Using Prussian blue staining, sideroblasts are visible under microscopic examination of bone marrow.

A blood test can indicate sideroblastic anemia. Indicative laboratory results of an iron panel test include:

• High levels for serum iron, serum ferritin, and transferrin iron saturation percentage.

• Low levels for total iron binding capacity and transferrin.

• Normal to high levels for serum transferrin receptor.

Additionally, other signs of sideroblastic anemia include:

• Hemoglobin is generally less than 10.0g/dL.

• Hypochromic (reduced color) cells coexist with normal cells.

• Stainable marrow and hemosiderin is increased.

• Ringed sideroblasts are visible with Prussian blue staining and observable under microscopic examination of bone marrow.

• Red cell distribution width is increased.

• White blood cells and platelets are normal.

Treatment and management

The main objective in treatment of X-linked sideroblastic anemia is to prevent the development of diabetes,

cirrhosis, and heart failure from iron overload (hemochromatosis).

X-linked sideroblastic anemia often improves with pyridoxine (vitamin B6) therapy. Dosage is 50–200 mg, however, pregnant or nursing mothers may wish to limit intake to 100 mg daily.

In cases of extreme anemia, whole red blood cell transfusion may be required. Repeated whole red blood cell transfusion, however, will contribute significantly to existing iron burden in sideroblastic anemia patients. It will likely require chelation therapy with desferrioxamine (Desferal), a drug with iron chelating properties. Desferrioxamine binds excess body iron and promotes excretion by the liver and kidneys. It is administered by intravenous infusion from a small portable pump. The pump is worn nine to twelve hours daily, usually at night while sleeping. Side effects vary and include pain and swelling at injection site.

Certain drugs are sometimes associated with acquired sideroblastic anemia: progesterone (found in oral contraceptives and hormone replacement therapy); copper chelating drugs like trientine, which is used in treating **Wilson disease**; and anti-tuberculosis drugs like isoniazid (a type of antibiotic), among others. In other cases, acquired sideroblastic anemia may be secondary to another disorder or disease. Other predisposing causes may be inflammatory disease such as **rheumatoid arthritis**, cancerous conditions such as leukemia and lymphoma, kidney disorders causing uremia, endocrine disorders such as hyperthyroidism, and metabolic disorders such as porphyria cutanea tarda. In these cases, it is important to treat the primary disease or disorder in order to reverse the anemia.

Development of leukemia is associated with the acquired form of the disease, often first showing up in the form of a myeloproliferative disorder. These disorders are characterized by abnormal growth of bone tissue and related cells.

Prognosis

The disorder can often be kept in check with regular medical supervision. Many individuals with X-linked sideroblastic anemia require chronic transfusion to maintain acceptable hemoglobin levels. Over a lifetime, problems related to iron overload, including congestive heart failure and cirrhosis, can become life-threatening issues.

Death can result from hemochromatosis (iron-overload) if the disease is untreated or if blood transfusions are inadequate to account for the iron overload.

KEY TERMS

Heme—The iron-containing molecule in hemoglobin that serves as the site for oxygen binding.

Hemochromatosis—Accumulation of large amounts of iron in the tissues of the body.

Hemoglobin—Protein-iron compound in the blood that carries oxygen to the cells and carries carbon dioxide away from the cells.

Mitochondria—Organelles within the cell responsible for energy production.

Myelodysplasia—A bone marrow disorder that can develop into aplastic anemia requiring bone marrow or stem cell transplantation.

Nucleus—The central part of a cell that contains most of its genetic material, including chromosomes and DNA.

Red blood cells—Hemoglobin-containing blood cells that transport oxygen from the lungs to tissues. In the tissues, the red blood cells exchange their oxygen for carbon dioxide, which is brought back to the lungs to be exhaled.

Resources

BOOKS

Current Medical Diagnosis & Treatment. Edited by Tierney, Lawrence M., Jr., et al. Stamford, CT: Appleton & Lange, 1998.

PERIODICALS

Sheth, Sujit, and Gary M. Brittenham. "Genetic disorders affecting proteins of iron metabolism: Clinical implications." *Annual Review of Medicine* 51 (2000): 443+.

ORGANIZATIONS

Leukemia & Lymphoma Society. 1311 Mamaroneck Ave., White Plains, NY 10605. (914) 949-5213. <http://www.leukemia-lymphoma.org>.

National Heart, Lung, and Blood Institute. PO Box 30105, Bethesda, MD 20824-0105. (301) 592-8573. nhlbiinfo@rover.nhlbi.nih.gov. <http://www.nhlbi.nih.gov>.

National Organization for Rare Disorders (NORD). PO Box 8923, New Fairfield, CT 06812-8923. (203) 746-6518 or (800) 999-6673. Fax: (203) 746-6481. <http://www.rarediseases.org>.

WEBSITES

Iron Disorders Institute. <http://www.irondisorders.org>.

National Center for Biotechnology Information. >http://www.ncbi.nlm.nih.gov>.

Jennifer F. Wilson, MS

Anencephaly

Definition

Anencephaly is a lethal birth defect characterized by the absence of all or part of the skull and scalp and malformation of the brain.

Description

Anencephaly is one of a group of malformations of the central nervous system collectively called **neural tube defects**. Anencephaly is readily apparent at birth because of the absence of the skull and scalp and with exposure of the underlying brain. The condition is also called acrania (absence of the skull) and acephaly (absence of the head). In its most severe form, the entire skull and scalp are missing. In some cases, termed "meroacrania" or "meroanencephaly," a portion of the skull may be present. In most instances, anencephaly occurs as an isolated birth defect with the other organs and tissues of the body forming correctly. In approximately 10% of cases, other malformations coexist with anencephaly.

Genetic profile

As an isolated defect, anencephaly appears to be caused by a combination of genetic factors and environmental influences that predispose to faulty formation of the nervous system. The specific genes and environmental insults that contribute to this multifactorial causation are not completely understood. It is known that nutritional insufficiency, specifically folic acid insufficiency, is one predisposing environmental factor and that mutations of genes involved in folic acid metabolism are genetic risk factors. The recurrence risk after the birth of an infant with anencephaly is 3-5%. The recurrence may be anencephaly or another neural tube defect, such as **spina bifida**.

Demographics

Anencephaly occurs in all races and ethnic groups. The prevalence rates range from less than one in 10,000 births (European countries) to more than 10 per 10,000 births (Mexico, China).

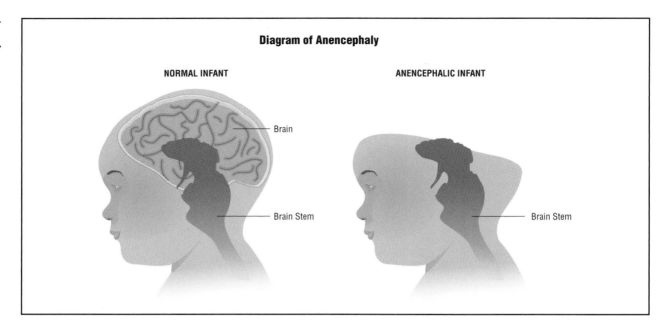

Diagram of Anencephaly

NORMAL INFANT

ANENCEPHALIC INFANT

Brain

Brain Stem

Brain Stem

Infants born with anencephaly have either a severely underdeveloped brain or total brain absence. A portion of the brain stem usually protrudes through the skull, which also fails to develop properly. *(Gale Group.)*

Signs and symptoms

Anencephaly is readily apparent at birth because of exposure of all or part of the brain. Not only is the brain malformed, but it is also damaged because of the absence of the overlying protective encasement. In about 10% of cases of anencephaly, other malformations are also present.

Diagnosis

Anencephaly is diagnosed by observation. Prenatal diagnosis may be made by ultrasound examination after 12 to 14 weeks' gestation. Prenatal diagnosis of anencephaly can also be detected through maternal serum alpha-fetoprotein screening. The level of alpha-fetoprotein in the maternal blood is elevated because of the leakage of this fetal protein into the amniotic fluid.

Treatment and management

No treatment is indicated for anencephaly. Affected infants are stillborn or die within the first few days of life. The risk for occurrence or recurrence of anencephaly may be reduced by half or more by the intake of folic acid during the months immediately before and after conception. Natural folic acid, a B vitamin, may be found in many foods (green leafy vegetables, legumes, orange juice, liver). Synthetic folic acid may be obtained in vitamin preparations and in

> **KEY TERMS**
>
> **Alpha-fetoprotein (AFP)**—A chemical substance produced by the fetus and found in the fetal circulation. AFP is also found in abnormally high concentrations in most patients with primary liver cancer.

certain fortified breakfast cereals. In the United States, all enriched cereal grain flours have been fortified with folic acid.

Prognosis

Anencephaly is uniformly fatal at birth or soon thereafter.

Resources

PERIODICALS

Czeizel, A. E., and I. Dudas. "Prevention of the first occurrence of neural tube defects by preconceptional vitamin supplementation." *New England Journal of Medicine* 327 (1992): 1832-1835.

Medical Research Council Vitamin Study Research Group. "Prevention of neural tube defects: results of the Medical

Research Council vitamin study." *Lancet* 338 (1991): 131-137.

Sells, C. J., and J. G. Hall, Guest Editors. "Neural Tube Defects." *Mental Retardation and Developmental Disabilities Research Reviews.* 4, no. 4, Wiley-Liss, 1998.

ORGANIZATIONS

March of Dimes Birth Defects Foundation. 1275 Mamaroneck Ave., White Plains, NY 10605. (888) 663-4637. resourcecenter@modimes.org. <http://www.modimes.org>.

National Birth Defects Prevention Network. Atlanta, GA (770) 488-3550. <http://www.nbdpn.org>.

Roger E. Stevenson, MD

Angelman syndrome

Definition

Angelman syndrome (AS) is a genetic condition that causes severe mental retardation, severe speech impairment, and a characteristic happy and excitable demeanor.

Description

Individuals with AS show evidence of delayed development by 6–12 months of age. Eventually, this delay is recognized as severe mental retardation. Unlike some genetic conditions causing severe mental retardation, AS is not associated with developmental regression (loss of previously attained developmental milestones).

Severe speech impairment is a striking feature of AS. Speech is almost always limited to a few words or no words at all. However, receptive language skills (listening to and understanding the speech of others) and non-verbal communication are not as severely affected.

Individuals with AS have a balance disorder, causing unstable and jerky movements. This typically includes gait ataxia (a slow, unbalanced way of walking) and tremulous movements of the limbs.

AS is also associated with a unique "happy" behavior, which may be the best-known feature of the condition. This may include frequent laughter or smiling, often with no apparent stimulus. Children with AS often appear happy, excited, and active. They may also sometimes flap their hands repeatedly. Generally, they have a short attention span. These characteristic behaviors led to the original name of this condition, the "Happy Puppet" syndrome. However, this name is no longer used as it is considered insensitive to AS individuals and their families.

Genetic profile

The genetics of AS are complex. There are at least five different genetic abnormalities that can cause the condition, all of which involve a specific region of the **chromosome** 15 inherited from the mother. This region is designated 15q11-13 (bands 11 through 13 on the long arm of chromosome 15). The fact that AS occurs only when there are abnormalities in this region of the maternal copy of chromosome 15 reflects a unique phenomenon known as **imprinting**. Imprinting is a chemical modification of **DNA** which acts as an "identification tag" indicating which parent contributed the chromosome. Imprinted genes or chromosome regions are expressed or not expressed depending on which parent transmitted the chromosome. Abnormalities in the paternally (from the father) inherited 15q11-13 region cause a different genetic condition called **Prader-Willi syndrome**.

Chromosome deletion

The most common cause of AS is a small deletion (missing piece) in the maternally inherited chromosome 15. Specifically, the deletion occurs within 15q11-13. Approximately 70% of AS individuals have this deletion.

UBE3A mutation

In approximately 11% of AS cases, there is a mutation within the maternally inherited UBE3A **gene**. All the genetic mechanisms leading to AS appear to compromise expression of this gene, which is located within the 15q11-13 region. This gene is considered to be the "critical gene" responsible for AS, although its specific function is unknown.

Uniparental disomy

Some cases of AS result from **inheritance** of both chromosomes in the 15 pair from the father, an unusual genetic phenomenon known as uniparental disomy. In this circumstance, there is no chromosome 15 from the mother. Approximately 7% of AS cases result from this mechanism.

Imprinting defect

Approximately 3% of AS cases result from an imprinting defect on the maternally inherited chromosome 15. As noted above, imprinting is a chemical modification to the DNA which serves as a marker indicating the parent of origin and controls gene expression. If there is defective imprinting on the maternally inherited 15, then the genes in the 15q11-15q13 region may not be expressed, leading to AS.

Chromosome rearrangement

Rarely, AS may be caused by chromosomal breaks that occur in the maternal inherited 15q11-13 region. The breaks may occur as the result of a translocation (in which two chromosomes break and exchange material) or an inversion (in which a piece of a chromosome breaks and rejoins in the opposite orientation), or other disturbance of the chromosome structure involving the maternal 15q11-15q13. This mechanism is responsible for about 1% of AS cases.

Unknown mechanism(s)

In about 8% of individuals with AS, no genetic cause can be identified. This may reflect misdiagnosis, or the presence of additional, unrecognized mechanisms leading to AS.

Demographics

AS has been reported in individuals of diverse ethnic backgrounds. The incidence of the condition is estimated at 1/10,000 to 1/30,000.

Signs and symptoms

The first abnormalities noted in an infant with AS are often delays in motor milestones (those related to physical skills, such as sitting up or walking), muscular hypotonia (poor muscle tone), and speech impairment. Some infants seem unaccountably happy and may exhibit fits of laughter. By age 12 months, 50% of infants with AS have microcephaly (a small head size). Tremulous movements are often noted during the first year of life.

Seizures occur in 80% of children with AS, usually by three years of age. No major brain lesions are typically seen on cranial imaging studies.

The achievement of walking is delayed, usually occurring between two-and-a-half and six years of age. The child with AS typically exhibits a jerky, stiff gait, often with uplifted and bent arms. About 10% of individuals with AS do not walk. Additionally, children may have drooling, protrusion of the tongue, hyperactivity, and a short attention span.

Many children have a decreased need for sleep and abnormal sleep/wake cycles. This problem may emerge in infancy and persist throughout childhood. Upon awakening at night, children may become very active and destructive to bedroom surroundings.

The language impairment associated with AS is severe. Most children with AS fail to learn appropriate and consistent use of more than a few words. Receptive language skills are less severely affected. Older children and adults are able to communicate by using gestures or communication boards (special devices bearing visual symbols corresponding to commonly used expressions or words).

Some individuals with AS caused by a deletion of the 15q11-q13 chromosomal region may have a lighter skin complexion than would be expected given their family background.

Diagnosis

The clinical diagnosis of AS is made on the basis of physical examination and medical and developmental history. Confirmation requires specialized laboratory testing.

There is no single laboratory test that can identify all cases of AS. Several different tests may be performed to look for the various genetic causes of AS. When positive, these tests are considered diagnostic for AS.

DNA methylation studies

DNA methylation studies determine if the normal imprinting pattern associated with the maternal (mother's) copy of the number 15 chromosome is present. The 15q11-q13 region is differently methylated (or "imprinted") depending on which parent contributed the chromosome. If an individual has a deletion of this region on the maternal chromosome 15, paternal uniparental disomy of the number 15 chromosomes (with no number 15 chromosome from the mother), or a defective imprinting mechanism, DNA methylation studies will be abnormal and indicate AS. This test detects the majority (approximately 78%) of cases of AS. Additional studies are then required to determine which of these three mechanisms lead to AS development.

UBE3A mutation analysis

Direct DNA testing of the UBE3A gene is necessary to detect cases of AS caused by mutations in this gene. Cases of AS caused by UBE3A mutations usually have a normal imprinting pattern.

Fluorescent in situ hybridization (FISH)

FISH studies may be necessary to detect chromosome rearrangements that disrupt the 15q11-q13 region on the maternal copy of chromosome 15. The FISH method is a special way of checking for the presence, absence, or rearrangement of very small

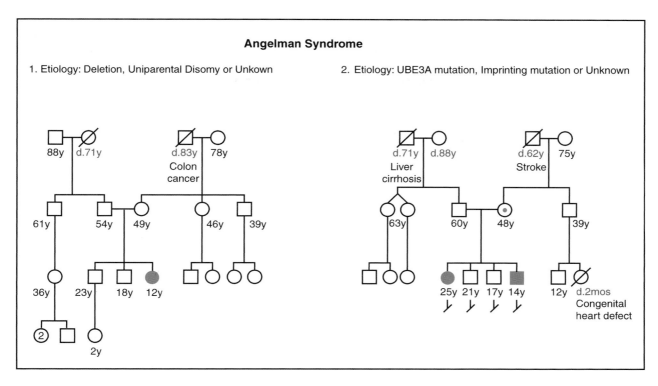

Angelman Syndrome

1. Etiology: Deletion, Uniparental Disomy or Unkown

2. Etiology: UBE3A mutation, Imprinting mutation or Unknown

(Gale Group.)

pieces of chromosomes. FISH testing can also readily detect AS caused by chromosome deletions, which account for approximately 70% of AS cases. FISH testing is often performed following an abnormal methylation study to determine if a chromosome deletion accounts for the abnormal methylation pattern.

Treatment and management

There is no specific treatment for AS. A variety of symptomatic management strategies may be offered for hyperactivity, seizures, mental retardation, speech impairment, and other medical problems.

The typical hyperactivity in AS may not respond to traditional behavior modification strategies. Children with AS may have a decreased need for sleep and a tendency to awaken during the night. Drug therapy may be prescribed to counteract hyperactivity or aid sleep. Most families make special accommodations for their child by providing a safe yet confining environment.

Seizures in AS are usually controllable with one or more anti-seizure medications. In some individuals with severe seizures, dietary manipulations may be tried in combination with medication.

Children with AS appear to benefit from targeted educational training. Physical and occupational therapy may improve the disordered, unbalanced movements typical of AS. Children with a severe balance disorder may require special supportive chairs. Speech therapy is often directed towards the development of nonverbal communication strategies, such as picture cards, communication boards, or basic signing gestures.

Individuals with AS may be more likely to develop particular medical problems which are treated accordingly. Newborn babies may have difficulty feeding and special bottle nipples or other interventions may be necessary. Gastroesophageal reflux (heartburn) may lead to vomiting or poor weight gain and may be treated with drugs or surgery. Constipation is a frequent problem and is treated with laxative medications. Many individuals with AS have strabismus (crossed eyes), which may require surgical correction. Orthopedic problems, such as tightening of tendons or **scoliosis**, are common. These problems may be treated with physical therapy, bracing, or surgery.

Prognosis

Individuals with AS have significant mental retardation and speech impairment that are considered to occur in all cases. However, they do have capacity to learn and should receive appropriate educational training.

Young people with AS typically have good physical health aside from seizures. Although life span data are not available, the life span of people with AS is expected to be normal.

Resources

PERIODICALS

"Angelman syndrome." *The Exceptional Parent* 30, no. 3 (March 2000): S2.

Lombroso, Paul J. "Genetics of Childhood Disorders: XVI. Angelman Syndrome: A Failure to Process." *Journal of the American Academy of Child and Adolescent Psychiatry* 39, no. 7 (July 2000): 931.

ORGANIZATION

Angelman Syndrome Foundation, Inc. 414 Plaza Drive, Suite 209, Westmont, IL 60559. (800) IF-ANGEL or (630) 734-9267. Fax: (630) 655-0391. Info@angelman.org. <http://www.angelman.org>.

WEBSITES

Williams, Charles A., M.D., Amy C. Lossie, Ph.D., and Daniel J. Driscoll, Ph.D. "Angelman Syndrome." (November 21, 2000). *GeneClinics.* University of Washington, Seattle. <http://www.geneclinics.org/profiles/angelman/details>.

Jennifer Ann Roggenbuck, MS, CGC

Ankylosing spondylitis

Definition

Ankylosing spondylitis (AS) is a relatively common disease that causes inflammation of the area where ligaments and tendons insert into the bone. The inflammatory process eventually leads to reduced mobility or immobility of affected joints. Specific joints are characteristically involved, notably in the spine and pelvis.

Description

Ankylosing spondylitis belongs to a group of disorders called the seronegative spondyloarthropathies. Each disease in this group is characterized by arthritis affecting the spine, as well as the absence of rheumatoid factor, a diagnostic marker that is present in **rheumatoid arthritis** and helps distinguish it from the group of diseases that includes AS. AS affects primarily the spine and the sacroiliac joint where the spine meets the hips. Progressive symptoms eventually result in fusion of these joints, pain, and markedly decreased joint mobility. AS is considered an autoimmune disease, meaning that symptoms are the result of the action of the immune system of the body against its own tissues. Although the exact mode of action is unknown, there is a strong association of AS with a specific type of human leukocyte antigen, HLA-B27. HLA are genetically-determined proteins that play an important role in the functioning of the immune response of the body, in that they enable the immune system to distinguish between its own cells and foreign cells. Therefore, HLA type is important in immunity, as well as organ and tissue transplantation.

Genetic profile

AS is considered a multifactorial disorder, or one that is the result of both genetic and environmental factors interacting. Two genes have been identified that confer susceptibility to AS, both of which are forms of an HLA **gene** on **chromosome** 6. Some HLA types have been implicated in various autoimmune diseases, meaning diseases in which the immune system attacks the body's own cells and tissues.

The association of HLA B-27 and AS has been clearly established. Ninety-five percent of individuals with AS are B-27 positive, and since AS appears to be a dominant trait, the presence of at least one B-27 allele (a form of the gene) confers a greatly increased chance of developing symptoms. While this population risk may seem relatively high, it is important to realize that only about 9% of the population carries the B-27 allele. Of these individuals who are B-27 positive, only 2-8% will develop AS.

Other environmental and genetic factors most certainly contribute to development of the disease. This becomes more evident when considering that B-27 positive individuals with an affected first-degree relative have a significantly higher chance of developing AS than a B-27 positive individual with no family history. In families with multiple affected members, studies estimate that no more than half of AS recurrence is explained by HLA type. Additionally, there are several B-27 subtypes that have been studied; some confer susceptibility and some do not. Importantly, about 5% of people with AS are B-27 negative. Other environmental and/or genetic factors must certainly be associated with disease in these individuals. Another HLA type—B-60—has also been shown to confer susceptibility, although the association appears to be much weaker and is not seen in all studies. Certain infections are suspected as being necessary for triggering AS in some individuals.

In the future, additional susceptibility genes and environmental factors can be expected to be identified.

Demographics

Approximately 0.25% to 1.5% of the population is affected with AS. Prevalence of the disease is comparable to the frequency of the HLA B-27 allele in the population, which varies among ethnic groups. Native North Americans, Alaskan Eskimos, and Norwegian Lapps all have relatively high levels of B-27 and AS. Low levels of B-27 and AS occur among individuals of most types of African ancestry, Australian aborigines, and Native South Americans. Generally, for every affected female, there are two to three affected males.

Signs and symptoms

The signs of AS vary, but a typical case involves progressive lower back pain and morning stiffness. The immune response at the point where the ligaments or tendons insert into the bones initially causes bone inflammation and fragility, followed by fibrosis, meaning the formation of fiber tissue. The area reacts by forming new bone, which eventually fuses, limiting motion. AS can also affect peripheral joints in a manner similar to other types of arthritis. The vertebral joints of everyone with AS are affected, and 50% of people will also have significant hip arthritis. **Osteoporosis** in advanced AS commonly results in fractures of the spine.

AS also affects areas other than the bones and joints. An eye complication called *anterior uveitis*, which is easily treated and generally does not affect vision, develops in 5-35% of people with AS. Rarely, the disease may affect the heart or aorta. Kidney failure is a rare complication. Lung function can be affected due to bone changes that affect the mechanics of breathing. Therefore, individuals with AS should refrain from smoking to avoid early respiratory failure. Ninety percent of affected individuals experience the first symptoms before age 45. Males are more commonly affected than females, who tend to be diagnosed later partly due to milder symptoms.

Diagnosis

Diagnostic criteria were established by the European Spondyloarthropathy Study Group in the early 1990s. A clinical diagnosis of AS requires the presence of spinal pain caused by inflammation or inflammation of the membrane surrounding the joints, which can be either asymmetric or involving primarily the lower limbs. One or more of the following conditions must also be present:

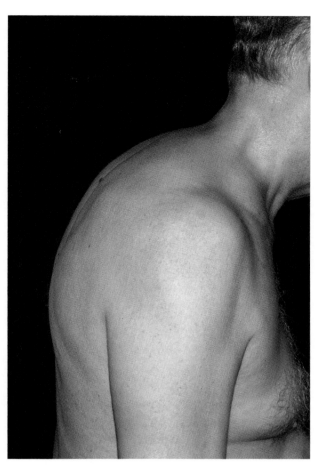

This 68-year old man has developed an outward curvature of his spine as a result of ankylosing spondylitis. Decreased mobility results as pain and stiffness of the joints between spinal vertebrae progresses. *(Photo Researchers, Inc.)*

- family history of AS
- sacroiliitis (inflammation of the sacroiliac joint) demonstrated by x ray
- acute diarrhea within one month before the appearance of symptoms
- inflammatory bowel disease
- psoriasis (a scaly skin disease)
- urethritis (inflammation of the urethra)
- cervicitis (inflammation of the cervix)
- alternating buttock pain
- enthesopathy (disorder of the ligament attachment to the bone)

This diagnostic description has close to an 87% sensitivity, meaning that 87% of those with AS are picked up using this description. Conversely, 13% of those with

KEY TERMS

Ankylosis—Immobility of a joint due to the formation of new bone at the site of inflammation.

Cervicitis—Inflammation of the cervix.

Enthesitis—Inflammation at the place where the ligaments insert into the bone.

Enthesopathy—Disorder of the ligament attachment to the bone.

HLA-B27—Stands for a specific form of human leukocyte antigen, the proteins involved in immune system function. Strongly associated with ankylosing spondylitis.

Human leukocyte antigens (HLA)—Proteins that help the immune system function, in part by helping it to distinguish "self" from "non-self."

Magnetic resonance imaging (MRI)—A technique that employs magnetic fields and radio waves to create detailed images of internal body structures and organs, including the brain.

Osteoporosis—Loss of bone density that can increase the risk of fractures.

Psoriasis—A common, chronic, scaly skin disease.

Rheumatoid arthritis—Chronic, autoimmune disease marked by inflammation of the membranes surrounding joints.

Rheumatoid factor—Antibodies present in the majority of individuals with rheumatoid arthritis. A diagnostic marker for rheumatoid arthritis that is absent from ankylosing spondylitis and other seronegative spondyloarthopathies.

Sacroiliac joint—The joint between the triangular bone below the spine (sacrum) and the hip bone (ilium).

Sacroiliitis—Inflammation of the sacroiliac joint.

Sensitivity—The proportion of people with a disease who are correctly diagnosed (test positive based on diagnostic criteria). The higher the sensitivity of a test or diagnostic criteria, the lower the rate of "false negatives," people who have a disease but are not identified through the test.

Specificity—The proportion of people without a disease who are correctly classified as healthy or not having the disease (test negative based on diagnostic criteria). The higher the specificity of a test or diagnostic criteria, the lower the number of "false positives," people who don't have a disease but who test positive.

Sponyloarthritis (spondylitis)—Inflammatory disease of the joints of the spine.

Urethritis—Inflammation of the urethra.

Uveitis—Inflammation of all or part of the uvea, which consists of the middle vascular portion of the eye including the iris, ciliary body, and choroid.

AS will not be identified as having the disease based on this description. The description has a specificity that is also approximately 87%, meaning that 87% of the time a person classified as having AS actually has AS, as opposed to another disease or no disease. Conversely, about 13% of the time this description will incorrectly classify someone who actually has a different disease as having AS.

This is a challenging diagnosis to make correctly. Testing for HLA B-27 can improve diagnosis by confirming specificity. In other words, when it looks like someone has AS based on the above description of conditions, a positive B-27 test will make the physician more certain that person is a true positive for AS. As imaging of the sacroiliac joint improves through the use of a technology called *magnetic resonance imaging (MRI)*, diagnosis of AS may also improve. Although, diagnosing a person with AS prior to the development of signs seen on x ray or MRI will continue to be very difficult.

Treatment and management

Phyical therapy plays a major role in maintaining flexibility, range-of motion, posture, and ultimately mobility. Surgery can improve joint function, as well as minimize associated pain, which may be treated with nonsteroidal anti-inflammatory medications. Other medications—sulfasalazine and methotrexate—can provide some relief for peripheral arthritis. Cycloplegics (medications that paralyze the ciliary muscle of the eye) and local steroids are effective at treating anterior uveitis. Rare complications are treated depending on their symptoms. Avoidance of smoking is encouraged to maintain lung function.

Prognosis

For most affected individuals, treatment and management is successful at maintaining quality of life. Quality can be significantly impacted, however, for the occasional individual with a severe, progressive course of the disease. Vision can be affected in some individuals with anterior uveitis that is not responsive to treatment, but this is rare. The rare complication of kidney failure can limit life-expectancy, as can respiratory failure that may result from smoking.

Resources

BOOKS

Wordsworth, P., and M. Brown. "Rheumatoid arthritis and allied inflammatory arthropathies." In *Emery and Rimoin's Principles and Practice of Medical Genetics.* 3rd ed. D. L. Rimoin, J. M. Connor, and R. E. Pyeritz, editors. New York: Churchill Livingston, 1997, pp. 2751–2771.

PERIODICALS

Benjamin, R., and P. Parham. "Guilt by association: HLA-B27 and ankylosing spondylitis." *Immunology Today* 11 (1990): 137–43.

Thomson, G. "HLA disease associations: models for the study of complex human genetic disorders." *Critical Reviews in Clinical Laboratory Sciences* 32 (1995): 183–219.

WEBSITES

"Arthritis associated with spondylitis." *The Merck Manual* <http://www.merck.com/pubs/mmanual/section5/chapter51/51a.htm>.

Spondylitis Association of America. (800) 777-8189. <http://www.spondylitis.org>.

Jennifer Denise Bojanowski, MS, CGC

Anxiety neurosis *see* **Panic disorder**

Apert syndrome

Definition

Premature closure of the skull bones leading to facial distortion with an unusually tall skull and fusion of the fingers and toes, known as syndactyly, are the major features of Apert syndrome (AS). Another name for this disorder is acrocephalysyndactyly.

Description

A French physician E. Apert first reported in 1906 the syndrome that bears his name. He detailed the skull malformation, midface hypoplasia (underdevelopment) and the hand abnormalities. The hand appears mitten-shaped because of the finger fusion. Intelligence varies from normal to severe mental retardation.

Genetic profile

Apert syndrome (AS) is an autosomal dominant disorder, meaning that a person only has to inherit one non-working copy of the **gene** to manifest the condition. In most cases, AS is sporadic meaning that the parents are usually unaffected, but a fresh mutation or gene change occurring in the egg or sperm was passed onto the affected child. For these families the chance to have another affected child is very low. An affected parent has a 50% chance of passing on the abnormal gene to their child, who will then also have Apert syndrome.

Two unique mutations in the fibroblast growth factor receptor 2 (FGFR2) gene located on **chromosome** 10 were discovered in 1995. This gene directs the development of bone formation. When parental studies were performed, genetic researchers determined that the father passed on the gene causing AS and was usually older than 30 years. No explanation has been found for this unusual finding.

After comparing the physical findings with **gene mutations** causing AS, researchers noted that one mutation resulted in a much more improved facial appearance after corrective surgery. The other mutation produced a more severe form of syndactyly.

Demographics

Apert syndrome has been estimated to occur in one of every 60,000-160,000 births. All races and both sexes are equally affected.

Signs and symptoms

At birth the craniofacial (pertaining to the skull and face) appearance is striking. Early or premature closure of the skull sutures (layer of fibrous tissue connecting the skull bones) makes the skull grow taller than normal with a short distance from the front to the back of the head. Always it is the coronal suture connecting the frontal and parietal bones that fuses early. The buildup of pressure on the brain is minimal because the fontanelles, or soft spots, and midline of the skull remain open. Due to the small space within the eye sockets, the eyeballs bulge outward and to the side. Also, the eyelids have a downward slant and cannot completely close.

From the middle of the eye sockets to the upper jaw, the face is sunken in or concave when viewed from the profile. This midfacial hypoplasia causes the upper jaw to slope backward pushing the lower teeth in front of the back teeth.

The mouth area has a prominent mandible (lower jaw), down-turned corners, high arched palate, cleft pal-

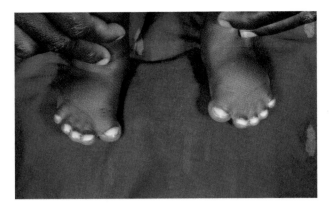

Webbing of the toes is a characteristic sign of Apert syndrome. *(Custom Medical Stock Photo, Inc.)*

ate (an opening in the roof of the mouth), crowded upper teeth, poor contact between the upper and lower teeth, delayed tooth eruption.

Syndactyly of the fingers and toes involves not only soft tissues but also the bones, nerves, and tendons. Flexing of the fingers and toes after the first digit is not usually possible. The thumb can be unattached or fused to the other fingers. Also, the other fingers may or may not be fused to each other in varying degrees. Fusion of the toes is less worrisome. Correction only becomes necessary when walking is difficult.

Most children with AS are noisy breathers. The nose and airways leading to the lungs are smaller than usual. These narrow passageways probably make breathing more difficult. At night if breathing is more troublesome, sleep apnea can occur. This stoppage of breathing while sleeping deprives the brain and body of oxygen. Mental impairment can occur as a result of oxygen deprivation.

Excessive sweating is often seen. Researchers do not know why the sweat glands are overactive. As the children reach puberty, they develop excessive acne. A skin specialist or dermatologist can help to control it.

The height and weight of children with AS is usually normal. However, their learning ability can be affected. A small number of children with Apert syndrome will have a normal level of intelligence while the majority will have some degree of mental retardation.

Diagnosis

During the newborn period most babies will be diagnosed after a geneticist examines them. This doctor specializes in diagnosing and explaining hereditary conditions. The unusual facial features and hand syndactyly

are unique to AS. Testing for the mutations known to cause AS should be arranged. If a mutation is found then the diagnosis can be made. When a mutation is not found, the physical findings alone can support the diagnosis.

Occasionally during an ultrasound examination, a fetus shows characteristics suggesting AS. This examination is best done after 16 weeks of pregnancy. Ultrasound is the use of sound waves to create a real time image of the fetus. Unlike x rays, ultrasound is not dangerous and the fetus can be examined for size, viability, and birth defects.

An experienced physician or ultrasound technician performing the examination may detect the caved in profile and syndactyly. More than one examination may be necessary to confirm the findings. If AS is suspected then **genetic testing** can be offered during the pregnancy. The pregnant woman can undergo an **amniocentesis** to obtain fetal cells that can be analyzed for the mutations causing AS. Amniocentesis is the removal of the amniotic fluid surrounding the fetus by inserting a needle through the uterus. Results may take as long as four weeks.

Treatment and management

The best treatment for AS begins at birth with the correct diagnosis. To provide better care, a craniofacial team should be involved. With the team approach all the specialists are in one center to minimize the number of appointments and corrective surgeries. More important, this team consists of specialists who understand the complex problems of AS and the family's concerns. Included on this team are a craniofacial surgeon, neurosurgeon, otolaryngologist (specialist of the ears, nose, and throat), ophthalmologist (eye specialist), orthodontist, speech therapist, and psychologist. A pediatric nurse, geneticist or genetic counselor, and social worker may also be part of the team during the first few years of the child's life. Many major medical centers will have a craniofacial team or the family can be referred to one.

Working together the craniofacial surgeon and neurosurgeon perform the multiple surgeries to reshape the tower skull. They reopen the prematurely closed sutures between the skull bones and then pull the front of the skull forward to create space within it and enlarge the eye orbits. Average age for these operations is about 4-8 months.

From ages five to nine the child will undergo a surgical procedure called a midface advancement. This technique will correct the concave profile that becomes

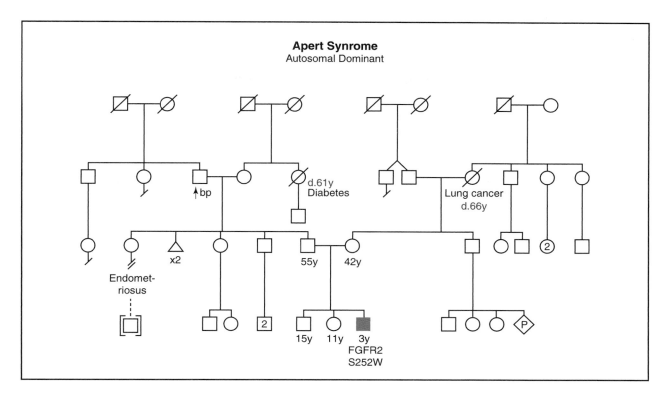

Apert Synrome
Autosomal Dominant

(Gale Group.)

pronounced because the upper and lower face grow normally while the middle of the face grows slowly. Corrective facial surgeries continue until the early adult years when growth is finally completed.

The neurosurgeon may perform the operations to unfuse and straighten the fingers. However, a completely normal hand cannot be created.

Frequent ear infections can decrease a child's hearing level. The otolaryngologist can monitor the hearing. Sometimes tiny plastic tubes are placed in the ears to prevent hearing loss from repeated infections.

The abnormal placement of the eyes and its muscles can sometimes prevent a child from looking straight ahead with both eyes. An ophthalmologist should examine the eyes regularly and correct a muscle imbalance of the eyes with surgery.

An orthodontist (dentist who specializes in correcting misaligned teeth) monitors the teeth because the abnormal jaw structure causes poor development and placement. An oral surgeon may correct the misalignment of the teeth. Proper positioning of the teeth improves speech and facial appearance.

Speech and language delay can result from decreased hearing and an unusual jaw shape. A speech

therapist works with the child to develop language skills through simple exercises.

The facial appearance of Apert syndrome can have a devastating emotional effect on the child and family. Support from a psychologist (a specialist in science of the mind) can help the child develop a positive self-image and help parents cope with feelings of guilt. Often parents will blame themselves for a child's condition even they in no way caused it or could have prevented it. The multiple doctors' visits and surgeries can create undue stress as well.

During the many hospitalizations, a pediatric nurse will care for the child. This nurse has received specialized training in the treatment of children with craniofacial disorders. Also, the nurse may introduce the child to the hospital.

Diagnosis of Apert syndrome will usually be made by the geneticist. The family will discuss with the genetic counselor how AS is inherited and the chance for future children to be affected.

Having a child with AS can place a tremendous financial strain on the family. A social worker gives the family important information about medical coverage. This person can also help coordinate medical care and special education services.

KEY TERMS

Amniocentesis—A procedure performed at 16-18 weeks of pregnancy in which a needle is inserted through a woman's abdomen into her uterus to draw out a small sample of the amniotic fluid from around the baby. Either the fluid itself or cells from the fluid can be used for a variety of tests to obtain information about genetic disorders and other medical conditions in the fetus.

Cleft palate—A congenital malformation in which there is an abnormal opening in the roof of the mouth that allows the nasal passages and the mouth to be improperly connected.

Craniofacial—Relating to or involving both the head and the face.

Dermatologist—A physician that specializes in disorders of the skin.

Fontanelle—One of several "soft spots" on the skull where the developing bones of the skull have yet to fuse.

Hypoplasia—Incomplete or underdevelopment of a tissue or organ.

Mandible—Lower jaw bone.

Mutation—A permanent change in the genetic material that may alter a trait or characteristic of an individual, or manifest as disease, and can be transmitted to offspring.

Ophthalmologist—A physician specializing in the medical and surgical treatment of eye disorders.

Orthodontist—Dentist who specializes in the correction of misaligned teeth.

Otolaryngologist—Physician who specializes in the care of the ear, nose, and throat and their associated structures.

Psychologist—An individual who specializes in the science of the mind.

Sleep apnea—Temporary cessation of breathing while sleeping.

Speech therapist—Person who specializes in teaching simple exercises to improve speech.

Suture—"Seam" that joins two surfaces together.

Syndactyly—Webbing or fusion between the fingers or toes.

Ultrasound—An imaging technique that uses sound waves to help visualize internal structures in the body.

Prognosis

Many factors affect the prognosis of a child with AS. The age at which the first surgery takes place to create spaces between the skull bones is important. Mental retardation can result from the buildup of pressure on the brain. Having a supportive, loving family environment increases the chances for normal development. Children with complex medical problems who lack a supportive setting often have delayed mental, social, and emotional development.

Although the hands will never be completely normal, surgeries to separate and straighten the fingers can be done. Tasks such as writing and manipulating buttons will be difficult. Adaptive devices in school and home will allow for more independence. Separation of the toes usually does not improve walking but may improve the child's self image.

Persons with AS who have a normal intelligence level can have full, productive lives. Vocational training will help those with borderline intelligence.

Resources

BOOKS

Dufresne, Craig, Benjamin Carson, and James Zinreich. *Complex Craniofacial Problems: A Guide to Analysis and Treatment.* New York, NY: Churchill Livingston, 1992.

Keene Nancy, Rachel Prentice, and Linda Lamb. *Your Child in the Hospital: A Practical Guide for Parents.* Cambridge, MA: O'Reilly and Associates, 1996.

Wilson, Golder N., and Carl W. Cooley. *Preventive Management of Children With Congenital Anomalies and Syndromes* New York, NY: Cambridge University Press, 2000.

PERIODICALS

Chang, C. C., et al. "Prenatal diagnosis of Apert syndrome." *Prenatal Diagnosis* 18 (1998): 621-625.

Ferreira, J. C., et al. "Second-trimester molecular prenatal diagnosis of sporadic Apert syndrome following suspicious ultrasound findings." *Ultrasound in Obstetrics and Gynecology* 14, no. 6 (December 1999): 426-30.

von Gernet, S., et al. "Genotype-phenotype analysis in Apert syndrome suggests opposite effects of the two recurrent mutations on syndactyly and outcome of craniofacial surgery." *Clinical Genetics* 57 (2000): 137-139.

Wilkie, A. O. M., et al. "Apert syndrome results from localized mutations of FGFR2 and is allelic with Crouzon syndrome." *Nature Genetics* 9 (1995): 165-172.

ORGANIZATIONS

Apert Syndrome Support Group. 8708 Kathy, St. Louis, MO 63126. (314) 965-3356.

Children's Craniofacial Association. PO Box 280297, Dallas, TX 75243-4522. (972) 994-9902 or (800) 535-3643. contactcca@ccakids.com. <http://www.ccakids.com>.

National Organization for Rare Disorders (NORD). PO Box 8923, New Fairfield, CT 06812-8923. (203) 746-6518 or (800) 999-6673. Fax: (203) 746-6481. <http://www.rarediseases.org>.

WEBSITES

FriendshipCenter.com. <http://www.friendshipcenter.com>.

Suzanne M. Carter, MS, CGC

Arginase deficiency

Definition

Arginase deficiency is an inborn error of metabolism that results from a defect in the urea cycle. This cycle is a series of biochemical reactions that occur in the body in order to remove ammonia from the bloodstream.

Description

During normal cellular function, proteins are broken down into nitrogen waste products and put into the blood stream as ammonia. The urea cycle transforms this toxin into urea, which can be safely removed by the kidneys as urine. Lack of an enzyme from the urea cycle, such as arginase, can result in the buildup of toxins in the body. There are six diseases that belong in the group of **urea cycle disorders**. Arginase is thought to be the rarest of these disorders.

The enzyme arginase is the last step of the urea cycle, where it turns arginine into ornithine and urea. If a person is born with arginase deficiency then they build up arginine in their blood. This is called argininemia. Since earlier steps in the urea cycle are left intact, patients may or may not build up ammonia in the blood. Commonly, the build up of arginine presents as a central nervous system disease or developmental delay in young children.

Genetic profile

Arginase deficiency is an autosomal recessive trait. Thus, both parents of an affected child would have to be carriers of the **gene**. There are two genetically distinct arginases in the human body. The arginase that is expressed in the liver and in red blood cells is the one that is lost in arginase deficiency. This gene has been mapped to the long arm of **chromosome** 6, specifically

6q23. Twenty different mutations have been found in patients with the disease.

Demographics

Like other autosomal recessive diseases, arginase deficiency remains rare. The first signs of this disease tend to occur while the patient is still very young. A child may have a normal birth, infancy, and may not show any signs of the disease for quite a few years. There is no gender or racial difference (men and women are both as likely to have the disease), but its absolute incidence rate cannot be known, due its rarity and the lack of statistics. Its incidence is well below one per 200,000.

Signs and symptoms

The onset of this disease tends to be subtle. While the first symptoms of this disease show up while the patient is still a baby, some infants are said to be normal before beginning to have the symptoms. In many cases, the disease is not found at first, and the child is labeled as having "cerebral palsy" (a general term for neurologic problems that result in altered development—often starting at birth). The symptoms include: loss of normal developmental milestones (the child does not perform tasks at the usual age—walking and speaking, for example); poor feeding; not being able to eat proteins (i.e. a high protein meal makes symptoms worse); fussy behavior; lessened alertness; choreoathetotic movements (strange, uncontrollable writhing movements of limbs); spasticity of lower limbs (weakness and stiffness of legs); poor coordination; tremors; seizures; and mental retardation. Affected children may also have an enlarged liver from the buildup of toxins.

Diagnosis

Diagnosis is made after children present with symptoms. The illness should be thought for children who have both a developmental delay and stiffness of the ankles and legs that interfere with walking. It should also be thought of anytime that other urea cycle disorders are considered. The lab test of choice is to measure arginase activity in red blood cells. If patients are truly deficient then they will have below normal activity levels. In patients in which there is a high chance of disease and only mildly elevated levels of arginine in the blood, more testing should be done. In other urea cycle disorders, patients tend to have hyperammonemia (a high amount of ammonia in the blood), but in arginase deficiency the ammonia levels are rarely raised. No prenatal diagnosis is currently done. If patients have one child with this disease, then they can be counseled about risk of disease in future children. Since this disease is

PERIODICALS

Lindor, Noralane, et al., "Initial Assessment of Infants and Children With Suspected Inborns Errors of Metabolism" *Mayo Clinical Proceedings* 70, no. 10 (October 1995): 987-988.

Scheuerle, Angela, et al., "Arginase Deficiency Presenting as Cerebral Palsy" *Pediatrics* 91, no. 5 (May 1993): 995-996.

WEBSITES

Roth, Karl. "Arginase Deficiency from Pediatrics/Genetics and Metabolic Disease." *eMedicine.* <http://www.emedicine.com/ped/GENETICS_AND_METABOLIC_DISEASE.htm.>.

Benjamin M. Greenberg

KEY TERMS

Autosomal recessive—A pattern of genetic inheritance where two abnormal genes are needed to display the trait or disease.

Urea cycle disorder—A disease that is caused by a lack of an enzyme that cleans the blood of ammonia.

inherited in an autosomal recessive pattern, each time carrier parents have a child there is a 25% chance that they will have an affected child.

Treatment and management

Treatment of arginase deficiency is similar to treatment methods for other urea cycle disorders. One would want to decrease, as much as one could, the amount of arginine that is building up. This is done through control of protein intake in foods. Arginine is one of the twenty amino acids that make up proteins, and if its intake is stopped, then the amount that can build up in a patient will be lessened. Supplements of essential amino acids (amino acids that cannot be made by the body and must be obtained through food) are given so that children do not become ill from malnourishment.

Other symptoms can also be controlled. For example, patients who have seizures should be treated with an anti-seizure medication. Also, physical therapy can be helpful for patients with stiff legs and problems walking.

Prognosis

The long-term effects of arginase deficiency are better than that for other urea cycle disorders. With proper food intake, children can have much milder symptoms. Often, though, the disease is not found until after severe problems have occurred. Data about patients that live until they are adults is limited, but many cases of patients living through teenage years have been reported. Hence, prognosis is clearly related to how early the disease can be found. This means that it is a very good idea for children to get tested when this group of symptoms are present.

Resources

BOOKS

Behrman, Richard, et al. *Nelson Textbook of Pediatrics.* Philadelphia, Pennsylvania: W. B. Saunders Company, 2000.

Argininemia *see* **Arginase deficiency**

Arnold-Chiari malformation

Definition

Arnold-Chiari malformation is a rare genetic disorder. In this syndrome, some parts of the brain are formed abnormally. Malformations may occur in the lower portion of the brain (cerebellum) or in the brain stem. Doctors are not sure of the cause of Arnold-Chiari malformation.

Description

A German pathologist named Arnold-Chiari was the first to describe Arnold-Chiari malformation in 1891. Normally, the brain stem and cerebellum are located in the posterior fossa, an area at the base of the skull attached to the spinal cord. In Arnold-Chiari malformation, the posterior fossa does not form properly. Because the posterior fossa is small, the brain stem, cerebellum, or cerebellar brain tissues (called the cerebellar tonsils) are squeezed downward through an opening at the bottom of the skull. The cerebellum and/or the brain stem may extend beyond the skull or protrude into the spinal column. The displaced tissues may obstruct the flow of cerebrospinal fluid (CSF), the substance that flows around the brain and spinal cord. CSF nourishes the brain and spinal cord.

Although this malformation is present at birth, there may not be any symptoms of a problem until adulthood. For this reason, Arnold-Chiari malformation is often not

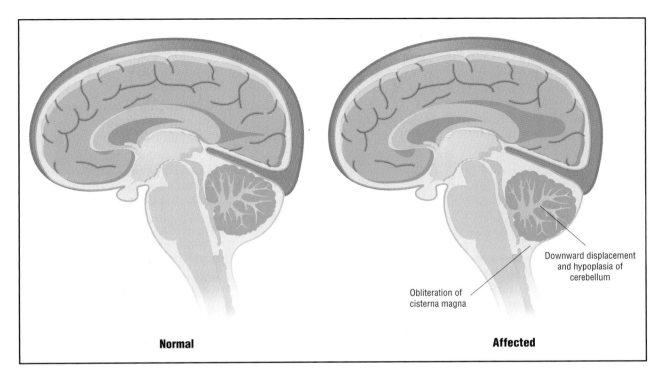

Normal

Affected

Downward displacement and hypoplasia of cerebellum

Obliteration of cisterna magna

A characteristic change that occurs in patients with Arnold-Chiari syndrome, type II, is the downward positioning of the cerebellum. This displacement destroys the area of the cisterna magna. *(Gale Group.)*

diagnosed until adulthood. Women have a higher incidence of this disorder than men.

Other names for Arnold-Chiari malformation are Arnold-Chiari malformation, Arnold-Chiari syndrome, herniation of the cerebellar tonsils, and cerebellomedullary malformation syndrome. When doctors diagnose Arnold-Chiari malformation, they classify the malformation by its severity. A Arnold-Chiari I malformation is the least severe. In a Arnold-Chiari I malformation, the brain extends into the spinal canal. Doctors measure the length of brain stem located in the spinal canal to further define the malformation.

A type II malformation is more severe than a type I. It is almost always linked with a type of **spina bifida**. A sac protrudes through an abnormal opening in the spinal column. The sac is called a myelomeningocele. It may be filled with part of the spinal cord, spinal membranes, or spinal fluid. Unlike many cases of Arnold-Chiari I malformation, Arnold-Chiari II malformation is diagnosed in childhood. Doctors have identified Arnold-Chiari III and IV malformations, but they are very rare.

Arnold-Chiari malformations may occur with other conditions. There may be excessive fluid in the brain (**hydrocephalus**), opening in the spine (spina bifida), or excessive fluid in the spinal cord (syringomyelia), but many people with Arnold-Chiari malformations do not have other medical problems.

Genetic profile

Doctors have not yet found the **gene** responsible for Arnold-Chiari malformations. There has not yet been a study that shows whether or not this disorder is inherited, but there are reports of several families where more than one family member has a Arnold-Chiari malformation.

Scientists do not know what causes Arnold-Chiari malformations. One hypothesis is that the base of the skull is too small, forcing the cerebellum downward. Another theory focuses on overgrowth in the cerebellar region. The overgrowth pushes the cerebellum downward into the spinal canal.

Demographics

Arnold-Chiari malformations are rare. There is no data that shows the incidence of Arnold-Chiari malformations. Arnold-Chiari malformations are the most common type of malformation of the cervico-medullary junction, the area where the brain and spine connect. About one percent of live newborns have a malformation in the cervico-medullary junction.

KEY TERMS

Cerebrospinal fluid—Fluid that circulates throughout the cerebral ventricles and around the spinal cord within the spinal canal.

Cervico-medullary junction—The area where the brain and spine connect.

Hydrocephalus—The excess accumulation of cerebrospinal fluid around the brain, often causing enlargement of the head.

Magnetic Resonance Imaging (MRI)—A technique that employs magnetic fields and radio waves to create detailed images of internal body structures and organs, including the brain.

Myelomeningocele—A sac that protrudes through an abnormal opening in the spinal column.

Posterior fossa—Area at the base of the skull attached to the spinal cord.

Spina bifida—An opening in the spine.

Syringomyelia—Excessive fluid in the spinal cord.

Signs and symptoms

Some people with Arnold-Chiari I malformations have no symptoms. Typically, with a Arnold-Chiari I malformation symptoms appear as the person reaches the third or fourth decade of life. Symptoms of this disorder vary. Most symptoms arise from the pressure on the cranial nerves or brain stem. The symptoms may be vague or they may resemble symptoms of other medical problems, so diagnosis may be delayed.

One of the most common symptoms of Arnold-Chiari malformations is a headache. The headache generally begins in the neck or base of the skull and may radiate through the back of the head. Coughing, sneezing, or bending forward may bring on these headaches. The headaches can last minutes or hours and may be linked with nausea.

There may be pain in the neck or upper arm with Arnold-Chiari malformations. Patients often report more pain on one side, rather than equal pain on both sides. There may also be weakness in the arm or hand. Patients may also report tingling, burning, numbness, or pins and needles. Balance can be affected as well. A person may be unsteady on their feet or lean to one side.

Some people with Arnold-Chiari malformation may have difficulty swallowing. They may say that food "catches" in their throat when they swallow. Another common complaint linked with Arnold-Chiari malformations is hoarseness.

People with Arnold-Chiari malformations may have visual problems, including blurred vision, double vision, or blind spots. There may be bobbing of the eyes.

Diagnosis

A Arnold-Chiari malformation is diagnosed with magnetic resonance imaging (MRI). An MRI uses magnetism and radio waves to produce a picture of the brain and show the crowding of the space between the brain and spinal cord that occurs with Arnold-Chiari malformations. In addition to an MRI, patients will also have a thorough neurologic examination.

Treatment and management

The recommended treatment for a Arnold-Chiari I malformation is surgery to relieve the pressure on the cerebellar area. During the surgery, the surgeon removes a small part of the bone at the base of skull. This enlarges and decompresses the posterior fossa. This opening is patched with a piece of natural tissue. In some people with Arnold-Chiari malformation, displaced brain tissue affects the flow of cerebrospinal fluid. Doctors may evaluate the flow of cerebrospinal fluid during surgery for Arnold-Chiari malformation. If they find that brain tissue is blocking the flow of cerebrospinal fluid, they will shrink the brain tissue during surgery.

Prognosis

Long-term prognosis for persons with Arnold-Chiari I malformations is excellent. Full recovery from surgery may take several months. During that time, patients may continue to experience some of the symptoms associated with Arnold-Chiari malformations.

Prognosis for Arnold-Chiari II malformations depends on the severity of the myelomeningocele and will be equivalent to that of spina bifida.

Resources

ORGANIZATIONS

American Syringomelia Project. PO Box 1586, Longview, Texas 75606-1586. (903)236-7079.

National Organization for Rare Disorders (NORD). PO Box 8923, New Fairfield, CT 06812-8923. ((203) 746-6518 or (800) 999-6673. Fax: (203) 746-6481. <http://www.raredisease.org>.

World Arnold-Chiari malformation Association. 31 Newton Woods Road, Newton Square, Philadelphia, PA19073. <http://presenter.com?~wacma/milhorat.htm>.

Lisa A. Fratt

Arteriohepatic dysplasia (AHD) *see* **Alagille syndrome**

Arthrogryposis multiplex congenita

Definition

Arthrogryposis multiplex congenita (AMC) is a term used to describe the presence of two or more (multiplex) joint contractures (arthrogryposis) present at birth (congenita). A joint contracture is a limitation of the normal range of motion of a joint.

Description

There are at least 21 recognized forms of AMC. Ten of these fall into a category called the distal arthrogryposes. Four of these are syndromes that include AMC as a set of symptoms. Each involves at least two joint contractures evident from birth. None of the AMC disorders are progressive, meaning the symptoms do not worsen with age.

Distal arthrogryposis (DAs) are all characterized by contractures of the fingers and toes. Each type can be distinguished by specific characteristics:

- Type 1a DA: club feet that point inward and down (talipes equinovarus).

- Type 2 DA: down slanting of the opening between the upper and lower eyelids (palpebral fissures), a small mouth with pursed lips and malformations of the nose that cause a whistling appearance upon breathing, a curvature of the spine (**scoliosis**), and some instances of mild developmental retardation. Type 2b DA, is characterized by those characteristics of type 2 DA accompanied by earlobes that are attached to the skin of the face and a permanent bending (flexion) of one or more fingers (camptodactyly).

- Type 3 DA: talipes equinovarus, camptodactyly, short stature, and vertebral abnormalities.

- Type 4 DA: short stature, an abnormally short neck, immobile facial expressions, camptodactyly, and the lack of the normal prominent creases (flexion creases) on the palms of the hands.

- Type 5 DA: contractures of the arms and legs, limited eye movement, deep set eyes, and abnormal coloring of the retina of the eye.

- Type 6 DA: camptodactyly, an abnormally small head (microcephaly), and hearing loss caused by an abnor-

mality of the auditory nerve (sensorineural hearing loss).

- Type 7 DA: camptodactyly when an affected individual attempts to open the hand, short stature, abnormally short muscles in the legs, and an inability to open the mouth completely (trismus).

- Type 8 DA: contractures of the wrist and/or ankles, short stature, and scoliosis.

- Type 9 DA: lack of muscle tone and development, abnormally low shoulder-to-shoulder width to body height ratio (marfanoid habitus), severe outward curvature of the spine in the neck and upper back (kyphoscoliosis), and contractures of the hips and shoulders.

The most serious forms of DA are types 6 and 9.

Signs and symptoms

The four syndromes that include arthrogryposis as a set of symptoms are cerebrooculofacioskeletal syndrome, adducted thumb-clubfoot syndrome, **Saethre-Chotzen syndrome**, and arthropathy-camptodactyly-pericarditis syndrome. Cerebrooculofacioskeletal (COFS) syndrome is characterized by an abnormally small head (microcephaly), a lack of muscle tone (hypotonia), eye defects, abnormally large ears and nose, a receding chin (micrognathia), and kyphoscoliosis. Adducted thumb-clubfoot syndrome is characterized by **clubfoot** (equinovarus talipes), clasped (adducted) thumbs, abnormally long fingers and toes (arachnodactyly), a prominent forehead, and psychomotor delay. Saethre-Chotzen syndrome is characterized by flattened facial features, wide set eyes (hypertelorism), abnormalities of the skull (**craniosynostosis**), abnormalities of the eyes, partially fused fingers or toes (syndactyly), congenital heart defects, and contractures of the elbows and knees. Arthropathy-camptodactyly-pericarditis syndrome is characterized by contractures of the elbows, wrists, and fingers; an abnormally elevated generalized stiffness upon waking; arthritis of the hips, shoulders, elbows, and knees; and, inflammation of the membranous sac that protects the heart (pericarditis).

The other forms of AMC include three relatively common forms: X-linked arthrogryposis, neurogenic arthrogryposis, **amyoplasia**; and four extremely rare forms that may or may not represent distinct disorders: spondylospinal thoracic dysostosis, Jarcho-Levin syndrome, prenatal growth retardation with pelvic hypolasia and arthrogryposis in the lower limbs, and lethal congenital contracture syndrome.

X-linked arthrogryposis is generally mild and affects only the legs. Neurogenic arthrogryposis is also relatively mild and affects only the elbows and the knees. Amyoplasia is the mildest form of arthrogryposis; it is generally sporadic in appearance. Amyoplasia is characterized by contractures of the wrists, elbows, and knees; club feet, and an abnormal internal rotation of the shoulders.

Spondylospinal thoracic dysostosis is characterized by a short, curved spine; a short neck; malformations of the bones of the mouth; abnormal ribs; and congenital heart defects. Jarcho-Levin syndrome is characterized by many of the same characteristics of spondylospinal thoracic dysostosis. These two disorders differ only in the presence of a fusion of certain spinal vertebrae in spondylospinal thoracic dysostosis that has not been observed in Jarcho-Levin syndrome. Prenatal growth retardation with pelvic hypoplasia and arthrogryposis in the lower limbs has only been described in a pair of sisters and four males and one female, all of whom were siblings. It seems likely that this disorder is one of the distal arthrogryposes. Lethal congenital contracture syndrome almost inevitably leads to prenatal death prior to week 32 of gestation. It appears to be a unique variant of AMC.

Genetic profile

Various forms of arthrogryposis have been traced to a variety of **gene mutations**. Type 1a DA has been linked as a non-sex linked (autosomal) dominant trait caused by a mutation on the short arm of **chromosome** 9 at location 9p21-q21. Type 2 DA has not been localized to a particular chromosome and it is not clear how this disorder is transmitted. Type 2b DA has been linked to an autosomal dominant trait caused by a mutation on a **gene** localized to the short arm of chromosome 11, specifically 11p15.5. Types 3, 4, 5, 6, 7, and 8 DA have also not been localized to specific genes, but are presumed to be autosomal dominant traits. Type 8 DA may also be transmitted as a recessive or an X-linked disorder. Type 9 DA has been linked to an autosomal dominant gene on the long arm of chromosome 5, localized to 5q23-q31.

Cerebrooculofacioskeletal syndrome is an autosomal recessive trait caused by a mutation on a gene that has been localized to the long arm of chromosome 10, 10q11 specifically. Adducted thumb-clubfoot syndrome has DA that has not been localized to a particular chromosome but it is transmitted through a recessive trait. Saethre-Chotzen syndrome has been linked to an autosomal dominant trait caused by a mutation in the TWIST gene that has been localized to 7p21 on the short arm of chromosome 7. Arthropathy-camptodactyly-pericarditis syndrome has been linked to an autosomal recessive trait caused by a mutation on a gene that has been localized to the long arm of chromosome 1 at 1q25-q31.

X-linked arthrogryposis is an X-linked trait caused by a mutation on a gene that has been localized to Xp11.3-p11.2. Neurogenic arthrogryposis has been linked to both an X-linked trait and a trait caused by a gene mutation on the long arm of chromosome 5. Amyoplasia is usually sporadic and any genetic cause of this type of arthrogryposis is in doubt though vascular disruptions have been postulated. A genetic cause of spondylospinal thoracic dysostosis has not been identified. Jarcho-Levin syndrome has been linked to an autosomal recessive trait caused by a gene mutation on chromosome 19, localized to 19q13. Lethal congenital contracture syndrome has been linked to an autosomal recessive trait caused by a mutation on a gene localized to 9q34 on chromosome 9.

Demographics

Arthrogryposis occurs in approximately one in every 3,000 live births. Most cases of arthrogryposis are caused by a lack normal joint movement during fetal development. For this reason, cases of non-genetic arthrogryposis are more frequent in multiple birth pregnancies than in single birth pregnancies.

Most forms of arthrogryposis are not known to affect one subpopulation more than another. However, Jarcho-Levin syndrome has been found almost exclusively in people of Puerto Rican decent. All forms of AMC appear to affect males with approximately twice the frequency seen in females.

Diagnosis

The symptoms of AMC are primarily immobility of two or more joints. The most common joints affected are the joints of the fingers and toes. Less commonly affected joints are the knees and elbows, and rarely affected joints are the jaws, hips and shoulders.

A diagnosis of AMC is indicated by the presence of two or more joint contractures present from birth. The symptoms that are present allow the differential diagnosis between one of the forms of distal arthrogryposis, a syndromic form of arthrogryposis, and the other forms of arthrogryposis.

Treatment and management

Physical therapy has proven an effective treatment for almost all forms of AMC. Splints, braces, and removable casts are often used to improve joint positioning. In most cases, these orthopedic devices are used only at night so that proper joint mobility can be encouraged during the waking hours. Occasionally, surgery to repair foot and ankle position may be necessary, especially in the case of talipes equinovarus. Much less frequently, orthopedic surgery of the hips, knees, elbows, shoulders, and wrists is required.

Tendon replacement surgery has also been successful in individuals affected with AMC.

In an informal Internet study on AMC and aging conducted in 2000, one-third of the 100 respondents replied that they had sought alternative therapies for symptoms related to AMC. The most common of these therapies being massage therapy, hydrotherapy, and acupuncture. Massage therapy was reported as providing excellent results for some, but the lack of medical coverage for these therapies combined with their cost prevented many from continuing these treatments. When asked what helped the most in relieving symptoms of AMC, 44% of respondents named pain or anti-inflammatory drugs, both prescription and over-the-counter types. Another 20% mentioned massage, and 18% mentioned heat treatments such as saunas, hot tubs, hot packs, or hot showers and/or baths. Most survey participants noted that if they decreased their physical activity, they felt a loss of both joint mobility and stamina.

Prognosis

In cases of AMC that do not involve complications of the central nervous system, the outlook is quite good. Most individuals can achieve a sufficient range of motion in their affected joints to live healthy, complete lives. AMC is non-progressive, therefore, once a joint contracture has been repaired through physical therapy and/or surgery, it will generally not return to a state of abnormal contracture.

When AMC is complicated by involvement of the central nervous system, approximately half of affected individuals die in infancy. Among the surviving half, many have varying degrees of mental retardation.

The informal Internet survey on AMC and aging conducted in 2000 found that 50% of the 100 respondents could walk without assistance. Twenty-five percent needed braces, canes, and/or crutches, while the remaining 25% used either a scooter or wheelchair. The number of people requiring assistance to walk is expected to decline over time since many of those individuals responding to this survey did not receive medical and physical therapy treatments that are now routinely available to children affected with AMC.

Two-thirds of these survey respondents also stated that they had arthritis or arthritis-like symptoms. An informal causal relationship was also made between those who had rigorous or painful childhood physical therapy and later suffered symptoms of arthritis.

KEY TERMS

Amniotic fluid—The fluid which surrounds a developing baby during pregnancy.

Amyoplasia—The mildest form of arthrogryposis muliplex congenita, characterized by sporadic and recurrent contractures of the wrists, elbows, and knees; club feet, and an abnormal internal rotation of the shoulders.

Arthrogryposis—Abnormal joint contracture.

Camptodactyly—An abnormal permanent bending of one or more fingers or toes.

Cell—The smallest living units of the body which group together to form tissues and help the body perform specific functions.

Contracture—A tightening of muscles that prevents normal movement of the associated limb or other body part.

Distal arthrogryposis—A disorder characterized by contractions of the muscles in the hands.

Flexion—The act of bending or condition of being bent.

Flexion creases—The lines present on the palms of the hands and the soles of the feet from normal bending of these body parts. Some individuals affected with arthrogryposis lack these characteristic lines.

Inheritance pattern—The way in which a genetic disease is passed on in a family.

Marfanoid habitus—An abnormally low weight to height ratio that is sometimes seen in extremely tall and thin people.

Neurologic—Pertaining the nervous system.

Palpebral fissures—The opening between the upper and lower eyelids.

Scoliosis—An abnormal, side-to-side curvature of the spine.

Talipes equinovarus—A type of club-foot characterized by a downward and inward pointing foot.

Trisomy 18—A chromosomal alteration where a child is born with three copies of chromosome number 18 and as a result is affected with multiple birth defects and mental retardation.

Ultrasound evaluation—A procedure which examines the tissue and bone structures of an individual or a developing baby.

Resources

BOOKS

Stahell, L., J. Hall, K. Jaffe, and D. Paholke (eds). *Arthrogryposis: A Text Atlas*. London: Cambridge University Press, 1998.

PERIODICALS

Bamshad, M., L. Jorde, L., and J. Carey. "A revised and extended classification of the distal arthrogryposes." *American Journal of Medical Genetics* (November 1996): 227-81.

Gordon, N. "Arthrogryposis multiplex congenita." *Brain & Development* (October 1998): 507-11.

Hall, J., S. Reed, S., E. Driscoll "Amyoplasia: a common, sporadic condition with congenital contractures." *American Journal of Medical Genetics* (August 1983): 571-90.

ORGANIZATIONS

Arthrogryposis Group (TAG). 1 The Oaks, Gillingham, Dorset, SP8 4SW. UK 01-747-822655. <http://tagonline.org.uk>.

AVENUES National Support Group for Arthrogryposis Multiplex Congenita. PO Box 5192, Sonora, CA 95370. (209) 928-3688. avenues@sonnet.com. <http://www.sonnet.com/avenues>.

WEBSITES

"Arthrogryposis." <http://members.aol.com/amcchat/amcinfo.htm>. (February 23, 2001).

"Entry 108120: Arthrogryposis multiplex congenita, distal, type 1; AMCD1." *OMIM—Online Mendelian Inheritance in Man.* <http://www.ncbi.nlm.nih.gov:80/entrez/dispomim.cgi?id=108120>. (February 23, 2001).

Paul A. Johnson

Arthropathy-camptodactyly syndrome

Definition

Arthropathy-camptodactyly syndrome is a disorder affecting the joints of the fingers. Arthropathy refers to a disease or disorder affecting a joint, and camptodactyly is a congenital condition, meaning present at birth, characterized by the bending of one or more fingers.

Description

In people with arthropathy-camptodactyly syndrome, one or more fingers are bent. Other joints may be affected as well–some children with arthropathy-camptodactyly syndrome also have swollen knees and ankles, and hip pain.

Problems with the pericardium, the sac that surrounds the heart, are also common in children with arthropathy-camptodactyly syndrome. In many cases the pericardium is removed, a surgical procedure called pericardiectomy.

Genetic profile

Arthropathy-camptodactyly syndrome typically occurs in children (both male and female) whose parents are related by blood. In one case, it was determined that the parents of children with arthropathy-camptodactyly syndrome shared the haplotype A1-Bw21. The **gene** map locus 1q24-q25 is also implicated.

Demographics

Cases of arthropathy-camptodactyly syndrome have been diagnosed in Canada, India, Mexico, Newfoundland, Pakistan, Saudi Arabia, and Turkey, as well as in African Americans.

Signs and symptoms

People with arthropathy-camptodactyly syndrome have a bend in the joint of one or more fingers. Other symptoms include swollen knees and ankles, and hip pain.

Inflammation of the sac lining the heart (pericarditis) is another observed symptom, often accompanied by chest pain. The pain is usually sharp, and felt behind the breast bone (sternum).

Diagnosis

Aside from the physical observation of bent fingers, no test is presently available to confirm diagnosis.

Treatment and management

Surgery can correct the bent fingers disorder that characterizes arthropathy-camptodactyly syndrome. Removal of the tendon sheaths in the affected fingers can help keep them mobile. Removal of the membranes surrounding a joint (synovectomy) of other body joints, such as knees, can also help maintain mobility.

In at least one case, a bent finger straightened without intervention.

KEY TERMS

Allele—One of two or more alternate forms of a gene.

Arthropathy—Any disease or disorder that affects joints.

Camptodactyly—A condition characterized by the bending of one or more fingers.

Chromosome—A microscopic thread-like structure found within each cell of the body and consists of a complex of proteins and DNA. Humans have 46 chromosomes arranged into 23 pairs. Changes in either the total number of chromosomes or their shape and size (structure) may lead to physical or mental abnormalities.

Congenital disorder—Refers to a disorder which is present at birth.

Deoxyribonucleic acid (DNA)—The genetic material in cells that holds the inherited instructions for growth, development, and cellular functioning.

Gene—A building block of inheritance, which contains the instructions for the production of a particular protein, and is made up of a molecular sequence found on a section of DNA. Each gene is found on a precise location on a chromosome.

Haplotype—The set of alleles on one chromosome.

Locus—The physical location of a gene on a chromosome.

Pericardiectomy is often performed to relieve the pericarditis often associated with the disorder.

Prognosis

Case studies show that children with arthropathy-camptodactyly syndrome have lived into their teens. There is reason to believe that with the proper treatment, the disorder is not life-shortening.

Resources

PERIODICALS

Athreya, B. H., and H. R. Schumacher. "Pathologic features of a familial arthropathy associated with congenital flexion contractures of fingers." *Arthritis and Rheumatism* 21 (1978): 429-437.

Bahabri, S. A., et al. "The camptodactyly-arthropathy-coxa vara-pericarditis syndrome: clinical features and genetic mapping to human chromosome 1." *Arthritis and Rheumatism* 41 (1998): 730-735.

Bulutlar, G., H. Yazici, H. Ozdogan, and I. Schreuder. "A familial syndrome of pericarditis, arthritis, camptodactyly, and coxa vara." *Arthritis and Rheumatism* 29 (1986): 436-438.

Martin, J. R., et al. "Congenital contractural deformities of the fingers and arthropathy." *Annals of the Rheumatic Diseases* 44 (1985): 826-830.

Suwairi, W. M., et al. "Autosomal recessive camptodactyly-arthropathy-coxa vara-pericarditis syndrome: clinical features and genetic mapping to chromosome 1q25-31." *(Abstract) American Journal of Human Genetics* 61 (supplement, 1997): A48.

WEBSITES

"Entry 208250: Arthropathy-Camptodactyly Syndrome." National Center for Biotechnology Information, *Online Mendelian Inheritance in Man* <http://www.ncbi.nlm.nih.gov/htbin-post/Omim/dispmim?208250>.

Sonya Kunkle

Asperger syndrome

Definition

Asperger syndrome (AS), which is also called Asperger disorder or autistic psychopathy, belongs to a group of childhood disorders known as **pervasive developmental disorders** (PDDs) or autistic spectrum disorders. The syndrome was first described by Hans Asperger, an Austrian psychiatrist, in 1944. Asperger's work was unavailable in English before the mid-1970s; as a result, AS was often unrecognized in English-speaking countries until the late 1980s. Before the American Psychiatric Association's *Diagnostic and Statistical Manual of Mental Disorders, Fourth Edition* (DSM-IV 1994), there was no official definition of AS.

Description

Children with AS learn to talk at the usual age and often have above-average verbal skills. They have normal or above-normal intelligence, and the ability to take care of themselves. The distinguishing features of AS are problems with social interaction, particularly reciprocating and empathizing with the feelings of others; difficulties with nonverbal communication (e.g., facial expressions); peculiar speech habits that include repeated words or phrases and a flat, emotionless vocal tone; an apparent lack of "common sense"; a fascination with obscure or limited subjects (e.g., doorknobs, railroad schedules, astronomical data, etc.), often to the exclusion of other interests; clumsy and awkward physical movements; and odd or eccentric behaviors (hand wringing or finger flapping; swaying or other repetitive whole-body movements; watching spinning objects for long periods of time).

Although less is known about adults with Asperger syndrome, they are often described as having rigid interests, social insensitivity, and a limited capacity for empathizing with others. However, many adults with Asperger have normal or even superior intelligence and can make great intellectual contributions due to their increased ability to focus and block out outside distractions. Many individuals are highly creative and excel in areas such as music, mathematics, and computer sciences. They tend to excel in fields that require little social interaction.

Genetic profile

There is some indication that AS runs in families, particularly in families with histories of **depression** and **bipolar disorder**. Dr. Asperger noted that his initial group of patients had fathers with AS symptoms. In addition, many reports now document the presence of Asperger-like behaviors in the extended families of individuals affected with Asperger syndrome. The presence of these behaviors contributes to the theory that Asperger syndrome is one end of a spectrum of defects that encompasses Asperger syndrome, **autism**, and pervasive developmental delay (NOS).

As of 2005, no single **gene** has been found to cause Asperger syndrome. Several genetic studies have identified genes or chromosomal regions that may be involved in Asperger syndrome, but it has become clear that there is more than one gene involved in the development of this complex syndrome. As of 2005, there are several candidate regions or areas of chromosomes involved in the development of this complex syndrome. These regions include the long arm of **chromosome** 1 (1q21-q22), the long arm of chromosome 3 (3q25-q27), the long arm of the X chromosome (Xq13), and the short arm of the X chromosome (Xp22.33). Further studies will need to be done to determine if any of these regions contains genes that contribute to the development of Asperger syndrome.

Demographics

Although the incidence of AS has been variously estimated between 0.024% and 0.36% of the general population in North America and northern Europe, further research is required to determine its true rate of occurrence—especially because the diagnostic criteria have been defined so recently. Previous research suggested that the overall rate of pervasive developmental disorders (PDDs) is 30 out of 10,000 people, but more recent research from 2003 revealed that the incidence of

PDD may be as high as 60 out of 10,000. The exact rate for Asperger syndrome has not been established, but it is thought to be approximately 2.5 out of 10,000.

It is unclear whether the rate of PDDs is actually increasing or if the increase that has been seen is due to wider diagnostic criteria and an increasing awareness of the diagnosis, leading to more individuals receiving the correct diagnosis. More research is necessary to answer this question completely.

AS appears to be much more common in boys. One Swedish study found the male/female ratio to be 4:1. Dr. Asperger's first patients were all boys, but girls have been diagnosed with AS since the 1980s. Asperger syndrome appears to affect all races equally.

Signs and symptoms

About 50% of patients with Asperger syndrome has a history of oxygen deprivation during the birth process, which has led to the hypothesis that the syndrome is caused by damage to brain tissue before or during childbirth. Another cause that has been suggested is an organic defect in the functioning of the brain. There are behavioral symptoms that are considered diagnostically significant.

Diagnosis

As of 2005, there are no blood tests or brain scans that can be used to diagnose AS. Until DSM-IV (1994), there was no official list of symptoms for the disorder, which made its diagnosis both difficult and inexact. Although most children with AS are diagnosed between five and nine years of age, many are not diagnosed until adulthood. Misdiagnoses are common; AS has been confused with such other neurological disorders as **Tourette syndrome**, or with attention-deficit disorder (ADD), oppositional defiant disorder (ODD), or obsessive-compulsive disorder (OCD). Some researchers think that AS overlaps with some types of learning disability, such as the nonverbal learning disability (NLD) syndrome identified in 1989. As of 2005, there is no clear answer to the question of whether AS is a distinct syndrome or a subtype of autism.

The inclusion of A syndrome as a separate diagnostic category in DSM-IV was justified on the basis of a large international field trial of more than 1,000 children and adolescents. Nevertheless, the diagnosis of AS is also complicated by confusion with such other diagnostic categories, such as high-functioning (IQ >70) autism (HFA) and schizoid personality disorder of childhood. With regard to schizoid personality disorder, Asperger syndrome does not have an unchanging set of personality traits, but has a developmental dimension. AS is distinguished from HFA by the following characteristics:

- later onset of symptoms (usually around three years of age)
- early development of grammatical speech (the AS child's verbal IQ is usually higher than performance IQ—the reverse being the case in autistic children)
- less severe deficiencies in social and communication skills
- presence of intense interest in one or two topics
- physical clumsiness and lack of coordination
- family is more likely to have a history of the disorder
- lower frequency of neurological disorders
- more positive outcome in later life

DSM-IV criteria for Asperger syndrome

DSM-IV specifies six diagnostic criteria for AS:

- The child's social interactions are impaired in at least two of the following ways: markedly limited use of nonverbal communication; lack of age-appropriate peer relationships; failure to share enjoyment, interests, or accomplishment with others; lack of reciprocity in social interactions.
- The child's behavior, interests, and activities are characterized by repetitive or rigid patterns, such as an abnormal preoccupation with one or two topics, or with parts of objects; repetitive physical movements; or rigid insistence on certain routines and rituals.
- The affected individual's social, occupational, or educational functioning is significantly impaired.
- The child has normal age-appropriate language skills.
- The child has normal age-appropriate cognitive skills, self-help abilities, and curiosity about the environment.
- The child does not meet criteria for another specific PDD or schizophrenia.

Other diagnostic scales and checklists

Other instruments that have been used to identify children with AS include Gillberg's criteria, a six-item list compiled by a Swedish researcher that specifies problems in social interaction, a preoccupying narrow interest, forcing routines and interests on the self or others, speech and language problems, nonverbal communication problems, and physical clumsiness; and the Australian Scale for Asperger Syndrome (ASAS), a detailed multi-item questionnaire developed in 1996.

Brain imaging findings

As of 2005, only a few structural abnormalities of the brain have been linked to AS. Findings include abnormally large folds in the brain tissue in the left frontal region, abnormally small folds in the operculum (a lid-like structure composed of portions of three adjoining brain lobes), and damage to the left temporal lobe. The first brain imaging study (using single-photon emission tomography [SPECT]) of patients with AS found a lower-than-normal blood supply in the left parietal area of the brain. Brain imaging studies on a larger sample of patients is the next stage of research.

Treatment and management

As of 2005, there is no cure for AS and no prescribed regimen for affected patients. Specific treatments are based on the individual's symptom pattern.

Medications

The drugs that are recommended most often for children with AS include psychostimulants (methylphenidate, pemoline), clonidine, or one of the tricyclic antidepressants (TCAs) for hyperactivity or inattention; beta blockers, neuroleptics, or lithium for anger or aggression; selective serotonin reuptake inhibitors (SSRIs) or TCAs for rituals and preoccupations; and SSRIs or TCAs for anxiety symptoms. One alternative herbal remedy that has been tried with AS patients is St. John's Wort.

Psychotherapy

Individuals with Asperger syndrome often benefit from psychotherapy, particularly during adolescence, in order to cope with depression and other painful feelings related to their social difficulties.

Educational considerations

Most patients with AS have normal or above-normal intelligence, and are able to complete their education up through the graduate or professional school level. Many are unusually skilled in music or good in subjects requiring rote memorization. On the other hand, the verbal skills of children with AS frequently cause difficulties with teachers, who may not understand why these "bright" children have social and communication problems. Some children with AS are dyslexic; others have difficulty with writing or mathematics. In some cases, these children have been mistakenly put in special programs either for children with much lower levels of functioning, or for children with conduct disorders. Children with AS do best in structured learning situations in which they learn problem-solving and life skills, as well as academic subjects. They frequently need protection from the teasing and

KEY TERMS

Autistic psychopathy—Hans Asperger's original name for Asperger syndrome, which is still used occasionally as a synonym for the disorder.

Gillberg's criteria—A six-item checklist for Asperger syndrome developed by Christopher Gillberg, a Swedish researcher, that is widely used as a diagnostic tool.

High-functioning autism (HFA)—A subcategory of autistic disorder consisting of children diagnosed with IQs of 70 or higher.

Nonverbal learning disability (NLD)—A learning disability syndrome identified in 1989 that may overlap with some of the symptoms of Asperger syndrome.

Pervasive developmental disorder (PDD)—The term used by the American Psychiatric Association for individuals who meet some but not all of the criteria for autism.

bullying of other children, and often become hypersensitive to criticism by their teen years.

Employment

Adults with AS are productively employed in a wide variety of fields. They do best, however, in jobs with regular routines or jobs that allow them to work in isolation. Employers and colleagues may need some information about Asperger syndrome in order to understand the employee's behavior.

Prognosis

AS is a lifelong but stable condition. The prognosis for children with AS is generally good as far as intellectual development is concerned, although few school districts as of 2005 are equipped to meet their special social needs; however, awareness of this unique disorder is growing. There is some research to suggest that people with AS have an increased risk of becoming psychotic in adolescence or adult life. Adult individuals with AS can make significant contributions to society and some marry and do well in their careers despite the social handicaps of their condition. In fact, there is a contingent of adults with AS who argue that AS is not a handicap or condition to be cured. They feel that their "differences" should be appreciated in a more positive light. However, some adults with AS live very socially isolated existences. While individuals with AS can be taught specific social guidelines, the underlying social impairment is lifelong.

Resources

BOOKS

American Psychiatric Association. *Diagnostic and Statistical Manual of Mental Disorders*, 4th edition. Washington, DC: American Psychiatric Association, 1994.

Ozonoff, Sally. *A Parent's Guide to Asperger Syndrome and High-Functioning Autism: How to Meet the Challenges and Help Your Child Thrive.* 1st Edition. New York, NY: The Guilford Press, 2002.

Romanowski Bashe, Patricia, and Barbara Kirby. *The OASIS Guide to Asperger Syndrome: Advice, Support, Insight, and Inspiration.* 1st Edition. New York, NY: Crown Publishing,2001.

Thoene, Jess G., editor. *Physicians' Guide to Rare Diseases.* Montvale, NJ: Dowden Publishing Company, 1995.

ORGANIZATIONS

Autism Research Institute. 4182 Adams Ave., San Diego, 92116. Fax: (619) 563-6840.

Families of Adults Afflicted with Asperger's Syndrome (FAAAS). PO Box 514, Centerville, MA 02632. (April 8, 2005.) <http://www.faaas.org>.

National Organization for Rare Disorders (NORD). PO Box 8923, New Fairfield, CT 06812-8923. (203) 746-6518 or (800) 999-6673. Fax: (203) 746-6481. (April 8, 2005.) <http://www.rarediseases.org>.

Yale-LDA Social Learning Disabilities Project. Yale Child Study Center, 230 South Frontage Road, New Haven, CT 06520-7900. (203) 785-3488. (April 8, 2005.) <http://info.med.Yale.edu/chldstdy/autism>.

WEB SITES

Autism and Asperger's Syndrome. (April 8, 2005.) <http://www.aspergerssyndrome.org/>.

Center for the Study of Autism Home Page. (April8, 2005.) <http://www.autism.org//asperger.html>.

MAAP Services for Autism and Asperger Spectrum. (April 8, 2005.)<http://maapservices.org>.

O.A.S.I.S. (Online Asperger Syndrome Information and Support). (April 8, 2005.) <http://www.udel.edu/bkirby/asperger/>.

Rebecca J. Frey, PhD
Kathleen A. Fergus, MS, CGC

Asplenia

Definition

The term "asplenia" literally means absent spleen. However, in the condition asplenia, the spleen is not always absent. Sometimes the spleen is present, but not fully developed (hypoplastic). In asplenia, the spleen is typically not the only organ affected. Individuals with this condition often have problems with other organs and organ systems. A related condition is polysplenia. The term "polysplenia" literally means multiple spleens. Both of these conditions affect the placement and development of the organs inside the body. There is controversy over whether asplenia and the other syndromes, like polysplenia, that affect the position of the internal organs are actually different aspects of the same condition, referred to as Heterotaxy syndrome, or separate and distinct syndromes. This issue has not been resolved.

Asplenia is just one of the names used to refer to this condition. Other names include Ivemark syndrome, right isomerism sequence, bilateral right-sideness sequence, splenic agenesis syndrome, and asplenia with cardiovascular anomalies.

Description

The human body can be viewed as having a right side and a left side. Normally, inside the human body, the right side and the left side are different with respect to the presence of certain organs. Several organs inside the body are placed asymmetrically, meaning that one organ may be located on one side of the body, but not the other. Furthermore, there are some organs that are found on both sides of the body, but have differences that distinguish the right organ from its partner on the left side. In asplenia, the position, location, appearance, and performance of some of the internal organs are altered. Organs can often be found on the wrong side of the body and/or have structural defects. Furthermore, in most people the right and left organs are different; in people with asplenia, both organs may appear to be structured the same.

Genetic profile

In most families, asplenia is believed to occur sporadically. In other words, it occurs for the first time in a family and has no known or identifiable pattern of **inheritance**.

There have been several couples described in the medical literature who have more than one child diagnosed with asplenia. In several of these families, the parents were related to each other. Individuals who are related to each other are more likely to carry some of the same non-working genes. Therefore, these families illustrate the possibility that asplenia can be inherited in an autosomal recessive manner. Individuals who have an autosomal recessive condition have both genes

in a pair that do not work as expected or are missing, thereby causing the disease. One non-working **gene** is inherited from the mother and the other is inherited from the father. These parents are called carriers of that condition. When two people are known carriers for an autosomal recessive condition, they have a 25% chance with each pregnancy of having a child affected with the disease.

There are a few families where asplenia appears to be inherited in an autosomal dominant or X-linked manner. In autosomal dominant inheritance, only one gene in the pair needs to be abnormal to cause symptoms of the condition. In families where asplenia appears to be inherited in an autosomal dominant manner, family members who carry the same non-working gene can have different symptoms and the severity of the condition may vary. In autosomal dominant inheritance, if an individual carries the non-working gene, he or she has a 50% chance of passing the gene on with each pregnancy.

In families where asplenia appears to be inherited in a X-linked manner, the gene causing the condition is located on the X **chromosome**. Since women have two X chromosomes, if a woman inherits the non-working gene on one of her X chromosomes, typically she will not have any symptoms of asplenia or will have a milder form of the condition. A woman who carries the X-linked form of asplenia will have a 50% chance of passing that non-working gene on with each pregnancy.

Since men tend to have one Y chromosome and one X chromosome, if it is a son that inherits the non-working gene, he will be affected with the condition. Men who have a X-linked form of asplenia will always pass their X chromosome containing the non-working gene on to all of their daughters, who would be carriers of the condition. In these families, asplenia will never be passed from the father to the son, since men give their sons a Y chromosome. If a woman who carries a X-linked condition passes the X chromosome containing the non-working gene to a daughter, then that daughter will be a carrier like her mother.

The pattern of inheritance of asplenia in a family is usually not obvious when there is only one individual diagnosed with the condition. Based on the families and studies performed on asplenia, the chance of a couple who have one child with asplenia having another child with the condition is approximately 5% or less. This chance may be higher if it is determined that asplenia is part of Heterotaxy syndrome, since there are a wider range of symptoms associated with that condition. Furthermore, if more than one family member has the diagnosis of asplenia, the chance of it occurring again in the family is based on the pattern of inheritance that the condition appears to be following.

Since asplenia appears to be inherited in different ways, it is theorized that there may be several different genes that could cause asplenia. This means that some families may have asplenia caused by one specific non-working gene, but in other families, a different non-working gene could cause the same condition to occur. The exact genes involved in causing asplenia have not been identified. However, there is ongoing research to identify the genes involved with this condition.

Demographics

It is estimated that the incidence of asplenia is low, approximately one in 10,000 to one in 20,000 live births. More males are affected with the condition than females. Asplenia also accounts for 1-3% of all congenital heart defects. Asplenia does not appear to occur more frequently in certain ethnic groups.

Signs and symptoms

Almost all individuals with asplenia have an abnormal or absent spleen. However, there are other organs and organ systems that can be affected.

Abdominal organs

SPLEEN As the name of the condition implies, the spleen is always affected in asplenia. The spleen in individuals with asplenia is either absent or does not develop completely (hypoplastic spleen). Since the spleen is involved in the body's immune system, these infants can have an abnormal immune system, which increases their risk for developing an infection.

DIGESTIVE TRACT DISORDERS There are several abnormalities that can occur with the digestive tract in individuals with asplenia. The most common digestive tract disorder associated with asplenia is malrotation of the intestine. Sometimes a digestive tract problem will present with symptoms of an obstruction in the digestive system, requiring emergency surgery.

STOMACH Most individuals with asplenia have their stomach located on the right side or in the center of the body instead of the left. In addition, individuals with asplenia can have a "twisted" stomach that could result in an obstruction in their digestive system and impair the blood supply to the stomach (gastric volvulus).

LIVER Normally, the liver is located on the right side of the body and the shape of the liver is not symmet-rical. In asplenia, there can be isomerism of the liver—it can be located in the middle of the body, or located on the left side with the larger half of the liver located in the upper left side of the abdominal area.

GALLBLADDER The gallbladder may also be located in the middle of the body in individuals with asplenia.

Heart

Many infants with asplenia first present with cyanosis and severe respiratory distress. These are symptoms often seen in individuals who have a heart defect. Most individuals with asplenia have a defect in the structure and/or the position of their heart.

Typically, the heart is divided into two sides, a left and right, with each side containing two chambers, called ventricle and atrium. The left and right sides of the heart are different from each other in their structure and function. The job of the right side of the heart is to pump blood to the lungs to receive oxygen. The job of the left side of the heart is to receive the oxygenated blood from the lungs and pump it to the rest of the body. In asplenia, sometimes the structures of the right side of the heart are duplicated on the heart's left side.

A common heart defect often seen in asplenia is anomalous pulmonary venous return, which occurs when the pulmonary veins (the blood vessels that carry blood containing oxygen from the lungs to the heart) are connected to the right atrium instead of the left atrium. This causes the oxygenated blood to be pumped back to the lungs instead of the body. Sometimes, there is a hole between the right and left atrium (called atrial septal defect or ASD) that allows some of the oxygenated blood into the left atrium and pumped to the rest of the body.

Other heart defects frequently seen in individuals with asplenia include: common atrioventricular canal, common atrial canal, persistent truncus arteriosus, pulmonary stenosis or atresia, single ventricle in the heart, and transposition of the great arteries. Often there is more than one heart defect present. Furthermore, in many individuals with asplenia, the heart is located on the right side of the body instead of the left.

Lungs

Normally, the lungs are divided into lobes. The lung on the right side of the body usually has three lobes and the left lung typically has two lobes. In asplenia, each lung usually has three lobes.

There can be abnormalities in other systems of the body as well, but they are not often seen in most individuals with asplenia. Other abnormalities associated with asplenia include kidney anomalies, extra fingers and toes, **scoliosis**, facial abnormalities, and central nervous system anomalies.

Diagnosis

The diagnosis of asplenia is typically made by imaging studies. An echocardiogram of the heart can help identify any structural abnormalities and its exact position within the body. A chest x ray can also be used to locate the position of the heart and some of the other organs in the body. Ultrasound and CT examinations can also help determine if there are any malformations with the abdominal organs, the position of the stomach, the presence, appearance, and number of spleens, and how many lobes each lung has. While a MRI can also detect the presence and position of organs inside the body, it is less commonly used because of the need for sedation and the high cost of the test, especially in children.

Testing for the presence of Heinz and Howell-Jolly bodies in the blood has been suggested as a method to screen for an absent spleen. Howell-Jolly bodies are unique cells that tend to be present in the blood of individuals who do not have a spleen, but they can also be seen in the blood of individuals who have certain types of anemia. Therefore, this test should not be used as the sole diagnostic test for an absent spleen.

Some of the abnormalities seen in asplenia can be detected prenatally. Often the position of the heart and some of the heart defects can be diagnosed by fetal echocardiogram (an ultrasound examination of the fetal heart) in the late second and third trimesters of pregnancy. A fetal echocardiogram should be performed during pregnancy when a couple already has a child with asplenia. Additionally, a level II ultrasound examination can detect some digestive system anomalies, such as the position of the stomach.

Treatment and management

Surgery can sometimes be performed on the heart to repair the defect or defects. There are limitations to heart surgery and it cannot always be performed. Additionally, heart surgery is not always successful. Surgery can also be used to correct many of the digestive tract disorders.

Additionally, because the spleen is involved in the body's immune system, it is recommended that all patients with the diagnosis of asplenia be given antibiotics and pneumococcal vaccination.

KEY TERMS

Anomalous—Irregular or different from normal.

Anomalous venous return—Normally, the veins that bring blood containing oxygen from the lungs to the heart (called pulmonary veins) are connected to the left atrium. In this situation, the pulmonary veins are connected to the right atrium.

Asplenia—The absence of the spleen in the body.

Atria/Atrium—The upper chamber of the heart. Typically, there are two atrias, one on the right side and one on the left side of the heart.

Atrial septal defect—An opening between the right and left atria of the heart.

Congenital—Refers to a disorder which is present at birth.

Cyanosis—The bluish color of the skin that occurs when there is very low oxygen in the blood that is being transported throughout the body.

Echocardiography/Echocardiogram—An ultrasound examination targeted at the heart and performed by a cardiologist or an individual trained at detecting differences in the structure of the heart.

Isomerism—Refers to the organs that typically come in pairs, but where the right organ is structurally different from the left organ. In a condition like asplenia, the organs are identical.

Malrotation—An abnormality that occurs during the normal rotation of an organ or organ system.

Pulmonary atresia—When there is no valve between the right ventricle and the pulmonary artery (the artery leading from the heart to the lungs). In the absence of this valve, the blood does not flow into the lungs well.

Pulmonary stenosis—Narrowing of the pulmonary valve of the heart, between the right ventricle and the pulmonary artery, limiting the amount of blood going to the lungs.

Syndrome—A group of signs and symptoms that collectively characterize a disease or disorder.

Transposition of the great arteries—A reversal of the two great arteries of the heart, causing blood containing oxygen to be carried back to the lungs and blood that is lacking in oxygen to be transported throughout the body.

Truncus arteriosus—Having only one artery coming from the heart instead of two. Often there is a ventricular septal defect (VSD) present.

Ventricular septal defect (VSD)—An opening between the right and left ventricles of the heart.

Prognosis

Without treatment, the prognosis of an infant diagnosed with asplenia is poor, with approximately 80% of these infants dying within the first year of life. The cause of death is usually complications from the heart defect. However, with advances in heart surgery and improvements in correcting many of the digestive tract anomalies, infants with asplenia are living much longer.

Resources

PERIODICALS

Applegate, K., et. al. "Situs Revisited: Imaging of the Heterotaxy Syndrome." *RadioGraphics* 19 (1999): 837-52.

Nakada, K., et. al. "Digestive Tract Disorders Associated with Asplenia/Polysplenia Syndrome." *Journal of Pediatric Surgery* 32 (1997): 91-94.

Splitt, M. P., et. al. "Defects in the Determination of Left-Right Asymmetry." *Journal of Medical Genetics* 33 (1996): 498-503.

ORGANIZATIONS

Ivemark Syndrome Association. 52 Keward Ave., Wells, Somerset, BAS-1TS. UK 1-(74)967-2603.

WEBSITES

Gee, Henry. "The Sources of Symmetry." *Nature: Science Update.* (1998) <http://www.nature.com.nsu/980806/980806-7.html>.

"OMIM# 208530: Asplenia with Cardiovascular Anomalies." *OMIM—Online Mendelian Inheritance in Man.* <http://www.ncbi.nih.gov/htbin-post/Omim/dispmim?208530>. (May 14, 1999).

Sharon A. Aufox, MS, CGC

Asplenia/polysplenia complex *see* **Asplenia; Laterality sequence**

Asthma

Definition

Asthma is a chronic inflammatory disease of the respiratory system that causes breathing difficulty. Asthma comes from the Greek word for panting. The disease is an over-responsiveness of the respiratory system to stimulating factors. It is characterized by repeated, temporary episodes of constriction and inflammation of the airways and lungs, along with excess mucous production. Asthma causes wheezing, coughing, and shortness of breath. Asthma attacks are characterized by severe difficulty breathing, especially when exhaling. Severe attacks that are left untreated may become fatal. An individual with asthma may be completely without symptoms between attacks.

Description

Asthma is a chronic, lifelong disease that affects the complex network of air passageways of the respiratory system. People with asthma may experience from mild discomfort to life-threatening attacks that require immediate emergency treatment. The respiratory system is made up of bronchial tubes (airways) and the lungs. Asthma involves the inflammation of the bronchial tubes and lining of the lungs. The inflammation causes the airways to be overly sensitive to irritating factors, which cause constriction and obstruction to the passage of air into the lungs. Asthmatics also produce excess amounts of mucous in the respiratory tract. Mucous is a normal component of respiratory function that aids in carrying irritating particles up and out of the respiratory system to be expectorated (coughed up) from the body. Asthmatics produce excessive, abnormally thick mucous that interferes with breathing and contributes to the problem. Severe asthma attacks can be fatal. Persistent or chronic inflammation of the airways can cause permanent damage, or airway "remodeling," and reduce lung function so that breathing becomes less efficient even outside of asthma attacks. Asthmatics may experience chronic wheezing, coughing, shortness of breath, and a feeling of a tightening of the chest. Medication and careful management of the disease is often necessary for maintaining normal function.

Chronic asthma has both a genetic and an environmental component. Research has demonstrated that some individuals inherit a strong genetic predisposition for asthma that can be triggered by a variety of environmental factors. Stimuli for triggering asthmatic symptoms include repeated exposure to irritants, such as dust mites, pet hairs, and tobacco smoke. These types of stimuli are considered allergens, or particles that trigger an allergic response. Asthma may also be induced by exercise, especially in cold climates where the respiratory system has to work harder to warm and moisten inhaled air. Some asthmatics only experience symptoms during viral infections. Asthma may also be stimulated by emotional stress. Both physical and psychological factors may precipitate an asthma attack.

Genetic profile

Asthma is a complex heritable disease in which a number of different genes contribute to asthmatic predisposition. While genes may cause a predisposition to asthma, actual asthma attacks are triggered by stimulating environmental factors. It has been clearly established that asthma tends to run in families. Research demonstrates increased risk of developing asthma for children of asthmatics. Studies also show that identical twins are more likely to share a genetic predisposition for asthma than are fraternal (non-identical) twins.

According to the National Institutes of Health (NIH) in 2005, chromosomes 5, 6, 11, 14, and 12 have all been implicated in asthmatic predisposition. However the relative role each of these genes has in asthma predisposition is not clear. One of the most likely candidates for further investigation is **chromosome** 5. Chromosome 5 is full of genes-encoding molecules involved in the inflammatory response that characterizes asthma.

Research studies show that specific symptoms experienced by asthma patients, such as the inflammation of the airways and lungs, are initiated by the action of genes that regulate the activity of the immune system. In other words, these genes control how the immune system responds to the presence of substances that can potentially trigger asthma symptoms. Like a microscopic army, the immune system consists of a wide array of specialized cells that work together to neutralize threats to the system. Antigens are any foreign agent invading the body that triggers such an immune response. Antigens include disease-producing organisms such as viruses, toxic chemicals in the environment, or allergens such as animal dander and dust mites. In response to the identification of foreign antigen particles, some immune cells produce antibodies to attack specific types of antigens. This immune response occurs after an initial encounter with an antigen and is known as a primary immune response. The immune system recognizes past contact with specific antigens by maintaining specific levels of the antibodies customized to attack specific antigens. When the same antigen is encountered again, the specific antibodies that have been maintained in the body multiply and mount a stronger immune response than the primary response. This process is known as the secondary immune response.

One of the specific antibodies produced in response to allergens is a protein known as immunoglobulin E (IgE), encoded by chromosome 5. In a normal inflammatory response, IgE recognizes foreign antigens and initiates immune reactions against the antigen by binding to other immune cells such as mast cells. Mast cells release chemical mediators that contribute to inflammation directly, but also recruit more immune cells to the site of inflammation. The recruited immune cells also release mediators of inflammation, such as histamine, that amplify the response and cause inflammation. Chromosome 5 encodes for multiple components of this immune response. In asthmatics, the IgE mast cells are highly excitable, making them hypersensitive to stimulation. When foreign antigens are breathed into the respiratory system, the entire inflammatory process, including the recruitment of other immune cells that release histamine, becomes exaggerated, resulting in asthma.

Research indicates that asthmatics produce higher levels of IgE antibodies, more hyperactive mast cells, and higher levels of consequent histamine than non-asthmatics. Histamine is a type of chemical signal that initiates the inflammatory response. Histamine stimulates the dilation of blood vessels walls and makes them more porous. As a result, blood fluid and proteins leak out of the blood vessels and into surrounding tissue, causing the swelling and reddening typical of inflammation. Inflammation involves increased blood flow to affected tissues to allow the passage of the recruited immune cells from the blood into the affected tissues. The immune cells may then dispose of the foreign particles. While this response is designed to defend the tissue from foreign invasion of harmful particles, an exaggerated response can be dangerous. In asthma, the resultant inflammation, along with the reactive constriction of the muscles in walls of the bronchial airways, narrows the air passages and causes an asthma attack.

Another component of the immune defense is the production of nitric oxide gas (NO) by an enzyme called inducible nitric oxide synthase (iNOS). Cells lining the bronchial tubes contain this enzyme that produces NO in response to chemical signals released from immune cells. Asthmatics produce an abnormally high level of iNOS in their respiratory cells than do non-asthmatics. Asthmatics have higher levels of NO in their lungs and bronchial tubes that contribute to the disease.

While chromosome 5 is implicated in asthma, there is conflicting evidence as to whether the genes responsible for the hyperactivity of the immune response in bronchial passages are distinct from the genes that regulate the action of the immune system. However, a region of chromosome 5 involved in the regulation of the immune system has been named bronchial hyperresponsiveness-1 (BHR1). Research on the BHR1 region is currently being performed by the NIH, in addition to other genetic regions. Another possible contributing factor for the overproduction of IgE antibodies could be a lack of exposure to common childhood illnesses. For example, cold viruses and other respiratory illnesses stimulate the human immune system to produce a certain type of immune cell, called a helper T cell, which specifically targets these disease agents. However, in the absence of stimuli, the immune system instead produces another type of helper T cell that initiates the production of the IgE antibody.

Demographics

In the United States, about 15 million people had asthma in 2004; approximately five million were children. Asthma affects individuals of all ages, but often starts in childhood. More than 50% of asthma cases occur in children between two and 17 years of age. Asthma is the most prevalent childhood chronic disease, and is more common in children than adults. In children, more males have asthma than females. Male children have a 30% higher prevalence of asthma compared to females. In adults, the trend is reversed, with more females having asthma than males. Adult females have a 30% higher prevalence of asthma than adult males. Within ethnic groups, non-Hispanic blacks have more asthma attacks and are more likely to be hospitalized and die from asthma than non-Hispanic whites. Asthma is distinct from, but closely linked to, allergies. Most, but not all, people with asthma have allergies.

The Centers for Disease Control (CDC) conducted a National Health Interview Survey in 2002 regarding asthma. At the time of the survey, 30.8 million individuals in the United States had been diagnosed with asthma during their lifetime: 21.9 million were adults and 8.9 million were children. Among all racial and ethnic groups, Puerto Ricans had the highest rate of lifetime asthma. Puerto Ricans were approximately 80% more likely than non-Hispanic whites to have been diagnosed with asthma.

Asthma attack prevalence is a crude indicator of how many individuals have uncontrolled asthma and are at risk for hospitalization. In 2002, 12 million people had experienced an asthma attack within the past year. Asthma attack prevalence decreased with age, being most prevalent in children. Puerto Ricans had the highest asthma attack prevalence, a full 100% higher than non-Hispanic whites. The prevalence of an asthma attack was about 30% higher in non-Hispanic blacks than in non-Hispanic whites. In this survey, Non-Hispanic blacks were the most likely to die from asthma, with an asthma death rate more than 200% higher than non-Hispanic whites. Females had an asthma death rate approximately 40% higher than males. Differences in male and female hormones may cause this disparity.

Asthma has been described as the fastest-growing chronic disease and a worldwide epidemic. According to Global Initiative for Asthma (GINA), an asthma research and education program, asthma accounts for about one in every 250 deaths worldwide. Many of the deaths are believed to be preventable and are caused by poor medical care. GINA estimates there are over three million asthmatic individuals worldwide. In most countries, asthmatic cases are increasing 20–50% every decade. The United States is one of the top countries for prevalence of asthma, along with England, Australia, parts of South America, and Canada. In Australia, the incidence of asthma is very high in Caucasian children, but much lower in aboriginal children.

It is speculated that lifestyle factors, such as a lack of physical activity, increased obesity, and more time spent indoors, may contribute to higher rates of asthma in highly developed countries. It is also possible that environmental irritants, such as poor indoor and outdoor air quality, along with the presence of potent irritants such as cockroach allergens, may contribute to higher rates of childhood asthma in poorer communities. Other factors that may prompt the onset of asthma are viral respiratory infections, low birth weight, and smaller-than-average air passageways in asthmatic patients.

Another area of research concerns the connection between common childhood infections and asthma. Many studies have shown that children who are exposed to viruses that cause the common cold and other respiratory infections at a very young age are less likely to develop asthma than peers living in a more hygienic environment. Children living at home with older siblings and those who spend time in daycare centers may be less likely to develop asthma than children who do not interact with others of their own age group. A related factor could be the overuse of antibiotics. Frequent use of antibiotic medications to treat relatively minor infections may produce changes in a person's immune system that increase the chance of developing asthma later in life.

Signs and symptoms

Asthmatics may experience coughing that is often worse at night or early in the morning, making sleep difficult. Wheezing is a common symptom, creating a whistling or squeaky sound when breathing. Asthmatics experience tightness in the chest region, as if it is being compressed. Shortness of breath and the feeling of breathlessness are common symptoms. There is difficulty getting enough air in or out of the lungs, especially during exhalation. If airflow to the lungs is inadequate, a lack of sufficient oxygen to the tissues causes the body to breathe faster, in an attempt to get more oxygen. Asthmatics often breathe faster as a result.

Asthmatics often have wheezing during a cold, flu, or other illness. Emotional stress may also result in asthmatic symptoms, such as coughing or wheezing from prolonged crying or laughing. Many indoor and outdoor factors can trigger or initiate typical symptoms of asthma, including allergies, viral respiratory infections, weather changes, and exercise. Medications containing aspirin also act as an asthma trigger in about 10–20% of adult asthmatics.

When allergies stimulate an asthma attack, it is known as allergic asthma. Allergic asthma is stimulated when an affected individual is physically near an allergen or irritant. Research has confirmed that allergies cause the majority of childhood asthma cases. Allergic asthma is the most common form of asthma and tends to run in families. Common allergens that may contribute to allergies and asthmatic reactions include dust mites, dust particles, animal dander, animal hair or bird feathers, mold, plant pollen, and substances found in food. Food products containing peanuts, eggs, dairy products, or seafood can cause asthma attacks in some children with allergies to these foods. Food additives, such as sulfites, can also act as asthma triggers. Synthetic (manmade) products like the latex material used in surgical gloves can also trigger asthma episodes in susceptible individuals. Non-allergic factors that can stimulate or aggravate asthma symptoms include tobacco smoke, chalk dust, talcum powder, car exhaust, and fumes from chemicals such as household cleaners. Auto pollution is a major factor in asthma prevalence.

Exercise is a common trigger for asthma in about 80% of asthmatic individuals. Some asthmatics have exercise-induced symptoms precipitated by brisk activity such as running, especially during cold weather. Pretreatment medications, such as short-acting bronchodilators, quickly widen air passages and thus help prevent the onset of asthma while an asthmatic participates in physical activities. Activities that allow for frequent breaks rather than prolonged endurance are most suitable. Asthma does not have to be a barrier to participating in athletic activities. Many Olympic athletes have exercise-induced asthma that is controlled by medication.

Changes in the weather, such as temperature and humidity variations, can also negatively affect asthma patients. Cold climates may exacerbate asthma because the lungs have to work harder to warm and moisten inhaled air. Asthmatics exercising in such conditions could wear a surgical mask that can trap the warm, moist air exhaled with each breath. Viral infections of the respiratory system that tend to increase in number during winter months may trigger severe asthma attacks. Additionally, unclean and poorly maintained forced-air heating systems release many pollutants that further aggravate asthmatic symptoms.

Every asthma patient is unique. Because there are so many environmental conditions that affect individuals with a genetic predisposition for asthma, it is often difficult to pinpoint the primary cause of the disease in individual cases.

An asthmatic may have any combination of symptoms, with symptoms varying from one asthma attack to another. Symptoms may exhibit a range of severity, from mildly irritating to life-threatening. Symptoms occur with varying frequency from once every few months to every day. Asthma classifications are based on symptom levels in the absence of medication. Mild intermittent asthma is defined as symptoms of wheezing, coughing, or breathing difficulty less than twice a week or less, with night symptoms twice a month or less. Mild persistent asthma is defined as symptoms of wheezing, coughing, or breathing difficulty once a day or less, but more than twice a week. Symptoms occur at night more than twice a month. Moderate persistent asthma is defined as daily symptoms that require daily medication. Symptoms at night occur more than once a week. Symptoms may be severe enough to interfere with normal physical activity. Severe asthma is described as ongoing, persistent symptoms with more serious asthma attacks. Symptoms may occur throughout the day, with night symptoms occurring often. In severe asthma, physical activity is likely to be limited.

All types of asthmatics may have severe asthma attacks. However, with appropriate treatment and avoidance of asthma stimulators, most asthmatics can achieve a general condition of minimal or no symptoms. Asthmatics are encouraged to learn to recognize their own specific asthma stimulators and avoid them, and to recognize their specific pattern of early warning signs that signal the start of an attack. The first signs of a mild or moderate attack may be a slight tightening of the chest, coughing or wheezing, and spitting up mucous. Severe attacks can bring on a feeling of extreme tightening of the neck and chest, making breathing increasingly difficult. Asthmatics may struggle to speak or breathe. In advanced stages of severe attacks, lips and fingernails may take on a grayish or bluish tinge, indicating declining oxygen levels in the blood. Such attacks can be fatal in the absence of prompt medical attention. Fortunately, asthma symptoms are usually reversible with medication.

Diagnosis

The first stage of asthma diagnosis is from a history of asthmatic symptoms. These symptoms include periods of coughing, wheezing, shortness of breath, or chest tightness that come on suddenly in response to specific stimulants or time periods. A history of head colds that evolve into chest congestion or take more than 10 days to recover from is pertinent. Family history of asthma or allergies may also be part of the diagnosis.

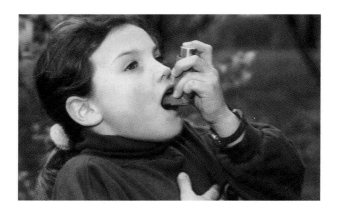

A young girl is using an inhaler to facilitate breathing. *(Custom Medical Stock Photo, Inc.)*

A physical exam may reveal wheezing in the chest that can be heard with a stethoscope. A device called a spirometer may be used to check the function of the airways in children over five years of age and in adults. The test measures the volume of air and the speed with which air can be blown out of the lungs after a deep breath. If the airways are narrowed from inflammation and the muscles around the airways tightening up from asthma, the results will be lower than normal. If spirometry results are normal but asthma symptoms are present, other tests are performed. A bronchial challenge test involves inhalation of a substance such as methacholine, which causes narrowing of the airways in asthma. The effect is measured by spirometry to determine is asthma is present. Children under five years of age usually cannot use a spirometer successfully. In such cases, asthma medications are often attempted as part of the diagnosis to determine if they are able to alleviate the symptoms.

Allergy testing may be performed to determine if there are specific allergens that the individual is reactive to. A device called a peak flow meter may be used every day for several weeks to measure breathing efficiency. Tests may be performed to determine the reaction of the airways to exercise. In some cases, a chest x ray or an electrocardiogram may be used to determine if a foreign object, other lung disease, or heart disease could be causing asthma-like symptoms. The results of the medical history, physical exam, and lung function tests are used to diagnose the severity of asthma and determine treatment.

Treatment and management

Asthma is treated by avoiding stimulating factors and by medication. There are two main types of asthma medi-

cation. Acute medications give rapid, short-term treatment, and are only used when asthma symptoms require immediate relief. Acute medications are bronchodilators that may be inhaled and take effect within minutes to dilate the airways and allow normal breathing. Bronchodilators may be used at the beginning of an asthma attack to provide relief. Bronchodilators may also be used before exercise to prevent exercise-induced asthma symptoms. Long-term control medications are taken daily over long periods of time to control chronic symptoms and prevent asthma attacks. The full effect of these medications requires several weeks of use. Individuals with persistent asthma require long-term control medications.

The most effective, long-term control medication for asthma is an inhaled corticosteroid. Corticosteroids reduce the swelling of airways and help to prevent asthma attacks from occurring. Inhaled corticosteroids are preferred for treatment of all levels of persistent asthma. In some cases, steroid tablets or liquid medications are used temporarily to control asthma. Other types of asthma medications inhibit the inflammatory mediators released in the asthma response. Some of these long-term control medications may be used in combination with inhaled corticosteroids to treat moderate persistent and severe persistent asthma. Long-term control medications are used in a preventative manner and will not stop a currently occurring asthma attack. Many asthmatics require both a short-acting bronchodilator to use when symptoms worsen and a long-term daily asthma control medication to treat ongoing inflammation.

Uncontrolled asthma during pregnancy can be very dangerous. Lowered oxygen levels to the fetus may cause damage. Many asthma treatments are considered safe to use during pregnancy. Older adults may need adjustments in asthma treatment because of other present diseases or conditions. Some medications, such as beta-blockers used for hypertension, aspirin, and nonsteroidal anti-inflammatory drugs such as ibuprofen, can interfere with some asthma medications or cause asthma attacks. The use of corticosteroids may also adversely affect bone density in adults.

Asthmatics can monitor the function of their respiratory system with the aid of peak flow meters and spirometers. These devices measure the amount of air exhaled with each breath. They are used to regularly monitor the severity of asthma symptoms and to evaluate and manage treatment procedures for individual patients. Maintaining control over asthma symptoms, combined with a healthy lifestyle, are key components of asthma treatment.

Emergency care may become necessary during a severe asthma attack. Emergency care takes place in a hospital setting and may include treatment with high levels of

KEY TERMS

Allergen—A substance or organism foreign to the body; allergens stimulate the immune system to produce antibodies.

Allergy—Condition in which immune system is hypersensitive to contact with allergens; an abnormal response by the immune system to contact with an allergen; condition in which contact with allergen produces symptoms such as inflammation of tissues and production of excess mucus in respiratory system.

Antibody—A protein produced by the mature B cells of the immune system that attach to invading microorganisms and target them for destruction by other immune system cells.

Antigen—A substance or organism that is foreign to the body and stimulates a response from the immune system.

Bronchi—Branching tube-like structures that carry air in and out of the lungs; walls of bronchi contain circular muscles that can constrict (tighten up to make airways narrower) or dilate (relax to make airways wider); bronchi divide into smaller bronchioles within the lung tissue.

Gene—A building block of inheritance, which contains the instructions for the production of a particular protein, and is made up of a molecular sequence found on a section of DNA. Each gene is found on a precise location on a chromosome.

Genetic disease—A disease that is (partly or completely) the result of the abnormal function or expression of a gene; a disease caused by the inheritance and expression of a genetic mutation.

Histamine—A substance released by immune system cells in response to presence of allergen; stimulates widening of blood vessels and increased porousness of blood vessel walls so that fluid and protein leak out from blood to surrounding tissue, causing inflammation of local tissues.

Hypersensitive—A process or reaction that occurs at above normal levels; overreaction to a stimulus.

IgE—An antibody composed of protein; specific forms of IgE produced by cells of immune system in response to different antigens that contact the body; major factor that stimulates the allergic response.

Immune system—A major system of the body that produces specialized cells and substances that interact with and destroy foreign antigens that invade the body.

Inflammation—Swelling and reddening of tissue; usually caused by immune system's response to the body's contact with an allergen.

---

bronchodilators and corticosteroids, additional medications, and oxygen administration in an attempt to restore normal respiratory activity. Delayed access to emergency treatment can lead to complete respiratory failure where the patient simply stops breathing and cannot be revived.

In cases of allergic asthma, allergy shots may also assist in reducing symptoms. Allergy shots, also known as allergen immunotherapy, are recommended for individuals who suffer from allergic asthma when it is not possible to avoid contact with the allergens that stimulate asthma. A series of shots with controlled and gradually increasing amounts of allergen may be given over a number of months or years. The shots are vaccines containing various allergens, such as pollen or dust mites. The increased exposure to the allergen desensitizes the immune system to allergen triggers. Allergy shots can diminish the severity of asthma symptoms and lower the dosage of required asthma medications.

Prognosis

There is currently no cure for asthma. Proper treatment and management has dramatically improved the quality of life for individuals with asthma. When medication is utilized properly, the prognosis for most asthmatics is excellent. An improvement in environmental conditions can reduce the number and severity of asthma attacks and improve the prognosis for asthmatics. Such improvement is also believed to affect the overall prognosis for a society, simply by decreasing the number of individuals sensitized to environmental triggers.

Resources

BOOKS

Katzung, B. G. *Basic and Clinical Pharmacology, Seventh Edition.* Stamford, CT: Appleton and Lange, 1998.

Roitt, I., J. Brostoff, and D. Male. *Immunology, Fifth Edition.* London, England: Mosby International, 1998.

PERIODICALS

"Clearing the Air: Asthma and Indoor Air Exposures." *The New England Journal of Medicine* 343 (December 14, 2000): 24.

"Day Care, Siblings, and Asthma—Please, Sneeze on My Child." *The New England Journal of Medicine* 343 (August 24, 2000): 8.

Folkerts, Gert, Gerhard Walzl, and Peter J. M. Openshaw. "Do Common Childhood Infections 'Teach' the Immune System Not to Be Allergic?" *Immunology Today* 21, no. 3 (2000): 118–120.

Herz, Udo, Paige Lacy, Harald Renz, and Klaus Erb. "The Influence of Infections on the Development and Severity of Allergic Disorders." *Current Opinion in Immunology* 12, no. 6 (2000): 632–640.

Illi, S., E. von Mutius, S. Lau, R. Bergmann, B. Niggemann, C. Sommerfeld, and U. Wahn. "Early Childhood Infectious Diseases and the Development of Asthma Up to School Age: A Birth Cohort Study." *British Medical Journal* 322 (February 17, 2001): 390–395.

Johnston, Sebastian L., and Peter J. M. Openshaw. "The Protective Effect of Childhood Infections—The Next Challenge Is to Mimic Safely This Protection Against Allergy and Asthma." *British Medical Journal* 322 (February 17, 2001): 376–377.

"Siblings, Day-Care Attendance, and the Risk of Asthma and Wheezing." *The New England Journal of Medicine* 343, no. 26 (December 28, 2000).

ORGANIZATIONS

Allergy and Asthma Network. Mothers of Asthmatics, Inc. 2751 Prosperity Ave., Suite 150, Fairfax, VA 22031. (800) 878-4403. Fax: (703) 573-7794.

American Academy of Allergy, Asthma & Immunology. 611 E. Wells St., Milwaukee, WI 53202. (414) 272-6071. Fax: (414) 272-6070. (April 18, 2005.) <http://www.aaaai.org/default.stm>.

American Lung Association. 1740 Broadway, New York, NY 10019. (212) 315-8700 or (800) 586-4872. (April 18, 2005.) <http://www.lungusa.org>.

Asthma and Allergy Foundation of America (AAFA). 1233 20th St. NW, Suite 402, Washington, DC 20036. (800) 7-ASTHMA. Fax: (202) 466-8940. (April 18, 2005.) <http://www.aafa.org>.

Division of Lung Diseases, National Heart, Lung and Blood Institute. Suite 10122, 6701 Rockledge Dr. MSC 7952, Bethesda, MD 20892-7952. (301) 435-0233. (April 18, 2005.) <http://www.nhlbi.nih.gov/index.htm>.

Global Initiative for Asthma (GINA). (207) 594-5008. Fax: (207) 594-8802. shurd@prodigy.net. (April 18, 2005.) <http://www.ginasthma.com>.

KidsHealth. Nemours Center for Children's Health Media. PO Box 269, Wilmington, DE 19899. (April 18, 2005.) <http://www.kidshealth.org>.

National Asthma Education and Prevention Program (NAEPP). School Asthma Education Subcommittee. (April 18, 2005.) <http://www.nhlbi.nih.gov/health/dci/Diseases/Asthma/Asthma_WhatIs.html>.

National Center for Environmental Health. Centers for Disease Control and Prevention, Mail Stop F-29, 4770 Buford Highway NE, Atlanta, GA 30341-3724. (April 18, 2005.) <http://www.cdc.gov/asthma/>.

National Institutes of Health (NIH). PO Box 5801, Bethesda, MD 20824. (800) 352-9424. (April 18, 2005.) <http://www.ninds.nih.gov>.

OTHER

Asthma. National Heart, Lung, and Blood Institute. (April 18, 2005.) <http://www.nhlbi.nih.gov/health/public/lung/index.htm>.

Asthma and Allergies. Centers for Disease Control and Prevention. (April 18, 2005.) <http://www.cdc.gov/niosh/topics/asthma>.

Asthma Basics. National Institutes of Health. (April 18, 2005.) <http://www2.niaid.nih.gov/newsroom/focuson/asthma01/basics.htm>.

Asthma Prevalence, Health Care Use and Mortality, 2002. National Center for Health Statistics. (April 18, 2005.) <http://www.cdc.gov/nchs/products/pubs/pubd/hestats/asthma/asthma.htm>.

Breath of Life Exhibition. National Library of Medicine. (April 18, 2005.) <http://www.nlm.nih.gov/hmd/breath/breath_exhibit/mainframe.html>.

"What Makes Asthma Worse?" medfacts 2000. Lung Line, National Jewish Medical and Research Center, 1400 Jackson Street, Denver, CO 80206. (303) 388-4461 (7700). (April 18, 2005.) <http://www.nationaljewish.org/medfacts/worse.html>.

Maria Basile, PhD

Ataxia-telangiectasia

Definition

Ataxia-telangiectasia (A-T) is a rare, genetic neurological disorder that progressively affects various systems in the body. Children affected with A-T appear normal at birth; however, the first signs of the disease—usually a lack of balance and slurred speech—often appear between one and two years of age.

Description

The onset of cerebellar ataxia (unsteadiness and lack of coordination) marks the beginning of progressive degeneration of the cerebellum, the part of the brain responsible for motor control (movement). This degeneration gradually leads to a general lack of muscle control, and eventually confines the patient to a wheelchair. Children with A-T become unable to feed or dress themselves without assistance. Because of the worsening ataxia, children with A-T lose their ability to write, and speech also becomes slowed and slurred. Even reading eventually becomes impossible, as eye movements become difficult to control.

Soon after the onset of the ataxia, an individual usually exhibits another symptom of the disease: telangiectases, or tiny red spider veins (dilated blood vessels). These telangiectases appear in the corners of the eyes—giving the eyes a blood-shot appearance—or on the surfaces of the ears and cheeks exposed to sunlight.

In about 70% of children with A-T, another symptom of the disease is present: an immune system deficiency that usually leads to recurrent respiratory infections. In many patients, these infections can become life threatening. Due to deficient levels of IgA and IgE immunoglobulins—the natural infection-fighting agents in the blood—children with A-T are highly susceptible to lung infections that are resistant to the standard antibiotic treatment. For these patients, the combination of a weakened immune system and progressive ataxia can ultimately lead to pneumonia as a cause of death.

Children with A-T tend to develop malignancies of the blood circulatory system almost 1,000 times more frequently than the general population. Lymphomas (malignant tumors of lymphoid tissues) and leukemias (abnormal overgrowth of white blood cells, causing tumor cells to grow) are particularly common types of **cancer**, although the risk of developing most types of cancer is high in those with A-T. Another characteristic of the disease is an increased sensitivity to ionizing radiation (high-energy radiation such as x rays), which means that patients with A-T frequently cannot tolerate the radiation treatments often given to cancer patients.

Genetic profile

Ataxia-telangiectasia is called a recessive genetic disorder because parents do not exhibit symptoms; however, each parent carries a recessive (unexpressed) **gene** that may cause A-T in offspring. The genetic path of A-T is therefore impossible to predict. The recessive gene may lie dormant for generations until two people with the defective gene have children. When two such A-T carriers have a child together, there is a 1-in-4 chance (25% risk) of having a child with A-T. Every healthy sibling of a child with A-T has a 2-in-3 chance (66% risk) of being a carrier, like his or her parents.

The A-T gene (called ATM, or A-T Mutated) was discovered by Tel Aviv researchers in 1995. The ATM protein is thought to prevent damaged **DNA** from being reproduced. However, the cells of patients with A-T lack the ATM protein, although the cells of those with the mild form of the disorder contain small amounts of it. It is thought that ATM is involved in sending messages to several other regulating proteins in the body. The absence of ATM severely disrupts the transmission of these messages, thereby affecting many different systems of the body.

Scientists have found that the ATM gene is often found with the p53 gene, which is defective in the majority of cancerous tumors. Tumor biologists, therefore, view A-T as one of the most explicit human models for studying inherited cancer susceptibility. In children who have A-T, the defective A-T gene blocks the normal development of the thymus, the organ most important for the development of the immune response. Understanding how immunodeficiencies develop in children with A-T may have relevance to research on other immunodeficiency disorders.

Demographics

Both males and females are equally affected by A-T. Epidemiologists estimate the frequency of A-T as between 1/40,000 and 1/100,000 live births. However, it is believed that many children with A-T, particularly those who die at a young age, are never properly diagnosed. Thus, the disease may occur much more often than reported.

It is also estimated that about 1% (2.5 million) of the American population carry a copy of the defective A-T gene. According to some researchers, these gene carriers may also have an increased sensitivity to ionizing radiation and have a significantly higher risk of developing cancer—particularly **breast cancer** in female carriers.

Signs and symptoms

Although there is much variability in A-T symptoms among patients, the signs of A-T almost always include the appearance of ataxia between the ages of two and five. Other, less consistent symptoms may include neurological, cutaneous (skin), and a variety of other conditions.

Neurological

Neurological symptoms of A-T include:

- progressive cerebellar ataxia (although ataxia may appear static between the ages of two and five)
- cerebellar dysarthria (slurred speech)
- difficulty swallowing, causing choking and drooling
- progressive apraxia (lack of control) of eye movements
- muscle weakness and poor reflexes

- initially normal intelligence, sometimes with later regression to mildly retarded range

Cutaneous

Cutaneous symptoms include:

- progressive telangiectases of the eye and skin develop between two to ten years of age
- atopic dermatitis (itchy skin)
- Café au lait spots (pale brown areas of skin)
- cutaneous atrophy (wasting away)
- hypo- and hyperpigmentation (underpigmented and overpigmented areas of skin)
- loss of skin elasticity
- nummular eczema (coin-shaped inflammatory skin condition)

Other symptoms

Other manifestations of A-T include:

- susceptibility to neoplasms (tumors or growths)
- endocrine abnormalities
- tendency to develop insulin-resistant **diabetes** in adolescence
- recurrent sinopulmonary infection (involving the sinuses and the airways of the lungs)
- characteristic loss of facial muscle tone
- absence or **dysplasia** (abnormal development of tissue) of thymus gland
- jerky, involuntary movements
- slowed growth
- prematurely graying hair

Diagnosis

For a doctor who is familiar with A-T, the diagnosis can usually be made on purely clinical grounds and often on inspection. But because most physicians have never seen a case of A-T, misdiagnoses are likely to occur. For example, physicians examining ataxic children frequently rule out A-T if telangiectases are not observed. However, telangiectases often do not appear until the age of six, and sometimes appear at a much older age. In addition, a history of recurrent sinopulmonary infections might increase suspicion of A-T, but about 30% of patients with A-T exhibit no immune system deficiencies.

The most common early misdiagnosis is that of static encephalopathy—a brain dysfunction, or ataxic cerebral palsy—paralysis due to a birth defect. Ataxia involving the trunk and gait is almost always the presenting symptom of A-T. And although this ataxia is slowly and steadily progressive, it may be compensated for—and masked—by the normal development of motor skills between the ages of two and five. Thus, until the progression of the disease becomes apparent, clinical diagnosis may be imprecise or inaccurate unless the patient has an affected sibling.

Once disease progression becomes apparent, **Friedreich ataxia** (a degenerative disease of the spinal cord) becomes the most common misdiagnosis. However, Friedreich ataxia usually has a later onset. In addition, the spinal signs involving posterior and lateral columns along the positive Romberg's sign (inability to maintain balance when the eyes are shut and feet are close together) distinguish this type of spinal ataxia from the cerebellar ataxia of A-T.

Distinguishing A-T from other disorders (differential diagnosis) is ultimately made on the basis of laboratory tests. The most consistent laboratory marker of A-T is an elevated level of serum alpha-fetoprotein (a protein that stimulates the production of antibodies) after the age of two years. Prenatal diagnosis is possible through the measurement of alpha-fetoprotein levels in amniotic fluid and the documentation of increased spontaneous chromosomal breakage of amniotic cell DNA. Diagnostic support may also be offered by a finding of low serum IgA, IgG and/or IgE. However, these immune system findings vary from patient to patient and are not abnormal in all individuals.

The presence of spontaneous **chromosome** breaks and rearrangements in lymphocytes in vitro (test tube) and in cultured skin fibroblasts (cells from which connective tissue is made) is also an important laboratory marker of A-T. And finally, reduced survival of lymphocyte (cells present in the blood and lymphatic tissues) and fibroblast cultures, after exposure to ionizing radiation, will confirm a diagnosis of A-T, although this technique is performed in specialized laboratories and is not routinely available to physicians.

When the mutated A-T gene (ATM) has been identified by researchers, it is possible to confirm a diagnosis by screening the patient's DNA for mutations. However, in most cases the large size of the ATM gene and the large number of possible mutations in patients with A-T seriously limit the usefulness of mutation analysis as a diagnostic tool or method of carrier identification.

Treatment and management

There is no specific treatment for A-T because **gene therapy** has not become an option. Also, the disease is usually not diagnosed until the individual has developed

KEY TERMS

Alpha-fetoprotein (AFP)—A chemical substance produced by the fetus and found in the fetal circulation. AFP is also found in abnormally high concentrations in most patients with primary liver cancer.

Atrophy—Wasting away of normal tissue or an organ due to degeneration of the cells.

Cerebellar ataxia—Unsteadiness and lack of coordination caused by a progressive degeneration of the part of the brain known as the cerebellum.

Dysarthria—Slurred speech.

Dysplasia—The abnormal growth or development of a tissue or organ.

Immunoglobulin—A protein molecule formed by mature B cells in response to foreign proteins in the body; the building blocks for antibodies.

Ionizing radiation—High-energy radiation such as that produced by x rays.

Leukemia—Cancer of the blood forming organs which results in an overproduction of white blood cells.

Lymphoma—A malignant tumor of the lymph nodes.

Recessive gene—A type of gene that is not expressed as a trait unless inherited by both parents.

Telangiectasis—Very small arteriovenous malformations, or connections between the arteries and veins. The result is small red spots on the skin known as "spider veins."

health problems. Treatment is therefore focused on the observed conditions, especially if neoplams are present. However, radiation therapy must be minimized to avoid inducing further chromosomal damage and tumor growth.

Supportive therapy is available to reduce the symptoms of drooling, twitching, and ataxia, but individual responses to specific medications vary. The use of sunscreens to retard skin changes due to premature aging can be helpful. In addition, early use of pulmonary physiotherapy, physical therapy, and speech therapy is also important to minimize muscle contractures (shortening or tightening of muscles).

Although its use has not been formally tested, some researchers recommend the use of antioxidants (such as vitamin E) in patients with A-T. Antioxidants help to reduce oxidative damage to cells.

Prognosis

A-T is an incurable disease. Most children with A-T depend on wheelchairs by the age of ten because of a lack of muscle control. Children with A-T usually die from respiratory failure or cancer by their teens or early 20s. However, some patients with A-T may live into their 40s, although they are extremely rare.

Resources

BOOKS

Vogelstein, Bert, and Kenneth E. Kinzler. *The Genetic Basis of Human Cancer.* New York: McGraw-Hill, 1998.

PERIODICALS

Brownlee, Shanna. "Guilty Gene." *U.S. News and World Report.* (July 3, 1995): 16.

Kum Kum, Khanna. "Cancer Risk and the ATM Gene." *Journal of the American Cancer Institute* 92, no. 6 (May 17, 2000): 795–802.

Stankovic, Tatjana, and Peter Weber, et al. "Inactivation of Ataxia Tlangiectasia Mutated Gene in B-cell Chronic Lymphocytic Leukaemia." *Lancet* 353 (January 2, 1999): 26–29.

Wang, Jean. "New Link in a Web of Human Genes." *Nature* 405, no. 6785 (May 25, 2000): 404–405.

ORGANIZATIONS

A-T Children's Project. 668 South Military Trail, Deerfield Beach, FL 33442. (800) 5-HELP-A-T. <http://www.atcp.org>.

A-T Medical Research Foundation. 5241 Round Meadow Rd., Hidden Hills, CA 91302. <http://pathnet.medsch.ucla.edu/people/faculty/gatti/gatsign.htm>.

National Ataxia Foundation. 2600 Fernbrook Lane, Suite 119, Minneapolis, MN 55447. (763) 553-0020. Fax: (763) 553-0167. naf@ataxia.org. <http://www.ataxia.org>.

National Organization to Treat A-T. 4316 Ramsey Ave., Austin, TX 78756-3207. (877) TREAT-AT. <http://www.treat-at.org>.

Genevieve T. Slomski, PhD

ATR-X syndrome *see* **Alpha-thalassemia X-linked mental retardation syndrome**

Attention deficit hyperactivity disorder

Definition

Attention deficit hyperactivity disorder (ADHD) is a neurological disorder that presents in various forms, with no two ADHD disorders having exactly the same characteristics. ADHD is classified as a disruptive behavior disorder characterized by ongoing difficulty with attention span, hyperactivity, and/or impulsivity. These difficulties occur more frequently and severely than is typical for individuals in the same stage of development.

Description

ADHD is a neurological condition, frequently familial, that affects specific types of brain functioning. The term ADHD is further divided into subcategories that describe the type of ADHD. The three categories recognized by the scientific community are ADHD inattentive type, ADHD impulsive-hyperactive type, or ADHD combined type. Some individuals, including many professionals, still refer to the condition as ADD (attention deficit disorder). However, this term is no longer in widespread use. For individuals who have been diagnosed with ADD in the past, the corresponding current terminology is most likely to be predominantly ADHD, inattentive type.

It is possible to meet the accepted diagnostic criteria for ADHD without displaying any symptoms of hyperactivity or impulsivity. Each ADHD individual will display a unique combination of symptoms. They will not necessarily have all of the symptoms associated with ADHD, and the levels of severity or impairment are varied from individual to individual. There are mild forms of ADHD in addition to the severe forms that result in significant impairment. Symptoms of ADHD usually begin before seven years of age, and can cause problems in school, jobs and careers, family life, and other relationships. ADHD can be managed through behavioral or medical interventions, or a combination of the two. Despite public controversy over the legitimacy of the disorder's existence, the National Institutes of Health (NIH), the Surgeon General of the United States, and the international community of clinical researchers and physicians have affirmed that ADHD is a valid disorder that may result in severe, lifelong consequences if left untreated. The Senate of the United States designated September 7, 2004, as National Attention Deficit Disorder Awareness Day.

Genetic profile

The exact cause of ADHD is unknown, although abnormal neurotransmitter levels, genetics, and complications occurring around the time of birth have been implicated. According to the National Resource Center on ADHD, heredity makes the largest contribution to the prevalence of ADHD in the population. ADHD occurs frequently in families, and **inheritance** is an important risk factor. Between 10–35% of children diagnosed with ADHD have a first-degree relative with ADHD. Approximately 50% of parents who have ADHD have a child with the disorder. ADHD is significantly more likely to be present in an identical (monozygotic) twin than in a fraternal (dizygotic) twin.

ADHD is not a form of gross brain damage. Because the symptoms of ADHD respond well to treatment with stimulants that increase the availability of the neurotransmitter dopamine, the dopamine hypothesis has gained acceptance. The dopamine hypothesis suggests that ADHD is due to inadequate availability of dopamine in the central nervous system. Dopamine plays a key role in initiating focused movement, increasing motivation and alertness, and preventing sleepiness in response to boredom. Multiple genes have been implicated in ADHD, including genes affecting dopamine usage by the brain.

The male to female ratio is 8:1. Despite the strong genetic linkage, research also suggests that non-genetic factors may play a role in ADHD. Hyperactivity and inattention are more common in children who have had exposure to toxins such as lead, alcohol, or cigarette smoke, or episodes of fetal oxygen deprivation during complications of pregnancy. These factors may adversely affect dopamine-rich areas of the brain.

In addition to dopamine, research has shown that glucose usage may also be involved in ADHD. Brain-imaging studies, using a technique called magnetic resonance imaging (MRI), have demonstrated differences between the brains of children with and without ADHD. A link has been established between an individual's ability to pay continued attention and the brain's use of glucose as a fuel. In adults with ADHD, the brain areas that control attention span may use less glucose and be less active, suggesting that a lower level of activity in this part of the brain may cause the inattention symptoms associated with ADHD.

By 2002, the NIMH Child Psychiatry Branch had performed a decade-long controlled study that demonstrated ADHD children having 3–4% smaller brain volumes in multiple critical brain regions affecting the types of behaviors associated with ADHD. The study also demonstrated that ADHD children receiving medication had developed volume of white matter that was the same as normal children. Individuals who had ADHD but were never medicated had an abnormally small volume of white matter. Whether or not genetic differences are responsible remains to be determined. As of 2004, the NIMH is conducting clinical trials examining the MRI of identical twins with ADHD.

Demographics

ADHD is the most commonly diagnosed behavioral disorder of childhood, affecting an estimated 3–5% of children, approximately two million in the United States. Males are considered up to eight times more likely to have ADHD than females. While it has been proven that males are more likely than females to develop ADHD, the difference in the numbers of male versus female may be due, in part, to males having a higher rate of hyperactivity symptoms that are easier to detect and diagnose. ADHD often occurs in conjunction with other problems such as depressive and anxiety disorders, conduct disorders, drug abuse, and antisocial behaviors. Children with untreated ADHD have increased rates of injury and co-morbid psychiatric disorders. Approximately 70–80% of children with ADHD exhibit significant symptoms into adolescence and adulthood. It is estimated that 2–6% of adolescents and 2–4% of adults have ADHD. Adults who had untreated ADHD in childhood have more severe symptoms and adverse risk factors later in life. Adverse factors both influence the expression of ADHD and increase the risk for associated disorders that reduce overall adjustment throughout life. ADHD is considered a lifelong disorder that requires appropriate diagnosis and treatment.

Signs and symptoms

Symptoms of ADHD often become apparent by the age of seven, but many adults remain undiagnosed. The three subtypes of ADHD recognized by the scientific community are a predominantly hyperactive-impulsive type that does not display significant symptoms of inattention, a predominantly inattentive type that does not display significant symptoms of hyperactive-impulsive behavior, and a combined type that displays both the inattentive and hyperactive-impulsive symptoms associated with ADHD. The predominantly inattentive type is sometimes still referred to as ADD, but this is an outdated term for the disorder.

Symptoms of inattention tend to persist through childhood into adulthood. The symptoms of inattention may include difficulty in paying attention to details, easy distractability and inability to concentrate, procrastination of tasks requiring sustained mental effort, frequent careless mistakes, disorganization, difficulty maintaining conversations, and difficulty completing appointed tasks. The symptoms of hyperactivity and impulsivity are nearly always present before the seventh year and tend to diminish with age. Hyperactivity symptoms may include restlessness, the perceived need to frequently walk or run during periods of prolonged sitting, excessive verbosity, and frequent inappropriate or uninhibited social interactions such as interrupting conversations or games. Hyperactive behavior is often associated with the development of other disruptive behavior disorders. It has been proposed that the impulsivity and inattention associated with ADHD may interfere with social learning in a way that predisposes the individual to the development of these disorders.

While many of these symptoms may sometimes occur in normal children, children with ADHD experience these behaviors more intensely and across several settings. Both children and adults with ADHD may experience these symptoms to a degree that interferes with normal functioning. Some individuals with moderate to severe ADHD may also experience periods of anxiety or **depression**. Individuals whose predominant symptom is inattention are most prone to depression. It follows that ADHD rarely occurs alone. It has been demonstrated that many people with ADHD also are subject to one or more co-morbid conditions such as depression, anxiety disorders, learning disabilities, or substance abuse disorders. Many conditions may have symptoms similar to, and be mistaken for, ADHD. It is critical that co-morbid disorders are diagnosed and treated or efforts to treat the ADHD may fail. When ADHD symptoms are present as a secondary to some other psychiatric disorder, the individual may be incorrectly treated for ADHD. However, when ADHD is the primary disorder, treating it often eliminates other dysfunctions.

There are many ADHD Internet sites available to the public. Many of these sites offer various questionnaires and descriptions of symptoms on the subject of ADHD. These Internet sites are not standardized or scientifically validated and should never be used to diagnose ADHD. A valid diagnosis can only be provided by a qualified, licensed medical professional.

Diagnosis

Well-established and research-validated clinical guidelines for the diagnosis of ADHD are provided in the American Psychiatric Association's *Diagnostic and Statistical Manual of Mental Disorders* (DSM-IV). The DSM-IV criteria for diagnosis include multiple symptoms of inattention or hyperactivity-impulsivity that persist for at least six months across multiple settings such as school or work and home. These symptoms must exist to a degree that is inconsistent with other individuals at the same developmental level. Some of the hyperactive-impulsive or inattentive symptoms must have been present before the age of seven years. The symptoms must not occur exclusively during the course of another developmental disorder, **schizophrenia**, or psychotic disorder and should not be better accounted for by any other mental disorder. Although fidgeting and inattentiveness are common childhood behaviors, the DSM-IV criteria indicate a diagnosis of ADHD for children in whom such behavior occurs so frequently that it produces continuing, pervasive dysfunction. A diagnostic evaluation requires histories from multiple sources, a medical evaluation of general and neurological health, and a full cognitive assessment. In practice, the diagnosis is often made in individuals who meet only some of the criteria established by the DSM-IV.

Treatment and management

The American Academy of Child and Adolescent Psychiatry (AACAP) established treatment as the support and education of family members, appropriate school placement, and pharmacology. Both pharmacological treatment and psychosocial treatment such as behavioral modification may be used.

Pharmacological treatment

Pharmacological treatment with psychostimulants is the most widely researched treatment for ADHD. This treatment has been used for childhood behavioral disorders since the 1930s. Psychostimulants are highly effective for approximately 75–90% of children with ADHD. There are four psychostimulant treatments that have been demonstrated by hundreds of randomized controlled trials to consistently reduce the primary symptoms of ADHD: methylphenidate, dextroamphetamine, pemoline, and a mixture of amphetamine salts. These medications are only effective for one to four hours and so must be administered with the individual's school or work schedule. The medications are most effective for symptoms of hyperactivity, impulsivity, inattention, and the associated features of rebelliousness, aggression, and argumentativeness. They promote improved overall performance. Individuals who do not respond to one stimulant may respond to another. Individuals in whom psychostimulant treatment has been indicated require an assessment to determine which, if any, psychostimulant may improve their symptoms with the least side effects. According to guidelines established by the AACAP, stimulants are usually started at a low dose and adjusted weekly. According to the NIMH, the stimulants most commonly prescribed for ADHD include methylphenidate (Ritalin), dextroamphetamine (Dexedrine), and amphetamine (Adderall).

In December 1999, the National Institutes of Mental Health (NIMH) began an ongoing Multimodal Treatment Study of Children with ADHD (MTA) that was one of the largest clinical studies ever conducted by the National Institutes of Health. The MTA utilized 18 nationally recognized authorities in ADHD at six different university medical centers and hospitals to evaluate the leading psychosocial and pharmacological treatments for ADHD. The MTA indicated that long-term combination treatments and pharmacological treatment alone are both significantly superior to intensive behavioral treatments and routine community care in reducing most ADHD symptoms. Combined treatment was equal in efficacy to medication alone in modifying the core ADHD symptoms of inattention, hyperactivity, impulsivity, and aggression. Combined treatment was superior to medication alone in treating anxiety symptoms and in improving academic performance and social skills. Combined treatment also allowed children to be successfully treated with lower doses of medication. The NIH ADHD Consensus Conference of 1998 reported that several decades of research have proven behavioral therapies to be very effective. However, the NIMH MTA study demonstrated that carefully monitored medication management is even more effective for the treatment of ADHD symptoms.

Some common side effects of psychostimulant therapy include insomnia, decreased appetite, stomachaches, headaches, and jitteriness. There may be rebound activation (a sudden increase in attention deficit and hyperactivity) after medication levels drop. Most side effects are mild, diminish over time, and respond to changes in dosage. There is no evidence that height or weight is affected by psychostimulant treatment, but precautionary monitoring of growth for children taking stimulants is still recommended. Atomoxetine (Strattera) is the only nonstimulant medication approved for the treatment of ADHD. Atomoxetine has effects on the neurotransmitter norepinephrine, which may also play a role in ADHD. Research contrasting atomoxetine with psychostimulants is being implemented. As of 2004, more than 70% of children with ADHD given Strattera have significant improvement in their symptoms.

Between 10–30% of individuals with ADHD do not respond to stimulant medication. For such non-responders and those who cannot tolerate the side effects, there are other useful medications. The antidepressant bupropion has been shown to be effective in a lower percentage of patients than stimulant medication. Certain types of antidepressants are sometimes used to augment psychostimulant treatment.

Psychosocial treatment

Psychosocial treatments may be used alone or in conjunction with pharmacological treatment to manage ADHD symptoms. Behavioral treatment for children typically involves using time-out, point systems, and contingent attention (adults reinforcing appropriate behavior by paying attention to it).

Children with ADHD can present a challenge that puts significant stress on the family. Skills training in psychosocial treatment for parents can help reduce this stress on the family. Systematic programs conducted in specialized classrooms or summer camps by highly trained individuals may be highly effective for some children. Adults may need treatment designed to train them in coping skills for management of ADHD symptoms. These skills may include list-making systems or other such reminders to assist in the completion of important tasks. Psychosocial treatment of ADHD symptoms has been proven to be less effective than pharmacological treatment when used alone, and needs to be consistently implemented in multiple settings to be fully effective. Behavioral interventions focus on improving targeted behaviors or skills, but are not as useful in reducing the core symptoms of inattention, hyperactivity, or impulsivity.

Educational accommodations for children with ADHD are federally mandated. Two federal laws that impact ADHD individuals are the Rehabilitation Act of 1973 and the Americans with Disabilities Act of 1990, which prohibit discrimination against individuals with disabilities in higher education and the workplace. Adults with ADHD are sometimes eligible for both protection and accommodation in higher education and the workplace under these laws. Organizations such as Children and Adults with Attention Deficit Disorder (CHADD) and the National Attention Deficit Disorder Association can provide information and support for individuals with ADHD.

Treatment controversies

Antidepressants known as selective serotonin reuptake inhibitors (SSRIs), such as fluoxetine, are not effective treatments for ADHD. Dietary manipulation has also been proven to be ineffective. In line with dietary research, controlled studies failed to demonstrate that sugar exacerbates the symptoms of children with ADHD. It is clear that research does not support the popularly held views that ADHD can be caused from excessive sugar intake, food additives, excessive television, poor parenting, or social and environmental factors such as poverty.

A highly controversial issue is whether there is over-diagnosis of ADHD and resultant over-prescription of stimulant medications. Special education legislation in the early 1990s increased general awareness of ADHD as a handicapping condition and provided the legal basis for accommodating ADHD-impaired students in the

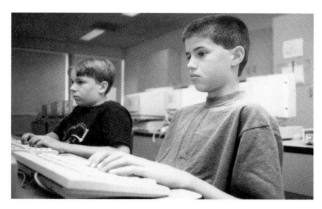

Students diagnosed with myopia have a difficult time concentrating for long periods of time. *(Field Mark Publications)*

school setting. These legal mandates have increased the awareness of ADHD within the school system and may have inadvertently led to the inaccurate conclusion that ADHD is a new disorder or that it is over-diagnosed. Despite the increased awareness, the Executive Summary on Mental Health, a supplement to the Surgeon General's Report in 2001, indicated that 75–80% of youths with mental health illnesses do not receive the needed treatments. Any increased use of stimulants in the 1990s is thought to reflect better diagnosis and more effective treatment of this prevalent disorder, which is still under-diagnosed. Most under-diagnosis is thought to be due to inadequate information supplied to the health care provider.

Prognosis

When properly diagnosed and treated, ADHD can be well managed. Treatment often leads to increased satisfaction in life and significant improvement in daily functioning. Many individuals with ADHD lead highly successful and happy lives. With proper treatment, the prognosis for ADHD can be very good. However, medications do not cure ADHD; they only temporarily control the symptoms. Although medications improve the prognosis and assist with symptom control, they cannot improve academic skills. The medications only help individuals to use those skills they already possess. Behavioral therapy and emotional counseling help individuals with ADHD to cope with their disorder.

Treatment may also mitigate risk factors for ADHD. A review of all long-term studies on stimulant medication and substance abuse, conducted by Researchers at Massachusetts General Hospital and Harvard Medical School, determined that teenagers with ADHD who remain on their medication have a lower probability of

KEY TERMS

Magnetic resonance imaging (MRI) scan—Noninvasive analysis of organs, large blood vessels, and soft tissues using magnetization without exposure to ionizing radiation.

White matter—Part of the brain that consists of fibers that establish long-distance connections between brain regions. It normally thickens as a child grows older and the brain matures.

substance abuse than those who do not remain on medication. Medications used properly where indicated at a young age may prevent additional later-onset emotional problems. ADHD individuals who do not receive any form of treatment, pharmacological or psychosocial, have a much poorer prognosis.

Resources

ORGANIZATIONS

Children and Adults with Attention/Hyperactivity Deficit Disorder. 8181 Professional Place, Suite 150, Landover, MD 20785. Toll-free: (800) 233-4050. <http://www.chadd.org>.

National Attention Deficit Disorder Association. P.O. Box 543 Pottstown, PA 19464. (484) 945-2101. <http://www.add.org>.

National Institutes of Health. 9000 Rockville PikeBethesda, Maryland 20892. (301) 496-4000. <http://www.nih.gov>.

OTHER

About AD/HD. National Resource Center on AD/HD. <http://www.help4adhd.org/en/about>.

Attention Deficit Hyperactivity Disorder. NIMH publication, 2003.

Attention Deficit Hyperactivity Disorder. Online Mendelian Inheritance in Man. <http://www.ncbi.nlm.nih.gov/entrez/dispomim.cgi?id=143465>.

Attention Deficit Hyperactivity Disorder (ADHD). <http://www.nimh.nih.gov/healthinformation/adhdmenu.cfm>.

Diagnosis and Treatment of Attention Deficit Hyperactivity Disorder. National Institutes of HealthConsensus Development Conference Statement,November 16–18, 1998. <http://odp.od.nih.gov/consensus/cons/110/110_statement.htm>.

Mental Health: A Report of the Surgeon General. <http://www.surgeongeneral.gov/library/mentalhealth/chapter3/sec4.html>.

National Institute of Mental Health. <http://www.nimh.nih.gov/nimhhome/index.cfm>.

Maria Basile, PhD

Autism

Definition

Autism is a potentially severe neurological condition affecting social functioning, communication skills, reasoning, and behavior. It is considered a spectrum disorder, meaning that the symptoms and characteristics of autism can present themselves in a variety of combinations, ranging from extremely mild to quite severe.

Description

Autism is a neurological disorder that affects a persons ability to communicate and form relationships. Individuals with autism have deficits in social interaction, communication, and understanding. Some individuals with autism have unusual repetitive behaviors, such as head banging, rocking, and hand-flapping. Up to 75–80% of individuals with autism are mentally retarded; only a small portion of this group (15–20%) have severe mental retardation. Additionally, over one-third of individuals with autism will develop seizures in early childhood or adolescence.

There is a wide degree of variability in the specific symptoms of autism. Because of this variability, autism is considered a spectrum disorder. There is no standard type or form of autism. Each individual is affected differently. This variability is reflected in some of the terms or names for autism. **Asperger syndrome** is a term used to describe individuals with autism with language skills. Pervasive developmental delay (PDD) is the term that is often used interchangeably with autism. The different terms for autism are partly due to the different individuals that first described this disorder.

Autism was first described by Leo Kanner in 1943. He observed and described a group of children with a pattern of symptoms. These children had some unique abilities and did not seem to be emotionally disturbed or mentally retarded. He invented the category early infantile autism (sometimes called Kanner's syndrome) to describe these children. In a strange coincidence, Hans Asperger made the same discoveries in the same year. He also described children with a unique behavioral profile and used the term autism to describe them. His original study was in German and was not translated into English until the late 1980s. Because the children that he identified all had speech, the term Asperger syndrome is often used to label autistic children who have speech.

While the effects of this disorder may vary in intensity, all individuals with autism have deficits in three key areas: social interaction, communication, and reasoning. In addition to these neurologic problems, individuals with autism often exhibit bizarre repetitive movements such as hand-flapping or head-banging. Other characteristics include a need for sameness or routine. While most individuals with autism have deficits, there are affected individuals that display unusual talents in areas such as math, music, and art. Some children have extraordinary talent in drawing and others learn to read before they learn to speak. These talents usually coexist with the other deficits of autism and are rare. These are usually referred to as *savant* skills.

Social interaction is the ability to interact, both verbally and nonverbally, with other humans. Individuals with autism have problems recognizing social cues such as facial expressions and tone of voice. Individuals with autism are often described as "being in their own world." This sense of isolation may arise from their inability to communicate effectively. They also lack the motivation for reciprocal communication.

Individuals with autism also have communication and language problems. They may or may not develop speech. Those individuals with autism that do speak use language in unusual ways. They may echo the comments of others (echolalia) or use phrases inappropriately. People with autism often use pronouns such as I, me, and you incorrectly. In addition to problems developing speech, individuals with autism have problems understanding the purpose of speech.

Individuals with autism can also have hyperacute senses. They may be very sensitive to bright lights, loud noises, or rough textures. The self-stimulating behaviors (head banging, hand flapping, rocking) sometimes seen in individuals with autism may be attempts to calm themselves due to over-stimulation. Other characteristic behaviors can include throwing temper tantrums for no apparent reason and developing fixations or obsessive interests.

The cause of autism is unknown. Originally, it was hypothesized that autism was a psychological problem caused by defective parenting. This hypothesis has been discredited as scientific information about neurological differences and biologic causes for autism have emerged.

Genetic profile

Although the search has been extensive, as of 2005, no single specific **gene** for autism has been discovered. Several candidate genes and chromosomal regions have been identified, but much research is needed before the exact roles that these genes play in the development of autism are understood.

Although the exact cause of autism is unknown, it is thought that autism occurs due to a combination of genetic and environmental causes. This combination of causative factors is often referred to as **multifactorial inheritance**. There are probably a number of different genes as well as unknown environmental factors involved in the development of autism. Multifactorial conditions tend to run in families, but the pattern of **inheritance** is not as predictable as with single-gene disorders. The chance of recurrence is also less than the risk for single-gene disorders and is usually derived from empiric or long-term studies of a large number of families.

Twins studies are used to determine the degree of heritability of a disorder. Identical twins have the exact same genes, while fraternal (non-identical) twins have only half of their genes in common. By examining the rates of concordance (the number of twin pairs that both have autism), it is possible to determine if there is a genetic component to autism. Studies that looked at the incidence of twins with autism determined that identical twins are more likely to be concordant (both affected) with autism than fraternal twins. This means that individuals with the same genes both have autism more often than twins with only half of the same genes. This finding suggests that genes play a role in the development of autism.

Identical twin pairs with autism reveal that there is a genetic component to autism. However, if autism was purely genetic, then all identical twins would be affected with autism (concordant). The fact that there are some identical twin pairs that are discordant for autism (one twin has autism and the other does not) means that other factors (possibly environmental) besides genes must also play a role in causing autism.

Speculations as to what other factors might influence or cause an individual to become autistic include viral, immunologic (including vaccinations), and environmental factors. While there are many theories about possible causes for autism, as of 2005, no specific non-genetic causes have been found and there is no scientific evidence for any specific environmental factor being a causative agent. Research in this area is ongoing.

Other scientific studies that point to the role of genes in the cause of autism look at the recurrence risk for autism. A recurrence risk is the chance that the same condition will occur for a second time in the same family. If a disease has no genetic component, then the recurrence risk should equal the incidence of the disorder. If autism had no genetic component, then it would not be expected to occur twice in the same family. However, studies have shown that autism does have an increased recurrence risk. In families with an affected son, the recurrence risk to have another child with autism is 7%. In families with an autistic daughter, the recurrence risk is 14%. In families with two children with autism, the chance that a subsequent child will also be affected is around 35%. Increased recurrence risks in families with one child with autism indicates that there is some genetic component to autism.

Genetic syndromes with autistic behaviors

While no specific gene has been found to cause isolated autism, there are some genetic syndromes in which the affected individual can have autistic behaviors. These genetic syndromes include untreated **phenylketonuria** (PKU), **fragile X syndrome**, tuberous sclerosis, **Rett syndrome**, and others.

Phenylketonuria is an inborn error of metabolism. Individuals with PKU are missing an enzyme necessary to break down phenylalanine, an amino acid found in protein-rich food. As these individuals eat protein, phenylalanine builds up in the bloodstream and nervous system, eventually leading to mental retardation and autistic behaviors. Most infants in the United States are tested at birth, and those affected with PKU are treated with a protein-free diet. This disorder is more common among individuals of northern European descent. The vast majority of infants in the Unites States are identified as having PKU through a newborn screening test done shortly after birth.

Fragile X syndrome is a mental retardation syndrome that predominantly (but not exclusively) affects males. Males with fragile X syndrome have long narrow faces, large cupped ears, enlarged testicles as adults, and varying degrees of mental retardation. Some individuals with fragile X syndrome also display autistic behaviors. The gene for fragile X syndrome, FMR1, is located on the X **chromosome**. **DNA** testing is available for this condition and will identify over 99% of individuals affected by fragile X syndrome.

Tuberous sclerosis is a variable disease characterized by hypopigmented skin patches, tumors, seizures, and mental retardation in some affected individuals. Up to 25% of individuals with tuberous sclerosis have autism. The genes for tuberous sclerosis have been identified as TSC1 and TSC2. DNA testing is available for this condition and will identify between 60–80% of individuals with tuberous sclerosis.

Rett syndrome is a progressive neurological disorder that almost exclusively affects females. Girls with Rett syndrome develop normally until the age of 18 months and then undergo a period of regression with loss of speech and motor milestones. Girls with Rett syndrome exhibit a nearly ceaseless hand-washing or hand-wringing motion. They also have mental retardation and can have autistic behaviors. The gene for Rett syndrome has been identified as MECP2. DNA testing is available for this syndrome and will identify approximately 80% of individuals with this syndrome.

While individuals with these genetic syndromes can have autistic behaviors, it is important to remember that 70–90% of individuals with autism do not have an underlying genetic syndrome as the cause of their disorder. Many studies are underway to try and determine the etiology or cause of autism.

Demographics

The exact incidence of autism is not known. Because the diagnostic criteria for autism has changed and broadened over the years, studies done to determine the incidence have yielded different estimates. Using the newer, more inclusive criteria, it is estimated that one in 500 individuals are affected with autism and that over half a million individuals in the United States fit the diagnostic criteria for autism, PDD, or Asperger syndrome.

Boys are affected with autism three times more often than girls. While boys may be affected more often, girls with autism tend to be more severely affected and have a lower IQ. The reasons for these differences are not known. Autism occurs in all racial, social, and economic backgrounds.

Signs and symptoms

One of the most frustrating aspects of autism is the lack of physical findings in individuals with autism. Most individuals with autism have normal appearances, and few, if any, medical problems. Because the specific cause of autism is unknown, there is no prenatal test available for autism.

Autism is a spectrum disorder. A spectrum refers to the fact that different individuals with a diagnosis of autism can have very different abilities and deficits. The spectrum of autism stretches from a socially isolated adult with normal IQ to a severally affected child with mental retardation and behavioral problems. The following is a partial list of behaviors seen in individuals with autism divided into main areas of concern. It is unlikely that any one individual would exhibit all of the following behaviors. Most affected people would be expected to exhibit some but not all of the behaviors.

In the area of communication skills, behaviors autistic individuals may display include:

• language delay or absence

- impaired speech
- meaningless repetition of words or phrases
- using gestures rather than words to communicate
- concrete or literal understanding of words or phrases
- inability to initiate or hold conversations

In the area of social interaction, behaviors autistic individuals may display include:

- unresponsiveness to people
- lack of attachment to parents or caregivers
- little or no interest in human contact
- failure to establish eye contact
- little interest in making friends
- unresponsiveness to social cues such as smiles or frowns

In the area of play, behaviors autistic individuals may display include:

- little imaginative play
- play characterized by repetition (e.g., endless spinning of car wheels)
- no desire for group play
- no pretend games

Autistic individuals may display behaviors that include:

- repetitive motions such as hand flapping and head banging
- rigid or flaccid muscle tone when held
- temper tantrums or screaming fits
- resistance to change
- hyperactivity
- fixates or develops obsessive interest in an activity, idea, or person
- overreaction to sensory stimulus such as noise, lights, and texture
- inappropriate laughing or giggling

Diagnosis

There is no medical test, such as a blood test or brain scan, to diagnose autism. The diagnosis of autism is very difficult to make in young children due to the lack of physical findings and the variable behavior of children. Because the primary signs and symptoms of autism are behavioral, the diagnosis usually requires evaluation by a specialized team of health professionals and occurs over a period of time. This team of specialists may include a developmental pediatrician, speech therapist, psychologist, geneticist, and other health professionals. Medical tests may be done to rule out other possible causes and may include a hearing evaluation, chromosome analysis, DNA testing for specific **genetic disorders**, and brain imaging scans, including magnetic resonance imaging (MRI), electroencephalogram (EEG), or computed tomography (CT), to rule out structural brain anomalies.

Once other medical causes have been excluded, the diagnosis for autism can be made using criteria from the fourth edition of the *Diagnostic and Statistical Manual of Mental Disorders* (DSM IV). This manual, developed by the American Psychiatric Association, lists abnormal behaviors in three key areas: impairment in social interaction, impairment in communication (language), and restrictive and repetitive patterns of behavior. These behaviors are usually seen in individuals with autism. If an individual displays enough distinct behaviors from the list, they meet the diagnostic criteria for autism. Most individuals will not exhibit all of the possible behaviors and, while individuals might exhibit the same behaviors, there is still a large degree of variability within this syndrome.

The DSM-IV criteria for a diagnosis of autistic disorder require a display total of at least six behaviors from items 1, 2, and 3, with at least two from 1, and one each from 2 and 3.

Under item 1 in the DSM-IV, the criteria are qualitative impairment in social interaction, as manifested by at least two of the following:

- marked impairment in the use of multiple nonverbal behaviors such as eye-to-eye gaze, facial expression, body postures, and gestures to regulate social interaction
- failure to develop peer relationships appropriate to developmental level
- markedly impaired expression of pleasure in other people's happiness

Under the DSM-IV's item 2, the criteria are qualitative impairments in communication, as manifested by at least one of the following:

- delay in, or total lack of, the development of spoken language (not accompanied by an attempt to compensate through alternative modes of communication such as gestures or mime)
- in individuals with adequate speech, marked impairment in the ability to initiate or sustain a conversation with others

- stereotyped and repetitive use of language or idiosyncratic language
- lack of varied spontaneous make-believe play or social imitative play appropriate to developmental level

Under item 3, the DSM-IV criteria are restricted repetitive and stereotyped patterns of behavior, interests, and activities, as manifested by as least one of the following:

- encompassing preoccupation with one or more stereotyped and restricted patterns of interest that is abnormal either in intensity or focus
- apparently compulsive adherence to specific nonfunctional routines or rituals
- stereotyped and repetitive motor mannerisms (e.g., hand or finger flapping or twisting, or complex whole-body movements)
- persistent preoccupation with parts of objects

Other criteria that help diagnosis autism include delays or abnormal functioning in at least one of the following areas, with onset prior to age three years:

- social interaction,
- language as used in social communication
- symbolic or imaginative play

Autism is the usual diagnosis when there is no findings of Rett disorder or childhood disintegrative disorder (CDD).

Using all these criteria, the diagnosis of autism is usually made in children by approximately the age of two and a half to three; they are originally seen for speech delay. Often these children are initially thought to have hearing impairments due to their lack of response to verbal cues and their lack of speech.

While speech delay or absence of speech might initially bring a child to the attention of medical or educational professionals, it soon becomes apparent that there are other symptoms in addition to the lack of speech. Children with autism are often noticed for their lack of spontaneous play and their lack of initiative in communication. These deficits become more obvious when these children are enrolled in school for the first time. Their inability to interact with their peers becomes highlighted. Behaviors such as hand flapping, temper tantrums, and head banging also contribute to the diagnosis.

Because the criteria to diagnose autism are based on observation, several appointments with health care providers may be necessary before a definitive diagnosis is reached. A specialist closely observes and evaluates the child's language and social behavior. In addition to observation, structured interviews of the parents are used to elicit information about early behavior and development.

Treatment and management

There is no cure for autism. However, autism is not a static disorder. Behaviors can and do modify over time, and educational treatments can be used to focus on appropriate behaviors. The treatments available for individuals with autism depend upon their needs, but are generally long and intensive. While treatments vary, and there is considerable controversy about some treatments, there is uniform agreement that early and intensive intervention allows for the best prognosis. A treatment plan is usually based upon an evaluation of the child's unique abilities and disabilities.

Standardized testing instruments are used to determine the child's level of cognitive development and interviews with parents and caregivers, as well as observation by health professionals, are used to gauge a child's social, emotional, and communications skills. Once a clear picture of the child's needs is developed, treatment is initiated. Studies have shown that individuals with autism respond well to a highly structured, specialized education program tailored to their individual needs. All treatments are best administered by trained professionals. Speech and language therapy may be used to develop and improve language skills. Occupational therapy may be used to develop fine motor skills and to teach basic self-help and functional skills such as grooming. Behavior modification, with positive reinforcement, plays a large role in the early treatment of some of the abnormal behaviors of individuals with autism. Other therapies may include applied behavioral analysis, auditory integration training, dietary interventions, medications, music therapy, physical therapy, sensory integration, and vision therapy.

Increasingly, medications are being used to treat some of the symptoms of autism. The drugs that are recommended most often for children with autism include psychostimulants (methylphenidate, pemoline), clonidine, or one of the tricyclic antidepressants (TCAs) for hyperactivity or inattention; beta blockers, neuroleptics, or lithium for anger or aggression; selective serotonin reuptake inhibitors (SSRIs) or TCAs for rituals and preoccupations; and SSRIs or TCAs for anxiety symptoms. One alternative herbal remedy that has been tried with AS patients is St. John's Wort.

KEY TERMS

Asperger syndrome—A term used to describe high-functioning individuals with autism. These individuals usually have normal IQ and some language skills.

Pervasive developmental disorder (PDD)—The term used to describe individuals who meet some but not all of the criteria for autism.

Savant skills—Unusual talents, usually in art, math, or music, that some individuals with autism have in addition to the deficits of autism.

In order to be effective, the treatments and therapies must be consistent and reinforced by the family. It is helpful if family members and caregivers receive training in working with and teaching individuals with autism. A team approach involving health care professionals, therapists, educators, and families is necessary for successful treatment of individuals with autism.

Prognosis

The prognosis for individuals with autism is variable but much brighter than it was a generation ago. Overall, the ultimate prognosis of an individual with autism is dependant on their IQ, their communicative abilities, and the extent of their behavioral problems.

Individuals with autism without mental retardation can develop independent living skills. Often these individuals do well and can become self-sufficient if they have good communication skills. Other individuals with autism develop some level of self-sufficiency but may never be able to live independently due to their severe communication or cognitive difficulties. Up to 60% of individuals with autism will require lifelong assistance.

Resources

BOOKS

Diagnostic and Statistical Manual of Mental Disorders, 4th Edition. Washington, DC: American Psychiatric Association, 1994.

Hart, C. *A Parent's Guide to Autism.* New York: Simon and Schuster, 1993.

Siegel, Byrna. *The World of the Autistic Child: Understanding and Treating Spectrum Disorders.* Oxford: Oxford University Press, 1998.

ORGANIZATIONS

Association for Science in Autism Treatment. 175 Great Neck Road, Suite 406, Great Neck, NY 11021.

(516) 466-4400. Fax: (516) 466-4484. asat@autism-treatment.org.

Autism Society of America. 7910 Woodmont Ave. Suite 300, Bethesda, MD 20814-3015. (301) 657-0881 or (800) 3-AUTISM. (April 8, 2005.) <http://www.autism-society.org>.

Cure Autism Now (CAN) Foundation. 5455 Wilshire Blvd. Suite 715, Los Angeles, CA 90036-4234. (500) 888-AUTISM. Fax: (323) 549-0547. info@cureautismnow.org. (April 8, 2005.) <http://www.cureautismnow.org>.

National Alliance for Autism Research (NAAR). 414 Wall Street Research Park, Princeton, NJ 08540. (609) 430-9160 or (888) 777-6227 CA: (310) 230-3568. Fax: (609) 430-9163. (April 8, 2005.) <http://www.naar.org>.

WEB SITES

The Autism/PDD Network. (April 8, 2005.) <http://www.autism-pdd.net/>.

Autism Resources. (April 8, 2005.) <http://www.autism-resources.com>.

National Research Council. (April 8, 2005.) <http://www.nap.edu/books/0309072697/html>.

O.A.S.I.S. Online Asperger Syndrome Information Society. (April 8, 2005.) <http://www.udel.edu/bkirby/asperger/>.

Kathleen A. Fergus, MS, CGC

Azorean disease

Definition

Azorean disease causes progressive degeneration of the central nervous system. Affected individuals experience deterioration in muscle coordination and other physical symptoms, but intelligence and mental function remain unaffected by the disease.

Description

Azorean disease is an inherited disorder that causes impaired brain functioning, vision problems, and loss of muscle control. It is named for the Azores, the group of nine Portuguese islands where the disease is prevalent. Many of the reported cases have been found in the direct descendants of William Machado, an Azorean native who immigrated to the New England area of the United States, and Atone Joseph, a Portuguese sailor from the island of Flores who came to California in 1845. Other names for Azorean disease include Machado-Joseph disease, Joseph disease, and **spinocerebellar ataxia** type III.

Azorean disease is classified into three types depending on the age of onset and the specific physical symptoms. In type I, the age of onset is usually before age 25 and the affected individuals experience extreme muscle stiffness and rigidity. In type II, the age of onset is typically in the mid-30s, and progressive loss of muscle coordination (ataxia) occurs, resulting in the inability to walk. In type III, the average age of onset is 40 or later, and the main symptoms are weakness and loss of sensation in the legs.

The symptoms of Azorean disease result from the loss of brain cells and the impairment of neurological connections in the brain and spinal cord. This degradation of the central nervous system is believed to be caused by the production of a destructive protein from a mutated **gene**.

Genetic profile

Azorean disease is inherited as an autosomal dominant trait. This means that only one parent has to pass on the gene mutation in order for the child to be affected with the syndrome.

Each gene in the human body is made up of units called nucleotides, abbreviated C (cytosine), A (adenine), T (thymine), and G (guanine). A sequence of three nucleotides is called a trinucleotide. Azorean syndrome is caused by a genetic mutation that results in the over-duplication of a CAG trinucleotide sequence. The location of the mutant gene in Azorean disease is 14q32, on the long arm of **chromosome** 14. This gene normally encodes the formation of a cellular protein called ataxin-3. In the general population, there are between 13 and 36 repeats of the CAG sequence, but in those individuals with Azorean disease, there may be between 61 and 84 repeats. The increased number of repetitions causes the gene to encode an abnormal protein product that is believed to cause cell death in the brain and spinal cord.

In successive generations, the number of the repetitions may increase, a phenomenon known as genetic anticipation. In addition, there appears to be a strong relationship between the number of repetitions and the age at onset of Azorean disease: the more repetitions, the sooner the disease presents and the more serious the symptoms are. Also, if the individual is homozygous for the mutated gene, meaning he or she inherits the gene from both parents, Azorean disease is more severe and the age of onset is as early as 16 years.

Demographics

Azorean disease is primarily found in people of Portuguese ancestry, particularly people from the Azores islands. In the Azores islands the incidence of Azorean disease is approximately one in every 4,000, while among those of Azorean descent, it is one in every 6,000. Azorean disease has also been identified in other ethnic groups, including Japanese, Brazilians, Chinese, Indians, Israelis, and Australian aborigines.

Signs and symptoms

The age of onset of Azorean disease is typically from the late teens to the 50s, although onset as late as the 70s has been reported. The first observable symptoms are difficulty in walking and slurred speech. There is wide variation in the range of observed symptoms, but they typically include problems with muscular coordination, eyes and vision, and other physical bodily functions such as speech and urination. Mental ability is not impaired by Azorean disease.

Muscular symptoms

Muscular symptoms observed in people with Azorean disease include difficulty in walking, including staggering or stumbling, weakness in arms or legs, involuntary jerking or spastic motions, cramping or twisting of the hands and feet, facial tics and grimaces, and twitching or rippling of the muscles in the face.

Eyes and vision

People with Azorean disease may experience double vision, bulging eyes, difficulty in looking upward, difficulty in opening the eyes, a fixed or staring gaze, or involuntary eye movements from side to side.

Other symptoms

Other symptoms reported with Azorean disease include difficulty in speech such as slurring; loss of feeling in arms or legs; frequent urination; infections of the lungs; **diabetes**; weight loss; and difficulty sleeping.

Diagnosis

Azorean disease can be diagnosed after observation of typical symptoms and a medical history that establishes a familial pattern to the disease. Brain imaging studies such as computerized tomography (CT) and magnetic resonance imaging (MRI) may be employed. Blood tests can show increased levels of blood sugar and uric acid. Genetic studies that reveal the presence of the increased number of CAG trinucleotide repeats in the affected individual will provide definite confirmation of the diagnosis of Azorean disease.

The symptoms of Azorean disease are similar to other degenerative neurological conditions such as **Parkinson disease**, **Huntington disease**, and **multiple**

KEY TERMS

Ataxia—A deficiency of muscular coordination, especially when voluntary movements are attempted, such as grasping or walking.

Genetic anticipation—The tendency for an inherited disease to become more severe in successive generations.

Homozygous—Having two identical copies of a gene or chromosome.

Nucleotides—Building blocks of genes, which are arranged in specific order and quantity.

Trinucleotide—A sequence of three nucleotides.

sclerosis. Careful diagnosis is required in order to distinguish Azorean disease from these other conditions.

Treatment and management

Treatment for Azorean disease is based on management of the symptoms. There is no treatment that stops or reverses the effects of the disease. A multidisciplinary team of specialists in neurology, ophthalmology, and endocrinology is often necessary. Medications that specifically treat movement disorders, such as dopamine agonists, may alleviate some of the symptoms of Azorean disease. Some experimental drugs and treatments under development for other neurological disorders may also benefit patients with Azorean disease. Genetic counseling is recommended for people with a family history of the disease since Azorean disease is an inherited disorder.

Prognosis

The prognosis for individuals with Azorean disease varies depending on the age of onset and severity of the symptoms. The muscular degeneration caused by the disease usually results in eventual confinement to a wheelchair. After onset of the symptoms, life expectancy ranges from 10 to 30 years.

Resources

PERIODICALS

Gaspar, C. et al. "Ancestral Origins of the Machado-Joseph Disease Mutation: A Worldwide Haplotype Study." *American Journal of Human Genetics* (February 2001): 523-8.

BOOKS

Hamilton, Patricia Birdsong. *A Balancing Act: Living with Spinal Cerebellar Ataxia.* Coral Springs, FL: Scripts Publishing, 1998.

Klockgether, Thomas (ed). *Handbook of Ataxia Disorders.* New York: Marcel Dekker, Inc., 2000.

ORGANIZATIONS

Ataxia MJD Research Project, Inc. 875 Mahler Rd., Suite 161, Burlingame, CA 94010-1621. (650) 259-3984. Fax: (650) 259-3983. <http://www.ataxiamjd.org>.

International Joseph Disease Foundation, Inc. PO Box 2550, Livermore, CA 94551-2550. (925) 461-7550. (925) 371-1288. <http://www.ijdf.net>.

MJD Family Network Newsletter. c/o Mike and Phyllis Cote, 591 Federal Furnace Rd., Plymouth, MA 02360-4761.

National Ataxia Foundation. 2600 Fernbrook Lane, Suite 119, Minneapolis, MN 55447. (763) 553-0020. Fax: (763) 553-0167. naf@ataxia.org. <http://www.ataxia.org>.

WEBSITES

Machado/Joseph's Disease. <http://www.lusaweb.com/machado.html> (April 20, 2001).

OMIM—Online Mendelian Inheritance in Man. <http://www.ncbi.nlm.nih.gov/htbin-post/Omim/dispmim?109150> (April 20, 2001).

Paul A. Johnson

B

Bardet-Biedl syndrome

Definition

Bardet-Biedl syndrome (BBS) is a condition that primarily affects vision, kidney function, limb development, growth, and intelligence.

Description

BBS expresses itself differently from person to person, even among members of the same family. However, certain features frequently appear.

Genetic profile

BBS is a genetically heterogeneous condition; this means that it has more than one known genetic cause. One of these causes is a mutation in the MKKS **gene**, located on **chromosome** 20. When working properly, this gene appears to produce a chaperonin, a factor needed to process proteins. Without the chaperonin, the proteins cannot work properly.

Using linkage analysis, researchers have connected some BBS cases to other chromosomes. Linkage analysis is a method of finding mutations based on their proximity to previously identified genetic landmarks. The specific genes responsible for these BBS cases remain unknown. However, several potential locations of BBS genes have been recognized. These sites are named for the number of the chromosome on which they are found, the arm of the chromosome ("q" for long arm, "p" for short arm), region of the arm, and band within the region. For example, "11q13" means chromosome number 11, long arm, region 1, band 3. In studies of families with BBS, researchers have found that a significant number of cases link either to 11q13, 15q22, or 16q21. In other families, researchers have linked BBS to either 2q31, 3p12, or 20p12. This last site is the location of the MKKS gene.

Regardless of the site involved, BBS displays an autosomal recessive **inheritance** pattern. This means

that the condition occurs only when an individual inherits two defective copies of a BBS gene. If one copy is normal, the individual does not have BBS. This individual is called a carrier of BBS and can pass the gene on to the next generation.

Research indicates that people who inherit one abnormal BBS gene and one normal gene may be at risk for some of the health problems seen in BBS. Compared to the general population, these BBS gene carriers are more likely to develop high blood pressure, **diabetes** mellitus, and kidney disease, including kidney **cancer**.

Demographics

BBS affects people around the world. However, it is most common in the Middle East, especially in the Arab and inbred Bedouin populations of Kuwait. In these groups, it may affect as many as 1 in 13,500 individuals. The incidence is almost as high in Newfoundland, where as many as 1 in 16,000 individuals has BBS. Outside of these areas, researchers estimate that BBS affects only 1 in 160,000 people.

The specific genetic cause of BBS differs by family and geographic location. For example, in the Middle East, BBS appears to link to 16q21 or 3p12. However, in patients of European descent, BBS appears to link to 11q13 or 15q22.

Signs and symptoms

If the newborn with BBS has finger or toe abnormalities, these are apparent at birth. However, these defects have a variety of congenital causes, meaning they originated during development of the fetus and were not inherited. For this reason, medical care providers may not immediately suspect BBS. It becomes a consideration as the child develops and additional abnormalities emerge. In boys, genital abnormalities become evident soon after birth. In almost all patients, obesity and retinal degeneration begin in early childhood. Learning disabilities, if present, are identified in school-aged children, if not earlier. Failure to menstruate leads to diagnosis of some adolescent girls. Infertility brings some young adults to medical attention. Kidney disease is progressive and may not become obvious until adulthood.

Due to progressive degeneration of the retina, vision damage occurs in all patients. Specific vision defects include poor night vision during childhood, severe **myopia** (nearsightedness), **glaucoma**, and cataracts. A few patients suffer from **retinitis pigmentosa**, a condition in which the field of vision progressively narrows. Most individuals affected with BBS are blind by age 30.

Many infants with BBS are born with a kidney defect affecting kidney structure, function, or both. The specific abnormality varies from patient to patient and may be aggravated by lifelong obesity, another common problem for BBS patients. The complications of obesity, such as high blood pressure (hypertension) and insulin-resistant diabetes mellitus, contribute to kidney disease.

BBS patients may have extra fingers or toes (**polydactyly**), short fingers (**brachydactyly**), or broad, short feet. Some patients have a combination of all three of these features. Alternately, polydactyly may be limited to one limb, hands only, or feet only. Syndactyly, the fusion of two or more fingers or toes, may also occur. In some BBS families, all affected members display at least some of these limb abnormalities.

Many individuals with BBS have genital abnormalities. Most boys with BBS have a very small penis and some also have undescended testes. Men with BBS are usually unable to have children. In women with BBS, the genitalia, ovaries, fallopian tubes, and uterus may or may not be underdeveloped. The vagina may not be completely formed. Though some women with BBS do not menstruate, others menstruate irregularly, and some women are able to have children. In both sexes, there may be birth defects in the urinary or gastrointestinal tract.

Some research indicates that people with BBS have characteristic facial features, including a prominent forehead, deep-set eyes, flat nasal bridge, and thin upper lip. Teeth are small and crowded, and a high, arched palate is common.

Occasionally, individuals with BBS have liver disease or heart abnormalities.

In addition to the physical effects of the condition, intelligence is sometimes affected. While some BBS patients show normal intelligence, others have mild to moderate learning disabilities. These patients are often developmentally delayed—they are slower than most children to walk, speak, or reach other developmental milestones. Difficulty with language and comprehension may continue into adulthood. In a few people with BBS, more severe mental retardation occurs. In some patients, vision handicap and developmental delay appear to be related.

Some parents report that their children with BBS have behavioral problems that continue into adulthood. These include lack of inhibition and social skills, emotional outbursts, and obsessive-compulsive behavior. Most people with BBS prefer fixed routines and are easily upset by a change in plans.

Diagnosis

Diagnosis of BBS is a challenge for medical professionals. Not only do the symptoms of BBS vary greatly from patient to patient, but some of these symptoms occur in other conditions, many of which are more common than BBS.

Though available on a research basis, **genetic testing** for BBS is not yet offered through clinical laboratories. Instead, it is the association of many BBS symptoms in one patient that generally leads to a clinical diagnosis. Therefore, patients must have a thorough genetic evaluation. This provides a chance to rule out other disorders with similar symptoms. Because symptoms emerge throughout childhood, patients diagnosed as infants require regular exams to confirm proper diagnosis. Some disorders historically confused with BBS include Lawrence-Moon syndrome, Kearns-Sayre syndrome, and **McKusick-Kaufman syndrome**. This last syndrome is also caused by mutation in the MKKS gene; in fact, the gene took its name from McKusick-Kaufman syndrome. While people with this syndrome show some of the same symptoms as BBS patients, the specific MKKS mutation differs between the conditions. This explains how one gene can be responsible for two distinct yet similar disorders.

Six major criteria form the basis of BBS diagnosis. These are retinal degeneration, polydactyly, obesity, learning disabilities, kidney abnormalities, and genital defects (in males). To confirm diagnosis, the patient should receive three particular diagnostic tests. An eye exam called an electroretinogram is used to test the electric currents of the retina. An ultrasound is used to examine the kidneys, as is an intravenous pyelogram (IVP). An IVP is an x-ray assessment of kidney function.

Treatment and management

Unless they have severe birth defects involving the heart, kidneys, or liver, patients with BBS can have a normal life span. However, obesity and kidney disease are major threats. If unchecked, obesity can lead to high blood pressure, diabetes mellitus, and heart disease. Untreated kidney disease can lead to renal failure, a frequent cause of early death in patients with BBS. Some

KEY TERMS

Brachydactyly—Abnormal shortness of the fingers and toes.

Electroretinogram (ERG)—A measurement of electrical activity of the retina.

Intravenous pyelogram—An x-ray assessment of kidney function.

Linkage analysis—A method of finding mutations based on their proximity to previously identified genetic landmarks.

Polydactyly—The presence of extra fingers or toes.

Retinitis pigmentosa—Degeneration of the retina marked by progressive narrowing of the field of vision.

Syndactyly—Webbing or fusion between the fingers or toes.

patients require dialysis and kidney transplant. Therefore, it is very important to monitor and manage patients with BBS, and to promptly treat any complications. Affected individuals should eat a well-balanced, low-calorie diet and should exercise regularly.

Because BBS carriers also appear prone to kidney disease, parents and siblings of patients with BBS should take extra precautions. These include baseline screening for kidney defects or cancer, as well as preventive health care on a regular basis.

In order to conserve vision to the extent possible, retinal degeneration should be carefully monitored. Therapy, education, and counseling help prepare the patient for progressive loss of vision. The Foundation Fighting Blindness, a support and referral group, offers help to BBS patients and their families.

Though not life-threatening, learning disabilities and reproductive dysfunction need attention in order to maximize the quality of life for patients with BBS. Affected people benefit greatly from special or vocational education, speech therapy, social skills training, and community support services. Some adult patients may never be able to live independently and may remain with their families. In these cases, families should plan future living arrangements in case the patients outlive their caregivers.

Genital abnormalities may require hormonal treatment or surgical attention. Sometimes removal of undescended testes is necessary to prevent cancer. Patients with genital and reproductive dysfunction may need counseling to help them deal with the personal, familial, social, and cultural impact of the condition. **Genetic**

counseling is available to help fertile BBS patients address their reproductive choices.

Prognosis

The outlook for people with BBS depends largely on the extent of the birth abnormalities, prompt diagnosis, and follow-up care. At this time there is no treatment for the extensive retinal damage caused by BBS. However, good health care beginning in childhood can help many people with BBS avoid other serious effects of this disorder. Researchers are actively exploring genetic causes, treatment, and management of BBS.

Resources

BOOKS

"Bardet-Biedl Syndrome." In *Smith's Recognizable Patterns of Human Malformation.* 5th ed. Philadelphia: W. B. Saunders, 1997, pp. 590-591.

PERIODICALS

Beales, P. L., et al. "New Criteria for Improved Diagnosis of Bardet-Biedl Syndrome: Results of a Population Survey." *Journal of Medical Genetics* 36 (1999): 437-446.

Foltin, Lynn. "Researchers Identify Inherited Obesity, Retinal Dystrophy Gene." *Texas Medical Center News* 22 (2000): 17.

Hrynchak, P. K. "Bardet-Biedl Syndrome." *Optometry and Vision Science* 77 (May 2000): 236-243.

ORGANIZATIONS

Foundation Fighting Blindness. Executive Plaza 1, Suite 800, 11350 McCormick Rd., Hunt Valley, MD 21031. (888) 394-3937. <http://www.blindness.org>.

Genetic Alliance. 4301 Connecticut Ave. NW, #404, Washington, DC 20008. (800) 336-GENE (Helpline) or (202) 966-5557. Fax: (888) 394-3937. info@geneticalliance. <http://www.geneticalliance.org>.

WEBSITES

"Bardet Biedl Syndrome." *NORD—National Organization for Rare Disorders.* <http://www.raredisorders.org>.

Avis L. Gibons

Batten disease

Definition

Batten disease is a disorder of the nervous system that begins in childhood. Symptoms of the disorder include mental impairment, seizures, and loss of sight and motor skills.

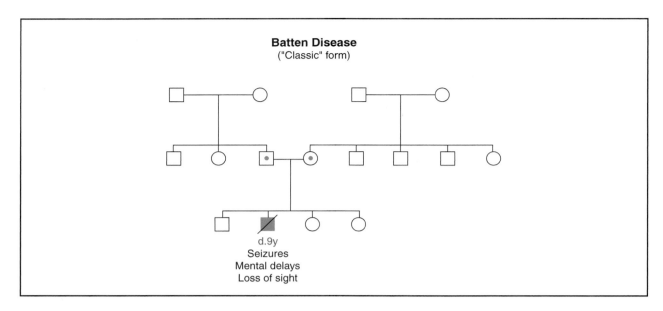

Batten Disease
("Classic" form)

d.9y
Seizures
Mental delays
Loss of sight

(Gale Group.)

Description

Batten disease is characterized by an abnormal buildup of lipopigments—substances made up of fats and proteins—in bubble-like compartments within cells. The compartments, called lysosomes, normally take in and break down waste products and complex molecules for the cell. In Batten disease, this process is disrupted, and the lipopigments accumulate. This breakdown is genetic. It is marked by vision failure and the loss of intellect and neurological functions, which begin in early childhood.

Batten disease is a form of a family of progressive neurological disorders known as neuronal ceroid lipofuscinoses (or NCLs). It is also known as Spielmeyer-Vogt-Sjögren-Batten disease, or juvenile NCL. There are three other disorders in the NCL family: Jansky-Bielchowsky disease, late infantile neuronal ceroid lipofuscinosis, and Kufs disease (a rare adult form of NCL). Although these disorders are often collectively referred to as Batten disease, Batten disease is a single disorder.

Genetic profile

Batten disease was named after the British pediatrician who first described it in 1903. It is an autosomal recessive disorder. This means that it occurs when a child receives one copy of the abnormal **gene** from each parent. Batten disease results from abnormalities in gene CLN3. This specific gene was identified by researchers in 1995.

Individuals with only one abnormal gene are known as carriers; they do not develop the disease but can pass

the gene on to their own children. When both parents carry one abnormal gene, their children have a one in four chance of developing Batten disease.

Demographics

Batten disease is relatively rare, occurring in two to four of every 100,000 births in the United States. NCLs appear to be more common in children living in Northern Europe and Newfoundland, Canada.

Signs and symptoms

Early symptoms of Batten disease include vision difficulties and seizures. There may also be personality and behavioral changes, slow learning, clumsiness, or stumbling. These signs typically appear between ages five and eight. Over time, the children experience mental impairment, worsening seizures, and the complete loss of vision and motor skills.

Batten disease, like other childhood forms of NCL, may first be suspected during an eye exam that displays a loss of certain cells. Because such cell loss can occur in other eye diseases, however, the disorder cannot be diagnosed by this sign alone. An eye specialist who suspects Batten disease may refer the child to a neurologist, who will analyze the medical history and information from various laboratory tests.

Diagnosis

Diagnostic tests used for Batten disease and other NCLs include:

KEY TERMS

Lipopigments—Substances made up of fats and proteins found in the body's tissues.

Lysosome—Membrane-enclosed compartment in cells, containing many hydrolytic enzymes; where large molecules and cellular components are broken down.

Neuronal ceroid lipofuscinoses—A family of four progressive neurological disorders.

- blood or urine tests that detect abnormalities that may indicate Batten disease

- skin or tissue sampling, which can detect the buildup of lipopigments in cells

- electroencephalogram, which displays electrical activity within the brain that suggests a person has seizures

- electrical studies of the eyes, which further detect various eye problems common in childhood NCLs

- brain scans, which spot changes in the brain's appearance

Treatment and management

There is no known treatment to prevent or reverse the symptoms of Batten disease or other NCLs. Anticonvulsant drugs are often prescribed to reduce or control seizures. Other medicines may be prescribed to manage other symptoms associated with the disorder. Physical and occupation therapy may also help people retain function for a longer period of time. Scientists' recent discovery of the genes responsible for NCLs may help lead to effective treatments.

There have been reports of the slowing of the disease among children who were given vitamins C and E and diets low in vitamin A. However, the fatal outcome of the disease remained the same.

Prognosis

People with Batten disease may become blind, confined to bed, and unable to communicate. Batten disease is typically fatal by the late teens or 20s. Some people with the disorder, however, live into their 30s.

Resources

ORGANIZATIONS

Battens Disease Support and Research Association. 2600 Parsons Ave., Columbus, OH 43207. (800) 448-4570. <http://www.bdsra.org.>.

Children's Brain Disease Foundation. 350 Parnassus Ave., Suite 900, San Francisco, CA 94117. (415) 566-5402.

Children's Craniofacial Association. PO Box 280297, Dallas, TX 75243-4522. (972) 994-9902 or (800) 535-3643. contactcca@ccakids.com. <http://www.ccakids.com>.

JNCL Research Fund. PO Box 766, Mundelein, IL 60060. <http://www.jnclresearch.org>.

National Organization for Rare Disorders (NORD). PO Box 8923, New Fairfield, CT 06812-8923. (203) 746-6518 or (800) 999-6673. Fax: (203) 746-6481. <http://www.rarediseases.org>.

WEBSITES

"Batten Disease Fact Sheet." (June 2000). *National Institute of Neurological Disorders and Stroke.* <http://www.ninds.nih.gov/health_and_medical/pubs/batten_disease.htm>.

"Gene for Last Major Form of Batten Disease Discovered." (September 18, 1997). *National Institute of Diabetes and Digestive and Kidney Disorders.* <http://www.niddk.nih.gov/welcome/releases/9_18_97.htm>

Michelle Lee Brandt

BBB syndrome *see* **Opitz syndrome**

Beals syndrome

Definition

Beals syndrome, also known as Beals contractural arachnodactyly (BCA), congenital contractural arachnodactyly, or Beals-Hecht syndrome, is a rare genetic disorder that involves the connective tissue of the skeleton.

Description

Individuals diagnosed with Beals syndrome usually have long, thin, fingers and toes that cannot be straightened out because of contractures, meaning a limited range of motion in the joints of their fingers, hips, elbows, knees, and ankles. They also have unusual external ears that appear crumpled. Contractures of the elbows, knees, and hips at birth are very common. Some babies also have **clubfoot**, causing one or both feet to be turned in towards each other at the ankles. In most individuals, the contractures improve with time and the clubfoot responds well to physiotherapy.

The condition occurs when fibrillin, an important component of the body's connective tissue (the glue and scaffolding of the body; for example, bones, cartilages, tendons, and fibers) is not made properly by the body. The **gene** responsible for making fibrillin is called FBN2 and it is located on **chromosome** 5. Any mutation (change) occurring in the FBN2 gene results in Beals syndrome.

Genetic profile

Beals syndrome is caused by a mutation occurring in a gene. Genes are units of hereditary material passed from a parent to a child through the egg and sperm. The information contained in genes is responsible for the development of all the cells and tissues of the body. Most genes occur in pairs: one copy of each pair is inherited from the egg cell produced by the mother and the other copy of each pair comes from the sperm cell of the father. One of these genes (called FBN2) tells the body how to make fibrillin-2, a specific type of protein. Proteins are substances made in the body that consist of chemicals called amino acids. Fibrillin-2 is an important part of connective tissue. Connective tissue provides structural support and elasticity to the body. It is made up of various components, including elastic-like fibers, and fibrillin-2 is thought to play a role in ensuring that the elastic fibers of the connective tissue are assembled properly early in development; however, the precise function of fibrillin-2 remains unknown. People with Beals syndrome have a mutation in one copy of their FBN2 gene. As a result, the fibrillin-2 they make is unable to work properly and this causes the BCA symptoms.

Beals syndrome is inherited as a dominant condition. In dominant conditions, a person needs to have only one altered gene copy to develop the condition. The mutation in the FBN2 gene that causes Beals syndrome can be inherited from a parent who is also affected with BCA. Individuals with Beals syndrome have a 50% chance in each pregnancy to have a child with Beals syndrome.

Sometimes Beals syndrome cannot be traced back to a parent with the condition. In these cases, the genetic change is said to be a spontaneous mutation. This means that some unknown event has caused the FBN2 gene (which functions normally in the parent) to mutate in either the sperm of the father or the egg of the mother. If fertilization occurs, the resulting individual will have Beals syndrome. A person who has Beals syndrome due to a spontaneous mutation can then pass on this altered FBN2 gene to his or her future children.

Demographics

Beals syndrome affects males and females of all ethnic groups. It is a rare condition and accurate estimates of the number of affected people are not available.

Signs and symptoms

Besides the general appearance displayed by persons with Beals syndrome (tall and thin, contractures, with typical crumpled ear), symptoms of the disorder vary from one affected individual to the next. Sometimes, arms are disproportionately long for the height of the person. Other less common features may include a small chin, protruding forehead, and a high arch in the roof of the mouth (palate).

An abnormal bending or twisting of the spine (kyphosis/scoliosis) is seen in about half of individuals diagnosed with Beals syndrome and can occur in early infancy. This bending and twisting of the spine tends to worsen over time. Some individuals may also have an abnormal indentation or protrusion of their chest wall. Decreased muscle bulk, especially in the lower legs, is also a common sign of Beals syndrome.

Less common symptoms of Beals syndrome include heart and eye problems. The most frequent heart problem involves one of the heart valves (mitral valve prolapse) and may necessitate medication prior to dental or other surgeries so as to prevent infection. More serious heart problems may occur but are rare. The aorta, the major blood vessel carrying blood away from the heart, may rarely enlarge. This condition usually requires medication to prevent further enlargement or occasionally, surgery. A small number of individuals with Beals syndrome may also be nearsighted and require eye glasses.

Diagnosis

The diagnosis of Beals syndrome is based on the presence of specific conditions. The diagnosis is suspected in anyone with the typical features of Beals syndrome such as tall, slender stature, contractures of many joints including the elbows, knees, hips, and fingers, abnormal curvature of the spine, decreased muscle bulk, and crumpled ears. A genetic test to confirm a BCA diagnosis has yet to become routinely available. **Genetic testing** for this syndrome remains limited to a few research laboratories around the world.

Testing during pregnancy (prenatal diagnosis) to determine whether the unborn child of at-risk parents may be affected by BCA is not routinely available. Also, because of the rather mild nature of the condition in most individuals, prenatal diagnosis is usually not requested. There has been at least one documented prenatal diagnosis for Beals syndrome. Using a procedure called **amniocentesis**, fluid surrounding the developing baby was removed and cells from that fluid were submitted to genetic testing in a research laboratory. The procedure allowed confirmation that the unborn child was affected with Beals syndrome.

KEY TERMS

Amniocentesis—A procedure performed at 16-18 weeks of pregnancy in which a needle is inserted through a woman's abdomen into her uterus to draw out a small sample of the amniotic fluid from around the baby. Either the fluid itself or cells from the fluid can be used for a variety of tests to obtain information about genetic disorders and other medical conditions in the fetus.

Chromosome—A microscopic thread-like structure found within each cell of the body and consists of a complex of proteins and DNA. Humans have 46 chromosomes arranged into 23 pairs. Changes in either the total number of chromosomes or their shape and size (structure) may lead to physical or mental abnormalities.

Connective tissue—A group of tissues responsible for support throughout the body; includes cartilage, bone, fat, tissue underlying skin, and tissues that support organs, blood vessels, and nerves throughout the body.

Contracture—A tightening of muscles that prevents normal movement of the associated limb or other body part.

Fibrillin-2—A protein that forms part of the body's connective tissue. The precise function of fibrillin-2 is not known.

Kyphosis—An abnormal outward curvature of the spine, with a hump at the upper back.

Mitral valve prolapse—A heart defect in which one of the valves of the heart (which normally controls blood flow) becomes floppy. Mitral valve prolapse may be detected as a heart murmur but there are usually no symptoms.

Mutation—A permanent change in the genetic material that may alter a trait or characteristic of an individual, or manifest as disease, and can be transmitted to offspring.

Protein—Important building blocks of the body, composed of amino acids, involved in the formation of body structures and controlling the basic functions of the human body.

Scoliosis—An abnormal, side-to-side curvature of the spine.

Treatment and management

There is no cure for Beals syndrome. Management of the disorder usually involves physiotherapy in early childhood to increase joint mobility and to lessen the effects of low muscle bulk. The contractures have been known to spontaneously improve, with surgery sometimes required to release them.

The abnormal curvature of the spine tends to worsen with time. A bone specialist should be consulted for advice on the appropriate treatment. Some individuals may require a back brace and/or surgery to correct the curvature.

A heart specialist should be consulted because some individuals with Beals syndrome have been known to have heart defects. Usually, an ultrasound of the heart is taken to assess whether there are any abnormalities. Medications may be used to treat some types of heart problems, if any. An eye specialist should also be consulted because of the possibility of eye problems such as **myopia** (nearsightedness). Prescription eye glasses may be necessary.

Individuals with Beals syndrome and their families may benefit from **genetic counseling** for information on the condition and recurrence risks for future pregnancies.

Prognosis

There tends to be gradual improvement in the joint contractures with time. The abnormal spinal curvature tends to get worse over time and may require bracing or surgery. The life span of individuals with Beals syndrome is not altered.

Resources

PERIODICALS

Robinson, Peter N., and M. Godfrey. "The molecular genetics of Marfan syndrome and related microfibrillinopathies." *Journal of Medical Genetics* 37 (2000): 9-25.

ORGANIZATIONS

AVENUES National Support Group for Arthrogryposis Multiplex Congenita. PO Box 5192, Sonora, CA 95370. (209) 928-3688. avenues@sonnet.com. <http://www.sonnet.com/avenues>.

National Marfan Foundation. 382 Main St., Port Washington, NY 11050-3121. (800) 862-7326. <http://www.marfan.org>.

National Organization for Rare Disorders (NORD). PO Box 8923, New Fairfield, CT 06812-8923. (203) 746-6518 or (800) 999-6673. Fax: (203) 746-6481. <http://www.rarediseases.org>.

WEBSITES

Godfrey, Maurice. "Congenital Contractural Arachnodactyly." *GeneClinics.* Univeristy of Washington, Seattle. <http://www.geneclinics.org>. (March 6, 2001)

Nada Quercia, Msc, CCGC CGC

Beals-Hecht syndrome *see* **Beals syndrome**

Bean syndrome *see* **Blue rubber bleb nevus syndrome**

Beare-Stevenson cutis gyrata syndrome

Definition

Beare-Stevenson Cutis gyrata syndrome is a serious, extremely rare inherited disorder affecting the skin, skull, genitals, navel, and anus. This condition often results in early death.

Description

Beare-Stevenson cutis gyrata syndrome is also known as Beare-Stevenson syndrome and cutis gyrata syndrome of Beare and Stevenson. This very rare inherited disease causes serious physical problems affecting many body parts. Cutis gyrata is characterized by an unusual ridging pattern in the skin resembling corrugation in cardboard. This skin corrugation is present from birth and commonly occurs on the head and arms.

All people with Beare-Stevenson cutis gyrata syndrome are mentally retarded or developmentally delayed. The brain, skull, face, respiratory system, and genitals are often malformed. Death at an early age is common.

Genetic profile

Beare-Stevenson cutis gyrata syndrome is an autosomal dominant disorder, meaning that a person needs a change, or mutation, in only one of two copies of the **gene** involved to manifest the disorder. All reported cases have been sporadic, or random, occurrences, happening in families with no family history of the disease. This syndrome is associated with mutations in FGFR2, a fibroblast growth factor receptor gene. The fibroblast growth factor receptor genes serve as blueprints for proteins important to inhibition of cell growth during and after embryonic development. FGFR2 is located on human **chromosome** 10 in an area designated as 10q26.

Demographics

Less than 10 cases of Beare-Stevenson cutis gyrata syndrome have been reported. Both males and females are affected. The few cases documented in the medical literature suggest that some cases of this disease might be associated with advanced paternal age, or older fathers.

KEY TERMS

Acanthosis nigricans—A skin condition characterized by darkly pigmented areas of velvety wart-like growths. Acanthosis nigricans usually affects the skin of the armpits, neck, and groin.

Amniocentesis—A procedure performed at 16-18 weeks of pregnancy in which a needle is inserted through a woman's abdomen into her uterus to draw out a small sample of the amniotic fluid from around the baby. Either the fluid itself or cells from the fluid can be used for a variety of tests to obtain information about genetic disorders and other medical conditions in the fetus.

Autosomal—Relating to any chromosome besides the X and Y sex chromosomes. Human cells contain 22 pairs of autosomes and one pair of sex chromosomes.

Chorionic villus sampling (CVS)—A procedure used for prenatal diagnosis at 10-12 weeks gestation. Under ultrasound guidance a needle is inserted either through the mother's vagina or abdominal wall and a sample of cells is collected from around the early embryo. These cells are then tested for chromosome abnormalities or other genetic diseases.

Sporadic—Isolated or appearing occasionally with no apparent pattern.

Signs and symptoms

All people with Beare-Stevenson cutis gyrata syndrome are developmentally delayed or mentally retarded. There may be excess fluid on the brain (**hydrocephalus**), and the nerve connection between the two halves of the brain (the corpus callosum) may be absent or underdeveloped.

A cloverleaf-shaped skull is a very unusual birth abnormality that is common in infants with Beare-Stevenson cutis gyrata syndrome. Abnormalities in skull shape happen when the sutures (open seams between the bony plates that form the skull) fuse before they typically would. Premature closure of the skull sutures is known as **craniosynostosis**. Growth of the brain pushes outward on skull plates that have not yet fused, causing characteristic bulges in those areas.

The characteristic face of someone with Beare-Stevenson cutis gyrata syndrome has prominent, bulging eyes that slant downward with droopy eyelids. The

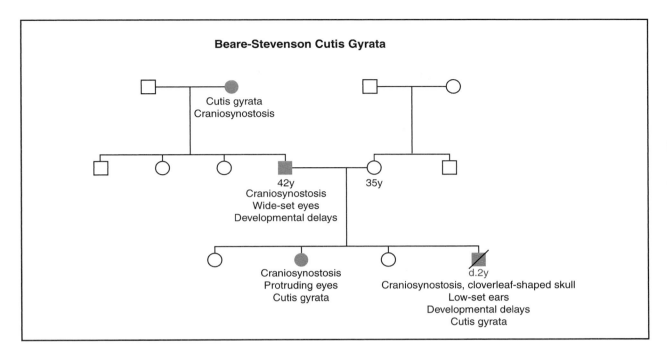

Beare-Stevenson Cutis Gyrata

Cutis gyrata
Craniosynostosis

42y
Craniosynostosis
Wide-set eyes
Developmental delays

35y

Craniosynostosis
Protruding eyes
Cutis gyrata

d.2y
Craniosynostosis, cloverleaf-shaped skull
Low-set ears
Developmental delays
Cutis gyrata

(Gale Group.)

middle third of the face is underdeveloped and may appear somewhat flattened. The ears are positioned lower and rotated backward from where they would typically be. Skin ridges may be found in front of the ear. Infants with this condition may be born with teeth.

The most recognizable physical symptom of this syndrome is the unusual ridging, or corrugation, of the skin. This cutis gyrata affects the skin on the scalp, face, ears, lips, and limbs and is usually evident at birth. Patches of skin on the armpits, neck, and groin may also display acanthosis nigricans, unusually dark, thickened patches of skin with multiple delicate growths. Skin tags may be present on the surface of the skin and on the tissues lining the mouth. Affected children usually have a prominent navel and may have extra nipples.

People with this disorder may not be able to fully straighten their arms at the elbow. The skin of the palms of the hands and the soles of the feet often show deep ridging. Affected individuals may have small, underdeveloped fingernails.

Children with Beare-Stevenson cutis gyrata syndrome may have breathing problems and narrowing of the roof of the mouth (cleft palate). The anus may be positioned more forward than normal. The genitals are often malformed and surrounded by corrugated skin.

An abnormal stomach valve may cause feeding problems.

Diagnosis

Diagnosis of Beare-Stevenson cutis gyrata syndrome is based on visible hallmark characteristics of the disease. All reported cases have shown hallmark characteristics from birth. **DNA** testing is available for Beare-Stevenson cutis gyrata syndrome. This testing is performed on a blood sample to confirm a diagnosis made on physical features. Prenatal **genetic testing** is also available. Beare-Stevenson cutis gyrata may be suspected in an unborn fetus if a hallmark characteristic, like a cloverleaf skull, is visible on **prenatal ultrasound**.

Treatment and management

There is no cure for Beare-Stevenson cutis gyrata syndrome. Of less than 10 reported cases in the literature, many died early in life. So few people have been diagnosed with this disease that there is no published information regarding its treatment and management.

Prognosis

Early death is common in people with Beare-Stevenson cutis gyrata syndrome, especially among those with a cloverleaf skull.

Resources

PERIODICALS

Hall, B. D., et al. "Beare-Stevenson Cutis Gyrata Syndrome." *American Journal of Medical Genetics* 44 (1992): 82- 89.

Krepelova, Anna, et al. "FGFR2 Gene Mutation (Tyr375Cys) in a New Case of Beare-Stevenson Syndrome." *American Journal of Medical Genetics* 76 (1998): 362-64.

ORGANIZATIONS

Children's Craniofacial Association. PO Box 280297, Dallas, TX 75243-4522. (972) 994-9902 or (800) 535-3643. contactcca@ccakids.com. <http://www.ccakids.com>.

FACES. The National Craniofacial Assocation. PO Box 11082, Chattanooga, TN 37401. (423) 266-1632 or (800) 332-2373. faces@faces-cranio.org. <http://www.faces-cranio.org/>.

WEBSITES

"Cutis Gyrata Syndrome of Beare and Stevenson." *OMIM— Online Mendelian Inheritance in Man.* <http://www.ncbi.nlm.nih.gov/entrez/dispomim.cgi?id=123790>.

Judy C. Hawkins, MS

Becker muscular dystrophy *see* **Duchenne muscular dystrophy**

Beckwith-Wiedemann syndrome

Definition

Beckwith-Wiedemann syndrome (BWS) refers to a disorder of overgrowth. This condition is usually characterized by large body size (macrosomia), large tongue (macroglossia), enlarged internal organs (visceromegaly), the presence of an abdominal wall defect (umbilical hernia or **omphalocele**), and low blood sugar in the newborn period (neonatal hypoglycemia).

Description

Beckwith and Wiedemann initially described Beckwith-Wiedemann syndrome in the 1960s. It is also known as Wiedemann-Beckwith syndrome and exomphalos macroglossia gigantism syndrome (EMG syndrome).

BWS syndrome will frequently present prenatally with fetal macrosomia, enlarged placentas, and often more than usual amniotic fluid (polyhydramnios) that may lead to premature delivery (a baby being born more than three weeks before its due date). In the first half of pregnancy, the majority of amniotic fluid is made by the movement of sodium, chloride, and water crossing the amniotic membrane and fetal skin to surround the fetus. During the second half of pregnancy, the majority of amniotic fluid is fetal urine that is produced by the fetal kidneys. Another major source of amniotic fluid is secretion from the fetal respiratory tract. This sterile fluid is not stagnant. It is swallowed and urinated by the fetus constantly and is completely turned over at least once a day. If the fetus has an enlarged tongue (macroglossia), and cannot swallow as usual, this can lead to build-up of excess amniotic fluid. Aside from swallowing difficulties in the newborn, macroglossia can also lead to difficulties with feeding and breathing.

Approximately 75% of infants who have BWS will have an omphalocele. An omphalocele occurs when the absence of abdominal muscles allows the abdominal contents to protrude through the opening in the abdomen. This is covered by a membrane into which the umbilical cord inserts. Omphaloceles are thought to be caused by a disruption of the process of normal body infolding at three to four weeks of fetal development. Although 25% of infants with BWS do not have omphaloceles, they may have other abdominal wall defects such as an umbilical hernia or even a less severe separation of the abdominal muscles, called diastasis recti.

Fifty to sixty percent of newborns with BWS present have low blood sugar levels within the first few days of life. This is called neonatal hypoglycemia and is caused by having more than the usual number of islet cells in the pancreas (pancreatic islet cell hyperplasia). The islet cells of the pancreas produce insulin. This cluster of cells is called the islets of Langerhans and make up about 1% of the pancreas. These cells are the most important sugar (glucose) sensing cells in the body. When an individual eats a meal high in glucose or carbohydrates, this leads to a rise in blood sugar, which is then a signal for the increased insulin secretion by the islet cells of the pancreas. If too much insulin is produced, then the blood glucose levels drop too low. This is called hypoglycemia. Since glucose is the primary fuel for brain function, if hypoglycemia lasts too long, it can lead to brain damage. For this reason, detection and treatment of the hypoglycemia is extremely important. Any child born with features of this syndrome should be carefully monitored for hypoglycemia, especially during the first week of life. Occasionally, onset of hypoglycemia is delayed until the first month after birth. For this reason, the parents of a child with BWS should be taught to watch for the symptoms of hypoglycemia so that they can seek care as soon as possible.

Children with BWS have an increased risk of mortality associated with tumor development. These tumors begin development during fetal life (embryonal tumors). These malignant tumors develop in approximately 8% of children who have BWS. The most frequently seen tumors in individuals who have BWS include Wilms tumor (nephroblastoma) and hepatoblastomas. Wilms tumor is a tumor that arises in the kidney and consists of several embryonic tissues. Wilms tumor accounts for 80% of all kidney tumors in children. The peak incidence occurs between two and three years of age, but can be present from infancy to adulthood.

Hepatoblasomas are tumors that arise in the liver during fetal development and is the most common primary liver tumor in infancy and childhood. A wide variety of other tumors, both malignant and benign, are also seen in individuals who have BWS and include, but are not limited to, nervous system tumors (neuroblastomas), adrenal gland tumors, and tumors that commonly occur in the head and neck (rhabdomyosarcoma). The increased risk for tumors appears to be concentrated in the first eight years of life, consistent with the embryonic nature of these tumors. In patients who have BWS, tumor development is not common after age eight.

Hemihyperplasia of a lower extremity or of the whole half of the body can be present. For example, one leg may be longer than the other leg. If hemihyperplasia is present, it may be recognized at birth and may become more or less obvious as a child grows. The risk of tumor development increases significantly when hemihyperplasia is present. While only 13% of affected individuals have hemihyperplasia, 40% of those with neoplasms have hyperplasia. Most patients with BWS remain at or above the 95th percentile for length through adolescence. Advanced bone age can be identified on x-ray examination. Growth rate usually slows down at around age seven or eight. After nine years of age, the average weight remains between the 75th and 95th percentile. Although height, weight, skeletal, and dental maturity may be above average for years, growth rate gradually slows down and eventually children reach average height and normal proportions. Puberty occurs at a usual time.

Another feature includes unusual linear grooves within the ear lobes and/or a groove or pit on the top of the outer ear. Facial characteristics may include prominent eyes (exophthalmos), "stork bite" birth marks (telangiectatic nevi) of the upper half of the face, and "port wine stain" birth marks (facial nevus flammeus) on the face.

Genetic profile

The genetics of BWS is complex. Approximately 85% of individuals who have BWS have no family history of BWS and have a normal **karyotype**. Of these patients, approximately 20% have paternal uniparental disomy for **chromosome** 11p15. Uniparental disomy occurs when an individual receives two copies of a chromosome, part of a chromosome, or a **gene** from one parent, as opposed to receiving one copy from each parent. In this situation, the amount of gene expression can be changed and cause a disease or disorder. Approximately 5-10% of patients who have no family history and a normal karyotype have a gene change identified near 11p15, called p57(KIP2). This gene region, p57(KIP2), is a tumor suppressor region, meaning that its presence suppresses tumor development, but that the loss of a normally functioning region could lead to tumor development and potentially lead to BWS. The IGF-2 (insulin-like growth factor-2) gene is also in this region. Both uniparental disomy and a gene mutation result in dosage changes of the normal functioning genes, resulting in overexpression and subsequently increased growth and tumor risk. When a gene change in the p57(KIP2) region is found in either of the parents of the affected child, the chance for a future child to have BWS could be as high as 50% with each future pregnancy. The remaining 70% of individuals who have BWS, no family history, and a normal karyotype, have no identifiable cause for BWS. The chance for other family members to be affected in this case is expected to be low.

Approximately 10-15% of individuals who have BWS have a positive family history and a normal karyotype. Of these families, up to 50% may have an identifiable gene change in the p57 region. If a female carries this gene change, then she has a 50% chance with each pregnancy for having a child with BWS. If a male carries the gene change, the chance for having an affected child is increased, but specific risks are not yet available. Up to 50% of individuals with a positive family history and a normal karyotype do not have an identifiable gene change in the p57 region. In this situation, the chance for the parents to have another affected child is as high as 50%.

Approximately 1-2% of patients with BWS have a detectable chromosome abnormality. In patients who have a translocation or a duplication of 11p15 detected on their karyotype, the parents' chromosome analysis should be analyzed. Depending upon the results of the parents' chromosome analysis, there could be up to a 50% chance of having an affected child with BWS.

Demographics

The reported incidence for BWS is approximately one in 14,000, although this is likely to be an underestimate because of undiagnosed cases. BWS is not found more commonly in any particular sex or geographic region and has been reported in a wide variety of ethnic backgrounds.

Signs and symptoms

Major signs or symptoms include: macrosomia, macroglossia, abdominal wall defect, visceromegaly, embryonal tumors, hemihyperplasia, ear lobe creases or ear pits, renal abnormalities, and rarely cleft palate.

Minor signs and symptoms include: polyhydramnios, prematurity, neonatal hypoglycemia, advanced bone age, heart defects, hemangioma, facial nevus flammeus, and the characteristic facial features, which include underdeveloped midface and possible soft-tissue folds under the eyes.

Diagnosis

BWS is diagnosed primarily by the identification of clinical signs and symptoms. Although there is no official diagnostic criteria for BWS, most would agree that a diagnosis requires the presence of three major findings, or at least two major findings and one minor finding. For the purposes of diagnosis, a major finding would also include a family history of BWS.

When considering the diagnosis of BWS, several other syndromes should also be considered (differential diagnosis). These include, but are not limited to, infant of a diabetic mother, **Simpson-Golabi-Behmel syndrome**, Perlman syndrome, **Sotos syndrome**, and **Costello syndrome**.

If a couple has had a child affected with BWS and an identifiable gene change in the p57 region has been identified, or if a chromosome abnormality is detected by chromosome analysis, then prenatal testing through chorionic villus sampling (CVS) or **amniocentesis** is possible. If this is not possible, then potentially, detailed ultrasound examination could help to reassure parents that the signs and symptoms of BWS are not present (such as omphalocele, macroglossia, and macrosomia). If any of these signs or symptoms are present, and the couple has had a previously affected child, then it would be very likely that the present pregnancy is affected as well.

If a couple has not had a previously affected child and has had an ultrasound examination that identifies an omphalocele, then chromosome analysis should be offered to rule out a chromosome abnormality and to look for the abnormal chromosome findings associated with BWS. If chromosome results are normal, BWS is still a possible cause for the ultrasound findings.

Treatment and management

Early treatment of hypoglycemia is important to reduce the risk of central nervous system damage. Most cases of hypoglycemia are mild and will resolve shortly with treatment, however, some cases may be more difficult. Treatment for hypoglycemia may include steroid therapy, which is usually required for only one to four months.

If an infant has an abdominal wall defect, such as an omphalocele, surgery is usually performed soon after birth to repair the defect. For very large omphaloceles, a several stage operation is performed. The treatment and management of the omphalocele depends upon the presence of other problems and is very specific to each individual.

A cardiac evaluation is recommended prior to surgery or if a heart defect is suspected by clinical evaluation. Cardiomegaly is frequently present, but usually resolves without treatment.

Non-malignant kidney abnormalities, including renal cysts and hydronephrosis, occur in approximately 25% of patients. A consult with a pediatric nephrologist would be recommended for patients who have structural renal abnormalities, including any evidence of renal calcium deposits on ultrasound examination.

To screen for tumors, a baseline MRI (magnetic resonance imaging) or CT (computed tomography) examination of the abdomen is recommended for individuals believed to have BWS. To screen for Wilms tumor and other embryonal tumors, abdominal ultrasound is recommended. Blood pressure should also be monitored, as approximately 50% of people with Wilms tumors may have associated hypertension. Because tumor development may occur at any time, though usually before eight years of age, the screening recommendations are that abdominal ultrasound be performed every three to six months until eight years of age, and then annually until growth is complete. In addition to ultrasound, screening for hepatoblastoma is accomplished by serial measurements of the serum alpha-fetoprotein (AFP) levels during these years as well. Elevated levels of serum AFP are present 80-90% of the time when a hepatoblastoma is present. Alpha-fetoprotein is a protein produced by the fetal liver. Concentrations of this protein fall rapidly during the first few weeks after birth and reach adult levels by six months of age. These adult levels are approximately 2-20 ng/ml. Thus, the presence of elevated levels in children and adults usually indicates tumor development. Abnormal AFP levels should be followed with an abdominal CT examination looking for evidence of a tumor in the liver.

Surgical removal is the primary treatment for hepatoblastoma; however, in tumors that cannot be removed, chemotherapy is performed.

Treatment for Wilms tumor is often only surgical removal of the tumor; however, in some cases chemother-

Amniocentesis—A procedure performed at 16-18 weeks of pregnancy in which a needle is inserted through a woman's abdomen into her uterus to draw out a small sample of the amniotic fluid from around the baby. Either the fluid itself or cells from the fluid can be used for a variety of tests to obtain information about genetic disorders and other medical conditions in the fetus.

Chorionic villus sampling (CVS)—A procedure used for prenatal diagnosis at 10-12 weeks gestation. Under ultrasound guidance a needle is inserted either through the mother's vagina or abdominal wall and a sample of cells is collected from around the early embryo. These cells are then tested for chromosome abnormalities or other genetic diseases.

Hemihyperplasia—A condition in which over development or excessive growth of one half of a specific organ or body part on only one side of the body occurs.

Neonatal—Neonatal refers to the first 28 days after birth.

Nevus flammeus—A flat blood vessel tumor present at birth, also known as a "port wine stain."

apy and radiation therapies are necessary, depending upon the stage of disease and the characteristics of the tumor.

Macroglossia may need to be addressed with the possibility of surgery. The large tongue may partially block the respiratory tract and lead to problems such as difficulty breathing and feeding. In most cases, the tongue growth slows over time and eventually the tongue can be accommodated. Dental malocclusion and a prominent jaw are secondary to the macroglossia. In rare cases, surgery to reduce tongue size is needed and is usually performed between two and four years of age.

Prognosis

After dealing with initial neonatal issues such as hypoglycemia, feeding, and respiratory problems, prognosis is usually good. Infants with BWS syndrome have an approximately 20% mortality rate. This is mainly due to complications stated above, and also includes complications of prematurity and omphalocele. The prognosis with repaired omphalocele is good. The majority of deaths in cases of omphalocele are usually associated with other anomalies or respiratory insufficiency. Respiratory insufficiency can occur in patients with omphaloceles if the omphalocele is so large that prenatal lung development cannot occur as usual. Respiratory insufficiency can also occur because of prematurity.

Tumor survival rates for Wilms tumor and for hepatoblastoma are as follows. In general, the four-year survival of all patients who have Wilms tumor with favorable histology approaches 90%. For hepatoblastomas, the combination of surgery and chemotherapy has achieved disease-free survival rates of 100% for stage I, 75% for stage II, and 67% for stage III hepatoblastomas.

In children who have BWS, development is usually normal if there is no history of significant, untreated hypoglycemia. After childhood, complications for patients with BWS are uncommon and prognosis is good.

Resources

BOOKS

Jones, Kenneth Lyons. *Smith's Recognizable Patterns of Human Malformation.* W. B. Saunders Company, 1997.

ORGANIZATIONS

Beckwith-Wiedemann Support Network. 2711 Colony Rd., Ann Arbor, MI 48104. (734) 973-0263 or (800) 837-2976. <http://www.beckwith-wiedemann.org>.

Renee A. Laux, MS

Berlin breakage syndrome *see* **Nijmegen breakage syndrome**

Beta thalassemia

Definition

Beta **thalassemia** is an inherited disorder that affects the beta globin (protein molecules) chains. These chains are required for the synthesis of hemoglobin A (a compound in the blood that carries oxygen to the cells and carbon dioxide away from the cells). A decrease of beta globin chains causes early destruction of the red blood cells. There are four types of the disorder and they range in severity of symptoms.

The thalassemias were first discovered by Thomas Cooley and Pearl Lee in 1975. Early cases of the disease were reported in children of Mediterranean descent and therefore the disease was named after the Greek word for sea, *thalasa*.

Description

Beta thalassemia results due to a defect in the beta globin **gene**. Shortly after birth, the body converts from producing gamma globin chains, which pair with alpha globin chains to produce fetal hemoglobin (HbF), to producing beta globin chains. Beta globin chains pair with alpha globin chains to produce adult hemoglobin (HbA). Due to the decreased amount of beta globin chains in individuals with beta thalassemia, there is an excess of free alpha globin chains. The free alpha globin chains become abnormal components in maturing red blood cells. This leads to destruction of the red blood cells by the spleen and a decreased number of red blood cells in the body. Individuals with beta thalassemia may continue producing gamma globin chains in an effort to increase the amount of HbF and compensate for the deficiency of HbA.

There are four types of beta thalassemias. These include beta thalassemia minima, minor, intermedia, and major. Beta thalassemia minima and beta thalassemia minor are less severe and usually asymptomatic. Beta thalassemia minima is known as the silent form of the disorder. There are no major hematologic (blood and blood forming tissue) abnormalities. The only noted abnormality is the decrease in beta globin production. Beta thalassemia minor is rare. A person with this type of the disorder inherits only one beta globin gene. Although children are usually asymptomatic, they do have abnormal hematologic (blood) findings.

Beta thalassemia intermedia and major often require medical treatment. Beta thalassemia intermedia is usually found during the toddler or preschool years. It is considered to be the mild form of thalassemia major and frequently does not require blood transfusions. Thalassemia major is typically diagnosed during the first year of life. There are two designations for beta thalassemia major, beta zero and beta positive. In type beta zero there is no adult hemoglobin (HbA) present due to the very small production of beta globin. In type beta positive there is a small amount of HbA detectable. In both forms of beta thalassemia major, individuals will experience severe fatigue due to the decrease or absence of adult hemoglobin (HbA), which is needed to carry oxygen to the cells, and is necessary for cellular survival.

Alternate names associated with beta thalassemia minor include thalassemia minor, minor hereditary leptocyosis, and heterozygous beta thalassemia. Alternate names associated with beta thalassemia intermedia include intermedia Cooley's anemia and thalassemia intermedia. Alternate names associated with beta thalassemia major include Cooley's anemia, erythroblastoic anemia of childhood hemoglobin lepore syndrome, major hereditary leptocytosis, Mediterranean anemia, mocrocythemia, target cell anemia, and thalassemia major.

Genetic profile

Beta thalassemia is an autosomal recessive disorder. A person who is a carrier will not develop the disorder but may pass the gene for the disorder onto their child. There is a 25% chance for each pregnancy that the disorder will be passed onto the children if both parents are carriers for the trait and a 100% chance if both parents have the trait.

Individuals with thalassemia minor are carriers for the beta globin gene and therefore possess only one of the genes necessary to express the disorder. These individuals are usually asymptomatic or have very few symptoms. Individuals with thalassemia major express both abnormal genes for beta globin and therefore will have the disease. These individuals show severe symptoms for the disorder.

The beta globin gene is found on **chromosome** 11. Mutations (inappropriate sequence of nucleotides, the building blocks of genes) resulting in beta thalassemia are usually caused by substitutions (switching one nucleotide for another) although some may be caused by deletions (part of a chromosome, a structure that places genes in order, is missing). Substitutions occur within the nucleotide and deletions occur on the chromosome that the beta globin gene is found on.

Demographics

Beta thalassemia affects males and females equally. It commonly occurs in people of Mediterranean heritage. It is also found in families descending from Africa, the Middle East, India, and Southeastern Asia.

Signs and symptoms

Symptoms for beta thalassemia vary in severity based on the type of the disorder.

Beta thalassemia minima

There are no symptoms for this type. It is considered to be a "silent" form of beta thalassemia.

Beta thalassemia minor

Individuals with this type of beta thalassemia may be asymptomatic or experience very few symptoms. Symptoms may be worse in individuals that are pregnant, under stress, or malnourished. Symptoms may include:

- Fatigue. This may be the only symptom that an individual with beta thalassemia minor exhibits. Fatigue is caused by the decreased oxygen carrying capacity of the red blood cells, resulting in lowered oxygenation for cells and tissues.

- Anemia. Anemia is a decrease in the amount of hemoglobin in the blood. Hemoglobin is needed to carry oxygen on the red blood cells. In beta thalassemia minor there is a decrease in adult hemoglobin (HbA) and an increase in hemoglobin A2. Hemoglobin A2 is a minor hemoglobin that contains delta globin chains in the place of beta globin chains. Anemia is most likely to occur during pregnancy.

- Splenomegaly. Enlargement of the spleen may occur due to increased removal of defective red blood cells. This is rarely seen in individuals with beta thalassemia minor and may be accompanied by pain in the upper left portion of the abdomen.

- Skin. The skin color of individuals with beta thalassemia minor may be pale (pallor) due to oxygen deprivation in blood.

Beta thalassemia intermedia

Individuals with this form of beta thalassemia usually begin to show symptoms during toddler or preschool years. These individuals present with many of the same symptoms as beta thalassemia major, however, symptoms for beta thalassemia intermedia are less severe and may include:

- Anemia. In individuals with beta thalssemia intermedia, hemoglobin levels are greater than 7g/dl but they are less than normal. Normal levels for hemoglobin are 13-18 for males and 12-16 for females.

- Hyperbilirubinemia. Bilirubin is a yellow pigment of bile that is formed by the breakdown of hemoglobin in the red blood cells. Excess amounts of bilirubin in the blood is caused by the increased destruction of red blood cells (hemolysis) by the spleen.

- Splenomegaly. Enlargement of the spleen is caused by increased removal of defective red blood cells. Red blood cells are defective due to the increased amount of inclusion bodies caused by circulation of free alpha globin chains.

- Hepatomegaly. Enlargement of the liver may be caused by a build-up of bile due to increased amounts of bilirubin in the blood.

- Additional abnormalities. Individuals with beta thalassemia intermedia may have a yellow discoloration (jaundice) of the skin, eyes, and mucous membranes caused by increased amounts of bilirubin in the blood. Individuals may also suffer from delayed growth and abnormal facial appearance.

Beta thalassemia major

Individuals with this form of beta thalassemia present with symptoms during the first year after birth. Symptoms are severe and may include:

- Severe anemia. Individuals with beta thalassemia major suffer from a hemoglobin level of less than 7 mg/dl.

- Hyperbilirubinemia. Individuals will have an increased amount of bilirubin in the blood. This is due to the increased destruction of red blood cells (hemolysis) by the spleen.

- Jaundice. Individuals may experience a yellow discoloration of the skin, eyes, and mucous membranes caused by increased amounts of bilirubin in the blood.

- Extramedullary hematopoiesis. Abnormal formation of red blood cells outside of the bone marrow may occur in the body's attempt to compensate for decreased production of mature red blood cells. This can cause masses or the enlargement of organs, which may be felt during physical examination.

- Splenomegaly. Enlargement of the spleen may result due to increased destruction of red blood cells and the occurrence of extramedullary hematopoiesis.

- Hepatomegaly. Enlargement of the liver may result due to accumulation of bile or the occurrence of extramedullary hematopoiesis.

- Cholithiasis. This is the presence of stones in the gallbladder, which may lead to blockage and cause bile to be pushed back into the liver.

- Bone marrow expansion. The bone marrow becomes expanded due to the increase of the production of red blood cells (erythropoiesis) in an attempt to produce more mature red blood cells and decrease the anemic state of the body.

- Facial changes. Due to expansion of the bone marrow, children will develop prominent cheekbones, depression of the nasal bridge, and protrusion of the upper jaw. These facial changes are a classic sign in children with untreated beta thalassemia.

- Iron overload. Iron overload of the tissues can be fatal and is due to erythroid (red blood cell) expansion. The increased destruction of a vast amount of red blood cells causes increased amounts of iron to be released from the hemoglobin.

- Cardiovascular abnormalities. Accumulation of iron deposits in the heart muscle can lead to cardiac abnormalities and possibly cardiac failure.

- Additional abnormalities. Individuals may also suffer from pale skin, fatigue, poor feeding, failure to thrive, and decreased growth and development.

Diagnosis

Completing a family history, performing a complete physical examination, and results of blood (hematological) tests can lead to a diagnosis of beta thalassemia. Bone abnormalities and masses or enlarged organs may be recognized during physical examination. Prenatal testing to detect beta thalassemia can be done by completing an **amniocentesis** (obtaining a sample of amniotic fluid, which surrounds the fetus during pregnancy). Lab results will vary depending on the type of beta thalassemia that an individual presents with.

Normal hemoglobin results are 13-18 g/dL for males and 12-16 g/dL for women. Normal red blood cell counts are 4.7-6.1 million for males and 4.2-5.4 million for females. In individuals with beta zero form of beta thalassemia major, there will be no HbA present in the blood.

Symptoms of beta thalassemia minor may be similar to those of sideroblastic anemia (a disorder characterized by low levels of hemoglobin, fatigue, and weakness) and **sickle cell disease** (a disease that changes red blood cell shape, rendering it incapable of functioning).

Symptoms of beta thalassemia major may be similar to those of hereditary spheocytic hemolytic anemia (presence of sphere shaped red blood cells).

Treatment and management

Beta thalassemia minima and minor usually require no treatment. Pregnant women that suffer from beta thalassemia minor may require blood transfusions to keep hemoglobin levels normal. Individuals with beta thalassemia intermedia and major can be treated with blood transfusions and iron chelation (binding and isolation of metal) therapy. Although individuals with beta thalassemia intermedia do not usually require transfusions, in certain cases it may be necessary.

Blood transfusions are performed in individuals that present with severe symptoms such as anemia and impaired growth and development. Children may receive transfusions every four to six weeks. A high risk associated with transfusions is iron overload, which is fatal. Iron overload results from inadequate amounts of serum transferring (a molecule that exchanges iron between body tissues), which is needed to bind and detoxify iron. Iron accumulation can lead to dysfunction of the heart, liver, and endocrine glands.

Monitoring iron levels in the body is essential. Individuals receiving blood transfusions should keep total body iron levels at 3-7 mg of iron per gram of body weight. There are three methods of measuring iron levels in the body. These include a serum ferritin test, liver biopsy, and radiological study performed by the Superconducting Quantum Interference Device (SQUID).

The serum ferritin (iron storage protein) test is completed by testing a blood sample for ferritin content. This method is the easiest and most affordable way of testing for body content of iron, but it is not reliable. A liver biopsy is an invasive procedure that requires removal of a small piece of the liver. Studies have shown that a liver biopsy is very accurate in measuring the level of iron stores in the body. The third method, which requires a Superconducting Quantum Interference Device, is also very accurate in measuring iron stores. The SQUID is a highly specialized machine and few centers in the world possess this advanced technology.

Iron overload can be prevented with the use of iron chelating therapy. Chelating agents attract the excess iron and assist with the process of binding and detoxifying this iron in the body. The drug deferoxamine (desferol) is one of the most widely used iron chelating agents. Treatment is completed through nightly infusions of deferoxamine by a pump or with daily intramuscular injections. Infusion by pump is used for the administration of high doses and low doses are given through injections. Iron chelation therapy by oral administration with a drug named deferiprone has been under experimental study and may be an alternative to deferoxamine.

Individuals receiving blood transfusions should pay close attention to iron intake in the diet. It is recommended that children under age 10 keep dietary iron intake at 10 mg/day or less. Individuals age 11 or older should keep dietary iron intake at 18 mg/day or less. Foods high in iron include: beef, beans, liver, pork, peanut butter, infant cereal, cream of wheat, prunes, spinach, raisins, and leafy green vegetables. Individuals should read food labels and avoid using cast iron cookware, which can provide more iron in food during cooking.

Increased amounts of iron in the body can cause a decrease in calcium levels, which impairs organs that aid in building strong bones. Individuals with beta thalassemia major are at risk for developing **osteoporosis** (disease resulting in weakened bones). Increased dietary intake of calcium and vitamin D can help increase the storage of calcium in the bones, thus making the bones stronger and decreasing the risk for osteoporosis.

Bone marrow transplantation is another form of treatment for beta thalassemia. Outcomes of transplantation are greatly influenced by the health of the individ-

KEY TERMS

Anemia—A blood condition in which the level of hemoglobin or the number of red blood cells falls below normal values. Common symptoms include paleness, fatigue, and shortness of breath.

Bone marrow—A spongy tissue located in the hollow centers of certain bones, such as the skull and hip bones. Bone marrow is the site of blood cell generation.

Globin—One of the component protein molecules found in hemoglobin. Normal adult hemoglobin has a pair each of alpha-globin and beta-globin molecules.

Hemoglobin—Protein-iron compound in the blood that carries oxygen to the cells and carries carbon dioxide away from the cells.

Hepatomegaly—An abnormally large liver.

Splenomegaly—Enlargement of the spleen.

ual. This form of treatment is only possible if the individual has a suitable donor.

Researchers are investigating the use of the drugs hydroxyurea and butyrate compounds to increase the amounts of fetal and total hemoglobin in individuals with beta thalassemia. Studies using **gene therapy**, such a stem cell replacement, are also being conducted.

Social and lifestyle issues

Children with beta thalassemia major that is not diagnosed and treated early may develop changes in the bone structure of the face due to the expansion of bone marrow. Supportive counseling may benefit children who feel inadequate or refuse to participate in social activities due to their appearance.

Adolescents may require counseling concerning the effects that blood transfusions and iron chelation therapy may have on their social lifestyle.

Parents may need to seek counseling or attend support groups that focus on the time demand and lifestyle changes of caring for a child diagnosed with beta thalassemia.

Prognosis

Prognosis for beta thalassemia is good for individuals diagnosed early and those who receive proper treatment. Children with beta thalassemia major live 20-30 years longer with treatment by blood transfusions and iron chelation therapy.

Resources

BOOKS

Bowden, Vicky R., Susan B. Dickey, and Cindy Smith Greenberg. *Children and Their Families: The continuum of care*. Philadelphia: W.B. Saunders Company, 1998.

"Thalassemias." In *Principles and Practice of Medical Genetics*, Volume 2, edited by Alan E.H. Emery, MD, PhD, and David L. Rimoin, MD, PhD. New York: Churchill Livingstone, 1983.

Thompson, M.W., R. R. McInnus, and H. F. Willard. *Thompson and Thompson Genetics in Medicine*, Fifth Edition. Philadelphia: W.B. Saunders Company, 1991.

PERIODICALS

Angelucci, E., et al. "Hepatic iron concentration and total body iron stores in Thalassemia Major." *The New England Journal of Medicine* 343, (2000): 327-331.

Mentzer, W. C., et al. "Prospects for research in hematologic disorders: sickle cell and thalassemia." *The Journal of The American Medical Association* 285 (2001): 640-642.

Olivieri, N. F. "The Beta Thalassemias." *The New England Journal of Medicine* 341 (1999): 99-109.

Olivieri, N. F. et al. "Treatment of thalassemia major with phenylbuyrate and hydroxyurea." *The Lancet* 350 (1997): 491-492.

ORGANIZATIONS

Children's Blood Foundation. 333 East 38th St., Room 830, New York, NY 10016-2745. (212) 297-4336. cfg@nyh.med.cornell.edu.

Cooley's Anemia Foundation, Inc. 129-09 26th Ave. #203, Flushing, NY 11354. (800) 522-7222 or (718) 321-2873. <http://www.thalassemia.org>.

March of Dimes Birth Defects Foundation. 1275 Mamaroneck Ave., White Plains, NY 10605. (888) 663-4637. resourcecenter@modimes.org. <http://www.modimes.org>.

National Heart, Lung, and Blood Institute. PO Box 30105, Bethseda, MD 20824-0105. (301) 592-8573. nhlbiinfo@rover.nhlbi.nih.gov. <http://www.nhlbi.nih.gov>.

National Organization for Rare Disorders (NORD). PO Box 8923, New Fairfield, CT 06812-8923. (203) 746-6518 or (800) 999-6673. Fax: (203) 746-6481. <http://www.rarediseases.org>.

Laith F. Gulli, MD
Tanya Bivens, BS

Beta-galactosidase-1 deficiency *see* Gm1 gangliosidosis

Bicuspid aortic valve

Definition

Bicuspid aortic valve is the most common malformation of the heart valves. In this type of deformity, the aortic valve has only two cusps, which are rigid points such as that seen on leaves, instead of the three cusps normally present. This condition may lead to abnormalities in the flow of blood from the heart to the aorta, leading to changes in the function of the heart and lungs. Treatment consists of surgical repair or replacement of the valve.

Description

A valve is a device that allows a fluid to flow in only one direction in a defined path, thereby preventing backflow of the fluid. The heart has four such valves, which allow the blood to flow in an orderly pattern through each of the four chambers of the heart and out into the largest artery of the body, the aorta. The aorta, in turn, branches into other blood vessels in the neck, limbs and organs of the body to supply it with oxygenated blood.

The aortic valve divides the left ventricle of the heart and the aorta. It is the last valve before blood leaves the heart and passes into the aorta. The valve is formed during pregnancy and is normally composed of three separate cusps or leaflets, which, when closed, form a tightly sealed barrier that prevents backflow of blood from the aorta into the heart. Thus, when the heart contracts or pumps, the aortic valve opens and allows blood to pass from the heart into the aorta, and when the heart relaxes, the aortic valve closes and prevents backflow of blood from the aorta into the heart.

The three-cusp structure of the valve is essential for its proper function, and was noted as far back as the fifteenth century when the great master of the High Renaissance, Leonardo da Vinci, reported on his observations of anatomy and blood circulation. In bicuspid aortic valve, the aortic valve fails to form properly during development in the womb; for reasons that are unclear, two of the three cusps fail to separate properly and remain attached along one edge, resulting in an aortic valve with only two cusps.

The bicuspid aortic valve is the most common heart valve defect at birth, and many people live a normal life without even being aware of this condition. Unfortunately, bicuspid aortic valves are also more prone to disease than the normal three cusped valves. Over the years, conditions such as restricted blood flow to the aorta (aortic stenosis), backflow of blood from the aorta into the heart (aortic regurgitation, or aortic insufficiency) and valve infection (endocarditis) are often detected with associated symptoms during the adult years as progressive damage is done to the bicuspid aortic valve.

Other conditions that may occur with bicuspid aortic valve include aneurysm of the aorta (ballooning out of the aorta wall), and aortic dissection (a life-threatening split in the layers of the aorta).

Genetic profile

Most occurrences of bicuspid aortic valve appear to be sporadic (i.e., random, and not associated with a inherited defect) and are not passed on from parent to child. However, there have been some reports that the valve malformation appears in multiple members of the same family. In at least one report, this familial occurrence appears to be inherited in an autosomal dominant pattern with reduced penetrance (not showing the malformation, despite possessing the genetic cause for it). However, if there is some sort of genetic or inherited cause in some patients with bicuspid aortic valve, it has not been identified. For purposes of **genetic counseling**, bicuspid aortic valve can be regarded as a sporadic condition with an extremely low risk of being transmitted from parent to child.

Demographics

Bicuspid aortic valve has been reported to occur in 1-2% of the general population, and is the most common valve defect diagnosed in the adult population, accounting for up to half of the operated cases of aortic stenosis. For reasons that are unclear, bicuspid aortic valve is three to four times more likely in males than in females, though some researchers suggest that the condition may simply be diagnosed more in males because of the higher rates of calcium deposits in men that bring the aortic valve to medical attention.

Interestingly, bicuspid aortic valve is also found with other conditions, including the genetic disorder Turner's syndrome, or in patients with a malformation called coarctation of the aorta (narrowing of the aorta). It has been reported that approximately 35% of patients with Turner's syndrome and up to 80% of patients with coarctation of the aorta have an associated bicuspid aortic valve. The significance of these associations is unclear.

Signs and symptoms

Many people with bicuspid aortic valve experience no symptoms and may live their entire lives unaware of the condition. However, progressive damage or infection of the valve may lead to three serious conditions: aortic stenosis, aortic regurgitation, or endocarditis.

As a person ages, calcium deposits on a bicuspid aortic valve making it stiff. Eventually, the valve may become so stiff that it does not open properly, making it more difficult for blood to leave the heart and pass into the aorta and resulting in aortic stenosis. When this blockage becomes serious enough, people may experience shortness of breath, chest pain, or fainting spells. These symptoms usually begin between the ages of 50 and 60 years old. Eventually, the blockage can become so bad that blood backs up in the heart and lungs instead of going out to supply the rest of the body with oxygen (congestive heart failure). Additionally, this condition can lead to thickening of the heart wall, which may cause abnormal heart rhythms leading to sudden death.

Aortic regurgitation results when the valve fails to close properly. People who develop this condition may become short of breath when exerting themselves. The extent of symptoms experienced by the patient depends on the severity of the aortic regurgitation.

Finally, bacteria may deposit on the malformed bicuspid aortic valve, causing endocarditis. People with endocarditis may have symptoms of lingering fevers, fatigue, weight loss, and sometimes damage to the kidneys or spots on their fingers and hands.

Other dangerous conditions associated with bicuspid aortic valve include aortic aneurysm and aortic dissection. People with aortic aneurysms usually do not experience symptoms unless the aneurysm ruptures, but people with aortic dissection experience tearing back pain. Aortic aneurysm rupture and aortic dissection are very dangerous and can rapidly lead to death if not promptly treated.

Diagnosis

Any of the symptoms of aortic stenosis, aortic regurgitation, or endocarditis should prompt a search for an underlying malformation of the aortic valve. Aortic stenosis or regurgitation is diagnosed by a combination of physical exam and cardiovascular tests and imaging. The earliest sign of aortic valve problems is a murmur (the sound of abnormal patterns of blood flow) heard with a stethoscope. When the valve has high levels of calcium deposits, a characteristic clicking sound can also be heard with the stethoscope just as the stiff valve attempts to open. Later signs include a large heart seen on x ray or by a special electrical test of the heart, called an ECG or EKG (electrocardiogram).

If these signs are present, it suggests that the aortic valve may be damaged. The next test to be performed is echocardiography, a method that uses ultrasound waves to look at the aortic valve, similar to the way in which ultrasound is used to look at a fetus during pregnancy. Often, only two cusps are seen on the aortic valve during the echocardiography, confirming a diagnosis of bicuspid aortic valve.

Endocarditis is diagnosed by demonstrating the presence of bacteria in the blood stream. This is performed by taking blood from the patient and growing

KEY TERMS

Aorta—The main artery located above the heart which pumps oxygenated blood out into the body. Many congenital heart defects affect the aorta.

Aortic regurgitation—A condition in which the aortic valve does not close tightly, allowing blood to flow backwards from the aorta into the heart.

Aortic stenosis—A condition in which the aortic valve does not open properly, making it difficult for blood to leave the heart.

Autosomal dominant—A pattern of genetic inheritance where only one abnormal gene is needed to display the trait or disease.

Coarctation—A narrowing of the aorta that is often associated with bicuspid aortic valve.

Echocardiogram—A non-invasive technique, using ultrasonic waves, used to look at the various structures and function of the heart.

Electrocardiogram (ECG, EKG)—A test used to measure electrical impulses coming from the heart in order to gain information about its structure or function.

Endocarditis—A dangerous infection of the heart valves caused by certain bacteria.

Heart valve—One of four structures found within the heart that prevents backwards flow of blood into the previous chamber.

Murmur—A noise, heard with the aid of a stethoscope, made by abnormal patterns of blood flow within the heart or blood vessels.

Reduced penetrance—Failing to display a trait or disease despite possessing the dominant gene that determines it.

Sporadic—Isolated or appearing occasionally with no apparent pattern.

Stethoscope—An instrument used for listening to sounds within the body, such as those in the heart or lungs.

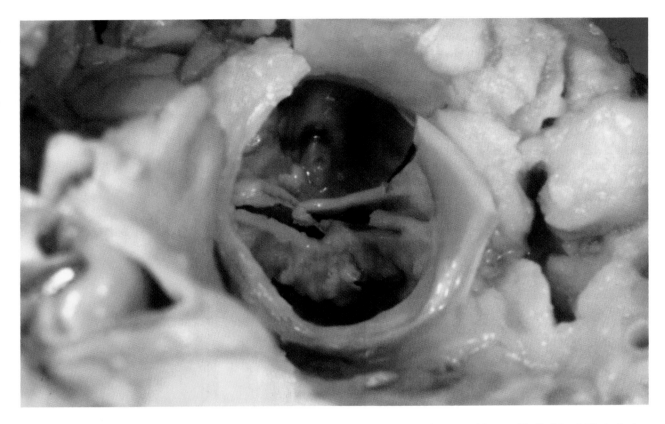

This view of a human heart specimen clearly shows the structure of a bicuspid aortic valve. (*Custom Medical Stock Photo, Inc.*)

the bacteria on plates with specialized nutrients. Skilled technicians can then use different tests to identify which species of bacteria is present so that appropriate treatment can be started. The diagnosis of endocarditis is also confirmed by using echocardiography to look for bacterial growths on the aortic valve. During the echocardiography, a bicuspid valve is often seen and explains the tendency to develop endocarditis.

Treatment and management

Most people with bicuspid aortic valve will not experience any complications or symptoms and will not require treatment. However, in patients with any complication of valve damage, as previously discussed, treatment may be necessary.

In younger patients who have aortic stenosis, a procedure can be performed in which a small balloon is inserted through one of the major blood vessels and into the aortic valve. The balloon is then inflated, creating a bigger opening for blood to pass. Alternatively, an "open heart" procedure can be performed to cut the valve into a more normal configuration. These treatments are usually temporary, and later in

life the patient, as well as any adult with advanced aortic stenosis, will most likely require aortic valve replacement.

Valve replacement is an "open heart" operation where the original malformed valve is removed and replaced with a new valve. This new valve can come from a human donor who has died, or from cows or pigs, or even from another part of the patient's heart. These valves function well, but may need to be replaced after 10 to 20 years, as they wear out. Another option is to use an artificial valve made of metal, plastic, or cloth. However, people who receive these artificial valves need to take blood thinners every day in order to prevent blood clots from forming on the new valve.

Patients with endocarditis need to be hospitalized and treated with high does of antibiotics given through a vein for several weeks. Damage done to the valve by the bacteria may make it necessary for a valve replacement procedure to be performed after the patient has recovered from the infection.

In any case, people who have been identified as having bicuspid aortic valve should be followed regularly by a cardiologist, with possible consultation with a cardio-thoracic surgeon. The function of the bicuspid aortic valve should be followed through the use of echocardiography, and the state of the heart itself should be followed by regular electrocardiograms.

It should be noted that children with aortic stenosis may not be able to engage in vigorous physical activity without the risk of cardiac arrest and should consult their physician. In addition, all people with bicuspid aortic valve should receive antibiotics prior to any dental procedure or surgery; these procedures may allow bacteria to enter the blood stream and could result in endocarditis if antibiotics are not given beforehand.

Prognosis

Most people born with bicuspid aortic valve experience no symptoms or complications, and their lives do not differ from someone born with a normal aortic valve. In patients who do experience complications and require valve replacement, risks of the operation generally depend on age, general health, specific medical conditions, and heart function. It is better to perform the operation before any of the advanced symptoms (shortness of breath, chest pain, fainting spells) develop; in patients without advanced symptoms, the risk of a bad outcome of surgery is only 4%. If a person with advanced symptoms chooses not to undergo surgery, the risk of death within three years is more than 50%. In general, valve replacement greatly reduces the amount and severity of symptoms and allows the patient to return to their normal daily activities without discomfort after they recover from the surgery.

Resources

PERIODICALS

Braunwald, E. *Heart Disease: A Textbook of Cardiovascular Medicine*. Philadelphia: Saunders, 1999.

Cotran, R. S. *Robbins Pathologic Basis of Disease*. Philadelphia: Saunders, 1999. pp. 566-570.

Friedman, W. F. "Congenital Heart Disease In The Adult." In *Harrison's Principles of Internal Medicine*, edited by A.S. Fauci. New York: McGraw-Hill, 1998.

ORGANIZATIONS

American Heart Association. 7272 Greenville Ave., Dallas, TX 75231-4596. (214) 373-6300 or (800) 242-8721. inquire@heart.org. <http://www.americanheart.org>.

Congenital Heart Anomalies Support, Education, and Resources. 2112 North Wilkins Rd., Swanton, OH 43558. (419) 825-5575. <http://www.csun.edu/~hfmth006/chaser>.

WEBSITES

"Bicuspid Aortic Valve." *OMIM—Online Mendelian Inheritance in Man*. National Center for Biotechnology Information. <http://www3.ncbi.nlm.nih.gov/htbin-post/Omim/dispmim?109730>.

Oren Traub, MD, PhD

Biotinidase deficiency

Definition

Biotinidase deficiency is a rare inherited defect in the body's ability to use dietary biotin, one of the B vitamins. The disease is also known as juvenile or late-onset multiple carboxylase deficiency.

Description

Biotin is essential as a co-factor (co-enzyme) for the reactions of four enzymes called carboxylases. These enzymes, in turn, play important roles in the metabolism of sugars, fats, and proteins within the human body. Another key enzyme, biotinidase, recycles biotin from these reactions so it can be used again. A defect in the biotinidase **gene** results in decreased amounts of normal enzyme, thus preventing the reuse of biotin. In turn, this leads to a disruption of the function of the four carboxylases that depend on biotin, and results in a variety of abnormalities of the nervous system and skin. Since symptoms usually do not appear immediately at birth, biotinidase deficiency is also referred to as late-onset or juvenile multiple carboxylase deficiency. A related disorder, early-onset or neonatal multiple carboxylase deficiency, is caused by the lack of a different enzyme, holocarboxylase synthetase, and, as the name suggests, results in symptoms in the newborn period.

Genetic profile

Inheritance pattern

Biotinidase deficiency is an autosomal recessive disorder affecting both males and females. In individuals with this disorder, both copies of the biotinidase gene are defective. Both parents of an affected child have one abnormal copy of the gene, but usually do not show symptoms because they also have one normal copy. The normal copy provides approximately 50% of the usual enzyme activity, a level adequate for the body's needs. Individuals with one abnormal copy of the gene and 50% enzyme activity are said to be carriers or heterozygotes. As is typical of autosomal recessive **inheritance**, their risk for having another

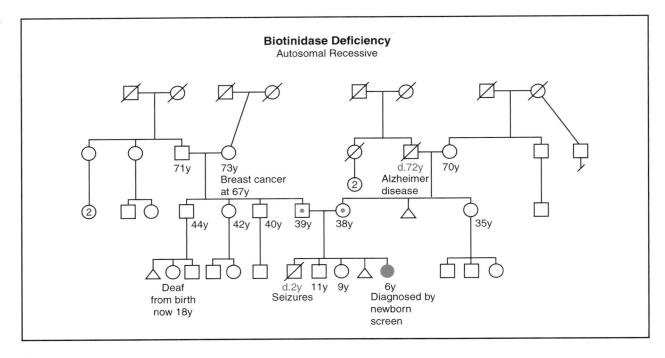

Biotinidase Deficiency
Autosomal Recessive

(Gale Group.)

child with the disorder is 25% in each subsequent pregnancy.

Gene location

The gene for biotinidase is located on the short arm of **chromosome** 3 (3p25). At least 40 different mutations in this gene have been identified in individuals with biotinidase deficiency. The fact that there are a number of different types of mutations helps explain why symptoms are variable from one individual to another. However, the presence of variability even within a family suggests there may be other, as yet unknown, factors that affect the severity of the disease.

Demographics

Individuals with biotinidase deficiency have been described in various ethnic groups worldwide. In the general population, the incidence of the disease is estimated at about one in 60,000 individuals and one in every 123 individuals is a carrier.

Signs and symptoms

The onset of symptoms is typically between three and six months of age but varies widely from one week to several years. The most common clinical features are hair loss (alopecia), skin rash (dermatitis), seizures (convulsions), decreased muscle tone (hypotonia), difficulty

walking (ataxia), breathing problems, redness of the eyes (conjunctivitis), hearing and vision loss, and developmental delay. Children with biotinidase deficiency are prone to fungal and bacterial infections, suggesting that the immune system is also affected. Symptoms are highly variable among affected individuals, even within a single family.

Biotinidase deficiency is classified as either partial or profound. If there is at least 10% enzyme activity, the deficiency is considered partial and is usually associated with minimal to mild symptoms. Profound biotinidase deficiency, defined as less than 10% of normal activity, is characterized by many of the symptoms mentioned above, and can, if left untreated, result in coma and death.

Diagnosis

Children with profound biotinidase deficiency may show general signs such as vomiting, seizures, and low muscle tone, all of which can be associated with a number of different disorders. Diagnosis can be difficult because of the many different enzyme deficiencies (inborn errors of metabolism) with similar symptoms and test results. For example, abnormally high amounts of certain acidic products in the blood and urine can be typical of a number of different metabolic disorders including biotinidase deficiency. Accurate diagnosis is made by measuring the activity of the enzyme in blood or skin cells. A number of states and countries test for

KEY TERMS

Amniocentesis—A procedure performed at 16-18 weeks of pregnancy in which a needle is inserted through a woman's abdomen into her uterus to draw out a small sample of the amniotic fluid from around the baby. Either the fluid itself or cells from the fluid can be used for a variety of tests to obtain information about genetic disorders and other medical conditions in the fetus.

Autosomal recessive—A pattern of genetic inheritance where two abnormal genes are needed to display the trait or disease.

Carrier—A person who possesses a gene for an abnormal trait without showing signs of the disorder. The person may pass the abnormal gene on to offspring.

Co-enzyme—A small molecule such as a vitamin that works together with an enzyme to direct a biochemical reaction within the body.

Enzyme—A protein that catalyzes a biochemical reaction or change without changing its own structure or function.

Gene—A building block of inheritance, which contains the instructions for the production of a particular protein, and is made up of a molecular sequence found on a section of DNA. Each gene is found on a precise location on a chromosome.

Immune system—A major system of the body that produces specialized cells and substances that interact with and destroy foreign antigens that invade the body.

Mutation—A permanent change in the genetic material that may alter a trait or characteristic of an individual, or manifest as disease, and can be transmitted to offspring.

this disorder at birth as part of a comprehensive newborn screening program. Infants whose tests indicate they have biotinidase deficiency can be started on treatment before symptoms appear. With regular treatment these infants usually remain symptom-free.

Carrier testing

Most carriers can be detected by measuring biotinidase activity in their blood. Fifty percent of normal enzyme activity is characteristic of carriers. Specific **DNA** tests can usually detect the particular gene mutation in any affected individual or carrier.

Prenatal diagnosis

If a couple has had one child with biotinidase deficiency, they can be offered prenatal testing in future pregnancies. Prenatal testing is accomplished by measuring biotinidase activity in amniotic fluid cells obtained by **amniocentesis** around the sixteenth week of pregnancy. Alternatively, if specific **gene mutations** have been identified in the parents, fetal DNA from amniotic fluid cells can be studied to test for these same mutations in the fetus. Carrier couples who are considering prenatal diagnosis should discuss the risks and benefits of this type of testing with a geneticist or genetic counselor.

Treatment and management

Treatment of the profound form of biotinidase deficiency consists of giving large doses of biotin orally. Partial deficiencies are usually treated with lower doses. The biotin must be in a free form; that is, not attached to other molecules as would be the case with the biotin found in food. Properly treated, biotinidase deficiency is not a life-threatening condition, but biotin treatment must continue throughout life. No treatment is needed before birth because the developing fetus is provided with sufficient free biotin from the mother.

Prognosis

Daily treatment with free biotin usually results in rapid improvement of the skin condition, hair regrowth, and a lessening or cessation of seizure activity. Many children whose development has been affected by biotinidase deficiency have shown some improvement after treatment. Hearing and vision losses are less reversible. Children who are diagnosed at birth through newborn screening programs rarely develop symptoms if they are started on biotin replacement therapy immediately.

Resources

BOOKS

Wolf, Barry. "Disorders of Biotin Metabolism." In *Metabolic and Molecular Bases of Inherited Disease,* edited by C. R. Scriver, et al. New York: McGraw-Hill, 2001.

PERIODICALS

Blanton, S. H., et al. "Fine Mapping of the Human Biotinidase Gene and Haplotype Analysis of Five Common Mutations." *Human Heredity* 50 (March-April 2000): 102-11.

Norrgard, K. J., et al. "Mutations Causing Profound Biotinidase Deficiency in Children Ascertained by Newborn Screening in the United States Occur at Different Frequencies Than in Symptomatic Children." *Pediatric Research* 46 (July 1999): 20-27.

ORGANIZATIONS

National Organization for Rare Disorders (NORD). PO Box 8923, New Fairfield, CT 06812-8923. (203) 746-6518 or (800) 999-6673. Fax: (203) 746-6481. <http://www.rarediseases.org>.

WEBSITES

"Biotinidase." *Online Mendelian Inheritance in Man.* <http://www.ncbi.nlm.nih.gov/entrez/dispomim.cgi?id=253260> (May 24, 2001).

Thibodeau, D. L., and B. Wolf. "Biotinidase Deficiency. A Booklet for Families and Professionals." <http://views.vcu.edu/biotin>.

Tyler for Life Foundation Home Page. <http://www.tylerforlife.com/biotinidase.htm>.

Sallie Boineau Freeman, PhD

Bipolar disorder

Definition

Bipolar disorder is characterized by severe and unusual changes in energy level, mood, and interactions with others. The mood swings associated with bipolar disorder are unpredictable, and range from mania (elevated or irritable mood) to **depression** (a mood characterized by loss of interest and sadness). Bipolar disorder causes significant impairment in social, occupational, and general functioning.

Description

Bipolar disorder is a manic-depressive psychiatric disorder that causes extreme fluctuations in mood and energy levels, which alternate over long time periods. These episodes are referred to as mania and depression, and appear in cycles throughout life. Between episodes, approximately two-thirds of bipolar patients are free of symptoms, with the remainder experiencing residual symptoms. A small percentage of patients experience chronic incessant symptoms despite treatment.

Bipolar disorder type I is the classic form of the illness, involving recurrent cycles of extreme manic and depressive episodes. Type II bipolar disorder patients never develop severe mania. Type II bipolar patients experience milder episodes called hypomania that alternate with depression. A third type, rapid-cycling bipolar disorder, involves four or more episodes of illness occur within a 12-month period. Multiple episodes may occur within one week or day. Rapid cycling tends to occur later in the course of illness and is most common in women.

Manic episodes are commonly associated with irritability, decreased need for sleep, euphoria (an exaggerated perception of feeling good), social extroversion (excessive friendliness), and feeling more important than one truly is (grandiosity). Depressive episodes are commonly associated with fatigue, impaired concentration and judgment, and altered sleep and appetite patterns. The depressive cycle can further progress to feelings of excessive shame and guilt, and lead to suicidal thoughts. Bipolar disorder is also called manic-depressive psychosis, and is a major affective disorder.

Genetic profile

There is no single **gene** or environmental factor that causes bipolar disorder. Like other mental illnesses, multiple factors together may contribute to the illness. Bipolar disorder has a strong genetic component. According to the Mayo Clinic, 60% of bipolar cases have a family history of the disease. The Child and Adolescent Bipolar Foundation (CABF) reports that the risk for a child of one bipolar parent to develop the disorder is 15–30%. If both parents have bipolar disorder, the risk for each child increases to 50–75%. The risk in siblings and fraternal twins is 15–25%. The risk in identical twins, who share the same genes, is approximately 70%. Research in identical twins indicates that both genes and other factors play a role in developing bipolar disorder.

No specific **gene mutations** have been identified that consistently show up in bipolar patients. However, there appears to be a potential genetic correlation between bipolar disorder and mutations in specific regions of chromosomes 13, 18, and 21. The building blocks of genes, called nucleotides, are normally arranged in a specific order and quantity. If these nucleotides are repeated in a redundant fashion, a genetic abnormality often results. Some evidence exists for a special type of nucleotide sequence (CAG/CTG repeats) in patients with type II bipolar disorder on **chromosome** 18. However, not all bipolar patients have this mutation and the presence of this sequence does not worsen the disorder or change the age of onset. Further research is needed to determine which genes are involved in bipolar disorder. The specific genetic defect for bipolar disorder has not yet been identified, and it is likely that both genetic and environmental factors contribute to the disease.

Demographics

According to the National Institutes of Mental Health (NIMH), approximately 1–1.3% of the United States adult population has bipolar disorder. It is estimated that approximately 2.3 million adult Americans are affected. Approximately 0.8% of the population has bipolar disorder type I, and 0.5% of the population has bipolar disorder type II. Approximately 25–50% of individuals with manic-depressive disorders attempt suicide, with 11% actually committing suicide. No racial predilection exists. While bipolar type I occurs equally in both sexes, type II and rapid-cycling bipolar disorder is more common in females than in males. Women may also be at increased risk of developing subsequent episodes in the immediate time period after giving birth. Bipolar disorder runs in families, with the rate disease in identical twins being higher than that in fraternal twins. The age of onset varies greatly. The age range of onset may be in early childhood or up to 50 years of age, with a mean of 21 years. The most frequent age of onset lies between 15 and 19 years of age. The second most frequent age of onset is between 20 and 24 years of age. Some patients previously diagnosed with recurrent major depression may have bipolar disorder and not develop a manic episode until 50 years of age. However, for most patients, mania onset after 50 years of age is due to other medical disorders such as cerebrovascular disease.

Signs and symptoms

Bipolar disorder causes recurrent dramatic mood swings that range from a manic high to a depressive low. There are often periods of normal mood in between episodes of mania and depression. Severe changes in energy and behavior accompany the swings in mood.

Manic episode symptoms include:

- increased energy, activity, and restlessness
- excessively high, euphoric mood
- extreme irritability and reactivity
- racing thoughts and fast speech that jump from one topic to another, known as flight of ideas
- distractibility due to unimportant events and the inability to concentrate
- reduced perceived need for sleep
- unrealistic beliefs in one's abilities, powers, or importance
- poor judgment and impulsive behaviors
- increased sexual drive
- provocative, intrusive, or aggressive behavior
- denial that anything is wrong

Depressive episode symptoms include:

- persistent sad, anxious, or empty mood
- feelings of irritability, hopelessness, or negative mood
- feelings of guilt, worthlessness, or helplessness
- inability to take pleasure in activities

- fatigue
- inability to concentrate and poor judgment
- extreme sleep patterns
- extreme appetite changes that result in weight change
- chronic pain or physical discomfort in the absence of physical illness or injury
- thoughts of or attempts at suicide

Some cases of type II bipolar disorder have depressive episodes concurrent with mood reactivity (mood improves with positive event), and can switch from depression to hypomania. Hypomania is characterized a mild or moderate level of mania. Because hypomania is less severe, it may be associated with increased functioning and enhanced productivity. However, hypomania is not a normal state of mind. Without proper treatment, hypomania may eventually progress into severe mania or switch into depression. Severe episodes of mania or depression may also include symptoms of psychosis. Psychotic symptoms include visual or auditory hallucinations and delusions (illogical, false, but strongly held beliefs). Psychotic symptoms in bipolar disorder tend to reflect the current extreme mood episode. During mania, psychotic delusions may include grandiosity, such as believing one has special powers of flight or extreme financial wealth. During depressive episodes, delusions may include paranoid fears of being poisoned or the belief that one has committed a terrible crime. Because of these psychotic symptoms, bipolar disorder is sometimes mistaken for **schizophrenia**.

Some bipolar cases present with a mixed state of symptoms. A mixed bipolar state is characterized by symptoms of agitation, sleeplessness, appetite changes, psychosis, and suicidal tendencies. A depressed and hopeless mood may occur in conjunction with extreme energy. Signs of bipolar disorder may also be demonstrated outside of mental illness symptoms in behaviors such as alcohol or drug abuse, poor work performance, strained interpersonal relationships, or excessive promiscuity. Symptoms of bipolar disorder with postpartum onset usually occur within four weeks after childbirth. Bipolar disorder with a seasonal pattern displays symptoms related to seasonal change and latitude. The prevalence of the season-specific bipolar symptoms increases with higher latitudes and winter months.

Children and young adolescents with bipolar disorder tend to have episodes that are less clearly defined than adults with the disorder. Young people often experience very fast swings (rapid cycle) between mania and depression within the same day. Children in a manic episode are more likely to be irritable and destructive than elated. Children and young adolescents are also more prone to mixed symptoms. Bipolar disorder in children and adolescents can be difficult to distinguish from other problems associated with this age group. Symptoms of irritability and aggressiveness may indicate bipolar disorder, or be symptoms of **attention deficit hyperactivity disorder**, conduct disorder, oppositional defiant disorder, other types of mental disorder, or drug abuse.

Diagnosis

Bipolar disorder is a manic-depressive psychiatric disorder that is difficult to diagnose. Like other mental illnesses, bipolar disorder cannot yet be identified through simple tools such as a blood test. A diagnosis of bipolar disorder is made on the basis of symptoms, course of illness, and family history. The diagnostic criteria for bipolar disorder are described in the *Diagnostic and Statistical Manual for Mental Disorders*, fourth edition (DSM-IV). A manic or hypomanic episode is diagnosed if elevated mood, including three or more associated symptoms, lasts one week or longer. A depressive episode is diagnosed if five or more of the associated symptoms last two weeks or longer. For a mixed episode, the criteria must be met for manic and depressive episodes, but the depressive episode need only last one week. The episodes must be of sufficient severity to cause impairment and not be due to substance abuse or some other illness. A mental status examination during an episode reveals obvious symptoms associated with bipolar disorder.

Bipolar manic depression should be distinguished from unipolar (major) depression. Individuals who exhibit bipolar disorder depressive episodes often present with signs of eating more (hyperphagia), sleeping more (hypersomnia), very low energy levels, are overweight, and experience worsening of mood during evening hours. The bipolar affected individual also tends to deny or minimize obvious signs of illness. Unipolar (major) depression usually presents with anxiety, difficulty sleeping, loss of appetite, loss of weight, and feeling worse during morning hours, which improves as the day progresses. Close friends, family members, and roommates are often very helpful in assisting the clinician make the correct diagnosis.

Suicide is the major complication of bipolar disorder, and is related to the duration of the depressive episode. The longer the depressive episode lasts, the higher the risk of suicidal tendencies. Alcoholics and patients with other chronic medical diseases are particularly prone to planning and implementing a suicide attempt.

The four main groups that are likely to carry out a suicide attempt include the following:

- Individuals who are overwhelmed by life problems. Suicide attempts in this group tend to be related to

aggression and impulsive behaviors, not significant depressive episodes.

- Individuals who are attempting to control others.

- Individuals who are chronically ill with another medical disease.

- Individuals with other severe types of psychotic illness, delusions, and paranoia.

Treatment and management

Most individuals with bipolar disorder can achieve substantial stabilization of mood swings and related symptoms with proper treatment. Treatment of bipolar disorder is achieved through medication and psychosocial interventions. Medications for bipolar disorder are prescribed by psychiatrists, medical doctors with expertise in the diagnosis and treatment of mental disorders. While primary care physicians may also prescribe medications used in bipolar disorder, it is recommended that bipolar patients see a psychiatrist for treatment.

Medications

Mood-stabilizing medications may be utilized for long-term maintenance and preventative treatment of bipolar disorder episodes. In the acute phase, the choice of medication for bipolar disorder is dependent on the stage or type of current episode. There are numerous drugs used to treat an acute manic episode, primarily the antipsychotics and benzodiazepines (lorazepam, clonazepam). In the presence of psychotic symptoms, atypical antipsychotics may be used to treat the psychotic symptoms and acute mania, and contribute to mood stabilization. For depressive episodes, antidepressants may be used. These may be added temporarily, to treat episodes of mania or depression that break through despite mood-stabilizer treatment.

Mood stabilizers have a stabilizing effect that dampens the extremes of manic and depressive episodes. Lithium was the first mood stabilizer approved by the U.S. Food and Drug Administration (FDA) for the treatment of mania and the prevention of both manic and depressive episodes. Lithium carbonate is a first-line medication used in the long-term preventative treatment of extreme mood episodes in bipolar disorder, and was demonstrated in 2003 to play a neuroprotective role in brain function. The beneficial effects of lithium carbonate usually appear one or two weeks after administration of oral doses. Lithium treatment has a high response rate, with 70–80% of patients experiencing acute manic attacks showing an improvement of symptoms. However lithium treatment has many side effects, including gastrointestinal discomfort, diarrhea, baldness, skin eruptions, and fluid retention. Lithium is primarily useful as a prophylactic (prevention) medication for future attacks.

Multiple anticonvulsant medications, such as valproate (Depakote), carbamazepine (Tegretol), and lamotrigine (Lamictal), also act as mood stabilizers. However, not all anticonvulsant medications have been FDA-approved for this use. Valproic acid is a second-line medication intended for patients who respond poorly to, or cannot tolerate the side effects of, lithium. Valproic acid has proven effective in treating and preventing mania. It can be used alone or in combination with lithium, and is especially useful in treating rapid-cycling bipolar disorder. For treatment of depressive bipolar episodes, mood stabilizers are preferred to antidepressants because antidepressants may cause a switch into a manic episode or aggravate irritability in mixed-symptom mania. Gabapentin (Neurontin) is not a mood stabilizer, but may have antidepressant and anti-anxiety effects.

Psychosocial interventions

Psychosocial interventions include both patient education and psychotherapy. It is important for patients to receive social support and illness management skills. Family and friends must be aware of the high rates of social dysfunction and marital discord. Involvement in national support groups is advisable (e.g., National Depressive and Manic-Depressive Association).

Psychoeducation usually focuses on all of the following:

- assessment of what parameters will have an impact on the outcome of patient's disease

- implementing the boundaries and requirements of treatment

- implementation of a personal cost-benefit analysis concerning specific treatment directions

- implementing a follow-up program

- implementing future directions, which may include adjustment or change interventions

Genetic counseling should be included in family education programs since the predisposition for this disorder has been genetically proven to increase among first-degree relatives.

Prognosis

Although the episodes of mania and depression appear in cycles, bipolar disorder is a long-term illness that currently has no cure. The long-term prognosis for bipolar disorder is variable. It is critical that bipolar patients maintain consistent and strict compliance with medications. Patients taking psychotropic medications must understand the importance of

> **KEY TERMS**
>
> **Neuroprotective**—Conveying some form of protection to the nervous system from injury.
>
> **Nucleotides**—Building blocks of genes, which are arranged in specific order and quantity.

regular dosing as prescribed and the necessity for constant psychiatric follow-up visits. In comparison to major depression (unipolar), bipolar disorder is usually associated with longer depression, more severe depressive symptoms, more relapses (having active symptoms return after a period of remission), and more incapacitation and hospitalization. Some studies have shown that early-onset bipolar disorder is associated with more recurrences, but not necessarily worse outcomes. Psychotherapy and education can improve prognosis by assisting the patient and family members with pertinent information concerning relapses, noncompliance with prescription medications, and specific adjustments necessary for the welfare of the affected individual.

Many individuals with bipolar disorder can lead productive lives when the illness is effectively treated. However, without treatment, the prognosis is very poor. The natural course of bipolar disorder tends to worsen over time, with increased frequency and severity of manic and depressive episodes. In most cases, proper treatment can reduce the frequency and severity of episodes and help to maintain a good quality of life. Remaining on medications, even during well times, is essential for keeping the disease under control and reducing the risk of recurrent, worsening episodes.

Resources

BOOKS

American Psychiatric Association. *Diagnostic and Statistical Manual of Mental Disorders*, fourth edition. Washington, DC: American Psychiatric Association, 1994.

Maxmen, J. S., and M. G. Ward. *Essential Psychopathology and Its Treatment.* New York, NY: W. W. Norton & Company, 1995.

Muench, K. H. *Genetic Medicine.* New York, NY: Elsevier Science Publishing Co., Inc., 1988.

PERIODICALS

Benazzi, F. "Early versus Late-onset Bipolar II Disorder." *Journal of Psychiatry and Neuroscience* 25 (2000): 53–56.

Callahan, A. M., and M. S. Bauer. "Psychosocial Interventions for Bipolar Disorder." *The Psychiatric Clinics of North America* 22 (1999): 675–686.

Parikh, S. V., J. B. Vincent, and J. L. Kennedy. "Clinical Characteristics of Bipolar Disorder Subjects with Large

CAG/CTG Repeat DNA." *Journal of Affective Disorders* 55 (1999): 221–224.

Sanchez, L., O. Hagino, E. Weller, and R. Weller. "Bipolarity in Children." *The Psychiatric Clinics of North America* 22 (1999): 629–639.

Schaffer, C. B., and L. C. Schaffer. "Open Maintenance Treatment of Bipolar Disorder Spectrum Patients Who Responded to Gabapentin Augmentation in the Acute Phase of Treatment." *Journal of Affective Disorders* 55 (1999): 237–240.

ORGANIZATIONS

National Depressive and Manic-Depressive Association. 730 N. Franklin, Suite 501, Chicago, IL 60610-7204. (800) 826-3632 or (312) 642-7243. (April 18, 2005.) <http://www.ndmda.org>.

WEBSITES

"About Pediatric Bipolar Disorder." Child & Adolescent Bipolar Foundation. (April 18, 2005.) <http://www.bpkids.org/learning/about.htm>.

American Psychological Association. (April 18, 2005.) <http://helping.apa.org/>.

Bipolar Disorder 2001. National Institutes of Mental Health. (April 18, 2005.) <http://www.nimh.nih.gov/publicat/bipolar.cfm>.

Bipolar Disorder Risk Factors. Mayo Clinic. (April 18, 2005.) <http://www.mayoclinic.com/invoke.cfm?objectid=B2138CDB-0C42-4B6F-8AF50CA8903055A7&dsection=4>.

E-medicine. "Bipolar Affective Disorder." (April 18, 2005.) <http://www.emedicine.com/med/topic229.htm>.

National Mental Health Organization. (April 18, 2005.) <http://www.nmha.org>.

"The Numbers Count." National Institutes of Health. (April 18, 2005.) <http://www.nimh.nih.gov/publicat/numbers.cfm>.

Maria Basile, PhD

Bloch-Sulzberger syndrome *see* Incontinentia pigmenti

Bloom syndrome

Definition

Bloom syndrome is a rare inherited disorder characterized primarily by short stature and a predisposition to various types of **cancer**. It is always associated with a decreased stability in the chromosomes that can be seen by cytogenetic laboratory techniques.

Description

Bloom syndrome (BS) was first described by D. Bloom in 1954. The clinical symptoms of BS include small body size, sun-sensitive skin that is prone to a reddish rash, patchy spots on the skin that are either lighter or darker than the expected skin color, severe immune deficiency, and an enormous predisposition to various types of cancer. The hallmark of the disorder is genetic instability that manifests itself in chromosomes that tend to exchange material with one another.

Genetic profile

BS is inherited in an autosomal recessive manner. The **gene** responsible for this disorder is known as BLM and it is located on **chromosome** 15, in band q26.1. Changes or mutations in the BLM gene lead to decreased stability in the chromosomes. Chromosomes of people with BS will show an increased amount of gaps, breaks, and structural rearrangements.

The most characteristic chromosomal abnormality in BS involves the tendency for **deoxyribonucleic acid (DNA)** strands to exchange material, most likely during replication. DNA is the molecule that encodes the genetic information and determines the structure, function and behavior of a cell. The exchange of DNA may occur between a *chromatid* of each of the two homologues of a chromosome pair, forming a unique structure called a *quadriradial*, or between the two sister chromatids of one chromosome, known as sister-chromatid exchange (SCE).

The BLM gene produces the BLM protein. The BLM protein is a member of the helicase family and is thus capable of unwinding DNA and **RNA**. This unwinding process provides single stranded templates for replication, repair, recombination, and transcription. Additionally, the BLM protein may function in a post-replication recombination process that resolves errors generated during replication. Mutations (changes) prevent the BLM gene from making BLM protein. Without adequate amounts of this protein, errors are likely to occur in these important processes and these errors are less likely to be repaired.

It is known that mutations in the BLM gene lead to the symptoms of BS. However, the precise relationship between these mutations and the symptoms seen in BS is still unknown.

Additionally, the DNA of individuals affected with BS is much more prone to spontaneous mutations, perhaps because the inadequate amount of BLM hinders the correction of these errors.

Demographics

BS is a very rare condition, thought to affect a very small proportion of the general population (approximately one in 6,330,000). However, in the Ashkenazi Jewish population, approximately one in 60,000 people are affected with BS. Approximately one in 100 people of this ethnic group are carriers of a mutation in the BLM gene. These carriers do not have BS but are capable of passing it on to their children if the other parent is also a carrier. If both parents are carriers, each pregnancy will have a 25% chance of being affected with the disorder. Carriers, or individuals with only one copy of the abnormal gene, do not appear to have an increased risk for cancer or other symptoms associated with BS. They have near normal or normal genetic stability.

Signs and symptoms

There are two characteristic signs that are seen in nearly all individuals with BS. The first is an overall small body size, which is usually noted at birth and continues throughout the person's lifetime. The growth deficiency is often accompanied by a small brain and head. The head may be dolichocephalic as well, meaning that is it elongated from the front to the back of the head. The average height for an adult with BS is 147.5 cm for males and 138.6 cm for females.

The second characteristic that is very common in individuals with this disorder is an enormous predisposition to cancer. Both benign (non-cancerous) and malignant (cancerous) tumors arise at an early age and with great frequency in a wide variety of body locations and cell types. Thirty-seven percent of patients have malignant tumors. The mean age at diagnosis of a cancer is 24 years with a range of 2–46 years. Lymphomas and leukemias are common and generally appear before the age of 25. Carcinomas are common as well, usually appearing after the age of 20, most often in the colon, skin, breast, or cervix. Cancer is the most common cause of death for individuals with BS. Radiation treatment or chemotherapy can lead to further complications in these patients due to the increased sensitivity to exposures that may damage their fragile chromosomes.

There are additional features that may or may not be present in individuals with BS and they vary in severity from person to person. In some cases of BS, the person may have some unique facial features, including a narrow, triangular face shape, a prominent nose, a small jaw, and protuberant ears. The voice may be high pitched and somewhat squeaky in tone.

Infants may experience repeated respiratory tract infections, ear infections, and vomiting and diarrhea that can lead to a life-threatening loss of body water (dehy-

dration). Additionally, after the first significant exposure to sunlight, an infant may develop a reddish "butterfly rash" on the cheeks and nose described as erythematous or telangiectatic. The severity of the rash can vary from a faint blush during the summertime to a severely disfiguring, flaming red lesion. Rarely, other areas of the body that are exposed to sunlight can show a similar rash. In childhood, the skin may begin to appear "patchy" showing some spots with less pigment than the rest of the skin (hypopigmentation) and some with more pigment than the rest of the skin (hyperpigmentation).

Men diagnosed with this disorder may have abnormally small testes and might be unable to produce sperm, making them infertile. Women can have early menopause and often have reduced fertility.

Individuals with BS have a higher incidence of **diabetes** mellitus when compared to the general population. The average age of onset of diabetes is 25 years, earlier than the usual age of onset of type II diabetes and later than that of type I. Additionally, this disorder can lead to a compromised immune system, resulting in an increased susceptibility to bacterial infections. Infections of the respiratory tract and ears are seen most commonly.

Intelligence in individuals with BS seems to be average to low average. When they exist, limitations in intellectual abilities range from minimal to severe. Even when intelligence is normal in these individuals, there tends to be a poorly defined and unexplained learning disability that is often accompanied by a short attention span. BS is often accompanied by a persistent optimistic attitude.

Diagnosis

BS can be suspected by the doctor but is generally confirmed by a cytogenetic study known as sister chromatid exchange (SCE) analysis. This disorder is the only one that features an increased risk of SCE. This analysis is indicated in any child or adult with unexplained growth deficiency regardless of whether or not other features of the BS are present.

SCE analysis involves taking a blood sample, treating it with a special process in the laboratory, and examining the chromosomes. In individuals with BS, the chromosomes will show an approximately 10-fold increased rate of sister chromatid exchange. Most likely, unique chromosome structures called quadriradials will also be visible in a higher frequency than expected. SCE and quadriradials are present in untreated cells from individuals without BS, although much less frequently.

In addition to examining the chromosomes, it is also possible to look for specific changes in the BLM gene. This type of evaluation is generally used only for those

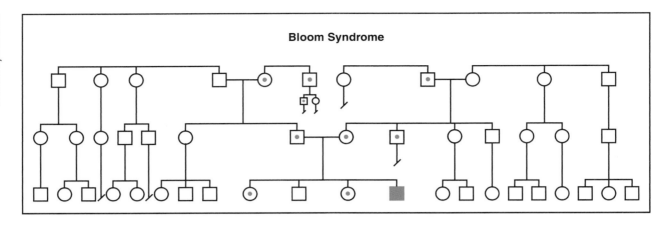

Bloom Syndrome

(Gale Group.)

who may be carriers of the gene mutation rather than those who are suspected to have the disorder. Carriers cannot be identified by SCE analysis because they do not show an increased rate of SCE.

Carrier testing is available for the Ashkenazi Jewish population. In these individuals, there is one particular mutation in the BLM gene that is responsible for most cases of BS. A blood sample can be tested for the presence of this mutation. Almost all Ashkenazi Jewish carriers of the BS gene can be identified in this manner. The great majority of carriers of the mutation causing BS are of Ashkenazi Jewish descent and, thus, this test is designed for that high-risk population. The test is not accurate for people from other ethnic populations in whom the specific changes of the BLM gene are not so well understood.

Prenatal diagnosis is available for carrier couples with previously identified mutations in the BLM gene.

It is thought that BS is highly underdiagnosed. Many affected individuals are treated for a symptom or are mistakenly considered to have another rare disorder.

Treatment and management

There is no treatment for BS—the underlying genetic defect cannot be repaired. However, early diagnosis and management can increase the life span of these individuals.

Babies and young children with BS are often poor eaters. Thus, nutritious food and multivitamins may help improve growth. Treatment with growth hormone has been attempted in several cases but has been generally unsuccessful. Further investigation into this possibility has been limited due to reports that cancer has developed in conjunction with growth hormone treatment.

The reddish skin lesions can be controlled by avoiding the sun, wearing a hat or bonnet, and by using a sunscreen. Avoidance of sun exposure is most critical in the first few years of life, since the severity of the skin lesion appears to be established at that time.

Cancer surveillance is of utmost importance in BS. After the age of 20, annual sigmoidoscopy and fecal blood testing are recommended, as well as breast self-examinations and pap smears for women. It is suggested that the individual be followed closely by a specialist or clinic knowledgeable about BS so that any subtle symptoms of carcinomas can be treated. Early surgical removal of these tumors provides the best chance of a cure. Individuals may wish to store their bone marrow early in life in case a later treatment diminishes their existing bone marrow. Unfortunately, early diagnosis of leukemia is not known to improve the chances of curative therapy; thus, surveillance of the blood and blood-forming tissues in children with BS is not recommended as a part of the cancer surveillance.

Additionally, individuals with this disorder are instructed to avoid x rays, chemotherapeutic drugs and other environmental exposures that may damage their unusually fragile chromosomes. Due to the immunodeficiencies often associated with BS, it is important to treat any bacterial infections promptly.

Prognosis

The mean age at death is 23 years with a range from 1–48 years. Cancer is the most common cause of fatalities in individuals with BS and is thought to be responsible for approximately 80% of deaths. Chronic respiratory infection is the next most common cause of death.

KEY TERMS

Carcinoma—Any cancer that arises in the epithelium, the tissue that lines the external and internal organs of the body.

Chromatid—Each of the two strands formed by replication of a chromosome. Chromatids are held together by the centromere until the centromere divides and separates the two chromatids into a single chromosome.

Erythema—Redness of the skin due to dilatation of capillaries.

Fecal blood testing—Examination of the stool for any evidence of blood, which may be a sign of cancers in the digestive tract.

Homologues—Chromosomes or chromosome parts identical with respect to their construction and genetic content (i.e., the pair of chromosome 1s are homologous, as are the two 2s, 3s, etc.).

Leukemia—Cancer of the blood forming organs which results in an overproduction of white blood cells.

Lymphoma—A malignant tumor of the lymph nodes.

Sigmoidoscopy—The visual examination of the inside of the rectum and sigmoid colon, using a lighted, flexible tube connected to an eyepiece or video screen for viewing.

Telangiectatic—A localized collection of distended blood capillary vessels.

Resources

PERIODICALS

Gennery, A. R., et al. "Immunodeficiency Associated With DNA Repair Defects." *Clinical and Experimental Immunology* 121 (2000): 1-7.

German, James. "Bloom's Syndrome." *Dermatologic Clinics* 13 (January 1995): 7-18.

Meyn, M. S. "Chromosome Instability Syndromes: Lessons for Carcinogenesis." *Current Topics in Microbiology and Immunology* 221 (1997): 71-148.

Nakura, J., et al. "Helicases and Aging." *Cellular and Molecular Life Sciences* 57 (2000): 716-730.

Rong, Suo-Bao, Valiaho Jouni, and Mauno Vihinen. "Structural Basis of Bloom Syndrome (BS) Causing Mutations in the BLM Helicase Domain." *Molecular Medicine* 6 (2000): 155-164.

Watt, Paul M., and Ian D. Hickson. "Genome Stability: Failure to Unwind Causes Cancer." *Current Biology* 6 (1996): 265-267.

Woods, C. Geoffrey. "DNA Repair Disorders." *Archives of Disease in Childhood* 78 (1998): 178-184.

WEBSITES

"Bloom Syndrome." *OMIM—Online Mendelian Inheritance in Man.* National Center for Biotechnology Information. <http://www3.ncbi.nlm.nih.gov/omim/>.

"Bloom Syndrome." Pediatric Database. *PEDBASE.* http://www.icondata.com/health/pedbase/index.htm.

"Bloom Syndrome." *University of Pittsburgh,* Department of Human Genetics. Genetics Education and Counseling Program. <http://www.pitt.edu/~edugene/>.

Mary E. Freivogel, MS

▌Blue rubber bleb nevus syndrome

Definition

Blue rubber bleb nevus syndrome (BRBNS) is a rare disorder characterized by hemangiomas of the skin and gastrointestinal (GI) tract. Hemangiomas are benign or noncancerous tumors of newly formed blood vessels and skin. This syndrome derives its name from these distinctive rubber-like skin lesions.

Description

In 1860 G. G. Gascoyen first reported the association of cutaneous or skin nevi and intestinal lesions with GI bleeding. William Bean in 1958 first used the term BRBNS to describe the rubber-like tumors. Because of his description, BRBNS is sometimes called Bean syndrome. Besides the skin and GI tract, nevi are found on all internal organs and even the brain. Nevi are birthmarks of the skin that are probably hereditary because they are not caused by external factors.

Genetic profile

To date, the **gene** that causes BRBNS has not been identified. The fact that it has not been discovered does not imply the gene does not exist. Some cases of BRBNS are familial and support an autosomal dominant form of **inheritance**, meaning that only one copy of the non-working gene is required to manifest the condition. An affected parent has a 50% chance of passing the disorder to his or her offspring. However, most cases are sporadic without a familial tendency.

Demographics

Less than 180 cases have been reported worldwide. BRBNS affects all races, both sexes, and may be present at birth. The effects on life expectancy are unknown because so few cases exist.

Signs and symptoms

The distinctive blue skin blebs are the hallmark of BRBNS and are not cancerous. Blebs are nevi that measure more than 5 mm around. Composed of skin and large dilated blood vessels, the nevi do not disappear and are found on internal organs such as the stomach, liver, spleen, heart, bone, muscle, bladder, and vulva. They are easily compressible and refill after compression. Occasionally, the nevi are painful. Ranging in size from millimeters to several centimeters, the nevi can number from a few to hundreds. As the patient ages, they can increase in size and number. In rare cases, large lesions can cause skeletal deformities that may lead to amputation.

Nevi are usually present at birth. Sometimes, however, they may not appear until ages two or three.

Patients with BRBNS develop an extreme paleness or pallor of the skin. This paleness results because anemia, a low blood count, decreases the amount of oxygen available to the surface skin. Often they complain of fatigue that results from low iron stores and the anemia.

Chronic or acute bleeding in the GI tract may be detected when blood is present in the stool. Chronic bleeding causes anemia, pallor, fatigue, and low iron stores. Iron supplements will help to increase the blood count. Acute bleeding in the GI tract happens quickly and can rapidly decrease a normal blood count. Immediate blood transfusion or surgery to remove the bleeding nevus can correct this condition.

Diagnosis

The first key to diagnosis of this condition is the appearance of the skin nevi. If they do not have the distinct rubbery texture, blue color, and refill after they have been compressed, another diagnosis should be considered. Endoscopy is required to examine the GI tract for nevi. If they are present, then the diagnosis is confirmed. However, lack of nevi in the GI tract does not completely rule out BRBNS, since they may not develop until adolescence.

KEY TERMS

Anemia—A blood condition in which the level of hemoglobin or the number of red blood cells falls below normal values. Common symptoms include paleness, fatigue, and shortness of breath.

Cutaneous—Of, pertaining to, or affecting the skin.

Endoscopy—A slender, tubular optical instrument used as a viewing system for examining an inner part of the body and, with an attached instrument, for biopsy or surgery.

Nevus—Any anomaly of the skin present at birth, including moles and various types of birthmarks.

During an endoscopy, a viewing instrument attached to a flexible tube is passed through the mouth to the small intestine. The tube can also be inserted through the rectum to the colon. The doctor can then examine the GI tract for nevi.

A patient will require blood tests to assess anemia and iron deficiency as well as a stool test for the presence of blood. Although nevi may be found on the brain, few patients have neurological signs such as seizures or partial paralysis.

Treatment and management

Treatment of BRBNS will depend upon the severity, number, size, and location of the nevi. Skin lesions that are life-threatening can be safely removed by surgery, or laser therapy. The severity of bleeding from GI lesions will determine how they are treated. Surgery can remove single lesions; however, the number may be too great to excise them all. Treatment methods that are less invasive than surgery use endoscopy to tie off bleeding nevi.

Patients who have neurological signs should have a magnetic resonance image (MRI) of the brain to discover the extent of nevi. Seizures can usually be controlled by medications. Physical therapy may improve paralysis.

Prognosis

Although BRBNS is a chronic, progressive disease it does not appear to be fatal. If the GI bleeding and anemia are treated, the patient will usually cope well. If a patient expresses concerns about his or her physical appearance psychological counseling should be considered.

Resources

BOOKS

Fry, L. *An Atlas of Dermatology.* New York: Parthenon Publications, 1997.

Helm, K. *Atlas of Differential Diagnosis in Dermatology.* New York: Churchill Livingston, 1997.

PERIODICALS

Ertem, D., et al. "Blue Rubber Bleb Nevus Syndrome." *Pediatrics* 107, no. 2 (February 2001): 418-20.

Fernandes, C., et al. "Blue Rubber Bleb Naevus: Case Report and Literature Review." *European Journal of Gastroenterology and Hepatology* 11, no. 4 (April 1999): 455-7.

Kim, S. J. "Blue Rubber Bleb Nevus Syndrome With Central Nervous System Involvement." *Pediatric Neurology* 22, no. 5 (May 2000): 410-2.

ORGANIZATIONS

Nevus Network, The Congenital Nevus Support Group. PO Box 1981, Woodbridge, VA 22193. (703) 492-0253. <http://www.nevus.org>.

Nevus Outreach, Inc. 1616 Alpha St., Lansing, MI 48910. (517) 487-2306. <http://www.nevus.org>.

WEBSITES

"Blue Rubber Bleb Nevus Syndrome." *University of Texas Southwestern Medical Center.* <http://www2.utsouthwestern.edu/brbns/>.

Fenske, Neil, and Basil Cherpelis. "Blue Rubber Bleb Nevus Syndrome" In *Dermatology/Diseases of the Vessels. E-Medicine* <http://emedicine.com/derm/topic56.htm>.

Suzanne M. Carter, MS, CGC

Brachmann–de Lange syndrome *see* Cornelia de Lange syndrome

Brachydactyly

Definition

Brachydactyly (BD) refers to shortening of the fingers or toes due to underdevelopment of the bones in the hands or feet.

Description

The word brachydactyly comes from the Greek terms *brachy,* meaning "short," and *daktylos,* meaning "digit." This term is used to describe the hands and feet of people who have shortened digits (fingers or toes). The digits themselves may be shorter than normal, or they may appear small because of shortening of the other bones in the hands or feet. This shortening occurs when one or more of the hand or foot bones fail to develop or grow normally.

BD is usually isolated, meaning that it is not associated with any other medical problems. BD may occur along with other physical differences or health problems, often as part of a "syndrome."

BD occurs in a variety of patterns, depending upon which hand or foot bones are affected and how severely they are shortened. It is important to know some basic information about the bone structure of the hands and feet in order to understand the various patterns of BD. Beyond the wrist and ankle, each hand and foot contains 19 tube-shaped (tubular) bones in a specific arrangement. For purposes of orientation, the fingers and toes are numbered from one (thumb or great toe) to five (little finger or little toe). When a fist is made, the bones in the hand that extend from the wrist to the knuckles are called metacarpals. There are five metacarpals, one for the thumb (first metacarpal) and each finger. Each thumb and finger contains several bones called phalanges. A single one of these bones is called a phalanx. The phalanges are arranged end to end and are separated by joints. The thumb has two phalanges and each finger has three phalanges. The phalanges within a particular finger are named according to their location. The phalanges closest to the metacarpals are called the "proximal" phalanges, those in the middle of the fingers are called the "middle" phalanges, and those at the ends of the fingers are called the "distal" or "terminal" phalanges. The thumbs have only proximal and distal phalanges.

The foot bones are very similar to the hand bones. Like the metacarpals, there are five metatarsal bones that extend from the ankle to each of the toes. The bones in the toes are also called phalanges. There are two phalanges in the great toe and three phalanges in each of the other toes.

BD can involve any of the phalanges, metacarpals, and metatarsals in many different combinations. The shortening of these bones may range from mild to severe. Sometimes certain bones are completely absent. Shortening of the bones may occur in one, several, or all of the digits. For a particular finger or toe, the entire digit may be short or only a particular phalanx may be underdeveloped. When BD involves the distal phalanges, the fingernails or toenails may be small or absent. A digit may also be of normal length but appear short due to shortening of its corresponding metacarpal or metatarsal bone. Reduced length of a metacarpal bone is often easiest to appreciate when the hand is held in a fist.

BD can also occur with other abnormalities of the hands and feet. When a phalanx is abnormally shaped, the finger or toe may be bent to one side (clinodactyly). Sometimes the digits have webbing between them (syndactyly). The phalanges may also be fused together at their ends (symphalangism). This makes it difficult to bend a digit at the joint where the phalanges are fused.

BD frequently occurs in characteristic patterns that can be inherited through families. These patterns are classified as particular types of BD, depending upon which bones and which digits of the hands and/or feet are shortened. There are several classification systems used to describe these different types of BD. The system that is used most frequently was developed by Dr. Julia Bell in 1951 and is called the "Bell Classification."

There are five main types of BD in the Bell Classification, which are designated types A through E. Their major features are as follows:

- In type A, the middle phalanges of one, several, or all of the fingers and/or toes are shortened. This form of BD is further divided into types A1, A2, and A3. In type A1, the middle phalanges of all digits and the proximal phalanges of the thumbs and great toes are shortened. People with this form of BD generally have hands and feet that appear small with relatively equal shortening of all digits. In type A2, the middle phalanges of the index finger and second toe are shortened and often abnormally shaped. In type A3, the middle phalanx of the fifth finger is shortened and this finger often bends toward the fourth finger. Several other forms of BD type A have also been described.

- In type B, the distal phalanges and nails of the fingers and/or toes are small or absent. The middle phalanges may also be shortened, and the tips of the thumbs and/or great toes may be broad or have a "duplicated" (double) appearance. In this type of BD, the digits typically look as though their tips have been amputated.

- In type C, the middle phalanges of all of the fingers may be shortened, but the fourth finger is least affected and is often the longest finger. The index and middle fingers may be bent toward the fourth finger. The first metacarpal bone can also be short, making the thumb appear small.

- In type D, the distal phalanges of the thumbs and/or great toes are shortened and broad.

- In type E, the metacarpals and/or metatarsals are shortened. The fourth and fifth metacarpals and metatarsals are most commonly shortened, but any of them may be affected.

Genetic profile

Many different genetic signals are required for normal formation of the hand and foot bones. BD is usually caused by abnormalities in these genetic blueprints. Sometimes

BD can be caused by exposure to drugs or medications taken during pregnancy. Problems with blood flow to the hands or feet during fetal life may also cause BD.

The types of BD in the Bell Classification are inherited in families from one generation to the next. Their pattern of **inheritance** is called autosomal dominant. This means that they are caused by abnormalities in only one copy of a **gene** from a particular gene pair. In fact, one form of BD (type A1) was the first human condition that was recognized to have this type of inheritance pattern. Autosomal dominant forms of BD can be inherited by a child of either sex from a parent of either sex. The gene change causing BD may also occur in a particular person for the very first time within a family. Each child born to a person having autosomal dominant BD has a 50% chance of also having BD. However, the degree of hand or foot abnormalities can be very different between people with the same type of BD, and even among members of the same family.

Until recently, nothing was known about the genes that cause BD. This has changed with the identification of the genes that cause two forms of autosomal dominant BD (types B and C) in the past several years. The gene causing BD type C was the first to be identified in 1997. The name of this gene is the "Cartilage Derived Morphogenetic Protein 1" gene, abbreviated as CDMP1. This gene is located on the long arm of **chromosome** 20 (at location 20q11.2) and provides an important genetic signal to the developing bones of the limbs. Most people with BD type C have abnormalities in one of their two copies of this gene.

The gene causing BD type B was identified in 2000. This gene is called ROR2 and is located on the long arm of chromosome 9. Like CDMP1, ROR2 also provides an important genetic blueprint for the normal development of bones. BD type B is caused by alterations in one copy of this gene.

One interesting feature of the CDMP1 and ROR2 genes is that they can also cause other medical conditions with bone problems that are much more severe than BD. This happens when both copies of either gene are altered in the same person. The genes for other types of autosomal dominant BD have not yet been discovered.

Demographics

BD occurs in people of many different racial and ethnic backgrounds. It is difficult to determine the overall frequency of BD in the general population because many people who have BD never seek medical attention for their shortened digits. Types A3 and D are the most common forms of BD, but their frequencies vary widely between groups of people from different backgrounds. For example, type A3 has been found in fewer than 1% of Americans, compared to 21% of Japanese people.

Because isolated forms of BD are generally inherited as autosomal dominant traits, they should affect males and females in equal numbers. However, several types of BD may be more common in females.

Signs and symptoms

BD is often evident at birth, but may also develop or become more obvious during childhood. It usually does not cause pain or other physical symptoms. In fact, many people who have BD consider it to be a normal family trait rather than a medical condition. When BD does cause problems, they are usually related to the size, appearance, or function of the hands or feet. The altered appearance of the hands or feet may make persons with BD feel self-conscious. Shortening of the digits may also make it difficult to find comfortable shoes or gloves. In its severe forms, BD may affect a person's ability to grip objects or participate in certain jobs or leisure activities. Hand function may be especially affected when BD is associated with clinodactyly, syndactyly, or symphalangism. When BD is associated with significant deformities of the feet, walking may be difficult or painful.

In some cases, BD occurs in combination with other physical changes or medical problems. For instance, people with autosomal dominant forms of BD are often shorter than expected and may have other alterations of the skeleton besides short digits. Some people with BD type E also have hypertension (high blood pressure). BD may also be present as one finding in a number of different genetic conditions (syndromes).

Diagnosis

The diagnosis of BD is made when a person has shortening of the digits due to lack of normal growth and development of one or more bones in the hands or feet. When the bones are significantly shortened, this is easily noticed in the appearance of the hands and feet. When the shortening is mild, it may only be apparent on x rays. Some people may not realize that they have BD until told by a physician who has carefully examined their hands and feet.

X rays of the hands and feet are used to look at the bones in detail. A special analysis of the hand x rays called a "metacarpophalangeal profile" is often performed for people with BD. This involves measuring the length of each hand and finger bone. These measurements are then compared to the normal range of sizes for each bone. The metacarpophalangeal profile is used to identify particular patterns of BD. X rays may also reveal other bone changes that help to pinpoint a specific type of BD or another genetic condition. If a person has short stature or other bone changes, a series of x rays of the entire skeleton (skeletal survey) may be recommended.

Since BD is often inherited, detailed information about a person's relatives can be very important in evaluating someone with BD. A geneticist may wish to examine other family members or obtain x rays of their hands and feet. Because BD can occur in a variety of genetic conditions, a geneticist evaluating someone with BD will usually review his or her medical history and perform a detailed physical examination. The presence of other physical differences or medical problems may indicate that the brachydactyly is part of another condition rather than an isolated finding.

Laboratory tests are usually not helpful in diagnosing BD when it is an isolated finding. Although the genes for BD types B and C are known, testing of these genes is not routinely available or usually necessary. If a person with BD has signs or symptoms of another underlying condition, certain laboratory tests may be recommended. These tests may identify other associated medical problems or help to pinpoint a specific diagnosis.

Treatment and management

Many people who have BD are perfectly healthy and do not require any specific treatment for their hands and feet. When use of the hands is impaired, physical therapy or hand exercises may improve grip strength or flexibility. Evaluation by an orthopedist or physical therapist may also be helpful for people who have trouble walking comfortably due to bone changes in the feet. Surgery can be used to lengthen the hand or foot bones in some severe forms of BD. Surgery may also be helpful for people who have significant clinodactyly, syndactyly, or symphalangism. For most people with BD, however, surgery is not needed. If BD is associated with other medical problems, such as hypertension, specific treatments for these problems may be indicated.

Prognosis

Isolated BD generally has an excellent prognosis. When BD is associated with other health problems or is part of another condition, the overall prognosis depends upon the nature of the associated condition.

Resources

BOOKS

Temtamy, Samia A., and Victor A. McKusick. *The Genetics of Hand Malformations.* New York: Alan R. Liss, 1978.

Winter, Robin M., Richard J. Schroer, and Leslie C. Meyer. "Hands and Feet." In *Human Malformations.* Vol. 2, edited by Roger E. Stevenson, Judith G. Hall, and Richard M. Goodman, New York: Oxford University Press, 1993, pp. 828–43.

PERIODICALS

Armour, C. M., D. E. Bulman, and A. G. W. Hunter. "Clinical and Radiological Assessment of a Family with Mild Brachydactyly Type A1: The Usefulness of Metacarpophalangeal Profiles." *Journal of Medical Genetics* 37 (April 2000): 292–296.

Oldridge, M., et al. "Dominant Mutations in ROR2, Encoding an Orphan Receptor Tyrosine Kinase, Cause Brachydactyly Type B." *Nature Genetics* 24 (March 2000): 275–78.

Polinkovsky, A., et al. "Mutations in CDMP1 Cause Autosomal Dominant Brachydactyly Type C." *Nature Genetics* 17 (September 1997): 18–19.

WEBSITES

Online Mendelian Inheritance in Man (OMIM). <http://www.ncbi.nlm.nih.gov/Omim/>.

David B. Everman, MD

Branchiootorenal syndrome

Definition

Branchiootorenal (BOR) syndrome is an autosomal dominant condition characterized by ear abnormalities, hearing loss, cysts in the neck, and kidney problems.

Description

The name branciootorenal syndrome describes the body systems most commonly affected by this genetic disorder. The term "branchio" refers to the abnormal-

ities of the neck found in individuals with this syndrome. Cysts (lump or swelling that can be filled with fluid) and fistulas (abnormal passage from the throat to the skin) in the neck occur frequently. The term "oto" refers to the ear disorders associated with the syndrome. For example, the outer ear can be unusual in appearance. Hearing loss is also common. Finally, the term "renal" stands for the kidney problems commonly seen in patients with this condition. These can be very mild or very severe, as can any of the symptoms associated with this disorder.

Dr. M. Melnick first described branchiootorenal (BOR) syndrome in 1975. Another name for BOR syndrome is Melnick-Fraser syndrome. Individuals with BOR syndrome typically have physical differences that are present at birth (congenital). These birth defects are caused by a change (mutation) in a **gene**.

Genetic profile

Scientists recently discovered that mutations in the EYA1 gene cause BOR syndrome. The EYA1 gene is located on **chromosome** 8. The exact function of the EYA1 gene is unknown, but mutations in this gene disrupt normal development, producing the physical differences common to BOR syndrome. A mutation in this gene can affect the normal development of the ear, kidney, and the branchial arches. The branchial arches are tissues that develop very early in pregnancy and are involved in the formation of the face and neck.

BOR syndrome is inherited in a dominant manner. This means that only one gene in the pair must be mutated in order for the individual to be affected. If a person has a mutation in one of their EYA1 genes, the disorder is typically present. The characteristics of the syndrome can be extremely variable in severity.

A mutation in the EYA1 gene may be inherited from a parent with BOR syndrome. A mutation can also occur by chance, in an individual without a family history of BOR syndrome. If a child inherits an abnormal gene from a parent, the signs of the disorder can be very different between the parent and the child. This is called *variable expressivity*. For example, a parent who has a very mild form of BOR syndrome can have a severely affected child. The reverse situation can also occur.

Once an individual has a mutation in the EYA1 gene, there is a 50/50 chance with each pregnancy that the gene will be passed on. This means that there is a 50/50 chance of having a child with BOR syndrome. Male and female children have the same risk. It does not matter if the gene is inherited from the mother or the father.

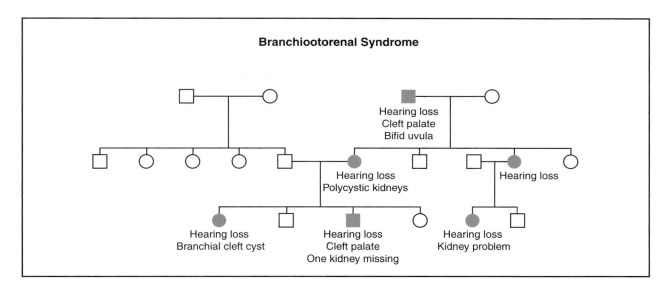

Branchiootorenal Syndrome

Hearing loss
Cleft palate
Bifid uvula

Hearing loss
Polycystic kidneys

Hearing loss

Hearing loss
Branchial cleft cyst

Hearing loss
Cleft palate
One kidney missing

Hearing loss
Kidney problem

(*Gale Group.*)

Demographics

BOR syndrome occurs one in every 40,000 live births. BOR syndrome is seen in all ethnic groups and cultures. It also affects males and females equally. One study suggested that 2% of individuals with severe hearing loss have BOR syndrome.

Signs and symptoms

The characteristics associated with BOR syndrome are highly variable. Some individuals with BOR syndrome have many physical deformations. Other individuals with BOR syndrome have a few minor physical differences. The birth defects can occur on only one side of the face (unilateral) or be present on both sides (bilateral).

Abnormal development of the ears is the most common characteristic of BOR syndrome. The ears may be smaller than normal (microtia) and may have an unusual shape. Ear tags (excess pieces of skin) may be seen on the cheek next to the ear. Preauricular pits (small pits in the skin on the outside of the ear) are found in 75% of patients with BOR syndrome. Hearing loss is present in 85% of individuals with BOR syndrome and this loss may be mild or severe.

The most distinctive finding in individuals with BOR syndrome is the presence of cysts or fistulas in the neck region due to abnormal development of the branchial arches. These cysts and fistulas can be filled with or discharge fluid.

Approximately two-thirds of individuals with BOR syndrome also have kidney abnormalities. These abnor-malities can be very mild and cause no health problems, or they can be very severe and life threatening. The kidneys can be smaller than normal (renal hypoplasia), abnormally shaped, malfunctioning, or totally absent (**renal agenesis**).

Other less common characteristics associated with BOR syndrome include cleft palate, facial nerve paralysis, and abnormalities of the tear ducts. The tear ducts (lacrimal ducts) may be absent or abnormal. Some patients with BOR syndrome uncontrollably develop tears while chewing (gustatory lacrimation).

Diagnosis

The diagnosis of BOR syndrome is made when an individual has the common characteristics associated with the condition. An individual does not need to have all three components of the disorder in order to be diagnosed with the condition.

There is no readily available genetic test that can diagnose BOR syndrome. Some laboratories are performing **DNA** testing for mutations in the EYA1 gene. However, this testing is currently being offered on a research basis only. Individuals interested in this type of testing should discuss it with their doctor.

Treatment and management

Once a child is diagnosed with BOR syndrome, additional tests should be performed. A hearing evaluation is necessary to determine if there is hearing loss. If

KEY TERMS

Autosomal dominant—A pattern of genetic inheritance where only one abnormal gene is needed to display the trait or disease.

Bilateral—Relating to or affecting both sides of the body or both of a pair of organs.

Cleft palate—A congenital malformation in which there is an abnormal opening in the roof of the mouth that allows the nasal passages and the mouth to be improperly connected.

Congenital—Refers to a disorder which is present at birth.

Cyst—An abnormal sac or closed cavity filled with liquid or semisolid matter.

Deoxyribonucleic acid (DNA)—The genetic material in cells that holds the inherited instructions for growth, development, and cellular functioning.

Ear tags—Excess pieces of skin on the outside of the ear.

Fistula—An abnormal passage or communication between two different organs or surfaces.

Gene—A building block of inheritance, which contains the instructions for the production of a particular protein, and is made up of a molecular sequence found on a section of DNA. Each gene is found on a precise location on a chromosome.

Gustatory lacrimation—Abnormal development of the tear ducts causing tears when chewing.

Lacrimal ducts—Tear ducts.

Microtia—Small or underdeveloped ears.

Mutation—A permanent change in the genetic material that may alter a trait or characteristic of an individual, or manifest as disease, and can be transmitted to offspring.

Preauricular pits—Small pits in the skin on the outside of the ear.

Renal agenesis—Absence or failure of one or both kidneys to develop normally.

Renal hypoplasia—Abnormally small kidneys.

Unilateral—Refers to one side of the body or only one organ in a pair.

Variable expressivity—Differences in the symptoms of a disorder between family members with the same genetic disease.

hearing loss is evident, the child should be referred to a hearing specialist. Hearing tests may need to be performed on a regular basis. Speech therapy may also be helpful. An ultrasound of the kidney may be necessary, due to the increased risk for birth defects in these areas. Finally, minor surgery may be required to correct the branchial cysts and fistulas commonly found in BOR syndrome.

Prognosis

The prognosis for individuals with BOR syndrome is very good. Individuals with BOR syndrome typically have a normal life span and normal intelligence.

Resources

BOOKS

Jones, Kenneth Lyons. "Melnick-Fraser Syndrome." In *Smith's Recognizable Patterns of Human Malformation.* 5th edition. Philadelphia: W.B. Saunders, 1997.

PERIODICALS

Chen, Achih, et al. "Phenotypic Manifestations of Branchiootorenal Syndrome." *American Journal of Medical Genetics* 58 (1995): 365-370.

ORGANIZATIONS

Alliance of Genetic Support Groups. 4301 Connecticut Ave. NW, Suite 404, Washington, DC 20008. (202) 966-5557. Fax: (202) 966-8553. <http://www.geneticalliance.org>.

National Kidney Foundation. 30 East 33rd St., New York, NY 10016. (800) 622-9010. <http://www.kidney.org>.

National Organization for Rare Disorders (NORD). PO Box 8923, New Fairfield, CT 06812-8923. (203) 746-6518 or (800) 999-6673. Fax: (203) 746-6481. <http://www.rarediseases.org>.

Research Registry for Hereditary Hearing Loss. 555 N. 30th St., Omaha, NE 68131. (800) 320-1171. <http://www.boystown.org/btnrh/deafgene.reg/waardsx.htm>

WEBSITES

"Branchio-Oto-Renal (BOR) Syndrome." *Boystown Research Registry.* <www.odc.state.or.us/tadoc/hloss3.htm>.

"Branchiootorenal Dysplasia." *OMIM—Online Mendelian Inheritance in Man.* <www.ncbi.nlm.nih.gov/entrez/dispomim.cgi?id=113650>.

"Branchiootorenal Syndrome." University of Washington, Seattle. *GeneClinics: Clinical Genetic Information Resource.* <www.geneclinics.org/profiles/bor/details.html>.

Holly Ann Ishmael, MS

Breast cancer

Definition

Breast **cancer** is a disease in which abnormal breast cells begin to grow uncontrollably, forming tumors. It often shows up as a breast lump, breast thickening, or skin change.

Description

The breasts are areas of tissue located on the front chest wall, and are essentially part of the skin. They are like "specialized sweat glands" in their structure and function, in that they can produce and secrete fluids, like milk. They are made of ductal tissue, supporting connective tissue, and fat. The breasts naturally drain fluid through the lymph channels to the axillary lymph nodes, located in the armpit areas. Within the breasts are intricate structures of ducts and lobules, which are channels and areas that create and transport milk during lactation.

Excluding skin cancers, breast cancer is the most common cancer among women and the leading cause of death in women in their middle years of life. Male breast cancer, though rare, accounts for less than 1% of all breast cancers. Both genetic and environmental factors are thought to cause breast cancer. Of all breast cancer diagnoses, only approximately 5-10% are caused by hereditary factors like specific alterations in breast cancer susceptibility genes, or by a genetic cancer syndrome. In these instances, individuals may have a strong family history of cancer and the cancers may be diagnosed at an earlier age than usual.

Breast cancers vary in their type and size, and this can be determined by a breast biopsy. Breast cancer may commonly be detected by a mammogram, a physician's clinical breast examination (CBE), or a patient's own breast self- examination (BSE). Breast cancer, if it is the first cancer diagnosed, may sometimes metastasize (spread) to other organs, such as the liver, bone, lungs, skin, or brain. The breasts may also be the site of metastasis from other primary cancers.

Breast cancer may present as a lump or other change within the breast. As with other types of cancer, the initial diagnosis may be unexpected. Each cancer has a unique prognosis, and this will affect the patient's concern. If an individual has a very strong family history of breast cancer, the diagnosis may be somewhat expected, but no less emotionally taxing. Treatment and management of the cancer may be extremely exhausting, painful, and stressful for the patient and his or her family.

Genetic profile

Cells in breast tissue normally divide and grow, according to controls and instructions of various genes. If these genes have changes within them, the instructions for cellular growth and division may go awry. Abnormal, uncontrolled cell growth may occur, causing breast cancer. Therefore, all breast cancers are genetic because they all result from changes within genes. However, most breast cancers occur later in life after years of exposure to various environmental factors that can cause alterations (such as the body's own hormones, asbestos exposure, or smoking).

A small proportion of breast cancers is caused by inherited genetic alterations. In 1994 a breast cancer susceptibility **gene**, known as BRCA1 (location 17q21), was identified. The discovery of BRCA2 (location 13q12) followed shortly in 1995. Women with alterations in these genes have an increased risk for breast and **ovarian cancer**, and men have an increased risk for **prostate cancer**. Men with a BRCA2 alteration have an increased risk for breast cancer. Slightly increased risks for colon and pancreatic cancers (in men and women) are associated with BRCA2 alterations.

BRCA1 and BRCA2 alterations are inherited in an autosomal dominant manner; an individual has one copy of a BRCA alteration and has a 50% chance of passing it on to each of his or her children, regardless of that child's gender. Nearly all individuals with BRCA alterations have a family history of the alteration, usually a parent. In turn, they also may have a very strong family history of breast, ovarian, prostate, colon, and/or pancreatic cancers. Aside from BRCA1 and BRCA2, there likely are other breast cancer susceptibility genes that are still unknown (such as BRCA3). Additionally, there may be other genes that convey increased risks solely for other cancers, such as ovarian cancer.

BRCA1 and BRCA2 are thought to function as "tumor-suppressor genes," meaning that their normal role is to prevent tumors from forming. Specifically, they control cellular growth and division, all the while preventing the over-growth that may lead to cancer. Alterations in tumor-suppressor genes, such as BRCA1 and BRCA2, would naturally lead to an increased risk of developing cancer. However, this risk is not 100%.

There are rare, genetic cancer syndromes that may include breast cancer. As a group, these comprise less than 1% of all breast cancer diagnoses. In these instances, an individual may have other health problems (unrelated to cancer) and a family history of a wide variety of cancers and symptoms. These health problems can initially appear unrelated, but may be caused by alterations in a specific gene. As an example, Cowden syndrome typically involves early-onset thyroid and breast cancers, as well as specific tissue growths on the face, limbs, and mouth. An individual with Cowden syndrome may have all or some of these symptoms. It is now known that alterations in the PTEN gene cause Cowden syndrome. Other known cancer syndromes are caused by specific alterations in different genes. These genes are responsible for the various symptoms and cancers in an individual.

Demographics

On average, a North American woman faces a lifetime risk of approximately one in nine (11%) to develop breast cancer. Most cases of breast cancer occur in women past the age of 50, and more commonly in individuals of North American descent.

The prevalence of BRCA alterations in the general population is estimated to be between one in 500 and one in 1,000. However, there are specific alterations that are commonly found in certain ethnic groups. In the Ashkenazi (Eastern European) Jewish population, two specific BRCA1 alterations and one BRCA2 alteration are commonly seen and range in prevalence from 0.1% to 1.0% in this group. As a result, hereditary forms of breast and ovarian cancer are more predominant in people of Ashkenazi Jewish ethnicity. A common BRCA1 alteration has been found in the Dutch population; a specific BRCA2 alteration exists in about 0.6% of people from Iceland. Additionally, common alterations have been identified in both BRCA1 and BRCA2 in French Canadians, and a BRCA1 alteration has often been seen in West Africans.

Signs and symptoms

Various symptoms may bring someone to medical attention in order to investigate the possibility of breast cancer. These may include a breast lump that persists, as opposed to one that only appears at certain times of a woman's menstrual cycle (which is more common). Other signs include changes from the normal breast shape, pain, itchiness, fluid leaking from the nipple (especially if a woman is not pregnant), a turned-in nipple, fatigue, or unexplained weight loss. Sometimes individuals may feel a breast lump or change while examining their own breasts, or a physician may note it on a CBE. Additionally, it may be seen on a screening mammogram. It is important to note not all breast lumps or breast changes signify cancer—they may be benign growths or cysts that need to be removed or drained.

Signs of a possible BRCA1 or BRCA2 alteration in a family, signifying hereditary breast or ovarian cancer, include:

- several relatives with cancer
- close genetic relationships between people with cancer, such as parent-child, sibling-sibling
- earlier ages of cancer onset, such as before ages 45-50
- an individual with both breast and ovarian cancer
- an individual with bilateral or multi-focal breast cancer
- the presence of ovarian, prostate, colon, or pancreatic cancers in the same family
- case(s) of breast cancer in men

Suspicion of a BRCA alteration may be raised if someone has the above features in their family and is of a particular ethnic group, such as an Ashkenazi Jew. This is because specific BRCA1 and BRCA2 alterations are known to be more common in this group of individuals.

Diagnosis

Once a suspicious breast abnormality has been found, the next step is determining if it is breast cancer. A mammogram can identify an area of increased breast density, which is a common sign of a malignant tumor. Women in their 20s to 30s naturally have denser breasts, so mammograms may not be as effective in this age group because the increased breast density associated with a tumor is difficult to see. Breast ultrasound, a way of visualizing the breast tissue using sound waves, can be helpful in younger women because breast density is not a large factor in its effectiveness. A breast biopsy can determine specifically whether the breast tissue has undergone a benign or malignant change because the breast tissue is studied directly under a microscope. Sometimes biopsies are performed with a very thin needle (known as fine needle aspiration), or with x ray guidance using a thicker needle (known as a core needle biopsy).

Newer techniques have improved breast cancer screening and diagnosis. Direct digital imaging in mammograms ends the need for film, and the digital images provide finer detail and allow the images to be rotated in order to get several different views of the breasts. Magnetic resonance imaging (MRI) uses magnetic energy to create an image. Its effectiveness is currently the subject of research studies, but MRI often provides very detailed imaging of tumors. MRI is expensive though, and this is another reason it is not widely used.

There is DNA-based **genetic testing** to identify a BRCA1 or BRCA2 alteration in an individual. In the United States, Myriad Laboratories in Utah is the only place to offer this costly testing. A blood sample is used and both BRCA genes are studied for alterations. There is also targeted testing for people in high-risk ethnic groups (such as the Ashkenazi Jews) in which only the common BRCA alterations can be tested; this testing is much less costly. Even with current technology, only certain regions of the BRCA genes can be studied, which leaves some alterations unlocated.

With either method of testing, it is best to begin the testing process with an individual who has survived breast and/or ovarian cancer. This is because tests are more likely to find an alteration a cancer survivor than someone who has not had cancer. A result is abnormal (or "positive") if a known cancer-causing BRCA alteration is found. If an alteration is found, it is assumed to have caused the cancer(s) in the tested, affected individual. That individual may also identify new cancer risks from the positive result. For example, if a woman survived breast cancer and was found to have a BRCA alteration through testing, she would now be at an increased risk to develop ovarian cancer, as well as a second breast cancer.

For people who go through testing and are not found to have a BRCA alteration (a "negative" result), this result is not informative. There are several possibilities for a negative result. First, there could be a BRCA alteration in the family and the person did not inherit it. In this case, the cancer would be due to reasons unrelated to BRCA1 and BRCA2. Additionally, they could have an alteration in an unknown gene (such as BRCA3), for which there is no testing available. Lastly, they could have a BRCA1 or BRCA2 alteration that is undetectable by available testing methods.

There is a possibility that individuals may have an "unknown alteration" in one of their BRCA genes. In this scenario, a change in the **DNA** is identified, but its significance is unclear. Therefore, it is unknown whether the gene change causes cancer. In these situations, the results are most often considered uninformative, until more information about the alteration becomes available in the future.

Once an alteration is identified, other at-risk relatives, both affected and unaffected, can pursue targeted analysis for the confirmed familial alteration. This is much quicker and far less expensive than the initial analysis.

Unaffected individuals who test positive for a known alteration in the family are at a significantly increased risk to develop the associated cancers. A woman's risks associated with a BRCA1 alteration are: 3-85% for breast cancer by age 70, 40–60% for ovarian cancer by age 70. A man's risk with a BRCA1 alteration is about 8% for prostate cancer by age 70. A woman's risks with a BRCA2 alteration are: 4–86% for breast cancer by age 70, and 16–27% for ovarian cancer by age 70. Less than 1% of men with BRCA 2 alteration develop

breast cancer but they are at a slight or moderate increased risk for prostate cancer. For BRCA2 in men and women, there is an increased risk for colon and pancreatic cancers. Cancers of the larynx (structure in neck that helps with breathing), esophagus (tube-like structure that connects mouth to stomach), stomach, gallbladder (structure that makes bile), bile duct (tube that transports bile between liver and intestine), blood, and melanoma (a form of skin cancer) have been seen in families with BRCA2 alterations.

When a person who has not had cancer tests negative for a known, familial BRCA alteration, they are lowered to the general risk to develop the associated cancers, such as the lifetime risk of 11% for a woman to develop breast cancer. This is because he or she did not inherit the genetic alteration causing cancer in his or her family.

Everyone should receive proper **genetic counseling** before pursuing any BRCA1 and BRCA2 testing. This should include asking them what they hope to learn from the testing. Many people are not aware of the testing limitations, and may be expecting a clear "yes/no" answer from the results. Asking people what they hope to learn from testing allows the opportunity to provide them with accurate facts, such as the possibility of a result that is not informative. Common motivations to be tested include the need to make informed medical decisions, financially planning for the future, or just "wanting to know" about cancer risk.

Genetic testing for cancer susceptibility often triggers strong emotional responses. It is important to find out about an individual's "support system" before they begin testing. Having a close friend, family member, or religious leader to talk with is often helpful for people pursuing testing. Someone who tests positive may be concerned because his or her risks for cancer are now higher than they were before the testing. Additionally, someone may feel "empowered" by the knowledge because they can better plan for medical procedures. Someone with a family history of a BRCA alteration may feel relief if they test negative, because they initially assumed they would develop cancer. Alternatively, someone who tests negative in this situation may feel "survivor guilt" for not having inherited the altered gene in the family. All of these feelings may change the way an individual interacts with his or her family and friends. People may not be aware of the emotional changes that can occur from learning about cancer risk through genetic testing.

It is important to discuss the possibility of insurance coverage for the testing, particularly because it is so expensive. Insurance companies may not routinely cover the testing unless a physician or genetic counselor

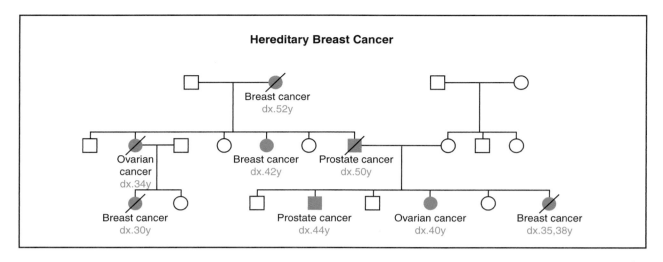

Hereditary Breast Cancer

(Gale Group.)

describes the need for testing in a letter. Some companies are willing to cover the testing without wanting to know the results.

Issues of potential "genetic discrimination" should be discussed. Unaffected individuals who test positive for a BRCA1 or BRCA2 mutation may face difficulty when trying to obtain health, life, and/or disability insurance. Fortunately, there are laws in place that can help protect American individuals who have group health insurance, but the exact laws vary by state. There are no laws to protect individuals from life and disability insurance discrimination, nor employer discrimination.

Treatment and management

Breast cancer treatment is determined by the exact size and type of cancer, so it is often unique to an individual. Treatment may include surgeries, such as a lumpectomy (removal of the breast lump) or mastectomy (removal of the entire breast). Breast reconstruction (recreation of the breast) by plastic surgery is an option some individuals may pursue.

Chemotherapy, or using strong chemicals to kill fast-growing cells, is a common treatment. Side effects from chemotherapy may include nausea, vomiting, hair loss, exhaustion, and sores in the mouth. Symptoms associated with menopause (such as "hot flashes" and the absence of menstrual periods) may occur, or menopause may actually begin because of chemotherapy. Radiation therapy is another common form of treatment, in which directed radioactive waves are used to kill fast-growing cells. Some side effects of radiation therapy are dry and itchy skin, rashes, exhaustion, nausea, and vomiting.

Sometimes, medications such as Tamoxifen are used to prevent a breast cancer from coming back. Tamoxifen is often used for five years following a breast cancer diagnosis to actively prevent a recurrence. Tamoxifen is only effective in specific types of breast cancer, which again are unique to each individual. Some side effects of Tamoxifen include beginning menopause, as well as an increased risk for uterine cancer. Other drugs, such as Raloxifene, are currently being studied for breast cancer prevention because it may be able to do the same things as Tamoxifen, without the side effects. Research studies are under way to determine whether Tamoxifen or Raloxifene can reduce the risk of breast cancer in women with BRCA alterations.

An example of a screening program for women at high risk to develop breast cancer includes:

- BSEs monthly starting in early adulthood (about 20–25 years of age)
- CBEs every six months or yearly starting at age 25–35
- mammograms yearly starting at age 25–35

Exact screening guidelines may vary between physicians. For men with a BRCA2 alteration, breast cancer screening is recommended, though no formal program is specifically recommended.

In addition to screening, women with BRCA1 or BRCA2 alterations should know about their preventive surgery options. They may consider having their healthy breasts and/or ovaries removed, in order to reduce their risks of developing breast and/or ovarian cancer. Women may be more agreeable to an oophorectomy because ovarian cancer is difficult to detect. Surgeries may

KEY TERMS

Alteration—Change or mutation in a gene, specifically in the DNA that codes for the gene.

Benign—A non-cancerous tumor that does not spread and is not life-threatening.

Bilateral breast cancer—Cancer of both breasts, caused by two separate cancer processes.

Bile—A substance produced by the liver, and concentrated and stored in the gallbladder. Bile contains a number of different substances, including bile salts, cholesterol, and bilirubin.

Breast biopsy—Small sample of tissue taken from the breast and studied, to diagnose and determine the exact type of breast cancer.

Breast self-exam (BSE)—Examination by an individual of their own breasts.

CA-125 (Carbohydrate antigen 125)—A protein that is sometimes high when ovarian cancer is present. A blood sample can determine the level of CA-125 present.

Clinical breast exam (CBE)—Examination of the breasts, performed by a physician or nurse.

Malignant—A tumor growth that spreads to another part of the body, usually cancerous.

Mammogram—A procedure in which both breasts are compressed/flattened and exposed to low doses of x rays, in an attempt to visualize the inner breast tissue.

Metastasis—The spreading of cancer from the original site to other locations in the body.

Multifocal breast cancer—Multiple primary cancers in the same breast.

Primary cancer—The first or original cancer site, before any metastasis.

Tumor—An abnormal growth of cells. Tumors may be benign (noncancerous) or malignant (cancerous).

greatly reduce a woman's cancer risk, but they can never eliminate the risk entirely.

For people with cancer or at high risk, there are support and discussion groups available. These may be invaluable to those who feel alone in their situation.

Prognosis

The type and size of breast cancer developed largely determines the overall prognosis for an individual. Those with larger tumors and those with a type of breast tumor that does not usually respond to treatment may have a poorer outcome. Additionally, once cancer has spread to other areas of the body the prognosis worsens because the cancer is more difficult to treat. The cancer may also be more likely to continue spreading to other areas of the body.

Those with BRCA alterations who develop breast cancer have a similar prognosis to those without BRCA alterations that have equivalent cancers. In addition, people with BRCA alterations are treated for their cancers using the same methods as those without alterations.

For cancer-free individuals identified to have BRCA alterations, it is important to remember that they are at an increased risk to develop the associated cancers, but that the risk is *not* 100%. Though people with BRCA alterations may feel "destined" to develop cancer, it is by no means a certainty. It is also important to emphasize that breast cancer screening techniques and treatments are constantly being evaluated and improved.

Resources

BOOKS

Chart, Pamela. *Breast Cancer: A Guide for Patients.* Toronto: Prospero Books, 2000.

ORGANIZATIONS

American Cancer Society. 1599 Clifton Rd. NE, Atlanta, GA 30329. (800) 227-2345. <http://www.cancer.org>.

Facing Our Risk of Cancer Empowered (FORCE). 934 North University Drive, PMB #213, Coral Springs, FL 33071. (954) 255-8732. info@facingourrisk.org. <http://www.facingourrisk.org>.

The National Alliance of Breast Cancer Organizations. 9 East 37th Street, 10th Floor, New York, NY 10016. (888) 806-2226 or (212) 889-0606. NABCOinfo@aol.com. <http://www.nabco.org>.

Susan G. Komen Breast Cancer Foundation. Occidental Tower, 5005 LBJ Freeway, Suite 370 LB74, Dallas, TX 75244. (800) 462-9273 (Hotline) or (214) 450-1777. helpline@komen.org. <http://www.breastcancerinfo.com>.

WEBSITES

"The Genetics of Breast and Ovarian Cancer." *CancerNet.* <http://cancernet.nci.nih.gov/clinpdq/cancer_genetics/Genetics_of_breast_and_ovarian_cancer>.

Deepti Babu, MS

Broad-thumb-hallux syndrome *see* Rubinstein-Taybi syndrome

Bruton agammaglobulinemia

Definition

Bruton agammaglobulinemia is an X-linked genetic condition caused by an abnormality in a key enzyme needed for proper function of the immune system. People who have this disorder have low levels of protective antibodies and are vulnerable to repeated and potentially fatal infections.

Description

An integral aspect of the body's ability to resist and fight off infections by microorganisms (bacteria, viruses, parasites, fungi) is the immune system. The immune system is comprised of specialized cells whose function is to recognize organisms that are foreign to the body and destroy them. One set of specialized cells used to fight infection is the B cells. B cells circulate in the bloodstream and produce organism-fighting proteins called antibodies.

Antibodies are made of different classes of immunoglobulin that are produced within a B cell and are then released into the bloodstream, where they attach to invading microorganisms. There are antibodies specifically designed to combine with each and every microorganism, very similar to a lock and key. Once the antibodies attach to the microorganism, it triggers other specialized cells of the immune system to attack and destroy the invader, thus preventing or fighting an existing infection.

In order for antibodies to be produced by the body, the B cells must develop and mature so they are capable of producing the infection-fighting antibodies. When this process does not occur normally, the immune system can not work properly to fight off infection, a state known as immunodeficiency. Bruton agammaglobulinemia (also called X-linked agammaglobulinemia, or congenital agammaglobulinemia) is an inherited immunodeficiency characterized by failure to produce mature B cells and thus to produce the antibodies needed to fight infections. The abnormality in this disorder resides in Bruton tyrosine kinase (BTK, also known as BPK or ATK), an enzyme needed for maturation of B cells. As a result, people with this condition have low levels of mature B cells and the antibodies that they produce, making them vulnerable to frequent and sometimes dangerous infections.

Bruton agammaglobulinemia was the first immunodeficiency disease to be identified, reported by the physician Colonel Ogden C. Bruton in 1952. Bruton patient, a four-year-old boy, was first admitted to Walter Reed Army Hospital because of an infected knee.

The child recovered well when Bruton gave him antibiotics, but over the next four years he had multiple infections. Just at that time, a new instrument was installed in the hospital's laboratory that was able to measure levels of antibodies in the bloodstream. At first the technician believed the machine was defective because it did not detect gammaglobulins (the building blocks of antibodies) in the boy, but Bruton recognized the significance of this finding, and remarked, "Things began to click then. No gammaglobulins; can't build antibodies."

Genetic profile

Bruton agammaglobulinemia is inherited in an X-linked recessive manner; thus, almost all persons with the disorder are male. Females have two X chromosomes, which means they have two copies of the BTK **gene**, whereas males only have one X **chromosome** and one copy of the BTK gene. If a male has an altered BTK gene, he will have Bruton agammaglobulinemia. If a female has one altered BTK gene, she will be a carrier and will be at risk to pass the altered gene on to her children. If her son inherits the altered gene, he will be affected; if her daughter inherits the altered gene, she will be a carrier like her mother. Alternatively, if her son does not inherit the altered gene, he will not be affected and will not pass the altered gene on to his children. Since fathers only pass a Y chromosome to their sons and an X chromosome to their daughters, none of an affected male's sons will develop the disorder, but all of the daughters will be carriers.

Mutations in the gene for BTK (located at Xq21.3-22) are responsible for the disease. Over 250 different mutations in BTK have been identified and they are spread almost evenly throughout the BTK gene. While this abnormal gene can be passed from parent to child, in half of the cases a child will show the disease without having a parent with the mutant gene. This is because new alterations in the BTK gene can occur. This new alteration can then be passed on to the affected individual's children.

Demographics

Bruton agammaglobulinemia occurs in all racial groups, with an incidence between one in 50,000 and one in 100,000 individuals.

Signs and symptoms

Bruton agammaglobulinemia is a defect in the B cells, leading to decreased antibodies in the blood and increased vulnerability to infection with certain types of bacteria and a few viruses. Children with Bruton agammaglobulinemia are born healthy and usually begin to show signs of infection in the first three to nine months of life, when antibodies that come from the mother during pregnancy and early breast-feeding disappear. In 20-30% of the cases, however, patients may have slightly higher levels of antibodies present, and symptoms will not appear until later in childhood.

Patients with Bruton agammaglobulinemia can have infections that involve the skin, bone, brain, gastrointestinal tract, sinuses, eyes, ears, nose, airways to the lung, or lung itself. In addition, the bacteria may migrate from the original site of infection and enter the bloodstream, leading to an overwhelming infection of the body that is potentially fatal.

Besides signs of recurrent infections, other physical findings in patients with Bruton agammaglobulinemia include slow growth, wheezing, small tonsils, and abnormal levels of tooth decay. Children may also develop unusual symptoms such as joint disease, destruction of red blood cells, kidney damage, and skin and muscle inflammation. Increased incidence of cancers, such as leukemia, lymphoma, and possibly colon **cancer**, have been associated with Bruton agammaglobulinemia in a small percentage of people.

Infections seen with Bruton agammaglobulinemia are caused by bacteria that are easily destroyed by a normal-functioning immune system. The most common bacterial species responsible for these infections include *Streptococcus pneumoniae*, *Streptococcus pyogenes*, *Staphylococcus aureus*, *Pseudomonas aeruginosa*, *Neisseria meningitides*, *Klebsiella pneumoniae*, *Hemophilus influenzae*, and *Mycoplasma* species. Chronic stomach and intestine infections are often linked to the parasite *Giardia lamblia*.

Patients with Bruton agammaglobulinemia can successfully defend themselves against infection from viruses and fungi because other aspects of the immune system are still functional. However, there are some notable exceptions—people with this disorder are still vulnerable to the hepatitis virus, poliomyelitis virus, and echovirus. Echovirus is particularly troubling, as it can lead to progressive and fatal infections of the brain, joints, and skin.

Diagnosis

Recurrent infections or infections that fail to respond completely or quickly to antibiotics should prompt a diagnostic search for immunodeficiency and Bruton agammaglobulinemia. Another helpful clue to a diagnosis of Bruton agammaglobulinemia is the presence of unusually small lymph nodes and tonsils. Additionally, many patients with this disorder have a history of continuous illness; that is, they do not have periods of well-being between bouts of illness.

When a patient is suspected of having Bruton agammaglobulinemia, the diagnosis is established by several tests. The amount of immunoglobulin is measured in a small amount of blood from the affected individual by a technique called immunoelectrophoresis. In Bruton agammaglobulinemia, all of the immunoglobulins will be markedly reduced or absent. It should be noted that there is some difficulty in diagnosing the disease in a young infant or newborn because immunoglobulins from the mother are still present in the child during the first few months of life.

For those patients in which the exact diagnosis is still unclear, tests can be performed to determine if there has been any response to normal childhood immunizations (such as the tetanus, diptheria, and pertussis vaccines). Patients with Bruton agammaglobulinemia are unable to respond with antibody formation following immunization. Confirmation of the diagnosis can be made by demonstrating abnormally low numbers of mature B cells in the blood or by genetic studies that look for mutations in the BTK gene. When a diagnosis of Bruton agammaglobulinemia is made in a child, **genetic testing** of the BTK gene can be offered to determine if a specific gene change can be identified. If a specific change is identified, carrier testing can be offered to the mother and female relatives. In families where the mother has been identified to be a carrier of a BTK gene change, diagnosis of Bruton agammaglobulinemia before birth is possible, if desired. Prenatal diagnosis is performed on cells obtained by **amniocentesis** (withdrawal of the fluid surrounding a fetus in the womb using a needle) at about 16-18 weeks of pregnancy or from the chorionic villi (a part of the placenta) at 10-12 weeks of pregnancy. In some families, a BTK gene change cannot be identified. Other laboratory techniques may be available to these families such as linkage studies or X chromosome inactivation studies.

Other diagnostic tests have been advocated to track the ongoing health of the patient with Bruton agammaglobulinemia. X rays of the sinuses and chest should be obtained at regular intervals to monitor for the early development of infections and to determine if proper treatment has been established. Lung function tests should also be performed on a regular basis, when the patient is old enough to cooperate. Patients who have ongoing gastrointestinal tract symptoms (diarrhea) should be tested for the parasite *Giardia lamblia*.

Treatment and management

Current research into a cure for Bruton agammaglobulinemia is focusing on the ability of bone marrow transplantation or **gene therapy** to correct the abnormal BTK gene, however, there is no cure at this time. Therefore the goals of treatment are threefold: to treat infection effectively, to prevent repeated infections, and to prevent the lung damage that may result from repeated infections.

The main abnormality in patients with Bruton agammaglobulinemia is a lack of immunoglobulins, which are the building blocks of antibodies. Thus, treatment focuses on replacing immunoglobulin, thereby providing patients with the antibodies they need to fight infection. Immunoglobulin can be obtained from the blood of several donors and given to a patient with Bruton agammaglobulinemia. Treatment with immunoglobulin is given every three to four weeks and is usually effective in preventing infection by various microorganisms.

Side effects from or allergic reactions to immunoglobulin are infrequent, but about 3-12% of people will experience shortness of breath, sweating, increased heart rate, stomach pain, fever, chills, headache, or nausea. These symptoms will usually subside if the immunoglobulin is given slowly, or the reactions may disappear after receiving the immunoglobulin several times. If the reactions continue, it may be necessary to use a special filtering process before giving the immunoglobulin to the patient.

If infection does occur in a patient with Bruton agammaglobulinemia, antibiotics (medications which kill bacteria) are also given to help fight off the infection. Recurrent or chronic infections will develop in some patients despite the use of immunoglobulin. In that case, antibiotics may be given every day, even when there is no infection present, in order to prevent an infection from forming. If chronic diarrhea is experienced by the patient, tests should be performed to look for the parasite *Giardia lamblia*, and proper antibiotics should be given to kill the organism.

Preventative techniques are also very important. Children with Bruton agammaglobulinemia should be treated promptly for even minor cuts and scrapes, and taught to avoid crowds and people with infections. People with this disorder and their family members should not be given vaccinations that contain live organisms (polio, or the measles, mumps, rubella vaccine) as the organism may result in the immunocompromised person contracting the disease that the vaccination is intended to prevent. Referral for **genetic counseling** is appropriate for female relatives seeking information about their carrier status and for family members making reproductive decisions.

KEY TERMS

Antibiotics—A group of medications that kill or slow the growth of bacteria.

Antibody—A protein produced by the mature B cells of the immune system that attach to invading microorganisms and target them for destruction by other immune system cells.

B cell—Specialized type of white blood cell that is capable of secreting infection-fighting antibodies.

Bruton tyrosine kinase (BTK)—An enzyme vital for the maturation of B cells.

Carrier—A person who possesses a gene for an abnormal trait without showing signs of the disorder. The person may pass the abnormal gene on to offspring.

Enzyme—A protein that catalyzes a biochemical reaction or change without changing its own structure or function.

Immune system—A major system of the body that produces specialized cells and substances that interact with and destroy foreign antigens that invade the body.

Immunodeficiency—A defect in the immune system, leaving an individual vulnerable to infection.

Immunoglobulin—A protein molecule formed by mature B cells in response to foreign proteins in the body; the building blocks for antibodies.

Mutation—A permanent change in the genetic material that may alter a trait or characteristic of an individual, or manifest as disease, and can be transmitted to offspring.

Vaccine—An injection, usually derived from a microorganism, that can be injected into an individual to provoke an immune response and prevent future occurrence of an infection by that microorganism.

X chromosome—One of the two sex chromosomes (the other is Y) containing genetic material that, among other things, determine a person's gender.

Prognosis

Without immunoglobulin treatment, 90% of patients with Bruton agammaglobulinemia will die by the age of eight years old. In most patients who have been diagnosed early and are receiving immunoglobulin on a regular basis, the prognosis is reasonably good. They should be able to lead a relatively normal childhood and need not be isolated to prevent dangerous infections. A full and active lifestyle is to be encouraged.

While current therapy allows most individuals with Bruton agammaglobulinemia to reach adulthood, the prognosis must be guarded. Paralysis of the legs may result from the poliomyelitis virus. Despite what may appear to be adequate immunoglobulin therapy, many patients develop severe, irreversible lung disease. Fatal brain infections have been reported even in patients receiving immunoglobulin therapy, and patients who recover from these infections may be left with severe brain damage. Finally, some patients may develop leukemia or lymphoma.

Resources

BOOKS

Ammann, A. J. "Antibody Immunodeficiency Disorders." In *Medical Immunology.* Stamford, CT: Appleton and Lange, 1997.

Buckley, R. H. "T, B, and NK Cells." In *Nelson Textbook of Pediatrics,* edited by R. E. Behrman. 16th ed. Philadelphia: W.B. Saunders, 2000.

Cooper, M. D. "Primary Immune Deficiencies." In *Harrison's Principles of Internal Medicine,* edited by A.S. Fauci. 14th ed. New York: McGraw-Hill, 1998.

PERIODICALS

Nonoyama, S. "Recent Advances in the Diagnosis of X-linked Agammaglobulinemia." *Internal Medicine* 38(September 1999): 687-688.

ORGANIZATIONS

Immune Deficiency Foundation. 40 W. Chesapeake Ave., Suite 308, Towson, MD 21204. (800) 296-4433. (410) 321-9165. <http://www.primaryimmune.org>.

WEBSITES

"Bruton Agammaglobulinemia Tyrosine Kinase." *Online Mendelian Inheritance in Man.* <http://www.ncbi.nlm.nih.gov/htbin-post/Omim/dispmim?300300> (May 24, 2001).

Oren Traub, MD, PhD

Bulldog syndrome *see* **Simpson-Golabi-Behmel syndrome**

C

CADASIL

Definition

CADASIL (cerebral autosomal dominant arteriopathy with subcortical infarcts and leukoencephalopathy) is an inherited cerebrovascular disease characterized by recurrent strokes, cognitive decline, and **dementia**.

Description

CADASIL (also known as familial vascular leukoencephalopathy, lacunar dementia, and multi-infarct dementia) is an inherited condition that varies widely in its symptoms, age of onset, and disease progression. The effects of CADASIL are primarily confined to the arteries in the brain. Due to a genetic defect, the smooth muscle cells that surround these arteries are gradually destroyed. Characteristic abnormalities in the brain can be seen on neuroimaging, such as magnetic resonance imaging (MRI).

The main clinical signs and symptoms of CADASIL are early ischemic (stroke-like) episodes, cognitive and behavioral disturbances, migraine headaches, and dementia. Psychiatric and mood disturbances may also be associated. These signs and symptoms usually appear between 30 and 40 years of age. Cognitive decline and migraine headaches are often the first manifestations. These are usually followed by transient ischemic attacks (TIAs) and stroke around the average age of 45. The majority of patients show severe cognitive defects and dementia by age 65.

Due to the autosomal dominant **inheritance** pattern, most individuals with CADASIL have a family history of the disease. However, even between family members, the severity and age of onset of clinical manifestations can vary widely.

Genetic profile

CADASIL is caused by mutations in the NOTCH3 **gene**, which resides on **chromosome** 19. The pene-

trance of the disease is approximately 100%. This means that anyone with a mutation in the NOTCH3 gene will show signs of the disorder, even though age of onset and severity of symptoms may vary. When the NOTCH3 gene does not function correctly, protein builds up in the smooth muscle cells that surround the arteries in the body. This leads to degeneration of these smooth muscle cells and a resulting loss of function of the arteries, specifically in the brain and, sometimes, in the heart.

CADASIL is inherited in an autosomal dominant fashion. Thus, the majority of affected individuals have a parent that is affected as well. However, this is not always the case as there may be a new (*de novo*) mutation in the affected individual that was not present in either parent. Additionally, there may appear to be a lack of family history due to the affected parent dying at a young age or the failure to recognize symptoms of the disorder in a parent.

Most often, one parent of the affected individual will have signs of CADASIL and/or a NOTCH3 mutation. In this case, siblings of the affected individual have a 50% chance of inheriting the same mutation and being affected as well. However, if a mutation is identified in the affected individual and both parents test negative for this mutation, it is likely that the NOTCH3 mutation is *de novo* and, therefore, recurrence risk to siblings is very low. For patients with a NOTCH3 mutation, each child is at a 50% risk to inherit the same mutation and, therefore, have a diagnosis of CADASIL.

Demographics

The exact prevalence of CADASIL is currently unknown. Approximately 500 affected families have been identified throughout the world. The majority of cases have been observed in European Caucasians and the number of reported cases in the United States and Canada has been lower than expected thus far. However, no formal conclusions can be drawn from this information since it is very likely that there are many affected families that have yet to be identified.

Signs and symptoms

In the vast majority of cases, patients affected with CADASIL will present with ischemic episodes, cognitive defects, migraine, or psychiatric disturbances. The onset and severity of these symptoms is highly variable, even within families.

In more than 80% of CADASIL cases, ischemic episodes are a recurrent problem. These include transient ischemic attacks (TIAs) and stroke. TIAs and stroke may have age of onset as early as the 20s or as late as the 60s. The average age of onset is 46 years. TIAs usually occur prior to a stroke, however, it is possible for a stroke to be the first sign of the CADASIL. Recurrent ischemic episodes can lead to severe disability, gait disturbance, and urinary incontinence.

In CADASIL, cognitive function worsens slowly over time due to the disturbances in blood flow to the brain that are caused by the disorder. There is variability in the onset and severity of cognitive impairment. It may onset as early as age 35 and is apparent in more than half of affected individuals by age 45. Approximately two-thirds of patients over age 65 demonstrate dementia and severe loss of cognitive function. The dementia is characterized by slowing of motor function, loss of memory, and decreased initiative. Dementia in CADASIL may actually result from recurrent TIAs or strokes that were undiagnosed.

Migraine headaches are seen in approximately 30–40% of patients with CADASIL and occur at the average age of 25. These headaches most often occur with aura, which is a fleeting visual disturbance that takes place prior to the onset of the headache. Migraines are the first sign of the disorder in about half of the cases and may be the most noticeable clinical manifestation. In some patients, migraines improve after the first stroke. Severe migraine headaches may be difficult to distinguish from TIAs.

Psychiatric disturbances, such as severe **depression**, **panic disorder**, or hallucinations, occur in approximately one-third of patients. It is unknown whether these disturbances are associated with CADASIL or whether they are a reaction to the disease.

In a few cases, acute encephalopathy has been described and manifests itself with headache, fever, confusion, seizures, and coma, which can be fatal. **Epilepsy**, although rare, has been observed in affected individuals and usually presents during middle age. Additionally, more recently, evidence supports an increased risk for cardiac problems, such as heart attacks, due to abnormalities in the smooth muscle cells surrounding the arteries in the heart. Other symptoms may include speech defects, insensitivity to pain, loss of vision, and deafness.

Clinical manifestations of CADASIL are always associated with symmetrical lesions in the white matter of the brain that can be seen on MRI. These lesions progress with time and their patterns evolve with age. Hyperintensities in the white matter can be seen on MRI in affected individuals as early as 21 years of age, long before clinical signs and symptoms occur. Additional MRI abnormalities may be associated with CADASIL as well, such as cerebral microbleeds and subcortical lacunar lesions (SLL), the latter of which may be a specific marker for the disease.

The overall course of CADASIL is variable. Some patients will be severely affected by the age of 50, whereas others will be asymptomatic until their 70s. Early onset of symptoms does not necessarily mean that the disorder will progress rapidly.

Diagnosis

CADASIL can be diagnosed via a skin or muscle biopsy. Electron microscope (EM) evaluation of the biopsy specimen will show characteristic abnormalities in smooth muscle cells. These abnormalities are very suggestive of CADASIL, however, the absence of them does not rule out the disorder.

Molecular **genetic testing** via sequencing of the NOTCH3 gene is also very helpful in the diagnosis of CADASIL. Approximately 95% of affected individuals will have an identifiable mutation in this gene. This testing is offered clinically and can be used to confirm a diagnosis in someone with clinical manifestations or as a predictive test in pre-symptomatic individuals. However, molecular genetic testing is only informative if a mutation can be found in a family. Once a NOTCH3 mutation has been found in an affected individual, family members can be tested for that particular mutation to determine whether or not they have a diagnosis of CADASIL.

Due to the severity of the disease and the lack of effective interventions, special considerations should be given to pre-symptomatic testing for CADASIL. Adequate counseling must be provided, including discussion of motivation for testing, impact of test results, and implications for family members and reproductive decisions. Due to the adult onset of symptoms, it is not recommended that children under the age of 18 are offered testing for CADASIL.

Prenatal diagnosis is possible via molecular genetic testing of the NOTCH3 gene in cells obtained from the fetus, however, this is not a common request due to the adult-onset nature of the disorder.

KEY TERMS

Arteriopathy—Any disease of the arteries.

Dementia—Impairment of brain functions, such as memory, reasoning, and judgment.

Encephalopathy—A degenerative disease of the brain that has a sudden onset.

Ischemic episode—A condition that occurs when blood flow to the brain is interrupted due to some type of blockage.

Leukoencephalopathy—Any disease that affects the white matter of the brain.

Magnetic resonance imaging (MRI)—A technique that uses a magnetic field and pulses of radio wave energy to provide pictures of organs and structures inside the body.

Subcortical infarct—An area of necrosis (tissue death) below the cerebral cortex of the brain resulting from obstruction of circulation to that area.

Transient ischemic attack (TIA)—A temporary interruption of blood flow to a part of the brain; causes symptoms that are similar to a stroke, but temporary.

Treatment and management

Unfortunately, there are no interventions that can effectively prevent CADASIL or its clinical manifestations. Certain signs and symptoms can be treated as they appear (i.e., treating migraine headaches with a drug called acetazolamide). Supportive care can be offered to affected individuals and their families, such as counseling and emotional support.

Prognosis

The prognosis of CADASIL is variable. In a large study, the length of time between onset of symptoms and death ranged from 3–43 years, with a mean of 23 years. The mean age of death in CADASIL patients is about 60 years.

Resources

PERIODICALS

Dichgans, Martin. "CADASIL: A Monogenic Condition Causing Stroke and Subcortical Vascular Dementia." *Cerebrovascular Diseases* 13 Supplement (2002): 37–41.

Dichgans, Martin. "Cerebral Autosomal Dominant Arteriopathy with Subcortical Infarcts and Leukoencephalopathy: Phenotypic and Mutational Spectrum." *Journal of the Neurological Sciences* 203–204 (2002): 77–80.

Kalimo, H., M. Ruchoux, M. Viitanen, and R. N. Kalaria. "CADASIL: A Common Form of Hereditary Arteriopathy Causing Brain Infarcts and Dementia." *Brain Pathology* 12 (2002): 371–384.

ORGANIZATIONS

National Organization for Rare Disorders (NORD), 55 Kenosia Avenue, PO Box 1968, Danbury, CT 06813-1968. (800) 999-6673. (April 4, 2005.) <http://www.rarediseases.org/search/zcat_search_results?allfields=cadasil&search_for=2>.

WEBSITES

"CADASIL." *Genetics Home Reference.* (April 4, 2005.) <http://ghr.nlm.nih.gov/condition=cadasil>.

Lesnik Oberstein, S. A. J, M. H. Breuning, and J. Haan. "CADASIL." *Gene Reviews.* (April 4, 2005.) <http://www.genetests.org/servlet/access?db=geneclinics&site=gt&id=8888891&key=n2v3Fs58ptTtr&gry=&fcn=y& fw=2TuG&filename=/profiles/cadasil/index.html>.

NINDS Multi-infarct Dementia Information Page. National Institute of Neurological Disorders and Stroke. (April 4, 2005.) <http://www.ninds.nih.gov/disorders/multi_infarct_dementia/multi_infarct_dementia.htm>.

Mary E. Freivogel, MS, CGC

Campomelic dwarfism *see* **Campomelic dysplasia**

Campomelic dysplasia

Definition

Campomelic **dysplasia** is a rare, often lethal, genetic condition characterized by multiple abnormalities including short limbs, bowed legs, distinctive facial features, and a narrow chest. It is also often associated with abnormal development of the sex (reproductive) organs in males.

Description

Campomelic dysplasia is also known as campomelic syndrome, campomelic dwarfism, CMD1, and CMPD1. This condition affects the bones and cartilage of the body, causing significantly short arms and legs, bowing of the legs, small chest size, and other skeletal (bony) and non-skeletal problems. Some genetic males with campomelic dysplasia have female sex organs. Death often results in the newborn period due to breathing problems related to the small chest size. Campomelic dysplasia is caused by an alteration (mutation) in a **gene** called SOX9. It usually occurs randomly in a family.

Genetic profile

Campomelic dysplasia is caused by an alteration in the SOX9 gene, which plays a role in bone formation and testes development. Genes are units of hereditary material found on chromosomes, which are passed from a parent to a child through the egg and sperm. The information contained in genes is responsible for the development of all the cells and tissues of the body.

The SOX9 gene is located on **chromosome** 17 (one of the 22 non-sex chromosomes) and it plays a role in both bone formation and testis development. The testes are responsible for producing male hormones. Every developing baby in the womb (fetus), whether genetically male (XY) or female (XX), starts life with the capacity to develop either male or female sex organs. After a few weeks, in an XY fetus, the genitals develop into male genitals if male hormones are present. In the absence of male hormones, a female body type with female genitals results.

In individuals with campomelic dysplasia, the SOX9 gene is altered such that it does not work properly. This causes the testes to form improperly and the male hormones are not produced; thus, individuals who are genetically male (XY) can develop as normal females. This is known as sex-reversal and occurs in about 66% of genetic males with campomelic dysplasia. Since SOX9 is also important for proper bone formation, the bones of the body are also affected causing short stature, bowed legs, and other problems.

There are usually two normal copies of the SOX9 gene: one copy of the gene is inherited from the mother and one copy is inherited from the father. Campomelic dysplasia is inherited as a dominant condition. In dominant conditions, a person only needs one altered gene copy to develop the condition. The alteration in the SOX9 gene that causes campomelic dysplasia is usually random. This means that some unknown event has caused the SOX9 gene (which functions normally in the parent) to become altered in either the sperm of the father or the egg of the mother. When this altered sperm or egg is fertilized, the child that results has campomelic dysplasia. The chance for parents of a child with campomelic dysplasia to have a second child with the same condition is slightly higher than it would be for another couple who has not had a child with this condition. A person who has campomelic dysplasia can pass on their altered SOX9 gene to his or her future children; however, there have not been any reports of individuals with campomelic dysplasia having children.

Demographics

Campomelic dysplasia is a rare condition that affects males and females of all ethnic groups. It is estimated that approximately one in 10,000 newborns are affected with this condition.

Signs and symptoms

Campomelic dysplasia can affect the body in several ways. Campomelic means "curved limb" and refers to the fact that individuals with campomelic dysplasia typically have curved or bowed legs. Usually there is a dimple in the leg just below the knee. The condition causes significantly short stature, which is evident from birth.

Other features include very small shoulder blades; a very small chest; a curved and twisted spine (kyphoscoliosis); feet that are often turned inwards (**clubfoot**); dislocated hips; short fingers and toes; and often there are 11 pairs of ribs instead of the usual 12. In some individuals, the pelvic bones and the bones of the spine can also be affected.

A large head size and distinctive facial features such as a high forehead; a flat, small face; small chin; low set ears; and widely spaced eyes are also common. Some individuals have an incomplete closure of the roof of the mouth (cleft palate). Breathing problems are common and are often the cause of death in newborns. The breathing problems usually result from the small chest size, small lungs, and narrow airway passages. Those who survive into early infancy frequently have feeding problems and difficulty breathing.

Individuals with campomelic dysplasia may also have heart defects and hearing loss. Some females with the condition have a Y chromosome. Females with campomelic dysplasia who have a Y chromosome are genetically male; however, their sex organs are female and thus they should be treated as normal females. The intellect of individuals with campomelic dysplasia is usually normal although there have been reports of some individuals who are mentally delayed.

Diagnosis

The diagnosis of campomelic dysplasia is based on the presence of certain clinical features. Some of the bony abnormalities are more obvious on x ray. The features that suggest a diagnosis of campomelic dysplasia include significantly short stature present from birth, small shoulder blades, 11 pairs of ribs instead of 12, small chest size, bowed legs, and a dimple on the leg below the knee.

The diagnosis of campomelic dysplasia can be confirmed through **genetic testing**, which requires a blood sample from the affected individual. The genetic test involves identifying the specific alteration in the SOX9 gene. Parents of an affected child may seek testing for campomelic dysplasia in future pregnancies. This can be performed on the developing baby before birth through **amniocentesis** or chorionic villus sampling if an alteration in the SOX9 gene is identified in the previously affected individual. Prenatal testing should only be considered after the gene alteration has been confirmed in the affected individual and the couple has been counseled regarding the risks of recurrence.

Treatment and management

Campomelic dysplasia is associated with a significant risk for death in the newborn period due to the small chest and small lungs. There is no effective treatment to expand the size of the chest. Those who survive into early infancy have feeding problems and often have difficulty breathing. An occupational therapist may be able to assist with the feeding issues. Breathing problems may necessitate that the child be placed on oxygen.

Some individuals with campomelic dysplasia have significant twisting and bending of their spine (kyphoscoliosis) which can interfere with breathing. A bone specialist (orthopedist) should be consulted for advice on potential treatments such as bracing or surgery. An orthopedist should also be consulted regarding the other bony problems such as clubfoot and bowed legs. Individuals with campomelic dysplasia should also have their hearing assessed and their heart examined because of the increased risk for hearing loss and heart defects, respectively.

In females with campomelic dysplasia who have a Y chromosome, the gonads (the organs that later become either testes or ovaries during fetal development) do not develop properly into ovaries. It is generally recommended that the they be surgically removed because there is an increased chance for tumors to occur in the gonads when they do not develop properly.

Very few individuals with campomelic dysplasia live beyond the newborn period but most who do are of normal intelligence. During the school years, it may be necessary to make some changes (such as providing the individual with a step-stool in the bathroom) to foster independence. For some, meeting other individuals of short stature may be beneficial. Groups, such as the Little People of America (LPA), serve as a source of information and offer opportunities to meet other people facing similar chal-

lenges. Individuals with campomelic dysplasia and their families may benefit from **genetic counseling**, which can provide them with further information on the condition itself and recurrence risks for future pregnancies.

Prognosis

Campomelic dysplasia is associated with a significant risk for death in the newborn period. Most newborns die during the first few hours after birth from breathing problems due to the small chest size and small, underdeveloped lungs. A few individuals with campomelic dysplasia have lived to be adults.

Resources

ORGANIZATIONS

Greenberg Center for Skeletal Dysplasias. 600 North Wolfe St., Blalock 1012C, Baltimore, MD 21287-4922. (410) 614-0977. <http://www.med.jhu.edu/Greenberg.Center/Greenbrg.htm>.

Johns Hopkins University—McKusick Nathans Institute of Genetic Medicine 600 North Wolfe St., Blalock 1008, Baltimore, MD 21287-4922. (410) 955-3071.

Little People of America, Inc. National Headquarters, PO Box 745, Lubbock, TX 79408. (806) 737-8186 or (888) LPA-2001. lpadatabase@juno.com. <http://www.lpaonline.org>.

National Organization for Rare Disorders (NORD). PO Box 8923, New Fairfield, CT 06812-8923. (203) 746-6518 or (800) 999-6673. Fax: (203) 746-6481. <http://www.rarediseases.org>.

WEBSITES

"Campomelic Dysplasia." *OMIM—Online Mendelian Inheritance in Man.* <http://www3.ncbi.nlm.nih.gov/>. (March 9, 2001).

Nada Quercia, MS

Campomelic syndrome *see* **Campomelic dysplasia**

Camunati-Englemann disease *see* **Engelmann disease**

Canavan disease

Definition

Canavan disease, which results when the body produces less than normal amounts of a protein called aspartoacylase, is a fatal inherited disorder characterized by progressive damage to the brain and nervous system.

Description

Canavan disease is named after Dr. Myrtelle Canavan who described a patient with the symptoms of Canavan disease but mistakenly diagnosed this patient with Schilder's disease. It was not until 1949, that Canavan disease was recognized as a unique genetic disease by Van Bogaert and Betrand. The credit went to Dr. Canavan, however, whose initial description of the disease dominated the medical literature.

Canavan disease, which is also called aspartoacylase deficiency, spongy degeneration of the brain, and infan-tile spongy degeneration, results from a deficiency of the enzyme aspartoacylase. This deficiency ultimately results in progressive damage to the brain and nervous system and causes mental retardation, seizures, tremors, muscle weakness, blindness and an increase in head size. Although most people with Canavan disease die in their teens, some die in childhood and some live into their twenties and thirties.

Canavan disease is sometimes called spongy degeneration of the brain since it is characterized by a sponginess or swelling of the brain cells and a destruction of the white matter of the brain. Canavan disease is an autosomal recessive genetic condition that is found in all ethnic groups, but is most common in people of Ashkenazi (Eastern European) Jewish descent.

Genetic profile

Canavan disease is an autosomal recessive genetic disease. A person with Canavan disease has changes (mutations) in both of the genes responsible for producing the enzyme aspartoacylase and has inherited one changed **gene** from his or her mother and one changed gene from his or her father. The aspartoacylase gene is called ASPA and is located on **chromosome** number 17. There are a number of different types of changes in the ASPA gene that can cause Canavan disease, although there are three common gene changes. When the ASPA gene is changed it does not produce any aspartoacylase or produces reduced levels of this enzyme. The amount of aspartoacylase produced depends on the type of gene alteration. Reduced production of aspartoacylase results in lower than normal amounts of this enzyme in the brain and nervous system. Aspartoacylase is responsible for breaking down a substance called N-acetylaspartic acid (NAA). When the body produces decreased levels of aspartoacylase, a build-up of NAA results. This results in the destruction of the white matter of the brain and nervous system and causes the symptoms of Canavan disease.

Parents who have a child with Canavan disease are called carriers, since they each possess one changed ASPA gene and one unchanged ASPA gene. Carriers usually do not have any symptoms since they have one unchanged gene that can produce enough aspartoacylase to prevent the build-up of NAA. Each child born to parents who are both carriers for Canavan disease, has a 25% chance of having Canavan disease, a 50% chance of being a carrier and a 25% chance of being neither a carrier nor affected with Canavan disease.

Demographics

Although Canavan disease is found in people of all ethnicities, it is most common in Ashkenazi Jewish individuals. Approximately one in 40 Ashkenazi Jewish individuals are carriers for Canavan disease and approximately one in 6,400 Ashkenazi Jewish people are born with Canavan disease.

Signs and symptoms

Most infants with Canavan disease appear normal for the first month of life. The onset of symptoms, such as a lack of head control and poor muscle tone, usually begins by two to three months of age, although some may have an onset of the disease in later childhood. Children with Canavan disease usually experience sleep disturbances, irritability, and swallowing and feeding difficulties after the first or second year of life. In many cases, irritability resolves by the third year. As the child with Canavan disease grows older there is a deterioration of mental and physical functioning. The speed at which this deterioration occurs will vary for each affected person. Children with Canavan disease are mentally retarded and most will never be able to sit, stand, walk or talk, although they may learn to laugh and smile and reach for objects. People with Canavan disease have increasing difficulties in controlling their muscles. Initially they have poor muscle tone but eventually their muscles become stiff and difficult to move and may exhibit spasms. Canavan disease can cause vision problems and some people with Canavan disease may eventually become blind. People with Canavan disease typically have disproportionately large heads and may experience seizures.

Diagnosis

Diagnostic testing

Canavan disease should be suspected in a person with a large head who has poor muscle control, a lack of head control and a destruction of the white matter of the brain, which can be detected through a computed tomography (CT) scan or magnetic resonance imaging (MRI). A diagnosis of Canavan disease can usually be confirmed by measuring the amount of NAA in a urine sample since a person with Canavan disease typically has greater than five to ten times the normal amount of NAA in their urine. Canavan disease can be less accurately diagnosed by measuring the amount of aspartocylase enzyme present in a sample of skin cells.

Once a biochemical diagnosis of Canavan disease is made, **DNA** testing may be recommended. Detection of an ASPA gene alteration in a person with Canavan disease can confirm an uncertain diagnosis and help facilitate prenatal diagnosis and carrier testing of relatives. Although there are a number of different ASPA gene changes responsible for Canavan disease, clinical laboratories typically test for only two to three common gene changes. Two of the ASPA gene changes are common in Ashkenazi Jews with Canavan disease and the other ASPA gene change is common in those of other ethnic backgrounds. Testing for other types of changes in the ASPA gene is only done on a research basis.

Carrier testing

DNA testing is the only means of identifying carriers of Canavan disease. If possible, DNA testing should be first performed on the affected family member. If a change in the ASPA gene is detected, then carrier testing can be performed in relatives such as siblings, with an accuracy of greater than 99%. If the affected relative does not possess a detectable ASPA gene change, then carrier testing will be inaccurate and should not be performed. If DNA testing of the affected relative cannot be performed, carrier testing of family members can still be performed but will be less accurate. Carrier testing for the three common ASPA **gene mutations** identifies approximately 97–99% of Ashkenazi Jewish carriers and 40–55% of carriers from other ethnic backgrounds.

Carrier testing of individuals without a family history of Canavan disease is only recommended for people of Ashkenazi Jewish background since they have a higher risk of being carriers. As of 1998, both the American College of Obstetricians and Gynecologists and the American College of Medical Genetics recommend that DNA testing for Canavan disease be offered to all Ashkenazi Jewish couples who are planning children or who are currently pregnant. If only one member of the couple is of Ashkenazi Jewish background than testing of the Jewish partner should be performed first. If the Jewish partner is a carrier, than testing of the non-Jewish partner is recommended.

Prenatal testing

Prenatal testing through chorionic villus sampling (CVS) and **amniocentesis** is available to parents who are both carriers for Canavan disease. If both parents possess an ASPA gene change, which is identified through DNA testing, then DNA testing of their baby can be performed. Some parents are known to be carriers for Canavan disease since they already have a child with Canavan disease, yet they do not possess ASPA gene changes that are detectable through DNA testing. Prenatal diagnosis can be performed in these cases by measuring the amount of NAA in the amniotic fluid obtained from an amniocentesis. This type of prenatal testing is less accurate than DNA testing and can lead to misdiagnoses.

KEY TERMS

Amniocentesis—A procedure performed at 16-18 weeks of pregnancy in which a needle is inserted through a woman's abdomen into her uterus to draw out a small sample of the amniotic fluid from around the baby. Either the fluid itself or cells from the fluid can be used for a variety of tests to obtain information about genetic disorders and other medical conditions in the fetus.

Amniotic fluid—The fluid which surrounds a developing baby during pregnancy.

Amniotic sac—Contains the fetus which is surrounded by amniotic fluid.

Biochemical testing—Measuring the amount or activity of a particular enzyme or protein in a sample of blood or urine or other tissue from the body.

Carrier—A person who possesses a gene for an abnormal trait without showing signs of the disorder. The person may pass the abnormal gene on to offspring.

Chorionic villus sampling (CVS)—A procedure used for prenatal diagnosis at 10-12 weeks gestation. Under ultrasound guidance a needle is inserted either through the mother's vagina or abdominal wall and a sample of cells is collected from around the early embryo. These cells are then tested for chromosome abnormalities or other genetic diseases.

Chromosome—A microscopic thread-like structure found within each cell of the body and consists of a complex of proteins and DNA. Humans have 46 chromosomes arranged into 23 pairs. Changes in either the total number of chromosomes or their shape and size (structure) may lead to physical or mental abnormalities.

Deoxyribonucleic acid (DNA)—The genetic material in cells that holds the inherited instructions for growth, development, and cellular functioning.

DNA testing—Analysis of DNA (the genetic component of cells) in order to determine changes in genes that may indicate a specific disorder.

Enzyme—A protein that catalyzes a biochemical reaction or change without changing its own structure or function.

Gene—A building block of inheritance, which contains the instructions for the production of a particular protein, and is made up of a molecular sequence found on a section of DNA. Each gene is found on a precise location on a chromosome.

Poor muscle tone—Muscles that are weak and floppy.

Prenatal testing—Testing for a disease such as a genetic condition in an unborn baby.

Protein—Important building blocks of the body, composed of amino acids, involved in the formation of body structures and controlling the basic functions of the human body.

White matter—A substance found in the brain and nervous system that protects nerves and allows messages to be sent to and from the brain to the various parts of the body.

Treatment and management

There is no cure for Canavan disease and treatment largely involves the management of symptoms. Seizures and irritability can often be controlled through medication. Children with loss of head control will often benefit from the use of modified seats that can provide full head support. When feeding and swallowing becomes difficult, liquid diets and/or feeding tubes become necessary. Feeding tubes are either inserted through the nose (nasogastric tube) or through a permanent incision in the stomach (gastrostomy). Patients with a later onset and slower progression of the disease may benefit from special education programs and physical therapy. Research trials of **gene therapy** are ongoing and involve the transfer of an unchanged ASPA gene into the brain cells of a patient. The goal of gene therapy is to restore normal amounts of aspartoclylase in the brain and nervous system and prevent the build-up of NAA and the symptoms of Canavan disease. The initial results of these early clinical trials have been somewhat promising but it will take time for gene therapy to become a viable treatment for Canavan disease.

Prognosis

The life span and progression of Canavan disease is variable and may be partially dependent on the type of medical care provided and other genetic risk factors. Most people with Canavan disease live into their teens although some die in infancy or survive into their 20s and 30s. There can be a high degree of variability even within families; some families report having one child die in infancy and another die in adulthood. Although different ASPA gene changes are associated with the production of different amounts of enzyme, the severity of the disease does not appear to be related to the type of ASPA gene change. It is, therefore, impossible to predict the life span of a particular individual with Canavan disease.

Resources

BOOKS

Scriver, C. R., et al., eds. *The Metabolic and Molecular Basis of Inherited Disease*. New York: The McGraw Hill Companies, 1995.

PERIODICALS

ACOG committee opinion. "Screening for canavan disease." Number 212, November 1998. Committee on Genetics. American College of Obstetricians and Gynecologists. *International Journal of Gynaecology and Obstetrics* 65, no. 1 (April 1999): 91–92.

Besley, G. T. N., et al. "Prenatal Diagnosis of Canavan Disease–Problems and Dilemmas." *Journal of Inherited Metabolic Disease* 22, no. 3 (May 1999): 263–66.

Matalon, Reuben, and Kimberlee Michals-Matalon. "Chemistry and Molecular Biology of Canavan Disease." *Neurochemical Research* 24, no. 4 (April 1999): 507–13.

Matalon, Reuben, and Kimberlee Michals-Matalon. "Recent Advances in Canavan Disease." *Advances In Pediatrics* 46 (1999): 493–506.

Matalon, Reuben, Kimberlee Michals-Matalon, and Rajinder Kaul. "Canavan Disease." *Handbook of Clinical Neurology* 22, no. 66 (1999): 661–69.

Traeger, Evelyn, and Isabelle Rapin. "The clinical course of Canavan disease." *Pediatric Neurology* 18, no. 3 (1999): 207–12.

ORGANIZATIONS

Canavan Foundation. 320 Central Park West, Suite 19D, New York, NY 10025. (212) 877-3945.

Canavan Research Foundation. Fairwood Professional Building, New Fairwood, CT 06812. (203) 746-2436. canavan_research@hotmail.com. <http://www.canavan.org>.

National Foundation for Jewish Genetic Diseases, Inc. 250 Park Ave., Suite 1000, New York, NY 10017. (212) 371-1030. <http://www.nfjgd.org>.

National Tay-Sachs and Allied Diseases Association. 2001 Beacon St., Suite 204, Brighton, MA 02135. (800) 906-8723. ntasd-Boston@worldnet.att.net. <http://www.ntsad.org>.

WEBSITES

American College of Medical Genetics. Position Statement on Carrier Testing for Canavan Disease. FASEB. <http://www.faseb.org/genetics/acmg/pol-31.htm>. (January 1998)

Matalon, Reuben. "Canavan disease." *GeneClinics*. <http://www.geneclinics.org/profiles/canavan/details.html?>. (20 July 1999).

Matalon, Reuben and Kimberlee Michals-Matalon. "Spongy Degeneration of the Brain, Canavan Disease: Biochemical and Molecular Findings." *Frontiers in Biosience*. <http://www.bioscience.org/2000/v5/d/matalon/fulltext.htm>. (March 2000)

McKusick, Victor A. "Canavan disease." *OMIM—Online Mendelian Inheritance in Man*. <http://www.ncbi.nlm.nih.gov/htbin-post/Omim/dispmim?271900>. (December 8, 1999).

Lisa Maria Andres, MS, CGC

Canavan-VanBogaert-Bertrand disease *see* Canavan disease

Cancer

Definition

Cancer is not just one disease, but a large group of diseases characterized by uncontrolled and abnormal growth of the cells in the human body and the ability of these cells to spread to distant sites (metastasis). If the spread is not controlled, cancer can result in death.

Description

Cancer, by definition, is a disease of the genes. Genes are formed from **deoxyribonucleic acid (DNA)** and located on chromosomes. They carry the hereditary instructions for the cell to make the proteins required for many body functions. Proteins are special chemical compounds that mostly contain carbon, hydrogen, oxygen, and nitrogen and that are required by our bodies to carry out all the processes that allow us to breathe, think, move, etc.

Throughout people's lives, the cells in their bodies are growing, dividing, and replacing themselves. Many genes produce proteins that are involved in controlling the processes of cell growth and division. A change (mutation) occurring in the DNA molecules can disrupt the genes and produce faulty proteins and cells. Abnormal cells can start dividing uncontrollably, eventually forming a new growth known as a "tumor" or "neoplasm" (medical term for cancer meaning "new growth"). In a healthy individual, the immune system can recognize the neoplastic cells and destroy them before they get a chance to divide. However, some abnormal cells may escape immune detection and survive to become cancerous.

Tumors are of two types, benign or malignant. A benign tumor is slow growing and does not spread or invade surrounding tissue. Once the tumor is removed, it will not usually start growing again. A malignant tumor, on the other hand, invades surrounding tissue and can spread to other parts of the body, often very distant from the location of the first tumor. Malignant tumors can be removed, but if the cancer cells have spread too much, the cancer becomes very difficult, if not impossible, to treat.

Most cancers are caused by changes in the cell's DNA that result from exposure to a harmful environment. Environmental factors responsible for causing the initial mutation in the DNA are called carcinogens. Other factors can cause cancer as well. For example, certain hormones have been shown to have an effect on the growth or control of a particular cell line. Hormones are substances made by one organ and passed through the bloodstream to affect the function of other cells in another organ.

While there is scientific evidence that both environmental and genetic factors play a role in most cancers, only 5-10% of all cancers are classified as hereditary. This means that a faulty **gene** that may cause cancer is passed from parent to child. This results in a greater risk for that type of cancer in the offspring of the family. However, if someone has a cancer-causing gene, this doesn't mean they will automatically get cancer. Rather, this person is thought to be "predisposed" to a type of cancer, or more likely to get this cancer when compared to the general population. Various cancers are known to have a hereditary component in some cases. A few examples are **breast cancer**, colon cancer, **ovarian cancer**, skin cancer and **prostate cancer**.

Aside from genes, certain physiological traits that are inherited can contribute to cancers as well. For example, fair skin makes a person more likely to develop skin cancer, but only if they also have prolonged exposure to intensive sunlight.

There are several different types of cancers. Some of the most common types include:

- *Carcinomas* These cancers arise in the epithelium (the layers of cells covering the body's surface and lining the internal organs and various glands). About 80% of human cancers fall into this category. Carcinomas can be subdivided into two subtypes: adenocarcinomas and squamous cell carcinomas. Adenocarcinomas are cancers that develop in an organ or a gland, while squamous cell carcinomas refer to cancers that originate in the skin.

- *Melanomas* This form also originates in the skin, usually in the pigment cells (melanocytes).

- *Sarcomas* These are cancers of the supporting tissues of the body, such as bone, muscle, cartilage, and fat.

- *Leukemias* Cancers of the blood or blood-forming organs.

- *Lymphomas* This type affects the lymphatic system, a network of vessels and nodes that acts as a filter in the body. It distributes nutrients to blood and tissue and prevents bacteria and other foreign substances from entering the bloodstream.

- *Gliomas* Cancers of the nerve tissue.

The most common cancers are skin cancer, lung cancer, colon and rectal (colorectal) cancer, breast cancer (in women), and prostate cancer (in men). In addition, cancer of the kidneys, ovaries, uterus, pancreas, bladder, and blood and lymph node cancer (leukemias and lymphomas) are also included among the 12 major cancers that affect most Americans.

Genetic profile

Three classes of genes are believed to play roles in the development of cancer. These are:

- Proto-oncogenes. These genes encourage and promote the normal growth and division of cells. When they are defective, they become oncogenes. Oncogenes are overactive proto-oncogenes and they cause excessive cell multiplication that can lead to tumors.

- Tumor suppressor genes. These act as brakes on cell growth. They prevent cells from multiplying uncontrollably. If these genes are defective, there is no control over cell growth and tumors can result.

- DNA repair genes. These genes ensure that each strand of DNA is correctly copied during cell division. When these genes do not function properly, the replicated DNA is likely to have mistakes. This causes defects in other genes and can also lead to tumor formation.

As stated above, approximately 5-10% of cancers have a hereditary component. In these cancers, a child does not inherit cancer from his parents. Rather, he inherits a predisposition to cancer. For example, he may inherit a faulty tumor suppressor gene. This gene is not able to control cell growth but the corresponding gene inherited from the other parent is still functional. Cell growth is then under control. However, as this child grows up, radiation, pollution, or any other harmful environmental factor could change the healthy gene, making it abnormal as well. When both of these tumor suppressor genes are not functioning, a tumor is most likely to develop. Defects in proto-oncogenes and DNA repair genes can be inherited as well, leaving a person more vulnerable to cancer than the general population.

Additionally, some cancers seem to be familial. In these cancers, there is not a specific gene that is responsible for the clustering of cancer in a family. However, a particular type of cancer may be seen more often than expected. It is suggested that this is due to a combination of genetic and environmental factors.

Demographics

One out of every four Americans will die from cancer. It is the second leading cause of death in this country, surpassed only by heart disease. Over 1.2 million new cases of cancer are diagnosed every year. The National Cancer Institute estimated that approximately 8.4 million Americans alive in 2001 had a history of cancer. Some of these people had been cured of their cancer while others were still affected with the disease and were undergoing treatment.

Anyone is at risk for developing cancer. Since the occurrence of cancer increases as a person ages, most of the cases are seen in adults who are middle-aged or older. Nearly 80% of cancers are diagnosed in people who are 55 years of age and older.

"Lifetime risk" is the term that cancer researchers use to refer to the probability that an individual will develop cancer over the course of their lifetime. In the United States, men have a one in two lifetime risk of developing cancer, and for women the risk is one in three. Overall, African-Americans are more likely to develop cancer than caucasians. They are also 33% more likely to die of cancer than caucasians.

The major risk factors for cancer are: tobacco, alcohol, diet, sexual and reproductive behavior, infectious agents, family history, occupation, environment, and pollution.

Tobacco

Eighty to ninety percent of the lung cancer cases occur in smokers. Smoking has also been shown to be a contributory factor in cancers of the mouth, pharynx, larynx, esophagus, pancreas, uterine cervix, kidney, and bladder. Smoking accounts for at least 30% of all cancer deaths. Recently, scientists have also shown that second-hand smoke (or passive smoking) can increase one's risk of developing cancer.

Alcohol

Excessive consumption of alcohol is a risk factor in some cancers, such as liver cancer and breast cancer. Alcohol, in combination with tobacco, significantly increases the chances that an individual will develop mouth, pharynx, larynx, and esophageal cancers. The combined effect of tobacco and alcohol is greater than the sum of their individual effects.

Diet and physical activity

One-third of all cancer deaths are due to a poor adult diet. High-fat diets have been associated with cancers of the colon and rectum, prostate, endometrium, and possibly breast. Consumption of meat, especially red meat, has been associated with increased cancer at various sites, such as the colon and prostate. Additionally, a high calorie diet and low level of physical activity can lead to obesity. This increases the risk for cancer at various sites including the breast, colon and rectum, prostate, kidney, and endometrium.

Sexual and reproductive behavior

The human papilloma virus, which is a sexually transmitted disease, has been shown to cause cancer of the cervix. Having many sexual partners and becoming sexually active early has been shown to increase a woman's chances of contracting this disease and, therefore, developing cervical cancer. In addition, it has also been shown that women who do not bear any children or those who become pregnant late in life have an increased risk for both ovarian and breast cancer.

Hormone replacement therapy

As women go through menopause, a doctor may recommend hormone replacement therapy. This involves taking female hormones (called estrogen and progesterone) to control certain symptoms that occur during this time of a woman's life, such as hot flashes and vaginal dryness. Taking estrogen alone can increase the risk for uterine cancer. However, progesterone is often prescribed at the same time to counteract the cancerous effects of estrogen. There is a questionable relationship between hormone replacement therapy and breast cancer as well. This relationship is not fully understood.

Family history

Some types of cancers tend to occur more frequently among members of a family. In most cases, this happens by chance or due to common family habits such as cigarette smoking or excessive sun exposure. However, this can also be due to a genetic predisposition that is passed from generation to generation. For example, if a certain gene called BRCA1 is defective in a given family, members of that family may have an increased risk to develop breast, colon, ovarian and prostate cancer. Other defective genes have been identified that can make a person susceptible to various types of cancer. Therefore, inheriting particular genes can increase a person's chance to develop cancer.

Childhood cancers associated with congenital syndromes or malformations

Syndrome or Anomaly	Tumor
Aniridia	Wilms tumor
Hemihypertrophy	Wilms tumor, hepatoblastoma, adrenocortical carcinoma
Genito-urinary abnormalities (including testicle maldescent)	Wilms tumor, Ewing sarcoma, nephroblastoma, testicular carcinoma
Beckwith-Wiedmann syndrome	Wilms tumor, neuroblastoma, adrenocortical carcinoma
Dysplastic naevus syndrome	Melanoma
Nevoid basal cell carcinoma syndrome	Basal cell carcinoma, medulloblastoma, rhabdomyosarcoma
Poland syndrome	Leukemia
Trisomy-21 (Down syndrome)	Leukemia, retinoblastoma
Bloom syndrome	Leukemia, gastrointestinal carcinoma
Severe combined immune deficiency disease	EBV-associated B-lymphocyte lymphoma/leukemia
Wiscott-Aldridge syndrome	EBV-associated B-lymphocyte lymphoma
Ataxia telangiectasia	EBV-associated B-lymphocyte lymphoma, gastric carcinoma
Retinoblastoma	Wilms tumor, osteosarcoma, Ewing sarcoma
Fanconi anemia	Leukemia, squamous cell carcinoma

Multiple endocrine neoplasia syndromes (MEN I, II, III)	Adenomas of islet cells, pituitary, parathyroids, and adrenal glands
	    Submucosal neuromas of the tongue, lips, eyelids
	Pheochromocytomas, medullary carcinoma of the thyroid,
	    malignant schwannoma, non-appendiceal carcinoid

Neurofibromatosis (von Recklinghausensyndrome)	Rhabdomyosarcoma, fibrosarcoma, pheochromocytomas, opticglioma, meningioma

Occupational hazards

There is strong evidence proving that occupational hazards account for 4% of all cancer deaths. For example, asbestos workers have an increased incidence of lung cancer. Similarly, bladder cancer is associated with dye, rubber and gas workers; skin and lung cancer with smelters, gold miners and arsenic workers; leukemia with glue and varnish workers; liver cancer with PVC manufacturers; and lung, bone and bone marrow cancer with radiologists and uranium miners.

Environment

High-frequency radiation has been shown to cause human cancer. Ultra-violet radiation from the sun accounts for a majority of melanoma. Other sources of radiation are x rays, radioactive substances, and rays that enter the Earth's atmosphere from outer space. Virtually any part of the body can be affected by these types of radiation, especially the bone marrow and the thyroid gland.

Additionally, being exposed to substances such as certain chemicals, metals, or pesticides can increase the risk of cancer. Asbestos is an example of a well-known carcinogen. It increases the risk for lung cancer. This risk is increased even further for a smoker who is exposed to asbestos over a period of time.

Signs and symptoms

Almost every tissue of the body can give rise to abnormal cells that cause cancer and each of these cancers is very different in symptoms and prognosis.

Cancer is also a progressive disease and goes through several stages. Each stage can produce a number of symptoms. Unfortunately, many types of cancer do not display any obvious symptoms or cause pain until the disease has progressed to an advanced stage. Early signs of cancer are often subtle and are easily mistaken for signs of other less-dangerous diseases.

Despite the fact that there are several hundred different types of cancers producing very different symptoms, the American Cancer Society (ACS) has established the following seven symptoms as possible warning signs of cancer:

- changes in the size, color, or shape of a wart or a mole

- a sore that does not heal

- persistent cough, hoarseness, or sore throat

- a lump or thickening in the breast or elsewhere

- unusual bleeding or discharge

- chronic indigestion or difficulty in swallowing

- any change in bowel or bladder habits

Many other diseases can produce similar symptoms. However, it is important to have these symptoms checked as soon as possible, especially if they do not stop. The earlier a cancer is diagnosed and treated, the better the chance of a cure. Many cancers, such as breast cancer, may not have any early symptoms. Therefore, it is important to undergo routine screening tests, such as breast self-exams and mammograms.

Diagnosis

If a person has symptoms of cancer, the doctor will begin with a complete medical history and a thorough physical examination. Different parts of the body will be examined to identify any variations from the normal

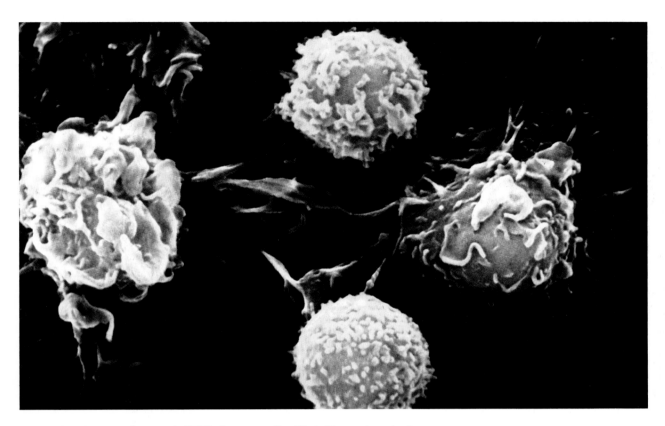

A scanning electron micrograph (SEM) of cancer cells. *(Photo Researchers, Inc.)*

size, feel and texture of the organ or tissue. Additionally, the doctor may order various other tests.

Laboratory tests on blood and urine are often used to obtain information about a person's health. If cancer is suspected, a special test can be done that measures the amount of certain substances, called tumor markers, in the blood, urine, or particular tissues. These proteins are released from some types of cancer cells. Thus, the levels of these substances may be abnormal when certain cancers are present. However, laboratory tests alone cannot be used to make a definitive diagnosis of cancer. Blood tests are generally more useful in monitoring the effectiveness of the treatment or in following the course of the disease and detecting any signs of recurrence.

The doctor may also look for tumors by examining pictures of areas inside the body. The most common way to obtain these images is by using x rays. Other techniques used to obtain pictures of the inside of the body include computed tomography scanning (CT scan), magnetic resonance imaging (MRI), and ultrasonography.

The most definitive diagnostic test is the biopsy. In this technique, a piece of tissue is surgically removed for examination under a microscope. A biopsy provides infor-

mation about the cellular nature of the abnormality, the stage it has reached, the aggressiveness of the cancer, and the extent of its spread. Further analysis of the tissue obtained by biopsy defines the cause of the abnormality. Since a biopsy provides the most accurate analysis, it is considered the gold standard of diagnostic tests for cancer.

Regular screening examinations conducted by healthcare professionals can result in the early detection of various types of cancer. If detected at an early stage, treatment is more likely to be successful. For example, the American Cancer Society recommends an annual mammogram (x ray of the breast) for women over the age of 40 to screen for breast cancer. It also recommends a sigmoidoscopy (procedure using a thin, lighted tube to view the inside of the colon) every five years for people over the age of 50. This technique can check for colorectal cancer. Self-examinations for cancers of the breast, testes, mouth and skin can also help in detecting tumors.

Recent progress in molecular biology and cancer genetics have led to the development of several tests designed to assess one's risk of developing certain types of cancer. This **genetic testing** involves looking closely at certain genes that have been linked to particular cancers. If these genes are abnormal, a person's risk for certain types of cancer increases. At present, there are many limitations to genetic testing. The tests may be uninformative and they are useful to a very small number of people. Additionally, there are concerns about insurance coverage and employment discrimination for someone who has an increased risk for cancer. These tests are reserved only for very specific people. A hereditary cancer clinic can help to assess who may benefit from this type of testing.

Treatment and management

The aim of cancer treatment is to remove all or as much of the tumor as possible and to prevent the metastasis of the primary tumor. While devising a treatment plan for cancer, the likelihood of curing the cancer must be weighed against the side effects of the treatment. For example, if the cancer is very aggressive and a cure is not possible, then the treatment should be aimed at relieving the symptoms and controlling the cancer for as long as possible.

Cancer treatment can take many different forms and it is always tailored to the individual patient. The decision on which type of treatment to use depends on the type and location of cancer and the extent to which it has already spread. The doctor will also consider the patient's age, sex, general health status, and personal treatment preferences. Treatment can be local, meaning that it seeks to destroy cancer cells in the tumor and the surrounding area. It can also be systemic, meaning that the treatment drugs will travel through the bloodstream and reach cancer cells all over the body. Surgery and radiation are local treatments. Chemotherapy, immunotherapy, and hormone therapy are examples of systemic treatments.

Surgery

Surgery can be used for many purposes in cancer therapy.

- Treatment surgery: This involves removal of the tumor to cure the disease. It is typically performed when the cancer is localized to a discrete area. Along with the cancer, some of the surrounding tissue may also be removed to ensure that no cancer cells remain in the area. Since cancer usually spreads via the lymphatic system, lymph nodes that are near the tumor site may be examined and removed as well.

- Preventive surgery: Preventive or prophylactic surgery involves removal of an abnormal area that is likely to become malignant over time. For example, 40% of people with a colon disease called ulcerative colitis ultimately die of colon cancer. Rather than live with the fear of developing colon cancer, these people may

choose to have their colons removed in order to reduce their risk of cancer.

- Diagnostic purposes: The most definitive tool for diagnosing cancer is a biopsy. Sometimes a biopsy can be performed by inserting a needle through the skin. In other cases, the only way to obtain a tissue sample for biopsy is by performing a surgical operation.

- Cytoreductive surgery: This is a procedure in which the doctor removes as much of the cancer as possible. He then treats the remaining cancer cells with radiation therapy, chemotherapy, or both.

- Palliative surgery: This type of surgery is aimed at relieving cancer symptoms or slowing the progression of disease. It is not designed to cure the cancer. For example, if the tumor is very large or has spread to many places in the body, removing the entire tumor may not be an option. However, by decreasing the size of the tumor, pain may be alleviated. This is known as "debulking surgery."

Radiation therapy

Radiation uses high-energy rays to kill cancer cells. This treatment may be used instead of surgery. It also may be used before surgery to shrink a tumor or after surgery to destroy any remaining cancer cells.

Radiation can be either external or internal. In the external form, the radiation comes from a machine that aims the rays at the tumor. In internal radiation (also known as brachytherapy), radioactive material is sealed in needles, seeds, or wires and placed directly in or near the tumor. Radiation may lead to various side effects, such as fatigue, hair loss, and a susceptibility to infections. However, these side effects can usually be controlled.

Chemotherapy

Chemotherapy is the use of drugs to kill cancer cells. The anticancer drugs are usually released into the entire body (systemic therapy) so as to destroy the hard-to-detect cancer cells that have spread and are circulating in the body. Chemotherapy is based on the principle that cancer cells are affected more dramatically than the normal cells because they are rapidly dividing. Chemotherapeutic drugs can be injected into a vein, the muscle, or the skin or they may be taken by mouth.

When chemotherapy is used before surgery, it is known as primary chemotherapy or "neoadjuvant chemotherapy." Its purpose is usually to reduce the size of the tumor. The more common use of chemotherapy is in "adjuvant therapy." In this form of treatment, chemotherapy is given after surgery to destroy any remaining cancer cells and to help prevent cancer from recurring. Chemotherapy can also be used in conjunction with radiation therapy.

The side effects of chemotherapy vary but can include susceptibility to infections, fatigue, poor appetite, weight loss, nausea, diarrhea, and hair loss. Decreased fertility can be a long-term side effect in some patients who undergo chemotherapy.

Immunotherapy

Immunotherapy, also called biological therapy, is the use of treatments that promote or support the body's immune system response to cancer. The side effects of this immunotherapy are variable but include flu-like symptoms, weakness, loss of appetite, and skin rash. These symptoms will subside after the treatment is completed.

Bone marrow failure is a complication of chemotherapy. When high dose chemotherapy is used, this failure is anticipated. Bone marrow transplantation (BMT) or peripheral stem cell transplantation (PSCT) are techniques used to treat this complication. Both techniques provide healthy stem cells for the patient. Stem cells are immature cells that mature into blood cells. They can replace the patient's own stem cells that have been damaged or destroyed by chemotherapy or radiation. It allows a patient to undergo very aggressive treatment for their cancer. Patients who receive BMT or PSCT have an increased risk of infection, bleeding, and other side effects due to the chemotherapy and radiation. Graft-versus-host disease may also occur as well. This complication occurs when the donated marrow reacts against a patient's tissues. It can occur any time after the transplant. Drugs may be given to reduce the risk of graft-versus-host disease and to treat the problem if it occurs.

Hormone therapy

Hormone therapy is used to fight certain cancers that depend on hormones for their growth. Drugs can be used to block the production of hormones or change the way they work. Additionally, organs that produce hormones may be removed. As a result of this therapy, the growth of the tumor slows and survival may be extended for several months or years.

Alternative and complementary therapies

There are certain cancer therapies that have not been scientifically tested and approved. If these unproven treatments are used instead of the standard therapy, this is known as "alternative therapy." If used along with standard therapy, this is known as "complementary therapy." The use of alternative therapies must be carefully considered because some of these unproven treatments may have life-threatening side effects. Additionally, if someone uses alternative therapy, they may lose the opportunity to benefit from the standard, proven therapy. However, some complementary therapies may help to relieve symptoms of cancer, decrease the magnitude of side effects from treatment, or improve a patient's sense of well-being. The American Cancer Society recommends that anyone considering alternative or complementary therapy consult a health care team.

Prevention

According to experts from leading universities in the United States, a person can reduce the chances of getting cancer by following these guidelines:

- eating plenty of fruits and vegetables
- exercising vigorously for at least 20 minutes every day
- avoiding excessive weight gain
- avoiding tobacco (including second hand smoke)
- decreasing or avoiding consumption of animal fats and red meats
- avoiding excessive amounts of alcohol
- avoiding the midday sun (between 11 a.m. and 3 p.m.) when the sun's rays are the strongest
- avoiding risky sexual practices
- avoiding known carcinogens in the environment or work place

Certain drugs that are currently being used for treatment can also be suitable for prevention. For example, the drug tamoxifen, also called Nolvadex, has been very effective against breast cancer and is now thought to be helpful in the prevention of breast cancer. Similarly, retinoids derived from vitamin A are being tested for their ability to slow the progression or prevent head and neck cancers.

Prognosis

Most cancers are curable if detected and treated at their early stages. A cancer patient's prognosis is affected by many factors, particularly the type of cancer the patient has, the stage of the cancer, the extent to which it has metastasized and the aggressiveness of the cancer. In addition, the patient's age, general health status and the effectiveness of the treatment being pursued are also important factors.

To help predict the future outcome of cancer and the likelihood of recovery from the disease, five-year survival rates are used. The five-year survival rate for all

KEY TERMS

Adenocarcinoma—A type of cancer which is in a gland-like form.

Adenomatous—Derived from glandular structures.

Aflatoxin—A substance produced by molds that grow on rice and peanuts. Exposure to aflatoxin is thought to explain the high rates of primary liver cancer in Africa and parts of Asia.

Alpha-fetoprotein (AFP)—A chemical substance produced by the fetus and found in the fetal circulation. AFP is also found in abnormally high concentrations in most patients with primary liver cancer.

Alteration—Change or mutation in a gene, specifically in the DNA that codes for the gene.

Alteration—Change or mutation in a gene, specifically in the DNA that codes for the gene.

Anti-androgen drugs—Drugs that block the activity of the male hormone.

Astrocytoma—Tumor of the central nervous system derived from astrocytes.

Barium—A chemical put into a solution and swallowed to help with outlining the gastrointestinal system during an x-ray study.

Benign—A non-cancerous tumor that does not spread and is not life-threatening.

Benign—A non-cancerous tumor that does not spread and is not life-threatening.

Benign—A non-cancerous tumor that does not spread and is not life-threatening.

Benign prostatic hyperplasia (BPH)—A noncancerous condition of the prostate that causes growth of the prostate tissue, thus enlarging the prostate and blocking urination.

Bilateral breast cancer—Cancer of both breasts, caused by two separate cancer processes.

Bile—A substance produced by the liver, and concentrated and stored in the gallbladder. Bile contains a number of different substances, including bile salts, cholesterol, and bilirubin.

Biopsy—The surgical removal and microscopic examination of living tissue for diagnostic purposes.

Bone marrow—A spongy tissue located in the hollow centers of certain bones, such as the skull and hip bones. Bone marrow is the site of blood cell generation.

BRCA2—Gene, when altered, known to cause increased risks of breast, ovarian and, possibly, pancreatic cancer.

Breast biopsy—Small sample of tissue taken from the breast and studied, to diagnose and determine the exact type of breast cancer.

Breast self-exam (BSE)—Examination by an individual of their own breasts.

CA-125 (Carbohydrate antigen 125)—A protein that is sometimes high when ovarian cancer is present. A blood sample can determine the level of CA-125 present.

Cancer—A disease caused by uncontrolled growth of the body's cells.

Carcinogen—Any substance capable of causing cancer by mutating the cell's DNA.

Cationic trypsinogen gene—Gene known to cause hereditary pancreatitis when significantly altered.

Central nervous system—In humans, the central nervous system is composed of the brain, the cranial nerves and the spinal cord. It is responsible for the coordination and control of all body activities.

CDKN2A or p16—Gene, when altered, known to cause Familial Atypical Multiple Mole Melanoma (FAMMM) syndrome and possibly increased pancreatic cancer risk.

Chemotherapy—Treatment of cancer with synthetic drugs that destroy the tumor either by inhibiting the growth of the cancerous cells or by killing the cancer cells.

Chronic atrophic gastritis—Irritation and break down of the stomach wall over a period of time.

Cirrhosis—A chronic degenerative disease of the liver, in which normal cells are replaced by fibrous tissue. Cirrhosis is a major risk factor for the later development of liver cancer.

Clinical breast exam (CBE)—Examination of the breasts, performed by a physician or nurse.

Computed tomography—An imaging procedure that produces a three-dimensional picture of organs or structures inside the body, such as the brain.

Computed tomography (CT) scan—An imaging procedure that produces a three-dimensional picture of organs or structures inside the body, such as the brain.

Desmoid tumor—Benign, firm mass of scar-like connective tissue.

Distal—Away from the point of origin.

(continued)

Dominant inheritance—A type of genetic inheritance pattern that results in one form of a gene being dominant over other forms. Therefore, the dominant allele can express itself and cause disease, even if only one copy is present.

Duct—Tube-like structure that carries secretions from glands.

Duodenum—Portion of the small intestine nearest the stomach; the first of three parts of the small intestine.

E-Cadherin/CDH1—A gene involved in cell-to-cell connection. Alterations in this gene have been found in several families with increased rates of gastric cancer.

Endoscopic retrograde cholangiopancreatography (ERCP)—A method of viewing the pancreas by inserting a thin tube down the throat into the pancreatic and bile ducts, injection of dye and performing x rays.

Endoscopy—A slender, tubular optical instrument used as a viewing system for examining an inner part of the body and, with an attached instrument, for biopsy or surgery.

Ependymoma—Tumor of the central nervous system derived from cells that line the central canal of the spinal cord and the ventricles of the brain.

Epidermoid cyst—Benign, cystic tumor derived from epithelial cells.

Epithelium—The layer of cells that cover the open surfaces of the body such as the skin and mucous membranes.

Esophagus—The part of the digestive tract which connects the mouth and stomach; the food pipe.

Estrogen—A female sex hormone.

Exocrine pancreas—The secreting part of the pancreas.

Familial adenomatous polyposis (FAP)—Inherited syndrome causing large numbers of polyps and increased risk of colon cancer and other cancers.

Familial gastric cancer—Gastric cancer that occurs at a higher rate in some families.

Fecal occult blood test—Study of stool (feces) to identify loss of blood in the gastrointestinal system.

Fine needle aspiration (FNA)—Insertion of a thin needle through the skin to an area of sample tissue.

Gastric—Associated with the stomach.

Gastrointestinal (GI) system—Body system involved in digestion, the breaking down and use of food.

Gene—A building block of inheritance, which contains the instructions for the production of a particular protein, and is made up of a molecular sequence found on a section of DNA. Each gene is found on a precise location on a chromosome.

Genetic counselor—A health professional with advanced training in genetics and psychology who educates people about genetic conditions and testing.

Glioblastoma multiforme—Tumor of the central nervous system consisting of undifferentiated glial cells.

***Helicobacter pylori* (*H. pylori*)**—Bacterium that infects humans and may be associated with an increased risk of gastric cancer.

Hepatitis—A viral disease characterized by inflammation of the liver cells (hepatocytes). People infected with hepatitis B or hepatitis C virus are at an increased risk for developing liver cancer.

Hereditary non-polyposis colon cancer (HNPCC)—A genetic syndrome causing increased cancer risks, most notably colon cancer. Also called Lynch syndrome.

Hereditary non-polyposis colon cancer (HNPCC)—A genetic syndrome causing increased cancer risks, most notably colon cancer. Also called Lynch syndrome.

Hormone therapy—Treatment of cancer by changing the hormonal environment, such as testosterone and estrogen.

Immunotherapy—Treatment of cancer by stimulating the body's immune defense system.

Insulin—A hormone produced by the pancreas that is secreted into the bloodstream and regulates blood sugar levels.

Jaundice—Yellowing of the skin or eyes due to excess of bilirubin in the blood.

Laparoscopy—A diagnostic procedure in which a small incision is made in the abdomen and a slender, hollow, lighted instrument is passed through it. The doctor can view the ovaries more closely through the laparoscope, and if necessary, obtain tissue samples for biopsy.

Laparotomy—An operation in which the abdominal cavity is opened up.

(continued)

Li-Fraumeni syndrome—Inherited syndrome known to cause increased risk of different cancers, most notably sarcomas.

Lymph node—A bean-sized mass of tissue that is part of the immune system and is found in different areas of the body.

Magnetic resonance imaging (MRI)—A technique that employs magnetic fields and radio waves to create detailed images of internal body structures and organs, including the brain.

Malignant—A tumor growth that spreads to another part of the body, usually cancerous.

Mammogram—A procedure in which both breasts are compressed/flattened and exposed to low doses of x rays, in an attempt to visualize the inner breast tissue.

Maori—A native New Zealand ethnic group.

Medulloblastoma—Tumor of the central nervous system derived from undifferentiated cells of the primitive medullary tube.

Melanoma—Tumor, usually of the skin.

Metachronous—Occurring at separate time intervals.

Metastasis—The spreading of cancer from the original site to other locations in the body.

Metastatic cancer—A cancer that has spread to an organ or tissue from a primary cancer located elsewhere in the body.

Multifocal breast cancer—Multiple primary cancers in the same breast.

Mutation—A permanent change in the genetic material that may alter a trait or characteristic of an individual, or manifest as disease, and can be transmitted to offspring.

Nitrates/nitrites—Chemical compounds found in certain foods and water that, when consumed, may increase the risk of gastric cancer.

Osteoma—A benign bone tumor.

Palliative—Treatment done for relief of symptoms rather than a cure.

Pancreas—An organ located in the abdomen that secretes pancreatic juices for digestion and hormones for maintaining blood sugar levels.

Pancreatitis—Inflammation of the pancreas.

Pelvic examination—Physical examination performed by a physician, often associated with a Pap smear. The physician inserts his/her finger into a woman's vagina, attempting to feel the ovaries directly.

Pernicious anemia—A blood condition with decreased numbers of red blood cells related to poor vitamin B12 absorption.

Peutz-Jeghers syndrome (PJS)—Inherited syndrome causing polyps of the digestive tract and spots on the mouth as well as increased risk of cancer.

Polyp—A mass of tissue bulging out from the normal surface of a mucous membrane.

Primary cancer—The first or original cancer site, before any metastasis.

Prophylactic—Preventing disease.

Prostatectomy—The surgical removal of the prostate gland.

Proximal—Near the point of origin.

Radiation—High energy rays used in cancer treatment to kill or shrink cancer cells.

Radiation therapy—Treatment using high-energy radiation from x-ray machines, cobalt, radium, or other sources.

Rectum—The end portion of the intestine that leads to the anus.

Semen—A whitish, opaque fluid released at ejaculation that contains sperm.

Seminal vesicles—The pouches above the prostate that store semen.

Sore—An open wound or a bruise or lesion on the skin.

Staging—A method of describing the degree and location of cancer.

Stomach—An organ that holds and begins digestion of food.

Synchronous—Occurring simultaneously.

Testicles—Two egg-shaped glands that produce sperm and sex hormones.

Testosterone—Hormone produced in the testicles that is involved in male secondary sex characteristics.

Trans-rectal ultrasound—A procedure where a probe is placed in the rectum. High-frequency sound waves that cannot be heard by humans are sent out from the probe and reflected by the prostate. These sound waves produce a pattern of echoes that are then used by the computer to create sonograms or pictures of areas inside the body.

(continued)

KEY TERMS (CONTINUED)

Transvaginal ultrasound—A way to view the ovaries using sound waves. A probe is inserted into the vagina and the ovaries can be seen. Color doppler imaging measures the amount of blood flow, as tumors sometimes have high levels of blood flow.

Tumor—An abnormal growth of cells. Tumors may be benign (noncancerous) or malignant (cancerous).

Ultrasound—An imaging technique that uses sound waves to help visualize internal structures in the body.

Whipple procedure—Surgical removal of the pancreas and surrounding areas including a portion of the small intestine, the duodenum.

X ray—An image of the body made by the passing of radiation through the body.

X rays—High energy radiation used in high doses, either to diagnose or treat disease.

---

cancers combined is 59%. This means that 59% of people with cancer are expected to be alive five years after they are diagnosed. These people may be free of cancer or they may be undergoing treatment. It is important to note that while this statistic can give some information about the average survival of cancer patients in a given population, it cannot be used to predict individual prognosis. No two patients are exactly alike. For example, the five-year survival rate does not account for differences in detection methods, types of treatments, additional illnesses, and behaviors.

Resources

BOOKS

American Cancer Society. *Cancer Facts & Figures 2000.* American Cancer Society, 2000.

Buckman, Robert. *What You Really Need to Know about Cancer: A Comprehensive Guide for Patients and Their Families.* Johns Hopkins University Press, 1997.

Murphy, Gerald P. *Informed Decisions: The Complete Book of Cancer Diagnosis, Treatment and Recovery.* American Cancer Society, 1997.

PERIODICALS

Ruccione, Kathy. "Cancer and Genetics: What We Need to Know." *Journal of Pediatric Oncology Nursing* 16 (July 1999): 156-171.

"What You Need to Know about Cancer." *Scientific American* 275, no. 3 (September 1996).

ORGANIZATIONS

American Cancer Society. 1599 Clifton Rd. NE, Atlanta, GA 30329. (800) 227-2345. <http://www.cancer.org>.

American Foundation for Urologic Disease, Inc. 1128 North Charles St., Baltimore, MD 21201-5559. (410)468-1808. <http://www.afud.org>.

American Liver Foundation. 75 Maiden Lane, Suite 603, New York, NY 10038. (800) 465-4837 or (888) 443-7222. <http://www.liverfoundation.org>.

National Cancer Institute. Office of Communications, 31 Center Dr. MSC 2580, Bldg. 1 Room 10A16, Bethesda, MD 20892-2580. (800) 422-6237. <http://www.nci.nih.gov>.

National Familial Pancreas Tumor Registry. Johns Hopkins Hospital, Weinberg Building, Room 2242, 401 North Broadway, Baltimore, MD 21231-2410. (410) 955-9132. <http://www.path.jhu.edu/pancreas>.

University of Texas M.D. Anderson Cancer Center. 1515 Holcombe Blvd., Houston, TX 77030. (800) 392-1611. <http://www.mdanderson.org>.

WEBSITES

American Cancer Society. *Cancer Resource Center.* <http://www3.cancer.org/cancerinfo/>.

National Cancer Institute. *CancerNet.* <http://cancernet.nci.nih.gov>.

University of Pennsylvania Cancer Center. *Oncolink.* <http://cancer.med.upenn.edu>.

Mary E. Freivogel, MS

Cardiofaciocutaneous syndrome

Definition

Cardiofaciocutaneous syndrome is an extremely rare genetic condition present at birth characterized by mental retardation, slow growth, and abnormalities of the heart, face, skin, and hair. There is no cure for cardiofaciocutaneous syndrome. Treatment centers on the correction of heart abnormalities and strategies to improve the quality of life of the affected individual.

Description

Cardiofaciocutaneous syndrome was first identified and described in 1986 by J. F. Reynolds and colleagues at the Shodair Children's Hospital in Helena, Montana and at the University of Utah. These physicians identified and described eight children with a characteristic set of mental and physical changes including abnormal skin conditions, an unusual face, sparse and curly hair, heart defects, and mental retardation. These physicians named the syndrome based on the changes of the heart (cardio), face (facio), and skin (cutaneous). Since that time, physicians have used the descriptions originally put forth by Dr. Reynolds to identify other children with cardiofaciocutaneous syndrome.

Scientific research conducted over the past decade suggests that cardiofaciocutaneous syndrome is associated with a change in the genetic material. However, it is still not known precisely how this change in the genetic material alters growth and development in the womb to cause cardiofaciocutaneous syndrome.

Cardiofaciocutaneous syndrome can sometimes be confused with another genetic syndrome, **Noonan syndrome**. Children with Noonan syndrome have abnormalities in the same genetic material as those with cardiofaciocutaneous syndrome, and the two syndromes share some similar physical characteristics. Many scientists believe that the two diseases are different entities and should be regarded as separate conditions, while others believe that Noonan syndrome and cardiofaciocutaneous syndrome may be variations of the same disease.

Genetic profile

Recent research has shown that people with cardiofaciocutaneous syndrome have changes in a **gene** located on a region of human **chromosome** 12 (locus 12q24), but the precise gene and genetic alteration is unknown.

In almost all cases of cardiofaciocutaneous syndrome, there is no family history of the disease. These cases are thought to represent new genetic changes that occur randomly and with no apparent cause and are termed sporadic. While the cause of the genetic change is still unclear, some studies suggest that the age of the father might be important in the genesis of the disease. In 20 cases for which information was available, scientists noted that fathers of affected children tended to be older (average age of 39 years) when the child was conceived. Therefore, it is believed that a change in the genetic material of the father's sperm may occur as the man ages, and that he may, in turn, pass this genetic change to the child, resulting in cardiofaciocutaneous syndrome.

Only one abnormal gene in a gene pair is necessary to display the disease. This is an example of a dominant gene (i.e. the abnormal gene of the gene pair dominates over the normal gene, resulting in the syndrome).

Demographics

Cardiofaciocutaneous syndrome is an extremely rare condition. Because the syndrome is relatively new and only a small number of physicians have actual first-hand experience with the diagnosis of the syndrome, some children with the syndrome may not be diagnosed, particularly if they are living in areas where sophisticated medical care is not available. As a result, it is difficult to know how many children are affected by cardiofaciocutaneous syndrome. However, scientists estimate that less than 200 children worldwide are presently affected by this condition.

Because the syndrome is so rare, it is not known whether the disease is distributed equally among different geographic areas or whether different ethnic groups have higher incidences of the syndrome.

Signs and symptoms

Individuals with cardiofaciocutaneous syndrome have distinct malformations of the head and face. An unusually large head (macrocephaly), a prominent forehead, and abnormal narrowing of both sides of the forehead (bitemporal constriction) are typical. A short, upturned nose with a low nasal bridge and prominent external ears that are abnormally rotated toward the back of the head are also seen. In most cases, affected individuals have downward slanting eyelid folds, widely spaced eyes, drooping of the upper eyelids, inward deviation of the eyes, and other eye abnormalities. In addition to having unusually dry, brittle, curly scalp hair, affected individuals may lack eyebrows and eyelashes.

Individuals with cardiofaciocutaneous syndrome may also have a range of skin abnormalities, varying from areas of skin inflammation to unusually dry, thickened, scaly skin over the entire body. Most affected individuals also have congenital heart defects, particularly obstruction of the normal flow of blood from the right chamber of the heart to the lungs and/or an abnormal opening in the wall that separates two of the heart chambers.

In addition, most individuals with the disorder experience growth delays, mild to severe mental retardation, and abnormal delays in the acquisition of skills requiring the coordination of muscular and mental activity. Other abnormalities encountered in children with cardiofaciocutaneous syndrome include seizures, abnormal movements of the eye, poor muscle tone, and poor digestion. In some cases, additional abnormalities may be present.

Diagnosis

The diagnosis of cardiofaciocutaneous syndrome relies on physical exam by a physician familiar with the condition and by radiographic evaluation, such as the use of x rays or ultrasound to define abnormal or missing structures that are consistent with the criteria for the condition (as described above). Although a diagnosis may be made as a newborn, most often the features do not become fully evident until early childhood.

There is no laboratory blood test or commercially available genetic test that can be used to identify people with cardiofaciocutaneous syndrome. However, because the condition is so rare, advanced genetic analysis may be available as part of a research study to determine if changes in regions of chromosome 12 are present.

Cardiofaciocutaneous syndrome can be differentiated from Noonan syndrome by the presence of nervous system abnormalities, such as low muscle tone, seizures, and abnormal movements of the eye, as well as by typical changes in the hair and skin.

Treatment and management

There is no cure for cardiofaciocutaneous syndrome. The genetic change responsible for cardiofaciocutaneous syndrome is present in every cell of the body and, at the current time, there is no means of correcting this genetic abnormality.

Treatment of the syndrome is variable and centers on correcting the different manifestations of the condition. For children with heart defects, surgical repair is often necessary. This may take place shortly after birth if the heart abnormality is life threatening, but often physicians will prefer to attempt a repair once the child has grown older and the heart is more mature. For children who experience seizures, lifelong treatment with anti-seizure medications is often necessary. Oral or topical medications may also be used to treat the inflammatory skin conditions and provide some symptomatic and cosmetic relief.

During early development and progressing into young adulthood, children with cardiofaciocutaneous should be educated and trained in behavioral and mechanical methods to adapt to their disabilities. This program is usually initiated and overseen by a team of health care professionals including a pediatrician, physical therapist, and occupational therapist. A counselor specially trained to deal with issues of disabilities in children is often helpful is assessing problem areas and encouraging healthy development of self-esteem. Support groups and community organizations for people with cardiofaciocutaneous syndrome or other disabilities

---

KEY TERMS

Autosomal dominant—A pattern of genetic inheritance where only one abnormal gene is needed to display the trait or disease.

Bitemporal constriction—Abnormal narrowing of both sides of the forehead.

Macrocephaly—A head that is larger than normal.

Noonan syndrome—A genetic syndrome that possesses some characteristics similar to cardiofaciocutanous syndromes. It is unclear whether the two syndrome are different or two manifestations of the same disorder.

Sporadic—Isolated or appearing occasionally with no apparent pattern.

---

often prove useful to the affected individual and their families. Specially-equipped schools or enrichment programs should also be sought.

Children with cardiofaciocutaneous syndrome should be seen regularly by a team of health care professionals, including a pediatrician, medical geneticist, pediatric cardiologist, dermatologist, and neurologist. Consultation with a reconstructive surgeon may be of use if some of the physical abnormalities are particularly debilitating.

Prognosis

The prognosis of children with cardiofaciocutaneous syndrome depends on the severity of the symptoms and the extent to which appropriate treatments are available. In addition to the physical disabilities, the mental retardation and other nervous system effects can be severe. Since cardiofaciocutaneous syndrome was discovered relatively recently, very little is known regarding the level of functioning and the average life span of individuals affected with the condition.

Resources

BOOKS

Behrman, R. E., ed. *Nelson Textbook of Pediatrics.* Philadelphia: W.B. Saunders, 2000.

PERIODICALS

Grebe, T. A., and C. Clericuzio. "Cardiofaciocutaneous syndrome." *Australiasian Journal of Dermatology* 40 (May 1999): 111–13.

Neri, G., and J. M. Opitz. "Heterogeneity of cardio-facio-cutaneous syndrome." *American Journal of Medical Genetics* 95 (November 2000): 135–43.

ORGANIZATIONS

Cardio-Facio-Cutaneous Syndrome Foundation. 3962 Van Dyke St., White Bear Lake, MN 55110. <http://www.cfcfoundation.com>.

CardioFacioCutaneous Support Network. 157 Alder Ave., McKee City, NJ 08232. (609) 646-5606.

Cardiofaciocutaneous Syndrome Family Network. 183 Brown Rd., Vestal, NY 13850. (607) 772-9666. <http://www.cfcsyndrome.org>.

National Organization for Rare Disorders (NORD). PO Box 8923, New Fairfield, CT 06812-8923. (203) 746-6518 or (800) 999-6673. Fax: (203) 746-6481. <http://www.rarediseases.org>.

WEBSITES

"Cardiofaciocutaneous syndrome." *OMIM—Online Mendelian Inheritance in Man.* National Center for Biotechnology Information. <http://www3.ncbi.nlm.nih.gov/htbin-post/Omim>.

Oren Traub, MD, PhD

Carnitine palmitoyltransferase deficiency

Definition

Carnitine palmitoyltransferase (CPT) deficiency refers to two separate, hereditary diseases of lipid metabolism, CPT-I deficiency and CPT-II deficiency. CPT-I deficiency affects lipid metabolism in the liver, with serious physical symptoms including coma and seizures. Two types of CPT-II deficiency are similar in age of onset and type of symptoms to CPT-I deficiency. The third, most common type of CPT-II deficiency involves intermittent muscle disease in adults, with a potential for myoglobinuria, a serious complication affecting the kidneys. Preventive measures and treatments are available for CPT-I deficiency, and the muscle form of CPT-II deficiency.

Description

Carnitine palmitoyltransferase (CPT) is an important enzyme required by the body to use (metabolize) lipids (fats). CPT speeds up the transport of long-chain fatty acids across the inner mitochondria membrane. This transport also depends on carnitine, also called vitamin B7.

Until the 1990s, discussion centered on whether defects in a single CPT enzyme were responsible for all the conditions resulting from CPT deficiency. Careful chemical and genetic analysis eventually pointed to two different enzymes: CPT-I and CPT-II. Both CPT-I and CPT-II were shown to play an important role in the metabolism of lipids. CPT deficiency of any type affects the muscles, so these disorders are considered to be metabolic myopathies (muscle diseases), or more specifically, mitochondrial myopathies, meaning myopathies that result from abnormal changes occurring in the mitochondria of the cells as a result of excessive lipid build-up.

Understanding the symptoms of CPT requires some familiarity with the basics of lipid metabolism in muscle cells. Fatty acids (FA) are the major component of lipids. FAs contain a chain of carbon atoms of varying length. Long-chain fatty acids (LCFAs) are the most abundant type, and have at least 12 carbon atoms. Lipids and glucose (sugar) are the primary sources of energy for the body. Both are converted into energy (oxidized) inside mitochondria, structures within each cell where numerous energy-producing chemical reactions take place. Each cell contains many mitochondria.

A single mitochondrion is enclosed by a double-layer membrane. LCFAs are unable to pass through the inner portion of this membrane without first being bound to carnitine, a type of amino acid. CPT-I chemically binds carnitine to LCFAs, allowing transfer through the inner membrane. However, LCFAs cannot be oxidized inside the mitochondrion while still attached to carnitine, so CPT-II reverses the action of CPT-I and removes carnitine. Once accomplished, LCFAs can proceed to be metabolized. Therefore, deficiency of either CPT-I or CPT-II results in improper transfer and utilization of LCFAs in the mitochondria.

CPT-I is involved in lipid metabolism in several tissues, most importantly the liver. There, LCFAs are broken down and ketone bodies are produced. Like lipids and glucose, ketone bodies are used by the body as fuel, especially in the brain and muscles. Deficiency of CPT-I in the liver results in decreased levels of ketone bodies (hypoketosis), as well as low blood-sugar levels (hypoglycemia). Hypoketosis combined with hypoglycemia in a child can lead to weakness, seizures, and coma. Symptoms can be reversed by glucose infusions, as well as supplementation with medium-chain fatty acids, which do not require CPT-I to produce energy.

As noted, glucose and fatty acids are important energy sources for the body. During exercise, the muscles initially use glucose as their primary fuel. After some time, however, glucose is depleted and the muscles switch to using fatty acids by a chemical process called oxidation. CPT-II deficiency results in a decrease in LCFAs that can be used by the mitochondria, and the muscles eventually exhaust their energy supply. This explains why prolonged exercise may cause an attack of muscle fatigue, stiffness, and pain in people with CPT-II deficiency. The ability to exercise for short periods is not affected. Infections, stress, muscle trauma, and exposure to cold also put extra demands on the muscles and can trigger an attack. Fasting, or a diet high in fats and low in carbohydrates (complex sugars), deplete glucose reserves in the muscles and are risk factors as well.

In some cases, CPT deficiency results in the breakdown of muscle tissue, a process called rhabdomyolysis, and it causes some components of muscle cells to "leak" into the bloodstream. Myoglobin, the muscle-cell equivalent of hemoglobin in the blood, is one of these components. Myoglobin is filtered from the blood by the kidneys and deposited in the urine, causing myoglobinuria. Dark-colored urine is the typical sign of myoglobinuria. Severe and/or repeated episodes of rhabdomyolysis and myoglobinuria can cause serious kidney damage.

Genetic profile

CPT-I deficiency is caused by defects in the CPT1 **gene** located on **chromosome** 11. CPT-II deficiency results from mutations in the CPT2 gene on chromosome 1.

Both CPT-I and CPT-II deficiency are considered autosomal recessive conditions. This means that both parents of an affected person carry one defective CPT gene, but also have a normal gene of that pair. Carriers of a single recessive gene typically do not express the deficiency because the second normal functioning gene, is able to compensate. A person with two mutated genes has no normal gene to make up for the deficiency, and thus expresses the disease. Parents who are both carriers for the same autosomal recessive condition face a 25% chance in each pregnancy that they will both pass on the defective gene and have an affected child.

Several individuals proven to be carriers of CPT-II deficiency have had mild symptoms of the disorder. Measurement of CPT-II enzyme levels (the protein coded for by CPT2) in most of the carriers tested show lower levels, as would be expected when one gene is mutated and the other is not. It is not yet clear why some carriers show mild symptoms, but this phenomenon occasionally occurs in other autosomal recessive conditions.

Demographics

CPT-I deficiency is rare, with fewer than 15 cases having been reported. CPT-II deficiency is more common, but its true occurrence is unknown. Muscle CPT-II deficiency makes up the majority of cases that have been reported; liver and multiorgan CPT-II deficiency are both quite rare. There seems to be no geographic area or ethnic group that is at greater risk for either type of CPT deficiency.

Approximately equal numbers of males and females with CPT-I deficiency have been seen, which is typical of autosomal recessive **inheritance**. However, about 80% of those individuals diagnosed with CPT-II deficiency are male. Males and females do have an equal likelihood of inheriting a defective CPT2 gene from a parent, but effects of the gene in each sex can be different. Hormonal differences between males and females may have some effect—a clue being the tendency of an affected woman to have more symptoms while pregnant.

Signs and symptoms

CPT-I deficiency

The CPT-I enzyme has two forms, coded for by different genes. CPT-IA is the form present in liver, skin, kidney, and heart cells, while CPT-IB functions in skeletal muscle, heart, fat, and testis cells. CPT-I deficiency refers to the CPT-IA form since a defective CPT-IB enzyme has not yet been described in humans. CPT-I deficiency has always been diagnosed in infants or children.

The brain and muscles use ketone bodies as a source of energy. The brain especially, relies heavily on ketone bodies for energy during times of stress, such as after fasting when low sugar levels (hypoglycemia) occur. In fact, children with CPT-I deficiency are usually first diagnosed after they have fasted due to an illness or diarrhea. Hypoketosis and hypoglycemia in CPT-I deficiency can become severe, and result in lethargy (lack of physical energy), seizures, and coma.

CPT-II deficiency

CPT-II deficiency is divided into three subtypes. "Muscle CPT deficiency" is the most common form of the condition. Onset of symptoms is usually in adolescence or adulthood, but varies. "Hepatic CPT-II deficiency" is rare and is diagnosed in childhood. The remaining cases are classified as "multiorgan CPT-II deficiency," and have been diagnosed in infants. Differences in the severity of symptoms between the groups, as well as within each group, are due in part to different mutations in the CPT2 gene. Environmental factors may assist the triggering of attacks and thus may contribute to the variety of observed symptoms.

MUSCLE CPT DEFICIENCY Muscle fatigue, stiffness, and pain are typically caused by prolonged exercise or exertion. Other possible triggers include fasting, infection, muscle injury, exposure to cold, and even emotional stress. Cases of adverse reactions to certain types of general anesthesia have also been reported.

These "muscle attacks" after a triggering event are the classic physical signs of muscle CPT-II deficiency. When an attack is associated with the breakdown of muscle tissue (rhabdomyolysis), myoglobinuria is the other classic sign. Unlike other metabolic myopathies, there are no obvious signs of an impending attack, and resting will not stop the symptoms once they have begun. Muscle symptoms may begin during or up to several hours after prolonged exercise or other triggering events. A specific muscle group may be affected, or generalized symptoms may occur. Muscle weakness between attacks is not a problem, unlike some other metabolic myopathies. In addition, muscle cells examined under the microscope typically appear normal. Some people with muscle CPT deficiency have only had a few attacks in their lifetime, while others may experience several attacks per week. Renal failure due to repeated episodes of myoglobinuria occurs in about 25% of individuals with muscle CPT deficiency.

HEPATIC CPT-II DEFICIENCY Symptoms and age of onset in hepatic CPT-II deficiency are similar to CPT-I deficiency, primarily coma and seizures associated with hypoketotic hypoglycemia. However, unlike CPT-I deficiency, most infants with liver CPT-II deficiency have had heart problems and have died.

MULTIORGAN CPT-II DEFICIENCY This type of CPT-II deficiency has only been reported a few times and involves the liver, skeletal muscles and heart. Infants with this type have all died.

Diagnosis

The symptoms of CPT-I deficiency can be dramatic, but the rare nature of the disease means that some time may elapse while other more common diseases are ruled out. Definitive diagnosis of CPT-I deficiency is made by measuring the activity of the CPT enzyme in fibroblasts, leukocytes, or muscle tissue. Abnormal results on several blood tests are also typical of CPT-I deficiency, but the most important finding is hypoketotic hypoglycemia. Analysis of the CPT1 gene on chromosome 11 may be possible, but is not yet considered a diagnostic test.

CPT-II deficiency is somewhat more common than CPT-I deficiency. However, the milder symptoms of muscle CPT deficiency and their similarity to other diseases often leads to a wrong diagnosis (misdiagnosis). For example, the symptoms of CPT-II deficiency are sometimes initially diagnosed as fibromyalgia or chronic fatigue syndrome. Misdiagnosis is a special concern for people with muscle CPT-II deficiency, since the use of available preventive measures and treatment are then delayed.

Analysis of the CPT-II enzyme levels can confirm the diagnosis, but must be done carefully if performed on any tissue other than a muscle specimen. Direct testing of the CPT2 gene is available and is probably the easiest method (simple blood sample) of making the diagnosis. If **genetic testing** shows two mutated CPT2 genes, the diagnosis is confirmed. However, not all disease-causing mutations in the gene have been discovered, so demonstration of only one mutated CPT2 gene, or a completely negative test, does not exclude the diagnosis. In those individuals in whom genetic testing is not definitive, the combination of clinical symptoms and a laboratory finding of low levels of CPT-II enzyme activity should be enough to confirm the diagnosis.

Treatment and management

While CPT-I and CPT-II deficiency differ in their typical age of onset and in the severity of their symptoms, treatment of both conditions is similar. Attacks may be prevented by avoiding those situations that lead to them, as noted above. Someone undergoing surgery should discuss the possibility of alternative anesthetics with their doctor. Most people with CPT deficiency find it necessary to carry or wear some type of identifying information about their condition such as a Medic-Alert bracelet.

Those who find that they cannot avoid a situation known to be a trigger for them should try to supplement their diet with carbohydrates. Since medium-chain fatty acids to not require carnitine to enter the mitochondrion, use of a dietary supplement containing them results in significant improvement in people with CPT-I deficiency and also helps prevent attacks in most people with CPT-II deficiency. The use of carnitine supplements (vitamin B7) is also helpful for some individuals diagnosed with the deficiency.

Anyone diagnosed with CPT deficiency, or anyone concerned about a family history of CPT deficiency, should be offered **genetic counseling** to discuss the most up-to-date treatment and testing options available to them.

Prognosis

Children with CPT-I deficiency improve significantly with treatment. So far, however, all have had some lasting neurological problems, possibly caused by damage to the brain during their first attack. The outlook at this point for infants and children with liver and multiorgan CPT-II deficiency is still poor.

Once a person with muscle CPT-II deficiency is correctly diagnosed, the prognosis is good. While it is impossible for many patients to completely avoid attacks, most people with the condition eventually find

KEY TERMS

Carnitine—An amino acid necessary for metabolism of the long-chain fatty acid portion of lipids. Also called vitamin B7.

Fatty acids—The primary component of fats (lipids) in the body. Carnitine palmitoyl transferase (CPT) deficiency involves abnormal metabolism of the long-chain variety of fatty acids.

Hypoglycemia—An abnormally low glucose (blood sugar) concentration in the blood.

Hypoketosis—Decreased levels of ketone bodies.

Ketone bodies—Products of fatty acid metabolism in the liver that can be used by the brain and muscles as an energy source.

Metabolic myopathies—A broad group of muscle diseases whose cause is a metabolic disturbance of some type.

Mitochondria—Organelles within the cell responsible for energy production.

Myoglobinuria—The abnormal presence of myoglobin, a product of muscle disintegration, in the urine. Results in dark-colored urine.

Myopathy—Any abnormal condition or disease of the muscle.

Rhabdomyolysis—Breakdown or disintegration of muscle tissue.

the right mix of preventive measures and treatments. CPT-II deficiency then has much less of a harmful impact on their lives. A number of excellent sources of information are available for families affected by CPT deficiency. Any new treatments in the future would likely attempt to directly address the enzyme deficiency, so that normal metabolism of lipids might occur.

Resources

ORGANIZATIONS

Fatty Oxidation Disorders (FOD) Family Support Group. Deb Lee Gould, MEd, Director, FOD Family Support Group, MCAD Parent and Grief Consultant, 805 Montrose Dr., Greensboro, NC 24710. (336) 547-8682. <http://www.fodsupport.org>.

Genetic Alliance. 4301 Connecticut Ave. NW, #404, Washington, DC 20008-2304. (800) 336-GENE (Helpline) or (202) 966-5557. Fax: (888) 394-3937 info@geneticalliance. <http://www.geneticalliance.org>.

March of Dimes Birth Defects Foundation. 1275 Mamaroneck Ave., White Plains, NY 10605. (888) 663-4637.

resourcecenter@modimes.org. <http://www.modimes.org>.

National Organization for Rare Disorders (NORD). PO Box 8923, New Fairfield, CT 06812-8923. (203) 746-6518 or (800) 999-6673. Fax: (203) 746-6481. <http://www.rarediseases.org>.

National Society of Genetic Counselors. 233 Canterbury Dr., Wallingford, PA 19086-6617. (610) 872-1192. <http://www.nsgc.org/GeneticCounselingYou.asp>.

United Mitochondrial Disease Foundation. PO Box 1151, Monroeville, PA 15146-1151. (412) 793-8077. Fax: (412) 793-6477. <http://www.umdf.org>.

OTHER

The Spiral Notebook—short takes on carnitine palmitoyl transferase deficiency. <http://www.spiralnotebook.org>

Scott J. Polzin, MS, CGC

Carpenter syndrome

Definition

Carpenter syndrome is a rare hereditary disorder resulting in the premature closing of the cranial sutures, which are the line joints between the bones of the skull, and in syndactyly, a condition characterized by the webbing of fingers and toes. The syndrome is named after G. Carpenter who first described this disorder in 1901.

Description

Carpenter syndrome is a subtype of a family of **genetic disorders** known as acrocephalopolysyndactyly (ACPS) disorders. Carpenter syndrome is also called Acrocephalopolysyndactyly Type II (ACPS II). There were originally five types of ACPS. This number has decreased because some of these conditions have been recognized as being similar to each other or to other genetic syndromes. For example, it is now agreed that ACPS I, or Noack syndrome, is the same as **Pfeiffer syndrome**. Researchers have also concluded that the disorders formerly known as Goodman syndrome (ACPS IV) and Summitt syndrome are variants (slightly different forms) of Carpenter syndrome.

All forms of ACPS are characterized by premature closing of the cranial sutures and malformations of the fingers and toes. Individuals diagnosed with Carpenter syndrome have short and broad heads (brachycephaly), the tops of which appear abnormally cone-shaped (acrocephaly). Webbing or fusion of the fingers or toes (syndactyly) and/or the presence extra fingers or toes (**polydactyly**) are also characteristic signs of Carpenter syndrome.

The human skull consists of several bony plates separated by a narrow fibrous joint that contains stem cells. These fibrous joints are called cranial sutures. There are six sutures: the sagittal, which runs from front to back across the top of the head; the two coronal sutures, which run across the skull parallel to and just above the hairline; the metopic, which runs from front to back in front of the sagittal suture; and the two lamboid sutures, which run side to side across the back of the head. The premature closing of one or more of these cranial sutures leads to skull deformations, a condition called **craniosynostosis**. There are seven types of craniosynostosis depending on which cranial suture or sutures are affected: sagittal, bicoronal (both coronal sutures), unicoronal (one coronal suture), coronal and sagittal, metopic, lambdoid and sagittal, and total, in which all the cranial sutures are affected. Individuals affected with Carpenter syndrome show sagittal and bicoronal types of skull malformations.

Genetic profile

Carpenter syndrome is inherited as a recessive non-sex linked (autosomal) condition. The **gene** responsible for the syndrome has not yet been identified, but it is currently believed that all ACPS syndromes may be the result of genetic mutations—changes occurring in the genes. Genetic links to other syndromes that also result in craniosynostosis have been identified. As of 1997, 64 distinct mutations in six different genes had been linked to craniosynostosis. Three of these genes, one located on the short arm of **chromosome** 8 (8p11), one on the long arm of chromosome 10 (10q26), and another on the short arm of chromosome 4 (4p16), are related to fibroblast growth factor receptors (FGFRs), which are molecules that control cell growth. Other implicated genes are the TWIST gene located on chromosome 7, the MSX2 gene on chromosome 5, and the FBN1 gene on the long arm of chromosome 15.

Demographics

Carpenter syndrome and the other ACPS disorders have an occurrence of approximately one in every one million live births. It is rare because both parents must carry the gene mutation in order for their child to have the disease. Therefore, Carpenter syndrome has been observed in cases where the parents are related by blood, though in most cases parents are not related. Parents with one child affected by Carpenter syndrome have a 25%

likelihood that their next child will also be affected with the disorder.

Signs and symptoms

Individuals diagnosed with Carpenter syndrome show various types of malformations and deformities of the skull. The two main examples are sagittal and bicoronal craniosynostosis. Sagittal craniosynostosis is characterized by a long and narrow skull (scaphocephaly). This is measured as an increase in the A-P, or anterior-to-posterior, diameter, which indicates that looking down on the top of the skull, the diameter of the head is greater than normal in the front-to-back orientation. Individuals affected with sagittal craniosynostosis also have narrow but prominent foreheads and a larger than normal back of the head. The so-called soft-spot found just beyond the hairline in a normal baby is very small or absent in a baby affected with sagittal craniosynostosis.

The other type of skull malformation observed, bicoronal craniosynostosis, is characterized by a wide and short skull (brachycephaly). This is measured as a decrease in the A-P diameter, which indicates that looking down on the top of the skull, the diameter of the head is less than normal in the front-to-back orientation. Individuals affected with this condition have poorly formed eye sockets and foreheads. This causes a smaller than normal sized eye socket that can cause eyesight complications. These complications include damage to the optic nerve, which can cause a loss of visual clarity; bulging eyeballs resulting from the shallow orbits (exophthalmus), which usually damages the eye cornea; widely spaced eyes; and a narrowing of the sinuses and tear ducts that can cause inflammation of the mucous membranes that line the exposed portion of the eyeball (conjunctivitis).

A further complication of bicoronal craniosynostosis is water on the brain (**hydrocephalus**), which increases pressure on the brain. Most individuals affected with this condition also have an abnormally high and arched palate that can cause dental problems and protrusion, the thrusting forward of the lower jaw. Coronal and sagittal craniosynostosis are characterized by a cone-shaped head (acrocephaly). The front soft-spot characteristic of an infant's skull is generally much larger than normal and it may never close without surgical intervention. Individuals with these skull abnormalities may also have higher than normal pressure inside the skull.

Individuals with Carpenter syndrome often have webbed fingers or toes (cutaneous syndactyly) or partial fusion of their fingers or toes (syndactyly). These individuals also tend to have unusually short fingers (bracydactyly) and sometimes exhibit extra toes, or more rarely, extra fingers (polydactyly).

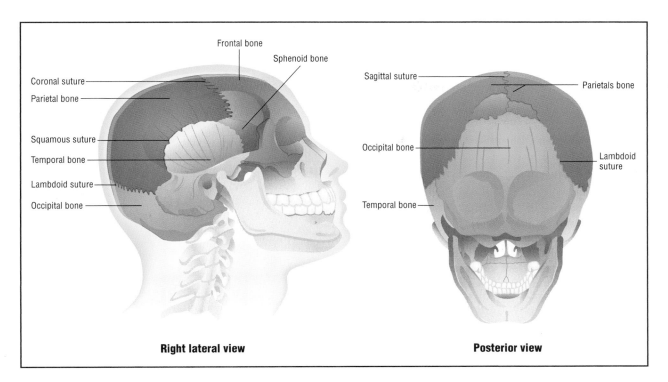

Frontal bone
Sphenoid bone
Coronal suture
Parietal bone
Squamous suture
Temporal bone
Lambdoid suture
Occipital bone

Right lateral view

Sagittal suture
Parietals bone
Occipital bone
Lambdoid suture
Temporal bone

Posterior view

Right lateral and posterior view of the skull with sutures identified. *(Gale Group.)*

Approximately one third of Carpenter syndrome individuals have heart defects at birth. These may include: narrowing of the artery that delivers blood from the heart to the lungs (pulmonary stenosis); blue baby syndrome, due to various defects in the structure of the heart or its major blood vessels; transposition of the major blood vessels, meaning that the aorta and pulmonary artery are inverted; and the presence of an extra large vein, called the superior vena cava, that delivers blood back to the heart from the head, neck, and upper limbs.

In some persons diagnosed with Carpenter syndrome, additional physical problems are present. Individuals are often short or overweight, with males having a disorder in which the testicles fail to descend properly (cryptorchidism). Another problem is caused by parts of the large intestine coming through an abnormal opening near the navel (umbilical hernia). In some cases, mild mental retardation has also been observed.

Diagnosis

The diagnosis of Carpenter syndrome is made based on the presence of the bicoronal and sagittal skull malformation, which produces a cone-shaped or short and broad skull, accompanied by partially fused or extra fingers or toes (syndactly or polydactyly). Skull x rays and/or a CT scan may also be used to diagnose the skull malformations correctly. Other genetic disorders are also characterized

by the same types of skull deformities and some genetic tests are available for them. Thus, positive results on these tests can rule out the possibility of Carpenter syndrome.

Before birth, ultrasound imaging, a technique used to produce pictures of the fetus, is generally used to examine the development of the skull in the second and third months of pregnancy, but the images are not always clear enough to properly diagnose the type of skull deformity, if present. New ultrasound techniques are being used in Japan however, that can detect skull abnormalities in fetuses with much higher image clarity.

Treatment and management

Operations to correct the skull malformations associated with Carpenter syndrome should be performed during the first year of the baby's life. This is because modifying the skull bones is much easier at that age and new bone growth, as well as the required bone reshaping, can occur rapidly. Also, the facial features are still highly undeveloped, so a greatly improved appearance can be achieved. If heart defects are present at birth, surgery may also be required. Follow-up support by pediatric, psychological, neurological, surgical, and genetic specialists may be necessary.

Individuals with Carpenter syndrome may have vision problems that require consultation with an ophthalmologist, or doctor specialized in the treatment of such problems. Speech and hearing therapy may also be

KEY TERMS

Acrocephalopolysyndactyly syndromes—A collection of genetic disorders characterized by cone shaped abnormality of the skull and partial fusing of adjacent fingers or toes.

Acrocephaly—An abnormal cone shape of the head.

Autosome—Chromosome not involved in specifying sex.

Brachycephaly—An abnormal thickening and widening of the skull.

Cranial suture—Any one of the seven fibrous joints between the bones of the skull.

Craniosynostosis—Premature, delayed, or otherwise abnormal closure of the sutures of the skull.

Cutaneous syndactyly—Fusion of the soft tissue between fingers or toes resulting in a webbed appearance.

Gene—A building block of inheritance, which contains the instructions for the production of a particular protein, and is made up of a molecular sequence found on a section of DNA. Each gene is found on a precise location on a chromosome.

Hydrocephalus—The excess accumulation of cerebrospinal fluid around the brain, often causing enlargement of the head.

Polydactyly—The presence of extra fingers or toes.

Scaphocephaly—An abnormally long and narrow skull.

Syndactyly—Webbing or fusion between the fingers or toes.

necessary if the ears and the brain have been affected. If the palate is severely malformed, dental consultation may also be necessary. In the most severe cases of Carpenter syndrome, it may be necessary to treat feeding and respiratory problems that are associated with the malformed palate and sinuses. Obesity is associated with Carpenter syndrome and dietary management throughout the patient's lifetime may also be recommended.

Webbed fingers or toes (cutaneous syndactyly) may be easily corrected by surgery. Extra fingers or toes (polydactyly) may often be surgically removed shortly after birth.

Surgical procedures also exist to correct some of the heart defects associated with Carpenter syndrome, as well as the testicles disorder of affected males. The abnormal opening of the large intestine near the navel (umbilical hernia or **omphalocele**) can also be treated by surgery. Additionally, intervention programs for developmental delays are available for affected patients.

Prognosis

Carpenter syndrome is not usually fatal if immediate treatment for the heart defects and/or skull malformations is available. In all but the most severe and inoperable cases of craniosynostosis, it is possible that the affected individual may attain a greatly improved physical appearance. Depending on damage to the nervous system, the rapidity of treatment, and the potential brain damage from excess pressure on the brain caused by skull malformation, certain affected individuals may display varying degrees of developmental delay. Some individuals will continue to have vision problems throughout life. These problems will vary in severity depending on the initial extent of their individual skull malformations, but most of these problems can now be treated.

Resources

PERIODICALS

Cohen, D., J. Green, J. Miller, R. Gorlin, and J. Reed. "Acrocephalopolysyndactyly type II—Carpenter syndrome: clinical spectrum and an attempt at unification with Goodman and Summit syndromes." *American Journal of Medical Genetics* (October 1987): 311-24.

Pooh, R., Y. Nakagawa, N. Nagamachi, K. Pooh, Y. Nakagawa, K. Maeda, R. Fukui, and T. Aono. "Transvaginal sonography of the fetal brain: detection of abnormal morphology and circulation." *Croation Journal of Medicine* (1998): 147-57.

Wilkie, A. "Craniosynostosis: genes and mechanisms." *Human Molecular Genetics* (1979): 1647-56.

ORGANIZATIONS

Children's Craniofacial Association. PO Box 280297, Dallas, TX 75243-4522. (972) 994-9902 or (800) 535-3643. contactcca@ccakids.com. <http://www.ccakids.com>.

Craniosynostosis and Parents Support. 2965-A Quarters, Quantico, VA 22134. (877) 686-CAPS or (703) 445-1078. <http://www.caps2000.org/>.

WEBSITES

Craniosupport. <http://www.craniosupport.com> (February 8, 2001).

Golwyn, D., T. Anderson, and P. Jeanty. "Acrocephalopolysyndactyly." *TheFetus.Net.* <http://www.thefetus.net> (February 8, 2001).

Paul A. Johnson

Cat cry syndrome *see* **Cri du chat syndrome**

Caudal dysplasia

Definition

Caudal **dysplasia** is a total or partial failure of development of the lower vertebrae, including the sacrum (tailbone), which results in associated abnormalities of the lower extremities (legs), spine, kidneys, gastrointestinal and genitourinary tracts.

Description

Caudal dysplasia is also known as sacral agenesis, sacral regression, caudal aplasia, caudal regression sequence, or **sirenomelia**. Caudal dysplasia results from a failure of the caudal or lower region of the spinal column to form correctly. This abnormal development of the lower spine causes a wide range, or spectrum, of other abnormalities. On the mild end of the spectrum, there may be a partial absence of the tailbone with no associated symptoms (sometimes picked up accidentally on x ray), and on the severe end of the spectrum, there can be complete absence of the kidneys, openings on the spinal cord, genitourinary, limb and bowel abnormalities. Some of these more serious abnormalities can be life-threatening. Most infants with caudal dysplasia fall in between the two ends of the spectrum. They may have kidney malformations, gastrointestinal malformations, spinal cord problems, heart abnormalities, and problems with their lower limbs.

Sirenomelia is a rare condition that was once thought to represent the most severe end of the caudal dysplasia sequence. Infants with sirenomelia may have complete fusion of the lower limbs, complete or partial **renal agenesis**, and severe bowel problems. There is often oligohydramnios, or a low amount of amniotic fluid, during pregnancy. Because of the severity of the defects in this condition, it is generally lethal. As of 2005, sirenomelia is now thought to be a separate syndrome.

Caudal dysplasia is caused by a problem with the formation of certain tissues early in pregnancy. The lower spine is usually completely formed by the seventh week of pregnancy. Caudal dysplasia is a primary defect of formation of the tissues that will become the sacrum, spinal cord, kidneys, and gastrointestinal system.

Genetic profile

The genetics of caudal dysplasia are not well understood. There is no convincing evidence that this is a genetic disorder. Some families have shown autosomal dominant **inheritance**, but more research will be necessary before the exact pattern of inheritance of this disorder is clear. In most cases, it occurs as an isolated event. In some families, there is evidence of an increased incidence of mild **scoliosis** and **spina bifida** occulta (opening on one or more of the vertebra without any physical effect) in the parents of children affected with caudal agenesis. This suggests that there may be some genetic factors that predispose some individuals to have caudal dysplasia but, as of 2005, these factors are not well understood.

Demographics

Estimates of the incidence of caudal dysplasia range between approximately one in 7,500 to one in 20,000 births. Caudal dysplasia occurs equally in males and females. There is an increased rate of caudal dysplasia among infants of diabetic mothers. As many as 16–22% of infants with caudal dysplasia are born to diabetic mothers, and the risk for a diabetic woman (with poor glucose control) to have an infant with caudal dysplasia is 200 times higher that the average population risk. **Diabetes** or impaired glucose metabolism is a common problem in pregnancy with 3–10% of all pregnancies affected by abnormal glucose metabolism. The exact mechanism by which diabetes causes caudal dysplasia in not well understood.

Caudal dysplasia is a defect of the mesodermal tissue, which develops early in the first trimester of pregnancy. Poor glucose control during the first trimester can lead to an increased risk for the fetus to develop caudal dysplasia. The interaction between poor glucose control and the defects that lead to problems in the mesodermal tissues is not well understood.

Most women with an increased risk to have a child with caudal regression have diabetes (often undiagnosed) prior to pregnancy. Gestational diabetes (or diabetes that develops during pregnancy) is a separate entity and should not be confused with diabetes in the first trimester. Gestational diabetes is not associated with an increased risk for caudal dysplasia.

Signs and symptoms

In order to understand the signs and symptoms of caudal dysplasia, it is important to understand early embryonic development. Very early in pregnancy, the cells that will develop into the embryo are organized as a small round ball. These cells eventually separate into three distinct layers: the endoderm, the mesoderm, and the ectoderm. The endoderm can be thought of as the inside layer. Cells from the endoderm will eventually form into the lining of the digestive tract and the respiratory tract. The mesoderm can be thought of as the middle layer, and the cells of the mesoderm will eventually become the muscles, bones, kidney, heart, and blood vessels. The endoderm can be thought of as the outside layer. The cells of the endoderm will eventually become the skin, hair, nails, brain, and nervous system. Caudal dysplasia is the result of an early insult to the tissues of the mesoderm. Since the mesoderm is the tissue that forms the bones, muscles, kidneys, and other tissues, individuals with caudal dysplasia will have problems with these tissues. Any disruption of the development of the mesoderm will lead to disruption of the organs formed from this layer. Impaired glucose metabolism early in pregnancy can lead to an insult, which results in the infant having caudal dysplasia. However, since only 16–22% of mothers of infants with caudal dysplasia have diabetes, there must be other factors that also cause caudal dysplasia. These other factors are not well understood at this time.

Caudal dysplasia is a disorder with a wide spectrum of defects. Some individuals are very mildly affected and some are much more severely affected. Individuals with caudal dysplasia can have some or all of the signs and symptoms.

Spinal cord abnormalities in infants affected with caudal dysplasia include:

- missing or malformed sacrum
- abnormal vertebrae
- cerebellum agenesis
- **hydrocephalus**
- spina bifida
- scoliosis

Kidney abnormalities include:

- hydronephrosis
- renal failure
- agenesis of the kidney
- hypoplasia of the kidney

Gastrointestinal abnormalities include:

- imperforate anus
- malformed or rotated gut

Heart abnormalities include:

- atrial septal defect
- coarctation of the aorta
- stenosis of the pulmonary valve

Lower limb abnormalities include:

- clubfeet
- missing reflexes
- paralysis or numbness of the legs

Neurological abnormalities include:

- neurogenic bladder (impaired bladder control)
- neurogenic bowel (impaired bowel control)
- motor and sensory nerve abnormalities

Other abnormalities include:

- cleft lip/palate
- diaphragmatic hernia
- hypoplastic lungs
- low-set ears
- tracheo-eosophageal fistula (connection between the trachea and eosophagus)

Diagnosis

The diagnosis of caudal dysplasia can be made during pregnancy, at birth, and during childhood, depending on the severity of the defects present.

Prenatal diagnosis

The diagnosis of caudal dysplasia can be made prenatally (during pregnancy) by **prenatal ultrasound** (a sonogram). Sonograms use sound waves to provide an image of a fetus. The structural abnormalities of caudal dysplasia, including absence of vertebra, kidney malformations, other spinal cord malformations, and limb abnormalities, can be seen during the second trimester of pregnancy. Because the bones of the sacrum do not ossify, or harden, until approximately 22 weeks of pregnancy, it may be difficult to diagnose caudal dysplasia before this time.

The diagnosis of caudal dysplasia can also be made by physical examination after birth. Physical signs can include flattening of the buttocks, shortening of the gluteal cleft, scoliosis, spina bifida, and hydrocephalus. X rays should be taken to look at the formation of the underlying bones and tissues.

Treatment and management

Pregnancy management

When caudal dysplasia is diagnosed by prenatal ultrasound, the mother should be tested for diabetes. Pregnancy termination may be an option. If the pregnancy continues, the parents may wish to consult with specialists to get more specific information about prognosis.

Delivery management

Because of the abnormalities seen and the possible complications, delivery should be at a tertiary care center or hospital able to provide specialized pediatric care. It is likely that an infant with caudal dysplasia will spend a significant amount of time in the hospital as a newborn.

KEY TERMS

Aplasia—Defective development resulting in absence of all or part of an organ or tissue.

Caudal—Pertaining to the tail (bone).

Dysplasia—Abnormal development of tissues, organs, or cells.

Sacrum—Triangular bone at the base of the spinal column.

If the tertiary care center is not located near the family, this can increase the burden of care for the family.

There is no cure for caudal dysplasia. Treatment is governed by the abnormalities present. If the abnormalities are severe (life-threatening), corrective surgery is not an option. The main goals of treatments include maintaining and improving kidney, lung, and gastrointestinal function. Orthopedic surgeries are done to correct malformation, and physical therapy is used to avoid secondary complications, such as scoliosis.

Many of the defects of caudal dysplasia can be surgically treated but not cured. For example, an opening on the spine (spina bifida) can be surgically closed, but if the nerves in that opening have been damaged, there is nothing that can be done to reverse this damage. Other surgeries include orthopedic surgeries to correct bone malformations and improve limb function. Surgery can also be done to correct hydrocephalus or imperforate anus.

Other treatments involve orthopedic devices and treatments for neurogenic bladder. Orthopedic devices may be used to help with problems of the hip, back, and legs. Neurogenic bladder is one of the more serious and debilitating problems in caudal dysplasia. Long-term bladder dysfunction can result in kidney damage and failure.

The treatments for caudal dysplasia often require lifelong medical attention. It is important to prepare the family for this and to stress the need for preventative care (i.e., prevention of infections) and vigilance in detecting complications.

Prognosis

The prognosis for caudal dysplasia is highly dependant on the severity of the malformation present. Those with extremely mild abnormalities may have no or few symptoms. Infants with more serious symptoms may require extensive urologic and orthopedic assistance, including multiple surgeries and lifelong therapies. Neu-

rogenic bladder is one of the more serious and debilitating problems in caudal dysplasia. Long-term bladder dysfunction can result is kidney damage and failure, and intensive efforts may be required to avoid this problem. Some infants with caudal dysplasia are born with lethal abnormalities that are incompatible with life. Infants that do survive generally have normal mental function.

Resources

WEB SITES

National Institute of Arthritis and Musculoskeletal and Skin Diseases. (April 8, 2005.) <http://www.nih.gov/niams>.

ORGANIZATIONS

National Institute of Arthritis and Musculoskeletal and Skin Diseases. 1 AMS Circle, Bethesda, MD 20892-3675. Telephone: (301) 496-8188. Fax: (877) 226-4267. E-mail: NAMSIC@mail.nih.gov. (April 8, 2005.) <http://www.nih.gov/niams>.

Kathleen A. Fergus, MS, CGC

Celiac disease

Definition

Celiac disease is a disease of the digestive system that damages the small intestine and interferes with the absorption of nutrients from food.

Description

Celiac disease occurs when the body reacts abnormally to gluten, a protein found in wheat, rye, barley, and possibly oats. When someone with celiac disease eats foods containing gluten, that person's immune system causes an inflammatory response in the small intestine, which damages the tissues and results in an impaired ability to absorb nutrients from foods. The inflammation and malabsorption create wide-ranging problems in many systems of the body. Since the body's own immune system causes the damage, celiac disease is classified as an "autoimmune" disorder. Celiac disease may also be called sprue, nontropical sprue, gluten sensitive enteropathy, celiac sprue, and adult celiac disease.

Genetic profile

Celiac disease can run in families and has a genetic basis, but the pattern of **inheritance** is complicated. The type of inheritance pattern that celiac disease follows is called multifactorial (caused by many factors, both genetic and environmental). Researchers think that several factors must exist in order for the disease to occur. First, the patient must have a genetic predisposition to develop the disorder. Then, something in their environment acts as a stimulus to trigger their immune system, causing the disease to become active for the first time. For conditions with **multifactorial inheritance**, people without the genetic predisposition are less likely to develop the condition with exposure to the same triggers. Or, they may require more exposure to the stimulus before developing the disease than someone with a genetic predisposition. Several factors may provoke a reaction including surgery, especially gastrointestinal surgery; a change to a low fat diet, which has an increased number of wheat-based foods; pregnancy; childbirth; severe emotional stress; or a viral infection. This combination of genetic susceptibility and an outside agent leads to celiac disease.

Demographics

Celiac disease may be discovered at any age, from infancy through adulthood. The disorder is more commonly found among white Europeans or in people of European descent. It is very unusual to find celiac disease in African or Asian people. The exact incidence of the disease is uncertain. Estimates vary from one in 5,000, to as many as one in every 300 individuals with this background. The prevalence of celiac disease seems to be different from one European country to another, and between Europe and the United States. This may be due to differences in diet and/or unrecognized disease. A recent study of random blood samples tested for celiac disease in the United States showed one in 250 testing positive. It is clearly underdiagnosed, probably due to the symptoms being attributed to another problem, or lack of knowledge about celiac disease by physicians and laboratories.

Because celiac disease has a hereditary influence, close relatives (especially first degree relatives, such as children, siblings, and parents) have a higher risk of being affected with the condition. The chance that a first degree relative of someone with celiac disease will have the disease is about 10%.

As more is learned about celiac disease, it becomes evident that there are many variations which may not produce typical symptoms. It may even be clinically "silent," where no obvious problems related to the disease are apparent.

Signs and symptoms

Each person with celiac disease is affected differently. When food containing gluten reaches the small intestine, the immune system begins to attack a substance called gliadin, which is found in the gluten. The resulting inflammation causes damage to the delicate finger-like structures in the intestine, called villi, where food absorption actually takes place. The patient may experience a number of symptoms related to the inflammation and the chemicals it releases, and or the lack of ability to absorb nutrients from food, which can cause malnutrition.

The most commonly recognized symptoms of celiac disease relate to the improper absorption of food in the gastrointestinal system. Many patients with gastrointestinal symptoms will have diarrhea and fatty, greasy, unusually foul-smelling stools. The patient may complain of excessive gas (flatulence), distended abdomen, weight loss, and generalized weakness. Not all people have digestive system complications; some people only have irritability or **depression**. Irritability is one of the most common symptoms in children with celiac disease.

Not all patients have these problems. Unrecognized and untreated celiac disease may cause or contribute to a variety of other conditions. The decreased ability to digest, absorb, and utilize food properly (malabsorption) may cause anemia (low red blood count) from iron deficiency or easy bruising from a lack of vitamin K. Poor mineral absorption may result in **osteoporosis**, or "brittle bones," which may lead to bone fractures. Vitamin D levels may be insufficient and bring about a "softening" of bones (osteomalacia), which produces pain and bony deformities, such as flattening or bending. Defects in the tooth enamel, characteristic of celiac disease, may be recognized by dentists. Celiac disease may be discovered during medical tests performed to investigate failure to thrive in infants, or lack of proper growth in children and adolescents. People with celiac disease may also experience lactose intolerance because they do not produce enough of the enzyme lactase, which breaks down the sugar in milk into a form the body can absorb. Other symptoms can include, muscle cramps, fatigue, delayed growth, tingling or numbness in the legs (from nerve damage), pale sores in the mouth (called aphthus ulcers), tooth discoloration, or missed menstrual periods (due to severe weight loss).

A distinctive, painful skin rash, called dermatitis herpetiformis, may be the first sign of celiac disease. Approximately 10% of patients with celiac disease have this rash, but it is estimated that 85% or more of patients with the rash have the disease.

Many disorders are associated with celiac disease, though the nature of the connection is unclear. One type of **epilepsy** is linked to celiac disease. Once their celiac disease is successfully treated, a significant number of these patients have fewer or no seizures. Patients with alopecia areata, a condition where hair loss occurs in sharply defined areas, have been shown to have a higher risk of celiac disease than the general population. There appears to be a higher percentage of celiac disease among people with **Down syndrome**, but the link between the conditions is unknown.

Several conditions attributed to a disorder of the immune system have been associated with celiac disease. People with insulin dependent **diabetes** (type I) have a much higher incidence of celiac disease. One source estimates that as many as one in 20 insulin-dependent diabetics may have celiac disease. Patients with juvenile chronic arthritis, some thyroid diseases, and IgA deficiency are also more likely to develop celiac disease.

There is an increased risk of intestinal lymphoma, a type of **cancer**, in individuals with celiac disease. Successful treatment of the celiac disease seems to decrease the chance of developing lymphoma.

Diagnosis

Because of the variety of ways celiac disease can manifest itself, it is often not discovered promptly. Its symptoms are similar to many other conditions including irritable bowel syndrome, Crohn's disease, ulcerative colitis, diverticulosis, intestinal infections, chronic fatigue syndrome, and depression. The condition may persist without diagnosis for so long that the patient accepts a general feeling of illness as normal. This leads to further delay in identifying and treating the disorder. It is not unusual for the disease to be identified in the course of medical investigations for seemingly unrelated problems. For example, celiac disease has been discovered during testing to find the cause of infertility.

If celiac disease is suspected, a blood test can be ordered. This test looks for the antibodies to gluten (called antigliadin, anti-endomysium, and antireticulin) that the immune system produces in celiac disease. Antibodies are chemicals produced by the immune system in response to substances that the body perceives to be threatening. Some experts advocate not just evaluating patients with symptoms, but using these blood studies as a screening test for high-risk individuals, such as those with relatives (especially first degree relatives) known to have the disorder. An abnormal result points towards celiac disease, but further tests are needed to confirm the diagnosis. Because celiac disease affects the ability of the body to absorb nutrients from food, several tests may be ordered to look for nutritional deficiencies. For example, doctors may order a test of iron levels in the blood because low levels of iron (anemia) may accompany celiac disease. Doctors may also order a test for fat in the stool, since celiac disease prevents the body from absorbing fat from food.

If these tests are suspicious for celiac disease, the next step is a biopsy (removal of a tiny piece of tissue surgically) of the small intestine. This is usually done by a gastroenterologist, a physician who specializes in diagnosing and treating bowel disorders. It is generally performed in the office, or in a hospital's outpatient department. The patient remains awake, but is sedated. A narrow tube, called an endoscope, is passed through the mouth, down through the stomach, and into the small intestine. A small sample of tissue is taken and sent to the laboratory for analysis. If it shows a pattern of tissue damage characteristic of celiac disease, the diagnosis is established.

The patient is then placed on a gluten-free diet (GFD). The physician will periodically recheck the level of antibodies in the patient's blood. After several months, the small intestine is biopsied again. If the diagnosis of celiac disease was correct (and the patient followed the rigorous diet), healing of the intestine will be apparent. Most experts agree that it is necessary to follow these steps in order to be sure of an accurate diagnosis.

Treatment and management

The only treatment for celiac disease is a gluten-free diet. This may be easy for the doctor to prescribe, but difficult for the patient to follow. For most people, adhering to this diet will stop symptoms and prevent damage to the intestines. Damaged villi can be functional again in three to six months. This diet must be followed for life. For people whose symptoms are cured by the gluten-free diet, this is further evidence that their diagnosis is correct.

Gluten is present in any product that contains wheat, rye, barley, or oats. It helps make bread rise, and gives many foods a smooth, pleasing texture. In addition to the many obvious places gluten can be found in a normal diet, such as breads, cereals, and pasta, there are many hidden sources of gluten. These include ingredients added to foods to improve texture or enhance flavor and products used in food packaging. Gluten may even be present on surfaces used for food preparation or cooking.

Fresh foods that have not been artificially processed, such as fruits, vegetables, and meats, are permitted as part of a GFD. Gluten-free foods can be found in health food stores and in some supermarkets. Mail-order food companies often have a selection of gluten-free products. Help in dietary planning is available from dieticians (health care professionals specializing in food and nutrition) or from support groups for individuals with celiac disease. There are many cookbooks on the market specifically for those on a GFD.

KEY TERMS

Antibodies—Proteins that provoke the immune system to attack particular substances. In celiac disease, the immune system makes antibodies to a component of gluten.

Gluten—A protein found in wheat, rye, barley, and oats.

Villi—Tiny, finger-like projections that enable the small intestine to absorb nutrients from food.

Treating celiac disease with a GFD is almost always completely effective. Gastrointestinal complaints and other symptoms are alleviated. Secondary complications, such as anemia and osteoporosis, resolve in almost all patients. People who have experienced lactose intolerance related to their celiac disease usually see those symptoms subside as well. Although there is no risk and much potential benefit to this treatment, it is clear that avoiding all foods containing gluten can be difficult.

Experts emphasize the need for lifelong adherence to the GFD to avoid the long-term complications of this disorder. They point out that although the disease may have symptom-free periods if the diet is not followed, silent damage continues to occur. Celiac disease cannot be "outgrown" or cured, according to medical authorities.

Prognosis

Patients with celiac disease must adhere to a strict GFD throughout their lifetime. Once the diet has been followed for several years, individuals with celiac disease have similar mortality rates as the general population. However, about 10% of people with celiac disease develop a cancer involving the gastrointestinal tract (both carcinoma and lymphoma).

There are a small number of patients who develop a refractory type of celiac disease, where the GFD no longer seems effective. Once the diet has been thoroughly assessed to ensure no hidden sources of gluten are causing the problem, medications may be prescribed. Steroids or immunosuppressant drugs are often used to try to control the disease. It is unclear whether these efforts meet with much success.

Prevention

There is no way to prevent celiac disease. However, the key to decreasing its impact on overall health is early diagnosis and strict adherence to the prescribed gluten-free diet.

Resources

BOOKS

Lowell, Jax Peters. *Against the Grain: The Slightly Eccentric Guide to Living Well without Wheat or Gluten.* New York: Henry Holt, 1996.

PERIODICALS

Gluten-Free Living (bimonthly newsletter) PO Box 105, Hastings-on-Hudson, NY 10706.

Guest, Jean. "Wheat's Your Problem?" *Diabetes Forecast* 49 (August 1996): 44–51.

Pruessner, H. "Detecting Celiac Disease in Your Patients." *American Family Physician* 57 (March 1998): 1023–34.

ORGANIZATIONS

American Celiac Society. 58 Musano Court, West Orange, NJ, 7052. (201) 325-8837.

Celiac Disease Foundation. 13251 Ventura Blvd., Suite 1, Studio City, CA 91604-1838. (818) 990-2354. <http://www.cdf@celiac.org>.

Celiac Sprue Association/United State of America (CSA/USA). PO Box 31700, Omaha, NE 68131-0700. (402) 558-0600.

Gluten Intolerance Group. PO Box 23053, Seattle, WA, 98102-0353. (206) 325-6980.

National Center for Nutrition and Dietetics. American Dietetic Association, 216 West Jackson Boulevard, Suite 800, Chicago, IL, 60606-6995. (800) 366-1655.

WEBSITES

National Institute of Diabetes & Digestive & Kidney Diseases. <http://www.niddk.nih.gov/health/digest/pubs/celiac/index.htm>.

Amy Vance, MS, CGC

Central core disease

Definition

Central core disease (CCD) is an inherited muscle disorder that affects many of the voluntary muscles necessary for movement. The hips and legs are particularly affected. Although central core disease is disabling, it is not fatal.

Description

First described in 1956, central core disease is one of a group of muscle disorders, or myopathies, named for certain abnormalities found in the muscle biopsies of people with the syndrome. CCD occurs when the central parts, or cores, of certain muscle cells are metabolically inactive, meaning they do not produce energy correctly. This happens because the cores lack a substance called mitochondria, the energy-producing parts of the muscle cells.

According to the **Muscular Dystrophy** Association, a muscle cell produces thousands of proteins during its lifetime. With all of the inheritable diseases of muscle, an altered **gene** leads to an absence of, or abnormality in, one of the proteins necessary for normal functioning of a muscle cell.

Scientists are pursuing a number of promising leads in their quest to understand the causes of CCD. New research suggests that muscle cells that have difficulty regulating calcium may cause central core disease.

Although CCD is not a progressive illness, different people experience varying degrees of weakness. Some children with CCD show mildly delayed motor milestones, then catch up and appear only slightly uncoordinated. Others have more severe delays, but also catch up somewhat and are able to walk and move about, although with more limitations. Some children use braces for walking, and a few use wheelchairs.

Genetic profile

Central core disease is inherited as a dominant trait, meaning that an individual with CCD has a 50% chance of passing the disorder on to each child. There are also occurrences of sporadic **inheritance**, which means that a gene alters spontaneously to cause the disorder in a person with no family history of the disease. In 1993, researchers identified the abnormal gene responsible for CCD. This finding has been important in understanding what causes central cores in the muscle and why the muscles of people with CCD are weak. According to scientific findings, an abnormality in a gene on **chromosome** 19 may lead to the disease.

Demographics

The disease becomes noticeable in early childhood, when muscle cramps are often present after exercising or performing other physical activities. Central core disease is often seen as "floppiness" in a newborn baby, followed by periods of persistent muscle weakness.

Signs and symptoms

Symptoms of central core disease are usually not severe; however, the disease can be disabling. A mild general weakness and hip displacement are key characteristics of the disease. Individuals with CCD reach motor

---

KEY TERMS

Dominant trait—A genetic trait where one copy of the gene is sufficient to yield an outward display of the trait; dominant genes mask the presence of recessive genes; dominant traits can be inherited from a single parent.

Malignant hyperthermia—A condition brought on by anesthesia during surgery.

Mitochondria—Organelles within the cell responsible for energy production.

Myopathy—Any abnormal condition or disease of the muscle.

Scoliosis—An abnormal, side-to-side curvature of the spine.

Sporadic inheritance—A status that occurs when a gene mutates spontaneously to cause the disorder in a person with no family history of the disorder.

---

skill milestones much later than those without the disorder. A child with the disease cannot run easily, and jumping and other physical activities are often impossible.

Other long-term problems caused by CCD include hip dislocation and curvature of the spine, a condition known as **scoliosis**. Central core disease also causes skin rash, muscular shrinkage, endocrine abnormalities, heart problems, or mental problems.

Diagnosis

The diagnosis of central core disease is made after several neurological tests are completed. These tests involve checking an individual's coordination, tendon reflexes such as the knee-jerk reaction, walking ability, and the ability to rise from a sitting position. A serum enzyme test might also be performed to measure how much muscle protein is circulating through the blood.

Treatment and management

Treatment measures greatly depend on the severity of the individual's symptoms, especially the degree of muscle weakness that is involved. Treatment measures include surgical procedures, pain management, muscle stimulation therapy, and physical therapy.

According to the Muscular Dystrophy Association, people who have central core disease are sometimes vulnerable to **malignant hyperthermia** (MH), a condition brought on by anesthesia during surgery. Malignant hyperthermia causes a rapid, and sometimes fatal, rise in body temperature, producing muscle stiffness. When susceptible individuals are exposed to the most commonly used general anesthetic, their muscles can become rigid and their body temperatures can rise to dangerous levels.

Prognosis

Fortunately, the outlook for children with this disease is generally positive. Although children with central core disease start their life with some developmental delays, many improve as they get older and stay active throughout their lives.

Resources

ORGANIZATIONS

Muscular Dystrophy Association. 3300 East Sunrise Dr., Tucson, AZ 85718. (520) 529-2000 or (800) 572-1717. <http://www.mdausa.org>.

WEBSITES

Central Core Disease. <http://www.mdausa.org/disease/ccd.html>.

Coping with Central Core Disease. <http://www.mdausa.org/publications/Quest/q62ccd.html>.

Bethanne Black

Central core disease of muscle *see* **Central core disease**

Cerebral giantism *see* **Sotos syndrome**

Cerebral palsy

Definition

Cerebral palsy (CP) is the term used for a group of nonprogressive disorders of movement and posture caused by abnormal development of, or damage to, motor control centers of the brain. CP is caused by events before, during, or after birth. The abnormalities of muscle control that define CP are often accompanied by other neurological and physical abnormalities.

Description

Voluntary movement (walking, grasping, chewing, etc.) is primarily accomplished using muscles that are attached to bones, known as the skeletal muscles. Control of the skeletal muscles originates in the cerebral cortex, the largest portion of the brain. Palsy means paraly-

sis, but may also be used to describe uncontrolled muscle movement. Therefore, cerebral palsy encompasses any disorder of abnormal movement and paralysis caused by abnormal function of the cerebral cortex. In truth, however, CP does not include conditions due to progressive disease or degeneration of the brain. For this reason, CP is also referred to as static (nonprogressive) encephalopathy (disease of the brain). Also excluded from CP are any disorders of muscle control that arise in the muscles themselves and/or in the peripheral nervous system (nerves outside the brain and spinal cord).

CP is not a specific diagnosis, but is more accurately considered a description of a broad but defined group of neurological and physical problems.

The symptoms of CP and their severity are quite variable. Those with CP may have only minor difficulty with fine motor skills, such as grasping and manipulating items with their hands. A severe form of CP could involve significant muscle problems in all four limbs, mental retardation, seizures, and difficulties with vision, speech, and hearing.

Muscles that receive abnormal messages from the brain may be constantly contracted and tight (spastic), exhibit involuntary writhing movements (athetosis), or have difficulty with voluntary movement (dyskinesia). There can also be a lack of balance and coordination with unsteady movements (ataxia). A combination of any of these problems may also occur. Spastic CP and mixed CP constitute the majority of cases. Effects on the muscles can range from mild weakness or partial paralysis (*paresis*), to complete loss of voluntary control of a muscle or group of muscles (*plegia*). CP is also designated by the number of limbs affected. For instance, affected muscles in one limb is monoplegia, both arms or both legs is diplegia, both limbs on one side of the body is hemiplegia, and in all four limbs is quadriplegia. Muscles of the trunk, neck, and head may be affected as well.

CP can be caused by a number of different mechanisms at various times—from several weeks after conception, through birth, to early childhood. For many years, it was accepted that most cases of CP were due to brain injuries received during a traumatic birth, known as birth asphyxia. However, extensive research in the 1980s showed that only 5–10% of CP can be attributed to birth trauma. Other possible causes include abnormal development of the brain, prenatal factors that directly or indirectly damage neurons in the developing brain, premature birth, and brain injuries that occur in the first few years of life.

Genetic profile

As noted, CP has many causes, making a discussion of the genetics of CP complicated. A number of hereditary/genetic syndromes have signs and symptoms similar to CP, but usually also have problems not typical of CP. Put another way, some hereditary conditions "mimic" CP. Isolated CP, meaning CP that is not a part of some other syndrome or disorder, is usually not inherited.

It might be possible to group the causes of CP into those that are genetic and those that are non-genetic, but most would fall somewhere in between. Grouping causes into those that occur during pregnancy (prenatal), those that happen around the time of birth (perinatal), and those that occur after birth (postnatal), is preferable. CP related to premature birth and multiple birth pregnancies (twins, triplets, etc.) is somewhat different and considered separately.

Prenatal causes

Although much has been learned about human embryology in the last couple of decades, a great deal remains unknown. Studying prenatal human development is difficult because the embryo and fetus develop in a closed environment—the mother's womb. However, the relatively recent development of a number of prenatal tests has opened a window on the process. Add to that more accurate and complete evaluations of newborns, especially those with problems, and a clearer picture of what can go wrong before birth is possible.

The complicated process of brain development before birth is susceptible to many chance errors that can result in abnormalities of varying degrees. Some of these errors will result in structural anomalies of the brain, while others may cause undetectable, but significant, abnormalities in how the cerebral cortex is "wired." An abnormality in structure or wiring is sometimes hereditary, but is most often due to chance, or a cause unknown at this time. Whether and how much genetics played a role in a particular brain abnormality depends to some degree on the type of anomaly and the form of CP it causes.

Several maternal-fetal infections are known to increase the risk for CP, including rubella (German measles, now rare in the United States), cytomegalovirus (CMV), and toxoplasmosis. Each of these infections is considered a risk to the fetus only if the mother contracts it for the first time during that pregnancy. Even in those cases, though, most babies will be born normal. Most women are immune to all three infections by the time they reach childbearing age, but a woman's immune status can be determined using the TORCH (Toxoplasmosis, Rubella, Cytomegalovirus, and Herpes) test before or during pregnancy.

Just as a stroke can cause neurologic damage in an adult, so too can this type of event occur in the fetus. A burst blood vessel in the brain followed by uncontrolled bleeding (coagulopathy), known as intracerebral hemorrhage, could cause a fetal stroke, or a cerebral blood vessel could be obstructed by a clot (embolism). Infants who later develop CP, along with their mothers, are more likely than other mother-infant pairs to test positive for factors that put them at increased risk for bleeding episodes or blood clots. Some coagulation disorders are strictly hereditary, but most have a more complicated basis.

A **teratogen** is any substance to which a woman is exposed that has the potential to harm the embryo or fetus. Links between a drug or other chemical exposure during pregnancy and a risk for CP are difficult to prove. However, any substance that might affect fetal brain development, directly or indirectly, could increase the risk for CP. Furthermore, any substance that increases the risk for premature delivery and low birth weight, such as alcohol, tobacco, or cocaine, among others, might indirectly increase the risk for CP.

The fetus receives all nutrients and oxygen from blood that circulates through the placenta. Therefore, anything that interferes with normal placental function might adversely affect development of the fetus, including the brain, or might increase the risk for premature delivery. Structural abnormalities of the placenta, premature detachment of the placenta from the uterine wall (abruption), and placental infections (chorioamnionitis) are thought to pose some risk for CP.

Certain conditions in the mother during pregnancy might pose a risk to fetal development leading to CP. Women with autoimmune anti-thyroid or anti-phospholipid (APA) antibodies are at slightly increased risk for CP in their children. A potentially important clue uncovered recently points toward high levels of cytokines in the maternal and fetal circulation as a possible risk for CP. Cytokines are proteins associated with inflammation, such as from infection or autoimmune disorders, and they may be toxic to neurons in the fetal brain. More research is needed to determine the exact relationship, if any, between high levels of cytokines in pregnancy and CP. A woman has some risk of developing the same complications in more than one pregnancy, slightly increasing the risk for more than one child with CP.

Serious physical trauma to the mother during pregnancy could result in direct trauma to the fetus as well, or injuries to the mother could compromise the availability of nutrients and oxygen to the developing fetal brain.

Perinatal causes

Birth asphyxia significant enough to result in CP is now uncommon in developed countries. Tight nuchal cord (umbilical cord around the baby's neck) and prolapsed cord (cord delivered before the baby) are possible causes of birth asphyxia, as are bleeding and other complications associated with placental abruption and placenta previa (placenta lying over the cervix).

Infection in the mother is sometimes not passed to the fetus through the placenta, but is transmitted to the baby during delivery. Any such infection that results in serious illness in the newborn has the potential to produce some neurological damage.

Postnatal causes

The remaining 15% of CP is due to neurological injury sustained after birth. CP that has a postnatal cause is sometimes referred to as acquired CP, but this is only accurate for those cases caused by infection or trauma.

Incompatibility between the Rh blood types of mother and child (mother Rh negative, baby Rh positive) can result in severe anemia in the baby (erythroblastosis fetalis). This may lead to other complications, including severe jaundice, which can cause CP. Rh disease in the newborn is now rare in developed countries due to routine screening of maternal blood type and treatment of pregnancies at risk. The routine, effective treatment of jaundice due to other causes has also made it an infrequent cause of CP in developed countries. Rh blood type poses a risk for recurrence of Rh disease if treatment is not provided.

Serious infections that affect the brain directly, such as meningitis and encephalitis, may cause irreversible damage to the brain, leading to CP. A seizure disorder early in life may cause CP, or may be the product of a hidden problem that causes CP in addition to seizures. Unexplained (idiopathic) seizures are hereditary in only a small percentage of cases. Although rare in infants born healthy at or near term, intracerebral hemorrhage and brain embolism, like fetal stroke, are sometimes genetic.

Physical trauma to an infant or child resulting in brain injury, such as from abuse, accidents, or near drowning/suffocation, might cause CP. Likewise, ingestion of a toxic substance such as lead, mercury, poisons, or certain chemicals could cause neurological damage. Accidental overdose of certain medications might also cause similar damage to the central nervous system.

Prematurity and multiple birth pregnancy

Advances in the medical care of premature infants in the last 20 years have dramatically increased the rate of survival of these fragile newborns. However, as gestational age at delivery and birth weight of a baby decrease, the risk for CP dramatically increases. A term

pregnancy is delivered at 37–41 weeks gestation. The risk for CP in a preterm infant (32–37 weeks) is increased about five-fold over the risk for an infant born at term. Survivors of extremely preterm births (less than 28 weeks) face as much as a fifty-fold increase in risk. About 50% of all cases of CP now being diagnosed are in children who were born prematurely.

Two factors are involved in the risk for CP associated with prematurity. First, premature babies are at higher risk for various CP-associated medical complications, such as intracerebral hemorrhage, infection, and difficulty in breathing, to name a few. Second, the onset of premature labor may be induced, in part, by complications that have already caused neurologic damage in the fetus. A combination of both factors almost certainly plays a role in some cases of CP. The tendency toward premature delivery tends to run in families, but the genetic mechanisms are far from clear.

An increase in multiple birth pregnancies in recent years, especially in the United States, is blamed on the increased use of fertility drugs. As the number of fetuses in a pregnancy increases, the risks for abnormal development and premature delivery also increase. Children from twin pregnancies have four times the risk of developing CP as children from singleton pregnancies, owing to the fact that more twin pregnancies are delivered prematurely. The risk for CP in a child of triplets is up to 18 times greater. Furthermore, recent evidence suggests that a baby from a pregnancy in which its twin died before birth is at increased risk for CP.

Demographics

Approximately 500,000 children and adults in the United States have CP, and it is newly diagnosed in about 6,000 infants and young children each year. The incidence of CP has not changed much in the last 20–30 years. Ironically, advances in medicine have decreased the incidence from some causes, Rh disease for example, but increased it from others, notably, prematurity and multiple birth pregnancies. No particular ethnic groups seem to be at higher risk for CP. However, people of disadvantaged background are at higher risk due to poorer access to proper prenatal care and advanced medical services.

Signs and symptoms

By definition, the defect in cerebral function causing CP is nonprogressive. However, the symptoms of CP often change over time. Most of the symptoms of CP relate in some way to the aberrant control of muscles. To review, CP is categorized first by the type of movement/postural disturbance(s) present, then by a description of which limbs are affected, and finally by the severity of motor impairment. For example, spastic diplegia refers to continuously tight muscles that have no voluntary control in both legs, while athetoid quadraparesis describes uncontrolled writhing movements and muscle weakness in all four limbs. These three-part descriptions are helpful in providing a general picture, but cannot give a complete description of any one person with CP. In addition, the various "forms" of CP do not occur with equal frequency—spastic diplegia is seen in more individuals than is athetoid quadraparesis. CP can also be loosely categorized as mild, moderate, or severe, but these are very subjective terms with no firm boundaries between them.

A muscle that is tensed and contracted is hypertonic, while excessively loose muscles are hypotonic. Spastic, hypertonic muscles can cause serious orthopedic problems, including **scoliosis** (spine curvature), hip dislocation, or contractures. A contracture is shortening of a muscle, aided sometimes by a weak-opposing force from a neighboring muscle. Contractures may become permanent, or "fixed," without some sort of intervention. Fixed contractures may cause postural abnormalities in the affected limbs. Clenched fists and contracted feet (equinus or equinovarus) are common in people with CP. Spasticity in the thighs causes them to turn in and cross at the knees, resulting in an unusual method of walking known as a "scissors gait." Any of the joints in the limbs may be stiff (immobilized) due to spasticity of the attached muscles.

Athetosis and dyskinesia often occur with spasticity, but do not often occur alone. The same is true of ataxia. It is important to remember that "mild CP" or "severe CP" refers not only to the number of symptoms present, but also to the level of involvement of any particular class of symptoms.

Mechanisms that can cause CP are not always restricted to motor-control areas of the brain. Other neurologically based symptoms may include:

• mental retardation/learning disabilities

• behavioral disorders

• seizure disorders

• visual impairment

• hearing loss

• speech impairment (dysarthria)

• abnormal sensation and perception

These problems may have a greater impact on a child's life than the physical impairments of CP, although not all children with CP are affected by other problems. Many infants and children with CP have growth impairment. About one-third of individuals with CP have moder-ate-to-severe mental retardation, one-third have mild mental retardation, and one-third have normal intelligence.

Diagnosis

The signs of CP are not usually noticeable at birth. Children normally progress through a predictable set of developmental milestones through the first 18 months of life. Children with CP, however, tend to develop these skills more slowly because of their motor impairments, and delays in reaching milestones are usually the first symptoms of CP. Babies with more severe cases of CP are normally diagnosed earlier than others.

Selected developmental milestones, and the ages for normally acquiring them, are given below. If a child does not acquire the skill by the age shown in parentheses, there is some cause for concern.

• Sits well unsupported—6 months (8–10 months)

• Babbles—6 months (8 months)

• Crawls—9 months (12 months)

• Finger feeds, holds bottle—9 months (12 months)

• Walks alone—12 months (15–18 months)

• Uses one or two words other than dada/mama—12 months (15 months)

• Walks up and down steps—24 months (24–36 months)

• Turns pages in books; removes shoes and socks—24 months (30 months)

Children do not consistently favor one hand over the other before 12–18 months, and doing so may be a sign that the child has difficulty using the other hand. This same preference for one side of the body may show up as asymmetric crawling or, later on, favoring one leg while climbing stairs.

It must be remembered that children normally progress at somewhat different rates, and slow beginning accomplishment is often followed by normal development. Other causes for developmental delay—some benign, some serious—should be excluded before considering CP as the answer. CP is nonprogressive, so continued loss of previously acquired milestones indicates that CP is not the cause of the problem.

No one test is diagnostic for CP, but certain factors increase suspicion. The Apgar score measures a baby's condition immediately after birth. Babies that have low Apgar scores are at increased risk for CP. Presence of abnormal muscle tone or movements may indicate CP, as may the persistence of infantile reflexes. Imaging of the brain using ultrasound, x rays, MRI, and/or CT scans may reveal a structural anomaly. Some brain lesions associated with CP include scarring, cysts, expansion of the cerebral

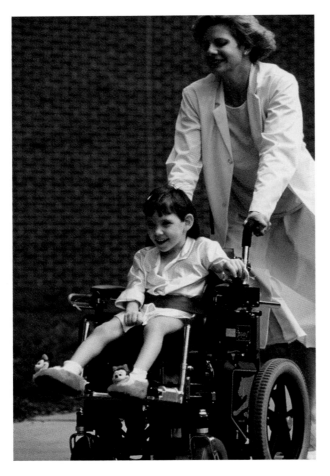

This nurse is taking a girl with cerebral palsy for a walk in her motorized wheelchair. Due to poor muscle control and coordination, many patients will require some form of assistive device. *(Photo Researchers, Inc.)*

ventricles (**hydrocephalus**), periventricular leukomalacia (an abnormality of the area surrounding the ventricles), areas of dead tissue (necrosis), and evidence of an intracerebral hemorrhage or blood clot. Blood and urine biochemical tests, as well as genetic tests, may be used to rule out other possible causes, including muscle and peripheral nerve diseases, mitochondrial and metabolic diseases, and other inherited disorders. Evaluations by a pediatric developmental specialist and a geneticist may be of benefit.

Cerebral palsy cannot be cured, but many of the disabilities it causes can be managed through planning and timely care. Treatment for a child with CP depends on the severity, nature, and location of the primary muscular symptoms, as well as any associated problems that might be present. Optimal care of a child with mild CP may involve regular interaction with only a physical therapist and occupational therapist, whereas care for a more severely affected child may include visits to multiple

medical specialists throughout life. With proper treatment and an effective plan, most people with CP can lead productive, happy lives.

Therapy

Spasticity, muscle weakness, coordination, ataxia, and scoliosis are all significant impairments that affect the posture and mobility of a person with CP. Physical and occupational therapists work with the patient and the family to maximize the ability to move affected limbs, develop normal motor patterns, and maintain posture. Assistive technology such as wheelchairs, walkers, shoe inserts, crutches, and braces are often required. A speech therapist and high-tech aids, such as computer-controlled communication devices, can make a tremendous difference in the life of those who have speech impairments.

Medications

Before fixed contractures develop, muscle-relaxant drugs such as diazepam (Valium), dantrolene (Dantrium), and baclofen (Lioresal) may be prescribed. Botulinum toxin (Botox), a newer and highly effective treatment, is injected directly into the affected muscles. Alcohol or phenol injections into the nerve controlling the muscle are another option. Multiple medications are available to control seizures, and athetosis can be treated using medications such as trihexyphenidyl HCl (Artane) and benztropine (Cogentin).

Surgery

Fixed contractures are usually treated with either serial casting or surgery. The most commonly used surgical procedures are tenotomy, tendon transfer, and dorsal rhizotomy. In tenotomy, tendons of the affected muscle are cut and the limb is cast in a more normal position while the tendon regrows. Alternatively, tendon transfer involves cutting and reattaching a tendon at a different point on the bone to enhance the length and function of the muscle. A neurosurgeon performing dorsal rhizotomy carefully cuts selected nerve roots in the spinal cord to prevent them from stimulating the spastic muscles. Neurosurgical techniques in the brain such as implanting tiny electrodes directly into the cerebellum, or cutting a portion of the hypothalamus, have very specific uses and have had mixed results.

Education

Parents of a child newly diagnosed with CP are not likely to have the necessary expertise to coordinate the full range of care their child will need. Although knowledgeable and caring medical professionals are indispensable for developing a care plan, a potentially more important source of information and advice is other

KEY TERMS

Asphyxia—Lack of oxygen. In the case of cerebral palsy, lack of oxygen to the brain.

Ataxia—A deficiency of muscular coordination, especially when voluntary movements are attempted, such as grasping or walking.

Athetosis—A condition marked by slow, writhing, involuntary muscle movements.

Cerebral palsy—Movement disability resulting from nonprogressive brain damage.

Coagulopathy—A disorder in which blood is either too slow or too quick to coagulate (clot).

Contracture—A tightening of muscles that prevents normal movement of the associated limb or other body part.

Cytokine—A protein associated with inflammation that, at high levels, may be toxic to nerve cells in the developing brain.

Diplegia—Paralysis affecting like parts on both sides the body, such as both arms or both legs.

Dorsal rhizotomy—A surgical procedure that cuts nerve roots to reduce spasticity in affected muscles.

Dyskinesia—Impaired ability to make voluntary movements.

Hemiplegia—Paralysis of one side of the body.

Hypotonia—Reduced or diminished muscle tone.

Quadriplegia—Paralysis of all four limbs.

Serial casting—A series of casts designed to gradually move a limb into a more functional position.

Spastic—A condition in which the muscles are rigid, posture may be abnormal, and fine motor control is impaired.

Spasticity—Increased muscle tone, or stiffness, which leads to uncontrolled, awkward movements.

Static encephalopathy—A disease of the brain that does not get better or worse.

Tenotomy—A surgical procedure that cuts the tendon of a contracted muscle to allow lengthening.

Prognosis

Cerebral palsy can affect every stage of maturation, from childhood through adolescence to adulthood. At each stage, those with CP, along with their caregivers, must strive to achieve and maintain the fullest range of experiences and education consistent with their abilities. The advice and intervention of various professionals remains crucial for many people with CP. Although CP itself is not considered a terminal disorder, it can affect a person's lifespan by increasing the risk for certain medical problems. People with mild cerebral palsy may have near-normal life spans, but the lifespan of those with more severe forms may be shortened. However, over 90% of infants with CP survive into adulthood.

The cause of most cases of CP remains unknown, but it has become clear in recent years that birth difficulties are not to blame in most cases. Rather, developmental problems before birth, usually unknown and generally undiagnosable, are responsible for most cases. The rate of survival for preterm infants has leveled off in recent years, and methods to improve the long-term health of these at-risk babies are now being sought. Current research is also focusing on the possible benefits of recognizing and treating coagulopathies and inflammatory disorders in the prenatal and perinatal periods. The use of magnesium sulfate in pregnant women with preeclampsia or threatened preterm delivery may reduce the risk of CP in very preterm infants. Finally, the risk of CP can be decreased through good maternal nutrition, avoidance of drugs and alcohol during pregnancy, and prevention or prompt treatment of infections.

Resources

BOOKS

Miller, Freema, and Steven J. Bachrach. *Cerebral Palsy: A Complete Guide for Caregiving.* Baltimore: Johns Hopkins University Press, 1995.

Peacock, Judith. *Cerebral Palsy.* Mankato, MN: Capstone Press, 2000.

Pimm, Paul. *Living With Cerebral Palsy.* Austin, TX: Raintree Steck-Vaughn Publishers, 2000.

Pincus, Dion. *Everything You Need to Know About Cerebral Palsy.* New York: Rosen Publishing Group, Inc., 2000

PERIODICALS

Chambers, Henry G. "Research in Cerebral Palsy." *The Exceptional Parent* 29 (July 1999): 50.

Myers, Scott M., and Bruce K. Shapiro. "Origins and Causes of Cerebral Palsy: Symptoms and Diagnosis." *The Exceptional Parent* 29 (April 1999): 28.

Seppa, Nathan. "Infections may underlie cerebral palsy." *Science News* 154 (October 17, 1998): 244.

parents who have dealt with the same set of difficulties. Support groups for parents of children with CP can be significant sources of both practical advice and emotional support. Many cities have support groups that can be located through the United Cerebral Palsy Association, and most large medical centers have special multidisciplinary clinics for children with developmental disorders.

Stephenson, Joan. "Cerebral Palsy Clues." *The Journal of the American Medical Association* 280 (21 October 1998): 1298.

ORGANIZATIONS

Epilepsy Foundation of America. 4351 Garden City Dr., Suite 406, Landover, MD 20785-2267. (301) 459-3700 or (800) 332-1000. <http://www.epilepsyfoundation.org>.

March of Dimes Birth Defects Foundation. 1275 Mamaroneck Ave., White Plains, NY 10605. (888) 663-4637. resourcecenter@modimes.org. <http://www.modimes.org>.

National Easter Seal Society. 230 W. Monroe St., Suite 1800, Chicago, IL 60606-4802. (312) 726-6200 or (800) 221-6827. <http://www.easter-seals.org>.

National Institute of Neurological Disorders and Stroke. 31 Center Drive, MSC 2540, Bldg. 31, Room 8806, Bethesda, MD 20814. (301) 496-5751 or (800) 352-9424. <http://www.ninds.nih.gov>.

National Society of Genetic Counselors. 233 Canterbury Dr., Wallingford, PA 19086-6617. (610) 872-1192. <http://www.nsgc.org/GeneticCounselingYou.asp>.

United Cerebral Palsy Association, Inc. (UCP). 1660 L St. NW, Suite 700, Washington, DC 20036-5602. (202)776-0406 or (800)872-5827. <http://www.ucpa.org>.

WEBSITES

"Cerebral Palsy: Hope Through Research." *National Institute of Neurological Disorders and Stroke.* <http://www.ninds.nih.gov/health_and_medical/pubs/cerebral_palsyhtr.htm>

"Cerebral Palsy Information Page." *National Institute of Neurological Disorders and Stroke.* <http://www.ninds.nih.gov/health_and_medical/pubs/cerebral_palsy.htm>

Scott J. Polzin, MS, CGC

▌Charcot-Marie-Tooth disease

Definition

Charcot-Marie-Tooth disease (CMT) is the name of a group of inherited disorders of the nerves in the peripheral nervous system (nerves throughout the body that communicate motor and sensory information to and from the spinal cord) causing weakness and loss of sensation in the limbs.

Description

CMT is named for the three neurologists who first described the condition in the late 1800s. It is also known as hereditary motor and sensory neuropathy and is sometimes called peroneal muscular atrophy, referring to the muscles in the leg that are often affected. The age of onset of CMT can vary anywhere from young childhood to the 50s or 60s. Symptoms typically begin by the age of 20. For reasons yet unknown, the severity in symptoms can also vary greatly, even among members of the same family.

Although CMT has been described for many years, it has only been since the early 1990s that the genetic cause of many types of CMT have become known. Therefore, knowledge about CMT has increased dramatically within a short time.

The peripheral nerves

CMT affects the peripheral nerves, those groups of nerve cells carrying information to and from the spinal cord and decreases their ability to carry motor commands to muscles, especially those furthest from the spinal cord located in the feet and hands. As a result, the muscles connected to these nerves eventually weaken. CMT also affects the sensory nerves that carry information from the limbs to the brain. Therefore, people with CMT also have sensory loss. This causes symptoms such as not being able to tell if something is hot or cold or difficulties with balance.

There are two parts of the nerve that can be affected in CMT. A nerve can be likened to an electrical wire, in which the wire part is the axon of the nerve and the insulation surrounding it is the myelin sheath. The job of the myelin is to help messages travel very fast through the nerves. CMT is usually classified depending on which part of the nerve is affected. People who have problems with the myelin have CMT type 1 and people who have abnormalities of the axon have CMT type 2.

Specialized testing of the nerves, called nerve conduction testing (NCV), can be performed to determine if a person has CMT1 or CMT2. These tests measure the speed at which messages travel through the nerves. In CMT1, the messages move too slow, but in CMT2 the messages travel at the normal speed.

Genetic profile

CMT is caused by changes (mutations) in any one of a number of genes that carry the instructions to make the peripheral nerves. Genes contain the instructions for how the body grows and develops before and after a person is born. There are probably at least 15 different genes that can cause CMT. However, as of early 2001, many have not yet been identified.

CMT types 1 and 2 can be broken down into subtypes based upon the **gene** that is causing CMT. The subtypes are labeled by letters. So there is CMT1A, CMT1B, etc. Therefore, the gene with a mutation that causes CMT1A is different from that which causes CMT1B.

Types of CMT

CMT1A

The most common type of CMT is called CMT1A. It is caused by a mutation in a gene called peripheral myelin protein 22 (PMP22) located on **chromosome** 17. The job of this gene is to make a protein (PMP22) that makes up part of the myelin. In most people who have CMT, the mutation that causes the condition is a duplication (doubling) of the PMP22 gene. Instead of having two copies of the PMP22 gene (one on each chromosome), there are three copies. It is not known how this extra copy of the PMP22 gene causes the observed symptoms. A small percentage of people with CMT1A do not have a duplication of the PMP22 gene, but rather have a point mutation in the gene. A point mutation is like a typo in the gene that causes it to work incorrectly.

Hereditary neuropathy with liability to pressure palsies (HNPP)

HNPP is a condition that is also caused by a mutation in the PMP22 gene. The mutation is a deletion resulting in only one copy of the PMP22 gene instead of two. People who have HNPP may have some of the signs of CMT. However, they also have episodes where they develop weakness and problems with sensation after compression of certain pressure point, such as the elbows or knee. These symptoms will often resolve after a few days or weeks, but sometimes they are permanent.

CMT1B

Another type of CMT, called CMT1B, is caused by a mutation in a gene called myelin protein zero (MPZ) located on chromosome 1. The job of this gene is to make the layers of myelin stick together as they are wrapped around the axon. The mutations in this gene are point mutations because they involve a change (either deletion, substitution, or insertion) at one specific component of a gene.

CMTX

Another type of CMT, called CMTX, is usually considered a subtype of CMT1 because it affects the myelin,

but it has a different type of **inheritance** than type 1 or type 2. In CMTX, the CMT causing gene is located on the X chromosome and is called connexin 32 (Cx32). The job of this gene is to code for a class of protein called connexins that form tunnels between the layers of myelin.

CMT2

There are at least five different genes that can cause CMT type 2. Therefore, CMT2 has subtypes A, B, C, D and E. Scientists have narrowed in on the location of most of the CMT2 causing genes. However, the specific genes and the mutations have not yet been found for most types. Very recently, the gene for CMT2E has been found. The gene is called neurofilament-light (NF-L). Because it has just been discovered, not much is known about how mutations in this gene cause CMT.

CMT3

In the past a condition called Dejerine-Sottas disease was referred to as CMT3. This is a severe type of CMT in which symptoms begin in infancy or early childhood. It is now known that this is not a separate type of CMT and in fact people who have onset in infancy or early childhood often have mutations in the PMP22 or MPZ genes.

CMT4

CMT4 is a rare type of CMT in which the nerve conduction tests have slow response results. However, it is classified differently from CMT1 because it is passed through families by a different pattern of inheritance. There are five different subtypes and each has only been described in a few families. The symptoms in CMT4 are often severe and other symptoms such as deafness may be present. There are three different genes that have been associated with CMT4. They are called MTMR2, EGR2, and NDRG1. More research is required to understand how mutations in these genes cause CMT.

Inheritance

Autosomal dominant inheritance

CMT1A and 1B, HNPP, and all of the subtypes of CMT2 have autosomal dominant inheritance. Autosomal refers to the first 22 pairs of chromosomes that are the same in males and females. Therefore, males and females are affected equally in these types. In a dominant condition, only one gene of a pair needs to have a mutation in order for a person to have symptoms of the condition. Therefore, anyone who has these types has a 50%, or one in two, chance of passing CMT on to each of their children. This chance is the same for each pregnancy and does not change based on previous children.

X-linked inheritance

CMTX has X-linked inheritance. Since males only have one X chromosome, they only have one copy of the Cx32 gene. Thus, when a male has a mutation in his Cx32 gene, he will have CMT. However, females have two X chromosomes and therefore have two copies of the Cx32 gene. If they have a mutation in one copy of their Cx32 genes, they will only have mild to moderate symptoms of CMT that may go unnoticed. This is because their normal copy of the Cx32 gene produces sufficient amounts of myelin.

Females pass on one or the other of their X chromosomes to their children—sons or daughters. If a woman with a Cx32 mutation passes her normal X chromosome, she will have an unaffected son or daughter who will not pass CMT on to their children. If the woman passes the chromosome with Cx32 mutation on she will have an affected son or daughter, although the daughter will be mildly affected or have no symptoms. Therefore, a woman with a Cx32 mutation has a 50%, or a one in two chance of passing the mutation to her children: a son will be affected, and a daughter may only have mild symptoms.

When males pass on an X chromosome, they have a daughter. When they pass on a Y chromosome, they have a son. Since the Cx32 mutation is on the X chromosome, a man with CMTX will always pass the Cx32 mutation on to his daughters. However, when he has a son, he passes on the Y chromosome, and therefore the son will not be affected. Therefore, an affected male passes the Cx32 gene mutation on to all of his daughters, but to none of his sons.

Autosomal recessive inheritance

CMT4 has autosomal recessive inheritance. Males and females are equally affected. In order for a person to have CMT4, they must have a mutation in both of their CMT causing genes—one inherited from each parent. The parents of an affected person are called carriers. They have one normal copy of the gene and one copy with a mutation. Carriers do not have symptoms of CMT. Two carrier parents have a 25%, or one in four chance of passing CMT on to each of their children.

Demographics

CMT has been diagnosed in people from all over the world. It occurs in approximately one in 2,500 people, which is about the same incidence as **multiple sclerosis**. It is the most common type of inherited neurologic condition.

Signs and symptoms

The onset of symptoms is highly variable, even among members of the same family. Symptoms usually progress very slowly over a person's lifetime. The main problems caused by CMT are weakness and loss of sensation mainly in the feet and hands. The first symptoms are usually problems with the feet such as high arches and problems with walking and running. Tripping while walking and sprained ankles are common. Muscle loss in the feet and calves leads to "foot drop" where the foot does not lift high enough off the ground when walking. Complaints of cold legs are common, as are cramps in the legs, especially after exercise.

In many people, the fingers and hands eventually become affected. Muscle loss in the hands can make fine movements such as working buttons and zippers difficult. Some patients develop tremor in the upper limbs. Loss of sensation can cause problems such as numbness and the inability to feel if something is hot or cold. Most people with CMT remain able to walk throughout their lives.

Diagnosis

Diagnosis of CMT begins with a careful neurological exam to determine the extent and distribution of weakness. A thorough family history should be taken at this time to determine if other people in the family are affected. Testing may be also performed to rule out other causes of neuropathy.

A nerve conduction velocity test should be performed to measure how fast impulses travel through the nerves. This test may show characteristic features of CMT, but it is not diagnostic of CMT. Nerve conduction testing may be combined with electromyography (EMG), an electrical test of the muscles.

A nerve biopsy (removal of a small piece of the nerve) may be performed to look for changes characteristic of CMT. However, this testing is not diagnostic of CMT and is usually not necessary for making a diagnosis.

Definitive diagnosis of CMT is made only by **genetic testing**, usually performed by drawing a small amount of blood. Testing is available to detect mutations in PMP22, MPZ, Cx32, and EGR2. However, research is progressing rapidly and new testing is often made available every few months. All affected members of a family have the same type of CMT. Therefore once a mutation is found in one affected member, it is possible to test other members who may have symptoms or are at risk of developing CMT.

Prenatal diagnosis

Testing during pregnancy to determine whether an unborn child is affected is possible if genetic testing in a family has identified a specific CMT-causing mutation. This can be done after 10-12 weeks of pregnancy using a procedure called chorionic villus sampling (CVS). CVS involves removing a tiny piece of the placenta and examining the cells. Testing can also be done by **amniocentesis** after 16 weeks gestation by removing a small amount of the amniotic fluid surrounding the baby and analyzing the cells in the fluid. Each of these procedures has a small risk of miscarriage associated with it, and those who are interested in learning more should check with their doctor or genetic counselor. Couples interested in these options should obtain **genetic counseling** to carefully explore all of the benefits and limitations of these procedures.

Treatment and management

There is no cure for CMT. However, physical and occupational therapy are an important part of CMT treatment. Physical therapy is used to preserve range of motion and minimize deformity caused by muscle shortening, or contracture. Braces are sometimes used to improve control of the lower extremities that can help tremendously with balance. After wearing braces, people often find that they have more energy because they are using less energy to focus on their walking. Occupational therapy is used to provide devices and techniques that can assist tasks such as dressing, feeding, writing, and other routine activities of daily life. Voice-activated software can also help people who have problems with fine motor control.

It is very important that people with CMT avoid injury that causes them to be immobile for long periods of time. It is often difficult for people with CMT to return to their original strength after injury.

There is a long list of medications that should be avoided if possible by people diagnosed with CMT such as hydralazine (Apresoline), megadoses of vitamin A, B6, and D, Taxol, and large intravenous doses of penicillin. Complete lists are available from the CMT support groups. People considering taking any of these medications should weigh the risks and benefits with their physician.

Prognosis

The symptoms of CMT usually progress slowly over many years, but do not usually shorten life expectancy. The majority of people with CMT do not need to use a wheelchair during their lifetime. Most people with CMT are able to lead full and productive lives despite their physical challenges.

KEY TERMS

Axon—Skinny, wire-like extension of nerve cells.

Myelin—A fatty sheath surrounding nerves in the peripheral nervous system, which help them conduct impulses more quickly.

Nerve conduction testing—Procedure that measures the speed at which impulses move through the nerves.

Neuropathy—A condition caused by nerve damage. Major symptoms include weakness, numbness, paralysis, or pain in the affected area.

Peripheral nerves—Nerves throughout the body that carry information to and from the spinal cord.

Resources

BOOKS

Parry, G. J., ed. *Charcot-Marie-Tooth Disorders: A Handbook for Primary Care Physicians.* Available from the CMT Association, 1995.

PERIODICALS

Keller. M. P., and P. F. Chance. "Inherited peripheral neuropathies." *Seminars in Neurology* 19, no. 4 (1999): 353–62.

Quest. A magazine for patients available from the Muscular Dystrophy Association.

Shy, M. E., J. Kamholz, and R. E. Lovelace, eds. "Charcot-Marie-Tooth Disorders." *Annals of the New York Academy of Sciences* 883 (1999).

ORGANIZATIONS

Charcot-Marie-Tooth Association (CMTA). 2700 Chestnut Parkway, Chester, PA 19013. (610) 499-9264 or (800) 606-CMTA. Fax: (610) 499-9267. cmtassoc@aol.com. <www.charcot-marie-tooth.org>.

CMT International. Attn: Linda Crabtree, 1 Springbank Dr. St. Catherine's, ONT L2S2K1. Canada (905) 687-3630. <www.cmtint.org>.

Muscular Dystrophy Association. 3300 East Sunrise Dr., Tucson, AZ 85718. (520) 529-2000 or (800) 572-1717. <http://www.mdausa.org>.

Neuropathy Association. 60 E. 42nd St. Suite 942, New York, NY 10165. (212) 692-0662. <www.neuropathy.org>.

WEBSITES

GeneClinics. University of Washington, Seattle. <www.geneclinics.org>.

HNPP—Hereditary Neuropathy with liability to Pressure Palsies. Online Support Group, <http://www.hnpp.org>.

OMIM—Online Mendelian Inheritance in Man. <www.ncbi.nlm.nih.gov/Omim>.

Karen M. Krajewski, MS, CGC

CHARGE syndrome

Definition

CHARGE syndrome, also known as CHARGE association, is a group of major and minor malformations that have been observed to occur together more frequently than expected by chance. The name of the syndrome is an acronym for some of its features, and each letter stands for the following conditions:

- C—Coloboma and/or cranial nerves
- H—Heart defects
- A—Atresia choanae,
- R—Retarded growth and development
- G—Genital anomalies
- E—Ear anomalies

While these features have classically been used for identification of affected individuals, many other malformations and medical problems have been observed to occur with this syndrome.

Description

CHARGE syndrome was first described in 1979 as an association of multiple congenital anomalies, all of which included choanal atresia, meaning the blocking of the choanae, the passages from the back of the nose to the throat which allow breathing through the nose. Soon after, several other papers were published describing similar patients who all had both choanal atresia and **coloboma**, that is a cleft or failure to close off the eyeball. It was in 1981 that the CHARGE acronym was proposed to describe the features of the condition. Due to the large number of patients described since 1979, many physicians now regard CHARGE association as a recognizable syndrome. However, the cause for the condition remains unclear. It is believed that perhaps a new dominant change in a **gene** is the cause for many cases. There have been a few familial cases but most cases are sporadic. Crucial development of the choanoa, heart, ear, and other organs occurs 35-45 days after conception and any disruption in development during this time is believed to lead to many of the features of the syndrome.

Infants with CHARGE syndrome generally have difficulty with feeding and most of those affected have mental retardation. About half die during the first year of life from respiratory insufficiency, central nervous system (CNS) malformations, and bilateral choanal atresia.

Genetic profile

Most cases of CHARGE syndrome are sporadic, meaning that they occur in a random or isolated way. However, reports of parent-to-child transmission of the condition indicate an autosomal dominant type of **inheritance**. There have also been cases in which a parent with one or two features of CHARGE had a child with enough features to fit the diagnosis. These families may demonstrate variable expressivity of a dominant gene. In addition, there have been a few cases of siblings affected, suggesting the possible presence of a mixture of cell types (germ line mosaicism) in a parent for a dominant mutation. Therefore, the recurrence risk for healthy parents of an affected child would be low, but not negligible.

Twin studies are often used to determine if the occurrence of a condition has a strong genetic component. One such study compared a pair of monozygotic twins, meaning identical twins resulting from a single **zygote** (fertilized egg that leads to the birth of two individuals), who were both affected with CHARGE syndrome and a pair of dizygotic twins, meaning twins that result from fertilization of two different eggs, of whom only one had the syndrome. Since monozygotic twins are roughly 100% genetically identical, this supports the idea that there is a strong genetic factor involved in CHARGE syndrome. Other interesting observations include slightly increased paternal age in sporadic cases. The mean paternal age in one study was 34 years as opposed to 30 years in a control group. Increased paternal age has been known to be associated with the increased occurrence of new dominant mutations in offspring.

Several patients with various **chromosome** defects have been diagnosed with CHARGE syndrome, again pointing to genetic factors as a cause. These cases of **chromosomal abnormalities** point to particular genes that should be further studied. In addition, some patients with CHARGE syndrome also have features of another condition called Di George sequence, which involves an immune deficiency, characteristic heart abnormalities and distinct craniofacial features. Many patients with Di George sequence have a missing chromosome 22q11. Therefore, newly diagnosed cases of CHARGE syndrome should have chromosome studies as well as molecular testing.

Demographics

The incidence of CHARGE syndrome is approximately one in 10,000. However, this is probably an underestimate of the true number of people affected. The incidence is likely to increase as the diagnostic features of the condition are refined and milder cases are diagnosed. CHARGE syndrome affects males more seriously than females, resulting in a higher number of females who survive. The cause of this is unclear. The syndrome has not been reported more often in any particular race or geographic area.

Signs and symptoms

CHARGE syndrome is believed to be caused by a disruption of fetal growth during the first three months of pregnancy and affecting many different organ systems undergoing development at that time.

Choanal atresia

Choanal atresia, the narrowing passages from the back of the nose to the throat, may occur on one or both sides (bilateral) of the nose. This condition usually leads to breathing difficulties shortly after birth. Bilateral choanal atresia may result in early death and surgery is often required to open up the nasal passages. Choanal atresia is also often accompanied by hearing loss. Since bilateral choanal atresia is rare, CHARGE syndrome should be considered in all babies with this finding. Fifty to sixty percent of children diagnosed with CHARGE syndrome have choanal atresia.

Heart abnormalities

Seventy-five to eighty-five percent of children with CHARGE syndrome have heart abnormalities. Many are minor defects, but many require treatment or surgery. Some of the heart problems seen in CHARGE Syndrome are very serious (e.g., Tetralogy of Fallot) and life threatening. Every child with a diagnosis of CHARGE syndrome should have an echocardiogram, a test that uses sound waves to produce pictures of the heart.

Coloboma and eye abnormalities

A coloboma is a cleft or failure to close off the eyeball properly. This can result in a keyhole shaped pupil or abnormalities in the retina of the eye or its optic nerve. The condition is visible during an ophthalmology exam. Colobomas may or may not cause visual changes. About 80% of children with CHARGE syndrome have colobomas and the effect on vision varies from mild to severe. Other eye abnormalities include microphthalmia (small eye slits) or anophthalmia (no eyes). Consistent eye examinations are recommended for children diagnosed with the syndrome.

Ear abnormalities and deafness

At least 90% of patients with CHARGE syndrome have either external ear anomalies or hearing loss. The most common external ear anomalies include low-set ears, asymmetric ears, or small or absent ear lobes. The degree of hearing loss varies from mild to severe. It is important for all patients to have regular hearing exams over time so that changes in sound perception can be detected. Hearing aids are used as soon as hearing loss is detected. Some patients require corrective surgery of the outer ear, so that a hearing aid can be worn. Children with CHARGE syndrome often develop ear infections and this can affect hearing over time as well.

Cranial nerve defects

Defects related to the formation of the cranial nerves during fetal development are common in patients with CHARGE syndrome. The defects include anosmia (inability to smell), facial palsy, hearing loss, and swallowing difficulty. Facial palsy is the inability to sense or control movement of part of the face. This usually occurs on one side of the face, which, in affected individuals, results in a characteristic asymmetric and expressionless look. Swallowing problems can also occur along with several different defects in the formation of the throat.

Facial features

The facial features of CHARGE syndrome are considered minor diagnostic signs because they are not as obvious as the facial features of other genetic syndromes. However, many patients have facial asymmetry, a small and underdeveloped jaw, a broad forehead, square face, arched eyebrows, and external ear malformations.

Growth and developmental delays

Most babies with CHARGE syndrome have normal length and weight at birth. Difficulty with feeding and the presence of other malformations often leads to weight loss, so that these babies usually weigh less for their age. Teenagers are also often shorter than average due to a delay in the onset of puberty. In a small number of patients, growth delay is due to a lack of growth hormone.

There are serious delays in motor development of children with CHARGE syndrome as well. Many children have low muscle tone and difficulty with balance that leads to delays in walking. Physical therapy is often helpful. Most children with CHARGE syndrome are classified as mentally retarded. However, successful treatment of other features of the condition can improve learning potential. Therefore, assessments made before other medical problems are addressed are often more pessimistic than later exams.

Urogenital abnormalities

Most obvious in males, underdevelopment of the genitals occurs in at least half of the male patients diagnosed with CHARGE syndrome and in some females as well. Abnormalities of genitalia in males include an underdeveloped penis (micropenis or microphallus) and testicles that fail to descend to the scrotum (cryptorchidism). In females, there may be overgrowth or underdevelopment of the labia or clitoris. Information concerning the fertility of patients is not available. About 25% of children have renal abnormalities that may lead to repeated infections. A renal ultrasound is indicated in children with the syndrome.

Central nervous system anomalies

In one series of tested patients, CNS anomalies were noted in 83% of the patients who underwent imaging tests that produce pictures of the brain such as MRI, CT scan, and ultrasound, or after autopsy. The CNS anomalies included diminution of the size of the brain (cerebral atrophy), asymmetry, and midline defects such as partial development (e.g., agenesis of the corpus callosum). In addition, brain stem dysfunction has also been observed after birth, a disorder that can cause respiratory and swallowing problems. These findings were associated with a poor prognosis.

Associated anomalies

Many other features have been reported in patients with CHARGE syndrome. Some of these include a cleft lip and/or palate, dental anomalies, absence of the thymus and parathyroid glands that leads to immunodeficiency (the inability of the body to produce a normal immune response), seizures, abnormally low levels of calcium (hypocalcaemia) or sugar (hypoglycemia) in the body, obstruction of the anal opening (imperforate anus), groin hernias, curvature of the spine (**scoliosis**), skeletal anomalies, body temperature regulation problems and umbilical hernias.

Diagnosis

Since there is currently no genetic test available for CHARGE syndrome, the diagnosis is based on clinical features. There is disagreement about the conditions required for diagnosis. Some suggest that one major malformation plus four of the other features suggested by the CHARGE acronym are sufficient. Others suggest that four major characteristics or three major characteristics plus three minor characteristics are sufficient for diagnosis.

The Charge Syndrome Foundation defines a specific set of birth defects and most common features to diagnose CHARGE syndrome. These major features include: choanal atresia, coloboma, cranial nerve abnormalities and conditions, such as swallowing problems (due to cra-

nial nerve IX/X defects), facial palsy (due to cranial nerve VII defects), hearing loss (due to cranial nerve VIII defects), heart defects, and retardation of growth and development.

Other minor features have also been reported that are either less common or less specific to CHARGE syndrome. These include genital abnormalities, cleft lip and/or palate, tracheoesophageal fistula and facial distortions.

Diagnosis of CHARGE syndrome before birth has not yet been reported. The condition may be suspected when a **prenatal ultrasound** reveals fetal growth restriction, CNS malformations, heart defects, and urinary tract malformations. In one series, 37.5% of patients diagnosed with CHARGE were noted to have an abnormal feature noted on ultrasound.

There are several other conditions that include signs similar to CHARGE syndrome. These include VACTERL association (for vertebral, anal, cardiac, tracheoesophageal, renal and limb abnormalities, velocardiofacial (VCF) syndrome (**deletion 22q11 syndrome**), and prenatal retinoic acid exposure (**Accutane embryopathy**).

Treatment and management

Treatment for CHARGE syndrome is specific to the features present in each child. Choanal atresia can be treated with dilatations of the choanoa or nasal passages. Heart defects may require surgery. Children with CHARGE syndrome should get ophthalmology and hearing screens every six months. Plastic surgery is sometimes needed for corrections of ear malformations or facial asymmetry. Medications are needed when seizures are present and growth hormone is sometimes taken for growth delay or underdeveloped genitalia.

A developmental evaluation and a plan for special education are required. Patients with CHARGE syndrome who have both hearing and vision difficulty should receive care from childhood educators experienced in dual sensory impairment. Once these children establish a system of mobility and communication, the degree of developmental retardation may improve. Lengthy hospital stays for children with CHARGE syndrome may limit the ability of specialists to work with the child in the early months. Once major hospitalizations are completed, development may improve as the result of regular care by the appropriate child specialists. Other learning problems have been noted and should also be addressed if present. These include attention deficit disorder, **autism**, and obsessive-compulsive disorder. Parents are often in the position of coordinating the many components of special education for their children.

The national and international support groups for CHARGE syndrome are able to provide information and assistance in this area.

Prognosis

It has been noted in several studies that about half of patients diagnosed with CHARGE syndrome die from complications of the condition. One study suggests that 40% of those die after birth. Factors that appear to influence survival include the presence of CNS malformations, bilateral choanal atresia, TE fistula, and male gender. Heart abnormalities and brain stem dysfunctions were not found to be related to poor prognosis. Significant hospitalizations are needed for most children with CHARGE syndrome.

Resources

BOOKS

Jones, Kenneth Lyons. *Smith's Recognizable Patterns of Human Malformation.* 5th ed. Philadelphia: W.B. Saunders Company, 1997.

McKusick, Victor. *Mendelian Inheritance in Man: A Catalog of Human Genes and Genetic Disorders.* 12th ed. Baltimore: The Johns Hopkins University Press, 1998.

PERIODICALS

Blake, K., et. al. "CHARGE Association: An Update and Review for the Primary Pediatrician." *Clinical Pediatrics* (1998): 159-173.

Tellier, A. L., et al. "CHARGE Syndrome: Report of 47 Cases and Review." *American Journal of Medical Genetics* (1998): 402-409.

ORGANIZATIONS

CHARGE Family Support Group. 82 Gwendolen Ave., London, E13 ORD. UK 020-8552-6961. <http://www.widerworld.co.uk/charge>.

CHARGE Syndrome Foundation. 2004 Parkade Blvd., Columbia, MO 65202-3121. (800) 442-7604. <http://www.chargesyndrome.org>.

Sonja Rene Eubanks, MS, CGC

Chediak-Higashi syndrome

Definition

Chediak-Higashi syndrome (CHS) is a very rare disease that affects almost every organ in the body. It is an autosomal recessive disease that results from an abnormality in lysosomes (a sac-like container of enzymes) that travel within cells. The problems that occur with this disease are quite varied and present in two stages.

Description

Chediak-Higashi syndrome was named for the two scientists who, in 1957, further detailed the disorder first described by a Cuban doctor in 1943. The disease progresses through two different stages: the "stable phase" and the "accelerated phase." This rare disease has both classic external signs and distinct cellular problems that always result in a fatal outcome.

Affected individuals have many kinds of immune system problems, making them more likely to get infections and cell proliferation problems. People with CHS have a lowered ability to target infectious organisms, and once their immune cells do become involved, they have a harder time killing the infectious organisms.

Affected individuals also have problems with their melanocytes, the cells that produce melanin, the compound that gives skin, hair, and eyes their color. Often, this can result in signs of **albinism** (lack of color in the skin, hair, and eyes).

Genetic profile

Chediak-Higashi is an autosomal recessive disease, which requires both parents to be carriers of altered, or mutated, genes. CHS often occurs in families with a history of marrying close relatives. Based on **genetic mapping** that was first done in a mouse model of Chediak-Higashi syndrome, a mutated **gene** found on **chromosome** 1q is thought to be the cause of the disease. This gene is called LYST.

Genetic tests of many different affected people with the disease have revealed strong signs of allelic variability (different mutations in the same gene). Some evidence suggests that the allelic variability accounts for the many different presentations of the disease, such as differing age of presentation, differences in the severity of symptoms, and different progression into the second stage of the disease.

Demographics

About 200 cases of CHS have been described in the world's literature. It is seen in the same number of males and females. Often there is a history of intermarriage.

Signs and symptoms

People with Chediak-Higashi syndrome will often have many different clinical problems such as recurrent bacterial infections without clear causes, fevers that cannot be explained, severe gingivitis (gum disease), peripheral and cranial neuropathies, vision problems, lack of coordination, weakness, easy bruising, and loss of coloring (hypopigmentation) of the hair, skin and eyes.

During the accelerated phase, affected people may show signs of enlargement of the liver and spleen (hepatosplenomegaly), low blood platelet counts (thrombocytopenia), low counts of a certain white blood cell group (neutropenia), and low red blood cell counts (anemia). Abnormal cells can cause bone marrow infiltration and suppression, and this may lower blood counts further, making affected individuals even more susceptible to get infections. The transformation to the accelerated phase of this disease tends to occur in the first or second decade of life.

Diagnosis

Diagnosis of CHS is based on microscopic examination of an affected person's blood, and possibly their bone marrow. Examiners look for giant lysosomal granules, which are abnormal groups of cellular sections inside certain white blood cells. At present, the carrier state of Chediak-Higashi syndrome cannot be diagnosed. Prenatal testing has been done using fetal blood samples and cells taken from the amniotic fluid around the fetus. **Genetic testing** is not yet available.

Since this disorder is passed on in an autosomal recessive fashion, parents who have one affected child should have **genetic counseling** before future pregnancies. With each pregnancy, these parents will have a 25% chance of having another affected child.

Treatment and management

The treatment of Chediak-Higashi syndrome differs based on the stage of the illness. During the stable phase, treatment is aimed at controlling infectious problems. Prophylactic antibiotics can be given to affected individ-

KEY TERMS

Allelic variability—Different mutations in the same gene, producing like outcomes.

Lysosome—Membrane-enclosed compartment in cells, containing many hydrolytic enzymes; where large molecules and cellular components are broken down.

Melanin—Pigments normally produced by the body that give color to the skin and hair.

Melanocyte—A cell that can produce melanin.

uals to reduce the risk of contracting the more common infections. Some evidence suggests that treatment with high doses of ascorbic acid (vitamin C) can help improve people clinically as well as improve immune system cell functions in laboratory tests.

During the accelerated phase of this disease, treatment is very difficult. Some affected people have done well with chemotherapy that is aimed at the abnormally growing cells. Some literature has claimed benefits from bone marrow transplants. Also, some literature has indicated that the vaccination of affected individuals against specific viruses may help prevent transformation of the disease from the stable phase into the accelerated phase.

Prognosis

Most affected people described in the medical literature died of infections during the accelerated phase of CHS. This occurred during their youth or teenage years. There are some reports of affected people living into their 30s.

Resources

BOOKS

Nathan, David, et al. "Disorders of Degranulation: Chediak-Higashi Syndrome." *Nathan and Oski's Hematology of Infancy and Childhood* Philadelphia, Pennsylvania: W. B. Saunders Company, 1998.

WEBSITES

Lo, Wilson, et al. "Entry 214500: Chediak-Higashi Syndrome; CHS1." *OMIM—Online Mendelian Inheritance In Man* <http://www3.ncbi.nlm.nih.gov/Omim/searchomim.html.>

Benjamin M. Greenberg

Chiari malformation *see* **Arnold-Chiari malformation**

Chondrodysplasia punctata

Definition

Chondrodysplasia punctata is a group of inherited disorders affecting the skeletal system, skin, eyes, and mental functioning.

Description

Chondrodysplasia punctata is characterized by shortened bones, punctated or dot-like calcification deposits in the cartilage, and abnormal peroxisomes. Peroxisomes are structures within cells that help remove toxins from the body.

There are three main variations of chondrodysplasia punctata: **rhizomelic chondrodysplasia punctata**, non-rhizomelic chondrodysplasia punctata, and Sheffield type. Within these variations, there are different syndromes characterized by distinct anomalies and modes of transmission.

Rhizomelic chondrodysplasia punctata is characterized by shortened long bones in the arms and legs, abnormalities of the spine, stippled or dotted appearance to the cartilage, scaling of the skin, cataract, and profound mental retardation. This type of chondrodysplasia punctata is caused by a single-gene mutation. Most fetuses with rhizomelic chondrodysplasia punctata die *in utero* or shortly after birth. Those that survive usually die within the first 10 years of life.

Non-rhizomelic chondrodysplasia punctata, sometimes called Conradi Hunermann disease, encompasses several distinct syndromes with unique characteristics and modes of transmission. Happle's chondrodysplasia is one type of non-rhizomelic chondrodysplasia characterized by asymmetry of the arms and legs, distinctive skin sores or scales, and cataract often affecting only one eye. Intelligence is usually normal. This type predominantly affects women and is usually lethal in males, generally resulting in miscarriage of male fetuses.

Another type of non-rhizomelic chondrodysplasia is brachytelephalangic chondrodysplasia punctata, which is characterized by severe facial abnormalities, abnormalities of the cartilage in the trachea and larynx, calcifications in the feet and legs, and hypoplastic, or small, little fingers and little toes. The abnormal facial features of this syndrome are called Binder's maxillonasal dystosis and include abnormalities of the upper jaw, flat nose, cleft palate, smooth or absent philtrum, and small teeth. These facial malformations and anomalies of the trachea and larynx can cause serious breathing difficulties for newborns. Infants with brachytelephalangic chondrodysplasia punctata often require respiratory therapy. This

syndrome primarily affects boys and may cause mental retardation.

Sheffield type of chondrodysplasia punctata is a mild form of the disorder affecting males and females equally. It is characterized by the abnormal dotted cartilage formations, flattened facial features, and mental retardation. This is considered a milder form of the disorder. The **inheritance** has not been determined, and the genetic mutation responsible has not been identified.

Genetic profile

The genetic cause of rhizomelic chondrodysplasia punctata is well documented. Many of the anomalies result from abnormalities of the perisomes and the resulting inability of the body to process and remove toxic enzymes and proteins. Perisomes are structures found within cells that remove toxins from cells and therefore from the body. Researchers have identified a genetic mutation of the peroxisome biogenesis factor 7 (PEX7) as causing these perisomal abnormalities. This mutation is transmitted as an autosomal recessive trait. Autosomal recessive conditions are carried on a **chromosome** that is not involved in determining sex and must be present in both parents to be transmitted to a child. In the case of rhizomelic chondrodysplasia, the PEX7 **gene** is found on chromosome 4 in the 4p16 locus.

Non-rhizomelic chondrodysplasia is an X-linked disorder, which means the mutations responsible for causing it are located on the X chromosome. There are two types of X-linked transmission: dominant and recessive. In X-linked dominant traits, the condition will manifest if only one copy of the genetic mutation is present. For this reason, many X-linked dominant conditions are milder in females than in males. Genetic material on the second X chromosome can reduce the effects of the mutation. X-linked dominant mutations can have more severe effects in females and may be lethal in males. Happle's chondrodysplasia is an X-linked dominate condition resulting from mutations in the emopamil binding protein (EBP) gene.

In X-linked recessive traits, the genetic mutation is recessive, meaning the characteristics of the mutation will be seen only when another normal copy of the gene is not present. For this reason, X-linked recessive mutations most frequently affect males. Females must have two mutated copies of the same gene to demonstrate the abnormalities the mutation causes. It is rare for females to be affected by X-linked recessive genetic mutations, but they may be carriers, passing the gene on to their offspring. Brachytelephalangic chondrodysplasia punctata is an X-linked recessive condition caused by a mutation of the arylsulfatase E (ARSE) gene and a deletion of the short arm of X chromosome.

Demographics

Chondrodysplasia punctata is a very rare condition. The exact prevalence is unknown.

The rhizomelic type of chondrodysplasia punctata is an autosomal recessive condition affecting males and females equally. In the non-rhizomelic types of the disorder, Happle's chondrodysplasia punctata affects females almost exclusively and is generally lethal to males. Brachytelephalangic chondrodysplasia punctata is seen more frequently in males; however, it may be seen in females. The milder form of the disorder, Sheffield type, affects females and males equally.

Signs and symptoms

The symptoms of chondrodysplasia punctata may involve the skeletal system, cartilage, face, eyes, and intellectual functioning. The specific signs and symptoms of this disorder depend on which type is present.

The symptoms of rhizomelic chondrodysplasia punctata can include:

- abnormal hair loss
- cataract
- cartilage abnormalities
- curvature of the spine
- facial abnormalities
- **ichthyosis** (scaly skin)
- mental retardation
- microcephaly
- short stature or dwarfism

The symptoms of non-rhizomelic chondrodysplasia punctata can include:

- abnormalities of the eye
- abnormalities of the cartilage in the larynx and trachea
- asymmetry of the body
- cartilage abnormalities
- dwarfism
- hearing impairment
- heart defects
- mental retardation
- mid-face abnormalities
- kidney malformations
- prematurity

- punctate vertebrae (dotted appearance in x rays)
- short and in-curving fingers
- shortened limbs

Diagnosis

For parents who know that they are carriers of the X-linked type of chondrodysplasia punctata, there is a prenatal procedure and test called preimplantation genetic diagnosis (PGD). After in vitro fertilization (IVF), PGD can test for genetic abnormalities, as well as gender before an embryo is implanted.

Prenatal ultrasound may be helpful in diagnosing chondrodysplasia punctata in the fetus. A second trimester ultrasound may detect the characteristic punctated calcifications of the spine and feet. Combined with evidence of shortened limbs, a diagnosis may be made. However, in milder cases of the disorder, the defects may be too subtle for detection by a routine prenatal ultrasound.

A physical examination may diagnose the external features of this disorder, including the facial abnormalities, shortened limbs, curvature of the spine, and ichthyosis.

A definitive diagnosis may be made by x ray of the limbs and spine. In children of one year or younger, punctated calcifications may be seen in the long bone and the feet in the areas of cartilage at the ends of growing bones. This cartilage disappears after the first year of age and is replaced with growth plates. These plates appear normal on x ray. In adults and older children, the diagnosis is based on shortened bones in the arms and legs and the presence of other physical characteristics of the disorder.

Treatment and management

The treatment and management of chondrodysplasia punctata is primarily orthopedic and dermatologic. The characteristic stippling or dotted cartilage will disappear as the child ages; however, shortened arms and legs and curvature of the spine require orthopedic treatment. In some cases, surgery may be necessary to help patients whose legs are different lengths.

In some individuals, bone growth may be induced by a surgical bone-lengthening procedure. This procedure involves several surgeries and an extensive recovery period. The bone to be lengthened is cut. Leaving a narrow gap between the two pieces of bone, metal pins are inserted into the bone and the skin is closed. An external frame is attached to the pins. Gradually, the bone is pulled apart just enough to provide a small gap

KEY TERMS

Asymmetry—Similar size, length, shape on both sides of the body.

Autosomal—Genetic trait found on a chromosome that is not involved in determining sex.

Cataract—Clouding of the lens in the eye.

Cleft palate—An abnormal opening or cleft between roof of the mouth and the nasal cavity.

Dermatologic—Pertaining to the field of dermatology, the science of the skin and diseases that affect the skin.

Calcification—The process by which tissue becomes hardened by the depositing of calcium.

Dominant—A genetic trait that is expressed when only one copy of the gene is present.

Hypoplastic—Small.

Ichthyosis—A skin condition characterized by a fish-scale appearance.

In vitro fertilization (IVF)—Sometimes referred to as "test tube baby," IVF is the fertilization of a human egg outside the body.

Larynx—The voice box.

Microcephaly—A birth defect in which the brain and head are too small.

Mutation—A permanent change in genetic material that is transmittable.

Orthopedic—Pertaining to the field of orthopedics, the science of the bones and diseases of the bones.

Peroxisomes—Structures within the cell that remove toxins from the cell.

Philtrum—The grooved space between the nose and the upper lip.

Prenatal ultrasound—An imaging test using high-frequency sound waves to create images of internal organs. Prenatal indicates the test is preformed on a fetus while still in the womb.

Prevalence—The number of individuals in a population that have a specific condition.

Punctated—Having a dotted pattern.

Vertebrae—Boney structures of the spine.

Recessive—A genetic trait that is only expressed when another identical recessive gene is present.

Trachea—The windpipe.

X-linked—A genetic trait that is carried on the X chromosome.

X ray—An imaging test that uses beams of energy to create images of structures within the body.

for the bone to grow into. As the bone grows, the space is widened and more bone grows. After the bone has healed, the pins are surgically removed.

Spinal abnormalities, such as spinal cord compression and **scoliosis**, may be treated surgically. A spinal column fusion can relieve the stress on the spinal cord caused by malformations of the spinal column. In a spinal fusion, two or more vertebrae are fused together using bone grafts or metal rods.

Ichthyosis is often most severe at birth and can resolve completely as the child ages. However, in some individuals, the skin lesions may be extensive and long lasting, leading to recurrent skin infections. Management of ichthyosis involves topical treatment and, in severe cases, bandaging to help prevent infection.

Prognosis

Prognosis of chondrodysplasia punctata depends on the type. The rhizomelic form of this disorder has a very poor prognosis. Most individuals with this type of chondrodysplasia punctata do not survive the fetal period or die shortly after birth. Of those that do survive, life expectancy is 10 years or less. Along with the skeletal anomalies, profound mental retardation is common as well.

The non-rhizomelic type, also known as Conradi Hunermann disease, can have a better prognosis. Though the condition is extremely rare, a range of outcomes has been reported from death to mildly affected adults. The X-linked dominant type, or Happle's type, is usually lethal to males, and they generally do not survive past the second trimester of pregnancy. However, females with this type usually survive and may have normal intelligence.

The X-linked recessive type called brachytelephalangic chondrodysplasia punctata can have a range of possible prognoses. Because a component of this type is a flat mid-face, small nose, and cartilage abnormalities of the larynx and trachea, these children may have breathing difficulties and may die shortly after birth. If these anomalies are not present or are mild, the prognosis is much better. Individuals with this type of the disorder usually have normal intelligence.

Resources

BOOKS

Rimoin, David, Ralph Lachman, and Shelia Unger. "Chrondrfodysplasia." In *Emery and Rimion's Principles and Practice of Medical Genetics,* 4th edition, edited by David L. Rimoin, J. Michael Connor, Reed Pyeritz, and Bruce R. Korf. London: Churchull Livingstone, 2002.

PERIODICALS

Has, Cristina, Leena Bruckner-Tuderman, Dietmar Muller, et al. "The Conradi-Hunerman-Happle Syndrome (CDPX2) and Emopamil Binding Protein: Novel Mutations, and Somatic and Gonadal Mosaicism." *Human Molecular Genetics* 9, no 13(2000): 1951–1955.

Unger, Sheila. "A Genetic Approach to the Diagnosis of Skeletal Dysplasia." *Clinical Orthopedics and Related Research* 401 (2002): 32–38.

ORGANIZATIONS

Human Growth Foundation. 997 Glen Cove Ave., Suite 5, Glen Head, NY, 11545. (800) 451-6434. (April 8, 2005.) <http://www.hgfound.org>.

Little People of America. 5289 NE Elam Young Parkway, Suite F-100, Hillsboro, OR 97124. Toll Free: (888) LPA-2001, Direct: (503) 846-1562. Fax: (503) 846-1590. (April 8, 2005.) <http://www.lpaonline.org/index.html>.

March of Dimes. 1275 Mamaroneck Ave., White Plaines, NY 10605. (April 8, 2005.) <http://www.marchofdimes.com>.

WEB SITES

Online Mendelian Inheritance in Man (OMIM). Johns Hopkins University, Baltimore, MD. December 22, 2004. (April 8, 2005.) <http://www.ncbi.nlm.nih.gov/omim>.

Rhizomelic Chondrodysplasia Punctata (RCP) Family Support Group. (Accessed April 1, 2005.) <http://www.angelfire.com/in/sassyshideout/RCP.html>.

Deborah L. Nurmi, MS

Chondroectodermal dysplasia
see Ellis-Van Creveld syndrome

▌Chondrosarcoma

Definition

Chondrosarcoma is a malignant tumor that produces a special type of connective tissue called cartilage. Malignant tumors have cells that have the ability to invade and are characterized by uncontrolled growth.

Description

Cartilage is a type of connective tissue that acts as a resistant surface. Cells called chondrocytes produce cartilage. Chondrosarcoma is a malignant growth arising in chondrocytes. There are two types of chondrosarcomas, either primary or secondary. Primary chondrosarcomas arise in areas of previously normal bone that are derived from cartilage. Secondary chondrosarcomas are lesions produced from pre-existing cartilage lesions. The chondrosarcoma tumors either produce enlargement or erosion of the area involved. The lesion is classified further as to where the lesion occurs and the grade of the lesion. It is graded from 1 (low-grade) to 3 (high-grade). This classification states that the higher the grade of the tumor, the higher the increased atypia, or abnormal cell growth.

Two non-cancerous diseases, Maffuci disease and Ollier disease, are similar to chondrosarcoma. Ollier disease, also known as enchondromatosis or dyschondroplasia, is a disorder affecting the growth plates of bone where new bone is deposited. The cartilage laid down is not reabsorbed and masses form near the ends of the long bones such as the thigh bone (femur) and upper arm bone (humerus). Maffucci disease has the same abnormalities as Ollier disease as well as soft tissue destruction including the skin. Patients with Maffucci or Ollier disease should have bone scans every three to five years to monitor potential malignant transformations.

Genetic profile

Anomalies of chromosomes 5, 7, 8, and 18 and structural alterations of chromosomes 1, 12, and 15 are commonly found in patients diagnosed with chondrosarcoma. Interestingly, the **gene** for the area of normal cartilage production, type II collagen, has been found in the same regions as chondrosarcoma. Studies on the tumor suppressor gene, EXT1, have shown that changes (mutations) of this gene may also be important in the growth of chondrosarcoma.

Demographics

In 2001, an estimated 2,900 new cases of bone and joint **cancer** were diagnosed. Primary cancer of bones accounts for less than 0.2% of all cancers. Chondrosarcoma is the second most common primary malignant bone tumor, meaning it did not originate at another site in the body. Osteosarcoma is the first most common.

There are conflicting reports as to how much more frequently men are diagnosed with chondrosarcoma than females. Findings range from twice as many males to only slightly more males than females. Chondrosarcoma occurs in people from the age of 30-70 years old, but it most commonly affects people over the age of 40. No ethnic group is affected more frequently than another.

Signs and symptoms

The signs and symptoms vary due to the type of tumor, but pain is typically the first symptom. If it is a fast growing, high grade form of chondrosarcoma, then the individual may have very severe pain. A low grade, slow growing, tumor usually has pain and swelling in the area of the tumor. If the tumor is located in the pelvis or hip area, the individual may have difficulty with urination or urinary urgency. The patient may also have the sensation of a groin pull if the tumor is in the pelvic area.

Diagnosis

Usually, chondrosarcoma is diagnosed with x ray radiography. X rays can show soft tissue calcification, where the muscles appear to be forming bone. The appearance of a soft tissue mass that has not yet calcified may also be visible. If the chondrosarcoma is secondary to another type of tumor, the chondrosarcoma may start to erode the edges of the other tumor. This is common where an enchondroma, a type of tumor within the bone shaft, is present. In this case, the chondrosarcoma produces areas of lysis, or destruction of the surrounding tissue.

Biopsy is used to determine the grade of the tumor. Grade 1 chondrosarcomas, or low-grade slow growing lesions, have a mild increase of new cell growth. Grade 3 chondrosarcomas are the opposite; they are high-grade, fast growing and have a dramatic increase in cellular growth. The more radiolucent or transparent to x rays the tumor appears, the greater the chance it is a higher grade.

Other imaging tests may also be used. Computed tomography scanning, CT, is an advanced form of x ray that can also produce bone pictures and help determine how much calcification the tumor is producing. Magnetic resonance imaging, MRI, will aid diagnosis since it can differentiate soft tissues such as muscle and fat. MRI will help determine the amount of malignant degeneration of the chondrosarcoma.

Treatment and management

The main course of therapy for chondrosarcoma is surgical removal of the tumor. The amount of surgery depends on the location and the stage of the tumor. Very low-grade tumors may be surgically removed. High-grade chondrosarcomas necessitate more radical operations where normal tissue is also removed due to the possibility of spread. If the tumor is located in an extremity such as an arm or leg, then amputation, or surgical

---

---

removal of the extremity, may be necessary in order to prevent metastasis, or spread of the cancer. Chemotherapy and radiotherapy may also be used depending on the type of tumor and the area of the body affected, but are usually not effective.

Prognosis

The higher the grade of a chondrosarcoma, the more likely the tumor will spread and thus worsen the prognosis. One study found the five year survival rate of patients with grades 1, 2, and 3 to be 90%, 83%, and 43% respectively. This means that five years after the diagnosis of the tumor, 90 out of 100 people with grade 1 were still alive. On the opposite spectrum, 43 out of 100 patients with grade 3 chondrosarcoma survived five years. Therefore the survival rate is very much dependent on the stage of the tumor and also on its location. Size of the tumor is also an important factor. Tumors greater than 4 in (10 cm) are more likely to become aggressive and spread. When they do spread, or metastasize, they often migrate to the lungs and skeleton.

Resources

BOOKS

Bridge, Julia A., et. al. "Sarcomas of Bone." In *Clinical Oncology*, 2nd ed. Edited by Martin D. Abeloff et. al. Philadelphia: Churchill Livingstone, 2000.

Levesque, Jerome, et al. *A Clinical Guide to Primary Bone Tumors.* Baltimore: Williams & Wilkins, 1998.

Rosenberg, Andrew E. "Skeletal System and Soft Tissue Tumors." In *Robbins Pathologic Basis of Disease,* 5th ed. Edited by Ramzi S. Cotran, Vinay Kumar, Stanley Robbins, and Frederick J. Schoen. Philadelphia: W. B. Saunders Company, 1994.

ORGANIZATIONS

American Cancer Society. Bone Cancer Resource Center. 1599 Clifton Road, NE, Atlanta, GA 30329. (800) 227-2345 or (404) 320-3333. <http://www.cancer.org/>.

Cancernet. National Cancer Institute, National Institutes of Health. NCI Public Inquiries Office, Building 31, Room 10A03, 31 Center Dr., MSC 2580, Bethesda, MD 20892-2580 USA.

WEBSITES

Bone Tumor Organization. <http://www.bonetumor.com/page39.html>.

Jason S. Schliesser, DC

Choroideremia

Definition

Choroideremia is a rare genetic disorder causing progressive eyesight loss due to the wasting away of retinal layers. It first affects the choroid and the retinal pigmented epithelium (RPE) layers and finally the photoreceptor cell layer. Atrophy (wasting) of the optic nerve is also observed in choroideremia.

Description

Formerly called tapetochoroidal dystrophy, choroideremia is a chronic form of retinal disease characterized by degeneration of the layers of the retina, which is the light-sensitive part of the eye. There are four main retinal layers: the outer neural retina, consisting of nerve cells and blood vessels; the retinal pigment epithelium (RPE); the choroid layer that contains connective eye tissue and a capillary layer (chorio capillaris); and the photorecep-

tor (light-sensitive) layer that contains the rods and cones, which function as detectors to process light, color and shape signals to the brain. Choroideremia is a progressive disease, meaning that the layers become affected one after the other over time.

The pigmentary changes in the RPE begin with fine spotting and continue with areas of depigmentation and increasing loss of the chorio capillaris. Chorio capillaris loss and degeneration of the larger choroidal blood vessels causes areas of bare sclera, the tough white fibrous tissue that covers the "white" of the eye. The disease begins in midperiphery of the choroid but then progresses to include the entire choroid.

Choroidal vessels provide oxygen and nutrients to both the RPE and the retina's photoreceptor cells. The RPE, which lies directly beneath the retina, supports the function of photoreceptor cells. Photoreceptor cells (rods and cones) convert light into the electrical impulses that transfer messages to the brain where "seeing" actually occurs. In the early stages of choroideremia, the choroid and the RPE begin to deteriorate. Eventually, photoreceptor cells also degenerate, resulting in a loss of central vision.

The age at which choroideremia first appears varies; initial symptoms (usually night blindness) may occur as early as three years of age and as late as 40 years. However, occurrence peaks between the ages of ten and 40. The visual field becomes progressively constricted, and patients usually reach legal blindness by 25 years of age. Loss of central vision usually occurs after the age of 35. However, in nearly all patients with choroideremia, visual acuity (acuteness or sharpness of vision) is well maintained until the late stages of the disease.

Genetic profile

Choroideremia is an X-linked, recessive disorder, or a condition that is transmitted on the X **chromosome.** Females have two X chromosomes; males have an X and a Y chromosome. Thus in females, the altered **gene** on one X chromosome can be masked by the normal gene on the other X chromosome. Female carriers—who may or may not be symptomatic—have a 50% chance of passing the X-linked abnormal gene to their daughters, who become carriers, and a 50% chance of passing the gene to their sons, who are then affected by the disease.

Choroideremia was the first of the retinal disorders to be mapped, the first to be cloned, and the first to have a simple protein test assigned to it. In 1991, Dr. Fran Cremers of the University of Nijmegen in the Netherlands isolated the gene believed to be responsible for choroiderermia. The gene for choroideremia was found on the Xq21 band of the X chromosome.

Although the choroideremia gene causes problems in the retina, choroid, and RPE, expression of this gene is not limited to the eyes. Choroideremia may also manifest as a generalized disorder. Choroideremia has been classified into two general types: isolated or associated.

Isolated choroideremia

In isolated choroideremia, which is the most common form of the disorder, affected individuals display only disease-related ocular symptoms.

Associated choroideremia

Although relatively rare, associated choroideremia with mental retardation occurs in patients with a deletion of part of the X chromosome, including the region called Xq21. Such a deletion may cause choroideremia with severe mental retardation or with mental retardation and congenital deafness. In these individuals, the mothers are the carriers, showing the same deletions but not the severe clinical manifestations.

Demographics

Choroideremia is believed to affect approximately one in 100,000 individuals—primarily men—although women who are carriers may exhibit mild symptoms as well. The disorder may be generally under-reported because there was no diagnostic test for choroideremia until the late 1990s.

In an area of northern Finland (the Sala region), for reasons that have yet to be determined, choroideremia has affected an unusually large number of people; about one in forty people have the disorder.

Signs and symptoms

A variety of other degenerations of the choroid may look like choroideremia. The decreased night and peripheral vision and diffuse pigmentary abnormalities seen in the early stages of the disorder are symptoms also seen in X-linked **retinitis pigmentosa** (one of a group of genetic vision disorders causing retinal degeneration). However, unlike retinitis pigmentosa, which starts in early childhood, the onset of choroideremia is variable and is rarely seen in childhood. The distinguishing feature of choroideremia is the diffuse choroidal atrophy that is uncommon in early retinitis pigmentosa.

Because the diffuse, progressive atrophy of the chorio capillaris and RPE layers begins peripherally and spreads centrally, central macular function is preserved until late in the course of the disease. **Myopia** occurs more frequently in men diagnosed with choroideremia. Although symptoms vary widely among affected individuals, men usually retain little or no useful vision beyond the age of 60.

Choroideremia is characterized by extensive abnormalities in the RPE layer. The initial symptoms include wasting of the retinal layers and choroid of the eye. The choroid (the vascular membrane located between the retina inside the eye and the sclera) contains large branched pigmented cells and prevents light rays from passing through areas of the eye outside of the pupils. Night blindness is usually the first noticeable symptom of choroideremia, usually occurring during childhood.

Degeneration of the vessels of the choroid and functional damage to the retina occur later in life and usually lead to progressive central vision field loss and eventual blindness. Small bony-like formations and scattered pigment clumps tend to accumulate in the middle portion and on the edges of the choroid. In addition, color vision is initially normal but may later evolve into tritanopia (**color blindness** in which there is an abnormality in the perception of blue).

Female carriers usually have no symptoms and have normal visual fields, normal electroretinograms (a measurement of electrical activity of the retina), and normal visual acuity. However, female carriers sometimes show abnormalities of the interior lining of the eye in the form of pigment spotting with tiny patches of RPE depigmentation. Brownish granular pigmentation and changes in the RPE and choroid may occur later. There is also some evidence to suggest that mild progression of symptoms—and even the full disease—may occur in a small number of female carriers.

Diagnosis

Although there is no treatment for choroideremia because the disorder is so rare and has received relatively little research attention, a diagnostic blood test developed by Canadian researchers allows early diagnosis of the disorder. Patients with the abnormal choroideremia gene lack a protein called Rab Escort Protein-1 (REP-1), which is involved in the lipid (any one of a group of fats or fat-like substances) modification of protein—a process called prenylation. The test uses a monoclonal antibody (an antibody of exceptional purity and specificity, derived from a single cell) to determine the presence or absence of the REP-1 protein in blood samples. The REP-1 test is unable to determine carrier status, however; the REP-1 protein is present in female carriers.

KEY TERMS

Choriocapillaris—Capillary layer of the choroid.

Choroid—A vascular membrane that covers the back of the eye between the retina and the sclera and serves to nourish the retina and absorb scattered light.

Electroretinogram (ERG)—A measurement of electrical activity of the retina.

Retina—The light-sensitive layer of tissue in the back of the eye that receives and transmits visual signals to the brain through the optic nerve.

Retinal pigment epithelium (RPE)—The pigmented cell layer that nourishes the retinal cells; located just outside the retina and attached to the choroid.

Retinitis pigmentosa—Progressive deterioration of the retina, often leading to vision loss and blindness.

Because no biochemical abnormality has been found in choroideremia, no single laboratory test is available for diagnosis. Rather, the diagnosis is based on the typical retinal abnormalities, abnormal electroretinogram findings, the progressive course of the disorder, and the combination of typical symptoms. Family history is also helpful in diagnosing the disorder. When the diagnosis is in doubt, examination of the mother usually reveals the pigmentary changes and other retinal abnormalities typically found in carriers.

Choroideremia is one of the few retinal degenerative disorders that may be detected before birth in some cases (in women who have been found to be carriers due to family history or abnormal ophthalmologic findings). All family members with a history of choroideremia are encouraged to consult an ophthalmologist and to seek **genetic counseling**. These professionals can explain the disease and the **inheritance** risk for all family members and for future offspring.

Treatment and management

There is no treatment for choroideremia because further research is needed to understand the exact mechanism causing this progressive loss of vision. It is not known whether any external environmental factors, such as light, contribute to the progression of the disease, or if genetic factors alone are responsible for the great variability observed. However, patients diagnosed with the disorder early are better able to make decisions regarding family planning and the onset of blindness.

Assistance for individuals with choroideremia is available through low-vision aids, including optical, electronic, and computer-based devices. Personal, educational, and vocational counseling, as well as adaptive training skills are also available through community resources.

Prognosis

Progression of the disease continues throughout the individual's life, although both the rate and degree of visual loss are variable among those affected, even within the same family.

Resources

BOOKS

Cremers, F.P.M., and F.F. Ropers. "Choroideremia." In *The Metabolic and Molecular Basis of Disease.* Ed. C.R. Scriver, A.L. Beaudet, W.S. Sly, and D. Valled, 4311–23, vol. 3. New York: McGraw Hill, 1995.

PERIODICALS

MacDonald, I. M., et al. "A Practical Diagnostic Test for Choroideremia." *Opthalmology* 105 (1998): 1637–40.

Majid, M. A., et al. "Unusual Macular Findings in a Known Choroideremia Carrier." *Eye* 12 (1998): 740–41.

Syed N., et al. "Evaluation of Retinal Photoreceptors and pigment epithelium in a female carrier of choroideremia." *Opthalmology* 108, no. 4 (April 2001): 711–20.

ORGANIZATIONS

American Foundation for the Blind. 11 Penn Plaza, Suite 300, New York, NY 10001. (800) 232-5463.

Choroideremia Research Foundation. 23 E. Brundreth St., Springfield, MA 01109. <http://www.choroideremia.org>.

National Association for Parents of the Visually Impaired. PO Box 317, Watertown, MA 02472. (617) 972-7441 or (800) 562-6265. <http://www.spedex.com/napvi>.

National Eye Institute. 31 Center Dr., Bldg. 31, Room6A32, MSC 2510, Bethesda, MD 20892-2510. <http://www.nei.nih.gov>.

National Federation for the Blind. 1800 Johnson St., Baltimore, MD 21230. (410) 659-9314. epc@roundley.com. <http://www.nfb.org>.

National Organization for Rare Disorders (NORD). PO Box 8923, New Fairfield, CT 06812-8923. (203) 746-6518 or (800) 999-6673. Fax: (203) 746-6481. <http://www.rarediseases.org>.

WEBSITES

The Choroideremia Group. <http://www.onelist.com/subscribe.cgi.choroideremia>.

Genevieve T. Slomski, PhD

Chromosomal abnormalities

Chromosomal abnormalities describe changes in the normal number of chromosomes or structural problems within the chromosomes themselves. These abnormalities occur when an egg or sperm with an incorrect number of chromosomes, or a structurally faulty **chromosome**, unites with a normal egg or sperm during conception. Some chromosome abnormalities occur shortly after conception. In this case, the **zygote**, the cell formed during conception that eventually develops into an embryo, divides incorrectly.

Chromosomal abnormalities can cause serious mental or physical disabilities. **Down syndrome**, for instance, is caused by an extra chromosome 21. People with Down syndrome are mentally retarded and may have a host of physical problems, including heart disorders. Other individuals, called Down syndrome *mosaics,* have a mixture of normal cells and cells with three copies of chromosome 21, resulting in a milder form of the disorder. Most abnormalities in chromosome number lead to the death of the embryo. Zygotes that receive a full extra set of chromosomes, a condition called polyploidy, usually do not survive inside the uterus and are spontaneously aborted (a process sometimes called a miscarriage).

Normal number and structure of human chromosomes

A chromosome consists of the body's genetic material, the **deoxyribonucleic acid**, or **DNA**, along with many kinds of proteins. Within the chromosomes, the DNA is tightly coiled around these proteins (called histones) allowing approximately 6 ft (2 m) strands of DNA to occupy a microscopic space within the nucleus of the cell. When a cell is not dividing, the chromosomes are invisible within the cell's nucleus. Just prior to cell division, the chromosomes begin to replicate and condense. As the replicated DNA condenses, each chromosome looks somewhat like a fuzzy "X" under the microscope. Chromosomes contain the genes, or segments of DNA that code for proteins, of an individual. When a chromosome is structurally faulty, or if a cell contains an abnormal number of chromosomes, the types and amounts of the proteins encoded by the genes is changed. When proteins are altered in the human body, the result can be serious mental and physical changes and disease.

Humans have 46 chromosomes—22 pairs of autosomal chromosomes and one pair of sex chromosomes. These chromosomes may be examined by constructing a **karyotype**, or organized depiction, of the chromosomes. To construct a karyotype, a technician stops cell division just after the chromosomes have replicated and condensed using a chemical, such as colchicine. The chromosomes are visible within the nucleus at this point. The image of the chromosomes seen through the microscope is photographed. Each chromosome is cut out of the picture, and arranged on another sheet in the correct sequence and orientation. The chromosome pairs are identified according to size, shape, and characteristic stripe patterns (called banding).

Normal cell division

In most animals, two types of cell division take place: mitosis and meiosis. In mitosis, each cell division produces two cells that are identical to the parent cell, i.e. one parent cell produces two daughter cells. Compared to its parent chromosome, each daughter cell has exactly the same number of chromosomes and identical genes. This preservation of chromosome number and structure is accomplished through the replication of the entire set of chromosomes just before mitosis.

Sex cells, such as eggs and sperm, undergo a different type of cell division called meiosis. Because sex cells each contribute half of a zygote's genetic material, sex cells must carry only half the full number of chromosomes. This reduction in the number of chromosomes within sex cells is accomplished during two rounds of cell division, called meiosis I and meiosis II. Before meiosis I, the chromosomes replicate. During meiosis I, a cell with 46 replicated chromosomes divides to form two cells that each contain 23 replicated chromosomes. Normally, the meiosis I division separates the 23 pairs of chromosomes evenly, so that each daughter cell contains one chromosome from each chromosome pair. No replication occurs between meiosis I and meiosis II. During meiosis II, the two daughter cells containing 23 replicated chromosomes divide to form four daughter cells, each containing 23 non-replicated chromosomes. Mistakes can occur during either meiosis I or meiosis II. Chromosome pairs may fail to separate during meiosis I, or a replicated chromosome may fail to separate during meiosis II.

Meiosis produces four daughter cells, each with half the normal number of chromosomes. These sex cells are called haploid cells (haploid means "half the number"). Non-sex cells in humans are called diploid (meaning "double the number") since they contain the full number of normal chromosomes. Human diploid cells normally each have 46 chromosomes, and haploid cells normally each have 23 chromosomes.

Alterations in chromosome number

Two kinds of chromosome number alterations can occur in humans: aneuploidy, an abnormal number of chromosomes, and polyploidy, more than two complete sets of chromosomes.

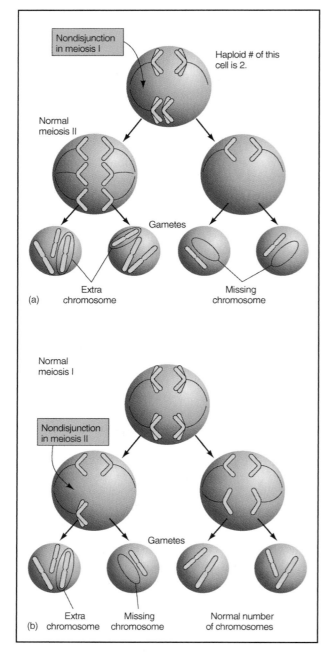

Normal meiosis II

Nondisjunction in meiosis I

Haploid # of this cell is 2.

Gametes

Extra chromosome

Missing chromosome

(a)

Normal meiosis I

Nondisjunction in meiosis II

Gametes

Extra chromosome

Missing chromosome

Normal number of chromosomes

(b)

Figure 1. *(Gale Group.)*

Aneuploidy

Most alterations in chromosome number occur during meiosis. During normal meiosis, chromosomes are distributed evenly among the four daughter cells. Sometimes, however, an uneven number of chromosomes are distributed to the daughter cells. As noted in the previous section, chromosome pairs may not move apart in meiosis I, or the chromosomes may not separate in meiosis II.

The result of both kinds of mistakes (called nondisjunction of the chromosomes) is that one daughter cell receives an extra chromosome, and another daughter cell does not receive any chromosome.

When an egg or sperm that has undergone faulty meiosis and has an abnormal number of chromosomes unites with a normal egg or sperm during conception, the zygote formed will have an abnormal number of chromosomes. This condition is called aneuploidy. There are several types of aneuploidy. If the zygote has an extra chromosome, the condition is called trisomy. If the zygote is missing a chromosome, the condition is called monosomy.

If the zygote survives and develops into a fetus, the chromosomal abnormality is transmitted to all of its cells. The child that is born will have symptoms related to the presence of an extra chromosome or absence of a chromosome.

Examples of aneuploidy include trisomy 21, also known as Down syndrome, and **trisomy 13**, also called Patau syndrome. Trisomy 13 occurs in one out of every 5,000 births, and its symptoms are more severe than those of Down syndrome. Children with trisomy 13 often have cleft palate and eye defects, and always have severe physical and brain malformations. **Trisomy 18**, known as Edwards syndrome, results in severe mutliple defects. Children with trisomy 13 and trisomy 18 usually survive less than a year after birth. (Figure 1).

Aneuploidy of sex chromosomes

Sometimes, nondisjunction occurs in the sex chromosomes. Humans have one set of sex chromosomes. These sex chromosomes are called "X" and "Y" after their approximate shapes in a karyotype. Males have both an X and a Y chromosome, while females have two X chromosomes. Disorders associated with abnormal numbers of sex chromosomes are less severe than those associated with abnormal numbers of autosomes. This is thought to be because the Y chromosome carries few genes, and extra X chromosomes are inactivated shortly after conception. Nevertheless, aneuploidy in sex chromosomes causes changes in physical appearance and in fertility. (Figure 2).

Individuals with **Klinefelter syndrome**, for instance, are men with two X chromosomes (XXY). This condition occurs in one out of every 600 male births. Men with Klinefelter syndrome have small testes and are usually sterile. Some men with Klinefelter develop enlarged breasts. Males who are XXY are of normal intelligence. However, mental retardation is not unusual in males with more than two X chromosomes, such as XXXY, XXXXY, or XXXXXY.

Males with an extra Y chromosome (XYY) have no physical defects, although they may be taller than average. XYY males occur in one out of every 1,000 male births.

Females with an extra X chromosome (XXX) are sometimes said to have "triple X syndrome" and were sometimes called metafemales. This defect occurs in one out of every 1,000 female births. Females with XXX do not usually have mental retardation; pubertal development and fertility are normal.

Females with only one X chromosome (XO) have **Turner syndrome**. Turner syndrome is also called monosomy X and occurs in one out of every 2,000-5,000 female births. The sex organs of females with Turner syndrome do not mature at puberty; therefore these women are usually sterile. They are of short stature and have no mental deficiencies. Heart defects are more common in girls with Turner syndrome.

Polyploidy

Polyploidy is lethal in humans. Normally, humans have two complete sets of chromosomes. Normal human cells, other than sex cells, are thus described as diploid. In polyploidy, a zygote receives more than two complete chromosome sets. Examples of polyploidy include **triploidy**, in which a zygote has three sets of chromosomes, and tetraploidy, in which a zygote has four sets of chromosomes. Triploidy could result from the fertilization of an abnormal diploid sex cell with a normal sex cell or from the fertilization of one egg by two sperm. Tetraploidy could result from the failure of the zygote to divide after it replicates its chromosomes. Human zygotes with either of these conditions usually die before birth, or soon after. Interestingly, polyploidy is common in plants and is essential for the proper development of certain stages of the plant life cycle. Also, some kinds of cancerous cells have been shown to exhibit polyploidy.

Alterations in chromosome structure

Another kind of chromosomal abnormality is changes of chromosome structure. Structural defects arise during replication of the chromosomes just before a meiotic cell division. Meiosis is a complex process that often involves the chromosomes exchanging segments with each other in a process called crossing-over. If the process is faulty, the structure of the chromosomes changes. Sometimes these structural changes are harmless to the zygote; other structural changes, however, can be lethal.

Four types of general structural alterations occur during replication of chromosomes. (Figure 3). All four

Klinefelter's syndrome	XXY
Extra Y	XYY
Metafemale	XXX
Turner's syndrome	XO

Figure 2. *(Gale Group.)*

types begin with the breakage of a chromosome during replication. In a deletion, the broken segment of the chromosome is "lost." Thus, all the genes that are present on this segment are also lost. In a duplication, the segment is inserted into the homologous chromosome as extra (duplicated) DNA. In an inversion, the segment attaches to the original chromosome, but in a reverse position. In a translocation, the segment attaches to an entirely different chromosome.

Because chromosomal structural changes cause the loss or misplacement of genes, the results can be quite severe. Deletions and duplications lead to missing and extra chromosomal material, meaning that there are too many or too few genes in that region. Translocations may or may not be harmful. If the translocation is balanced, meaning that all of the DNA is present and none is missing, the only effect may be a higher risk for abnormal sperm or eggs. If the translocation is not balanced, the chance of associated physical and cognitive abnormalities increases. Inversions of DNA may also be harmless except for a risk of abnormal sperm or eggs. However, both inversions and balanced translocations may have clinical consequences, depending on where the breakage and rejoining of DNA occurred.

A structural abnormality in chromosome 21 occurs in about 4% of people with Down syndrome. In this abnormality, a translocation, a piece of chromosome 21 breaks off during meiosis of the egg or sperm cell and attaches to chromosome 13, 14, or 22. The parents of a child with Down syndrome due to this type of translocation could be balanced carriers for the translocation, and if so, are at increased risk to have another child with Down syndrome.

Some structural chromosomal abnormalities have been implicated in certain cancers. For instance, myelogenous leukemia is a **cancer** of the white blood cells. Researchers have found that the cancerous cells contain

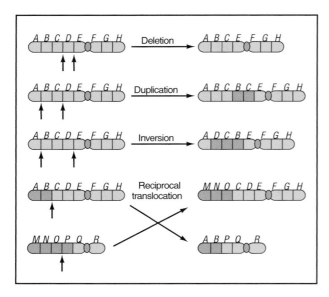

Figure 3. *(Gale Group.)*

a translocation of chromosome 22, in which a broken segment switches places with the tip of chromosome 9.

Syndromes associated with chromosomal deletions

Many syndromes are associated with chromosomal deletions. These include **Cri du chat syndrome**, velocardiofacial syndrome, **Prader-Willi syndrome**, **Angelman syndrome**, **Wolf-Hirschhorn syndrome**, **Smith-Magenis syndrome**, **Miller-Dieker syndrome**, Langer-Giedion syndrome, and the trichorhinophalangeal syndromes.

Cri du chat means "cat cry" in French. Children with this syndrome have an abnormally developed larynx that makes their cry sound like the meowing of a cat in distress. They also have a small head, misshapen ears, and a rounded face, as well as other systemic abnormalities and mental retardation. Cri du chat syndrome is caused by a deletion of a segment of DNA in chromosome 5.

Velocardiofacial syndrome is also called DiGeorge syndrome or Shprintzen syndrome. More recently, it has been called **deletion 22q11 syndrome** because it is caused by a deletion of part of chromosome 22. Individuals with velocardiofacial syndrome may have **congenital heart disease**, cleft palate, learning difficulties, and subtle characteristic facial features.

Two syndromes caused by a chromosome abnormality illustrate an interesting concept: the severity or type of symptoms associated with a chromosomal defect may depend upon whether the child receives the changed **gene** from the mother or the father. Both Prader-Willi

syndrome and Angelman syndrome are usually caused by a deletion in chromosome 15. Prader-Willi syndrome is characterized by mental retardation, obesity, short stature, and small hands and feet. Angelman syndrome is characterized by jerky movements and neurological symptoms. People with this syndrome also have an inability to control laughter, and may laugh inappropriately at odd moments. If a child inherits the changed chromosome from its father, the result is Prader-Willi syndrome. But if the child inherits the changed chromosome from its mother, the child will have Angelman syndrome.

A person may have Prader-Willi or Angelman syndrome, but not have the chromosomal deletion usually associated with these conditions. This may be due to a chromosomal error called uniparental disomy. Usually, one of each chromosome pair is inherited from each parent, and every section of DNA has two copies–one maternally inherited and the other paternally inherited. Uniparental disomy refers to the mistake of both copies of a section of DNA being inherited from one parent. Two copies of a maternally inherited chromosome 15 (no paternal gene present) causes Prader-Willi syndrome, and two copies of a paternally inherited chromosome 15 causes Angelman syndrome.

The sequence of events leading to Prader-Willi and Angelman syndrome is unknown. Researchers have determined that the genes in this region on chromosome 15 may be "turned off," depending on which parent contributed the chromosome. This process of gene inactivation is called **imprinting**. Some people have Prader-Willi and Angelman syndrome because the mechanism controlling the imprinting malfunctions.

Expansion of chromosomal material

Not only can the sex of the parent from whom a gene is inherited determine whether it is turned "on" or turned "off," but the sex of the parent may also influence whether certain abnormal sections of chromosomes become more abnormal. For example, the sex of the parent contributing the X chromosome may increase or decrease the chance that a child will be affected with **fragile X syndrome**.

Fragile X syndrome occurs in one out of 1,000 male births and one out of 2,000 female births. Males are affected more severely than females and the syndrome may be more pronounced if the child inherits the disorder from his/her mother. Part of this is explained by the fact that fragile X syndrome is caused by an abnormality of the X chromosome. Remember that a male is XY and a female is XX. A male child receives a Y chromosome from the father and an X

Amniocentesis—A procedure performed at 16-18 weeks of pregnancy in which a needle is inserted through a woman's abdomen into her uterus to draw out a small sample of the amniotic fluid from around the baby. Either the fluid itself or cells from the fluid can be used for a variety of tests to obtain information about genetic disorders and other medical conditions in the fetus.

Aneuploidy—An abnormal number of chromosomes in a cell. Trisomy 18 and trisomy 13 are examples of aneuploid conditions.

Angelman syndrome—A syndrome caused by a deletion in the maternally inherited chromosome 15 or uniparental disomy of the paternal chromsome 15.

Chorionic villus sampling (CVS)—A procedure used for prenatal diagnosis at 10-12 weeks gestation. Under ultrasound guidance a needle is inserted either through the mother's vagina or abdominal wall and a sample of cells is collected from around the early embryo. These cells are then tested for chromosome abnormalities or other genetic diseases.

Chromosome—A microscopic thread-like structure found within each cell of the body and consists of a complex of proteins and DNA. Humans have 46 chromosomes arranged into 23 pairs. Changes in either the total number of chromosomes or their shape and size (structure) may lead to physical or mental abnormalities.

Cri du chat syndrome—A syndrome caused by a deletion in chromosome 5; characterized by a strange cry that sounds like the mewing of a cat.

Deletion—The absence of genetic material that is normally found in a chromosome. Often, the genetic material is missing due to an error in replication of an egg or sperm cell.

Deoxyribonucleic acid (DNA)—The genetic material in cells that holds the inherited instructions for growth, development, and cellular functioning.

Diploid—Means "double number." The normal number of chromosomes (two) for all cells of the human body, except for the sex cells.

Down syndrome—A genetic condition characterized by moderate to severe mental retardation, a characteristic facial appearance, and, in some individuals, abnormalities of some internal organs.

Down syndrome is always caused by an extra copy of chromosome 21, or three rather than the normal two. For this reason, Down syndrome is also known as *trisomy 21*.

Duplication—A type of chromosomal defect in which a broken segment of a chromosome attaches to the chromosome pair resulting in extra chromosomal material.

Edwards syndrome—A syndrome caused by trisomy 18; characterized by multi-system defects; and usually lethal by age 1.

Fragile X syndrome—A condition caused by an abnormality of a region on the X chromosome which may be expressed in males or females, and may increase in severity when inherited from the mother.

Gene—A building block of inheritance, which contains the instructions for the production of a particular protein, and is made up of a molecular sequence found on a section of DNA. Each gene is found on a precise location on a chromosome.

Haploid—Means "half the number"; the number of chromosomes in a sex cell.

Inversion—A type of chromosomal defect in which a broken segment of a chromosome attaches to the same chromosome, but in reverse position.

Klinefelter syndrome—A syndrome that occurs in XXY males; characterized by sterility and small testes; normal intelligence.

Meiosis—The process in which a cell in the testes or ovaries undergoes chromosome separation and cell division to produce sperms or eggs.

Metafemale—An out of date term for XXX females, also called triple X syndrome.

Mitosis—The process by which a somatic cell—a cell not destined to become a sperm or egg—duplicates its chromosomes and divides to produce two new cells.

Monosomy—Missing an entire copy of a chromosome or a piece of one copy of a chromosome.

Nucleus—The central part of a cell that contains most of its genetic material, including chromosomes and DNA.

Patau syndrome—A syndrome caused by trisomy 13; characterized by cleft palate, severe mental retardation, and many other physical defects; usually lethal by age 1.

(continued)

KEY TERMS (CONTINUED)

Polyploidy—A condition in which a cell receives more than two complete sets of chromosomes.

Prader-Willi syndrome—A syndrome caused by a deletion in the paternally inherited chromosome 15 or by uniparental disomy of the maternal chromosome 15.

Tetraploidy—A form of polyploidy; four sets of chromosomes.

Translocation—The transfer of one part of a chromosome to another chromosome during cell division. A balanced translocation occurs when pieces from two different chromosomes exchange places without loss or gain of any chromosome material. An unbal-

anced translocation involves the unequal loss or gain of genetic information between two chromosomes.

Triploidy—A form of polyploidy; three sets of chromosomes.

Trisomy—The condition of having three identical chromosomes, instead of the normal two, in a cell.

Turner syndrome—Chromosome abnormality characterized by short stature and ovarian failure, caused by an absent X chromosome. Occurs only in females.

Zygote—The cell formed by the uniting of egg and sperm.

chromosome from the mother. A female child, however, can receive an X from either the mother or the father. Girls with fragile X syndrome are less severely affected than boys because they have a normal X chromosome that helps to protect them from the abnormal X chromosome. However, it was somewhat perplexing that girls were affected at all.

This mystery was solved when researchers learned that there is a range of abnormality in the fragile X chromosome. If the abnormality of the fragile X region of the chromosome is severe, the influence can be strong enough to affect females. If the abnormality is mild, females will not have symptoms of fragile X syndrome. Furthermore, the fragile X region of the X chromosome may become more severe when it is maternally inherited. The sex of the parent that the region is inherited from affects whether the chromosome abnormality remains stable or becomes greater.

Many other conditions are associated with similar chromosome abnormalities and may remain stable or become more severe depending upon whether the chromosome region is inherited from the mother or the father. In some of these conditions, the region becomes more abnormal when it is paternally inherited. **Huntington disease**, an adult onset neurological disease, is one such condition.

Maternal age and prenatal diagnosis

Currently, no cures exist for any of the syndromes caused by chromosomal abnormalities. For most of the conditions caused by aneuploidy, the risk to give birth to a child with a chromosomal abnormality increases with the mother's age. The risk for Down syndrome, for

instance, jumps from one in 1,000 when the mother is age 15-30 to one in 350 at age 35. This is most likely because the risk for nondisjunction as the eggs finish forming increases as maternal age increases. A man's age does not increase the nondisjunction risk because of differences in the way eggs and sperms develop. Sperm are maturing and reproducing throughout a man's adult life. Women, on the other hand, are born with all of the eggs they will ever have. At birth these eggs are part way through meiosis I, and each month as a woman ovulates one egg finishes meiosis I and begins meiosis II.

People at high risk for chromosomal abnormalities may opt to know whether the fetus they have conceived has one of these abnormalities. **Amniocentesis** is a procedure in which some of the amniotic fluid that surrounds and cushions the fetus in the uterus is sampled with a needle placed in the uterus. Real-time ultrasound is used to guide the procedure. The amniotic fluid contains fetal cells that can be tested for chromosomal, DNA, and biochemical abnormalities. Another test, chorionic villi sampling (CVS), involves taking a piece of tissue from the developing placenta. Undergoing either amniocentesis or CVS increases the risk of miscarriage slightly. Women and couples considering the procedure should be fully informed of the risks, benefits, and limitations of each procedure. If an abnormality is detected, the prenatal care provider discusses the options available with the woman or couple. Chromosomal abnormalities cannot be corrected. Some parents may terminate the pregnancy. Other parents choose to continue the pregnancy and use the time to prepare for the birth of a child with special needs.

Many resources are available to parents learning of abnormalities before or after birth. In the case of a sex chromosome abnormality, it is common for people to learn of the abnormality as a teenager or even as an adult. A primary care physician, obstetrician, or support group can recommend a specialist from whom more information may be obtained. This specialist is often a medical geneticist, perinatologist, or genetic counselor. Many organizations also provide resources and information to individuals and families.

In conclusion, the division of chromosomes during developmental and during sperm and egg formation is a complex process. Most of the time, however, the process occurs normally. Mistakes that are made can result in changes in chromosome number as well as abnormal chromosomes. Extra or missing chromosomal material usually leads to physical and congitive defects. Changes in sex chromosome compliment are often associated with milder problems. Some problems with chromosomes are relatively common and are associated with well defined syndromes. Other problems with chromosomes occur rarely and problems associated with the change are only seen in a few individuals.

Resources

BOOKS

Baker, Diane, et al. *Chromosome Abnormalities and Genetic Counseling.* New York: Wiley-Liss, 1998.

Gardner, R. J. M., et al. *A Guide to Genetic Counseling.* New York: Oxford University Press, 1996.

PERIODICALS

Bos, A. P., et. al. "Avoidance of emergency surgery in newborn infants with trisomy 18." *The Lancet* 339 no. 8798, (April 11, 1992): 913-6.

Kubas, C. "Noninvasive means of identifying fetuses with possible Down syndrome: a review." *The Journal of Perinatal and Neonatal Nursing* 13 no. 2, (September 1999): 27-46.

Newberger, D. S. "Down syndrome: prenatal risk assessment and diagnosis." *American Family Physician* 62 no.4, (August 2000): 837-8.

Sanders, Roger C. *Structural Fetal Abnormalities: The Total Picture.* St. Louis: Mosby, 1996.

ORGANIZATIONS

American Association for Klinefelter Syndrome Information and Support (AAKSIS) 2945 W. Farwell Ave., Chicago, IL 60645-2925. (773) 761-5298 or (888) 466-5747. Fax: (773) 761-5298. aaksis@aaksis.org>. <http://www.aaksis.org.

Angelman Syndrome Foundation. 414 Plaza Dr., Suite 209, Westmont, IL 60559-1265. (630) 734-9267 or (800) 432-6435. Fax: (630) 655-0391. info@angelman.org. <http://www.angelman.org>.

Chromosome Deletion Outreach, Inc. PO Box 724, Boca Raton, FL 33429-0724. (561) 391-5098 or (888) 236-6880. Fax: (561) 395-4252. cdo@worldnet.att.net. <http://members.aol.com/cdousa/cdo.htm>.

Genetic Alliance. 4301 Connecticut Ave. NW, #404, Washington, DC 20008-2304. (800) 336-GENE (Helpline) or (202) 966-5557. Fax: (888) 394-3937 info@geneticalliance. <http://www.geneticalliance.org>.

Klinefelter Syndrome and Associates, Inc. PO Box 119, Roseville, CA 95678-0119. (916) 773-2999 or (888) 999-9428. Fax: (916) 773-1449. ksinfo@genetic.org. <http://www.genetic.org/ks>.

National Down Syndrome Congress. 7000 Peachtree-Dunwoody Rd., Bldg 5, Suite 100, Atlanta, GA 30328-1662. (770) 604-9500 or (800) 232-6372. Fax: (770) 604-9898. ndsccenter@aol.com. <http://www.ndsccenter.org>.

National Down Syndrome Society. 666 Broadway, New York, NY 10012-2317. (212) 460-9330 or (800) 221-4602. Fax: (212) 979-2873. <http://www.ndss.org info@ndss.org>.

National Fragile X Foundation. PO Box 190488, San Francisco, CA 94119-0988. (800) 688-8765 or (510) 763-6030. Fax: (510) 763-6223. natlfx@sprintmail.com. <http://nfxf.org>.

Prader-Willi Syndrome Association. 5700 Midnight Pass Rd., Suite 6, Sarasota, FL 34242-3000. (941) 312-0400 or (800) 926-4797. Fax: (941) 312-0142. <http://www.pwsausa.org PWSAUSA@aol.com>.

Triple X syndrome support. 231 W. Park Ave., Sellersville, PA 18960. (215) 453-2117. <http://www.voicenet.com/~markr/triple.html edr@starbyte.com>.

Velo-Cardio-Facial Syndrome Research Institute. Albert Einstein College of Medicine, 3311 Bainbridge Ave., Bronx, NY 10467. (718) 430-2568. Fax: (718) 430-8778. rgoldber@aecom.yu.edu. <http://www.kumc.edu/gec/vcfhome.html>.

WEBSITES

"Angelman Syndrome" *NCI Genes and Disease.* <http://www.ncbi.nlm.nih.gov/disease/angelman.html>.

"Fragile X Syndrome" *NCI Genes and Disease.* <http://www.ncbi.nlm.nih.gov/disease/FMR1.html>.

"Velocardiofacial Syndrome" *NCI Genes and Disease.* <http://www.ncbi.nlm.nih.gov/disease/DGS.html>.

Michelle Bosworth, MS, CGC

Chromosome

Chromosomes are microscopic units containing organized genetic information, located in the nuclei of diploid and haploid cells (e.g. human somatic and sex cells), and are also present in one-cell non-nucleated organisms (unicel-

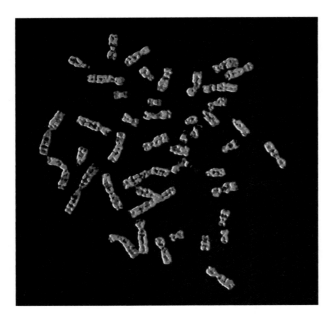

False-color light micrograph of normal human chromosomes, obtained by amniocentesis. *(Photo Researchers, Inc.)*

lular microorganisms), like bacteria, which do not have an organized nucleus. The sum-total of genetic information contained in different chromosomes of a given individual or species are generically referred to as the genome.

In humans, chromosomes are structurally made of roughly equal amounts of proteins and **DNA**. Each chromosome contains a double-strand DNA molecule, arranged as a double helix, and tightly coiled and neatly packed by a family of proteins called histones. DNA strands are comprised of linked nucleotides. Each nucleotide has a sugar (deoxyribose), a nitrogenous base, plus one to three phosphate groups. Each nucleotide is linked to adjacent nucleotides in the same DNA strand by phosphodiester bonds. Phosphodiester is another sugar, made of sugar-phosphate. Nucleotides of one DNA strand link to their complementary nucleotide on the opposite DNA strand by hydrogen bonds, thus forming a pair of nucleotides, known as a base pair, or nucleotide base. Genes contain up to thousands of sequences of these base pairs. What distinguishes one **gene** from another is the sequence of nucleotides that code for the synthesis of a specific protein or portion of a protein. Some proteins are necessary for the structure of cells and tissues. Others, like enzymes, a class of active (catalyst) proteins, promote essential biochemical reactions, such as digestion, energy generation for cellular activity, or metabolism of toxic compounds. Some genes produce several slightly different versions of a given protein through a process of alternate transcription of bases pairs segments known as codons.

Amounts of autosomal chromosomes differ in cells of different species; but are usually the same in every cell of a given species. Sex determination cells (mature ovum and sperm) are an exception, where the number of chromosomes is halved. Chromosomes also differ in size. For instance, the smallest human chromosome, the sex chromosome Y, contains 50 million base pairs (bp), whereas the largest one, chromosome 1, contains 250 million base pairs. All three billion base pairs in the human genome are stored in 48 chromosomes. Human genetic information is therefore stored in 24 pairs of chromosomes (totaling 48), 24 inherited from the mother, and 24 from the father. Two of these chromosomes are sex chromosomes (chromosomes X and Y). The remaining 46 are autosomes, meaning that they are not sex chromosomes and are present in all somatic cells (i.e., any other body cell that is not a germinal cell for spermatozoa in males or an ovum in females). Sex chromosomes specify the offspring gender: normal females have two X chromosomes and normal males have one X and one Y chromosome.

Each set of 24 chromosomes constitutes one allele, containing gene copies inherited from one of the progenitors. The other allele is complementary or homologous, meaning that it contains copies of the same genes and on the same positions, but originated from the other parent. As an example, every normal child inherits one set of copies of gene BRCA1, located on chromosome 13, from the mother and another set of BRCA1 from the father, located on the other allelic chromosome 13. Allele is a Greek-derived word that means "one of a pair," or any one of a series of genes having the same locus (position) on homologous chromosomes.

The first chromosome observations were made under light microscopes, revealing rod-shaped structures in varied sizes and conformations, commonly J- or V-shaped in eukaryotic cells and ring-shaped in bacteria. Staining reveals a pattern of light and dark bands. Today those bands are known to correspond to regional variations in the amounts of the two nucleotide base pairs: adenine-thymine (A-T or T-A) in contrast with amounts of guanine-cytosine (G-C or C-G).

Genetic abnormalities and diseases occur when one of the following events happens: a) one chromosome copy is missing, b) extra copies of a chromosome are present, c) a chromosome breaks and its fragment is fused into another chromosome (insertion), d) a fragment is deleted, e) a gene is transferred from one chromosome to another (translocation), f) duplication of a chromosomal segment occurs, g) inversion of a chromosomal segment occurs. **Down syndrome**, for instance, is caused by the presence of a third copy of chromosome 21.

In non-dividing cells, it is not possible to distinguish morphological details of individual chromosomes, because they remain elongated and entangled to each other. However, when a cell is dividing, i.e., undergoing mitosis, chromosomes become highly condensed and each individual chromosome occupies a well-defined spatial location.

Mitotic chromosomes present a constricted region, to which the spindle fibers attach during cellular division. Such constricted region, known as centromere or primary constriction, may be located in three different positions in chromosomes. Centromeric position allows the classification of chromosomes in three groups: a) acrocentric: centromere lies very near one end; b) metacentric: centromere at the middle, dividing the chromosome in two equal parts or arms; and c) submetacentric: centromere near middle, but dividing chromosome in two unequal arms.

When a chromosome loses its centromere, it is known as acentric. As the centromere is essential for both division and retention of chromosome copies in the new cells, acentric chromosomes will not pass to the daughter cells during the parental cell division. Therefore, daughter cells will miss one chromosome in their **karyotype**. A karyotype map shows mitotic chromosomes in the mitotic phase, known as metaphase. In metaphase, chromosomes align in pairs. In a normal human karyotype, there are 22 pairs of autosomal chromosomes and two sex chromosomes (X and Y). Each pair of autosomal chromosomes contains two complementary or homologous chromosomes, a maternal and a paternal copy.

Some chromosomes also present a secondary constriction that always appears at the same site. They are also useful, along with centromere position and chromosome size, for identifying and characterizing individual chromosomes, in a karyotype.

Karyotype analysis was the first genetic screening utilized by geneticists to assess inherited abnormalities, like additional copies of a chromosome or a missing copy, as well as DNA content and gender of the individual. With the development of new molecular screening techniques and the growing number of identified individual genes, detection of other more subtle chromosomal mutations is now possible (e.g., determinations of **gene mutations**, levels of gene expression, etc.). Such data allow scientists to better understand disease causation and to develop new therapies and medicines for those diseases.

Sandra Galeotti, MS

Chromosome mapping *see* **Gene mapping**

Chronic pancreatitis *see* **Hereditary pancreatitis**
Cleft lip *see* **Cleft lip and palate**

Cleft lip and palate

Definition

A cleft is a birth defect that occurs when the tissues of the lip and or palate of the fetus do not fuse very early in pregnancy. A cleft lip, sometimes referred to as a harelip, is an opening in the upper lip that can extend into the base of the nostril. A cleft palate is an opening in the roof of the mouth.

Description

Infants born with cleft lips will have an opening involving the upper lip. The length of the opening ranges from a small notch, to a cleft that extends into the base of the nostril. Cleft lips may involve one or both sides of the lip.

Cleft palates are openings in the palate, which is the roof of the mouth. The size and position of the opening varies. The cleft may only be in the hard palate, the bony portion of the roof of the mouth opening into the floor of the nose or it may only occur in the soft palate, the soft portion of the roof of the mouth. The cleft palate may involve both the hard and soft palate and may occur on both sides of the center of the palate.

Cleft lips can develop with or without cleft palates. Cleft palates may also occur without cleft lips.

Genetic profile

Cleft lip and palates not associated with a syndrome are caused by a combination of genetic and environmental factors. **Inheritance** caused by such a combination is called multifactorial. The embryo inherits genes that increase the risk for cleft lip and or palate. When an embryo with such genes is exposed to certain environmental factors, the embryo develops a cleft.

The risk of a baby being born with a cleft lip or palate increases with the number of affected relatives and increases with relatives that have more severe clefts.

Environmental factors that increase the risk of cleft lip and palate include cigarette and alcohol use during pregnancy. Some drugs also increase the incidence of clefting, such as phenytoin, sodium valproate, and

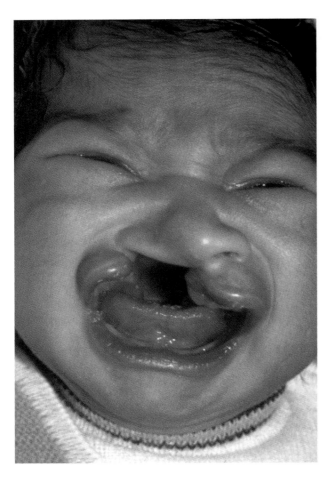

An infant with a unilateral cleft lip. *(Custom Medical Stock Photo, Inc.)*

methotrexate. The pregnant mother's nutrition may affect the incidence of clefting as well.

Demographics

The incidence of cleft lip and palate not associated with a syndrome is one in 700 newborns. Native Americans have an incidence of 3.6 in 1,000 newborns. The incidence among Japanese newborns is two in 1,000. The incidence among caucasians is one in 1,000 newborns. African Americans have an incidence of 0.3 in 1,000 newborns.

Signs and symptoms

Babies born with a cleft lip will have an elongated opening in the upper lip. The size of this opening may range from a small notch in the upper lip to an opening that extends into the base of the nostril. The cleft lip may be below the right or left nostril or below both nostrils.

Babies born with a cleft palate will have an opening into the roof of the mouth. The size and position of the cleft varies and it may involve only the hard palate, or only the soft palate and may occur on both sides of the center of the palate.

In some cases the cleft palate will be covered with the normal lining of the mouth and can only be felt by the examiner.

Infants with cleft lips and palates have feeding difficulties, which are more severe in those with cleft palates. The difficulty in feeding is due to the baby being unable to achieve complete suction. In the case of clefts of the hard palate, liquids enter the nose from the mouth through the opening in the hard palate.

A cleft palate also affects a child's speech, since the palate is necessary for speech formation. The child's speech pattern may still be affected despite surgical repair.

Ear infections are more common in babies born with cleft palates. The infections occur because the muscles of the palate do not open the Eustachian tubes which drain the middle ear. This allows fluid to collect and increases the risk of infection and hearing loss.

Teeth may also erupt misaligned.

Diagnosis

Cleft lip and palate can be diagnosed before birth by ultrasound. After birth, cleft lip and palate are diagnosed by physical exam.

Treatment and management

If cleft lip and/or palate are diagnosed by ultrasound before birth, further testing may be required to diagnose associated abnormalities if present. Referral to a cleft team is essential. A cleft team consists of specialists in the management of patients with clefts and includes surgeons as well as nurses and speech therapists. Members of the team inform the parents of all aspects of management. Feeding methods are also discussed, since feeding is the first problem that must be dealt with. It may be possible to breast feed a baby born with only a cleft lip, but babies born with cleft palates usually have more problems with feeding and frequently require special bottles and teats. A palatal obturator is a device that fits into the roof of the mouth, thus blocking the cleft opening and allowing easier suckling.

Surgery to repair cleft lips is sometimes performed after orthodontic treatment to narrow the gap in the upper lip. Orthodontic treatment can involve acrylic splints with or without screws or may involve the use of adhesive tape placed across the gap in the lip. The orthodontic treatment for cleft lip should begin within the first three weeks of life and continue until the cleft lip is repaired.

The timing of surgical cleft lip repair depends on the judgement of the surgeon who will perform the operation. The procedure is usually performed between one and three months of age. The goals of the operation are to close the gap in the upper lip, place scars in the natural skin curves and to repair muscle so that the lip appears normal during movement. The closure is done in the three layers (skin, muscle, and mucosa) that line the inside of the lip. At the time of the procedure, if the nose is shaped abnormally due to the cleft lip, it is also corrected. Sometimes further surgery may be needed on the lip and or nose to refine the result.

The goals of the surgeon repairing a cleft palate are normal speech, normal facial growth, and hearing for the affected infant. The repair of the cleft palate is usually performed between three and 18 months of age. The timing may extend beyond this and varies with the type of cleft plate and center where the procedure is being performed. Depending on the type of cleft palate, more than one operation may be needed to close the cleft and improve speech.

Nonsurgical treatment of a cleft palate is available for patients who are at high risk for surgery and consists of a prosthetic appliance worn to block the opening in the palate.

Babies born with cleft palates are vulnerable to ear infections. Their Eustachian tubes do not effectively drain fluid from the middle ear so fluid accumulates and infection sets in. This may lead to hearing loss. These children require drainage tubes to be inserted to prevent fluid accumulation.

Babies born with clefts usually require orthodontic treatment between 13 and 18 years of age. They also require speech therapy.

Prognosis

Individuals born with cleft lip and palate have a good prognosis, and approximately 80% will develop normal speech. There is no known means of preventing clefting. Good prenatal care is essential and avoiding harmful substances appear to reduce the risk.

Resources

PERIODICALS

Bender, Patricia L. "Genetics of Cleft lip and Palate" *Journal of Pediatric Nursing* 15 (August 2000): 242-249.

Christensen, Karr "The 20th Century Danish Facial cleft Population–Epidemiological and Genetic-Epidemiolical Studies" *Cleft Palate–Craniofacial Journal* 36 (March 1999): 96-104.

Chung, Kevin C. "Maternal Cigarette Smoking during Pregnancy and the risk of having a child with Cleft Lip/Palate." *Plastic and Reconstructive Surgery* 105 (February 2000): 458-491.

Cockell, Anna. "Prenatal Diagnosis and Management of orofacial Clefts." *Prenatel Diagnosis* 20 (February 2000): 149-151.

Denk, Michael J. "Topics in Pediatric Plastic Surgery." *Pediatric Clinics of North America* 45 (December 1998)

Litwak-Saleh, Kim. "Practical Points in the case of the Patient with post-Cleft lip repair." *Journal of Post Anesthesia Nursing* 8 (February 1993): 35-37.

Rohrich, Rod J. "Optimal Timing of Cleft Palate Closure." *Plastic and Reconstructive Surgery* 106 (August): 413-421.

ORGANIZATIONS

Cleft Palate Foundation. (800) 24-CLEFT. <http://www.cleftline.org>.

Farris F. Gulli, MD

Cleft palate *see* **Cleft lip and palate**

Cleidocranial dysostosis *see* **Cleidocranial dysplasia**

Cleidocranial dysplasia

Definition

Cleidocranial **dysplasia** (CCD), also known as cleidocranial dysostosis, is a hereditary condition characterized by abnormal clavicles, delayed fusion of the bones in the skull, extra teeth, short stature, and other skeletal changes.

Description

Cleidocranial dysplasia is one of the **skeletal dysplasia** conditions, a large family of disorders involving abnormal growth and development of the skeleton.

CCD involves a characteristic group of abnormalities affecting primarily the skull, teeth, and clavicles. Other bones, such as the ribs, pelvis, and bones of the hands and feet may also be affected. Older children and adults with CCD are typically shorter than average. Most individuals with this condition do not have significant physical or mental disability.

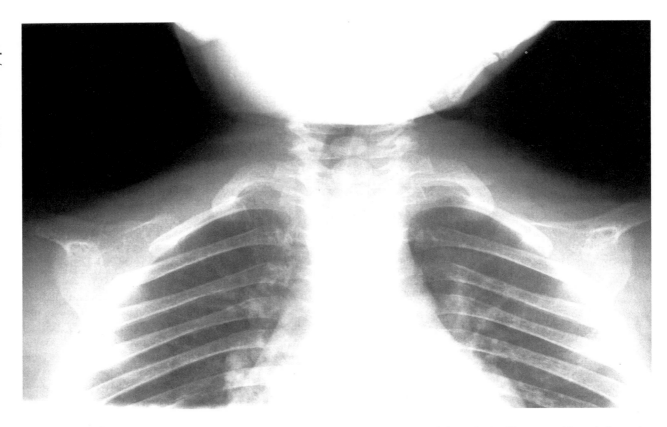

This chest x ray shows the absence of collar bones, a feature common in cleidocranial dysplasia. *(Greenwood Genetic Center.)*

Genetic profile

CCD is an autosomal dominant condition with variable expressivity (variable symptoms) and complete penetrance (meaning that all individuals who carry the **gene** for CCD have some symptoms). It is estimated that one third of cases represent new mutations, or genetic changes. The gene responsible for CCD has been mapped to the short arm of **chromosome** 6 and is called CBFA1. This gene encodes a transcription factor, meaning a protein that regulates **DNA** transcription, and is specifically expressed in the bone. Mutations in CBFA1 have been identified in many individuals and families with CCD.

Demographics

More than 500 cases of CCD among individuals of various ethnic backgrounds have been described in the medical literature. The incidence of CCD is reported to be highest around Cape Town, South Africa. The number of affected individuals in this area was estimated to exceed 1,000 as of 1996. These individuals descended from an affected Chinese sailor who settled in the area in 1896 and had seven wives. Study of this large family helped localize the gene responsible for the condition.

Signs and symptoms

Individuals with CCD typically show a delay or failure of the fusion of the calvarial sutures, the openings between the bones of the skull in infants. In some cases, the anterior fontanelle (the "soft spot" on an infant's head) or other areas of the skull may remain unfused through life. A typical facial appearance in persons with CCD includes a broad forehead and widely spaced eyes. The overall head size is usually at the upper limit of normal.

Almost all persons with CCD have some degree of hypoplasia, or underdevelopment, of the clavicles (collar bones). In severe cases, both clavicles may be absent. More commonly, there is hypoplasia of the outside end of the clavicles. Depending on the degree of severity of clavicular hypoplasia, the external appearance of the shoulder may be affected. Some persons with CCD appear to have narrow, sloping shoulders, and some have the unusual ability to bring their shoulders together beneath their chin. This defect usually does not result in physical disability for the individual.

Dental abnormalities are very frequent among persons with CCD and are considered characteristic of the disorder. Almost all individuals are slow to lose their deciduous teeth (baby teeth), with a delay in the eruption of the permanent teeth. Some persons with CCD describe "living without teeth" until their permanent teeth started growing. Additionally, there may be a large number of extra teeth present. These extra teeth are so numerous so as to constitute a more or less complete third set of teeth. Additionally, the enamel of the teeth may be abnormal and prone to decay.

Other signs of CCD include a small rib cage with short or abnormal ribs. The vertebra of the spine may be malformed. The pelvis may be underdeveloped, with an increased space between the pubic bones. The growth of the bones in the hands and feet are often abnormal; most are shorter but others are longer than normal. Final height in adults with CCD is usually shorter than expected given the family background.

More unusual complications associated with CCD include **scoliosis** (curvature of the spine), bone fragility, deafness, cleft palate, and a small jaw.

Diagnosis

The diagnosis of CCD is typically made by the doctor following review of the information obtained from physical exams, history, and x ray or other studies. The clavicular hypoplasia may only be seen on x rays.

The combination of hypoplastic clavicles, open fontanelles, and extra teeth is considered typical of CCD. The multiple dental anomalies in CCD are also quite specific and the diagnosis is evident in any individual with normal deciduous teeth, delayed eruption of permanent teeth, and multiple extra teeth.

Testing of the CBFA1 gene for mutations may also be performed. Identification of a mutation may confirm the initial diagnosis, or allow diagnosis before birth.

In a few cases, recognition of the features of CCD by ultrasound imaging, a technique that produces pictures of the fetus, has led to diagnosis of the condition before birth.

Treatment and management

There is no specific treatment for cleidocranial dysplasia. Typically, a course of treatment is designed to manage the specific symptoms.

Children with CCD may be screened for deafness.

Long term dental treatment is often required. Surgery may be performed to remove the baby teeth and open the bony coverings surrounding the permanent teeth, with the goal of promoting their eruption. Orthodontic procedures may be required to align the teeth.

> ## KEY TERMS
>
> **Clavicle**—Also called the collarbone. Bone that articulates with the shoulder and the breast bone.
>
> **Deciduous teeth**—The first set of teeth or "baby teeth."
>
> **Fontanelle**—One of several "soft spots" on the skull where the developing bones of the skull have yet to fuse.
>
> **Hypoplasia**—Incomplete or underdevelopment of a tissue or organ.
>
> **Mutation**—A permanent change in the genetic material that may alter a trait or characteristic of an individual, or manifest as disease, and can be transmitted to offspring.

In pregnant females with CCD, the hypoplastic pelvis often necessitates a caesarian section delivery.

Prognosis

CCD is not expected to affect life expectancy in most cases and most diagnosed persons enjoy good overall health.

In some newborns, the small rib cage and reduced lung capacity may lead to respiratory distress. Height is often lower compared to that of other family members. The clavicular hypoplasia does not appear to significantly impair function, and some individuals with hypoplastic or absent clavicles have worked as manual laborers without difficulty. Dental problems are expected, and are sometimes severe enough so as to become a "dental disability." Intelligence is usually normal.

Resources

BOOKS

Jones, K. L. *Smith's Recognizable Patterns of Human Malformation.* W. B. Saunders Company, Philadelphia, 1997.

PERIODICALS

Mundlos, S. "Cleidocranial Dysplasia: Clinical and Molecular Genetics." *Journal of Medical Genetics* 36 (1999):177-182.

Ramesar, Rajkumar S. et al. "Mapping the Gene for Cleidocranial Dysplasia in the historical Cape Town (Arnold) Kindred and Evidence for Locus Homogeneity." *Journal of Medical Genetics* 33 no. 6 (1996): 511-514.

Jennifer Roggenbuck, MS, CGC

Clubfoot

Definition

Clubfoot is a condition in which one or both feet are twisted into an abnormal position at birth. The condition is also known as talipes.

Description

True clubfoot is characterized by abnormal bone formation in the foot. There are four variations of clubfoot, including talipes varus, talipes valgus, talipes equines, and talipes calcaneus. In talipes varus, the most common form of clubfoot, the foot generally turns inward so that the leg and foot look somewhat like the letter J. In talipes valgus, the foot rotates outward like the letter L. In talipes equinus, the foot points downward, similar to that of a toe dancer. In talipes calcaneus, the foot points upward, with the heel pointing down.

Clubfoot can affect one foot or both. Sometimes an infant's feet appear abnormal at birth because of the intrauterine position of the fetus birth. If there is no anatomic abnormality of the bone, this is not true clubfoot, and the problem can usually be corrected by applying special braces or casts to straighten the foot.

Genetic profile

Experts do not agree on the precise cause of clubfoot. The exact genetic mechanism of **inheritance** has been extensively investigated using family studies and other epidemiological methods. No definitive conclusions have been reached, although a Mendelian pattern of inheritance is suspected. This may be due to the interaction of several different inheritance patterns, different patterns of development appearing as the same condition, or a complex interaction between genetic and environmental factors. The MSX1 **gene** has been associated with clubfoot in animal studies. But these findings have not been replicated in humans.

A family history of clubfoot has been reported in 24.4% of families in a single study. These findings suggest the potential role of one or more genes being responsible for clubfoot.

Several environmental causes have been proposed for clubfoot. Obstetricians feel that intrauterine crowding causes clubfoot. This theory is supported by a significantly higher incidence of clubfoot among twins compared to singleton births. Intrauterine exposure to the drug, misoprostol, has been linked with clubfoot. Misoprostol is commonly used when trying, usually unsuccessfully, to induce abortion in Brazil and in other countries in South and Central America. Researchers in Norway have reported that males who are in the printing trades have significantly more offspring with clubfoot than men in other occupations. For unknown reasons, **amniocentesis**, a prenatal test, has also been associated with clubfoot. The infants of mothers who smoke during pregnancy have a greater chance of being born with clubfoot than are offspring of women who do not smoke.

Demographics

The ratio of males to females with clubfoot is 2.5 to 1. The incidence of clubfoot varies only slightly. In the United States, the incidence is approximately one in every 1,000 live births. A 1980 Danish study reported an overall incidence of 1.20 in every 1,000 children; by 1994, that number had doubled to 2.41 in every 1,000 live births. No reason was offered for the increase.

Signs and symptoms

True clubfoot is usually obvious at birth. The four most common varieties have been described. A clubfoot has a typical appearance of pointing downward and being twisted inwards. Since the condition starts in the first trimester of pregnancy, the abnormality is quite well established at birth, and the foot is often very rigid. Uncorrected clubfoot in an adult causes only part of the foot, usually the outer edge, or the heel or the toes, to touch the ground. For a person with clubfoot, walking becomes difficult or impossible.

Diagnosis

True clubfoot is usually recognizable and obvious on physical examination. A routine x ray of the foot that shows the bones to be malformed or misaligned supplies a confirmed diagnosis of clubfoot. Ultrasonography is not always useful in diagnosing the presence of clubfoot prior to the birth of a child.

Treatment and management

Most orthopedic surgeons agree that the initial treatment of congenital (present at birth) clubfoot should be non-operative. Non-surgical treatment should begin in the first days of life to take advantage of the favorable fibro-elastic properties of the foot's connective tissues, those forming the ligaments, joint capsules, and tendons. In a common treatment, a series of casts is applied over a period of months to reposition the foot into a normal alignment. In mild cases, splinting and wearing braces at night may correct the abnormality.

When clubfoot is severe enough to require surgery, the condition is usually not completely correctable, although significant improvement is possible. In the

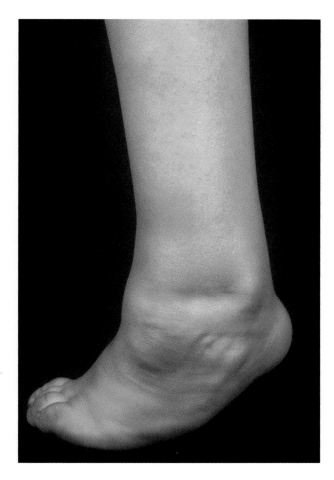

A clubbed foot. *(Photo Researchers, Inc.)*

ately treated, the abnormality becomes fixed. This has an effect on the growth of the leg and foot, and some degree of permanent disability usually results.

Resources

BOOKS

Hall, Judith G. "Chromosomal Clinical Abnormalilties." In *Nelson Textbook of Pediatrics.* 16th ed. Edited by Richard E. Behrman et al., 325–34. Philadelphia: Saunders, 2000.

Jones, KL. "XO Syndrome." In *Smith's Recognizable Patterns of Human Malformation.* 5th ed. Edited by Kenneth L. Jones and Judy Fletcher, 81–7. Philadelphia: Saunders, 1997.

Thoene, Jess G., ed. *Physicians' Guide to Rare Diseases.* 2nd ed. Montvale, NJ: Dowden Publishing Co., 1995.

Van Allen, Margot I., and Judith G. Hall. "Congenital Anomalies." In *Cecil Textbook of Medicine.* 21st ed. Edited by Lee Goldman, et al., 150–52. Philadelphia: Saunders, 2000.

PERIODICALS

Chesney, D., et al. "Epidemiology and Genetic Theories in the Etiology of Congenital Talipes Equinovarus." *Bulletin of the Hospital for Joint Diseases* 58, no. 1 (1999): 59–64.

Gonzalez, C. H., et al. "Congenital Abnormalities in Brazilian Children Associated with Misoprostol Misuse in First Trimester of Pregnancy." *Lancet* 351, no. 9116 (May 30, 1998): 1624–27.

Honein, M. A., L. J. Paulozzi, and C. A. Moore. "Family History, Maternal Smoking, and Clubfoot: An Indication of a Gene-Environment Interaction." *American Journal of Epidemiology* 157, no. 7 (October 1, 2000): 658–65.

Lochmiller, C., et al. "Genetic Epidemiology Study of Idiopathic Talipes Equinovarus." *American Journal of Medical Genetics* 79, no. 2 (September 1, 1998): 90–6.

Rebbeck, T. R., et al. "A Single-Gene Explanation for the Probability of Having Idiopathic Talipes Equinovarus." *American Journal of Human Genetics* 53, no. 5 (November 1993): 1051–63.

Robertson, W. W., and D. Corbett. "Congenital Clubfoot. Month of Conception." *Clinics in Orthopedics* 340, no. 338 (May 1997): 14–18.

most severe cases, surgery may be required, especially when the Achilles tendon, which joins the muscles in the calf to the bone of the heel, needs to be lengthened. Because an early operation induces fibrosis, a scarring and stiffness of the tissue, surgery should be delayed until an affected child is at least three months old.

Much of a clubfoot abnormality can be corrected by the use of manipulation and casting during the first three months of life. Proper manipulative techniques must be followed by applications of appropriately molded plaster casts to provide effective and safe correction of most varieties of clubfoot. Long-term care by an orthopedist is required after initial treatment to ensure that the correction of the abnormality is maintained. Exercises, corrective shoes, or night-time splints may be needed until the child stops growing.

Prognosis

With prompt, expert treatment, clubfoot is usually correctable. Most individuals are able to wear regular shoes and lead active lives. If clubfoot is not appropri-

ORGANIZATIONS

March of Dimes/Birth Defects Foundation. 1275 Mamaroneck Ave., White Plains, NY 10605. (888) 663-4637. resourcecenter@modimes.org. <http://www.modimes.org>.

National Easter Seal Society. 230 W. Monroe St., Suite 1800, Chicago, IL 60606-4802. (312) 726-6200 or (800) 221-6827. <http://www.easter-seals.org>.

National Organization for Rare Disorders (NORD). PO Box 8923, New Fairfield, CT 06812-8923. (203) 746-6518 or (800) 999-6673. Fax: (203) 746-6481. <http://www.rarediseases.org>.

WEBSITES

"Clubfoot." *National Library of Medicine.* <http://www.nlm.nih.gov/medlineplus/ency/article/001228.htm>.

Clubfoot.net. <http://www.clubfoot.net/treatment.php3>.

Ponseti, Ignacio, MD. "Treatment of Congenital Clubfoot." Revised January 1998. *University of Iowa Health Care.* <http://www.vh.org/Providers/Textbooks/Clubfoot/Clubfoot.html>.

Schopler, Steven A., MD. "Clubfoot." *Southern California Orthopedic Institute.* <http://www.scoi.com/clubfoot.htm>.

L. Fleming Fallon, Jr., MD, DrPH.

Cobblestone dysplasia *see* **Lissencephaly syndrome**

Cockayne syndrome

Definition

Cockayne syndrome (CS) is a rare inherited disorder that results in an extreme sensitivity to ultraviolet (UV) irradiation, mental retardation, and precocious (premature) aging.

Description

Since first reported in 1936 by Dr. Edward A. Cockayne, less than 200 cases of this disorder have been documented in medical literature. At birth, newborns with CS may have microcephaly (small-sized head) and low birth weight. During the first year of life they do not feed well and, as a result, they suffer from growth failure and delayed development. Ultimately, the disease usually results in death during the teenage years.

Genetic profile

CS results from mutations in the CSA **gene** (also known as the ERCC8 gene) located on **chromosome** 5. An affected person has inherited one abnormal or non-working gene from each parent, a pattern that is consistent with autosomal recessive **inheritance**. When functioning normally, the CSA gene helps cells remove and destroy **deoxyribonucleic acid** (**DNA**) errors from strands undergoing active transcription. Also, the CSA gene allows cells to synthesize **ribonucleic acid** (**RNA**) after exposure to UV light. Although the parents of an affected child are normal, each of them carries an abnormal gene for CS. Therefore, they have a 25% risk with each pregnancy of having another affected child.

Demographics

CS occurs in less than one in 250,000 births and does not affect any one ethnic group more than another. Males and females are equally affected.

Signs and symptoms

The symptoms of CS are very striking. Failure to grow begins during the first year of life and results in the appearance of dwarfism. The patient's weight is affected more than height. Also, some babies do not feed well and require feeding through a gastrostomy tube (a tube inserted through the abdominal wall into the stomach) to prevent malnutrition. As the infant grows, a delay in developmental milestones becomes apparent around the time that walking and talking should occur. Mental retardation in the mild to moderate range is found in all patients with CS. A small number of patients will have severe to profound mental retardation and some never have more than a few words of speech.

Other physical features include sun-sensitive skin, degeneration of retinal pigment, cataracts, and hearing loss. With exposure to sunlight, skin rashes appear and patients develop dry, scaly skin and thin hair. As part of the disease process, the skin develops an aged, leathery appearance. Although the eyes appear normal early in life, the retina later loses its pigment or color and develops a "salt-and-pepper" appearance. If cataracts appear within the first three years of life, the patient usually has the more severe form of CS that leads to death before adolescence. More than half the patients with CS have sensorineural hearing loss. The range of loss is from mild to severe.

Another finding of CS is an unusual gait (walk), caused by a combination of leg spasticity and contractures of the hips, knees, and ankles. The stooped posture often seen in CS results from kyphosis and joint contrac-

KEY TERMS

Cataract—A clouding of the eye lens or its surrounding membrane that obstructs the passage of light resulting in blurry vision. Surgery may be performed to remove the cataract.

Contracture—A tightening of muscles that prevents normal movement of the associated limb or other body part.

Fibroblast—Cells that form connective tissue fibers like skin.

Gastrostomy—The construction of an artificial opening from the stomach through the abdominal wall to permit the intake of food.

Kyphosis—An abnormal outward curvature of the spine, with a hump at the upper back.

Microcephaly—An abnormally small head.

Mutation—A permanent change in the genetic material that may alter a trait or characteristic of an individual, or manifest as disease, and can be transmitted to offspring.

Myelin—A fatty sheath surrounding nerves in the peripheral nervous system, which help them conduct impulses more quickly.

Spasticity—Increased muscle tone, or stiffness, which leads to uncontrolled, awkward movements.

Transcription—The process by which genetic information on a strand of DNA is used to synthesize a strand of complementary RNA.

tures. Some of the first signs of neurologic changes are increased or decreased muscle tone and reflexes.

The most notable sign of CS is precocious senility (premature memory loss and confusion). Patients undergo neurological changes that resemble normal aging; the central and peripheral nervous systems lose myelin and neurons disappear from the central cortex and cerebellum. However, these changes occur at an extremely accelerated pace leading to death during early adolescence.

Diagnosis

Any child who displays these signs should have a genetic examination. CS is diagnosed by excluding other disorders. Specialized testing such as chromosome analysis, chromosome breakage studies, and DNA mutation analysis will rule out other **genetic disorders** such as **Bloom syndrome**, **Werner syndrome**, and **xeroderma**

pigmentosum. A person with CS will have a normal complement of 46 chromosomes. Their chromosomes also will not show any breakage when subjected to specialized laboratory analysis. DNA testing to look for the specific mutations in the CSA gene is also possible.

Only a very limited number of laboratories can perform the specialized testing that exposes cultured skin fibroblasts to UV irradiation. The fibroblasts of an affected person will lack the ability to form colonies.

Treatment and management

No specific treatment exists for CS. Patients should be treated according to the symptoms they have. Physical therapy will help prevent joint contractures that limit walking. Poor feeders may require a gastrostomy tube to prevent malnutrition. Patients should use sunscreen liberally and limit their exposure to sunlight. Special education will help to maximize the child's learning potential.

Prognosis

The prognosis for CS is grim. Most patients die during the early adolescent years. Some survive until early adulthood. However, some patients have a more severe form and may die during early childhood.

Prevention

Since carriers of the gene that causes CS appear normal, and routine testing before pregnancy is not yet available, couples will not be aware of their risk until they have an affected child. For future pregnancies, prenatal diagnosis can determine whether or not the baby has CS.

Resources

PERIODICALS

Cleaver, J. E., et al. "A Summary of Mutations in the UV-sensitive Disorders: Xeroderma Pigmentosum, Cockayne Syndrome, and Trichothiodystrophy." *Human Mutation* 14, no.1 (1999): 9-22.

Greenhaw, G. A., et al. "Xeroderma Pigmentosum and Cockayne Syndrome: Overlapping Clinical and Biochemical Phenotypes." *American Journal of Human Genetics* 50, no.4 (April 1992): 677-89.

Higginbottom, M. C., et al. "The Cockayne Syndrome: An Evaluation of Hypertension and Studies of Renal Pathology." *Pediatrics* 64, no. 6 (December 1979): 929-34.

Mathur, R., M. R. Chowdhury, and G. Singh. "Recent Advances in Chromosome Breakage Syndromes and Their Diagnosis." *Indian Pediatrics* 37, no. 6 (June 2000): 615-25.

Nance, M. A., and S. A. Berry. "Cockayne Syndrome: Review of 140 cases." *American Journal of Medical Genetics* 42, no. 1 (January 1, 1992): 68-84.

Sugita, T., et al. "Prenatal Diagnosis of Cockayne Syndrome Using Assay of Colony-forming Ability in Ultraviolet Light Irradiated Cells." *Clinical Genetics* 22, no. 3 (September 1982): 137-42.

Suzanne M. Carter, MS, CGC

Coffin-Lowry syndrome

Definition

Coffin-Lowry syndrome (CLS) is an inherited syndrome characterized by mental retardation, slow growth, distinctive facial appearance, large soft hands, loose joints, minor skeletal changes, and low muscle tone (hypotonia). Full expression of the disorder is seen only in males, although females may have some of the physical features and learning disability.

Description

Coffin-Lowry syndrome is one of a large number of mental retardation syndromes caused by abnormalities (mutations) of genes on the X **chromosome**. The pattern of physical findings, combined with mental retardation, makes the condition readily recognizable and its frequency makes it one of the well-known **X-linked mental retardation** syndromes. Although CLS was initially considered to be two separate syndromes, Coffin syndrome and Lowry syndrome, the two entities were recognized as the same disease in 1975.

Genetic profile

The **gene** for Coffin-Lowry syndrome, RSK2, is located on the short arm of the X chromosome designated as Xp22. Mutation of the RSK2 gene leads to full expression of the Coffin-Lowry syndrome in males since they only have a single X chromosome. If one of the two RSK2 genes is altered, it leads to some expression of the condition in the form of physical features and learning disabilities. Because females have two X chromosomes, CLS is considered inherited as an X-linked semidominant.

Demographics

Coffin-Lowry syndrome appears to occur in all populations. The full syndrome is seen in males with lesser expression in carrier females. A prevalence range of one in 50,000-100,000 males has been cited, but no studies with complete case findings have been conducted.

Signs and symptoms

Although the findings in Coffin-Lowry change with age, some manifestations are present from birth. Low muscle tone (hypotonia) and distinctive facial features that include prominent forehead, increased space between the eyes, forward direction of the nostrils, arching of the upper lip, and simple ear structure may be present in infancy. With the passing years, the face elongates, the ears become notably large, the lips and nasal structures thicken, and the mouth is usually open and agape. The hands are large and soft with thick fingers that narrow at their ends. There is generalized looseness at the joints. The central part of the chest may bow outward, the knees are flexed, and the feet flat.

Growth is slow, as manifest by low birth weight, a small head, and short stature during childhood and adult life. All developmental milestones in infancy and childhood are delayed, and intellectual function is severely impaired.

Milder findings consisting of short stature, increased space between the eyes, thick nasal tissues, prominent lips, and soft fleshy hands with thick fingers are consistently seen in carrier females. Intellectual function may be normal or mildly impaired.

Diagnosis

The diagnosis is usually based on the presence of the distinctive facial appearance and mental retardation. In many cases there will be a family history of other affected males or carrier females. X rays may show a number of minor features including delayed maturation of the bones, expansion at the ends of the bones of the digits, notching of the bones of the spine and narrowing of the space between the bones of the spine. The RSK2 gene responsible for Coffin-Lowry syndrome has been isolated, but gene testing is currently available only in research laboratories.

Treatment and management

There is no cure for Coffin-Lowry syndrome. There are no major malformations or specific health problems that pose complications. Because of severe mental retardation, lifelong supervision is generally required. Developmental progress can be promoted by early intervention, speech therapy, and physical therapy.

Prognosis

Long-term survival is the expectation, since individuals with Coffin-Lowry do not have any particular dis-

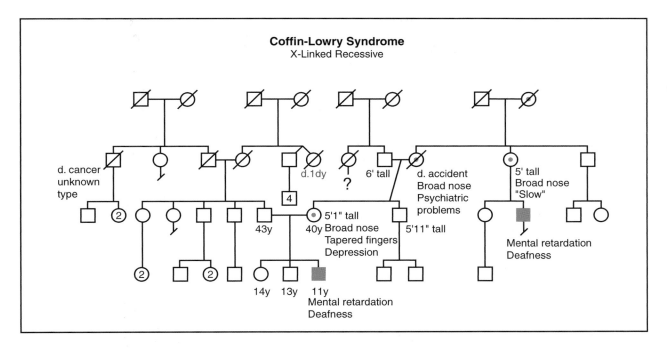

Coffin-Lowry Syndrome
X-Linked Recessive

d. cancer
unknown
type

4

d.1dy

?

6' tall

d. accident
Broad nose
Psychiatric
problems

5' tall
Broad nose
"Slow"

43y

40y

5'1" tall
Broad nose
Tapered fingers
Depression

5'11" tall

Mental retardation
Deafness

14y 13y 11y
Mental retardation
Deafness

2 2

(Gale Group.)

ease susceptibilities, nor do they have any major malformations. However, although there is an overall decrease in longevity in persons with severe mental retardation, specific information on survival in the Coffin-Lowry syndrome is not available.

Resources

PERIODICALS

Coffin, G. S., E. Siris, and L. C. Wegienka. "Mental Retardation with Osteocartilaginous Anomalies." *American Journal of Diseases of Children* 112 (1966): 205.

Lowry, B., and J. R. Miller. "A New Dominant Gene Mental Retardation Syndrome." *American Journal of Diseases of Children* 121 (1971): 496,.

Temtamy, S. A., J. D. Miller, and I. Hussels-Maumenee. "The Coffin-Lowry Syndrome: An Inherited Faciodigital Mental Retardation Syndrome." *Pediatrics* 86 (1975): 724.

Trivier, E., et al. "Mutations in the Kinase RSK-2 Associated with Coffin-Lowry Syndrome." *Nature* 384 (1996): 567.

Roger E. Stevenson, MD

Coffin-Siris syndrome

Definition

Coffin-Siris syndrome is a rare congenital disorder that affects more females than males. Individuals with this syndrome have some degree of mental retardation or developmental delay, a coarse facial appearance, incompletely formed or absent fifth fingernails, and absent fifth fingers (distal phalanges). The cause of this disorder is unknown, and the severity of symptoms varies by individual.

Description

Coffin-Siris syndrome was first described in 1970 by Dr. Grange S. Coffin and Dr. Evelyn Siris. It may also be known as fifth digit syndrome. The cause of the disorder is unknown, and the combination of symptoms may vary by individual. All affected children have some form of mental retardation or developmental delay, and incompletely formed (hypoplastic) or absent fifth fingernails and tips of the fifth fingers (distal phalanges). There are some reports of fingers other than the fifth being affected, and affected toes and toenails. The face of a child with Coffin-Siris syndrome is usually described as coarse. This includes a flat nasal bridge, broad nose, wide mouth, thick lips, and in some cases, thick eyebrows, long eyelashes, palate malformations, a large tongue (macroglossia), and a small head (microcephaly). While some infants have an abnormal facial appearance, most of the facial features become more prominent as the child grows. Typically, there is sparse scalp hair in the infant and excessive growth of body hair (hirsutism). Reduced muscle tone (hypotonia), lax joints, delay in bone maturation, and short stature are commonly found. There are reports of frequent upper respiratory and ear infections. Occasionally, children with this disorder have cardiac or spinal abnormalities, hernias, vision or hearing problems, or delayed tooth development (dentition).

Infants with Coffin-Siris syndrome typically have sucking problems and feeding difficulties that may continue as they age. The extent of growth and mental retardation varies by individual. Mental retardation is usually reported as moderate. There are delays in motor activities such as rolling over, sitting up, and walking. Speech is usually delayed. Most children are more capable of responding to speech, rather than verbally expressing themselves.

Genetic profile

At present, the cause of Coffin-Siris syndrome is unknown. Most children reported with this disorder have a normal **chromosome** set (**karyotype**). There are a few cases in which a transfer of genetic material between chromosomes (translocation) has occurred. This may provide information about a specific chromosome site responsible for Coffin-Siris syndrome, but it has not been found in many individuals.

The majority of cases are sporadic, or random, in which the parents and siblings of an affected child are all healthy. However, there are some cases of affected siblings, and parental relatedness (consanguinity). Coffin-Siris syndrome was originally thought to follow an autosomal recessive pattern of **inheritance**. This would mean that both healthy parents were carriers for the disorder, and the affected child inherited the affected **gene** from both parents. However, there are some reported cases that do not follow this pattern. An exact pattern of inheritance is unknown. The recurrence risk may be as high as 25%.

Demographics

At present, there are reports of more than 60 individuals affected with Coffin-Siris syndrome. It is more common in females, and the female to male ratio may be as high as a 3:1. There are cases of affected siblings, and parental relatedness. In general, cases are random, with affected children having healthy siblings and parents.

Signs and symptoms

At birth, infants with Coffin-Siris syndrome will have an absence or incomplete formation of the fifth fingernail and tip of the fifth finger (distal phalanx). This absence may also occur in the toes or in other fingers. Infants may have an abnormal facial appearance at birth. As the child grows, the facial abnormalities characteristic of Coffin-Siris syndrome become more apparent. Sparse scalp hair in an infant usually becomes more dense with age and excessive hair growth (hirsutism) develops. Infants typically have sucking problems and feeding difficulties that may continue with age.

There is a delay in both gross and fine motor skills. Developments such as sitting up and walking may be delayed or not possible, depending upon the severity of the disorder. Speech is usually delayed and most children are better able to respond to language rather than express it. Some older children are able to form short sentences and answer simple questions. Mental retardation is usually moderate. Social adaptation is usually delayed.

Diagnosis

At present, the diagnosis of Coffin-Siris syndrome is based upon clinical findings. There are no laboratory tests that can confirm the disorder. The combination of symptoms such as coarse facial appearance, fifth finger appearance, and developmental delay would suggest Coffin-Siris syndrome. X ray of the hands to reveal the absence of the fifth finger bone is usually the best indicator of this syndrome. Neonatal ultrasounds for cardiac, kidney (renal), and other malformations that may be present with this disorder can also be informative.

Prenatal ultrasound may show intrauterine (occurring within the uterus) growth retardation, and can reveal the condition of the fifth finger. However, these symptoms alone cannot conclusively lead to a prenatal diagnosis of Coffin-Siris syndrome.

Due to the rarity, range of symptoms, and variability of Coffin-Siris syndrome, a definitive diagnosis may be difficult. It is important to exclude other disorders that may have similar symptoms. These include **Coffin-Lowry syndrome**, **Cornelia de Lange syndrome**, fetal hydantoin syndrome, trisomy 9p, and Brachymorphism-onychodysplasia-dysphalangism syndrome.

Treatment and management

The treatment or therapy required for children with Coffin-Siris syndrome is based on the particular symptoms of each individual. Some children may require surgery to repair malformations that may be seen with this disorder. This ranges from cleft palate repair to cardiac, renal, or other surgery. Speech therapy and special education may be considered depending upon the degree of mental retardation, developmental delay, and motor impairment.

Prognosis

Infants born with Coffin-Siris syndrome may experience a delay or absence of motor and mental activities, but with support can live into adulthood. The lifestyle of an individual with Coffin-Siris syndrome is dependent to a large extent upon the degree of mental retardation and developmental delay.

Resources

PERIODICALS

Braun-Quentin, C., et al. "Variant of Coffin-Siris Syndrome or Previously Undescribed Syndrome?" *American Journal of Medical Genetics* 64 (1996): 568-572.

Coffin, G. S., and E. Siris. "Mental Retardation with Absent Fifth Fingernail and Terminal Phalanx." *American Journal of Diseases of Children* 119 (1970): 433-439.

Dimaculangan, D. P., et al. "Difficult Airway in a Patient with Coffin-Siris Syndrome." *Anesthesia and Analgesia* 92(2001): 554-555.

Fleck, B. J., et al. "Coffin-Siris Syndrome: Review and Presentation of New Cases From A Questionnaire Study." *American Journal of Medical Genetics* 99 (2001): 1-7.

McPherson, E. W., et al. "Apparently Balanced t(1;7)(q21.3;q34) in an Infant With Coffin-Siris Syndrome." *American Journal of Medical Genetics* 71 (1997): 430-433.

Rabe, P., et al. "Syndrome of Developmental Retardation, Facial and Skeletal Anomalies, and Hyperphosphatasia in Two Sisters: Nosology and Genetics of the Coffin-Siris Syndrome." *American Journal of Medical Genetics* 41(1991): 350-354.

ORGANIZATIONS

National Organization for Rare Disorders (NORD). PO Box 8923, New Fairfield, CT 06812-8923. (203) 746-6518 or (800) 999-6673. Fax: (203) 746-6481. <http://www.rarediseases.org>.

WEBSITES

Coffin-Siris Syndrome. <http://members.aol.com/CoffinSiri/index.html>.

Maureen Teresa Mahon, BS, MFS

Cohen syndrome

Definition

Cohen syndrome is a very rare genetic disorder characterized by infantile hypotonia (a weakening of the skeletal muscles), childhood obesity and several malformations.

Description

Cohen syndrome was first described in 1973 by Dr. M. M. Cohen, Jr. in three children with distinct physical and developmental observations. Since then, over 100 cases have been reported throughout the world, offering the picture of an extremely rare disease with a wide range of clinical characteristics. The initial description given by Cohen included obesity, mental retardation, low muscle tone, narrow hands and feet, and distinctive facial features with prominent upper central teeth. The underlying cause of the disease remains unknown.

Cohen syndrome has also been referred to as Pepper syndrome, hypotonia-obesity-prominent incisors syndrome, obesity-hypotonia syndrome, and Mirhosseini-Holmes-Walton syndrome.

Genetic profile

Research has suggested that the **gene** for Cohen syndrome lies between 8q21.3 and 8q22.1. This refers to a location on the long arm of **chromosome** 8 between positions 21.3 and 22.1 and is a rough estimate of where the gene may lie. This region was originally referred to as CHS1 but has since become known as COH1. The phrase "COH1 gene region" is often used due to the fact that the exact location of the gene remains to be discovered.

Chromosomes are the genetic material passed down from generation to generation that tell a person's body how to work and how to grow. Each chromosome is composed of smaller pieces known as genes. A person inherits one set of 23 chromosomes from both the egg and the sperm of the parents. These chromosomes can then be matched into pairs, giving two copies of each chromosome and likewise two copies of each gene.

Cohen syndrome is an autosomal recessive disorder. Recessive means that both copies of the COH1 gene region must have a change or mutation for a person to be affected. An individual with only one changed COH1 gene region is not affected by the disease but can pass the disease on to a future child. These individuals are called carriers. If two carriers have a child there is a 25% chance with each pregnancy that the child will be affected. At this time prenatal diagnosis is not available.

Demographics

While Cohen syndrome affects all races and genders, several small samplings of affected populations have been studied around the world. Interestingly, it has been found that Cohen syndrome manifests in these populations in distinctly different ways, with certain clinical findings being family- or ethnic-specific.

For example, Cohen syndrome has been studied extensively in Finland. In the populations studied, individuals diagnosed with the syndrome typically have fewer white blood cells than normal (granulocytopenia), a specific eye abnormality called mottled retina, and mental retardation. As a rule, they do not have truncal obesity, a common characteristic of Cohen syndrome in other populations. Although the symptoms of Cohen syndrome are known to vary widely between affected individuals within the same family, affected people within the Finnish populations are very similar to each other in their presentation.

Due to the extreme rarity of the disease, the exact incidence of Cohen syndrome is not known. A relatively high frequency of the disease has also been noted in Israel. However, earlier reports suggesting a possible increase in the frequency of Cohen syndrome among Ashkenazi Jews no longer seems to be true.

Signs and symptoms

Four main areas are affected by Cohen syndrome: physical appearance, mental function, vision, and hematology (blood function). The list of possible conditions is extensive however, and it is important to remember that each case is different. While a given characteristic may be common to the syndrome, not all affected individuals have been found to have it.

Physical appearance

When they are born, babies with Cohen syndrome usually look just like babies without the syndrome, although they are typically born at a low birth weight. As they grow, the various physical signs associated with the syndrome become increasingly obvious.

Narrow hands and feet with long slender fingers are a hallmark feature, found in approximately 89% of diagnosed individuals. Truncal obesity, or the abnormal deposition of fat around the mid-section of the body, has been observed in roughly 70% of patients. Most individuals with Cohen syndrome have large and rather noticeable front teeth, referred to as prominent upper central incisors. In general, the teeth are abnormal in shape and position. A majority of individuals with Cohen syndrome are also short, with many experiencing growth deficiency at all stages of life. Microcephaly (small head) is another common feature of the syndrome.

In addition, there are many other associated physical characteristics that occur less often. The palate (roof of the mouth) may be overly high, arched, and narrow. The mid-face can have an underdeveloped appearance and the area below the nose to the upper lip (philtrum) may be very short. The eyes can be down-slanting and thick hair and eyebrows may be observed.

Mental dysfunction

It is thought that every individual with Cohen syndrome experiences some level of developmental delay. Mental retardation can range from mild to severe. Even from infancy many are obviously behind in developmental milestones and are not able to sit up or roll over within the same time frame as their peers.

Most children with Cohen syndrome do learn to walk, although there have been a few reported cases of individuals who were wheelchair-bound. There is usually a noticeable delay, with affected children not learning to walk independently until much later than their peers (the normal average age for walking independently is 12 months).

Language deficiencies are also a common occurrence. Many affected individuals never learn to talk or have a vocabulary limited to a few singular words and two-word phrases. In general an IQ of less than 50 is considered average for Cohen syndrome.

Visual deficiencies

Vision is affected to varying degrees. Severe limitation in eyesight due to **myopia** is often observed. Several other dysfunctions and defects of the eyes causing low visual clarity have been reported including retinal dystrophy, strabismus, astigmatism, microphthalmia, and **coloboma** of the iris.

Hematologic abnormalities

Cohen syndrome can have a profound effect on the composition of the blood. Abnormally low counts of white blood cells, referred to as granulocytopenia, was once thought to be a standard symptom. It was hoped that it could help in early diagnosis because it can be tested for at birth. However, further studies have shown that not all affected individuals suffer from granulocytopenia. Some individuals have no blood disorders associated with their disease at all while others have various forms of white blood cell problems, such as a reduction in the number of white blood cells in the blood (leucopenia) or of neutrophils, which are specialized white blood cells (neutropenia).

Other deficiencies

Hypotonia, or low muscle tone, is found in 90-100% of the persons diagnosed with Cohen syndrome. Babies with hypotonia are described as "floppy" due to their lack of muscle strength. Although the observed hypotonia is not thought to be associated with any nervous system disorder, it does delay the overall development of the child, most notably in slowing the development of motor skills.

Social skills

Many studies have described Cohen syndrome patients as being outgoing and friendly with mild hyperactivity and severe attention deficits. There are a few reports of diagnosed individuals showing signs of **autism**, an extreme form of centering attention and interest on the self only.

Diagnosis

In 1972, Dr. Mirhosseini and others described two patients with symptoms similar to those observed in Cohen syndrome. These patients and a few subsequent cases were given a diagnosis of Mirhosseini-Holmes-Walton syndrome. Over the years, scientific opinion has come to consider Mirhosseini-Holmes-Walton syndrome and Cohen syndrome as different manifestations of the same disease.

Diagnosis of Cohen syndrome is difficult due to the varied nature of the symptoms. Most features of Cohen syndrome are not evident in the newborn and many symptoms, such as truncal obesity and visual deficits are not easily observed until early childhood. In the past, the average age of diagnosis was approximately 6-8 years. However, as physicians become more aware of the disorder it is hoped that diagnosis will occur at earlier ages, offering affected individuals the opportunity for rapid intervention and treatment.

Incorrect diagnosis is not uncommon in patients with Cohen syndrome. Affected individuals may be misdiagnosed with **Marfan syndrome**, **Sotos syndrome**, hypothyroidism, **Prader-Willi syndrome**, or mental retardation of an unknown nature.

A correct and early diagnosis is important to ensure the favorable prognosis of the patient and so that the family can receive appropriate **genetic counseling** concerning the affected child or the risks involved in future pregnancies.

Treatment and management

Treatment of Cohen syndrome is focused on improving or alleviating symptoms as they arise. There is no cure for Cohen syndrome.

Early correction of vision problems, usually with glasses, often leads to general improvement to cognitive skills, an area of marked deficit in affected individuals.

As is the case for many disorders involving hypotonia and slowed development, physical and occupational therapy are invaluable tools. These treatment strategies are important at any age, but should be started as early as possible. There is no need to wait for a definitive diagnosis of Cohen syndrome as any child with hypotonia can benefit from physical and occupational therapy.

Prognosis

Varying symptoms lead to varying prognosis. Mental retardation can range from mild to severe. However, there is no way to predict the level of developmental delay a specific child will experience. Language deficiencies also vary a lot, with some children never learning to speak at all and others speaking full sentences. The hypotonia observed in infancy may persist and moderate obesity usually develops in mid-childhood.

In 2001, there was one reported case of a woman with Cohen syndrome giving birth. The child had some developmental delays but was thought not to have Cohen syndrome.

Resources

PERIODICALS

Kivitie-Kallio, S., J. Rajantie, E. Juvonen, and R. Norio. "Granulocytopenia in Cohen syndrome." *British Journal of Haematology* 98 (1999): 308-311.

Young, I. D., and J. Moore. "Intrafamilial variation in Cohen syndrome." *Journal of Medical Genetics* 24 (1987): 488-492.

ORGANIZATIONS

International Cohen Syndrome Support Group. 7 Woods Court, Brackley, Northants, NN13-6HP. UK (012) 80–704515.

WEBSITES

The Arc: A National Organization on Mental Retardation. <http://www.thearc.org>.

NORD—National Organization for Rare Diseases, Inc. <http://www.rarediseases.org>.

Java O. Solis, MS

Coloboma

Definition

Coloboma, also known as keyhole defect of the iris, is a congenital genetic disorder that affects the iris of the eye. Present at birth, coloboma implies the absence of tissue.

Description

A coloboma describes a condition wherein a portion of a structure of the eye is absent, usually the iris, retina, or the optic nerve. The disorder is often referred to as a keyhole defect of the iris because the shape of the coloboma appears as the shape of a keyhole or an upside-down pear. There are many different types of colobomas, as described below.

Types of colobomas:

- Optic disc coloboma. This disorder occurs when the coloboma covers the optic nerve and may involve the macula, a structure in the eye that is responsible for visual acuity.

- Iris coloboma. This type of coloboma may be in one eye (unilateral) or in both eyes (bilateral). The pupil is often described as an upside-down pear shape when an individual has an iris coloboma.

- Retinal coloboma. In this disorder, a notch or cleft of the retina or part of the retina is missing. For example, 35% or more of the retina may be missing.

- Choroidal coloboma. This condition is similar to a retinal coloboma. The choroid is a structure in the eye that lies between the sclera and the retina.

- Morning glory syndrome. This condition, a type of optic nerve coloboma, affects the shape of the optic nerve. The syndrome is aptly named because it describes the appearance of the optic nerve, which looks like the inside of a morning glory flower.

Genetic profile

Colobomas may be isolated abnormalities in otherwise normal individuals or they may occur as part of a syndrome. As isolated findings, they are generally sporadic (not inherited). Some families, however, have shown an autosomal dominant **inheritance** pattern, meaning only one copy of the abnormal **gene** needs to be present for the disorder to occur. Some of the **genetic disorders** thought to contribute to coloboma include cat-eye syndrome, **trisomy 13**, **trisomy 18**, **Sturge-Weber syndrome**, and basal cell nevus syndrome.

Demographics

The condition occurs in about one in 10,000 births. Coloboma may be associated with hereditary or genetic conditions, trauma to the eye, or eye surgery.

Signs and symptoms

Chorioretinal colobomas are those that affect the choriod (light impermeable lining consisting primarily of blood vessels) and the retina (the photosensitive lining inside the eye). The extent to which vision would be impaired depends on the size of the coloboma, and its impact on the optic nerve and macula. A coloboma can appear as a black indentation of varying depth at the edge of the pupil, and gives the pupil an odd or irregular shape. It may also appear as a split in the iris from the pupil to the edge of the iris.

Symptoms usually present as blurred or decreased vision, and an appearance of a hole or odd-shaped pupil in the individual's eye. A smaller colboma, especially if it is not attached to the pupil, often causes a secondary image to focus on the back of the eye, producing blurred vision or decreased visual sharpness.

Diagnosis

A diagnosis is made by a physical exam and includes a detailed eye examination by an ophthalmologist. The ophthalmologist will also ask the individual when the symptoms were first noticed, determine what part of the eye is affected, the size and shape of the dark area in the eye, and ask for reports of any changes in the individual's vision.

Certain diagnostic tests are often used to diagnose coloboma. These include a visual acuity test, refraction test, and an in-depth history of symptoms.

Treatment and management

Colobomas may be accompanied by other problems that may be neurological or chromosomal in nature. In addition, some genetic syndromes also include coloboma

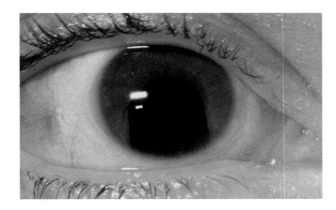

The pupil in this eye is enlarged, extending to the lower edge of the cornea. Colobomas form because of a failure of the rudimentary eye to join the optic fissure during embryonic development. *(Photo Researchers, Inc.)*

as part of the disorder's potential findings. More importantly, a specific combination of abnormalities identified by the acronym CHARGE must also be considered when a diagnosis of coloboma is made.

The medical condition known as CHARGE association is a very rare and serious condition. Individuals that have the condition will require attention from several specialists and treatment from an early age. Colobomas are usually one of the findings in individuals with CHARGE. The disorder includes these problems:

- (C)oloboma
- (H)eart defects
- (A)tresia of the choanae, which is a blockage of the nasal passages
- (R)etarded growth and development
- (G)enital hypoplasia, which occurs when the testes do not descend properly
- (E)ar abnormalities

While there is no specific treatment for coloboma, some treatments are available that can manage vision problems associated with the disorder. For example, physicians often recommend cosmetic contact lenses and sunglasses for individuals whose eyesight is adversely affected. Additional optical aids are often helpful such as eye patching. Since many individuals with coloboma are highly sensitive to light, ophthalmologists often recommend special lights or other personalized visual aids.

Prognosis

The effects of coloboma can be mild or severe, depending upon the extent and location of the gap or cleft. The gap itself is usually located at the bottom of the eye, but it may occur in the iris, choroid, macula or optic nerve.

A coloboma of the lens, particularly if it is large, may also include abnormalities of the iris and choroids, which increases the risk of retinal tearing. In severe cases of coloboma, the eye may be reduced in size. This condition is called microphthalmous, a disorder that can arise with or without coloboma.

The specific gene or genes responsible for coloboma have not yet been identified, but research continues throughout the United States, Scotland, and England.

Resources

ORGANIZATIONS
Royal National Institute for the Blind. PO Box 173, Peterborough PE2 6WS. <http://www.rnib.org.uk>.

WEBSITES
Coloboma. <http://www.coloboma.org/whatis.html>.

Medlineplus. <http://www.medline.adam.com/ency/article/003318.htm>.

Bethanne Black

Coloboma-obesity-hypogenialism-mental retardation syndrome *see* **Coloboma**

Color blindness

Definition

Color blindness is an abnormal condition characterized by the inability to clearly distinguish different colors of the spectrum. The difficulties can be mild to severe. It is a misleading term because people with color blindness are not blind. Rather, they tend to see colors in a limited range of hues; a rare few may not see colors at all.

Description

Normal color vision requires the use of specialized receptor cells called cones, which are located in the retina of the eye. There are three types of cones, termed red, blue, and green, which enable people to see a wide spectrum of colors. An abnormality, or deficiency, of any of the types of cones will result in abnormal color vision.

There are three basic variants of color blindness. Red/green color blindness is the most common deficiency, affecting 8% of Caucasian males and 0.5% of Caucasian females. The prevalence varies with culture.

Blue color blindness is an inability to distinguish both blue and yellow, which are seen as white or gray. It is quite rare and has equal prevalence in males and females. It is common for young children to have blue/green confusion that becomes less pronounced in adulthood. Blue color deficiency often appears in people who have physical disorders such as liver disease or **diabetes** mellitus.

A total inability to distinguish colors (achromatopsia) is exceedingly rare. These affected individuals view the world in shades of gray. They frequently have poor visual acuity and are extremely sensitive to light (photophobia), which causes them to squint in ordinary light.

Genetic profile

Red/green and blue color blindness appear to be located on at least two different **gene** locations. The majority of affected individuals are males. Females are carriers but are not normally affected. This indicates that the X **chromosome** is one of the locations for color blindness. Male offspring of females who carry the altered gene have a fifty-fifty chance of being colorblind. The rare female that has red/green color blindness, or rarer still, blue color blindness, indicates there is an involvement of another gene. The location of this gene has not been identified.

Achromatopsia, the complete inability to distinguish color, is an autosomal recessive disease of the retina. This means that both parents have one copy of the altered gene but do not have the disease. Each of their children has a 25% chance of not having the gene, a 50% chance of having one altered gene (and, like the parents, being unaffected), and a 25% risk of having both the altered gene and the condition. In 1997, the achromatopsia gene was located on chromosome 2.

Demographics

Researchers studying red/green color blindness in the United Kingdom reported an average prevalence of only 5% in one group. Only 1% of Eskimo males are color blind. Approximately 3% of boys from Saudi Arabia and 4% from India were found to have deficient color vision. Red/green color blindness may slightly increase an affected person's chances of contracting leprosy. Pre-term infants exhibit an increased prevalence of blue color blindness. Achromatopsia has a prevalence of about one in 33,000 in the United States and affects males and females equally.

Color blindness is sometimes acquired. Chronic illnesses that can lead to color blindness include **Alzheimer disease**, diabetes mellitus, **glaucoma**, leukemia, liver disease, chronic **alcoholism**, macular degeneration, **multiple sclerosis**, **Parkinson disease**, sickle cell anemia, and **retinitis pigmentosa**. Accidents or strokes that damage the retina or affect particular areas of the brain can lead to color blindness. Some medications such as antibiotics, barbiturates, anti-tuberculosis drugs, high blood pressure medications, and several medications used to treat nervous disorders and psychological problems may cause color blindness. Industrial or environmental chemicals such as carbon monoxide, carbon disulfide, fertilizers, styrene, and some containing lead can cause loss of color vision. Occasionally, changes can occur in the affected person's capacity to see colors after age 60.

Signs and symptoms

The inability to correctly identify colors is the only sign of color blindness. It is important to note that people with red/green or blue varieties of color blindness use other cues such as color saturation and object shape or location to distinguish colors. They can often distinguish red or green if they can visually compare the colors. However, most have difficulty accurately identifying colors without any other references. Most people with any impairment in color vision learn colors, as do other young children. These individuals often reach adolescence before their visual deficiency is identified.

Diagnosis

There are several tests available to identify problems associated with color vision. The most commonly used is the American Optical/Hardy, Rand, and Ritter Pseu-

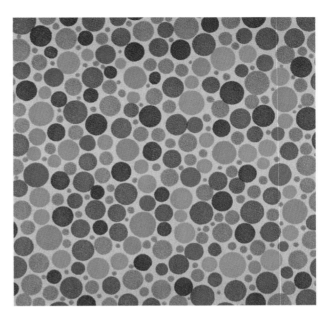

A common test used to detect color blindness. The number "hidden" in the image will not be visible to an individual with red/green color blindness. *(Corbis.)*

doisochromatic test. It is composed of several discs filled with colored dots of different sizes and colors. A person with normal color vision looking at a test item sees a number that is clearly located somewhere in the center of a circle of variously colored dots. A color-blind person is not able to distinguish the number.

The Ishihara test is comprised of eight plates that are similar to the American Optical Pseudoisochromatic test plates. The individual being tested looks for numbers among the various colored dots on each test plate. Some plates distinguish between red/green and blue color blindness. Individuals with normal color vision perceive one number. Those with red/green color deficiency see a different number. Those with blue color vision see yet a different number.

A third analytical tool is the Titmus II Vision Tester Color Perception test. The subject looks into a stereoscopic machine. The test stimulus most often used in professional offices contains six different designs or numbers on a black background, framed in a yellow border. Titmus II can test one eye at a time. However, its value is limited because it can only identify red/green deficiencies and is not highly accurate.

Treatment and management

There is no treatment or cure for color blindness. Most color vision deficient persons compensate well for their abnormality and usually rely on color cues and

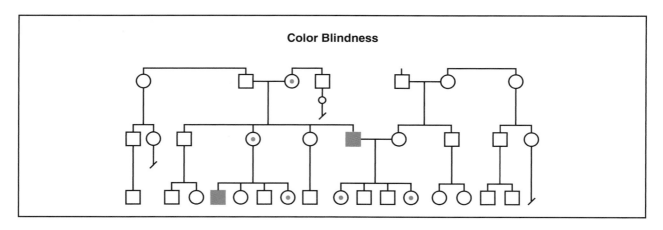

Color Blindness

(Gale Group.)

KEY TERMS

Achromatopsia—The inability to distinguish any colors.

Cones—Receptor cells that allow the perception of colors.

Photophobia—An extreme sensitivity to light.

Retina—The light-sensitive layer of tissue in the back of the eye that receives and transmits visual signals to the brain through the optic nerve.

Rod—Photoreceptor that is highly sensitive to low levels of light and transmits images in shades of gray.

---

details that are not consciously evident to persons with typical color vision.

Inherited color blindness cannot be prevented. In the case of some types of acquired color deficiency, if the cause of the problem is removed, the condition may improve with time. But for most people with acquired color blindness, the damage is usually permanent.

Prognosis

Color blindness that is inherited is present in both eyes and remains constant over an individual's entire life. Some cases of acquired color vision loss are not severe, may appear in only one eye, and can last for only a short time. Other cases tend to be progressive, becoming worse with time.

Resources

BOOKS

Rosenthal, Odeda, and Robert H. Phillips. *Coping with Color Blindness*. Garden City Park, NY: Avery Publishing Group, 1997.

Sacks, Oliver. *The Island of the Colorblind*. New York, Knopf, 1997.

Wiggs, Janey L. Color Vision. In: *Ophthalmology,* edited by Myron Yanoff and Jay S. Duker. St. Louis, Mosby, 2000, pp. 8-10.

PERIODICALS

Arbour, N. C., et al. "Homozygosity Mapping of Achromatopsia to Chromosome 2 Using DNA Pooling." *Human Molecular Genetics* 6, no. 5 (May 1997): 689-694.

Dobson, V., et al. "Color Vision Measured with Pseudoisochromatic Plates at Five-and-a-Half Years in Eyes of Children from the CRYO-ROP Study." *Investigations in Ophthalmology and Visual Science* 37, no. 12 (November 1996): 2467-2474.

Holroyd, E., and D. M. Hall. "A Re-Appraisal of Screening for Colour Vision Impairments." *Child Care Health Developments* 23, no. 5 (September 1997): 391-398.

Osuobeni, E. P. "Prevalence of Congenital Red-Green Color Vision Defects in Arab Boys from Riyadh, Saudi Arabia." *Ophthalmic Epidemiology* 3, no. 3 (December 1996): 167-170.

ORGANIZATIONS

Achromatopsia Network. C/O Frances Futterman, PO Box 214, Berkeley, CA 94701-0214. <http://www.achromat.org/how_to_join.html>.

American Academy of Ophthalmology. PO Box 7424, San Francisco, CA 94120-7424. (415) 561-8500. <http://www.eyenet.org>.

International Colour Vision Society: Forschungsstelle fuer Experimentelle Ophthalmologie. Roentgenweg 11, Tuebingen, D-72076. Germany <http://orlab.optom.unsw.edu.au/ICVS>.

National Society to Prevent Blindness. 500 East Remington Rd., Schaumburg, IL 60173. (708) 843-2020 or (800) 331-2020. <http://www.preventblindness.org>.

WEBSITES

"Breaking the Code of Color." *Seeing, Hearing and Smelling the World.* <http://www.hhmi.org/senses/b/b130.htm>.

"Color Blindness." *Geocities.* <http://www.geocities.com/Heartland/8833/coloreye.html>.

"Medical Encyclopedia: Colorblind." *MEDLINEplus.* <http://medlineplus.adam.com/ency/article/001002sym.htm>.

University of Manchester. <http://www.umist.ac.uk/UMIST_OVS/welcome.html>.

University of Nevada–Reno. <http://www.delamare.unr.edu/cb/>.

L. Fleming Fallon, Jr., MD, MPH

Cone-rod dystrophy

Definition

Cone-rod dystrophy (CRD) is a progressive retinal degenerative disease that causes deterioration of the cones and rods in the retina and frequently leads to blindness. Cone-rod dystrophy is also accompanied by amelogenesis imperfecta, an abnormality affecting the teeth.

Description

Cone-rod dystrophy is characterized by all of the following elements: skin pigmentation abnormality, involuntary, rhythmic movements of the eyes (nystagmus), degeneration of vision (optic atrophy), and sensitivity to light (photophobia).

Cone-rod dystrophy can be inherited as either an autosomal dominant or autosomal recessive trait. In its most common form, however, it is usually inherited as an autosomal recessive trait, which means that both parents have one copy of the cone-rod dystrophy **gene** but do not have the disease. Autosomal recessive cone-rod dystrophy (arCRD) is a genetically heterogeneous disease with changes (mutations) in the ABCR gene. These mutations cause an abnormality in rod outer segment function that ultimately leads to dysfunction or death of the photoreceptor cells in the retina.

Genetic profile

The CRX gene has been shown to contain mutations that cause an autosomal dominant form of cone-rod dystrophy. This means that only one parent has to pass on the gene mutation in order for the child to be affected

with the disease. This genetic form of CRD is clinically known as CORD2, or cone-rod dystrophy 2. Mutations in the CRX gene interfere in the development process of embryonic photoreceptor cells during the early stages of life. The result is abnormal photoreceptor cells with reduced function.

Demographics

Inherited retinal degeneration dystrophies have an incidence of approximately one in 4,000 people. Cone-rod dystrophy is an uncommon entity. The prevalence is estimated to be in the range of one in 10,000 to one in 100,000.

Signs and symptoms

The earliest symptom of CRD is loss of night vision that usually begins after the age of 20. The vision loss is progressive and unrelenting. Over the next decade, loss of all vision begins and by age 50, most people with cone-rod dystrophy have gone completely blind.

Cone-rod dystrophy is occasionally accompanied by amelogenesis imperfecta, which is characterized by abnormally shaped teeth and abnormalities in the tooth enamel.

Diagnosis

The earliest symptom of cone-rod dystrophy is decreased visual acuity. However, the diagnosis of cone-rod dystrophy is usually established with loss of the peripheral visual fields. Cone-rod dystrophy must be distinguished from **retinitis pigmentosa** (RP). In CRD, rods and cones are lost at approximately the same rate. It is further distinguished from RP by the absence of night blindness as a presenting symptom.

Treatment and management

There are no known treatments or cures for cone-rod dystrophy. It has been suggested, however, that people with cone-rod dystrophy may be able to slow the progression of their blindness by wearing sunglasses and avoiding bright light.

Prognosis

Studies of individuals thought to have cone-rod dystrophy reveal that central vision loss begins in the first decade of life with the onset of night blindness occurring sometime after age 20. Little visual function remains after the age of 50. There is no cure for this syndrome.

Resources

BOOKS

McKusick, Victor A. *Mendelian Inheritance in Man: A Catalog of Human Genes and Genetic Disorders.* 12th ed. Baltimore: Johns Hopkins University Press, 1998.

Yanoff, Myron, and Jay S. Duker. *Ophthalmology.* St. Louis: Mosby, 2000.

PERIODICALS

Downes, Susan M., et al. "Autosomal Dominant Cone and Cone-Rod Dystrophy With Mutations in the Guanylate Cyclase Activator 1A Gene-Encoding Guanylate Cyclase Activating Protein-1." *Archives of Ophthalmology* 119, no. 1 (2001): 96–105.

ORGANIZATIONS

American Academy of Ophthalmology. PO Box 7424, San Francisco, CA 94120-7424. (415) 561-8500. <http://www.eyenet.org>.

Association for Macular Diseases, Inc. 210 East 64th St., New York, NY 10021. (212) 605-3719. 2020@nei.nih.gov. <http://www.macula@macula.org>.

Foundation Fighting Blindness. Executive Plaza 1, 11350 McCormick Rd, Suite 800, Hunt Valley, MD 21031. (888) 394-3937. jchader@blindness.org. <http://www.blindness.org>.

National Eye Institute. 31 Center Dr., Bldg. 31, Rm 6A32, MSC 2510, Bethesda, MD 20892-2510. (301) 496-5248. 2020@nei.nih.gov. <http://www.nei.nih.gov>.

Retinitis Pigmentosa International. 23241 Ventura Blvd., Suite 117, Woodland Hills, CA 91364. (818) 992-0500 or (800) 344-4877. rpint@pacbell.net. <http://www.rpinternational.org>.

WEBSITES

Foundation Fighting Blindness: <http://www.blindness.org/html/science/wcord2.html>.

Retina Foundation of the Southwest. <http://www.retinafoundation.org/eyeinfo2.html>.

Southeastern Eye Center. <http://www.southeasterneyecenter.com/cases/bulls_eye.htm>.

L. Fleming Fallon , Jr, MD, DrPH

Congenital adrenal hyperplasia

Definition

Congenital adrenal hyperplasia (CAH) refers to a group of autosomal recessive genetic conditions that result from an abnormality in one of the enzymes required by the adrenal glands to convert cholesterol into cortisol, aldosterone, and androgens.

Description

The first likely description of congenital adrenal hyperplasia (CAH) occurred in 1865 when an anatomist named Luigi De Crecchio reported on a cadaver who had what appeared to be a penis with the urinary opening on its underside and undescended testicles. What was remarkable about this cadaver was that it also had a vagina, a uterus, fallopian tubes, ovaries, and very enlarged adrenal glands. From four years of age until his death, this person had lived his life as a male although at birth he was declared a female. He died in his 40s after many episodes of vomiting, diarrhea, and prostration. This genetic female with masculinized external genitals and abnormalities in regulating the amount of salt in her body had all the symptoms of a textbook case of a severe and untreated CAH.

Congenital adrenal hyperplasia (CAH), formerly called adrenogenital syndrome, results from an abnormality in one of the enzymes required by the adrenal glands to convert cholesterol into cortisol, aldosterone, and androgens such as testosterone. These three hormones are very necessary for normal health. Cortisol helps the body to cope with stress such as injury or illness, aldosterone helps to insure that the body retains normal amounts of salt, and androgens such as testosterone are involved in the production of masculine traits such as body hair and the development of male sex organs.

There are many different enzymes necessary for the normal production of cortisol, aldosterone, and testosterone. Each type of CAH results from a deficiency in one of these enzymes. One of the most important enzymes involved in the breakdown of cholesterol is 21-hydroxylase. 21-hydroxylase is involved in the conversion of cholesterol to cortisol and aldosterone but is not involved in the conversion of cholesterol to testosterone. Ninety to ninety-five percent of people with CAH have a deficiency or absence of 21-hydroxylase (21-hydroxylase deficiency).

A deficiency or absence of 21-hydroxylase (CAH21) results in the production of decreased levels of cortisol and aldosterone, which prompts the body to compensate by forcing the adrenal glands to increase the conversion of cholesterol. This does not result in significantly increased levels of cortisol and aldosterone, but does result in increased levels of testosterone, which is produced by another enzyme. Both men and women normally produce some testosterone, although men typically produce larger amounts of this hormone.

Increased levels of testosterone can result in premature puberty in males and females and can cause the absence of a menstrual period and increased amounts of body hair in women. Females who produce high levels of this hormone in utero can be born with masculinized external genitals. Decreased levels of cortisol can also result in increased levels of two other hormones called 17-hydroxyprogesterone and androstenedione. Increased levels of 17-hydroxyprogesterone in conjunction with decreased levels of aldosterone can result in an inability of the body to retain normal amounts of salt.

The three major types of 21-hydroxylase deficiency (CAH21) are: (1) the classic salt-losing form, (2) the classic non-salt-losing form, and (3) the non-classical form (later onset form). The classic forms of the disorder, if untreated, can result in premature puberty in boys and can cause girls to be born with an enlarged clitoris or external male genitals. Men and women with untreated classical CAH21 can have increased growth in childhood but short adult height. The salt-losing form of CAH21 results in reduced levels of salt in the body, which can sometimes result in an adrenal crisis. An adrenal crisis is a life threatening condition characterized by severe dehydration, very low blood pressure, and vomiting. The non-classic form, which is milder and has a later onset, can cause women to have an absence of menstruation and increased body hair and can cause a low sperm count in men.

Genetic profile

All types of CAH are autosomal recessive genetic conditions. An autosomal recessive condition is caused by a change in both genes of a pair. A person with CAH, has changes in both copies of the **gene** responsible for producing one of the enzymes involved in the breakdown of cholesterol. He or she has inherited one changed gene from his or her mother and one changed gene from his or her father. CAH21 results from changes in a gene, called CYP21, which creates the enzyme 21-hydroxylase, and is found on **chromosome** 6. When the CYP21 gene is changed it does not produce any 21-hydroxylase or it produces small amounts of this enzyme. There are a number of different types of gene changes that can result in reduced levels of 21-hydroxylase. The amount of 21-hydroxylase produced depends on the type and combination of CYP21 gene changes and partially determines the severity of CAH21.

Parents who have a child with CAH are called carriers, since they each possess one changed CAH gene and one unchanged CAH gene. Carriers usually do not have any symptoms since they have one unchanged gene that produces enough enzyme to prevent the symptoms of CAH. Each child born to parents who are both carriers for the same type of CAH, has a 25% chance of having CAH, a 50% chance of being a carrier, and a 25% chance of being neither a carrier nor affected with CAH disease.

Demographics

Approximately one in 10,000 infants is born with CAH, making it the most common disorder of the adrenal glands. CAH affects both females and males of all ethnic backgrounds. CAH21 is the most common form of CAH affecting 90–95% of people with CAH. Approximately one in 60 people are carriers for CAH21.

Signs and symptoms

The type of symptoms experienced by a person with CAH depends on their particular enzyme deficiency. CAH can cause congenital masculinization of the female external genitals or can cause feminization of the male genitals. CAH does not, however, affect the internal sexual organs of either males or females. CAH can cause women to have an absence of menstrual periods and increased body hair and is associated with premature puberty in both males and females. In some cases CAH can result in an inability of the body to retain normal amounts of salt.

CAH21 has a range of symptoms and the severity of the disorder is partially related to the amount of 21-hydroxylase that the body produces. The three major types of 21-hydroxylase deficiency (CAH21) are: (1) the classic salt-losing form, (2) the classic non-salt-losing form, and (3) the non-classical form (later onset form).

Classic salt-losing form of CAH21

The classic salt-losing form is the most severe form of CAH21 and results when very little or no 21-hydroxylase is produced. Untreated girls may be mistaken for boys at birth since they are typically born with fairly masculinized external genitals. Their internal sexual organs are, however, normal. Males with untreated CAH21 have normal external genitals but may experience premature puberty. Signs of puberty such as pubic hair, enlarged penis, deepened voice, and increased muscle strength can occur long before normal puberty and can sometimes occur as early as two to three years of age. This form of CAH21, if untreated, results in a loss of salt that can trigger an adrenal crisis. An adrenal crisis is a life-threatening condition characterized by severe dehydration, very low blood pressure, weakening of the heart muscles, and vomiting. The adrenal crisis typically occurs by six to twelve weeks. On occasion, salt loss is not noticed until precipitated by an infection in early childhood. This form of CAH21, if untreated, can also cause increased growth in childhood but short adult height in men and women.

Classical non-salt-losing form of CAH21

The classical non-salt-losing form of CAH21 results when a low amount of 21-hydroxylase is produced. In this form of CAH21 enough enzyme is present to prevent abnormally low levels of salt in the body and to prevent an adrenal crisis. Girls are born with slightly masculinized external genitals such as an enlarged clitoris and a partial fusion of the labia. If untreated, they may also experience early puberty and the lack of a menstrual period. Untreated boys have normal genitals but may have premature puberty. This form of CAH21, can also cause increased growth in childhood but short adult height in men and women.

Non-classical form of CAH21

The non-classical form is the mildest form of CAH21 and results from mildly decreased levels of 21-hydroxylase. Males and females with this form of CAH21 appear normal at birth and do not exhibit a salt deficiency. Untreated women may have an increase in body hair, irregular or absent menstrual periods, and/or cysts on their ovaries. Many men do not have any symptoms even if untreated. Some men and woman have short stature, severe acne, and decreased fertility.

Diagnosis

Diagnostic testing

Most forms of CAH can be diagnosed by measuring the amount of specific hormones in a urine sample. The type of hormone that is found in excess amounts in the urine depends on the type of CAH. CAH21 can be diagnosed by measuring the amount of 17-hydroxyprogesterone in a urine sample since people with CAH21 typically have elevated amounts of this hormone in their urine.

CAH21 is however, best diagnosed through a blood test called an ACTH (adrenocorticotropic hormone) stimulation test. ACTH is a hormone that stimulates the adrenal glands to convert cholesterol to cortisol. The ACTH stimulation test measures the amount of 17-hydroxyprogesterone in the blood before and after stimulation with ACTH. People with CAH21 have an exaggerated production of 17-hydroxyprogesterone after stimulation with ACTH. The ACTH stimulation test can usually identify what type of CAH21 a person is affected with.

Once a biochemical diagnosis of CAH is made, **DNA** testing may be recommended. DNA testing is available for some but not all types of CAH. Detection of a CYP21 gene alteration in a person with CAH21 can confirm an uncertain diagnosis and can help facilitate prenatal diagnosis and carrier testing of relatives. Some people with CAH21 may possess DNA changes that are not detectable through DNA testing.

Carrier testing

A person who has a relative with CAH or parents who have a child with CAH21 should consider undergoing carrier testing. Carriers for CAH21 can sometimes be identified through the ACTH stimulation test, although DNA testing is more accurate and is usually the recommended test. If possible, DNA testing should be first performed on the family member who is affected with CAH21. If a change in the CYP21 gene is detected, then carrier testing can be performed in relatives such as siblings and parents, with an accuracy of greater than 99%. If the affected relative does not possess detectable CYP21 gene changes, then DNA carrier testing will be inaccurate and should not be performed. In these cases ACTH stimulation testing of the potential carrier can be considered. If DNA testing of the affected relative cannot be performed, DNA carrier testing of family members can still be performed but will only identify approximately 95% of carriers.

Carrier testing should also be considered by someone who has a partner who is a carrier or is affected with CAH. DNA testing, which identifies approximately 95% of carriers for CAH21, is the recommended test for people who choose to undergo carrier testing but who do not themselves have a family history of CAH21.

Prenatal testing

If both parents are carriers for the same type of CAH or one parent is a carrier for CAH and one parent is affected with the same type of CAH, then prenatal testing should be considered. Prenatal testing is available for CAH21 and some of the other types of CAH. DNA testing is the recommended method of prenatal testing for CAH21 but it can only be performed if both parents have detectable mutations (gene changes) in CYP21. Prenatal testing cannot always identify what type of CAH21 a fetus has.

Some parents are known to be carriers for CAH21 since they already have a child with CAH21, yet they do not possess CYP21 gene changes that are detectable through DNA testing. Prenatal diagnosis can be performed in these cases by measuring the amount of 17-hydroxyprogesterone in the amniotic fluid, obtained from an **amniocentesis**. This type of prenatal testing can only detect the salt-losing form of CAH21.

Prenatal testing is especially important for mothers who are undergoing dexamethasone therapy to help prevent their daughters from being born with masculine genitalia. Although treatment must be started before prenatal testing can be performed, treatment can be discontinued if the baby is found to be a male or female who does not have CAH21.

Newborn screening

Many states offer newborn screening for CAH21. If newborn screening is available, hospitals in that state will automatically screen for CAH21 by measuring the amount of 17-hydroxyprogesterone in a drop of blood obtained from a newborn baby. More precise testing should be done if the initial test indicates that the infant has CAH21.

Treatment and management

Medications

Most people with CAH are treated with cortisol-like medications and in most cases this therapy is life-long. The goal of treatment is to return cortisol, aldosterone, and testosterone to near normal levels. People with the salt-losing and non-salt-losing forms of CAH21 are treated with injections of cortisol-like steroid medications or oral steroid medications. People with the salt-losing form are also given a form of oral aldosterone. Babies with the salt-losing form of CAH21 need to have salt added to their formula or breast milk. Children and adults do not need a salt supplement provided they have a high salt diet. An adrenal crisis is treated by intravenous administration of fluids containing sugars and salt. People with the non-classical form of CAH21, who require treatment, are treated with oral steroids. Medical therapy achieves hormonal balance most of the time, but CAH patients can have periods of fluctuating hormonal

control. These fluctuations often require modifications in the amount of steroid required for treatment.

Some people with the salt-losing form of CAH21 are resistant to standard therapy. In 2001, the National Institutes of Health began conducting clinical trials determining the efficacy of a new combination drug treatment for CAH21. This experimental therapy involves treatment with a combination of four medications—flutamide, testolactone, reduced hydrocortisone dose, and fludrocortisone. The goal of these trials is to see whether this type of medical therapy is able to effectively treat CAH21 and still allow treated individuals to obtain a normal adult stature. Preliminary results are encouraging, but further research trials are necessary before the safety and effectiveness of this therapy is fully known.

Surgery

Adrenalectomy, a surgical procedure to remove the adrenal glands, is a more radical treatment for people with the salt-losing form of CAH21 who have little or no enzyme activity. This surgery allows people with CAH21 to be treated with lower dose steroids.

Girls born with masculinized genitals may undergo a surgery to create female genitals. This surgery is often performed at about six to twelve weeks of age. Sometimes an initial surgery is performed at that time followed by a surgery to correct the opening to the vagina when the girl becomes sexually active. Some people believe that any genital surgery should be delayed until the individual is old enough to decide whether they want the surgery.

Prenatal treatment

Some mothers who are at risk for having a child with CAH21 choose to take a type of steroid called dexamethasone while they are pregnant. This treatment can often prevent the masculinization of external genitals in female fetuses. To be fully effective this treatment needs to be started at approximately five to six weeks of gestation prior to the formation of the external genitals. Treatment can be stopped if prenatal testing finds that the baby is male or is an unaffected female, otherwise treatment continues until birth. Although this treatment does not appear to have many adverse effects on the fetus, the long-term risks are not known. The mother may, however, experience side effects such as weight gain, fluid accumulation, sugar intolerance, high blood pressure, gastrointestinal problems, and mood swings.

Prognosis

If appropriately treated, the prognosis for CAH and particularly CAH21 is good and most people have a nor-

KEY TERMS

Adrenal gland—A triangle-shaped endocrine gland, located above each kidney, that synthesizes aldosterone, cortisol, and testosterone from cholesterol. The adrenal glands are responsible for salt and water levels in the body, as well as for protein, fat, and carbohydrate metabolism.

Amniocentesis—A procedure performed at 16-18 weeks of pregnancy in which a needle is inserted through a woman's abdomen into her uterus to draw out a small sample of the amniotic fluid from around the baby. Either the fluid itself or cells from the fluid can be used for a variety of tests to obtain information about genetic disorders and other medical conditions in the fetus.

Autosomal recessive—A pattern of genetic inheritance where two abnormal genes are needed to display the trait or disease.

Carrier—A person who possesses a gene for an abnormal trait without showing signs of the disorder. The person may pass the abnormal gene on to offspring.

Carrier testing—Testing performed to determine if someone possesses one changed copy and one unchanged copy of a particular gene.

Chromosome—A microscopic thread-like structure found within each cell of the body and consists of a complex of proteins and DNA. Humans have 46 chromosomes arranged into 23 pairs. Changes in either the total number of chromosomes or their shape and size (structure) may lead to physical or mental abnormalities.

Congenital—Refers to a disorder which is present at birth.

Deoxyribonucleic acid (DNA)—The genetic material in cells that holds the inherited instructions for growth, development, and cellular functioning.

Diagnostic testing—Testing performed to determine if someone is affected with a particular disease.

DNA testing—Analysis of DNA (the genetic component of cells) in order to determine changes in genes that may indicate a specific disorder.

Enzyme—A protein that catalyzes a biochemical reaction or change without changing its own structure or function.

Gene—A building block of inheritance, which contains the instructions for the production of a particular protein, and is made up of a molecular sequence found on a section of DNA. Each gene is found on a precise location on a chromosome.

Hormone—A chemical messenger produced by the body that is involved in regulating specific bodily functions such as growth, development, and reproduction.

In utero—While in the uterus; before birth.

Labia—Lips of the female genitals.

Mutation—A permanent change in the genetic material that may alter a trait or characteristic of an individual, or manifest as disease, and can be transmitted to offspring.

Prenatal testing—Testing for a disease such as a genetic condition in an unborn baby.

---

mal life span. The prognosis for patients with the salt-losing form of CAH21 is, however, dependent on early identification and treatment. Some women and men with CAH 21, even if treated, have a short adult stature and may have decreased fertility. Women surgically treated for masculinized genitals may experience physical and/or psychological difficulties with sexual intercourse. They may also experience gender confusion and sexual identity difficulties.

Resources

BOOKS

"Congenital Adrenal Hyperplasia." In *The Metabolic and Molecular Basis of Inherited Disease.* Edited by C. R. Scriver, et al. New York: McGraw Hill, 1995.

"Fetal Adrenal Development." In *Williams Obstetrics.* 20th ed. Stamford, CT: Appleton & Lange, 1997.

PERIODICALS

New, Maria, and Robert Wilson. "Steroid Disorders in Children: Congenital Adrenal Hyperplasia and Apparent Mineralocorticoid Excess." *Proceedings of the National Academy of Science (USA)* 96, no. 2 (October 1999): 12790–97.

Speiser, P. W. "Prenatal Treatment of Congenital Adrenal Hyperplasia." *The Journal of Urology* 162 (August 1999): 594–36.

Speiser, P.W., et al. "A Multicenter Study of Women with Nonclassical Congenital Adrenal Hyperplasia: Relationships Between Genotype and Phenotype." *Molecular Genetics and Metabolism* 71, no. 3 (November 2000): 527–34.

ORGANIZATIONS

Ambiguous Genitalia Support Network. PO Box 313, Clements, CA 95227-0313. (209) 727-0313. Fax: (209) 727-0313. agsn@jps.net. <http://www.stepstn.com>.

Congenital Adrenal Hyperplasia <http://congenitaladrenalhyperplasia.org>.

National Adrenal Diseases Foundation. 510 Northern Blvd., Great Neck, NY 11021. (516) 487-4992. <http://medhlp.netusa.net/www/nadf.htm>.

WEBSITES

McKusick, Victor. "Adrenal Hyperplasia, Congenital, Due to 21-hydroxylase Deficiency." *Online Mendelian Inheritance in Man.* <http://www3.ncbi.nlm.nih.gov/htbin-post/Omim/dispmim?201910>. (February 16, 2001).

Speiser, Phyllis W. "New Developments in the Treatment and Diagnosis of Congenital Adrenal Hyperplasia." National Adrenal Diseases Foundation. (June 16, 2005.) <http://www.medhelp.org/nadf/nadf5.htm>.

Lisa Andres, MS, CGC

Congenital contractural arachnodactyly *see* **Beals syndrome**

Congenital familial hypertrophic synovitis *see* **Arthropathy-camptodactyly syndrome**

Congenital heart disease

Definition

Congenital heart disease, also called congenital heart defect, includes a variety of malformations of the heart or its major blood vessels that are present at the birth of a child.

Description

Congenital heart disease occurs when the heart or blood vessels near the heart do not develop properly before birth. Some infants are born with mild types of congenital heart disease, but most need surgery in order to survive. Patients who have had surgery are likely to experience other cardiac problems later in life.

Most types of congenital heart disease obstruct the flow of blood in the heart or the nearby vessels, or cause an abnormal flow of blood through the heart. Rarer types of congenital heart disease occur when the newborn has only one ventricle, when the pulmonary artery and the aorta come out of the same ventricle, or when one side of the heart is not completely formed.

Patent ductus arteriosus

Patent ductus arteriosus refers to the opening of a passageway—or temporary blood vessel (ductus)—to carry the blood from the heart to the aorta before birth, allowing blood to bypass the lungs, which are not yet functional. The ductus should close spontaneously in the first few hours or days after birth. When it does not close in the newborn, some of the blood that should flow through the aorta then returns to the lungs. Patent ductus arteriosus is common in premature babies, but rare in full-term babies. It has also been associated with mothers who had German measles (rubella) while pregnant.

Hypoplastic left heart syndrome

Hypoplastic left heart syndrome, a condition in which the left side of the heart is underdeveloped, is rare, but it is the most serious type of congenital heart disease. With this syndrome, blood reaches the aorta, which pumps blood to the entire body, only from the ductus, which then normally closes within a few days of birth. In hypoplastic left heart syndrome, the baby seems normal at birth, but as the ductus closes, blood cannot reach the aorta and circulation fails.

Obstruction defects

When heart valves, arteries, or veins are narrowed, they partly or completely block the flow of blood. The most common obstruction defects are pulmonary valve stenosis, aortic valve stenosis, and coarctation of the aorta. **Bicuspid aortic valve** and subaortic stenosis are less common.

Stenosis is a narrowing of the valves or arteries. In pulmonary stenosis, the pulmonary valve does not open properly, forcing the right ventricle to work harder. In aortic stenosis, the improperly formed aortic valve is narrowed. As the left ventricle works harder to pump blood through the body, it becomes enlarged. In coarctation of the aorta, the aorta is constricted, reducing the flow of blood to the lower part of the body and increasing blood pressure in the upper body.

A bicuspid aortic valve has only two flaps instead of three, which can lead to stenosis in adulthood. Subaortic stenosis is a narrowing of the left ventricle below the aortic valve, which limits the flow of blood from the left ventricle.

Septal defects

When a baby is born with a hole in the septum (the wall separating the right and left sides of the heart),

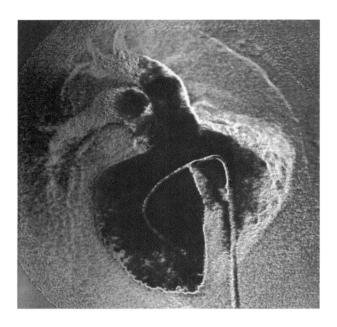

An angiogram showing a hole in the heart of a young patient.
(Photo Researchers, Inc.)

blood leaks from the left side of the heart to the right, or from a higher pressure zone to a lower pressure zone. A major leakage can lead to enlargement of the heart and failing circulation. The most common types of septal defects are atrial septal defect, an opening between the two upper heart chambers, and ventricular septal defect, an opening between the two lower heart chambers. Ventricular septal defect accounts for about 15% of all cases of congenital heart disease in the United States.

Cyanotic defects

Heart disorders that cause a decreased, inadequate amount of oxygen in blood pumped to the body are called cyanotic defects. Cyanotic defects, including truncus arteriosus, total anomalous pulmonary venous return, tetralogy of Fallot, transposition of the great arteries, and tricuspid atresia, result in a blue discoloration of the skin due to low oxygen levels. About 10% of cases of congenital heart disease in the United States are tetralogy of Fallot, which includes four defects. The major defects are a large hole between the ventricles, which allows oxygen-poor blood to mix with oxygen-rich blood, and narrowing at or beneath the pulmonary valve. The other defects are an overly muscular right ventricle and an aorta that lies over the ventricular hole.

In transposition (reversal of position) of the great arteries, the pulmonary artery and the aorta are reversed, causing oxygen-rich blood to re-circulate to the lungs while oxygen-poor blood goes to the rest of the body. In tricuspid atresia, the baby lacks a triscupid valve and

blood cannot flow properly from the right atrium to the right ventricle.

Other defects

Ebstein's anomaly is a rare congenital syndrome that causes malformed tricuspid valve leaflets, which allow blood to leak between the right ventricle and the right atrium. It also may cause a hole in the wall between the left and right atrium. Treatment often involves repairing the tricuspid valve. Ebstein's anomaly may be associated with maternal use of the psychiatric drug lithium during pregnancy.

Brugada syndrome is another rare congenital heart defect that appears in adulthood and may cause sudden death if untreated. Symptoms, which include rapid, uneven heart beat, often appear at night. Scientists believe that Brugada syndrome is caused by mutations in the **gene** SCN5A, which involves cardiac sodium channels.

Infants born with DiGeorge sequence can have heart defects such as a malformed aortic arch and tetralogy of Fallot. Researchers believe DiGeorge sequence is most often caused by mutations in genes in the region 22q11.

Marfan syndrome is a connective tissue disorder that causes tears in the aorta. Since the disease also causes excessive bone growth, most Marfan syndrome patients are over six-feet-tall. In athletes, and others, it can lead to sudden death. Researchers believe the defect responsible for Marfan syndrome is found in gene FBN1, on **chromosome** 15.

Genetic profile

Scientists have made much progress in identifying some of the genes that are responsible for congenital heart defects, but others remain a mystery. When possible, **genetic testing** can help families determine the risk that their child will be born with a heart defect.

Demographics

About 32,000 infants are born every year with congenital heart disease, which is the most common birth defect. About half of these patients require medical treatment. More than one million people with heart defects are currently living in the United States.

Signs and symptoms

In most cases, the causes of congenital heart disease are unknown. Genetic and environmental factors and lifestyle habits can all be involved. The likelihood of having a child with a congenital heart disease increases if the mother or father, another child, or another relative had congenital heart disease or a family history of sudden death. Viral infections, such as German measles, can produce congenital heart disease. Women with **diabetes** and **phenylketonuria** also are at higher risk of having children with congenital heart defects. Many cases of congenital heart disease result from the mother's excessive use of alcohol or illegal drugs, such as cocaine, while pregnant. The mother's exposure to certain anticonvulsant and dermatologic drugs during pregnancy can also cause congenital heart disease. There are many genetic conditions, such as **Down syndrome**, which affect multiple organs and can cause congenital heart disease.

Symptoms of congenital heart disease in general include: shortness of breath, difficulty feeding in infancy, sweating, cyanosis (bluish discoloration of the skin), heart murmur, respiratory infections that recur excessively, stunted growth, and limbs and muscles that are underdeveloped.

Symptoms of specific types of congenital heart disease are as follows:

• Patent ductus arteriosus: quick tiring, slow growth, susceptibility to pneumonia, rapid breathing. If the ductus is small, there are no symptoms.

• Hypoplastic left heart syndrome: ashen color, rapid and difficult breathing, inability to eat.

• Obstruction defects: cyanosis (skin that is discolored blue), chest pain, tiring easily, dizziness or fainting, congestive heart failure, and high blood pressure.

• Septal defects: difficulty breathing, stunted growth. Sometimes there are no symptoms.

• Cyanotic defects: cyanosis, sudden rapid breathing or unconsciousness, and shortness of breath and fainting during exercise.

Diagnosis

Echocardiography and cardiac magnetic resonance imaging are used to confirm congenital heart disease when it is suggested by the symptoms and physical examination. An echocardiograph will display an image of the heart that is formed by sound waves. It detects valve and other heart problems. Fetal echocardiography is used to diagnose congenital heart disease in utero, usually after 20 weeks of pregnancy. Between 10 and 14 weeks of pregnancy, physicians also may use an ultrasound to look for a thickness at the nuchal translucency, a pocket of fluid in back of the embryo's neck, which may indicate a cardiac defect in 55% of cases. Cardiac magnetic resonance imaging, a scanning method that

uses magnetic fields and radio waves, can help physicians evaluate congenital heart disease, but is not always necessary. Physicians may also use a chest x ray, to look at the size and location of the heart and lungs, or an electrocardiograph (ECG), which measures electrical impulses to create a graph of the heart beat.

Treatment and management

Congenital heart disease is treated with drugs and/or surgery. Drugs used include diuretics, which aid the baby in excreting water and salts, and digoxin, which strengthens the contraction of the heart, slows the heartbeat, and removes fluid from tissues.

Surgical procedures seek to repair the defect as much as possible and restore circulation to as close to normal as possible. Sometimes, multiple surgical procedures are necessary. Surgical procedures include: arterial switch, balloon atrial septostomy, balloon valvuloplasty, Damus-Kaye-Stansel procedure, Fontan procedure, pulmonary artery banding, Ross procedure, shunt procedure, and venous switch or intra-atrial baffle.

Arterial switch, to correct transposition of the great arteries, involves connecting the aorta to the left ventricle and connecting the pulmonary artery to the right ventricle. Balloon atrial septostomy, also done to correct transposition of the great arteries, enlarges the atrial opening during heart catheterization. Balloon valvuloplasty uses a balloon-tipped catheter to open a narrowed heart valve, improving the flow of blood in pulmonary stenosis. It is sometimes used in aortic stenosis. Transposition of the great arteries can also be corrected by the Damus-Kaye-Stansel procedure, in which the pulmonary artery is cut in two and connected to the ascending aorta and the farthest section of the right ventricle.

For tricuspid atresia and pulmonary atresia, the Fontan procedure connects the right atrium to the pulmonary artery directly or with a conduit, and the atrial defect is closed. Pulmonary artery banding, narrowing the pulmonary artery with a band to reduce blood flow and pressure in the lungs, is used for ventricular septal defect, atrioventricular canal defect, and tricuspid atresia. Later, the band can be removed and the defect corrected with open-heart surgery.

To correct aortic stenosis, the Ross procedure grafts the pulmonary artery to the aorta. For tetralogy of Fallot, tricuspid atresia, or pulmonary atresia, the shunt procedure creates a passage between blood vessels, sending blood into parts of the body that need it. For transposition of the great arteries, venous switch creates a tunnel inside the atria to re-direct oxygen-rich blood to the right ventricle and aorta and venous blood to the left ventricle and pulmonary artery.

KEY TERMS

Aorta—The main artery located above the heart which pumps oxygenated blood out into the body. Many congenital heart defects affect the aorta.

Congenital—Refers to a disorder which is present at birth.

Cyanotic—Marked by bluish discoloration of the skin due to a lack of oxygen in the blood. It is one of the types of congenital heart disease.

Ductus—The blood vessel that joins the pulmonary artery and the aorta. When the ductus does not close at birth, it causes a type of congenital heart disease called patent ductus arteriosus.

Electrocardiograph (ECG, EKG)—A test used to measure electrical impulses coming from the heart in order to gain information about its structure or function.

Hypoplastic—Incomplete or underdevelopment of a tissue or organ. Hypoplastic left heart syndrome is the most serious type of congenital heart disease.

Neuchal translucency—A pocket of fluid at the back of an embryo's neck visible via ultrasound that, when thickened, may indicate the infant will be born with a congenital heart defect.

Septal—Relating to the septum, the thin muscle wall dividing the right and left sides of the heart. Holes in the septum are called septal defects.

Stenosis—The constricting or narrowing of an opening or passageway.

When all other options fail, some patients may need a heart transplant. Children with congenital heart disease require lifelong monitoring, even after successful surgery. The American Heart Association recommends regular dental check-ups and the preventive use of antibiotics to protect patients from heart infections, or endocarditis. Since children with congenital heart disease have slower growth, nutrition is important. Physicians may also limit their athletic activity.

Prognosis

The outlook for children with congenital heart disease has improved markedly in the past two decades. Many types of congenital heart disease that would have been fatal can now be treated successfully. Research on diagnosing heart defects when the fetus is in the womb may lead to future treatment to correct defects before birth. Promising new prevention methods and treatments include genetic screening and the cultivation of cardiac tissue in the laboratory that could be used to repair congenital heart defects.

Resources

BOOKS

Mayo Clinic Heart Book. New York: William Morrow and Company, 2000.

Wild, C. L., and M. J. Neary. *Heart Defects in Children: What Every Parent Should Know.* Chronimed Publishing, Minneapolis, 2000.

Williams, R. A. *The Athlete and Heart Disease.* Lippincott Williams & Wilkins, Philadelphia, 1999.

PERIODICALS

"Coping with Congenital Heart Disease in Your Baby." *American Family Physician* 59 (April 1, 1999): 1867.

Hyett, Jon, et. al. "Using fetal nuchal translucency to screen for major congenital cardiac defects at 10-14 weeks: population based cohort study." *Lancet* 318 (January 1999): 81-85.

ORGANIZATIONS

American Heart Association. 7272 Greenville Ave., Dallas, TX 75231-4596. (214) 373-6300 or (800) 242-8721. inquire@heart.org. <http://www.americanheart.org>.

Congenital Heart Disease Information and Resources. 1561 Clark Dr., Yardley, PA 19067. <http://www.tchin.org>.

Texas Heart Institute Heart Information Service. PO Box 20345, Houston, TX 77225-0345. (800) 292-2221. <http://www.tmc.edu/thi/his.html>.

Melissa Knopper

Congenital hypothyroid syndrome

Definition

Congenital hypothyroid syndrome is a condition in which a child is born with a deficiency in thyroid gland activity or thyroid hormone levels.

Description

The thyroid gland is a small gland in the front of the neck that secretes thyroid hormones called thyroxine (T4) and triiodothyronine (T3) into the bloodstream. Some of the T4 is converted into T3 by the liver and kidney. These thyroid hormones help regulate a great number of proc-

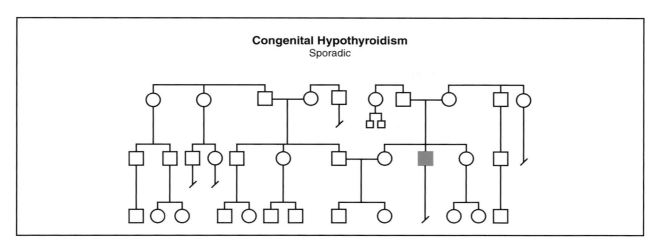

Congenital Hypothyroidism
Sporadic

(Gale Group.)

esses. A deficiency in the level of these hormones can affect the brain, heart, muscles, skeleton, digestive tract, kidneys, reproductive function, blood cells, other hormone systems, heat production, and energy metabolism.

In most cases of congenital hypothyroidism, the thyroid gland is either completely absent or severely underdeveloped. Sometimes thyroid tissue is located in ectopic, or abnormal, locations along the neck.

Other abnormalities can lead to congenital hypothyroidism including:

- abnormal synthesis of thyroid hormones;
- abnormal synthesis of thyroid-stimulating hormone (TSH) or thyrotropin-releasing hormone (TRH), which are regulatory hormones that affect the production of thyroid hormones;
- abnormal response to thyroid hormones, TSH or TRH;

- inadvertent administration of harmful drugs or substances to the pregnant mother, possibly resulting in temporary congenital hypothyroidism in the newborn;
- dietary deficiency of iodine, a raw component vital to the manufacture thyroid hormones.

Genetic profile

Most causes of congenital hypothyroidism are not inherited. Some abnormalities in thyroid hormone synthesis (TSH synthesis), or the response to TSH, are inherited in autosomal recessive fashion. This means that both parents have one copy of the changed (mutated) **gene** but do not have the condition. Abnormal response to thyroid hormone may be an autosomal dominant condition, meaning that only one parent has to pass on the gene mutation in order for the child to be affected with the syndrome.

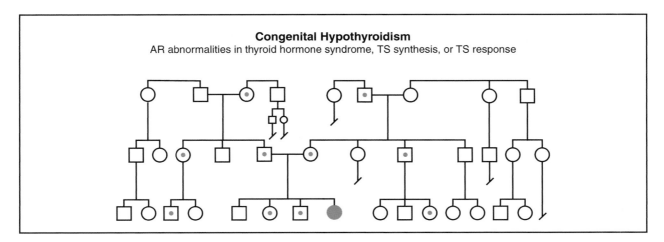

Congenital Hypothyroidism
AR abnormalities in thyroid hormone syndrome, TS synthesis, or TS response

(Gale Group.)

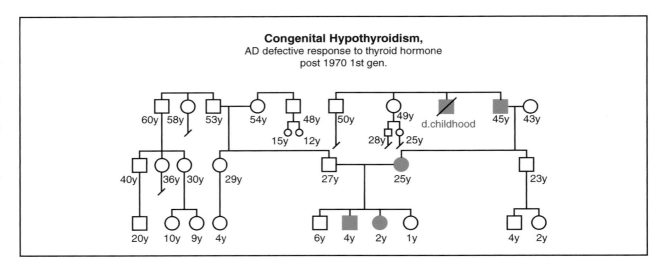

Congenital Hypothyroidism,
AD defective response to thyroid hormone
post 1970 1st gen.

(Gale Group.)

Demographics

Congenital hypothyroidism occurs in one in every 4,000 newborns in the United States. It is twice as common in girls as in boys. The condition is less common in African Americans and more common in Hispanics and Native Americans.

Signs and symptoms

The signs and symptoms of congenital hypothyroidism are difficult to observe because the mother passes along some of her thyroid hormones to the fetus during pregnancy. Even if the newborn is completely lacking a thyroid gland, it may not be obvious in the early stages of life. Ectopic thyroid tissue may also provide enough thyroid hormones for a short period of time.

Rarely, the affected newborn will exhibit jaundice (yellow skin), noisy breathing, and enlarged tongue. If hypothyroidism continues undetected and untreated, the infant may gradually demonstrate feeding problems, constipation, sluggishness, sleepiness, cool hands and feet, and failure to thrive. Other signs include protruding abdomen, slow pulse, enlarged heart, dry skin, delayed teething, and coarse hair. Affected children may also have myxedema, which is swelling of the face, hands, feet, and genitals. Hypothyroidism eventually leads to marked retardation in physical growth, mental development, and sexual maturation.

Diagnosis

Prompt diagnosis and treatment are critical to avoid the profound consequences of hypothyroidism. The signs and symptoms of hypothyroidism are often subtle in newborns, only to manifest themselves later in life when permanent damage has been done. Before the implementation of screening for hypothyroidism in the 1970s, most children with the disease suffered growth and mental retardation, as well as neurological and psychological deficits.

Most cases of congenital hypothyroid syndrome are now detected by a screening test performed during a newborn's first few days of life. Every state offers testing, and most states require it. The test for hypothyroidism is part of a battery of standard screening tests designed to diagnose important conditions. A sample of the child's blood is analyzed for levels of thyroxine (T4), thyroid-stimulating hormone (TSH), or both, depending on the individual state or country. Some states also require a second round of screening performed one to four weeks later.

Once the diagnosis of congenital hypothyroidism is made, other tests can pinpoint the nature of the abnormality. X rays of the hip, shoulder, or skull often reveal characteristically abnormal patterns of bone development. Scintigraphy is a method by which images of the thyroid gland and any ectopic thyroid tissue are obtained to determine if the thyroid is absent or ectopic. But treatment should not be delayed for these other tests. Early treatment offers a good probability of normal development.

Treatment and management

Treatment of congenital hypothyroidism requires replacement of deficient thyroid hormones with levothyroxine, an oral tablet form of T4. There is no need to

KEY TERMS

Congenital—Refers to a disorder which is present at birth.

Ectopic—Tissue found in an abnormal location.

Hypothyroid—Deficiency in thyroid gland activity or thyroid hormone levels.

Jaundice—Yellowing of the skin or eyes due to excess of bilirubin in the blood.

Levothyroxine—A form of thyroxine (T4) for replacement of thyroid hormones in hypothryoidism.

Myxedema—Swelling of the face, hands, feet, and genitals due to hypothyroidism.

Scintigraphy—Injection and detection of radioactive substances to create images of body parts.

Thyroxine (T4)—Thyroid hormone.

Triiodothyronine (T3)—Thyroid hormone.

directly replace T3, since T4 is converted to T3 by the liver and kidney. Hypothyroid children usually require more levothyroxine per pound of body weight than hypothyroid adults do. The importance of prompt and adequate treatment cannot be overemphasized. Delays in treatment result in permanent stunting of physical, mental, and sexual development.

Blood levels of T4 should be checked regularly to ensure appropriate replacement. The blood levels of TSH should also be monitored since TSH is an indicator of the effectiveness of T4 replacement. As the child develops, the physical growth rate also provides a good measure of treatment.

Prognosis

If congenital hypothyroidism is detected and treated early in life, the prognosis is quite good. Most children will develop normally. However, the most severely affected infants may have mild mental retardation, speech difficulty, hearing deficit, short attention span, or coordination problems.

Resources

BOOKS

"Hypothyroidism." In *Nelson Textbook of Pediatrics*, edited by Richard E. Behrman, et al. 16th ed. Philadelphia: W.B. Saunders Company, 2000.

"The Thyroid." In *Cecil Textbook of Medicine*, edited by Lee Goldman, et al. 21st ed. Philadelphia: W.B. Saunders Company, 2000.

"Thyroid Hormone Deficiency." In *Williams Textbook of Endocrinology*, edited by Jean D. Wilson, et al. 19th ed. Philadelphia: W.B. Saunders Company, 1998.

ORGANIZATIONS

U.S. Preventive Services Task Force, Guidelines from Guide to Clinical Preventive Services. Williams and Wilkins, 1996.

Kevin O. Hwang, MD

Congenital ichthyosis-mental retardation-spasticity syndrome *see* **Sjögren Larsson syndrome**

Congenital isolated hemihypertrophy *see* **Hemihypertrophy**

Congenital megacolon *see* **Hirschsprung disease**

Congenital retinal blindness *see* **Leber amaurosis congenita**

Conjoined twins

Definition

Conjoined twins are an extremely rare type of identical twins who are physically joined at birth.

Description

Scientists believe conjoined twins form because of a delay in the fertilized egg's division. In normal identical twins, the egg splits at four to eight days after fertilization. In conjoined twins, however, the split occurs sometime after day 13. Instead of forming two separate embryos, the twins remain partially attached as they develop inside the womb. In most cases, conjoined twins do not survive more than a few days past birth because of a high rate of malformed organs and other severe birth abnormalities. However, surgical separations have been successful in conjoined twins that have a superficial physical connection.

Conjoined twins are commonly referred to as Siamese twins, although this is now considered a derogatory term. The phrase Siamese twins originated from the famous conjoined twins Eng and Chang Bunker, who were born in Siam (Thailand) in 1811.

Some conjoined twins are attached at the upper body, others may be joined at the waist and share a pair

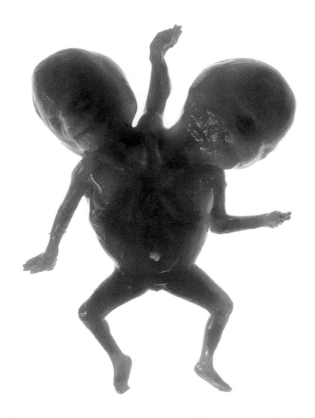

These conjoined twins developed until the seventeenth week of pregnancy. It is difficult for conjoined twins to survive when they share the same key organs such as these siblings. (Custom Medical Stock Photo, Inc.)

of legs. Conjoined twins often share major organs such as a heart, liver, or brain. Medical experts have identified several types of conjoined twins. They are classified according to the place their bodies are joined. Most of the terms contain the word pagus, which means "fastened" in Greek.

Upper body

Cephalopagus: A rare form that involves conjoined twins with fused upper bodies and two faces on opposite sides of a single head.

Craniopagus: Conjoined twins with separate bodies and one shared head is a rare type and only occurs in 2% of cases.

Thoracopagus: About 35% of conjoined twin births have this common form of the condition, which joins the upper bodies. These twins usually share a heart, making surgical separation nearly impossible.

Lower body

Ischopagus: About 6% of conjoined twins are attached at the lower half of the body.

Omphalopagus: The type of conjoined twins that are attached at the abdomen and that often share a liver accounts for approximately 30% of all cases.

Parapagus: About 5% of conjoined twins are joined along the side of their lower bodies.

Pygopagus: About 19% of conjoined twins are joined back to back with fused buttocks.

Rare types

Dicephalus: Twins that share one body, but have two separate heads and necks.

Parasitic twins: This occurs when one smaller, malformed twin is dependent on the larger, stronger twin for survival.

Fetus in fetu: In this unusual case, one fetus grows inside the body of the other twin.

Genetic profile

Scientists are still searching for the cause of conjoined twins. They believe a combination of genetic and environmental factors may be responsible for this rare condition.

Demographics

Conjoined twins occur in one out of every 50,000 births. Many such pregnancies are terminated before birth, or the infants are stillborn. Conjoined twins are always identical and of the same sex. They are more often female than male, by a ratio of 3:1. Conjoined twins are more likely to occur in Africa, India, or China than in the United States. Conjoined twins have appeared in triplet and quadruplet births, but no cases of conjoined triplets or quadruplets have ever been reported. Most parents of conjoined twins are younger than 35 years old.

Signs and symptoms

Approximately 50% of women who are pregnant with conjoined twins will develop excess fluid surrounding the fetuses, which can lead to premature labor and an increased risk of miscarriage. Conjoined twins joined at the abdomen (omphalopagus) are more likely to be breech babies. In breech births, infants are born feet or buttocks first instead of head first. Most omphalopagus conjoined twins are born by cesarean section to increase their odds of survival.

Conjoined twins can be born with a complication called hydrops, which causes excessive fluid to build up in an infant's body and can be life-threatening. Those who survive past birth may experience **congenital heart disease**, liver or kidney disease, physical or mental disabilities, and intestinal blockages.

Diagnosis

Physicians typically try to determine if a woman is having conjoined twins at an early stage so that the parents can have an option to terminate the pregnancy if the odds of survival are low. Ultrasound imaging is a technique in which high-frequency sound waves create a picture of a developing fetus inside the womb and is often used to make the diagnosis. Initial diagnosis is possible at 10-12 weeks of gestation, but it is difficult to determine which body structures are involved until 20 weeks of gestation.

In utero, the three-dimensional magnetic resonance imaging (MRI) test is another important diagnostic tool that helps more precisely define which body parts of the conjoined twins are connected. An abdominal x ray of the mother is used to look for connected bones in conjoined twin embryos.

Treatment and management

Early diagnosis is key so that families and health-care providers can begin to plan for the birth of conjoined twins. Because of the high rate of miscarriage and difficult labor, most conjoined twins are delivered by cesarean section. Some conjoined twins have survived and lived full lives without serious medical interventions. If the twins do not share a large number of organs, however, physicians typically will recommend a surgical separation.

A large medical team must be assembled for a surgical separation. Physicians prefer to wait for a few months after birth, but that may not be possible if the twins are born with life-threatening congenital abnormalities. The type of surgery that is performed is determined by where the twins are connected. Doctors will often insert tissue expansion devices into the twins' skin before the operation to promote better healing at the site of separation.

Conjoined twins who survive a surgical separation will have many ongoing health-care needs, from wound care to prosthetic limbs and special diets. As the twins grow up and start school, they also may need counseling to help them adjust.

Prognosis

The majority of conjoined twin pregnancies are not successful. However, most conjoined twins who undergo a planned surgical separation several months after birth do survive. The survival rate for conjoined twins who need an emergency separation at birth is approximately 44%.

KEY TERMS

Breech delivery—Birth of an infant feet or buttocks first.

Craniopagus—Conjoined twins with separate bodies and one shared head.

Dicephalus—Conjoined twins who share one body but have two separate heads and necks.

Fetus in fetu—In this case, one fetus grows inside the body of the other twin.

Ischopagus—Conjoined twins who are attached at the lower half of the body.

Omphalopagus—Conjoined twins who are attached at the abdomen.

Parapagus—Conjoined twins who are joined at the side of their lower bodies.

Parasitic twins—Occurs when one smaller, malformed twin is dependent on the larger, stronger twin for survival.

Pygopagus—Conjoined twins who are joined back to back with fused buttocks.

Thoracopagus—Conjoined twins joined at the upper body who share a heart.

Zygote—The cell formed by the uniting of egg and sperm.

Resources

BOOKS

Martel, Joanne. *Millie-Christine: Fearfully and Wonderfully Made*. John F. Blair, 2000.

Segal, Nancy L. *Entwined Lives: Twins and What They Tell Us about Human Behavior*. Dutton, 1999.

Strauss, Darin. *Chang and Eng*. EP Dutton, 2000.

PERIODICALS

Johnson, Kimberly. "I Had Siamese Twins." *Ladies' Home Journal*. 110, Issue 3 (March 1993): 24-27.

Paden, Cheryl Sacra, and Sondra Forsyth. "Miracle Babies." *Ladies' Home Journal* 116, Issue 11 (November 1999): 145-151.

ORGANIZATIONS

Center for Loss in Multiple Birth, Inc. (CLIMB). PO Box 1064, Palmer, AK 99654. (907) 222-5321.

Center for Study of Multiple Birth. 334 E. Superior St., Suite 464, Chicago, IL 60611. (312) 266-9093. <http://www.multiplebirth.com>.

Conjoined Twins International. PO Box 10895, Prescott, AZ 86304-0895.

National Organization of Mothers of Twins Clubs. PO Box 438, Thompson Station, TN 37179. (615) 595-0936. <http://www.nomotc.org>.

Twins Foundation. PO Box 6043, Providence, RI 02940-6043. (401) 751-8946. Twins@twinsfoundation.com.

WEBSITES

Conjoined Twins fact sheet from Children's Hospital of Columbus. <www.childrenscolumbus.org/gen/twinsfact.html>.

"Conjoined Twins." (April 30, 2001). *TwinStuff.com.* <http://www.twinstuff.com/conjoined.htm>.

OTHER

Twin Falls Idaho. Videotape. Sony Pictures Classics, 1990.

Melissa Knopper

Cooley's anemia *see* **Beta-thalassemia**

Corneal dystrophy

Definition

Corneal dystrophy is a condition that causes a layer of the cornea to cloud over and impair visual clarity. It is usually a bilateral problem, which means it occurs in both eyes equally. There are more than 20 different forms of inherited corneal dystrophies. A corneal dystrophy can occur in otherwise healthy individuals. Depending on the type of condition and the age of the individual, a corneal dystrophy may either cause no problems, moderate vision impairment, or severe difficulties that require surgery.

Description

The cornea is the outside layer of the eye, and comprises five layers itself, including the outer epithelium, the Bowman's layer, the stroma, or middle, layer that takes up about 90% of the entire cornea, the Descemet's membrane, and the endothelium. In most cases, the central (stromal) layer of the cornea is involved.

Some corneal dystrophies are named after the individual who discovered them, while others are descriptive of the pattern seen with the dystrophy or the location of the disease. The key forms of corneal dystrophy are congenital hereditary endothelial dystrophy (CHED), epithelial basement membrane dystrophy, Fuchs' endothelial dystrophy, granular dystrophy, lattice dystrophy, macular corneal dystrophy, Meesmann's corneal dystro-phy, posterior polymorphous dystrophy (PPD), and Reis-Bucklers' dystrophy.

Genetic profile

Genetic alterations (mutations) causing corneal dystrophies have been mapped to 10 different chromosomes. Some dystrophies have not yet been mapped, including Fuchs' dystrophy.

Some corneal dystrophies have the same genetic address. Mutations on the BIGH3 **gene** of **chromosome** 5q31 cause granular corneal dystrophy and Reis-Bucklers' dystrophy. Macular corneal dystrophy has been mapped to an altered gene on chromosome 16. The mutation causing congenital hereditary endothelial dystrophy has been mapped to 20p11-20q11. Lattice type I is linked to the 5q31 locus (location), while lattice type II dystrophy is linked to the 9q34 locus. Posterior polymorphous corneal dystrophy has been linked to the 20q11 locus.

Most corneal dystrophies, with the exception of congenital endothelial corneal dystrophy and macular dystrophy, are autosomal dominant. In dominant disorders, a single copy of the mutated gene (received from either parent) dominates the normal gene and results in the appearance of the disease. The risk of transmitting the disorder from parent to offspring is 50% for each pregnancy.

Both congenital endothelial corneal dystrophy and macular dystrophy are autosomal recessive. This means the affected person inherits the same abnormal gene for the same trait from both parents; each parent is a carrier for the disease but usually does not have symptoms of the disease. The risk of transmitting the disease to each pregnancy is 25%.

Demographics

The diversity of corneal dystrophies diseases makes it difficult to provide specific demographic data. Some dystrophies appear in early childhood or even infancy, such as Reis-Bucklers' dystrophy. Others may not appear until middle age or beyond, as with Fuchs' dystrophy. Women are at greater risk for Fuchs' dystrophy, especially those over age 40. However, most corneal dystrophies present before age 20.

Signs and symptoms

The symptoms vary with the type of corneal dystrophy and the location of the site. Most experts categorize these diseases based on whether they are located on the anterior (outer) layer, stromal (middle) layer, or endothelial (inner) layer.

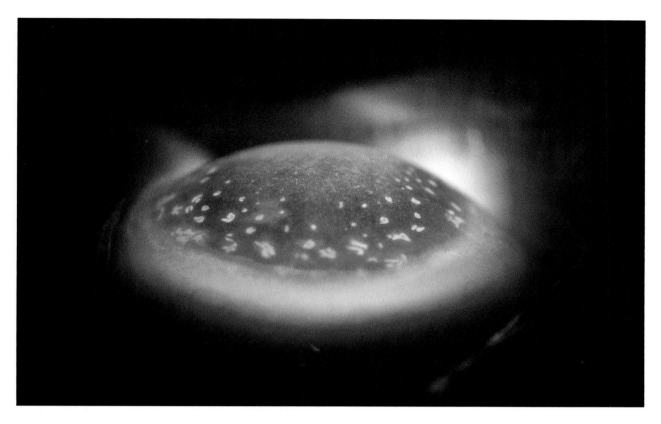

Gradual deterioration of the corneal tissue layers results in corneal dystrophy. As the tissue deteriorates, a gritty appearance such as that shown above, becomes apparent. *(Custom Medical Stock Photo, Inc.)*

Anterior corneal dystrophies

The epithelium, or the "basement membrane," and the Bowman's layer together comprise the anterior, or outer part, of the cornea. Epithelial basement membrane dystrophy, also known as Cogan's map-dot-fingerprint dystrophy, is a disorder that causes errors in refractions of the eye and may also present with microscopic cysts. This disease results from excessive fluid (edema) and swelling of the basement membrane into the epithelium. Symptoms of this disease are map-like dots, opaque circles, or thin lines that are formed in a swirled pattern like fingerprints. Individuals with this disorder feel like they have something irritating in the eye and experience pain and light sensitivity (photophobia).

The tiny opaque collagen fibers that cause Reis-Bucklers' dystrophy create a linear or ring-like pattern. People with this disease have recurrent painful erosions of the cornea and may also suffer from severe visual impairment. Reis-Bucklers' is usually noticed in an infant or young child who suddenly has very red eyes. To the ophthalmologist, the cornea looks like frosted glass. This disorder may recur several times per year and disappear when affected individuals are in their 20s or 30s.

Stromal dystrophies

The primary dystrophies found in the stromal layer are granular dystrophy, lattice dystrophy, and macular dystrophy. Granular dystrophy is so named because of the small opaque areas caused by deposits of hyaline, a substance that accumulates as cells deteriorate. Lattice dystrophy is caused by deposits of amyloid, the same substance that accumulates in the brain in people with **Alzheimer disease**. Both granular dystrophy and lattice dystrophy have been identified in family members in Avellino, Italy, and these dystrophies are sometimes grouped together and called Avellino corneal dystrophy. Lattice and granular dystrophies can cause severe eye pain. With lattice dystrophy, by about age 40, an affected person's vision can be very obscured and a corneal transplant is required.

Endothelial dystrophies

Fuchs' dystrophy is the most common of the endothelial dystrophies and is inherited as an autosomal dominant trait. It is characterized by blurred vision, hypersensitivity to light (photophobia), and two to eight acute inflammatory attacks per year. It may also cause ulceration and erosion of the cornea. Fuchs' can cause deterioration of endothelial cells and result in corneal guttata, which are thickenings or leakages from the Descemet's membrane of the cornea. These guttata eventually cause edema (excessive fluid) to leak into the stromal or epithelial areas.

Posterior polymorphous dystrophy (PPD), an autosomal dominant disease, also causes edema, although it affects a larger area than Fuchs' dystrophy. It usually does not cause vision impairment.

Congenital hereditary endothelial dystrophy (CHED) comprises two types. The autosomal dominant form is CHED 1 and the recessive form is CHED 2. CHED 1 can occur in early childhood and may also cause hearing loss. The key symptoms of CHED 1 are sensitivity to light and excessive tearing. CHED 2 is present at birth and is more severe than CHED 1. In both CHED 1 and 2, the cornea presents with a milky haze or the appearance of ground glass.

Macular dystrophy is inherited as an autosomal recessive trait. It can present as early as age three and up to about age nine and is very debilitating. This disorder is caused by deposits of keratin sulfate (sulfur-containing fibrous proteins) and becomes increasingly painful. The child will have a feeling of something in the eye and also experience photophobia (sensitivity to light).

Diagnosis

Corneal dystrophy may be identified by an optometrist and diagnosed by an ophthalmologist. The findings determine the existence and type of corneal dystrophy. The presence, size, and shape of any opaque material in the eyes are considered.

The affected cornea of a person with lattice dystrophy will have a ground glass appearance, while granular deposits indicate granular dystrophy. The examination can also reveal the presence of amyloid deposits, which are typical of individuals with lattice dystrophy.

Treatment and management

Treatment depends on the severity of the disease. If the affected person is in acute pain, treatment with eye drops, antibiotics, and other solutions is necessary. Some doctors advise affected people with eye edema to use a hair dryer at arm's length to dry some of the edema. Soft contact lenses may also help. Individuals with increasingly severe vision problems may need a corneal transplant.

KEY TERMS

Basement membrane—Part of the epithelium, or outer layer of the cornea.

Bowman's layer—Transparent sheet of tissue directly below the basement membrane.

Corneal transplant—Removal of impaired and diseased cornea and replacement with corneal tissue from a recently deceased person.

Descemet's membrane—Sheet of tissue that lies under the stroma and protects against infection and injuries.

Edema—Extreme amount of watery fluid that causes swelling of the affected tissue.

Endothelium—Extremely thin innermost layer of the cornea.

Epithelium—The layer of cells that cover the open surfaces of the body such as the skin and mucous membranes.

Hyaline—A clear substance that occurs in cell deterioration.

Stroma—Middle layer of the cornea, representing about 90% of the entire cornea.

For other forms of corneal dystrophy, affected people may need artificial tears and other medications. Some individuals may need laser treatment, such as phototherapeutic keratectomy (PK), which is the removal of part of the corneal stroma, or they may need a corneal transplant.

Prognosis

With most forms of corneal dystrophy, the disease progresses as the affected person ages. The severity of the conditions varies and a particular form of the disease may cause few or no problems or may also cause severe visual difficulties requiring surgery. Cases must be evaluated individually.

Resources

PERIODICALS

Akimune, Chika, et al. "Corneal Guttata Associated with the Corneal Dystrophy Resulting from a Big-h3 R124H Mutation." *British Journal of Ophthalmology* 84 (January 2000).

Bass, Sherry J. "Unraveling the Genetic Mysteries of the Corneal Dystrophies." *Review of Optometry* 138 (January 15, 2001).

Kabat, Alan G., and Joseph W. Sowka. "How to Detect and Deal with Dystrophies and Degenerations." *Review of Optometry* 136 (November 1999).

Korvatska, E., et al. "Mutation Hot Spots in 5q31-Linked Corneal Dystrophies." *American Journal of Human Genetics* 62 (1998).

National Eye Institute. "Fact Sheet: The Cornea and Corneal Disease." April 2000.

ORGANIZATIONS

Eye Bank Association of America. 1015 18th St. NW, Suite 1010, Washington, DC 20036. (202) 775-4999. <http://www.restoresight.org/>.

National Association for Visually Handicapped. 22 West 21st Street, New York, NY 10010. (212) 889-3141. <http://www.navh.org>.

National Eye Institute. 31 Center Dr., Bldg. 31, Rm 6A32, MSC 2510, Bethesda, MD 20892-2510. (301) 496-5248. 2020@nei.nih.gov. <http://www.nei.nih.gov>.

National Organization for Rare Disorders (NORD). PO Box 8923, New Fairfield, CT 06812-8923. (203) 746-6518 or (800) 999-6673. Fax: (203) 746-6481. <http://www.rarediseases.org>.

WEBSITES

"Corneal Dystrophies." *National Eye Institute, National Institutes of Health* <http://www.nei.nih.gov/publications/asptest/c.htm>.

"Report of the Corneal Diseases Panel: Program Overview and Goals." *National Eye Institute, National Institutes of Health.* <http://www.nei.nih.gov/publications/plan/NEIPlan/corneal.htm>.

Christine Adamec

Cornelia de Lange syndrome

Definition

Cornelia de Lange syndrome is a congenital syndrome of unknown origin diagnosed on the basis of facial characteristics consisting of synophrys (eyebrows joined at the midline), long eyelashes, long philtrum (area between the upper nose and the lip), thin upper lip, and a downturned mouth. It is a multisystemic disease that most often affects the gastrointestinal tract and the heart. Patients also present with mental retardation as well as many skeletal system malformations. It is estimated that this syndrome affects one in 10,000 newborns.

Description

This syndrome was named after the physician who described the condition in Amsterdam in 1933. It is also known as Amsterdam Dwarf Syndrome of de Lange. In 1916, another physician named Brachmann first described a more severe form of this syndrome and therefore it is also known as Brachmann-de Lange syndrome. It is known that there are three distinct categories of this condition.

The most severe form of this condition is the Type I or "classic form." Patients with this form have a prenatal growth deficiency that is also noticeable after birth. In addition these patients are marked with a distinct face and moderate to profound mental retardation. These individuals often have major deformities in the gastrointestinal tract and heart which may lead to severe incapacity or death.

The mild form of this condition is known as the Type II form. This is characterized by similar facial features to that of Type I, however, they may not become apparent until later in life. Along with a less severe pre- and postnatal growth deficiency, major malformations are seen at a decreased rate or may be absent completely.

Type III Cornelia de Lange syndrome, also called phenocopy, includes patients who have phenotypic manifestations of the syndrome that are related to chromosomal aneuplodies or teratogenic factors.

Genetic profile

The syndrome is suspected to be genetic in origin but the mode of transmission is unknown. Most cases are sporadic and are thought to result from a new mutation (an abnormal sequence of the components that make a **gene**). There is also evidence that this may be transmitted in an autosomal dominant fashion, thus if only one parent is affected there exists a 50% chance of transmitting the abnormal gene to each child. A gene of **chromosome** 3 may be responsible for the syndrome.

Demographics

Cornelia de Lange syndrome appears to affect males and females in equal numbers. It is more common to see affected females transmitting the trait, however, these women seem to transmit only the mild form to their offspring. It has also been noted that consanguineous relations, or relations within families, may result in an affected child. The recurrence risk has been estimated to be between two and six percent.

Signs and symptoms

Musculoskeletal abnormalities

- Microcephaly. Microcephaly is the term used to describe individuals with an abnormally small head. People with microcephaly have an accompanying small brain, resulting in mild to profound mental retardation.

- Micrognathia. This term is used when characterizing people with an abnormally small mandible or lower jaw bone.

- Nasal. Individuals with Cornelia de Lange syndrome often have a small nose. Anteversion, or turning, of the nostrils is also seen. A long philtrum (area between the nose and the upper lip) is also characteristic of a patient with Cornelia de Lange syndrome.

- Limb and digit malformations. Limb abnormalities sometimes include relatively short limbs. Limitations of elbow extension is often seen in mild forms. In addition, relative smallness of the hands and/or feet is almost always universal. Oligodactyly (presence of less than five digits on hand or feet), and clinodactyly or bending of the fifth finger and thumbs are also sometimes seen. Webbing of the toes (syndactyly) is also not rare in patients with Cornelia de Lange syndrome.

- Characteristic facial features. Facial features are possibly the most diagnostic of the physical signs. Patients look similar to each other with the bushy eyebrows joined at the midline, which is known as synophrys. Patients also have long eyelashes, a thin upper lip, and a downturned mouth. In mild cases, this classical appearance may not be present at birth and may take two or three years before becoming obvious. These individuals also have hypertrichosis, which is excessive facial (as well as body) hair.

- Other symptoms. Most patients are also of low birth weight, have a cleft palate, and a low-pitched growl or cry.

Gastrointestinal abnormalities

A number of gastrointestinal (GI) problems can manifest and are by far the most common system involved. Both the upper and lower GI tract can be involved.

- Gastroesophageal reflux. This is caused when acid from the stomach refluxes back into the esophagus. This can lead to severe heartburn and, if left untreated, can cause damage to the esophagus (reflux esophagitis) due to repeated irritations. Gastroesophageal reflux can also cause symptoms of pulmonary congestion and irritation due to chemical pneumonitis (inflammation of the lung).

- Barrett's esophagus. Barrett's esophagus is a change from the normal tissue type of the lower esophagus to a different type. This is normally a complication on gastroesophageal reflux and is significant because it may develop into an adenocarcinoma (carcinoma of glandular tissue).

- Esophageal stenosis. A narrowing of the esophagus which may decrease esophageal motility and make feeding difficult.

- Gastric ulcers. The majority of ulcers of the stomach are caused by bacteria. Ulcers of this nature may lead to abdominal discomfort.

- **Pyloric stenosis**. A narrowing of the pyloric canal that leads from the stomach to the duodenum. This may result in vomiting and diarrhea complicated by electrolyte imbalances.

- Intestinal malrotation. This is a failure during fetal development of normal rotation of the small intestine. This can cause a volvulus—a twisting of the intestine back on itself—cutting-off blood supply to the tissue or possibly an intestinal obstruction.

- Meckel diverticulum. In this condition, there are tiny pouches that protrude in the small intestine. Sometimes ulceration develops and bleeding occurs.

Cardiac abnormalities

Heart problems are not uncommon in patients with Cornelia de Lange syndrome.

- Ventricular septal defect. In this condition the septum of the ventricles (wall between the lower chambers of the heart) is not fully closed. This results in a murmur and can possibly lead to congestive heart failure. Other complications may include infective endocarditis, which is an infection of the endothelium, the tissue that lines the heart.

- Atrial septal defect. This is a defect of the septum between the upper chambers of the heart. This is caused by the persistence of the foramen ovale which is a hole normally present in the fetus that closes at birth. Individuals with this condition may also have a heart murmur.

- Symptoms are normally not present in patients with atrial septal defects but they are at an increased risk of infective endocarditis.

- **Patent ductus arteriosus**. This is a failure of the ductus arteriosus, a blood vessel between the pulmonary artery and the aorta found only in the fetus, to close. Normally there are symptoms, but severe cases may require surgery to close.

- Pulmonary valve stenosis. In this condition, the valve that allows blood to go from the right ventricle to the lungs becomes narrowed. This may result in right-sided heart enlargement and heart failure.

- Tetralogy of Fallot. This is a condition consisting of pulmonary stenosis, ventricular septal defect, enlarged right ventricle, and a displaced aorta. This condition results in a decrease in oxygenated blood that is pumped to the body. It can normally be corrected by surgery.

Growth and developmental deficiency

Most people afflicted with Cornelia de Lange syndrome have both prenatal and postnatal growth deficiencies as well as a developmental delay. This may be due to endocrine system involvement concerning a growth hormone delivery problem. Most patients have a characteristically short stature, but often have a pubertal growth spurt at a comparable age to normal individuals.

Developmental delays are numerous and are found in most patients with Cornelia de Lange syndrome. Some of the delays include walking alone, speaking, toilet training, and dressing. In some instances these patients never reach these milestones. Other developmental delays include IQ, which is within the mild to moderate range for mental retardation and averages 53.

Disorders of ears and eyes

Many patients with Cornelia de Lange syndrome often have some form of hearing loss. Cases may range from mild to severe, and may affect either one or both ears. This loss can be attributed to a lack of prenatal development of some of the important bony structures associated with the inner ear. In addition, development failure of important neural elements play a role in this hearing loss.

A significant number of Cornelia de Lange syndrome patients have eye and/or vision problems including:

- Myopia. Nearsightedness or shortsightedness is often seen in children diagnosed with Cornelia de Lange syndrome.

- Nystagmus. This is the term used to describe the rhythmical oscillations of the eyes slowly to one side followed by a rapid reflex movement in the opposite direction. It is usually horizontal, although rotatory or vertical nystagmus may also occur.

- Ptosis. Ptosis is the medical term used to characterize patients having a drooping eyelid(s). This may result from lesions either in the brainstem or in the nerves supplying the muscles that raise the eyelid.

- Nasolacrimal duct fistula. The lacrimal gland secretes tears to keep the eyeball moist and protected. In a naso-

lacrimal duct fistula the tears do not get drained from the eyeball and therefore the patient may develop chronic tearing and discharge from the eyes.

Other symptoms

Other malformations include undescended testicles, which can cause fertility problems. Diaphragmatic hernia is another complication that may lead to GI difficulties. Patients may also have a cleft palate and a low-pitched growl or cry.

Diagnosis

Cornelia de Lange syndrome has no set criteria that can indicate with absolute certainty whether or not a child is afflicted. This is due in part to a lack of specific biochemical markers postnatally that would lead a clinician to a definitive diagnosis. However, diagnosis is made subjectively from the characteristic symptoms that are present in this condition including the ones listed above. Perhaps the most diagnostic tool is the distinguishing face that a patient has, combined with facial hypertrichosis.

Prenatal diagnosis is possible through the use of ultrasound. The association of intrauterine growth retardation, oligodactyly, an absent ulna, underdevelopment of hands, diaphragmatic hernia, and cardiac defects lead to the differential diagnosis. When uncertain, the presence of long eyelashes or unusually long hair on the back restrict the diagnosis to Cornelia de Lange syndrome.

Researchers have also found that maternal serum samples collected from women who gave birth to a child with Cornelia de Lange syndrome revealed low levels of a pregnancy associated plasma protein-A (PAPP-A) during the second trimester. In addition, it has been noted that an amniotic molecule (5-OH-indole-3-acetic acid), and a fetal serum protein (galactose-1-phosphate-uridyltrasferase) were increased in afflicted individuals.

Treatment and management

The treatment and management of patients with Cornelia de Lange syndrome is strictly symptomatic. This means that treatment is prescribed according to presenting symptoms.

Musculoskeletal concerns

For patients with limb and digit malformations a variety of prosthesis are advised if necessary. Physical and occupational therapy may also be needed. Surgery may be necessary to correct more severe deformities.

Gastrointestinal treatment

Gastroesophageal reflux disease (GERD) can be treated with special diets and a number of different drugs that either block acid secretion from the stomach or neutralize acid once it is produced. Drugs may include antacids, histamine receptor blockers, and proton pump inhibitors. If these treatments prove unsuccessful, surgery my be performed to eliminate the possibility of further complications such as Barrett's esophagus or esophageal stenosis.

Patients with Cornelia de Lange syndrome should have endoscopic evaluation with biopsies for Barrett's esophagus. If this occurs, treatment will include the aforementioned drugs to reduce stomach acid and removal of the precancerous tissue may be indicated. Surgery to shorten the esophagus may also be performed.

Esophageal stenosis treatment may include a procedure done in order to dilate the esophagus. Some patients may require surgery to implant a stent or to replace part of the esophagus.

Gastric ulcers are often treated by the same means used to treat GERD. In addition, antibiotics are used in order to eliminate any bacteria that may be the cause of the ulcer. Sucralfate may be used to form a barrier over the ulcer that protects it from stomach acid allowing it to heal.

Patients with pyloric stenosis normally require surgery in order to widen the canal leading from the stomach to the duodenum. In addition, those with intestinal malrotation may require surgery depending on the severity of the condition. Surgery may also be required for patients with Meckel diverticulum if bleeding is a problem.

Cardiovascular treatment

In mild cases of cardiovascular involvement, no treatment plan is initiated other than to monitor the dysfunctions. Some of the septal defects may be asymptomatic and heal on their own. Since most of these abnormalities can lead to infective endocarditis, patients should be given antibiotics before undergoing dental procedures or surgeries. Most often penicillin or amoxicillin are used.

For patients who develop congestive heart failure, a regiment of drugs known as beta blockers may be useful to slow down the heart. Other drugs that may be used are diuretics to prevent fluid retention or ACE inhibitors.

For more serious cardiac involvement surgery is recommended. Surgery for tetralogy of Fallot involves widening the pulmonary valve and repairing the ventricular septal defect. This surgery is normally performed on patients between the ages of eight months and three

---

KEY TERMS

Chromosomal aneuplodies—A condition in which the chromosomal number is either increased or decreased.

Clinodactyly—An abnormal inward curving of the fingers or toes.

Consanguineous—Sharing a common bloodline or ancestor.

Fistula—An abnormal passage or communication between two different organs or surfaces.

Hypertrichosis—Growth of hair in excess of the normal. Also called hirsutism.

Infective endocarditis—An infection of the endothelium, the tissue lining the walls of the heart.

Oligodactyly—The absence of one or more fingers or toes.

Syndactyly—Webbing or fusion between the fingers or toes.

Synophrys—A feature in which the eyebrows join in the middle. Also called blepharophimosis.

Teratogenic factor—Any factor that can produce congenital abnormalities.

---

years. Ventricular septal defects can be repaired usually with a synthetic patch. Atrial septal defects are normally performed by catherization by placing a device between the atria in the septum. Patent ductus arteriosus correction is done by either ligating the vessel or cutting it off.

Hearing and visual concerns

Patients diagnosed with Cornelia de Lange syndrome should be examined for hearing loss as soon as possible due to the possibility of speech delay that may be experienced because of this loss. Patients should be fitted with hearing aids and may be considered for pharyngeal-esophageal tubes.

It is also important to identify vision problems early. Glasses may be necessary for nearsightedness. Children should be seen by an opthamologist in order to assess limitations and to develop a treatment plan.

Other issues

Since development of speech is often delayed, people affected with Cornelia de Lange syndrome should be seen by a speech pathologist at an early age. Alternative communication strategies, such as sign language, may be employed depending on the level of speech development.

Children and family members may also benefit from therapy available from a number of organizations. Patients may qualify for health related support services from a variety of national support services for retarded persons.

Prognosis

Patients with Cornelia de Lange syndrome can live well into adulthood, however, it is typical for most to have a shortened life span. In 1976, a nationwide survey in Denmark revealed the oldest patient was found to be 49 years old.

A patient's prognosis can be improved by early diagnosis and intervention. These two factors can influence not only the patients life expectancy, but also their quality of life and those lives of the family and caregivers.

Resources

BOOKS

Behrman, Richard, ed. "Intestinal Atresia, Stenosis, and Malrotation." In *Nelson Textbook of Pediatrics.* 16th ed. Philadelphia: W. B. Saunders Company, 2000.

Oski, Frank A., ed. "Cornelia de Lange's Syndrome." In *Principles and Practice of Pediatrics.* 2nd ed. Philadelphia: Lippincott, 1994.

Thoene, Jess G., ed. "Cornelia de Lange Syndrome." In *Physicians' Guide to Rare Diseases.* 2nd ed. Montvale, N.J.: Dowden Publishing Company, 1995.

PERIODICALS

Aitken, D.A., et al. "Second-trimester pregnancy associated plasma protein-A levels are reduced in Cornelia de Lange Syndrome pregnancies." *Prenatal Diagnosis* 19 (1999): 706–10.

Akhtar, M.I., et al. "Cornelia de Lange Syndrome and Barrett's Esophagus:123." *Journal of Pediatric Gastro and Nutrition* 25 (1997): 473.

Boog, G., et al. "Brachmann-de Lange syndrome: a cause of early symmetric fetal growth delay." *European Journal of Obstetrics & Gynecology and Reproductive Biology* 85 (1999): 173–77.

Jackson, L., et al. "de Lange Syndrome: a clinical review of 310 individuals." *American Journal of Medical Genetics* 47 (1993): 940–46.

Kimitaka, K., et al. "Auditory brainstem responses in children with Cornelia de Lange Syndrome." *International Journal of Pediatric Otorhinolaryngology* 31 (1995): 137–46.

Kline, A.D., et al. "Developmental data on individuals with the Brachmann-de Lange syndrome." *American Journal of Medical Genetics* 47 (1993): 1053–58.

Kousseff, B.G., et al. "Physical growth in Brachmann-de Lange Syndrome." *American Journal of Medical Genetics* 47 (1993): 1050–52.

Mehta, A.V., et al. "Occurrence of congenital heart disease in children with Brachmann-de Lange Syndrome." *American Journal of Medical Genetics* 71 (1997): 434–35.

Sasaki, T., et al. "Temporal bone and brain stem histopathological findings in Cornelia de Lange syndrome." *International Journal of Pediatric Otorhinolaryngology* 36 (1996): 195–204.

Scaillon, M., et al. "Oesophageal motility disorders in Cornelia de Lange Syndrome original feature or oesophagitis related abnormalities?" *Journal of Pediatric Gastro and Nutrition.* 25, supplement 1 (1997): 46.

ORGANIZATIONS

Alliance of Genetic Support Groups. 4301 Connecticut Ave. NW, Suite 404, Washington, DC 20008. (202) 966-5557. Fax: (202) 966-8553. <http://www.geneticalliance.org>.

Cornelia de Lange Syndrome Foundation, Inc. 302 West Main St., Suite 100, Avon, CT 06001. (860) 676-8166 (800) 223-8355. Fax: (860) 676-8337.

March of Dimes Birth Defects Foundation. 1275 Mamaroneck Ave., White Plains, NY 10605. (888) 663-4637. resourcecenter@modimes.org. <http://www.modimes.org>.

National Organization for Rare Disorders (NORD). PO Box 8923, New Fairfield, CT 06812-8923. (203) 746-6518 or (800) 999-6673. Fax: (203) 746-6481. <http://www.rarediseases.org>.

WEBSITES

Cornelia de Lange Syndrome USA Foundation. <http://www.Cornelia de Lange Syndromeoutreach.org>.

MD Consult. <http://www.mdconsult.com>.

Medscape. <http://www.medscape.com>.

OMIM—Online Mendelian Inheritance in Man. National Center for Biotechnology Information. <http://www.ncbi.nlm.nih.gov:80/entrez/query.fcgi?cmd=&db=OMIM&term=>.

NORD—National Organization for Rare Disorders Inc. <http://www.rarediseases.org/>.

United States National Library of Medicine. <http://www.nlm.nih.gov>.

WebMD. <http://www.webmd.com>.

Laith F. Gulli, MD
Robert Ramirez, BS

Corpus callosum, agenesis

Definition

Agenesis of the corpus callosum is the complete or partial absence of the corpus callosum, the structure within the brain that connects the two hemispheres.

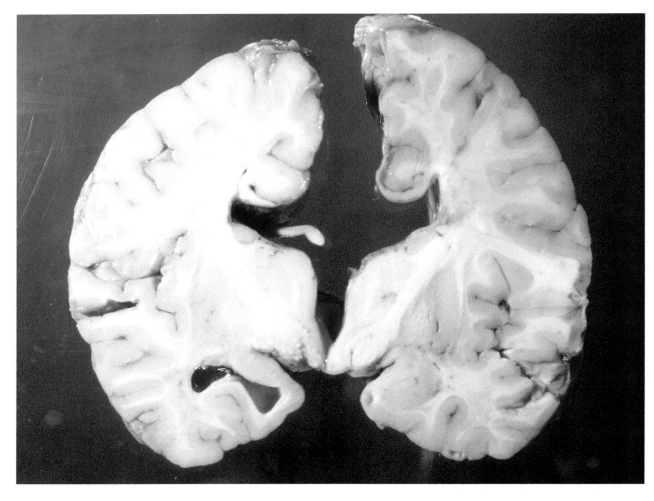

Agenesis of the corpus callosum is the complete or partial absence of the corpus callosum, the structure that connects the two hemispheres of the brain. *(© Jan Leestma, M.D./Custom Medical Stock Photo.)*

Description

Agenesis of the corpus callosum is a congenital anomaly occurring during the first trimester of pregnancy. During this time, the fetal brain is developing, and bundles of nerve fibers that create the corpus callosum are forming. This process may be interrupted if the mother is exposed to toxic substances or certain medications during pregnancy. Genetic abnormalities in the fetus may prevent the nerve fibers from growing correctly. In most cases, the exact cause of agenesis of the corpus callosum is unknown.

In some people with agenesis of the corpus callosum, these nerve fibers are formed, but grow from front to back rather than from side to side. When the anomaly forms from front to back, groups of nerve fibers known as bundles of Probst form. These bundles stay within each hemisphere, never crossing the midline, and the two sides of the brain cannot share information. This

lack of communication causes the symptoms of agenesis of corpus callosum.

The term agenesis of the corpus callosum usually refers to a complete absence of the corpus callosum. In some individuals, the corpus callosum is partially formed, and the condition is referred to as dysgenesis of the corpus callosum. There are two types of dysgenesis of the corpus callosum, partial and atypical. Partial dysgenesis occurs when the front, or anterior, portion of the corpus callosum does not form. In atypical dysgenesis of the corpus callosum, the rear, or posterior, portion the corpus callosum is not formed.

The corpus callosum is not essential for life or for normal intellectual functioning. Many people who have agenesis of the corpus callosum as an isolated condition have no symptoms at all, and some may only experience mild difficulties with skills that required matching visual patterns. Since the two hemispheres of the brain cannot communicate, images seen by one eye cannot be connected to images processed by the other.

The more severe symptoms experienced by people with agenesis of the corpus callosum are most often caused by other brain malformations, **chromosomal abnormalities**, and genetic syndromes of which agenesis of the corpus callosum is only one component. Especially in children who have agenesis of the corpus callosum in addition to other brain malformations, the effects can be severe, including mental retardation, seizures, **hydrocephalus**, and impairment of motor functioning.

Agenesis of the corpus callosum often occurs along with other brain malformations, such as **Arnold-Chiari malformation**, **Dandy-Walker malformation**, and other defects of the midbrain. It may also be found in patients with defects of the size and shape of the brain, such as schizencephaly **lissencephaly**, pachygyria, and hydrocephalus.

Individuals with anomalies of the formation of the forebrain, such as frontal **encephalocele** and **holo-prosencephaly**, will usually have agenesis of the corpus callosum as well. In this case, the forebrain does not develop into two distinct hemispheres and the corpus callosum does not form. These are severe birth defects and are usually incompatible with life.

Agenesis of the corpus callosum may occur as an isolated birth defect; in such cases, a genetic cause has not been identified. However, it often occurs as part of a syndrome. Agenesis of the corpus callosum has been associated with more than 30 inherited syndromes caused by chromosomal and single-gene anomalies and may result from prenatal exposure to anticoagulant medication during the first trimester of pregnancy.

Agenesis of the corpus callosum may also be known as absent corpus callosum, corpus callosum hypoplasia, ACC, CCA, collasal agenesis, or collasal dysgenesis.

Genetic profile

Agenesis of the corpus callosum is a component of many different genetic syndromes and chromosomal abnormalities, most of which are extremely rare.

Examples of autosomal malformation syndromes that include agenesis of the corpus callosum are:

• acrocallosal syndrome

• Andermann syndrome

• craniofacial dysmorphism-absent corpus callosum-iris colobomas-connective tissue **dysplasia** syndrome

• Fryns syndrome

• Joubert syndrome

• Larsen syndrome

• Miller-Dieker syndrome

• Rubinstein-Taybi syndrome

• Seckel syndrome

• Varadi-Papps syndrome

Agenesis of the corpus callosum is found in X-linked malformation syndromes such as:

• Acardi syndrome

• Berry-Kravis and Israel syndrome

• Brooks syndrome

• CRASH syndrome

• Opitz-Kaveggia syndrome (FG syndrome)

• Proud syndrome

• Toriello-Carey syndrome

• X-linked hydrocephalus

Agenesis of the corpus callosum occurs more frequently in individuals with trisomies, such as trisomy 3, **trisomy 13**, trisomy 15, and **trisomy 18**. It has also been associated with chromosomal rearrangements, such as **Wolf-Hirschhorn syndrome** (del(4)(p16)). It is also part of syndromes whose exact cause is still unknown, such as Bohring syndrome, congenital thrombocytopenia-Robin sequence-agenesis of corpus callosum-distinctive facies-developmental delay syndrome, Curry-Jones syndrome, **Proteus syndrome**, and agenesis of corpus callosum-mental retardation-osseous lesions syndrome.

Demographics

Researchers estimate the frequency of individuals affected with agenesis of the corpus callosum in the United States to be approximately 5.3%. It is more common in females than males and is often seen in individuals with other brain malformations and as a part of many complex chromosomal and genetic syndromes.

Signs and symptoms

The symptoms of agenesis of the corpus callosum can range from virtually no difficulties to significant delays in reaching developmental milestones, mental retardation, and limited mobility.

Agenesis of the corpus callosum may be asymptomatic if occurring as an isolated brain malformation. With the increased use of imaging studies, many cases of absence of the corpus callosum are inadvertently discovered when a patient has a test to diagnose an unrelated condition. For many people with agenesis of the corpus callosum, however, symptoms of other clinical and genetic syndromes and brain malformations can be severe, especially in infants.

Symptoms of agenesis of the corpus callosum may include:

- seizures
- delays in reaching developmental milestones, such as sitting up, crawling, and walking
- mental retardation
- poor hand-to-eye coordination
- impairments in auditory and visual memory

Although agenesis of the corpus callosum can be asymptomatic, it is considered a risk factor for neurological impairment. Agenesis of the corpus callosum may be suspected in children who have seizures, especially a specific type of seizures called infantile spasms. Agenesis of the corpus callosum may also be suspected in children with feeding problems, poor muscle control, and difficulties sitting, standing, and walking. It may be diagnosed later in children who experience other symptoms, such as frequent headaches or repetitive speech, in addition to seizures.

Diagnosis

Agenesis of the corpus callosum is diagnosed primarily by computed tomography (CT) scan and magnetic resonance imaging (MRI). MRI is the preferred imaging method for identifying abnormalities of the structures of the brain.

Agenesis of the corpus callosum may be diagnosed prenatal after week 20 of gestation, using **prenatal ultrasound**.

Treatment and management

There is no treatment for agenesis of the corpus callosum; however, the symptoms may be managed. Most symptoms associated with agenesis of the corpus callosum are caused by other anomalies that occur along with the defect.

Symptoms, such as seizures, may be treated with anticonvulsant medications. Another common associated condition, hydrocephalus, may be treated by the surgical installation of a medical device called a shunt. A shunt relieves the pressure of access fluid in the brain by draining that fluid away from the brain.

For infants and young children with agenesis of the corpus callosum and syndromes that include agenesis of the corpus callosum, early intervention programs may be

---

KEY TERMS

Autosomal—Pertaining to one or more of the 22 chromosomes that are not involved in determining gender.

Arnold-Chiari malformation—A congenital anomaly in which parts of the brain protrude through the opening in the base of the skull into the spinal column.

Bundles of Probst—Abnormally developed nerve fibers in the brain.

Congenital anomaly—A defect that is present at birth.

Computed tomography (CT) scan—A diagnostic imaging procedure in which x ray and computer technology are used to generate slices or cross-sectional images of the body.

Dandy-Walker malformation—A congenital anomaly of the brain that causes a specific type of hydrocephalus.

Encephalocele—A congenital anomaly in which part of the brain is herniated through the skull.

Forebrain—The anterior of the front section of the brain.

Holoprosencephaly—A congenital anomaly of the front sections of the brain.

Hydrocephalus—The excess accumulation of cerebrospinal fluid within the skull.

Lissencephaly—Abnormality of the brain in which the surface is smooth, lacking the normal folds and grooves known as gyria.

Magnetic resonance imaging (MRI)—A diagnostic procedure that uses a combination of high powered magnets, radio frequencies, and computers to generate detailed images of structures within the body.

Pachygyria—Abnormality of the surface of the brain in which the gyria, or folds and grooves, in the surface of the brain are too large.

Schizencephaly—Abnormality of the brain in which there are deep ruts and clefts in the surface of the brain.

Trisomy—Three copies of an individual chromosome as opposed to the normal set of two chromosomes.

X-linked—Located on the X chromosome.

---

helpful in assisting these children to reach developmental milestones. Other treatments, such as occupational therapy, physical therapy, and speech therapy, may help individuals improve deficits caused by the accompanying malformations.

Prognosis

The prognosis for individuals with agenesis of the corpus callosum varies widely. If agenesis of the corpus callosum occurs alone, the prognosis is usually excellent. Depending on the other associated birth defects and the severity of the syndrome affecting the patient, mental retardation, impaired neuromuscular functioning, and a shortened life expectancy may result. In rare cases, syndromes that may include agenesis of the corpus callosum are incompatible with life.

Resources

PERIODICALS

Shevell, Michael. "Clinical and Diagnostic Profile of Agenesis the Corpus Callosum." *Journal of Child Neurology* 17, no 12 (December 2002): 895–899.

ORGANIZATIONS

March of Dimes. 1275 Mamaroneck Ave., White Plains, NY 10605. (April 9, 2005.) <http://www.marchofdimes.com>.

National Organization of Disorders of the Corpus Callosum. 18032-C Lemon Drive, PMB 363, Yorba Linda, CA 92886. (April 9, 2005.) <http://www.corpuscallosum.org>.

WEB SITES

Online Mendelian Inheritance in Man, OMIM. Johns Hopkins University, Baltimore, MD. (April 9, 2005.) <http://www.ncbi.nlm.nih.gov/entrez/query.fcgi?CMD=search&DB=omim>.

Deborah L. Nurmi, MS

Costello syndrome

Definition

Newborn feeding problems, poor growth, loose, wrinkled skin, and mental retardation are some of the recognizable features of Costello syndrome. Although the genetic basis is unknown, the unusual skin features have given an important clue as to the cause of the disorder.

Description

The first sign of Costello syndrome may be seen even before birth. Many mothers carrying these babies have polyhydramnios (an excess of amniotic fluid in the womb). This may be due to the fact that the baby has poor swallowing ability, even in the womb. Many of these babies are large at birth, especially with respect to their weight. Their head size is usually larger too. Most significant, all of these babies begin life with severe feeding problems. They do not grow and thrive as most babies do. As this continues, they lose weight and become quite ill. Their height also tapers off. This poor growth continues until about two years of age. Then, for reasons unknown, their growth, especially weight gain, becomes more normal. However, these children continue to grow more slowly in height, and remain short throughout life. Most adults with Costello syndrome are approximately 4.5 ft (1.5 m) tall. X-ray studies done at different ages show that bone growth is delayed. The delay in normal bone growth leads to reduced height.

Some interesting features of the face and loose, soft skin add to the clinical picture. Even as babies, individuals with Costello syndrome have a slight downward slant of their eyes, full cheeks, and thick lips. The neck is short, and they have an upturned nose. The ears are low set (below the level of the nose) with large, fleshy ear lobes. These features seem to coarsen and become more noticeable over time. However, the signature feature of Costello syndrome is the soft, deeply wrinkled skin, especially on the hands and feet. This is evident at birth and becomes even more striking in the first few months of life. All individuals with Costello syndrome have these deep creases and looseness of the skin. Some physicians have described the distinct, deep creases in the skin as resembling "bath tub hands," i.e., similar to the puffiness seen after soaking one's hands in water for awhile.

Other features of Costello syndrome include skin markings, sparse, curly hair, and a hoarse voice. Individuals with Costello syndrome have unusual skin growths called papillomatous papules, which are skin-colored, raised bumps (not warts). These papules are found on the skin inside the nose and mouth, on the tongue, and around the anus. The papules form in late childhood or early teenage years. Most of these growths are benign (non-cancerous) and rarely become malignant (cancerous). Other skin markings may include dark colored moles on the palms of the hands and on the bottom of the feet; brownish colored skin marks (birthmarks) found almost anywhere on the body; and small, red marks which are broken blood vessels on the surface of their skin.

Most individuals with Costello syndrome also have sparse, curly hair. The hair turns gray in color at a much earlier age than expected (sometimes even in teenage years). Along with the loose, wrinkled skin, the graying of the hair makes them look much older than their age. The last feature of note is their voice, many times described as being low and hoarse. It has been suggested that the hoarse voice may possibly be due to weakness in the tissues or muscles of the larynx.

Cardiovascular problems are common in children with Costello syndrome. Among the congenital heart defects seen are atrial or ventricular septal defects, **bicuspid aortic valve**, **patent ductus arteriosus**, and mitral valve prolaspe. More than half of the reported cases of Costello syndrome included heart rhythm disturbances and abnormalities in the structure and functions of the heart muscle (hypertrophic cardiomyopathy).

Genetic profile

The genetic basis of Costello syndrome is unknown. There have been two instances where siblings (brother and sister) each had Costello syndrome. The syndrome has also occurred in a few families where the parents were said to be closely related (i.e., may have shared the same altered **gene** within the family). For these reasons, the possible involvement of an autosomal recessive gene in Costello syndrome was raised. An autosomal recessive condition is caused by a change in both genes of a pair.

As more individuals with Costello syndrome were described, the evidence began to suggest autosomal dominant **inheritance**. This means only one altered copy of a gene pair is needed to cause the disorder. The cases of Costello syndrome that occur for the first time in a family are probably due to a new, sporadic (non-inherited) gene mutation. To explain the two families with more than one child with Costello syndrome, the concept of germ line mosaicism was proposed.

Germ line mosaicism occurs when one parent carries an altered gene mutation that affects his or her germ line cells (either the egg or sperm cells) only. The gene mutation does not affect the somatic (body) cells. Therefore, the parent does not express the disease and **DNA** testing does not show that the parent carries an altered gene. However, parents with germ line mosaicism can have more than one child with a disorder (like Costello syndrome) since the syndrome occurs whenever an egg or sperm carrying the altered gene mutation is passed on. Germ line mosaicism occurs very rarely. However, it has been seen in other autosomal dominant conditions, such as **osteogenesis imperfecta** (brittle bone disease). Based on the available evidence, Costello syndrome is probably an autosomal dominant condition. In some families, germ line mosaicism explains the pattern of expression of the condition.

Most individuals with Costello syndrome have undergone extensive testing to look for a cause for their growth and developmental problems. For the most part these tests have been normal. The underlying problem appears to be complex. However, some researchers had the idea to look more closely at the makeup of the skin cells for clues to the disorder.

Stretchable tissues like the skin require not only strength but also the ability, once stretched, to return to their original form. Human skin is made up of a network of fibers that give the skin its flexibility. The fibers themselves are made out of different proteins. One such protein is called elastin. Elastin acts like a rubber band in the skin. It can be stretched and then returns to its original form. Within our skin cells, the elastin protein is randomly twisted and tied to form elastin fibers. A study of the skin cells of individuals with Costello syndrome shows that the elastin fibers do not appear to be formed in the normal way. The skin cells seem to stretch but do not have the ability to snap back, as do normal skin cells. Thus, the skin has a loose and wrinkled appearance. Specifically, a protein called the elastin binding protein seems to play a role in forming the elastin fibers. In Costello syndrome, this protein is abnormal causing the elastin fibers themselves to become loose and disrupted.

The defect in the elastin building pathway explains many of the clinical features of Costello syndrome, especially the loose and wrinkled skin. Elastin fibers make up tissues of the heart, the larynx, even the developing skeleton. Therefore, the heart disease, the hoarse voice, even the short height may be explained by abnormal formation of the elastin fibers.

Demographics

In 1971, and later in 1977, Dr. J. Costello first described a syndrome of mental and growth delays, and distinct features of the face and skin that bear his name. After the initial description, there were no further reports of individuals with Costello syndrome until 1991. It was then that the term Costello syndrome was used to describe the features seen in a Canadian child. Further cases from several countries have since been reported. In all, at least 40 individuals with Costello syndrome have been described in medical literature. The condition may be more common than previously thought, and may be under diagnosed. It affects both males and females equally, and most likely occurs in every racial and ethnic group.

Signs and symptoms

All individuals with Costello syndrome have fairly significant mental retardation. This impairment leads to early delays in walking and talking. They are usually a few years behind other children their age. These learning problems continue as they get older, and require a special education environment. IQ testing in some individuals with Costello syndrome has shown a range from mild to moderate retardation (IQ from 30 to 68). Although they have special needs, their outgoing and friendly personality is an asset, and helps them make the most of their abilities.

Diagnosis

The pattern of overgrowth in the womb, poor growth after birth, and short height is typical of individuals with Costello syndrome. Other clinical features, especially the loose, wrinkled skin and graying, curly hair give them an aged appearance that is quite distinct. The skin papules found in the nose, mouth and on the anus add to the picture. Taking these features together, the diagnosis can be made.

Treatment and management

Heart disease is seen in almost half of the individuals with Costello syndrome. The heart problems are sometimes found at birth. The heart problems include holes in the muscle wall of the heart; abnormal thickening of the walls of the heart; and an abnormal heart beat or arrhythmia. An echocardiogram (ultrasound of the heart) is usually done early in life to assess heart function. Heart function is also closely monitored as these individuals get older.

At least eight individuals (of the 40 or so now described) with Costello syndrome have developed rare types of **cancer**. The cancers have occurred early in life, and a few cases have occurred in infancy. The tumors seen include two cases of ganglioneuroblastoma, a tumor of the nerve fibers; three cases of rhabdomyosarcoma, a tumor of the skeletal muscle; and two cases of bladder cancer in teenagers, a cancer usually seen in the elderly.

Prognosis

The severe problems with feeding and growth that characterize Costello syndrome can be life-threatening. Most of these infants need to be fed with a feeding tube in order to survive. Complications of heart disease are another cause for concern, even early in life. For most individuals, however, the heart problems are not severe, and usually can be successfully treated without heart sur-

---

KEY TERMS

Arrhythmia—Abnormal heart rhythm, examples are a slow, fast, or irregular heart rate.

Elastin—A protein that gives skin the ability to stretch and then return to normal.

Ganglioneuroblastoma—A tumor of the nerve fibers and ganglion cells.

Germ line mosaicism—A rare event that occurs when one parent carries an altered gene mutation that affects his or her germ line cells (either the egg or sperm cells) but is not found in the somatic (body) cells.

Larynx—The voice box, or organ that contains the vocal cords.

Papillomatous papules—Skin-colored, raised bumps (not warts) found on the skin. Most of these growths are benign (non-cancerous) and rarely become malignant (cancerous).

Polyhydramnios—A condition in which there is too much fluid around the fetus in the amniotic sac.

Rhabdomyosarcoma—A malignant tumor of the skeletal muscle.

---

gery. Unfortunately, some individuals with Costello syndrome have experienced heart failure and sudden death. Lastly, there may be an increased risk for developing cancer. Since some of these individuals have died from complications of their cancer, increased screening may be important to detect cancer at an early stage.

Resources

PERIODICALS

Costello, J. "A New Syndrome: Mental Submormality and Nasal Papillomata." *Australian Pediatric Journal* (July 1977): 114-118.

Hinek, Aleksander. "Decreased Elastin Deposition and High Proliferation of Fibroblasts from Costello Syndrome Are Related to Funtional Deficiancy in the 67-kD Elastin-Binding Protein." *American Journal of Human Genetics* (March 2000): 859-872.

Johnson, John. "Costello Syndrome: Phenotype, Natural History, Differential Diagnosis, and Possible Causes." *The Journal of Pediatrics* (September 1998): 441-448.

Lurie, I. "Genetics of the Costello Syndrome." *American Journal of Medical Genetics* (September 1994): 358-359.

Van Eeghen, A. "Costello Syndrome: Report and Review." *American Journal of Medical Genetics* (January 1999): 187-193.

WEBSITES

"Costello Syndrome." *Online Mendelian Inheritance in Man.* <http://www.ncbi.nlm.nih.gov/htbin-post/Omim/getmim>

Kevin M. Sweet, MS, CGC

CPT II deficiency *see* **Carnitine palmitoyl transferase deficiency**

Crane-Heise syndrome

Definition

Crane-Heise syndrome is a lethal genetic disorder first defined in 1981. Some of the features of Crane-Heise syndrome are similar to those of another genetic disorder called aminopterin syndrome sine aminopterin (or pseudoaminopterin syndrome), indicating that the two conditions may be part of a spectrum of symptoms.

Description

Aminopterin syndrome is an established disorder resulting from the use of aminopterin as an abortifacient. Surviving infants who had been exposed to this chemical had severe developmental abnormalities, especially those of the skull. Crane-Heise is distinct from aminopterin syndrome in that the mothers of infants with Crane-Heise syndrome were not exposed to aminopterin.

Genetic profile

There are very few documented cases of Crane-Heise syndrome, and therefore, little is known about the genetic basis of the disorder. No specific **chromosome** or **gene** location has been identified.

Since Crane-Heise syndrome has affected more than one sibling in a family, and has been seen in both males and females, it is most likely transmitted through autosomal recessive **inheritance**. This means that two copies of the abnormal gene would have to be inherited, one from each parent, in order for the disorder to occur.

Demographics

Males and females are at equal risk for inheriting Crane-Heise syndrome since it is assumed to be an autosomal trait, meaning it is not inherited on one of the sex-determining chromosomes. No one ethnic group has been shown to be at higher risk, primarily due to the few

number of reported cases. Of the cases reported, there tends to be a frequent reoccurrence of the disease with each pregnancy.

Signs and symptoms

Many distinct characteristics are seen in infants with Crane-Heise syndrome. Some of these include:

- large head with a relatively small face
- depressed nose with nasal openings turned forward
- underdeveloped jaw
- a narrow nose bridge with eyes close together
- low-set ears that are turned to the back
- short neck
- partially fused fingers or toes
- clubfoot

The most definitive features of Crane-Heise syndrome and aminopterin syndrome are the cranial and bone abnormalities. Infants born with these syndromes typically have absent or underdeveloped brains (**anencephaly**), underdeveloped shoulder blades, and absent collarbones and vertebrae.

Diagnosis

Since the signs of Crane-Heise syndrome are nearly identical to those observed in infants with aminopterin syndrome, it is important to identify whether or not the mother was exposed to aminopterin for differential diagnosis. Some fetuses have been diagnosed with Crane-Heise syndrome in the uterus via ultrasonography, however most diagnoses are based on physical examination at the time of birth.

Treatment and management

No treatment has been developed. Further research to better understand the cause and genetic basis of this disorder is necessary.

Prognosis

Crane-Heise syndrome is a lethal disorder and infants are usually stillborn or survive only a few days after birth. Malformations of the brain and vertebrae are usually severe and cannot be corrected surgically.

Resources

PERIODICALS

Barnicoat, A. J., M. J. Seller, and C. P. Bennett. "Fetus with features of Crane-Heise syndrome and aminopterin syndrome sine aminopterin (ASSAS)." *Clinical Dysmorphology* 3 (1994): 353-357.

Crane, J. P., R. L. Heise. "New syndrome in three affected siblings." *Pediatrics* 68 (1981): 235-237.

WEBSITES

"Entry 218090: Crane-Heise Syndrome." *OMIM—Online Mendelian Inheritance in Man*. National Center for Biotechnology Information. <http://www.ncbi.nlm.nih.gov/htbin-post/Omim/dispmim?218090>.

Sonya Kunkle
Stacey L. Blachford

Craniofrontonasal dysplasia *see* **Otopalatodigital syndrome**

Craniostenosis *see* **Craniosynostosis**

Craniosynostosis

Definition

Craniosynostosis is a congenital abnormality of the central nervous system that involves the premature closing of one or more of the fibrous joints between the bones of the skull (cranial sutures).

Description

Craniosynostosis is a birth defect that affects the shape of the skull. Individuals born with craniosynostosis have abnormally shaped heads and a prominent bony ridge over the affected suture or sutures. All affected individuals also are likely to experience water on the brain (**hydrocephalus**) that can cause enlargement of the head and increased pressure inside the skull. Developmental delay is commonly experienced by those individuals affected by craniosynostosis.

There are two major classifications of craniosynostosis: primary and secondary. There are multiple causes of primary craniosynostosis, which involves abnormal cranial suture development. The premature closure of one or more of the sutures causes the skull bones to grow parallel to the affected suture but not perpendicular to it. At other sutures there may be too much growth. The disrupted growth patterns cause a misshapen skull. The cause of secondary craniosynostosis is failure of the brain to grow and expand. This results in uniform premature suture closure, so that the head is symmetric and abnormally small (microcephalic).

The human skull consists of several bony plates separated by a narrow gap that contains stem cells. These fibrous joints are referred to as cranial sutures. There are six cranial sutures: the sagittal, which runs from front to back across the top of the head; the two coronal sutures, which run across the skull parallel to and just above the hairline; the metopic, which runs from front to back in front of the sagittal suture; and the two lambdoid sutures, which run side to side across the back of the head. There are seven types of primary craniosynostosis divided by the cranial suture or sutures that are affected: sagittal, bicoronal (both coronal sutures), unicoronal (one coronal suture), coronal and sagittal, metopic, lambdoid and sagittal, and total, in which all the cranial sutures are affected. Approximately 40% of all cases of craniosynostosis are sagittal, 20% are bicoronal, 15% are unicoronal, 10% are coronal and sagittal, 4% are metopic, 1% are lambdoid and sagittal, and 10% are total.

Genetic profile

Craniosynostosis does not have a single genetic cause, but it has been demonstrated to have a genetic component in that it is sometimes passed from one generation to another. It has been associated with over 150 different genetic syndromes. Genetic **inheritance** of craniosynostosis is not sex-linked (it is autosomal), and has been tied to both dominant and recessive traits. The overall occurrence rates are equivalent between males and females, but sagittal craniosynostosis is seen four times as often in males as in females, while coronal craniosynostosis is observed twice as often in females as in males.

At least 64 distinct mutations in six different genes have been linked to craniosynostosis. Three of these genes, at **chromosome** locations 8p11, 10q26, and 4p16, are related to fibroblast growth factor receptors (FGFRs), which are molecules that control cell growth. Other implicated genes are the TWIST **gene** (7p21), the MSX2 gene (5q34-35), and the FBN1 gene (15q21.1).

Not all instances of craniosynostosis appear to have a genetic origin. The most common cause of non-genetic craniosynostosis is constraint of the fetal head during pregnancy. This is believed to account for between 50 and 60% of all cases of craniosynostosis.

Known genetic syndromes account for another 10 to 20% of the cases of craniosynostosis. These syndromes include Muenke syndrome, **Apert syndrome**, **Pfeiffer syndrome**, **Carpenter syndrome**, and **Crouzon syndrome**, among others.

Demographics

Craniosynostosis has an incidence of approximately one in every 2,000 live births. Genetic-based craniosynostosis is most commonly a dominant trait, but in some cases has also been shown to be recessive. Therefore, while it is more likely to occur in children with a family history of craniosynostosis, it may not occur in the children of such families and it may also occur in children with no family history of the disorder. Nongenetic craniosynostosis has a higher occurrence among the children of malnourished or drug-abusing mothers. It is also more likely to occur in the children of teenage mothers because of the lack of development of an appropriately sized uterus for fetal growth in many of these cases.

Signs and symptoms

The most obvious symptom of craniosynostosis is an abnormally shaped head that is not the result of the birth process. Craniosynostosis may be confirmed by the presence of a bony ridge over the affected cranial suture. Associated symptoms include unusual facial features such as wide-set, down-slanting, or protruding eyes and a prominent jaw; visual impairment; hearing loss; breathing problems; water on the brain (hydrocephalus); and developmental delay.

Each type of craniosynostosis has different physically observable symptoms and results in a different head shape. Sagittal craniosynostosis is characterized by a long and narrow skull (scaphocephaly). This is referred to as an increase in the A-P, or anterior-to-posterior, diameter. Thus, looking down on the top of the skull, the diameter of the head is greater than normal in the front-to-back direction. Individuals born with sagittal craniosynostosis have broad foreheads and a larger than normal back of the head. The so-called soft spot found just beyond the hairline in a normal baby (the anterior fontanelle) is missing or very small in a baby affected with sagittal craniosynostosis. The result of neurological testing is generally normal for individuals with sagittal craniosynostosis.

Bicoronal craniosynostosis is characterized by a wide and short skull (brachycephaly) or by a cloverleaf-shaped skull. This is referred to as a decrease in the A-P diameter. Individuals affected with bicoronal craniosynostosis have poorly formed eye sockets and fore-

heads. This causes a lower than normal sized eye-socket that can cause complications of vision. These complications include damage to the optical nerve, which can cause a loss of visual clarity; bulging eyeballs (a condition called proptosis), which usually results in damage to the cornea; widely spaced eyes; and a narrowing of the sinuses and tear ducts that can cause inflammation of the mucous membranes lining the exposed portion of the eyeball (conjunctivitis). Bicoronal craniosynostosis can be further complicated by water on the brain (hydrocephalus) and increased intracranial pressure. Most individuals affected with bicoronal craniosynostosis also have an abnormally high and arched palate that can cause dental problems and protrusion of the lower jaw. Bicoronal craniosynostosis is associated with the Acrocephalosyndactyly syndromes (genetic syndromes that involve abnormalities of the head and webbed fingers or toes), which include Apert syndrome, Apert-Crouzon syndrome, Chotzen syndrome, and Pfeiffer syndrome.

Unicoronal craniosynostosis is characterized by a skull that is more developed in the front on one side than it is on the other side (frontal plagiocephaly). This leads to a distinct asymmetry between the sides of the face, a flattening of the forehead on the side affected by the premature suture closure, and a misalignment of the eyes such that the eye on the affected side is higher than the eye on the unaffected side.

Coronal and sagittal craniosynostosis is characterized by a cone-shaped head (acrocephaly). The front soft-spot (the anterior fontanelle) is generally much larger than normal and it may never close without surgical intervention. Individuals affected with coronal and sagittal craniosynostosis may have higher than normal intracranial pressure. Pfeiffer syndrome is closely associated with coronal and sagittal craniosynostosis.

Total craniosynostosis is characterized by a normally shaped but small skull (microcephaly). Individuals affected with total craniosynostosis have higher than normal intracranial pressures and they are the most likely of all craniosynostosis affected individuals to suffer from developmental delay.

Metopic craniosynostosis is characterized by a triangular shaped forehead (trigonocephaly) and thickened bones in the forehead and narrowly spaced eyes. Individuals affected with metopic craniosynostosis tend to have developmental abnormalities associated with processes that are known to be controlled by the front of the brain (the forebrain). Lambdoid and sagittal craniosynostosis is the most rare type of craniosynostosis. It is characterized by a flattening of the back of the skull (the occipital bone) and a bulging of the front of the skull (the frontal bone). This condition may occur symmetrically or asymmetrically.

Diagnosis

Prenatal, transabdominal, or traditional ultrasound is generally used to assess fetal skull development in the second and third trimesters of pregnancy. The resolution of such images is not always clear enough for a confident diagnosis of craniosynostosis. A transvaginal ultrasonic test to detect skull abnormalities in fetuses has been conducted in Japan and it offers much higher image clarity, allowing for the direct observation of cranial suture development as early as the second trimester, particularly of the sagittal and coronal sutures. Bicoronal and unicoronal craniosynostosis associated with one of the acrocephalosyndactyly syndromes may be detected via two different genetic tests now available that are able to identify the underlying mutations in the FGFR or TWIST genes. The sensitivity of this test is very high for certain genetic syndromes associated with coronal craniosynostosis: 100% for Muenke syndrome and 98% for Apert syndrome.

Almost all cases of craniosynostosis are evident at birth; however, the cranial sutures are not fully closed at this time so instances of craniosynostosis have been diagnosed later in infancy as well. Skull x rays and/or a CT scan may also be used after birth to diagnose craniosynostosis.

Treatment and management

Since craniosynostosis is associated with other conditions and may require multiple treatments of the skull, face, eyes, and ears, a multidisciplinary team of doctors and specialists is often required. The skull abnormalities of craniosynostosis should be surgically corrected within the first year of life. In the first year of life, changing the elevation and contours of the skull bones is much easier and new bone growth and reshaping occur rapidly. Also, at this point, the facial features are still highly undeveloped, so significant improvement in appearance can be achieved. Multiple surgeries may be required over the patient's lifetime, depending on the circumstances of the case. Follow-up support by pediatric, psychological, neurological, surgical and genetic specialists may be necessary.

In the types of craniosynostosis that involve the eyes, consultation with an ophthalmologist is often recommended and eye surgery may also be necessary. Speech and hearing therapy may also be needed when the ears and the frontal lobe have been affected. In the case of bicoronal craniosynostosis where the palate is severely malformed, dental consultation may also be required. In the most severe cases of coronal craniosynostosis, it will be necessary to address feeding and respiratory problems that are associated with the abnormally formed palate and sinuses.

Families with a history of craniosynostosis can participate in **genetic counseling** in order to learn whether

genetic testing can identify the likelihood that their children might be affected.

Prognosis

In all but the most severe and inoperable cases of craniosynostosis, it is possible that considerable improvement in physical appearance can be achieved via surgery. Depending on the neurological damage resulting from certain types of craniosynostosis versus the rapidity of treatment, certain affected individuals may suffer developmental disabilities ranging from the extremely mild to very severe. Most individuals with craniosynostosis that involves coronal sutures will continue to have vision problems throughout life. These problems vary in severity and many are now amenable to fully corrective treatments.

Resources

PERIODICALS

Pooh, R., et al. "Transvaginal sonography of the fetal brain: Detection of abnormal morphology and circulation." *Croatian Journal of Medicine* (1998): 147-57.

Wilkie, A. "Craniosynostosis: genes and mechanisms." *Human Molecular Genetics* (1979): 1647-56.

ORGANIZATIONS

Children's Craniofacial Association. PO Box 280297, Dallas, TX 75243-4522. (972) 994-9902 or (800) 535-3643. contactcca@ccakids.com. <http://www.ccakids.com>.

Craniosynostosis and Parents Support. 2965-A Quarters, Quantico, VA 22134. (877) 686-CAPS or (703) 445-1078. <http://www.caps2000.org/>.

WEBSITES

Craniosupport. <http://www.craniosupport.com/>.

Pediatric Database (PEDBASE) Homepage. <http://www.icondata.com/health/pedbase/files/CRANIOSY.HTM>.

Robin, N. "Craniosynostosis Syndromes (FGFR-Related)." *GeneClinics*. <http://www.geneclinics.org/profiles/craniosynostosis/details.html>.

Paul A. Johnson

Creutzfeldt-Jakob disease *see* **Prion diseases**

Cri du chat syndrome

Definition

Cri du chat syndrome occurs when a piece of chromosomal material is missing from a particular region on **chromosome** 5. Individuals with this syndrome have unusual facial features, poor muscle tone (hypotonia), small head size (microcephaly), and mental retardation. A classic feature of the syndrome is the cat-like cry made by infants with this disorder.

Description

Dr. Jerome Lejeune first described cri du chat syndrome in 1963. The syndrome is named for the cat-like cry made by infants with this genetic disorder. *Cri du chat* means "cry of the cat" in French. This unusual cry is caused by abnormal development of the larynx (organ in the throat responsible for voice production). Cri du chat syndrome is also called "5p minus syndrome" because it is caused by a deletion, or removal, of genetic material from chromosome 5. The deletion that causes cri du chat syndrome occurs on the short or "p" arm of chromosome 5. This deleted genetic material is vital for normal development. Absence of this material results in the features associated with cri du chat syndrome.

A high-pitched mewing cry during infancy is a classic feature of cri du chat. Infants with cri du chat also typically have low birth weight, slow growth, a small head (microcephaly) and poor muscle tone (hypotonia). Infants with cri du chat may have congenital heart defects. Individuals with cri du chat syndrome have language difficulties, delayed motor skill development, and mental retardation. Behavioral problems may also develop as the child matures.

Genetic profile

Cri du chat is the result of a chromosome abnormality. Human beings have 46 chromosomes in the cells of the their body. Chromosomes contain genes, which regulate the function and development of the body. An individual's chromosomes are inherited from their parents, 23 chromosomes from the egg and 23 chromosomes from the sperm. The 46 chromosomes in the human body are divided into pairs based on their physical characteristics. Chromosomes can only be seen when viewed under a microscope and appear identical because they contain the same genes.

Most chromosomes have a constriction near the center called the centromere. The centromere separates the chromosome into long and short arms. The short arm of a chromosome is called the "p arm." The long arm of a chromosome is called the "q arm."

Individuals should have two copies of chromosome 5. Cri du chat is caused when a piece of material is deleted, or erased, from the "p" arm of one chromosome 5. The piece of chromosomal material deleted contains many genes necessary for normal development. When these genes are missing, the larynx, brain, and other parts of the body do not develop as expected. This is what causes the symptoms associated with cri du chat.

In 90% of patients with cri du chat syndrome, the deletion is sporadic. This means that it happens randomly and is not hereditary. If a child has cri du chat due to a sporadic deletion, the chance the parents could have another child with cri du chat is 1%. In approximately 10% of patients with cri du chat, there is a hereditary chromosomal rearrangement that causes the deletion. If a parent has this rearrangement, the risk for them to have a child with cri du chat is greater than 1%.

Demographics

It has been estimated that cri du chat syndrome occurs in one of every 50,000 live births. According to the 5p minus Society, approximately 50-60 children are born with cri du chat syndrome in the United States each year. It can occur in all races and in both sexes.

Signs and symptoms

An abnormal larynx causes the unusual cat-like cry made by infants that is a hallmark feature of the syndrome. As children with cri du chat get older, the cat-like cry becomes less noticeable. This can make the diagnosis more difficult in older patients. In addition to the cat-like cry, individuals with cri du chat also have unusual facial features. These facial differences can be very subtle or more obvious. Microcephaly (small head size) is common. During infancy, many patients with cri du chat do not gain weight or grow normally. Approximately 30% of infants with cri du chat have a congenital heart defect. Hypotonia (poor muscle tone) is also common, leading to problems with eating, and slow normal development. Mental retardation is present in all patients with cri du chat but the degree of mental retardation varies between patients.

Diagnosis

During infancy the diagnosis of cri du chat syndrome is strongly suspected if the characteristic cat-like cry is heard. If a child has this unusual cry or other features seen in cri du chat syndrome, chromosome testing should be performed. Chromosome analysis provides the definitive diagnosis of cri du chat syndrome and can be performed from a blood test. Chromosome analysis, also called "karyotyping," involves staining the chromosomes and examining them under a microscope. In some cases the deletion of material from chromosome 5 can be easily seen. In other cases, further testing must be performed. FISH (fluorescence in-situ hybridization) is a special technique that detects very small deletions. The majority of the deletions that cause cri du chat syndrome can be identified using the FISH technique.

Cri du chat syndrome can be detected before birth if the mother undergoes **amniocentesis** testing or chorionic villus sampling (CVS). This testing would only be recommended if the mother or father is known to have a chromosome rearrangement, or if they already have a child with cri du chat syndrome.

Treatment and management

Currently, there is no cure for cri du chat syndrome. Treatment consists of supportive care and developmental therapy.

Prognosis

Individuals with cri du chat have a 10% mortality during infancy due to complications associated with congenital heart defects, hypotonia, and feeding difficulties. Once these problems are controlled, most individuals with cri du chat syndrome have a normal life span. The degree of mental retardation can be severe. However, a recent study suggested that the severity is somewhat affected by the amount of therapy received.

Resources

BOOKS

Gardner, R., J. McKinlay, and Grant R. Sutherland. *Chromosome Abnormalities and Genetic Counseling.* New York: Oxford University Press, 1996.

Jones, Kenneth. *Smith's Recognizable Patterns of Human Malformation,* 5th Edition. Philadelphia: W.B. Saunders Company, 1997.

Rimoin, David, Michael Connor, and Reed Pyeritz. *Emery and Rimoin's Principles and Practice of Medical Genetics,* Third Edition. New York: Churchill Livingstone, 1996.

PERIODICALS

Van Buggenhout, G. J. C. M., et al. "Cri du Chat Syndrome: Changing Phenotype in Older Patients." *American Journal of Medical Genetics* 90 (2000): 203-215.

ORGANIZATIONS

5p- Society. 7108 Katella Ave. #502, Stanton, CA 90680. (888) 970-0777. <http://www.fivepminus.org>.

Alliance of Genetic Support Groups. 4301 Connecticut Ave. NW, Suite 404, Washington, DC 20008. (202) 966-5557. Fax: (202) 966-8553. <http://www.geneticalliance.org>.

Cri du Chat Society. Dept. of Human Genetics, Box 33, MCV Station, Richmond VA 23298. (804) 786-9632.

Cri du Chat Syndrome Support Group. <http://www.criduchat-net.com>.

National Organization for Rare Disorders (NORD). PO Box 8923, New Fairfield, CT 06812-8923. (203) 746-6518 or (800) 999-6673. Fax: (203) 746-6481. <http://www.rarediseases.org>.

WEBSITES

OMIM—Online Mendelian Inheritance in Man. <http://www.ncbi.nlm.nih.gov/Omim/>.

Holly Ann Ishmael, MS, CGC

Crouzon craniofacial dysostosis *see*
Crouzon syndrome

Crouzon syndrome

Definition

Crouzon syndrome is a genetic condition that causes early closure of the bones in the skull. This event is

called **craniosynostosis** and causes the skull to be formed differently in affected individuals. Because of the craniosynostosis, individuals affected with Crouzon syndrome will have the characteristic facial features described below.

Description

Other features of Crouzon syndrome include wide-set and prominent eyes. Individuals with this syndrome may also have a condition called strabismus, which means the eyes have difficulty focusing on objects. Other facial features may include an underdeveloped upper jaw, which causes tooth abnormalities. Individuals with Crouzon syndrome often have a beak-shaped nose and hearing loss. A skin condition, called acanthosis nigricans, occurs in approximately 5% of individuals with Crouzon syndrome. It is important to note that there is a wide range of severity in Crouzon syndrome. No two individuals with the condition will necessarily have all the listed features.

It is rare for individuals with Crouzon syndrome to have learning delays or mental impairments. Affected individuals often undergo several corrective surgeries, increasing the need for continual medical care throughout their lives. This can be very stressful and difficult for individuals and their families. Additionally, since people with Crouzon syndrome have significant facial differences, it may be difficult for them (and their parents) to feel accepted by society. There may be psychological implications, ranging from the affected person feeling bad for "looking different" to the parents having trouble bonding to their child for similar reasons. The psychological impact may be less if there are others in the family with Crouzon syndrome. Having more than one family member with this syndrome may help those affected feel less isolated and give them a stronger support system.

Genetic profile

Crouzon syndrome is caused by mutations in the FGFR2 (location 10q25.3-q26) and FGFR3 (location 4p16.3) genes. Crouzon syndrome is inherited in an autosomal dominant manner. An affected individual has one copy of the FGFR mutation and has a 50% chance to pass it on to each of his or her children, regardless of that child's gender. As of 1997, about 75% of affected people have a family history of Crouzon syndrome, which is typically a parent with the condition. In the remaining 25%, the genetic mutation occurs as a new event in the affected individual, and there is no one in their family with the disease. These new mutations are thought to occur because of advancing paternal age, i.e. the age of the patient's father is a factor. Additionally, there is no increased recurrence risk for Crouzon syndrome above the general population risk when there is no family history of the condition.

FGFR2 and FGFR3 are responsible for the proper growth, movement, and creation of specific cells in the body, known as fibroblasts. Fibroblasts are often part of the bony structures in the body (such as the skull), so problems in fibroblast growth and movement would naturally lead to skull/bone problems. As of 1998, about 95% of patients have an FGFR2 mutation, and 5% have an FGFR3 mutation. However, nearly all of the affected individuals that also have acanthosis nigricans have one common FGFR3 mutation.

Demographics

As of 2000, Crouzon syndrome occurs in about one per 25,000 live births. It affects all ethnic groups equally.

Signs and symptoms

There commonly is bilateral (two-sided) coronal craniosynostosis in Crouzon syndrome. A cloverleaf skull may be present if the sagittal (long suture going from front to back of the head) and/or lambdoidal (short suture at very back of the head) sutures are involved. This causes the skull shape to be taller than usual, often described as "tower-shaped." The pattern looks like a cloverleaf because the skull is taller, and the sides of the skull and face bulge slightly from right to left. Additionally, the eye orbits are very shallow, causing the eyes to protrude significantly. This eye finding is always present in the condition. Strabismus may be present and eyes may be wide-set, making vision poor. Some individuals may have unexplained difficulties with their vision. The nose can be narrow and beak-shaped, forcing the individual to breathe through their mouth as a result.

The upper jaw may not be formed properly and can cause dentition problems, most commonly a missing tooth. The palate (upper ridge of the mouth) may be high and narrow, causing crowding of the existing teeth. Occasionally, clefting (improper closure) of the lip and palate may occur. Mild to moderate conductive hearing loss (due to abnormal ear structure formation) may occur in a proportion of cases.

Intellectual development is typically within normal limits. Only rare cases have been reported with significant mental deficiency. In about 30% of patients, **hydrocephalus** can occur. Hydrocephalus is an accumulation of fluid in the brain and skull, and this may progress or worsen with time. This typically shows up as a general enlarging of the skull. Sometimes the fluid can put increased pressure on various structures of the brain, lim-

iting their growth and development. Hydrocephalus may be an explanation for the few reported cases of Crouzon syndrome with learning problems. Occasionally, seizures may occur in the condition.

Individuals with Crouzon syndrome may be shorter than the normal expected height. This seems to affect females with the condition more than males.

Diagnosis

Historically, Crouzon syndrome has been diagnosed after careful physical examination and further studies. A diagnosis of Crouzon syndrome can be made through observing several of the following features. The abnormally shaped head is typically seen right away, in the newborn period. It may sometimes be seen in the prenatal period with an ultrasound examination. X-ray or physical examination of the skull can diagnose craniosynostosis. Once craniosynostosis is seen, it is important to determine whether it occurred because of abnormal biology of the cranial suture, possibly caused by an FGFR mutation. This is known as primary craniosynostosis and would make Crouzon syndrome a possibility. Craniosynostosis may also be caused by abnormal outside forces (known as secondary craniosynostosis) such as decreased brain growth or abnormal fetal head positioning. This may have occurred in the prenatal period, and in these cases the abnormal head shape may correct itself with time. The next step is to determine the type of craniosynostosis. A cloverleaf skull makes Crouzon syndrome a possibility, but it is also seen more commonly in other genetic craniosynostosis syndromes.

Some babies with Crouzon syndrome have breathing problems in the newborn period, due to narrowed nasal passages. Protruding eyes are a hallmark feature for the condition, and can be seen almost immediately after birth. The lack of abnormalities in the extremities (hands and feet) are also considered part of the diagnosis of Crouzon syndrome versus another type of craniosynostosis.

Molecular (DNA-based) **genetic testing** to diagnose Crouzon syndrome is available at a few laboratories. This testing is specific for the condition, separating it from other craniosynostosis syndrome possibilities. A blood or other type of sample (such as fetal cells from amniotic fluid) from the affected individual is provided, and the FGFR2 **gene** is analyzed.

Abnormal results occur when a mutation in the sequence of the FGFR2 **DNA** is identified from genetic analysis. This means that the mutation caused the symptoms in the individual, confirming the diagnosis of Crouzon syndrome. As mentioned earlier, not every person with Crouzon syndrome will have an FGFR2 mutation. Therefore, one could conceivably go through genetic testing and have no mutation found. This could mean that the person's symptoms are not caused by Crouzon syndrome.

Only a little more than 50% of the mutations that cause Crouzon syndrome are known. Therefore, a negative result could also mean that the patient has a genetic mutation that is unable to be found by current technology. Once a mutation is found in a family, it is much easier (and less time-consuming) to test others in the same family. For people with the features of Crouzon syndrome and acanthosis nigricans, there is DNA-based testing to determine if they have the common FGFR3 mutation.

Prenatal testing is available for both FGFR2 and FGFR3 mutations, done via **amniocentesis** or chorionic villus sampling (CVS). This is only offered when there is a parent with a *known* mutation. However, knowing prenatally that an individual has a mutation tells nothing about the extent of the disease. The only way to determine the severity of Crouzon syndrome is by seeing the individual after birth, not by molecular testing. A **prenatal ultrasound** can sometimes make a possible diagnosis of a syndrome involving craniosynostosis, but it is not as accurate as direct DNA testing. Additionally, a cloverleaf skull seen on a prenatal ultrasound usually implies a more severe outcome for the baby than other types of craniosynostosis.

Treatment and management

Treatment of individuals with Crouzon syndrome often involves the coordinated efforts of several medical specialists in a team setting. The specialists may include a pediatrician, plastic surgeon, neurosurgeon, geneticist, genetic counselor, dentist, social worker, audiologist, speech pathologist, psychologist, and otolaryngologist.

Craniosynostosis is typically repaired through a series of operations. There is a major surgery performed as early as the first three months of life, followed by several others that may extend over the life span. Each series of operations is tailored to the individual, but it is rare for the correction to be "perfect" despite the interventions. Because the skull is continually growing in the early part of life, timing of these surgeries is critical for proper brain formation and better results. Surgeries after the skull has stopped growing rarely yield good results. Surgeries performed before various portions of the facial region have stopped growing also have a poor prognosis, and will require additional follow-up procedures.

For individuals with hydrocephalus, sometimes a shunt, or tube, needs to be placed in order to allow the fluid to drain from the affected area(s) of the brain.

KEY TERMS

Acanthosis nigricans—A skin condition characterized by darkly pigmented areas of velvety wart-like growths. Acanthosis nigricans usually affects the skin of the armpits, neck, and groin.

Amniocentesis—A procedure performed at 16-18 weeks of pregnancy in which a needle is inserted through a woman's abdomen into her uterus to draw out a small sample of the amniotic fluid from around the baby. Either the fluid itself or cells from the fluid can be used for a variety of tests to obtain information about genetic disorders and other medical conditions in the fetus.

Chorionic villus sampling (CVS)—A procedure used for prenatal diagnosis at 10-12 weeks gestation. Under ultrasound guidance a needle is inserted either through the mother's vagina or abdominal wall and a sample of cells is collected from around the fetus. These cells are then tested for chromosome abnormalities or other genetic diseases.

Coronal suture—Skull suture that lies behind the forehead area, across the head from left side to the right side.

Craniosynostosis—Premature, delayed, or otherwise abnormal closure of the sutures of the skull.

Mutation—A permanent change in the genetic material that may alter a trait or characteristic of an individual, or manifest as disease, and can be transmitted to offspring.

Otolaryngologist—Physician who specializes in the care of the ear, nose, and throat and their associated structures.

Strabismus—An improper muscle balance of the ocular musles resulting in crossed or divergent eyes.

Suture—"Seam" that joins two surfaces together.

For babies with respiratory distress, oxygen and ventilation are often provided. Occasionally, a tracheostomy (opening in the windpipe) is created to help the individual breathe.

Because their eyes protrude so significantly, people with Crouzon syndrome sometimes have trouble closing their eyes. Surgical eye closure may be necessary, which allows the eye and its various structures (such as the cornea) to remain protected.

Occasionally, surgeries to correct structural ear abnormalities (resulting in hearing loss) are necessary.

Prognosis

The most problematic complication in Crouzon syndrome is the craniosynostosis. Prognosis primarily depends upon the severity and extent of this skull abnormality. Consequently, the success of corrective surgeries often determines prognosis.

Resources

BOOKS

Charkins, Hope. *Children with Facial Difference: A Parent's Guide.* Bethesda, MD: Woodbine House, 1996.

ORGANIZATIONS

AboutFace USA. PO Box 458, Crystal Lake, IL 60014. (312) 337-0742 or (888) 486-1209. aboutface2000@aol.com. <http://www.aboutface2000.org>.

American Cleft Palate-Craniofacial Association. 104 South Estes Dr., Suite 204, Chapel Hill, NC 27514. (919) 993-9044. Fax: (919) 933-9604. <http://www.cleftline.org>.

Children's Craniofacial Association. PO Box 280297, Dallas, TX 75243-4522. (972) 994-9902 or (800) 535-3643. contactcca@ccakids.com. <http://www.ccakids.com>.

Crouzon Support Network. PO Box 1272, Edmonds, WA 98020. penny@crouzon.org. <http://www.crouzon.org>.

Crouzon's/Meniere's Parent Support Network. 3757 North Catherine Dr., Prescott Valley, AZ 86314-8320. (800) 842-4681. katy@northlink.com.

WEBSITES

"Craniofacial Anomalies." *Columbia Presbyterian Medical Center Neurological Institute.* <http://cpmcnet.columbia.edu/dept/nsg/PNS/Craniofacial.html>.

Deepti Babu, MS

Cryptophthalmos syndactyly syndrome *see* **Fraser syndrome**

Cutis-gyrata syndrome of Beare and Stevenson *see* **Beare-Stevenson cutis gyrata syndrome**

Cystathionine beta-synthetase *see* **Homocystinuria**

Cystic fibrosis

Definition

Cystic fibrosis (CF) is an inherited disease that affects the lungs, digestive system, sweat glands, and male fertility. Its name derives from the fibrous scar tissue that develops in the pancreas, one of the principal organs affected by the disease.

Description

Cystic fibrosis affects the body's ability to move salt and water in and out of cells. This defect causes the lungs and pancreas to secrete thick mucus, blocking passageways and preventing proper function.

CF affects approximately 30,000 children and young adults in the United States, and about 3,000 babies are born with CF every year. CF primarily affects people of white northern European descent; rates are much lower in non-white populations.

Many of the symptoms of CF can be treated with drugs or nutritional supplements. Close attention to and prompt treatment of respiratory and digestive complications have dramatically increased the expected life span of a person with CF. Several decades ago most children with CF died by age two years; today, about half of all people with CF live past age 31. That median age is expected to grow as new treatments are developed, and it is estimated that a person born in 1998 with CF has a median expected life span of 40 years.

Genetic profile

Cystic fibrosis is a genetic disease, meaning it is caused by a defect in the person's genes. Genes, found in the nucleus of all the body's cells, control cell function by serving as the blueprint for the production of proteins. Proteins carry out a wide variety of functions within cells. The **gene** that, when defective, causes CF is called the CFTR gene, which stands for cystic fibrosis transmembrane conductance regulator. A simple change in this gene leads to all the consequences of CF. There are over 500 known defects in the CFTR gene that can cause CF. However, 70% of all people with an abnormal CFTR gene have the same defect, known as delta-F508.

Genes can be thought of as long strings of chemical words, each made of chemical letters, called nucleotides. Just as a sentence can be changed by rearranging its letters, genes can be mutated, or changed, by changes in the sequence of their nucleotide letters. The gene changes in CF are called point mutations, meaning that the gene is mutated only at one small spot along its length. In other words, the delta-F508 mutation is a loss of one "letter" out of thousands within the CFTR gene. As a result, the CFTR protein made from its blueprint is made incorrectly, and cannot perform its function properly.

The CFTR protein helps to produce mucus. Mucus is a complex mixture of salts, water, sugars, and proteins

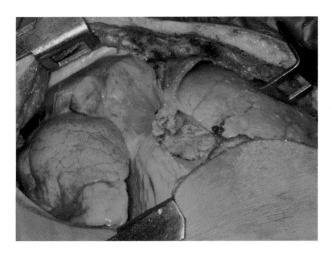

Accumulation of mucus in the smaller passageways of the lungs can plug them up, decreasing functional lung volume. As the air is exhaled, much of it becomes trapped in the small pores of the lungs. This leads to expansion of the lung and swollen appearance seen in the left lung above. *(Custom Medical Stock Photo, Inc.)*

that cleanses, lubricates, and protects many passageways in the body, including those in the lungs and pancreas. The role of the CFTR protein is to allow chloride ions to exit the mucus-producing cells. When the chloride ions leave these cells, water follows, thinning the mucus. In this way, the CFTR protein helps to keep mucus from becoming thick and sluggish, thus allowing the mucus to be moved steadily along the passageways to aid in cleansing.

In CF, the CFTR protein does not allow chloride ions out of the mucus-producing cells. With less chloride leaving, less water leaves, and the mucus becomes thick and sticky. It can no longer move freely through the passageways, so they become clogged. In the pancreas, clogged passageways prevent secretion of digestive enzymes into the intestine, causing serious impairment of digestion—especially of fat—which may lead to malnutrition. Mucus in the lungs may plug the airways, preventing good air exchange and, ultimately, leading to emphysema. The mucus is also a rich source of nutrients for bacteria, leading to frequent infections.

To understand the **inheritance** pattern of CF, it is important to realize that genes actually have two functions. First, as noted above, they serve as the blueprint for the production of proteins. Second, they are the material of inheritance: parents pass on characteristics to their children by combining the genes in egg and sperm to make a new individual.

Each person actually has two copies of each gene, including the CFTR gene, in each of his or her body cells. During sperm and egg production, however, these two

copies separate, so that each sperm or egg contains only one copy of each gene. When sperm and egg unite, the newly created cell once again has two copies of each gene.

The two gene copies may be the same or they may be slightly different. For the CFTR gene, for instance, a person may have two normal copies, or one normal and one mutated copy, or two mutated copies. A person with two mutated copies will develop cystic fibrosis. A person with one mutated copy is said to be a carrier. A carrier will not have symptoms of CF, but can pass on the mutated CFTR gene to his or her children.

When two carriers have children, they have a one in four chance of having a child with CF each time they conceive. They have a two in four chance of having a child who is a carrier, and a one in four chance of having a child with two normal CFTR genes.

Approximately one in every 25 Americans of northern European descent is a carrier of the mutated CF gene, while only one in 17,000 African-Americans and one in 30,000 Asian-Americans are carriers. Since carriers are symptom-free, very few people will know whether or not they are carriers, unless there is a family history of the disease. Two white Americans with no family history of CF have a one in 2,500 chance of having a child with CF.

It may seem puzzling that a mutated gene with such harmful consequences would remain so common; one might guess that the high mortality of CF would quickly lead to loss of the mutated gene from the population. Some researchers now believe the reason for the persistence of the CF gene is that carriers, those with only one copy of the gene, are protected from the full effects of cholera, a microorganism that infects the intestine, causing intense diarrhea and eventual death by dehydration. It is believed that having one copy of the CF gene is enough to prevent the full effects of cholera infection, while not enough to cause the symptoms of CF. This so-called "heterozygote advantage" is seen in some other **genetic disorders**, including sickle-cell anemia.

Signs and symptoms

The most severe effects of cystic fibrosis are seen in two body systems: the gastrointestinal (digestive) system and the respiratory tract, from the nose to the lungs. CF also affects the sweat glands and male fertility. Symptoms develop gradually, with gastrointestinal symptoms often the first to appear.

Gastrointestinal system

Ten to fifteen percent of babies who inherit CF have meconium ileus at birth. Meconium is the first dark stool that a baby passes after birth; ileus is an obstruction of

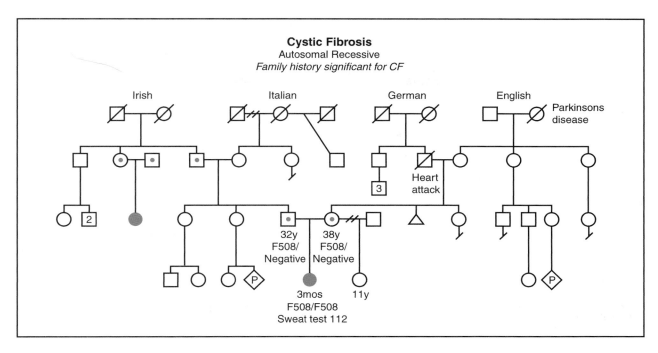

Cystic Fibrosis
Autosomal Recessive
Family history significant for CF

(Gale Group.)

the digestive tract. The meconium of a newborn with meconium ileus is thickened and sticky, due to the presence of thickened mucus from the intestinal glands. Meconium ileus causes abdominal swelling and vomiting, and often requires surgery immediately after birth. Presence of meconium ileus is considered highly indicative of CF. Borderline cases may be misdiagnosed, however, and attributed instead to a "milk allergy."

Other abdominal symptoms are caused by the inability of the pancreas to supply digestive enzymes to the intestine. During normal digestion, as food passes from the stomach into the small intestine, it is mixed with pancreatic secretions, which help to break down the nutrients for absorption. While the intestines themselves also provide some digestive enzymes, the pancreas is the major source of enzymes for the digestion of all types of foods, especially fats and proteins.

In CF, thick mucus blocks the pancreatic duct, which is eventually closed off completely by scar tissue formation, leading to a condition known as pancreatic insufficiency. Without pancreatic enzymes, large amounts of undigested food pass into the large intestine. Bacterial action on this rich food source can cause gas and abdominal swelling. The large amount of fat remaining in the feces makes it bulky, oily, and foul-smelling.

Because nutrients are only poorly digested and absorbed, the person with CF is often ravenously hungry, underweight, and shorter than expected for his age.

When CF is not treated for a longer period, a child may develop symptoms of malnutrition, including anemia, bloating, and, paradoxically, appetite loss.

Diabetes becomes increasingly likely as a person with CF ages. Scarring of the pancreas slowly destroys those pancreatic cells which produce insulin, producing type I, or insulin-dependent, diabetes.

Gallstones affect approximately 10% of adults with CF. Liver problems are less common, but can be caused by the build-up of fat within the liver. Complications of liver enlargement may include internal hemorrhaging, abdominal fluid (ascites), spleen enlargement, and liver failure.

Other gastrointestinal symptoms can include a prolapsed rectum, in which part of the rectal lining protrudes through the anus; intestinal obstruction; and rarely, intussusception, in which part of the intestinal tube slips over an adjoining part, cutting off blood supply.

Somewhat fewer than 10% of people with CF do not have gastrointestinal symptoms. Most of these people do not have the delta-F508 mutation, but rather a different one, which presumably allows at least some of their CFTR proteins to function normally in the pancreas.

Respiratory tract

The respiratory tract includes the nose, the throat, the trachea (or windpipe), the bronchi (which branch off

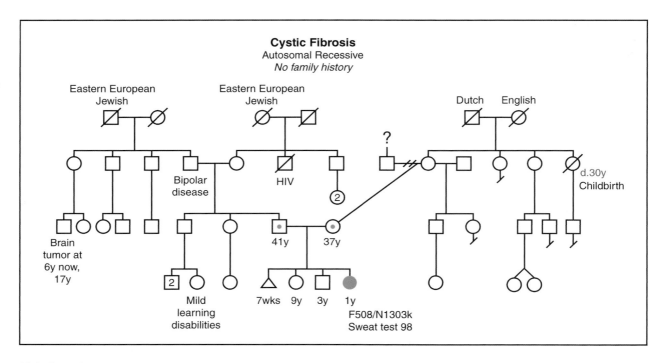

Cystic Fibrosis
Autosomal Recessive
No family history

Eastern European Jewish

Eastern European Jewish

Dutch   English

Bipolar disease

HIV

d.30y
Childbirth

Brain tumor at 6y now, 17y

41y   37y

Mild learning disabilities

7wks   9y   3y   1y

F508/N1303k
Sweat test 98

(Gale Group.)

from the trachea within each lung), the smaller bronchioles, and the blind sacs called alveoli, in which gas exchange takes place between air and blood.

Swelling of the sinuses within the nose is common in people with CF. This usually shows up on x ray, and may aid the diagnosis of CF. However, this swelling, called pansinusitis, rarely causes problems, and does not usually require treatment.

Nasal polyps, or growths, affect about one in five people with CF. These growths are not cancerous, and do not require removal unless they become annoying. While nasal polyps appear in older people without CF, especially those with allergies, they are rare in children without CF.

The lungs are the site of the most life-threatening effects of CF. The production of a thick, sticky mucus increases the likelihood of infection, decreases the ability to protect against infection, causes inflammation and swelling, decreases the functional capacity of the lungs, and may lead to emphysema. People with CF will live with chronic populations of bacteria in their lungs, and lung infection is the major cause of death for those with CF.

The bronchioles and bronchi normally produce a thin, clear mucus, which traps foreign particles including bacteria and viruses. Tiny hair-like projections called cilia on the surface of these passageways slowly sweep the mucus along, out of the lungs and up the trachea to

the back of the throat, where it may be swallowed or coughed up. This "mucociliary escalator" is one of the principal defenses against lung infection.

The thickened mucus of CF prevents easy movement out of the lungs, and increases the irritation and inflammation of lung tissue. This inflammation swells the passageways, partially closing them down, further hampering the movement of mucus. A person with CF is likely to cough more frequently and more vigorously as the lungs attempt to clean themselves out.

At the same time, infection becomes more likely since the mucus is a rich source of nutrients. Bronchitis, bronchiolitis, and pneumonia are frequent in CF. The most common infecting organisms are the bacteria *Staphylococcus aureus*, *Haemophilus influenzae*, and *Pseudomonas aeruginosa*. A small percentage of people with CF have infections caused by *Burkholderia cepacia*, a bacterium which is resistant to most current antibiotics (*Burkholderia cepacia* was formerly known as *Pseudomonas cepacia*). The fungus *Aspergillus fumigatus* may infect older children and adults.

The body's response to infection is to increase mucus production; white blood cells fighting the infection thicken the mucus even further as they break down and release their cell contents. These white blood cells also provoke more inflammation, continuing the downward spiral that marks untreated CF.

As mucus accumulates, it can plug up the smaller passageways in the lungs, decreasing functional lung volume. Getting enough air can become difficult; tiredness, shortness of breath, and intolerance of exercise become more common. Because air passes obstructions more easily during inhalation than during exhalation, over time, air becomes trapped in the smallest chambers of the lungs, the alveoli. As millions of alveoli gradually expand, the chest takes on the enlarged, barrel-shaped appearance typical of emphysema.

For unknown reasons, recurrent respiratory infections lead to "digital clubbing," in which the last joint of the fingers and toes becomes slightly enlarged.

Sweat glands

The CFTR protein helps to regulate the amount of salt in sweat. People with CF have sweat that is much saltier than normal, and measuring the saltiness of a person's sweat is the most important diagnostic test for CF. Parents may notice that their infants taste salty when they kiss them. Excess salt loss is not usually a problem except during prolonged exercise or heat. While most older children and adults with CF compensate for this extra salt loss by eating more salty foods, infants and young children are in danger of suffering its effects (such as heat prostration), especially during summer. Heat prostration is marked by lethargy, weakness, and loss of appetite, and should be treated as an emergency condition.

Fertility

Ninety-eight percent of men with CF are sterile, due to complete obstruction or absence of the vas deferens, the tube carrying sperm out of the testes. While boys and men with CF form normal sperm and have normal levels of sex hormones, sperm are unable to leave the testes, and fertilization is not possible. Most women with CF are fertile, though they often have more trouble getting pregnant than women without CF. In both boys and girls, puberty is often delayed, most likely due to the effects of poor nutrition or chronic lung infection. Women with good lung health usually have no problems with pregnancy, while those with ongoing lung infection often do poorly.

Diagnosis

The decision to test a child for cystic fibrosis may be triggered by concerns about recurring gastrointestinal or respiratory symptoms, or salty sweat. A child born with meconium ileus will be tested before leaving the hospital. Families with a history of CF may wish to have all children tested, especially if there is a child who already

has the disease. Some hospitals now require routine screening of newborns for CF.

Sweat test

The sweat test is both the easiest and most accurate test for CF. In this test, a small amount of the drug pilocarpine is placed on the skin. A very small electrical current is then applied to the area, which drives the pilocarpine into the skin. The drug stimulates sweating in the treated area. The sweat is absorbed onto a piece of filter paper, and is then analyzed for its salt content. A person with CF will have salt concentrations that are one-and-one-half to two times greater than normal. The test can be done on persons of any age, including newborns, and its results can be determined within an hour. Virtually every person who has CF will test positively on it, and virtually everyone who does not will test negatively.

Genetic testing

The discovery of the CFTR gene in 1989 allowed the development of an accurate genetic test for CF. Genes from a small blood or tissue sample are analyzed for specific mutations; presence of two copies of the mutated gene confirms the diagnosis of CF in all but a very few cases. However, since there are so many different possible mutations, and since testing for all of them would be too expensive and time-consuming, a negative gene test cannot rule out the possibility of CF.

Couples planning a family may decide to have themselves tested if one or both have a family history of CF. Prenatal **genetic testing** is possible through **amniocentesis**. Many couples who already have one child with CF decide to undergo prenatal screening in subsequent pregnancies. Siblings in these families are also usually tested, both to determine if they will develop CF, and to determine if they are carriers, to aid in their own family planning. If the sibling has no symptoms, determining his or her carrier status is often delayed until the teen years or later, when he or she is closer to needing the information to make decisions.

Newborn screening

Some states now require screening of newborns for CF, using a test known as the IRT test. This is a blood test which measures the level of immunoreactive trypsinogen, which is generally higher in babies with CF than those without it. This test gives many false positive results immediately after birth, and so requires a second test several weeks later. A second positive result is usually followed by a sweat test.

Treatment and management

There is no cure for cystic fibrosis. Treatment has advanced considerably in the past several decades, increasing both the life span and the quality of life for most people affected by CF. Early diagnosis is important to prevent malnutrition and infection from weakening the young child. With proper management, many people with CF engage in the full range of school and sports activities.

Nutrition

People with CF usually require high-calorie diets and vitamin supplements. Height, weight, and growth of a person with CF are monitored regularly. Most people with CF need to take pancreatic enzymes to supplement or replace the inadequate secretions of the pancreas. Tablets containing pancreatic enzymes are taken with every meal; depending on the size of the tablet and the meal, as many as 20 tablets may be needed. Because of incomplete absorption even with pancreatic enzymes, a person with CF needs to take in about 30% more food than a person without CF. Low-fat diets are *not* recommended except in special circumstances, since fat is a source of both essential fatty acids and abundant calories.

Some people with CF cannot absorb enough nutrients from the foods they eat, even with specialized diets and enzymes. For these people, tube feeding is an option. Nutrients can be introduced directly into the stomach through a tube inserted either through the nose (a nasogastric tube) or through the abdominal wall (a gastrostomy tube). A jejunostomy tube, inserted into the small intestine, is also an option. Tube feeding can provide nutrition at any time, including at night while the person is sleeping, allowing constant intake of high-quality nutrients. The feeding tube may be removed during the day, allowing normal meals to be taken.

Respiratory health

The key to maintaining respiratory health in a person with CF is regular monitoring and early treatment. Lung function tests are done frequently to track changes in functional lung volume and respiratory effort. Sputum samples are analyzed to determine the types of bacteria present in the lungs. Chest x rays are usually taken at least once a year. Lung scans, using a radioactive gas, can show closed off areas not seen on the x ray. Circulation in the lungs may be monitored by injection of a radioactive substance into the bloodstream.

People with CF live with chronic bacterial colonization; that is, their lungs are constantly host to several species of bacteria. Good general health, especially good nutrition, can keep the immune system healthy, which

decreases the frequency with which these colonies begin an infection, or attack on the lung tissue. Exercise is another important way to maintain health, and people with CF are encouraged to maintain a program of regular exercise.

In addition, clearing mucus from the lungs helps to prevent infection, and mucus control is an important aspect of CF management. Bronchial drainage is used to allow gravity to aid the mucociliary escalator. For this technique, the person with CF lies on a tilted surface with head downward, alternately on the stomach, back, or side, depending on the section of lung to be drained. An assistant thumps the rib cage to help loosen the secretions. A device called a "flutter" offers another way to loosen secretions: it consists of a stainless steel ball in a tube. When a person exhales through it, the ball vibrates, sending vibrations back through the air in the lungs. Some special breathing techniques may also help clear the lungs.

Several drugs are available to prevent the airways from becoming clogged with mucus. Bronchodilators can help open up the airways; steroids reduce inflammation; and mucolytics loosen secretions. Acetylcysteine (Mucomyst) has been used as a mucolytic for many years but is not prescribed frequently now, while DNase (Pulmozyme) is a newer product gaining in popularity. DNase breaks down the **DNA** from dead white blood cells and bacteria found in thick mucus.

People with CF may pick up bacteria from other CF patients. This is especially true of *Burkholderia cepacia*, which is not usually found in people without CF. While the ideal recommendation from a health standpoint might be to avoid contact with others who have CF, this is not usually practical (since CF clinics are a major site of care), nor does it meet the psychological and social needs of many people with CF. At a minimum, CF centers recommend avoiding prolonged close contact between people with CF, and scrupulous hygiene, including frequent hand washing. Some CF clinics schedule appointments on different days for those with and without *B. cepacia* colonies.

Some doctors choose to prescribe antibiotics only during infection, while others prefer long-term antibiotic treatment against *S. aureus*. The choice of antibiotic depends on the particular organism or organisms found. Some antibiotics are given as aerosols directly into the lungs. Antibiotic treatment may be prolonged and aggressive.

Supplemental oxygen may be needed as lung disease progresses. Respiratory failure may develop, requiring temporary use of a ventilator to perform the work of breathing.

Lung transplantation is another option for people with CF, although the number of people who receive them is still much lower than those who want them. Transplantation is not a cure, however, and has been likened to trading one disease for another. Long-term immunosuppression is required, increasing the likelihood of other types of infection. About 50% of adults and more than 80% of children who receive lung transplants live longer than two years. Some CF patients whose livers have been damaged by fibrosis also undergo liver transplants.

Long-term use of ibuprofen has been shown to help some people with CF; presumably by reducing inflammation in the lungs. Close medical supervision is necessary, however, since the effective dose is high and not everyone benefits. Ibuprofen at the required doses interferes with kidney function, and together with aminoglycoside antibiotics, may cause kidney failure.

A number of experimental treatments are currently the subject of much research. Some evidence indicates that aminoglycoside antibiotics may help overcome the genetic defect in some CF mutations, allowing the protein to be made normally. While promising, these results would apply to only about 5% of those with CF.

Gene therapy is currently the most ambitious approach to curing CF. In this set of techniques, non-defective copies of the CFTR gene are delivered to affected cells, where they are taken up and used to create the CFTR protein. While elegant and simple in theory, gene therapy has met with a large number of difficulties in trials so far, including immune resistance, very short duration of the introduced gene, and inadequately widespread delivery.

Alternative treatment

In homeopathic medicine, the symptoms of the disease would be addressed to enhance the quality of life for the person with cystic fibrosis. Treating the cause of CF, because of the genetic basis for the disease, is not possible. Homeopathic medicine seeks to treat the whole person, however, and in cystic fibrosis, this approach might include:

- Mucolytics to help thin mucous.

- Supplementation of pancreatic enzymes to assist in digestion.

- Respiratory symptoms can be addressed to open lung passages.

- Hydrotherapy techniques to help ease the respiratory symptoms and help the body eliminate mucus.

- Immune enhancements can help prevent the development of secondary infections.

KEY TERMS

Carrier—A person who possesses a gene for an abnormal trait without showing signs of the disorder. The person may pass the abnormal gene on to offspring.

CFTR—Cystic fibrosis transmembrane conductance regulator. The protein responsible for regulating chloride movement across cells in some tissues. When a person has two defective copies of the CFTR gene, cystic fibrosis is the result.

Emphysema—A chronic lung disease that begins with breathlessness during exertion and progresses to shortness of breath at all times, caused by destructive changes in the lungs.

Mucociliary escalator—The coordinated action of tiny projections on the surfaces of cells lining the respiratory tract, which moves mucus up and out of the lungs.

Mucolytic—An agent that dissolves or destroys mucin, the chief component of mucus.

Pancreatic insufficiency—Reduction or absence of pancreatic secretions into the digestive system due to scarring and blockage of the pancreatic duct.

- Dietary enhancements and adjustments to treat digestive and nutritional problems.

Prognosis

People with CF may lead relatively normal lives. The possible effect of pregnancy on the health of a woman with CF requires careful consideration before beginning a family, as do issues of longevity, and their children's status as carriers. Although most men with CF are functionally sterile, new procedures for removing sperm from the testes are being tried, and may offer more men the chance to become fathers.

Approximately half of people with CF live past the age of 30. Because of better and earlier treatment, a person born today with CF is expected, on average, to live to age 40.

Resources

BOOKS

Gehehrter, Thomas, Francis Collins, and David Ginsburg. *Principles of Medical Genetics.* Baltimore: Williams & Wilkins, 1998.

Harris, Ann, and Maurice Super. *Cystic fibrosis: The facts.* New York; Oxford, UK: Oxford University Press, 1995.

Orenstein, David. *Cystic fibrosis: A guide for patient and family.* Philadelphia; New York: Lippincott-Raven, 1997.

ORGANIZATIONS

Cystic Fibrosis Foundation. 6931 Arlington Rd., Bethesda, MD 20814. (301) 951-4422. <http://www.cff.org>.

WEBSITES

Cystic Fibrosis Information. <http://cf-web.mit.edu/index.html>.

Edward Rosick, DO, MPH, MS

Cystinosis

Definition

Cystinosis is a rare genetic metabolic disease that causes cystine, an amino acid, to accumulate in lysosomes of various organs of the body such as the kidneys, liver, eyes, muscles, pancreas, brain, and white blood cells. Although cystinosis primarily affects children, a form of the disease also occurs in adults.

Description

In cystinosis, the cystine content of cells increases to an average of 50 to 100 times its normal value. This increase is caused by an abnormality in the transport of cystine out of a sac-like compartment of the cell called the lysosome. Because of cystine's low solubility in water, this amino acid forms crystals that accumulate within the lysosomes of cells. The accumulation of cystine is believed to destroy the cells.

There are three basic forms of cystinosis: infantile nephropathic cystinosis; late-onset nephropathic cystinosis; and benign non-nephropathic cystinosis.

Infantile nephropathic cystinosis

Children with infantile cystinosis usually appear normal at birth and during the first six to eight months of life. As Fanconi syndrome (a tubular dysfunction of the kidneys causing an impairment in the kidneys' ability to reabsorb minerals and nutrients back into the bloodstream) develops, sodium and water depletion occurs, leading to polyuria (excessive urination) and polydipsia (excessive thirst). Affected children become especially vulnerable to dehydration. This tubular abnormality, in addition to an abnormality in sweat production, often leads to recurrent fevers as a presenting symptom.

By one year of age, children generally exhibit growth retardation, rickets (inadequate deposition of minerals in developing cartilage and newly formed bone, causing abnormalities in shape and structure of bones), metabolic acidosis (excessive acid in the blood), and other chemical evidence or renal tubular abnormalities of the kidney, such as increased renal (kidney) excretion of glucose, amino acids, phosphate, and potassium. However, more subtle clinical and biochemical evidence of the disease can be detected at a much earlier age by careful examination of at-risk children (those with a sibling or other relative with the disease). As a child with infantile nephropathic cystinosis ages, failure to thrive is apparent.

Without therapeutic intervention, children remain below the norm in both height and weight throughout life. The typical patient with infantile nephropathic cystinosis has short stature, retinopathy (retinal disorder), photophobia (light sensitivity), and onset of Fanconi's syndrome in the first year of life. By one to two years of age, corneal cystine crystals and rickets are evident. Glomerular failure (the glomerulus is a small structure in the kidney made up of a cluster of capillaries) progresses, and end-stage renal disease occurs by about nine to ten years of age.

Late-onset cystinosis

In late-onset nephropathic cystinosis, the age of onset ranges from 2–26 years; however, the typical age at which this condition presents is 12–13 years. If more than one sibling develops late-onset cystinosis, their age of onset and symptoms are generally similar. Patients with this condition develop crystalline deposits in the cornea and conjunctiva (mucous membrane lining the eyelids) as well as in the bone marrow. Although patients with late-onset cystinosis often do not develop full-blown Fanconi's syndrome, renal failure progresses to such a degree that kidney transplantation is necessary, as in the case of infantile nephropathic cystinosis. These individuals are usually in end-stage renal failure within a few years of diagnosis.

Benign non-nephropathic cystinosis

Formerly known as adult cystinosis, benign non-nephropathic cystinosis is usually discovered by chance when an ophthalmologic (eye) examination reveals crystalline opacities within the cornea and conjunctiva. As in patients with infantile nephropathic cystinosis, those with benign cystinosis may also have photophobia; however, light sensitivity may not develop until middle age and is usually not as debilitating. Because the only patients diagnosed with benign cystinosis are those who undergo slit-lamp (a lamp constructed such that intense light is emitted through a slit) eye examination, it is possible that many individuals with this form of the disease never experience eye symptoms and are never diagnosed. Patients with benign cystinosis develop crystalline deposits in their bone marrow and white blood cells but do not develop renal dysfunction or retinopathy.

Genetic profile

Cystinosis is an autosomal recessive genetic disease. The term "autosomal" refers to a **gene** situated on one of the 22 of the 23 pairs of chromosomes other than a sex **chromosome** (or the X or Y chromosome). The term "recessive" refers to an allele, or a form of a gene that may be expressed and/or active; however, the "dominant" form of the gene on the other chromosome usually takes over enough of the gene's normal function to prevent symptoms of a disorder. Each parent of a child with cystinosis carries one abnormal (recessive) gene and one normal gene. Thus, the child must inherit an abnormal (or altered) gene from each parent to develop the disease. In addition, when a child develops cystinosis, the parents are almost always surprised because they never exhibited any symptoms of the disease. The recessive gene may lie dormant for generations until two people with the abnormal gene come together and have children.

Each time two such cystinosis carriers—persons with one copy of the altered gene and one copy of a normal or functioning gene—have a child together, there is a one-in-four chance (25% risk) of having a child with cystinosis; two-in-four (50% risk) the child will not have cystinosis but will be a carrier; and a one-in-four chance the child will not have cystinosis or be a carrier. Also, every unaffected sibling of a child with cystinosis has a two-in-three (67%) chance of being a carrier (having one copy of the abnormal gene and one copy of a normal gene), like his or her parents.

Scientists have mapped the cystinosis gene, CTNS, to the short arm of chromosome 17 (at location 17p13). Mutations (changes) in the cystinosis gene (specifically, a deletion of a particular part of the gene) have been found to cause all three types of cystinosis. However, this deletion is difficult to identify in some individuals for reasons that are uncertain. In these individuals, extensive and very sophisticated laboratory work (molecular **genetic testing**) to identify and prove the existence of the deletion would be necessary.

In patients of Northern European descent, for example, there is about a 50/50 probability that an individual with cystinosis has the deletion. Genetic testing is under investigation for populations of these regions, but until details of the methodology are refined, measurement of lysosomal cystine in white cells and fibroblasts (any cell or corpuscle from which connective tissue is developed)

will remain the state-of-the art and the most broadly based general method for diagnosing cystinosis.

Demographics

It is estimated that 2,000 individuals worldwide have cystinosis, although exact figures are difficult to obtain because the disease often remains undiagnosed. In the United States, the disease is believed to affect approximately 400 individuals.

Signs and symptoms

Although the symptoms of cystinosis vary, depending on the type of disease present, general symptoms include:

- acidosis
- dehydration
- rickets
- growth retardation
- renal glomerular failure
- corneal ulcerations and retinal blindness
- delayed puberty
- swallowing difficulties

Diagnosis

Cystinosis may be diagnosed prenatally by examining cystine levels in chorionic villi (obtained by chorionic villus sampling, usually done at 10–12 weeks gestation) or in cells contained in amniotic fluid (obtained by **amniocentesis**, usually done at 16–18 weeks gestation). In early infancy, cystinosis is usually diagnosed by measuring free cystine in white blood cells and skin fibroblasts.

Chorionic villus sampling

Chorionic villus sampling (tissue sample of tiny pieces of placental tissue obtained by inserting a thin needle or narrow tube into the uterus) is performed at 10–12 weeks of gestation. Intracellular cystine levels are measured. The values in a fetus with cystinosis are more than 10 times greater than normal.

Amniocentesis

Amniocentesis (sample of amniotic fluid obtained by inserting a thin needle into the uterus) can be performed at 16–18 weeks of gestation.

White blood cell testing

When diagnosed early, the progressive kidney failure, retarded growth, and vision problems can be prevented or delayed by proper management and medication. The metabolic abnormality in cystinosis is the failure of the cellular lysosomes to release cystine. As a result, the free cystine in the lysosomes accumulates to many times the normal value. The diagnosis of cystinosis is therefore based in part on the measurement of free cystine in the tissues that accumulate this amino acid. This measurement is most easily accomplished in white blood cells. Whole blood contains red cells, which are rich in glutathione, a compound that can react with cystine. To prevent this reaction, white cells are separated from red cells. The white cells are kept cold to slow down reactions, then broken open, and frozen. Freezing prevents the reaction of cystine with compounds such as glutathione and precipitates the cell protein. These steps stabilize the cystine content of the preparation.

Skin fibroblast testing

Cultured skin fibroblasts may also be used to diagnose cystinosis. Because of the increased time and costs, white blood cells are usually sent for testing first. Skin fibroblast testing (biopsy) is also more invasive than a blood sample. On rare occasions the expression of the abnormality in white cells is borderline for diagnosis. Thus, confirmation using fibroblasts is definitive.

Treatment and management

Cystinosis is treated by a variety of pharmacologic and nonpharmacologic therapies as well as by surgical transplantation.

Pharmacologic therapy

The aim of specific treatment for cystinosis is to reduce cystine accumulation within the cells. This goal is achieved by cysteamine treatment, which has proven effective in delaying or preventing renal failure. Cysteamine treatment also improves growth in children with cystinosis. The growth improvement with cysteamine bitartrate usually allows the patient to maintain growth along a percentile but does not usually aid in achieving "catch-up" growth.

The Food and Drug Administration (FDA) approved a capsule form of cysteamine bitartrate called Cystagon in August 1994. However, oral cysteamine does not prevent the progression of ocular lesions and has many potential side effects. Little is known about the drug's long-term effects. The main disadvantage of cysteamine treatment is the need for four daily capsules (every six hours) and the sulfurous breath it causes. Cysteamine treatment is also expensive.

Many children with cystinosis receive growth hormone, and some have had improvements in height. There is also evidence that indomethacin (Indocin) increases appetite, decreases urine volume, decreases water consumption, and improves growth in pretransplanted patients with cystinosis.

Vitamin/mineral supplementation

The symptomatic treatment of the Fanconi's syndrome is essential in patients with cystinosis. The urinary losses of water, salts, bicarbonate, and minerals must be replaced. Most children receive a solution of sodium and potassium citrate, as well as phosphate. Some also receive extra vitamin D.

Organ transplantation

Kidney transplantation has proven useful in patients with cystinosis. If a patient with cystinosis receives a kidney transplant and reaches adulthood, the new kidney will not be affected by the disease. However, without cysteamine treatment, kidney transplant recipients can develop complications in other organs due to the continued cystine accumulation in the body. These complications can include muscle wasting, difficulty swallowing, **diabetes**, hypothyroidism, and blindness. Not all older patients, however, develop these symptoms.

In both young children with cystinosis and older patients with a kidney transplant, cysteamine eye drops may be useful in removing the corneal cystine crystals and reduce photophobia. However, the drops have not yet received FDA approval.

Prognosis

Since 1980, the prognosis of a child with cystinosis has greatly improved. However, if children with the disease receive no treatment, they rarely survive past the age of nine or ten.

Resources

BOOKS

Milunsky, Aubrey, ed. *Genetic Disorders and the Fetus.* Baltimore: Johns Hopkins University Press, 1998.

Moreman, Kelley, and Dag Malm. *Human Genetic Disease: A Layman's Approach.* <http://mcrcr2.med.nyu.edu/ murphy01/lysosome/hgd.htm>. (1997).

PERIODICALS

Cherqui, S., V. Kalatzis, L. Forester, I. Poras, and C. Antignac. "Identification and Characterization of the Murine Homologue for the Gene Responsible for Cystinosis, CTNS." *BMC Genomics* 1 (2000): 2. <http:// biomedcentral.com/1471-2164/1/2>.

McDowell G., M. M. Town, W. van't Hoff, and W. A. Gahl. "Clinical and molecular aspects of nephropathic cystinosis." *Journal of Molecular Medicine* 76 (1998): 295–302.

Vester U., M. Schubert, G. Offneer, and J. Brodehl. "Distal myopathy in nephropathic cystinosis." *Pediatric Nephrology* 14 (January 2000): 36–38.

ORGANIZATIONS

Cystinosis Foundation. 2516 Stockbridge Dr., Oakland, CA 94611. (800) 392-8458. <http:// www.cystinosisfoundation.org>.

Cystinosis Research Network. 8 Sylvester Rd., Burlington, MA 01803. (866) CURE NOW. Fax: (781) 229-6030. <http:// www.cystinosis.org>.

National Center for Biotechnology Information. National Library of Medicine, Building 38A, Room 8N805, Bethesda, MD 20894. (301) 496-2475. <http:// www3.ncbi.nlm.nih.gov>.

National Organization for Rare Disorders (NORD). PO Box 8923, New Fairfield, CT 06812-8923. (203) 746-6518 or (800) 999-6673. Fax: (203) 746-6481. <http:// www.rarediseases.org>.

WEBSITES

Cystinosis Pediatric Database (PEDBASE). <http:// icondata.com/health/pedbase/files/CYSTINOS.HTM>.

"What Is Cystinosis?" *The Cystinosis Research Network.* <http://cystinosis.org./what_is_cystinosis.htm>.

Genevieve T. Slomski, PhD

Cystinuria

Definition

Cystinuria is a relatively common inherited disorder characterized by the formation of cystine urinary tract stones that can lead to obstruction, infection, and eventual loss of renal function.

Description

In cystinuria there is a defect in the movement of cystine and the dibasic amino acids (lysine, arginine, and ornithine) across the epithelial cells of the kidneys and the small intestine. In the kidney, most amino acids are filtered by the glomerulus and reabsorbed by the proximal tubules with little residual amino acid in the urine. In cystinuria, cystine and the dibasic amino acids are not reabsorbed by the tubules of the kidney and eventually build up in the urine. Cystine in high concentrations is insoluble in urine and will form stones (calculi) in the kidneys, bladder, and ureters. The transport defect in the small intestine leads to the accumulation of digestion breakdown products of cystine and the dibasic amino acids in the stool, urine, and plasma. The intestinal defect does not appear to result in any adverse symptoms for the affected individual.

Cystinuria has been classified into three types (I, II, and III) based on the urinary excretion of cystine and the dibasic amino acids among carriers of the disease (heterozygotes) and on the nature of the intestinal transport defect among affected individuals (homozygotes).

The name cystine is derived from the Greek word for bladder, *kystis.* When the disease was first described in the 1800's, it was thought that the origin of the cystine stones was the bladder. Historically, cystinuria is important because it was one of the four inborn errors of metabolism reported by Sir Archibald Garrod in his famous Croonian lectures in 1908. Although alternate names for the disorder include: cystine-lysinuria, cystine-lysine-arginine-ornithinuria and cystinuria dibasic amnioaciduria, the term cystinuria is used most often to describe the disease.

Genetic profile

Cystinuria is a complex autosomal recessive disorder. Type I cystinuria is completely recessive; carriers have no manifestations. Types II and III cystinuria are incompletely recessive; carriers can display symptoms. Two amino acid transporter genes, SLC3A1 (solute carrier family 3, member 1) located on **chromosome** 2p, and SLC7A9 (solute carrier family 7 member 9) located on chromosome 19q are known to cause cystinuria. The proteins produced by these two genes apparently interact with one another. An individual with two mutations in the SLC3A1 **gene** (homozygote) has type I disease. Mutations in the SLC7A9 gene lead to types II and III cystinuria. Types II and III cystinuria are allelic; different changes (mutations) in the same gene lead to alternative forms of the disease. There are some patients who are genetic compounds, they have a type II mutation on one copy of the gene and a type III mutation on the other copy. There are also individuals who may have mutations in both the SLC3A1 gene and the SLC7A9 gene.

Demographics

Cystinuria is considered one of the more common **genetic disorders** with an estimated prevalence of one in 7,000. Most affected individuals have type I disease. Type II disease is relatively rare. Due to a founder effect, an increased incidence of cystinuria exists among individuals of Libyan Jewish ancestry. Approximately one in 2500 persons of Libyan Jewish descent has type II disease. The carrier frequency in this population is around one in 25.

Signs and symptoms

Symptoms of cystinuria develop due to the high level of cystine in the urine. Since cystine at high concentrations is insoluble in urine, undissolved cystine accumulates in the urine and affected individuals are prone to recurrent urinary tract stone formation (nephrolithiasis). Also, hexagonal-shaped crystals form in the urine; these crystals signify the presence of cystine in potentially stone-forming concentrations. The onset of cystinuria is variable and symptoms can appear anytime between the first year of life and the ninth decade. Most cystinurics develop symptoms in the second and third decades of life. In many affected individuals the first sign of the disorder is renal colic, a painful condition caused by obstruction of the urinary tract. Obstruction of the urinary tract due to calculi can lead to infection and eventually to renal insufficiency. Less often, complaints such as infection, hypertension, and renal failure are the first reasons cystinuric patients seek medical attention.

Unlike most autosomal recessive disorders, carriers for types II and III cystinuria can be symptomatic. Type II carriers have high urinary excretion of cystine and lysine and type II carriers have moderate excretion of cystine, lysine, arginine, and ornithine. Both type II and type III carriers are at-risk to develop stones. Type I carriers have no excess cystine or dibasic amino acids in their urine and are without symptoms of the disorder.

Although there are reports of an association between cystinuria and neurologic abnormalities, little is known about the mechanism responsible for this nor is the prevalence of this complication among affected individuals known.

Diagnosis

The diagnosis of cystinuria is made at the biochemical level. Molecular (genetic) testing is also available but is generally not the first means of making a cystinuria diagnosis. The simplest approach to diagnosis of this condition is microscopic examination of the urine for the characteristic hexagonal-shaped crystals. Urinary microscopic examination was the primary means of cystinuria diagnosis for many years since the discovery of these crystals by Stromeyer in 1824, and it remains a useful aid in the diagnosis of this condition today. Another widely used screening procedure is the cyanide-nitroprusside test, a test that measures the amount of cystine excreted in the urine in comparison to the amount of creatinine (a protein normally found in urine). In those patients who display crystals and have a positive nitroprusside test, further diagnostic tests such as thin-layer chromatography or high-voltage electrophoresis can identify the specific amino acids (cystine, lysine, arginine, ornithine), and other techniques such as ion-exchange chromatography, liquid chromatography-mass spectrophotometer, and high-performance liquid chromatography may be performed to measure the amounts of these amino acids in the urine.

The type (I, II, or II) of cystinuria in an affected patient can be determined by family studies and/or by study of the intestinal transport defect in an affected individual. Type I obligate carriers have normal amounts of urinary cystine and dibasic amino acids. Type II carriers have between nine and fifteen times the normal amount of cystine and lysine in their urine. Type III carriers have up to twice the normal range of cystine and the dibasic amino acids in their urine. The intestinal absorption defect in an affected individual can be demonstrated by oral loading tests and/or by study of the transport of cystine and the dibasic amino acids in an intestinal biopsy specimen from an affected individual.

Testing for mutations in the SLC3A1 gene and the SLC7A9 gene is possible. Over forty mutations in the SLC3A1 gene have been found and almost as many have been detected in the SLC7A9 gene.

Treatment and management

Prevention

The primary goal of treatment of cystinuria is prevention of existing cystine stones through non-invasive means. There are three main categories of treatment: increase cystine solubility, reduce cystine production

KEY TERMS

Alkalinization—The process of making a solution more basic, rather than more acidic, by raising the pH.

Allelic—Related to the same gene.

Amino acid—Organic compounds that form the building blocks of protein. There are 20 types of amino acids (eight are "essential amino acids" which the body cannot make and must therefore be obtained from food).

Carrier—A person who possesses a gene for an abnormal trait without showing signs of the disorder. The person may pass the abnormal gene on to offspring.

Catheter—A narrow, flexible tube used to create a pathway for introducing drugs, nutrients, fluids, or blood products into the body and/or for removing fluid or other substances from the body.

Chromosome—A microscopic thread-like structure found within each cell of the body and consisting of a complex of proteins and DNA. Humans have 46 chromosomes arranged into 23 pairs. Changes in either the total number of chromosomes or their shape and size (structure) may lead to physical or mental abnormalities.

Cystine—A sulfur-containing amino acid, sometimes found as crystals in the kidneys or urine, that forms when proteins are broken down by digestion.

Epithelial cells—The layer of cells that cover the open surfaces of the body such as the skin and mucous membranes.

Founder effect—Increased frequency of a gene mutation in a population that was founded by a small ancestral group of people, at least one of whom was a carrier of the gene mutation.

Glomerulus—A structure in the kidney composed of blood vessels that are actively involved in the filtration of the blood.

Homozygote—Having two identical copies of a gene or chromosome.

Obligate carrier—An individual who, based on pedigree analysis, must carry a genetic mutation for a particular genetic disease. Parents of a child with an autosomal recessive disorder are obligate carriers.

Oral loading test—A procedure in which cystine is administered orally to a patient and plasma levels of cystine are measured. Under normal circumstances, amino acids are absorbed by the intestine and result in an increase in plasma amino acid levels. However, in cystinuria, there is a problem in the absorption process and blood levels of amino acids do not rise or rise slowly after eating.

Plasma—The liquid part of the blood and lymphatic fluid that contains antibodies and other proteins.

Renal—Related to the kidneys.

Renal colic—A spasmodic pain, moderate to severe in degree, located in the back, side and/or groin area.

Small intestine—The part of the digestive tract in-between the stomach and the large intestine.

Tubule—A small tube lined with glandular epithelium in the kidney.

Ureters—Tubes through which urine is transported from the kidneys to the bladder.

and excretion, and convert cystine into a more soluble compound. The first step in treatment is to increase cystine solubility via hydration therapy. It is recommended that patients increase their fluid intake such that the concentration of cystine is 200-250 mg/liter of urine. This therapy prevents stone formation approximately two-thirds of the time. Another therapy that increases cystine solubility is known as oral alkalinization. Medications such as sodium citrate, potassium citrate, or sodium bicarbonate increase the pH of urine to levels at which cystine becomes a more soluble compound. To reduce cystine excretion and production, individuals with cystinuria may follow a diet low in sodium and protein.

If the above measures are not successful in preventing stones and/or dissolving existing ones, drug therapy may be necessary. Tiopronin and d-penicillamine are two drugs that are known to bind excess cystine into a form that is more soluble than cystine alone and thus reduce the excessive urinary excretion of this amino acid. Since both tiopronin and d-penicillamine can have adverse side effects, patients on these regimens require follow-up to monitor the efficacy and tolerance of the medication. Other medications that reduce cystine excretion include mercaptopropionylglycine (MPG) and captopril. Although they are not as effective as tiopronin or d-penicillamine, MPG and captopril have fewer side effects.

If stones form despite the above therapeutic regimens, surgical intervention may be required. Surgical management of cystine stones may include dissolution of calculi by irrigation through a catheter, removal of cystine stones by lithotripsy or lithotomy, and renal transplantation. Catheter irrigation is a minimally invasive procedure in which catheters are placed into the ureters and the urinary tract is irrigated with a solution that dissolves the stones over a period of one week to several months. Lithotripsy is a medical procedure used to break a kidney stone into small pieces that can be passed in the urine. In extracorporeal shock wave lithotripsy, a shock wave produced outside the body is used to break up the stone and a catheter placed in the ureter facilitates passage of the stone fragments. In percutaneous nephrolithotripsy, an opening (port) is created by puncturing the kidney through the skin; a specialist then inserts instruments via this opening into the kidney to break up the stone and remove the debris. Lithotomy is the surgical removal of a (kidney) stone.

Prognosis

The prognosis of cystinuria is variable and depends on the level of renal function at the time of diagnosis and initiation of therapy, and the success of preventative measures and surgical management. It is known that males tend to have a more severe course and a higher mortality rate.

Resources

BOOKS

Holton, John B. *The Inherited Metabolic Diseases*. New York, New York: Churchill Livingstone, 1994.

Rimoin, David, et. al. *Emery and Rimoin's Principles and Practice of Medical Genetics*. New York, New York: Churchill Livingstone, 1997.

Scriver, Charles R., et. al. *The Metabolic and Molecular Basis of Inherited Disease*. McGraw-Hill, Inc., 1995.

PERIODICALS

ORGANIZATIONS

National Organization for Rare Disorders (NORD). PO Box 8923, New Fairfield, CT 06812-8923. (203) 746-6518 or (800) 999-6673. Fax: (203) 746-6481. <http://www.rarediseases.org>.

WEBSITES

Cystinuria Support Network homepage. <http://www.cystinuria.com/>.

Dawn Cardeiro, MS, CGC

Cytogenetic mapping *see* **Genetic mapping**

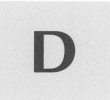

Dandy-Walker malformation

Definition

Dandy-Walker malformation is a congenital (present at birth) condition involving several abnormalities in the development of the brain. The malformation appears to result from destructive processes, such as inflammation or trauma, which block the circulation of cerebrospinal fluid (CSF) inside the head after the brain has been formed in the embryo.

Description

Dandy-Walker malformation was first described in 1914 by Drs. Dandy and Blackfan. The disorder typically includes the following abnormalities in brain structure:

- Absence or incomplete formation of the vermis, the middle portion of the cerebellum, which is the part of the human brain that lies behind the two cerebral hemispheres.

- Enlargement of the fourth ventricle, one of the human brain's four interconnected ventricles (inner cavities or chambers) that produce cerebrospinal fluid (CSF). In Dandy-Walker malformation, the CSF cannot circulate freely through the ventricles and the rest of the central nervous system (CNS), so it builds up inside the fourth ventricle and causes it to enlarge.

- Cysts (sacs) containing CSF are formed in the posterior fossa, which is a hollow at the back of the skull that covers the cerebellum.

- Absence or incomplete formation of the three foramina (small openings or holes) in the fourth ventricle.

In Dandy-Walker malformation, the CSF produced by the ventricles of the brain is not fully reabsorbed by the body; thus, the excess fluid accumulates in the fourth ventricle and the posterior fossa. As cysts in these areas grow, pressure from the fluid rises, producing a condition known as obstructive, or non-communicating, **hydrocephalus** (excess fluid on the brain).

This type of hydrocephalus develops in 90% of children diagnosed with Dandy-Walker malformation. The size of the head may or may not be affected by the fluid pressure.

Genetic profile

The genetic transmission of Dandy-Walker malformation is not fully understood because the disorder often occurs with other birth abnormalities including cleft palate, extra fingers (**polydactyly**) or fingers joined together (syndactyly), cataracts, and malformations of the face or heart. An abnormality in the central nervous system that often occurs together with Dandy-Walker malformation is agenesis (absence or failure to develop) of the corpus callosum, the thick band of nerve fibers that joins the two cerebral hemispheres. It is not yet clear whether these and other abnormalities in CNS development are determined by the same **gene** or whether they are inherited separately.

Dandy-Walker malformation appears to be transmitted in some families in an autosomal, or X-linked, recessive pattern, which means that both parents have one copy of the changed (mutated) gene but do not have the malformation. These families have a high risk of recurrence of the malformation. Families in which there has been inbreeding among close relatives also appear to transmit Dandy-Walker in an autosomal recessive pattern. Several **chromosomal abnormalities** have been associated with Dandy-Walker.

Demographics

Dandy-Walker malformation is a rare disorder. It is estimated to occur in about 3% of children with hydrocephalus, which occurs in 1–2 per 1,000 births. It appears to affect both sexes equally. While there is no known association with specific races or ethnic groups, recent genetic case studies of Dandy-Walker malformation include cases from Argentina, Poland, Germany, Brazil, Austria, and Japan.

Signs and symptoms

Some signs of Dandy-Walker malformation may appear before birth. It is possible to detect hydrocephalus by ultrasound as early as 15-18 weeks after conception. A newborn with hydrocephalus may have difficulty breathing, dilated veins visible on the scalp, and rapid head growth. Infants with Dandy-Walker may be slow to develop motor (movement) skills, and may have abnormally large skulls as a result of the fluid pressure inside the head.

Older children with Dandy-Walker malformation may have symptoms associated with fluid pressure inside the head including vomiting, convulsions, and emotional irritability. If the cerebellum has been damaged, the child's sense of balance and coordination will be affected. About 20% of older children with Dandy-Walker have difficulty coordinating movements of the hands or feet (ataxia) or have involuntary jerking movements of the eyes (nystagmus). Developmental delays and mental retardation are more common. In some cases Dandy-Walker may be associated with an abnormal pituitary gland and delayed puberty. Other symptoms that sometimes appear in this group include unusually large head size, a bulge at the back of the head caused by fluid pressure in the posterior fossa, and abnormal breathing patterns.

Diagnosis

About 80% of children with Dandy-Walker malformation are diagnosed before the end of the first year, usually as a result of the signs of hydrocephalus. Following birth, the newborn's head circumference is measured to determine whether it has been enlarged by the development of cysts. As has already been mentioned, ultrasound screening before birth can detect some signs of hydrocephalus. Ultrasound screening is recommended if the family has a history of congenital neurologic abnormalities. **Genetic counseling** is recommended for parents who have already had a child with Dandy-Walker malformation as there is an increased risk that the malformation will reoccur in later pregnancies.

Imaging studies used to diagnose and monitor Dandy-Walker include:

- x rays of the skull to determine that the posterior fossa has been enlarged;

- CT scan or magnetic resonance imaging (MRI) tests to evaluate the size and shape of the fourth ventricle, the presence and size of the vermis, and the displacement of other parts of the brain by fluid pressure;

- cranial ultrasound to evaluate the size of the ventricle or to assess the progression of hydrocephalus; or

- transillumination, a technique that shines a strong light through an organ or body part to assist in diagnosis.

KEY TERMS

Agenesis—Failure of an organ, tissue or cell to develop or grow.

Congenital—Refers to a disorder which is present at birth.

Corpus callosum—A thick bundle of nerve fibers deep in the center of the forebrain that provides communications between the right and left cerebral hemispheres.

Cyst—An abnormal sac or closed cavity filled with liquid or semisolid matter.

Foramen—A small opening or hole in a body part or tissue. Dandy-Walker malformation is characterized by the absence or failure to develop the three foramina in the fourth ventricle of the brain.

Hydrocephalus—The excess accumulation of cerebrospinal fluid around the brain, often causing enlargement of the head.

Posterior fossa—Area at the base of the skull attached to the spinal cord.

Shunt—A small tube placed in a ventricle of the brain to direct cerebrospinal fluid away from the blockage into another part of the body.

Trisomy—The condition of having three identical chromosomes, instead of the normal two, in a cell.

Ventricle—The fluid filled spaces in the center of the brain that hold cerebral spinal fluid.

Vermis—The central portion of the cerebellum, which divides the two hemispheres. It functions to monitor and control movement of the limbs, trunk, head, and eyes.

The posterior fossa may be transilluminated as part of the differential diagnosis of Dandy-Walker.

Treatment and management

Treatment of Dandy-Walker malformation is usually focused on managing hydrocephalus when it is present. Hydrocephalus cannot be cured, but it can be treated surgically by placing a shunt in the ventricles of the brain to reduce fluid pressure. The shunt carries some of the CSF into another part of the body where it can be reabsorbed.

Another important part of managing Dandy-Walker is treatment of conditions or abnormalities associated with it—such as giving anticonvulsant medications for seizures or hormones to bring on puberty that has been delayed.

Prognosis

The prognosis for children with Dandy-Walker malformation is usually not encouraging because of the associated multiple abnormalities. Children with other congenital abnormalities occurring together with Dandy-Walker often do not survive. The affected person's chances of normal intellectual development depend on the severity of the malformation and the presence of other abnormalities.

Resources

BOOKS

Martin, John H., PhD. *Neuroanatomy: Text and Atlas*, 2nd ed. Norwalk, CT: Appleton & Lange, 1996.

"Neurologic Abnormalities." *The Merck Manual of Diagnosis and Therapy*, edited by Mark H. Beers, MD, and Robert Berkow, MD. Whitehouse Station, NJ: Merck Research Laboratories, 1999.

PERIODICALS

Cavalcanti, D. P., and M. A. Salomao. "Dandy-Walker malformation with postaxial polydactyly: further evidence for autosomal recessive inheritance." *American Journal of Medical Genetics* 16 (July 1999): 183-184.

Kawame, H., et al. "Syndrome of microcephaly, Dandy-Walker malformation, and Wilms tumor caused by mosaic variegated aneuploidy with premature centromere division (PCD): report of a new case and review of the literature. *Journal of Human Genetics* 44, no. 4 (1999): 219-224.

Macmillin, M. D., et al. "Prenatal diagnosis of inverted duplicated 8p." *American Journal of Medical Genetics* 17 (July 2000): 94-98.

Marszal, E., et al. "Agenesis of corpus callosum: clinical description and etiology." *Journal of Child Neurology* 15, no. 6 (June 2000): 401-405.

Rittler, M., and E. E. Castilla. "Postaxial polydactyly and Dandy-Walker malformation. Further nosological comments." *Clinical Genetics* 56 (1999): 462-463.

Ulm, B., et al. "Isolated Dandy-Walker malformation: prenatal diagnosis in two consecutive pregnancies." *American Journal of Perinatology* 16, no. 2 (1999): 61-63.

von Kaisenberg, C. S., et al. "Absence of 9q22-9qter in trisomy 9 does not prevent a Dandy-Walker phenotype." *American Journal of Medical Genetics* 18 (December 2000): 425-428.

ORGANIZATIONS

Dandy-Walker Syndrome Network. 5030 142nd Path West, Apple Valley, MN 55124. (612) 423-4008.

Guardians of Hydrocephalus Research Foundation. 2618 Avenue Z, Brooklyn, NY 11235-2023. (718) 743-4473 or (800) 458-865. Fax: (718) 743-1171. ghrf2618@aol.com.

Hydrocephalus Association. 870 Market St. Suite 705, San Francisco, CA 94102. (415) 732-7040 or (888) 598-3789. (415) 732-7044. hydroassoc@aol.com. <http://neurosurgery.mgh.harvard.edu/ha>.

National Institute of Neurological Disorders and Stroke. 31 Center Drive, MSC 2540, Bldg. 31, Room 8806, Bethesda, MD 20814. (301) 496-5751 or (800) 352-9424. <http://www.ninds.nih.gov>.

National Organization for Rare Disorders (NORD). PO Box 8923, New Fairfield, CT 06812-8923. (203) 746-6518 or (800) 999-6673. Fax: (203) 746-6481. <http://www.rarediseases.org>.

WEBSITES

Hydrocephalus Association. <http://www.HydroAssoc.org> or <http://www.neurosurgery.mgh.harvard.edu/ha>.

Rebecca J. Frey, PhD

Deletion *see* Chromosomal abnormalities

Deletion 22q11 syndrome

Definition

Deletion 22q11 syndrome is a relatively common genetic disorder characterized by congenital heart defects, palate abnormalities, distinct facial features, immune problems, learning disabilities and other abnormalities. This syndrome is caused by a deletion of chromosomal material from the long arm of **chromosome** 22 (22q) that leads to a wide spectrum of effects.

Description

Deletion 22q11 syndrome is also known as velocardiofacial syndrome, DiGeorge syndrome, Sphrintzen syndrome, conotruncal anomaly face syndrome, and the CATCH-22 syndrome. Because of the wide variability in the features of this syndrome, medical professionals originally thought that deletion 22q11 syndrome was more than one syndrome and it was separately described by a number of physicians—Dr. DiGeorge, Dr. Sphrintzen, and others. Dr. DiGeorge described the more severe end of deletion 22q11 syndrome (infants with congenital heart defects, unusual facial features and immune system abnormalities). The term velocardiofacial (VCF) syndrome was used for the milder end of deletion 22q11 syndrome. These individuals usually had palate anomalies, distinct facial features, and learning disabilities.

Deletion 22q11 syndrome is an extremely variable syndrome. The main features are congenital heart defects, distinctive facial features and palate (roof of the mouth) problems. Other problems include immune system abnormalities, thyroid problems, kidney abnormalities and learning difficulties including mild developmental delay. Very rarely do individuals have all of the problems associated with this syndrome. Most individuals with deletion 22q11 syndrome have only a few of the associated features. Some individuals with 22q11 deletion syndrome are very mildly affected and others are more severely affected. The reason for the wide variability in this syndrome is not known.

Genetic profile

Deletion 22q11 syndrome is a genetic disorder caused by a deletion of chromosomal material from the long arm of chromosome 22. A series of genes are located in this region. Individuals with deletion 22q11 syndrome may have some or all of these genes deleted. This syndrome is sometimes called a microdeletion syndrome or a contiguous **gene** syndrome. Contiguous refers to the fact that these genes are arranged next to each other. The size of the deletion can be large or small, which may explain why some individuals with deletion 22q11 syndrome are more severely affected than others. The exact genes responsible for this syndrome are not known.

Deletion 22q11 syndrome is an autosomal dominant disorder. Genes always come in pairs and in an autosomal dominant disorder only one gene needs too be missing or altered for an individual to have the disorder. About 10–15% of the time, deletion of the long arm of chromosome 22 that causes this syndrome is inherited from a parent. If a parent has deletion 22q11 syndrome, then there is a 50% chance they will pass the deletion on to each of their children who will also be affected with 22q11 syndrome. For reasons that are not understood, it is possible for a parent with mild features of deletion 22q11 syndrome to have a child with severe features of the syndrome.

Although deletion 22q11 syndrome is an autosomal dominant disorder, over 85–90% of individuals with this disorder are the only individuals in their family with this disorder. When this is the case, the chromosome deletion that causes deletion 22q11 syndrome is called *de novo*. A *de novo* deletion is one that occurs for the first time in the affected individual. The causes of *de novo* chromosome deletions are not known. Parents of a child with deletion 22q11 syndrome due to a *de novo* deletion are very unlikely to have a second child with deletion 22q11 syndrome.

Demographics

Deletion 22q11 syndrome is one of the most common chromosomal deletion syndromes. It is estimated that approximately one in 2,000 to one in 6,000 individuals has a deletion of chromosome 22q11. Approximately 130,000 individuals in the United States have deletion 22q11 syndrome. Because of the extreme variability of this syndrome, it is possible that individuals with milder features are under diagnosed and the exact incidence of this disorder is not known. As more physicians become familiar with this syndrome, it is likely that more individuals will be correctly diagnosed.

Individuals with deletion 22q11 syndrome are diagnosed based upon physical findings. Of infants born with congenital heart defects, 5% will be found to have a deletion of chromosome 22q11. Of infants with a cleft palate, approximately 5–8% of them will be found to a have a 22q11 deletion.

Signs and symptoms

Deletion 22q11 syndrome is a multisystem disorder. It is also sometimes referred to as velocardiofacial syndrome. This name reflects the organ systems that are most commonly affected in deletion 22q11 syndrome. Velo is from the Latin word *velum*, which means "palate" and back of the throat, cardio refers to the heart and facial refers to the distinctive facial features of individuals with deletion 22q11 syndrome. While it may seem unusual that these three separate areas are affected, a possible explanation lies in the early development of the embryo. Very early in development, the cells that will become the heart, face and thyroid lie next to each other in a region called the neural crest. As the embryo continues to develop, these cells migrate or move to become organs (the heart, face and palate). It is believed that the deletion of chromosomal material from chromosome 22q causes a problem in the migration of these cells leading to the variability of features or problems seen in deletion 22q11 syndrome.

In addition to the heart, palate, and face, many other organ systems can also be affected including the kidneys, the immune system, the brain, the throat, the skeletal system, the skin, the genitourinary system and the endocrine (hormone) system. It is not possible to cover every possible feature of deletion 22q11 syndrome but the following is an overview of the most common features.

The characteristic facial features seen in individuals with deletion 22q11 syndrome include a long face with narrow palpebral fissures (the opening for the eyes), a prominent nasal bridge (the arch of the nose between the eyes), a slightly bulbous nasal tip, a long nose, small ears with thick helical folds, and a small jaw. None of these features individually is abnormal but the combination of features is characteristically seen in individuals with deletion 22q11 syndrome. These features may not be present or as easily noticeable in African-American individuals with deletion 22q11 syndrome.

Approximately 70% of individuals with deletion 22q11 syndrome have palate abnormalities. These may include complete cleft palate (an opening of the bones and skin of the roof of the mouth) or a submucous cleft palate (an opening of only the bones of the roof of the mouth covered by skin). Other individuals with deletion 22q11 syndrome have more subtle palate and throat abnormalities including velopharyngeal insufficiency, which is a problem in the coordination between the tongue, palate, and throat muscles. All of these problems can lead to feeding problems in infancy and speech problems such as hypernasal speech.

Cardiac or congenital heart defects are one of the more serious symptoms of deletion 22q11 syndrome and affect about 75% of individuals. There is a wide range of cardiac abnoramlities seen in deletion 22q11 syndrome. Some are minor and may require no treatment, some are correctable by surgery, and others are invariably fatal. The most common heart defects seen in individuals with deletion 22q11 syndrome are truncus arteriosus, interrupted aortic arch, tetralogy of Fallot, ventricular septal defects (VSDs), pulmonary stenosis and **patent ductus arteriosus**. Many of these heart defects are known as conotruncal heart defects. Conotruncal refers to the type of embryonic cells that were involved in the development of these regions of the heart.

Immune problems are another of the serious problems associated with this syndrome. Because of the underdevelopment of the thymus gland, individuals with deletion 22q11 syndrome can have reduced amounts of the cells necessary to fight infections—T cells. Because of this reduction in T cells, individuals with deletion 22q11 syndrome are more prone to getting infections and less able to fight them off. The degree of immune deficiency can be variable with some individuals having life threatening infections and others having much milder problems.

Growth problems may be seen in children with deletion 22q11 syndrome. Infants with deletion 22q11 syndrome are often diagnosed as having failure to thrive. This may result from feeding problems due to their palate abnormalities but they can also have gastroesophageal reflux and vomiting problems. It also appears that individuals with deletion 22q11 syndrome have generalized growth problems. Most adult individuals with deletion 22q11 syndrome have short stature.

Individuals with deletion 22q11 syndrome can also have specific learning disabilities and possibly mild developmental delay. The learning disabilities are specific. Most individuals with learning disabilities have a discrepancy between their performance IQ score (higher) and their verbal IQ score (lower) that indicates a nonver-

bal learning disability. Simple IQ testing may not reveal this learning disability and it is important to evaluate the components of IQ scores separately. Individuals with deletion 22q11 syndrome seem to do better at verbal learning and do well in subjects such as reading. They have more trouble with abstract concepts such as math.

Individuals with deletion 22q11 syndrome are also at risk to develop psychological problems and mental illness. Deletion 22q11 syndrome has been associated with higher rates of bipolar affective disorder, manic-depressive illness, and schizoaffective disorder when compared to individuals who do not have deletion 22q11 syndrome. Other mood disorders, such as **depression**, also occur at a higher incidence in individuals with deletion 22q11 syndrome. Most of these disorders appear during adolescence or adulthood. Some individuals with deletion 22q11 syndrome are mildly mentally retarded. Others have learning disabilities and some are diagnosed as having **attention deficit hyperactivity disorder**.

Endocrine problems are also commonly seen. The endocrine system is the hormone producing system of the body and is composed of glands such as the thyroid and parathyroid. Individuals with deletion 22q11 syndrome may either be missing one or more of these glands or have underactive glands. An underactive thyroid is called hypothyroidism and an underactive parathyroid is called hypoparathyroidism. Because the parathyroids help to regulate the level of calcium in the body, individuals with deletion 22q11 syndrome also have problems with their calcium levels. Low levels of calcium can lead to seizures.

Individuals with deletion 22q11 syndrome may also have kidney problems such as a cystic kidney, missing (aplastic) kidney, or malformed kidney. They can have limb differences such as extra fingers, ribs, or problems with the vertebrae in the back that might lead to **scoliosis**.

Diagnosis

The diagnosis of deletion 22q11 syndrome is usually made by a physician familiar with the syndrome and based upon a physical examination of the individual and a review of the patient's medical history. It is often made in infants after a heart problem is diagnosed. In children without significant heart problems, the possibility of a diagnosis may first be raised by preschool teachers or by other medical professionals such as plastic surgeons and speech therapists. These medical professionals may be seeing the child for one of the features of deletion 22q11 syndrome and may be the first ones to become suspicious about the diagnosis. In rare cases, the diagnosis is made in a parent after they have had an affected child.

While a diagnosis can be made based upon physical examination and medical history, the diagnosis is now confirmed by a **DNA** test.

Sometimes the 22q11 deletion is large enough that it can be seen during a **karyotype** analysis. A karyotype is a microscopic analysis of an individual's chromosomes. However, many 22q11 deletions are too small to be seen by microscopic examination and another specific technique called **fluorescent in situ hybridization** testing, or FISH testing, can determine whether genetic material is missing. A FISH test will be positive (detect a deletion) in over 95% of individuals with deletion 22q11 syndrome. A negative FISH test for deletion 22q11 syndrome means that no genetic material is missing from the critical region on chromosome 22. Research testing on these individuals usually reveals that up to 5% of individuals with deletion 22q11 syndrome will have a smaller deletion that is not picked up by the routine FISH test.

Prenatal testing (testing during pregnancy) for deletion 22q11 syndrome is possible using the FISH test on DNA sample obtained by chorionic villus sampling (CVS) or by **amniocentesis**. Chorionic villus sampling is a prenatal test that is usually done at 10–12 weeks of pregnancy and involves removing a small amount of tissue from the placenta. Amniocentesis is a prenatal test that is usually performed at 16–18 weeks of pregnancy and involves removing a small amount of the amniotic fluid that surrounds the fetus. DNA is obtained from these samples and tested to see if the deletion responsible for deletion 22q11 syndrome is present. While prenatal testing is possible, it is not routinely performed. Typically, the test is done only if there is a family history of deletion 22q11 syndrome or if a congenital heart defect has been seen on a sonogram (ultrasound).

A sonogram uses sound waves to provide an image of a fetus. During the second trimester of pregnancy, it becomes possible to evaluate the fetal heart. If a heart defect is detected, DNA testing may be offered to the parents (along with other tests) to determine the cause of the heart defect. Unfortunately, congenital heart defects are common and there are many other syndromes that also cause congenital heart defects.

Treatment and management

Because of the incredible variability seen in deletion 22q11 syndrome, there is no one plan of treatment for all affected individuals. The treatment and management of an individual with deletion 22q11 syndrome depends on his or her age and symptoms. Because deletion 22q11 syndrome is a multisystem disorder, it is important to have multiple evaluations. Individuals with deletion

22q11 syndrome may see geneticists, plastic surgeons, immunologists, cardiologists, rheumatologists, endocrinologists, ophthalmologists, neurosurgeons, pediatricians, audiologists, and specialists in feeding, speech, and child development.

It is important that all individuals with deletion 22q11 syndrome have a cardiac evaluation by a cardiologist. An evaluation may include special tests such as a chest x ray, electrocardiogram, and echocardiogram (ultrasound of the heart). Some cardiac defects do not require treatment and others may require surgery.

Because of the wide variety of cleft palate and velopharyngeal problems, all individuals with deletion 22q11 syndrome should be evaluated by a cleft palate team. Cleft palate teams may include a plastic surgeon, ENT (ear, nose, and throat) specialist, genetic counselor and other staff. Because of the effect of cleft palate abnormalities on speech, all children with deletion 22q11 should have a speech evaluation and speech therapy if necessary. A referral to a feeding specialist may also be helpful if there is a cleft problem or other medical problem that interferes with feeding.

Because of the possibility and serious nature of immune problems, individuals with deletion 22q11 syndrome should have an immune evaluation. This can be done by an immunologist and usually requires blood tests to check immune function.

Individuals with deletion 22q11 syndrome should also have an endocrinology examination to check the function of their thyroid, parathyroid, and pituitary glands. They may also see an endocrinologist if they are having growth problems.

Neurologists can help with issues such as seizures and other neurology problems. Psychiatrists can help with psychiatric illness and problems arising from having a chronic illness.

Individuals with deletion 22q11 syndrome should be seen by a geneticist to confirm the diagnosis and to discuss issues such as the **inheritance** of deletion 22q11 syndrome, the recurrence risks and the availability of prenatal diagnosis. Geneticists can also help arrange the necessary medical consults.

Prognosis

The prognosis for individuals with deletion 22q11 syndrome is highly dependant on the medical complications of the specific individual. Because this is such a variable syndrome, it is impossible to give one prognosis. The cardiac defects associated with deletion 22q11 syndrome are a major variable in determining prognosis. Those with serious heart defects have a guarded progno-

KEY TERMS

Cleft palate—A congenital malformation in which there is an abnormal opening in the roof of the mouth that allows the nasal passages and the mouth to be improperly connected.

Conotruncal heart abnormality—Congenital heart defects particularly involving the ventricular (lower chambers) outflow tracts of the heart includes subarterial ventricular septal defect, pulmonic valve atresia and stenosis, tetralogy of Fallot and truncus arteriosus.

Velo—Derived from the Latin word *velum*, meaning palate and back of the throat.

sis. Individuals with deletion 22q11 syndrome with minor or treatable cardiac defects have a good prognosis. Good medical care and treatment of problems allows most individuals with deletion 22q11 syndrome to have a normal life span.

While the physical features and medical complications of deletion 22q11 syndrome can affect prognosis, the degree of intellectual and psychological can also have an effect. Those individuals with normal IQ and no mental illness have a good prognosis. Those with learning disabilities can benefit from specific educational interventions. Individuals with developmental delay need more help but can do well in sheltered environments. Individuals with mental illness may or may not do well. Some individuals benefit from psychiatric counseling and medication.

The range of abilities among individuals with deletion 22q11 syndrome is very wide and the ultimate functioning of an individual is dependent on his or her abilities.

Resources

ORGANIZATIONS

National Institute on Deafness and Other Communication Disorders. 31 Center Dr., MSC 2320, Bethesda, MD 20814. <http://www.nidcd.nih.gov>.

Velo-Cardio-Facial Syndrome Educational Foundation. VCFS Educational Foundation, Inc., Upstate Medical University Hospital, 708 Jacobsen Hall (C.D.U.), 750 East Adams St., Syracuse, NY 13210.

Velo-Cardio-Facial Syndrome Research Institute. Albert Einstein College of Medicine, 3311 Bainbridge Ave., Bronx, NY 10467. (718) 430-2568. Fax: (718) 430-8778. rgoldber@aecom.yu.edu. <http://www.kumc.edu/gec/vcfhome.html>.

WEBSITES

McDonald-McGinn, Donna M., Beverly S. Emanuel, and Elaine H Zackai. "22q11 deletion syndrome." *GeneClinics.* <http://www.geneclinics.org/profiles/22q11deletion/index.html>.

National Institute on Deafness and Other Communication Disorders. <http://www.nidcd.nih.gov/health/pubs_vsl/velocario.htm>.

The VCFS Educational Foundation. <http://www.vcfsef.org/>.

Kathleen Fergus, MS, CGC

Delta storage pool disease *see* Hermansky-Pudlak syndrome

Dementia

Definition

Dementia is not a specific disorder or disease. It is a syndrome (group of symptoms) associated with a progressive loss of memory and other intellectual functions that is serious enough to interfere with the tasks of daily life. Dementia can occur to anyone at any age from an injury or oxygen deprivation, although it is most commonly associated with aging.

Description

The definition of dementia has become more inclusive over the past several decades. Whereas earlier descriptions of dementia emphasized memory loss, the last two editions of the *Diagnostic and Statistical Manual of Mental Disorders* (DSM-III-R in 1987 and DSM-IV in 1994) define dementia as an overall decline in intellectual function, including difficulties with language, simple calculations, planning and judgment, and motor (muscular movement) skills as well as loss of memory. Although dementia is not caused by aging itself—most researchers regard it as resulting from injuries, infections, brain diseases, tumors, or other disorders—it is quite common in older people. Common estimates are that over 15% of people in North America over the age of 65 suffer from dementia, and 40% of people over 80. Surveys indicate that dementia is the condition most feared by older adults in the United States.

Dementia can be caused by nearly forty different diseases and conditions, ranging from dietary deficiencies and metabolic disorders to head injuries and inherited diseases. The possible causes of dementia can be categorized as follows:

- Primary dementia. These dementias are characterized by damage to or wasting away of the brain tissue itself. They include **Alzheimer disease** (AD), Pick disease, and frontal lobe dementia (FLD).

- Multi-infarct dementia (MID). Sometimes called vascular dementia, this type is caused by blood clots in the small blood vessels of the brain. When the clots cut off the blood supply to the brain tissue, the brain cells are damaged and may die.

- Lewy body dementia. Lewy bodies are areas of injury found on damaged nerve cells in certain parts of the brain. They are associated with Alzheimer and **Parkinson disease**, but researchers do not yet know whether dementia with Lewy bodies is a distinct type of dementia or a variation of Alzheimer or Parkinson disease.

- Dementia related to **alcoholism** or exposure to heavy metals (arsenic, antimony, bismuth).

- Dementia related to infectious diseases. These infections may be caused by viruses (HIV, viral encephalitis); spirochetes (Lyme disease, syphilis); or prions (Creutzfeldt-Jakob disease).

- Dementia related to abnormalities in the structure of the brain. These may include a buildup of spinal fluid in the brain (**hydrocephalus**); tumors; or blood collecting beneath the membrane that covers the brain (subdural hematoma).

Dementia may also be associated with **depression**, low levels of thyroid hormone, or niacin or vitamin (B12) deficiency. Dementia related to these conditions is often reversible.

Genetic profile

Genetic factors play a role in several types of dementia, but the importance of these factors in the development of the dementia varies considerably. Alzheimer disease (AD) is known, for example, to have an autosomal (non-sex-related) dominant pattern in most early-onset cases as well as in some late-onset cases, and to show different degrees of penetrance (frequency of expression) in late-life cases. Moreover, researchers have not yet discovered how the genes associated with dementia interact with other risk factors to produce or trigger the dementia. One non-genetic risk factor presently being investigated is toxic substances in the environment.

Early-onset Alzheimer disease

In early-onset AD, which accounts for 2-7% of cases of AD, the symptoms develop before age 60. It is usually caused by an inherited genetic mutation. Early-onset AD is also associated with **Down syndrome**, in that persons with trisomy 21 (three forms of human **chromosome** 21 instead of a pair) often develop early-onset AD.

Late-onset Alzheimer disease

Recent research indicates that late-onset Alzheimer disease is a polygenic disorder; that is, its development is influenced by more than one **gene**. It has been known since 1993 that a specific form of a gene for apolipoprotein E (APOE) on human chromosome 19 is a genetic risk factor for late-onset AD. In 1998 researchers at the University of Pittsburgh reported on another gene that controls the production of bleomycin hydrolase (BH) as a second genetic risk factor that acts independently of the APOE gene. In December 2000, three separate research studies reported that a gene on chromosome 10 that may affect the processing of amyloid-beta protein is also involved in the development of late-onset AD.

Multi-infarct dementia (MID)

While the chief risk factors for MID are high blood pressure, advanced age, and male sex, there is an inherited form of MID called **CADASIL**, which stands for cerebral autosomal dominant arteriopathy with subcortical infarcts and leukoencephalopathy. CADASIL can cause psychiatric disturbances and severe headaches as well as dementia.

Frontal lobe dementias

Researchers think that between 25% and 50% of cases of frontal lobe dementia involve genetic factors. Pick's dementia appears to have a much smaller genetic component than FLD. It is not yet known what other risk factors combine with inherited traits to influence the development of frontal lobe dementias.

Familial British dementia (FBD)

FBD is a rare autosomal dominant disorder that was first reported in the 1940s in a large British family extending over nine generations. FBD resembles Alzheimer in that the patient develops a progressive dementia related to amyloid deposits in the brain. In 1999 a mutated gene that produces the amyloid responsible for FBD was discovered on human chromosome 13. Studies of this mutation may yield further clues to the development of Alzheimer disease as well as FBD itself.

Creutzfeldt-Jakob disease

Although Creutzfeldt-Jakob disease is caused by a prion, researchers think that 5-15% of cases may have a genetic component.

Demographics

The demographic distribution of dementia varies somewhat according to its cause. Moreover, recent research indicates that dementia in many patients has overlapping causes, so that it is not always easy to assess the true rates of occurrence of the different types. For example, AD and MID are found together in about 15-20% of cases.

Alzheimer disease

AD is by far the most common cause of dementia in the elderly, accounting for 60-80% of cases. It is estimated that 4 million adults in the United States suffer from AD. The disease strikes women more often than men, but researchers do not know yet whether the sex ratio simply reflects the fact that women tend to live longer than men, or whether female sex is itself a risk factor for AD. One well-known long-term study of Alzheimer in women is the Nun Study, begun in 1986 and presently conducted at the University of Kentucky.

Multi-infarct dementia

MID is responsible for between 15% and 20% of cases of dementia (not counting cases in which it coexists with AD). Unlike AD, MID is more common in men than in women. **Diabetes**, high blood pressure, a history of smoking, and heart disease are all risk factors for MID. Researchers in Sweden have suggested that MID is underdiagnosed, and may coexist with other dementias more frequently than is presently recognized.

Dementia with Lewy bodies

Dementia with Lewy bodies is now thought to be the second most common form of dementia after Alzheimer disease. But because researchers do not completely understand the relationship between Lewy bodies, AD, and Parkinson disease, the demographic distribution of this type of dementia is also unclear.

Other dementias

FLD, Pick disease, **Huntington disease**, Parkinson's disease, HIV infection, alcoholism, head trauma, etc. account for about 10% of all cases of dementia. In FLD and Pick dementia, women appear to be affected slightly more often than men.

Signs and symptoms

DSM-IV specifies that certain criteria must be met for a patient to be diagnosed with dementia. One criterion is significant weakening of the patient's memory with regard to learning new information as well as recalling previously learned information. In addition, the patient must be found to have one or more of the following disturbances:

- Aphasia. Aphasia refers to loss of language function. A person with dementia may use vague words like "it" or "thing" a lot because they cannot recall the exact name of an object; they may echo what other people say, or repeat a word or phrase over and over. People in the later stages of dementia may stop speaking at all.

- Apraxia. Apraxia refers to loss of the ability to perform intentional movements even though the person is not paralyzed, has not lost their sense of touch, and knows what they are trying to do. For example, a patient with apraxia may stop brushing their teeth, or have trouble tying their shoelaces.

- Agnosia. Agnosia refers to loss of the ability to recognize objects even though the person's sight and sense of touch are normal. People with severe agnosia may fail to recognize family members or their own face reflected in a mirror.

- Problems with abstract thinking and complex behavior. This criterion refers to the loss of the ability to make plans, carry out the steps of a task in the proper order, make appropriate decisions, evaluate situations, show good judgment, etc. For example, a patient might light a stove burner under a saucepan before putting food or water in the pan, or be unable to record checks and balance his or her checkbook.

DSM-IV also specifies that these disturbances must be severe enough to cause problems in the person's daily life, and that they must represent a decline from a previously higher level of functioning.

The following sections will focus on the signs and symptoms that are used to differentiate among the various types of dementia during a diagnostic evaluation.

Alzheimer disease

Dementia related to AD often progresses slowly; it may be accompanied by irritability, wide mood swings, and personality changes in the early stage. In second-stage AD, the patient typically gets lost easily, is completely disoriented with regard to time and space, and may become angry, uncooperative, or aggressive. In final-stage AD, the patient is completely bedridden, has lost control over bowel and bladder functions, and may be unable to swallow or eat. The risk of seizures increases as the patient progresses from early to end-stage Alzheimer disease. Death usually results from an infection or malnutrition.

Multi-infarct dementia

In MID, the symptoms are more likely to occur after age 70. In the early stages, the patient retains his or her personality more fully than a patient with AD. Another distinctive feature of this type of dementia is that it often progresses in a stepwise fashion; that is, the patient shows rapid changes in functioning, then remains at a plateau for awhile rather than showing a continuous decline. The symptoms of MID may also have a "patchy" quality; that is, some of the patient's mental functions may be severely affected while others are relatively undamaged. Other symptoms of MID include exaggerated reflexes, an abnormal gait (manner of walking), loss of bladder or bowel control, and inappropriate laughing or crying.

Dementia with Lewy bodies

This type of dementia may combine some features of AD, such as severe memory loss and confusion, with certain symptoms associated with Parkinson disease, including stiff muscles, a shuffling gait, and trembling or shaking of the hands. Visual hallucinations may be one of the first symptoms of dementia with Lewy bodies.

Frontal lobe dementias

The frontal lobe dementias are gradual in onset. Pick's dementia is most likely to develop in persons between 40 and 60, while FLD typically begins before the age of 65. The first symptoms of the frontal lobe dementias often include socially inappropriate behavior (rude remarks, sexual acting-out, lack of personal hygiene, etc.). Patients are also often obsessed with eating and may put non-food items in their mouths as well as making frequent sucking or smacking noises. In the later stages of frontal lobe dementia or Pick's disease, the patient may develop muscle weakness, twitching, and delusions or hallucinations.

Creutzfeldt-Jakob disease

The dementia associated with Creutzfeldt-Jakob disease occurs most often in persons between 40 and 60. It is typically preceded by a period of several weeks in which the patient complains of unusual tiredness, anxiety, loss of appetite, or difficulty concentrating. This type of dementia also usually progresses much more rapidly than other dementias, usually over a span of a few months.

Diagnosis

In some cases, a patient's primary physician may be able to diagnose the dementia; in many instances, however, the patient will be referred to a neurologist or a specialist in geriatric medicine. The differential diagnosis of dementia is complicated because of the number of possible causes; because more than one cause may be present;

and because dementia can coexist with other conditions such as depression and delirium. Delirium is a temporary disturbance of consciousness marked by confusion, restlessness, inability to focus one's attention, hallucinations, or delusions. In elderly people, delirium is frequently a side effect of surgery, medications, infectious illnesses, or dehydration. Delirium can be distinguished from dementia by the fact that delirium usually comes on fairly suddenly (in a few hours or days) and may vary in severity—it is often worse at night. Dementia develops much more slowly, over a period of months or years, and the patient's symptoms are relatively stable. It is possible for a person to have delirium and dementia at the same time. Another significant diagnostic distinction in elderly patients is the distinction between dementia and age-associated memory impairment (AAMI). Older people with AAMI have a mild degree of memory loss; they do not learn new information as quickly as younger people, and they may take longer to recall a certain fact or to balance their checkbook. But they do not suffer the degree of memory impairment that characterizes dementia, and they do not get progressively worse.

Patient history

The doctor will begin by taking a full history, including the patient's occupation and educational level as well as medical history. The occupational and educational history allows the examiner to make a more accurate assessment of the extent of the patient's memory loss and other evidence of intellectual decline. In some cases the occupational history may indicate exposure to heavy metals or other toxins. A complete medical history allows the doctor to assess possibilities such as delirium, depression, alcohol-related dementia, dementia related to head injury, or dementia caused by infection. It is particularly important for the doctor to have a list of all the patient's medications, including over-the-counter preparations, because of the possibility that the patient's symptoms are related to side effects.

Mental status examination

A mental status examination (MSE) evaluates the patient's ability to communicate, follow instructions, recall information, perform simple tasks involving movement and coordination, as well as his or her emotional state and general sense of space and time. The MSE includes the doctor's informal evaluation of the patient's appearance, vocal tone, facial expressions, posture, and gait as well as formal questions or instructions. A common form that has been used since 1975 is the so-called Folstein Mini-Mental Status Examination, or MMSE. Questions that are relevant to diagnosing dementia include asking the patient to count backward from 100 by 7s, to make change, to name the current President, to repeat a short phrase after the examiner (e.g., "no ifs, ands, or buts") to draw a clock face or geometric figure, and to follow a set of instructions involving movement (e.g., "Show me how to throw a ball" or "Fold this piece of paper and place it under the lamp on the bookshelf"). The examiner may test the patient's abstract reasoning ability by asking him or her to explain a familiar proverb (e.g., "People who live in glass houses shouldn't throw stones") or test the patient's judgment by asking about a problem with a common-sense solution, such as what one does when a prescription runs out.

Neurological examination

A neurological examination includes an evaluation of the patient's cranial nerves and reflexes. The cranial nerves govern the ability to speak as well as sight, hearing, taste, and smell. The patient will be asked to stick out the tongue, follow the examiner's finger with the eyes, raise the eyebrows, etc. The patient is also asked to perform certain actions (e.g., touching the nose with the eyes closed) that test coordination and spatial orientation. The doctor will usually touch or tap certain areas of the body, such as the knee or the sole of the foot, to test the patient's reflexes. Failure to respond to the touch or tap may indicate damage to certain parts of the brain.

Laboratory tests

Blood and urine samples are collected in order to rule out such conditions as thyroid deficiency, niacin (vitamin B12) deficiency, heavy metal poisoning, liver disease, HIV infection, syphilis, anemia, medication reactions, or kidney failure. A lumbar puncture (spinal tap) may be done to rule out neurosyphilis.

Diagnostic imaging

The patient may be given a CT (computed tomography) scan or MRI (magnetic resonance imaging) to detect evidence of strokes, disintegration of the brain tissue in certain areas, blood clots or tumors, a buildup of spinal fluid, or bleeding into the brain tissue. PET (positron-emission tomography) or SPECT (single-emission computed tomography) imaging is not used routinely to diagnose dementia, but may be used to rule out Alzheimer disease or frontal lobe degeneration if a patient's CT scan or MRI is unrevealing.

Treatment and management

Reversible and responsive dementias

Some types of dementia are reversible, and a few types respond to specific treatments related to their

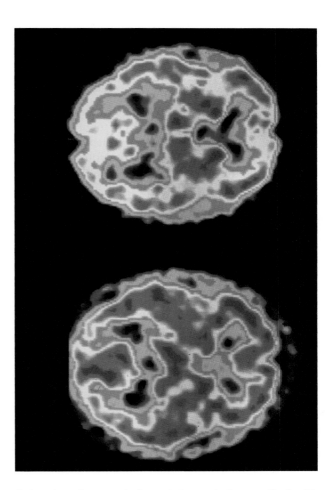

Colored positron emission of dementia in a patient with AIDS. *(Photo Researchers, Inc.)*

causes. Dementia related to dietary deficiencies or metabolic disorders is treated with the appropriate vitamins or thyroid medication. Dementia related to HIV infection often responds well to zidovudine (Retrovir), a drug given to prevent the AIDS virus from replicating. Multi-infarct dementia is usually treated by controlling the patient's blood pressure and/or diabetes; while treatments for these disorders cannot undo damage already caused to brain tissue, they can slow the progress of the dementia. Patients with alcohol-related dementia often improve over the long term if they are able to stop drinking. Dementias related to head injuries, hydrocephalus, and tumors are treated by surgery.

It is important to evaluate and treat elderly patients for depression, because the symptoms of depression in older people often mimic dementia. This condition is sometimes called pseudodementia. In addition, patients who suffer from both depression and dementia often show some improvement in intellectual functioning when the depression is treated.

KEY TERMS

Age-associated memory impairment (AAMI)—A condition in which an older person suffers some memory loss and takes longer to learn new information. AAMI is distinguished from dementia in that it is not progressive and does not represent a serious decline from the person's previous level of functioning.

Agnosia—Loss of the ability to recognize objects by use of the physical senses.

Amyloid—A waxy translucent substance composed mostly of protein, that forms plaques (abnormal deposits) in the brain.

Aphasia—Loss of previously acquired ability to speak, or to understand written or spoken language.

Apraxia—Impairment of the ability to make purposeful movements, but not paralysis or loss of sensation.

Creutzfeldt-Jakob disease—A degenerative disease of the central nervous system caused by a prion, or "slow virus."

Delirium—A disturbance of consciousness marked by confusion, difficulty paying attention, delusions, hallucinations, or restlessness. It can be distinguished from dementia by its relatively sudden onset and variation in the severity of the symptoms.

Hematoma—An accumulation of blood, often clotted, in a body tissue or organ, usually caused by a break or tear in a blood vessel.

Huntington disease—A midlife-onset inherited disorder characterized by progressive dementia and loss of control over voluntary movements. It is sometimes called Huntington's chorea.

Hydrocephalus—The excess accumulation of cerebrospinal fluid around the brain, often causing enlargement of the head.

Lewy bodies—Areas of injury found on damaged nerve cells in certain parts of the brain associated with dementia.

Multi-infarct dementia—Dementia caused by damage to brain tissue resulting from a series of blood clots or clogs in the blood vessels. It is also called vascular dementia.

Parkinson disease—A disease of the nervous system most common in people over 60, characterized by a shuffling gait, trembling of the fingers and hands, and muscle stiffness. It may be related in some way to Lewy body dementia.

Pick's disease—A rare type of primary dementia that affects the frontal lobes of the brain. It is characterized by a progressive loss of social skills, language, and memory, leading to personality changes and sometimes loss of moral judgment.

Pseudodementia—A term for a depression with symptoms resembling those of dementia. The term dementia of depression is now preferred.

Irreversible dementias

There are no medications or surgical techniques that can cure Alzheimer disease, the frontal lobe dementias, MID, or dementia with Lewy bodies. There are also no "magic bullets" that can slow or stop the progression of these dementias. Patients may be given medications to ease the depression, anxiety, sleep disturbances, and similar symptoms that accompany dementia, but most physicians prescribe relatively mild dosages in order to minimize the troublesome side effects of these drugs. Dementia with Lewy bodies appears to respond better to treatment with the newer antipsychotic medications than to treatment with such older drugs as haloperidol (Haldol).

Patients in the early stages of dementia can often remain at home with some help from family members or other caregivers, especially if the house or apartment can

be fitted with safety features (handrails, good lighting, locks for cabinets containing potentially dangerous products, nonslip treads on stairs, etc.). Patients in the later stages of dementia, however, usually require skilled care in a nursing home or hospital.

Prognosis

The prognosis for reversible dementia related to nutritional or thyroid problems is usually good once the cause has been identified and treated. The prognoses for dementias related to alcoholism or HIV infection depend on the patient's age and the severity of the underlying disorder.

The prognosis for the irreversible dementias is gradual deterioration of the patient's functioning ending in death. The length of time varies somewhat. Patients with Alzheimer disease may live from two to 20 years with the disease, with an average of seven years. Patients with frontal lobe dementia or Pick's disease live on average between five and 10 years after diagnosis. The course of Creutzfeldt-Jakob disease is much more rapid, with patients living between five and 12 months after diagnosis.

Resources

BOOKS

American Psychiatric Association. *Diagnostic and Statistical Manual of Mental Disorders*, 4th edition. Washington, DC: American Psychiatric Association, 1994.

"Delirium and Dementia." Section 5 in *The Merck Manual of Geriatrics*. Whitehouse Station, NJ: Merck Research Laboratories, 1995.

"Dementia." *The Merck Manual of Diagnosis and Therapy*, edited by Mark H. Beers, MD, and Robert Berkow, MD. Whitehouse Station, NJ: Merck Research Laboratories, 1999.

Lyon, Jeff, and Peter Gorner. *Altered Fates: Gene Therapy and the Retooling of Human Life*. New York and London: W. W. Norton & Co., Inc., 1996.

Morris, Virginia. *How to Care for Aging Parents*. New York: Workman Publishing, 1996. A good source of information about caring for someone with dementia as well as information about dementia itself.

ORGANIZATIONS

Alzheimer's Association. 919 North Michigan Ave., Suite 1000, Chicago, IL 60611-1676. (800) 272-3900.

Alzheimer's Disease International. 45/46 Lower Marsh, London, SE1 7RG. UK (+44 20) 7620 3011. adi@alz.co.uk. <http://www.alz.co.uk.>.

National Institute of Mental Health. 6001 Executive Blvd., Rm. 8184, MSC 9663, Bethesda, MD 20892-9663. (301) 443-4513. Fax: (301) 443-4279. <http://www.nimh.nih.gov/publicat/index.cfm>.

National Institute of Neurological Disorders and Stroke. 31 Center Drive, MSC 2540, Bldg. 31, Room 8806, Bethesda, MD 20814. (301) 496-5751 or (800) 352-9424. <http://www.ninds.nih.gov>.

National Institute on Aging Information Center. PO Box 8057, Gaithersburg, MD 20898. (800) 222-2225 or (301) 496-1752.

National Organization for Rare Disorders (NORD). PO Box 8923, New Fairfield, CT 06812-8923. (203) 746-6518 or (800) 999-6673. Fax: (203) 746-6481. <http://www.rarediseases.org>.

WEBSITES

Alzheimer's Disease Education and Referral (ADEAR): <http://www.alzheimers.org>.

National Institute of Mental Health (NIMH): <http://www.nimh.nih.gov>.

National Institute of Neurological Disorders and Stroke (NINDS): <http://www.ninds.nih.gov>.

National Institute on Aging (NIA): <http://www.nih.gov/nia>.

The Nun Study: <http://www.coa.uky.edu/nunnet>.

Rebecca J. Frey, PhD

▌ Dentatorubral-pallidoluysian atrophy

Definition

Dentatorubral-pallidoluysian atrophy (DRPLA) is a disorder of ataxia (loss of balance), choreoathetosis (involuntary rapid, irregular, jerky movements or slow, writhing movements that flow into one another), and **dementia** (inability to clearly think; confusion, poor judgement; failure to recognize people, places, and things; personality changes) in adults, and ataxia, myoclonus (involuntary spasms of a muscle or muscle group), **epilepsy** (seizures), and loss of intellectual function (mental retardation) in children.

Description

DRPLA has also been referred to as Haw River syndrome and Natito-Oyanagi disease. The typical age of onset of DRPLA is 30, but it can present in people as young as one year of age and as late as 62 years of age, with differences in presentation between children and adults. In patients under the age of 20, DRPLA presents as seizures, ataxia, myoclonus, as well as progressive (worsening) mental deterioration. In patients over the age of 20, DRPLA is suspected when a person develops ataxia, choreoathetosis, dementia, and psychiatric disturbances (delusions, hallucinations). A positive family history (a relative with similar symptoms or one already diagnosed) confirms the diagnosis. DRPLA is sometimes initially thought to be **Huntington disease**.

A possible diagnosis of DRPLA can be devastating for a family to experience—their once healthy child, or young adult, will begin to have seizures, involuntary movements, loss of control over voluntary movement, and delusions—perhaps no longer being able to identify family members. Diagnosing DRPLA is complicated and requires a knowledgeable physician with expertise in both neurology and genetics. Usually an individual diagnosed with DRPLA already has a parent with the disease, however, if the disorder was not diagnosed properly, or the parent died prior to the onset of symptoms, or the parent has very late onset of the disease, there may not be a documented family history of DRPLA.

Genetic profile

DRPLA is an autosomal dominant condition which means that both males and females are equally likely to have the disease, and an individual with the variant **gene** has a 50/50 chance to pass the condition to any child. The DRPLA gene is located on **chromosome** number 12 and has a section of **DNA** where the DNA alphabet is repeated in triplets, called CAG repeats. Normally a person has 6 to 35 CAG repeats in the DRPLA gene. In patients with DRPLA, there are 49 to 88 repeats which causes the gene's protein product, Atrophin 1, to be toxic to cells. Although scientists do not understand the exact mechanism, the number of repeats expands when the gene is transmitted from parent to child. The size of the repeat transmitted to the next generation depends upon the size of the parent's repeat and the sex of the transmitting parent.

There is an inverse correlation between the age of onset and the size of the expanded CAG repeats. In other words, the younger the age of onset, the larger the number of CAG repeats:

- Onset before age 21—repeat range of 63–69 (average of 68).

- Onset from 21–40 years—repeat range of 61–69 (average of 64).

- Onset after 40 years—repeat range of 54–63 (average of 63). Although there is significant overlap, the inverse correlation exists.

DRPLA as well as other genetic conditions, exhibits a phenomenon known as anticipation. Anticipation means that the disease increases in severity and presents at a younger age of onset with each successive generation. For example, when the CAG repeat is inherited from the father, DRPLA can manifest itself 28 years earlier than the father began having symptoms, while if transmitted from the mother, DRPLA can present 15 years earlier than the previous generation.

Demographics

DRPLA has been reported to occur most often in the Japanese population, although it has been described in other ethnic groups including those in Europe and North America. The prevalence of DRPLA in the Japanese population is estimated to be 2–7 in 1,000,000, which is similar to the prevalence of Huntington disease in this population. A CAG repeat size of 17 or higher (usually 20–35) is more common in healthy Japanese individuals than Caucasians, which may explain why DRPLA is more common in the Japanese. In other words, a larger repeat size in a parent increases the possibility that the DNA will become unstable and expand when transmitted

to the next generation. Even though DRPLA is rare in the United States, a large African-American family in North Carolina has DRPLA, where the condition is also called the Haw River syndrome.

Signs and symptoms

The cardinal features of DRPLA are involuntary movements (usually in the face, neck, tongue and hands) and dementia (inability to clearly think; confusion; poor judgement; failure to recognize people, places, and things; personality changes) regardless of the age of onset. A history of ataxia, epilepsy, and mental retardation in children, combined with a positive family history, are often the presenting signs of this condition in an individual under 20 years of age. Seizures are always present in patients under 20, but are not as common in patients age 20–40, and rarely seen in patients with onset after 40. Adult onset DRPLA (after 20) presents with ataxia, choreoathetosis, dementia, and psychiatric disturbances.

Diagnosis

A diagnosis of DRPLA exists when there is a positive family history of the disease, characteristic clinical findings, and DNA testing that reveals an expansion in the CAG repeat of the DRPLA gene. **Genetic testing** to examine the CAG repeats in the DRPLA gene can be performed from a small blood sample. A few reports have described DRPLA as sporadic (occurring by chance) in some families. Upon closer examination, the asymptomatic fathers had a mildly expanded CAG repeat size. Therefore, it is always important to evaluate both parents of an affected individual even if they appear to have no symptoms of DRPLA. Testing of asymptomatic children is not appropriate since it takes away the child's right to want to know, or not know this information, raises the possibility of stigmatization (labeling someone a certain way and making assumptions about them) within a family, as well as the threat of educational and employment discrimination. Children *with* symptoms, however, usually benefit from having a diagnosis established.

For pregnancies at 50% risk, prenatal diagnosis is available via either CVS (chorionic villus sampling) or **amniocentesis**. CVS is a biopsy of the placenta performed in the first trimester of pregnancy under ultrasound guidance. Ultrasound is the use of sound waves to visualize the developing pregnancy. The genetic makeup of the placenta is identical to the fetus (developing baby) and therefore the DRPLA gene can be studied from this tissue. There is approximately a 1 in 100 chance for miscarriage with CVS. Amniocentesis is a procedure done under ultrasound guidance where a long thin needle is inserted into the mother's abdomen, into the uterus, to withdraw a couple of tablespoons of amniotic fluid (fluid

KEY TERMS

Amniocentesis—A procedure performed at 16-18 weeks of pregnancy in which a needle is inserted through a woman's abdomen into her uterus to draw out a small sample of the amniotic fluid from around the baby. Either the fluid itself or cells from the fluid can be used for a variety of tests to obtain information about genetic disorders and other medical conditions in the fetus.

Amniotic fluid—The fluid which surrounds a developing baby during pregnancy.

Anticipation—Increasing severity in disease with earlier ages of onset, in successive generations; a condition that begins at a younger age and is more severe with each generation

Ataxia—A deficiency of muscular coordination, especially when voluntary movements are attempted, such as grasping or walking.

Autosomal dominant—A pattern of genetic inheritance where only one abnormal gene is needed to display the trait or disease.

Choreoathetosis—Involuntary rapid, irregular, jerky movements or slow, writhing movements that flow into one another.

Chorionic villus sampling (CVS)—A procedure used

for prenatal diagnosis at 10-12 weeks gestation. Under ultrasound guidance a needle is inserted either through the mother's vagina or abdominal wall and a sample of cells is collected from around the fetus. These cells are then tested for chromosome abnormalities or other genetic diseases.

Dementia—A condition of deteriorated mental ability characterized by a marked decline of intellect and often by emotional apathy.

DNA repeats—A three letter section of DNA, called a triplet, which is normally repeated several times in a row. Too many repeats often cause the gene to not function properly, resulting in disease.

DRPLA—Dentatorubral-pallidoluysian atrophy; also called Haw River syndrome and Natito-Oyanagi disease. DRPLA is a disorder of ataxia, choreoathetosis, and dementia in adults, and ataxia, myoclonus, epilepsy, and mental retardation in children.

Epilepsy—A seizure disorder.

Myoclonus—Twitching or spasms of a muscle or an interrelated group of muscles.

Sporadic—Isolated or appearing occasionally with no apparent pattern.

surrounding the developing baby) to study. The DRPLA gene can be studied using cells from the amniotic fluid. Other genetic tests, such as a chromosome analysis, may also be performed on either a CVS or amniocentesis. A small risk of miscarriage (1 in 200 to 1 in 400) is associated with amniocentesis.

Treatment and management

There is currently no cure for DRPLA; treatment is supportive. Epilepsy is treated with anti-seizure medication.

Prognosis

Patients with DRPLA have progressive disease, which means symptoms become worse over time.

Resources

WEBSITES

International Network of Ataxia Friends (INTERNAF). <http://www.internaf.org>.

National Ataxia Foundation. <http://www.ataxia.org>.

WE MOVE (Worldwide Education and Awareness for Movement Disorders). <http://www.wemove.org>.

Catherine L. Tesla, MS, CGC

Deoxyribonucleic acid *see* **DNA**

Depression

Definition

Depression is the general name for a family of illnesses known as depressive disorders. Depression is an illness that affects not only the mood and thoughts, but also the physical functions of affected individuals. Depressive disorders usually result from a combination of genetic, environmental, and psychological factors.

Description

Everyone feels sadness, grief, or despair at some point in their lives. However, unlike these normal, transient emotional states, a depressive disorder is not a temporary bout of "feeling down" but rather a serious disease that should be recognized and treated as a medical condition. Without treatment, a depressive disorder can persist and its symptoms can go on for weeks, months, or years. The three most common types of depression are dysthymia or dysthymic disorder, major depression, and **bipolar disorder**.

Depression is quite widespread and one of the leading causes of disability in the world. Commonly recognized symptoms of all types of depressive disorders are recurring feelings of sadness and guilt, changes in sleeping patterns such as insomnia or oversleeping, changes in appetite, decreased mental and physical energy, unusual irritability, the inability to enjoy once-favored activities, difficulty in working, and thoughts of death or suicide. If only these "down" symptoms are experienced, the individual may suffer from a unipolar depressive disorder such as dysthymia or major depression. If the depressed periods alternate with extreme "up" periods, the individual may have a bipolar disorder.

Dysthymia is a relatively mild depressive disorder that is characterized by the presence of two or more of the symptoms listed above. The symptoms are not severe enough to disable the affected individual, but are long-term (chronic), and may last for several years. Dysthymia is a compound word originating in Greek that means ill, or bad, (dys-) soul, mind, or spirit (thymia). Individuals affected with dysthymia often also experience episodes of major depression at some point in their lives.

In major depression, the affected individual has five or more symptoms and experiences one or more prolonged episodes of depression that last longer than two weeks. These episodes disrupt the ability of the affected individual to the point that the person is unable to function. Individuals experiencing an episode of major depression often entertain suicidal thoughts, the presence of which contribute to this disorder being quite serious. Major depression should not be confused with a *grief reaction* such as that associated with the death of a loved one. Some individuals affected by major depression may experience only a single bout of disabling depression in their lifetimes. More commonly, affected individuals experience recurrent disabling episodes throughout their lives.

Bipolar disorder, formerly called manic depression or manic-depressive illness, is not nearly as common as major depression and dysthymia. Bipolar disorder is associated with alternating periods of extreme excitement (mania) and periods of extreme sadness (depression). The rate of the transition between cycles is usually gradual, but the mood swings may also be severe and dramatically rapid. When in the depressive state, the bipolar disorder affected individual may show any or all of the common symptoms of depression. In the manic state, the bipolar disorder affected individual may feel restless and unnaturally elated, have an overabundance of confidence and energy, and be very talkative. Mania can distort social behavior and judgment, causing the affected individual to take excessive risks and perhaps make imprudent decisions that can have humiliating or damaging consequences. Without medical treatment, bipolar disorder may progress into psychosis.

Depressive disorders are believed to be related to imbalances in brain chemistry, particularly in relation to the chemicals that carry signals between brain cells (neurotransmitters) as well as the hormones released by parts of the brain. Serotonin and neuroepinephrine are two important neurotransmitters. Disruption of the brain's circuits in areas involved with emotions, appetite, sexual drive, and sleep is a likely cause of the dysfunctions associated with depressive disorders. Thus, some of the newest treatments for depression are drugs that are known to have an effect on brain chemistry.

Genetic profile

Depression is known to be genetically linked because it often runs in families and has been studied in identical twins, but the specific **gene** markers for depression remain elusive. In 2000, the National Institutes of Mental Health began enrolling patients in what became the largest clinical psychiatric genetic study ever attempted to investigate how recurrent depression is transmitted across generations. This study primarily focused on major depression and dysthymia.

In familial cases of bipolar disorder, the most widely implicated genetic regions are those of **chromosome** 18 and chromosome 21. However, other researchers have mapped bipolar disorder to chromosomes 11p, Xq28, 6p, and many others. From this evidence, it is possible that bipolar disorder is a multi-gene (polygenic) trait requiring a combination of 3 or more genes on separate chromosomes for the condition to be expressed. Further research is also ongoing to determine the genetic marker, or markers, for bipolar disorder.

It is understood that there are also many non-genetic factors that cause depression, including stressful environmental conditions, certain illnesses, and precipitating conditions such as the loss of a close relationship. Alcohol abuse and the use of sedatives, barbiturates, narcotics, or other drugs can cause depression due to their effect on brain chemistry.

Demographics

It is estimated that the likelihood of experiencing an episode of major depression during one's lifetime is 5%. Approximately 9.5% of the American population, or 19 million people, are affected by depression in any given year. Depression occurs worldwide, but more Americans are diagnosed with depression than inhabitants of any other country. These lower occurrences of diagnosis in other parts of the world might indicate a higher incidence of depression in Americans than in all other peoples, but it may also be the result of the stigma, or shame, often associated with the diagnosis of a psychological disorder. Depression is not generally linked to any particular race of people.

In the United States, women experience depression at a rate that is almost twice that of men. This may be partially explained by the greater willingness of women to seek psychological treatment, but this does not explain the entire discrepancy. Many physical events specific to women, such as menstruation, pregnancy, miscarriage, the post-partum period, and menopause are recognized as factors contributing to depression in women. Women in the United States may face environmental stresses with a higher frequency than men. Most single parent households are headed by women; women still provide the majority of child and elder care, even in two-income families; and women are generally paid less than men so financial concerns may be greater.

Particular demographic problems associated with depression are depression in the elderly and depression in children and adolescents. A common belief is that depression is normal in elderly people. This is not the case, although increasing age and the absence of interpersonal relationships are associated with higher rates of depression. Because of this misconception, depressive disorders in the elderly population often go undiagnosed and untreated. Similarly, many parents often ignore the symptoms of a depressive disorder in their children, assuming that these symptoms are merely a phase that the child will later outgrow.

Signs and symptoms

Individuals affected with depressive disorders display a wide range of symptoms. These symptoms vary in severity from person to person and vary over time in a single affected individual.

Symptoms that characterize a depressive state are: feelings of hopelessness, guilt, or worthlessness; a persistent sad or anxious mood; restlessness or irritability; a loss of interest in activities that were once considered pleasurable; difficulty concentrating, remembering, or making decisions; sleep disorders, including insomnia, early morning awakening, and/or oversleeping; constant fatigue; eating disorders, including weight loss or overeating; suicidal thoughts and/or tendencies; and persistent physical symptoms that do not respond to the normal treatments of these symptoms, such as headaches, digestive problems, and chronic pain.

Symptoms that characterize a manic state are: increased energy accompanied by a decreased need for sleep, a loss of inhibitions accompanied by inappropriate social behavior, excessive enthusiasm and verve, increased talking, poor judgment, a feeling of invincibility, grandiose thinking and ideas, unusual irritability, and increased sexual desire.

Diagnosis

Depression is notoriously difficult to diagnose because its symptoms are not readily apparent to the medical professional unless the patient first recognizes and admits to them. Once the individual seeks help for his or her symptoms, the first step in the diagnosis of a depressive disorder is a complete physical examination to rule out any medical conditions, viral infections, or currently used medications that may produce the effects also seen in depression. Alcohol or other drug abuse as a possible cause of the observed symptoms should also be investigated. Once a physical basis for these symptoms is eliminated, a complete psychological exam should be undertaken. This examination consists of a mental status examination; a complete history of both current and previously experienced symptoms; and a family history.

The mental status examination is used to determine if a more severe psychotic condition is evident. This mental status examination will also determine whether the depressive disorder has caused changes in speech or thought patterns or memory that may indicate the presence of a depressive disorder. The complete psychological exam also includes a complete history of the symptoms being experienced by the affected individual. This history includes the onset of the symptoms, their duration, and whether or not the affected individual has had similar symptoms in the past. In the case of past symptoms, a treatment history should be completed to assess whether these symptoms previously responded to treatment, and if so, which treatments were effective. The final component of the complete psychological exam is the family history. In cases where the affected individual has had similarly affected family members a treatment history should also be completed, as much as possible, for these family members.

Treatment and management

Treatment of depression is on a case-by-case basis that is largely dependent on the outcome of the psy-

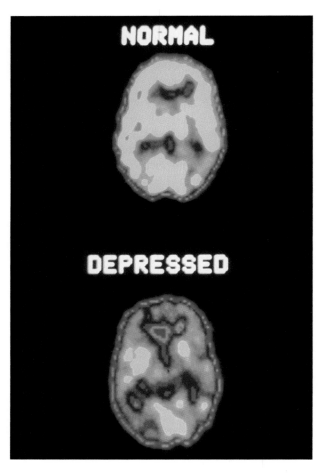

Clinical depression can be detected by a CAT scan. These two images demonstrate the difference between normal brain activity and depressed brain activity. *(Photo Researchers, Inc.)*

chological examination. Some mildly affected individuals respond fully to psychotherapy and do not require medication. Some individuals affected with moderate or severe depression benefit from antidepressant medication. Most affected individuals respond best to a combination of antidepressant medication and psychotherapy: the medication to provide relatively rapid relief from the symptoms of depression and the psychotherapy to learn effective ways to manage and cope with problems and issues that may cause the continuation of symptoms or the onset of new symptoms of depression.

Various types of antidepressant medications are available for the treatment of depressive disorders. Many individuals affected by depression will go through a variety of antidepressants, or antidepressant combinations, before the best medication and dosage

for them is identified. Almost all antidepressant medications must be taken regularly for at least two months before the full therapeutic effects are realized. A full course of medication is generally no shorter than six to nine months to prevent recurrence of the symptoms. In individuals affected with bipolar disorder or chronic major depression, medication may have to be continued throughout the remainder of their lives. These time-related conditions often pose problems in the management of individuals affected with depressive disorder. Many individuals who have a depressive disorder discontinue their medications before the fully prescribed course, for a variety of reasons. Some affected individuals feel side effects of the medications prior to feeling any benefits; others do not feel that the medication is helping because of the delay between the initiation of the treatment and the feelings of symptom relief; and, many feel better prior to the full course and so cease taking the medication.

The three most commonly prescribed antidepressant drug classes consist of the older tricyclics (TCAs) and the two relatively new drug classes: the selective serotonin reuptake inhibitors (SSRIs) and the monoamine oxidase inhibitors (MAOIs). The most common TCAs are amitriptyline (Elavil), clomipramine (Anafranil), desipramine (Norpramin, Pertofrane), doxepin (Sinequan, Adapin), imipramine (Tofranil, Janimine), nortriptyline (Pamelor, Aventyl), protriptyline (Vivactil), and trimipramine (Surmontil). The most common SSRIs are: citalopram (Celexa), fluoxetine (Prozac), fluvoxamine (Luvox), paroxetine (Paxil), and sertraline (Zoloft). The most common MAOIs are: phenelzine (Nardil) and tranylcypromine (Parnate).

Many antidepressant medications cause side effects such as agitation, bladder problems, blurred vision, constipation, drowsiness, dry mouth, headache, insomnia, nausea, nervousness, or sexual problems. Most of these side effects wear off as the treatment course progresses. The tricyclics cause more severe side effects than the newer SSRIs or MAOIs.

St. John's wort is an herbal remedy that has been widely used to treat depressive disorders. In Germany, this herbal remedy is used more than any other antidepressant. No scientific studies have been completed on the long-term effects of St John's wort in the treatment of depression. In 2000, the National Institutes of Health (NIH) completed patient enrollment in a three-year clinical study to study this herbal treatment of depression.

In the most severely affected individuals, or where antidepressant medications either have not worked or cannot be taken, electroconvulsive therapy (ECT) may be considered. In the ECT procedure, electrodes are put on specific locations on the head to deliver electrical stimulation to the brain. This electrical stimulation is designed to trigger a brief seizure within the brain. These seizures generally last approximately 30 seconds and are not consciously felt by the patient. ECT has been much improved in recent years; it is no longer the electro-shock treatment of nightmares, and its deleterious effects on long-term memory have been reduced. ECT treatments are generally administered several times a week as necessary to control the symptoms being experienced.

Several short-term (10 to 20 week) psychotherapies have also been demonstrated to be effective in the treatment of depressive disorders. These include interpersonal and cognitive/behavioral therapies. Interpersonal therapies focus on the interpersonal relationships of the affected individual that may both cause and heighten the depression. Cognitive/behavioral therapies focus on how the affected individual may be able to change his or her patterns of thinking or behaving that may lead to episodes of depression. Psychodynamic therapies, which generally are not short-term psychotherapies, seek to treat the individual with a depressive disorder through a resolution of internal conflicts. Psychodynamic therapies are generally not initiated during major depression episodes or until the symptoms of depression are significantly improved by medication or one of the short-term psychotherapies.

Prognosis

Over 80% of individuals affected with a depressive disorder have demonstrated improvement after receiving the appropriate combination of treatments. A significant tragedy associated with depression is the failure of many affected individuals to realize that they have a treatable medical condition. Some affected individuals who do not receive treatment may recover completely on their own, but most will suffer needlessly. A small number of individuals with depressive disorder do not respond to treatment.

Resources

BOOKS

Appleton, William. *Prozac and the New Antidepressants: What You Need to Know About Prozac, Zoloft, Paxil, Luvox, Wellbutrin, Effexor, Serzone, and More.* New York: Plume, 2000.

Beck, Aaron, and Brian Shaw. *Cognitive Theory of Depression.* New York: Guilford Press, 1987.

Papolos, Demitri, and Janice Papolos. *Overcoming Depression,* 3rd ed. New York: Guilford Press, 1997.

KEY TERMS

Bipolar disorder—Formerly called "manic depression," this psychological disorder is characterized by periods of mania followed by periods of depression.

Cognitive/behavioral therapies—Psychological counseling that focuses on changing the behavior of the patient.

Dysthymia—A psychological condition of chronic depression that is not disabling, but prevents the sufferer from functioning at his or her full capacity.

Electroconvulsive therapy—A psychological treatment in which a series of controlled electrical impulses are delivered to the brain in order to induce a seizure within the brain.

Grief reaction—The normal depression felt after a traumatic major life occurrence such as the loss of a loved one.

Interpersonal therapies—Also called "talking therapy," this type of psychological counseling is focused on determining how dysfunctional interpersonal relationships of the affected individual may be causing or influencing symptoms of depression.

Major depression—A psychological condition in which the patient experiences one or more disabling attacks of depression that lasts two or more weeks.

Polygenic—A trait, characteristic, condition, etc. that depends on the activity of more than one gene for its emergence or expression.

Psychodynamic therapies—A form of psychological counseling that seeks to determine and resolve the internal conflicts that may be causing an individual to be suffering from the symptoms of depression.

Psychotherapy—Psychological counseling that seeks to determine the underlying causes of a patient's depression. The form of this counseling may be cognitive/behavioral, interpersonal, or psychodynamic.

PERIODICALS

Cytryn, L. "The cutting edge of sadness." *Psychiatric Times* (October 1996).

Kelsoe, G. "An update on the search for genes for bipolar disorder." *Psychiatric Times* (September 1996).

Nemeroff, C. "The neurobiology of depression." *Scientific American* (June 1998): 42-9.

ORGANIZATIONS

National Depressive and Manic Depressive Association. 730 N. Franklin, Suite 501, Chicago, IL 60610-7204. (800) 826-3632 or (312) 642-7243. <http://www.ndmda.org>.

National Foundation for Depressive Illness, Inc. PO Box 2257, New York, NY 10016. (212) 268-4260 or (800) 239-1265. <http://www.depression.org>.

National Institute of Mental Health. 6001 Executive Blvd., Rm. 8184, MSC 9663, Bethesda, MD 20892-9663. (301) 443-4513. Fax: (301) 443-4279. <http://www.nimh.nih.gov/publicat/index.cfm>.

WEBSITES

Depression—Information and Support. (June 17, 2005.) <http://depression.about.com>.

Medical Health InfoSource—Depression. (June 17, 2005.) <http://www.mhsource.com/depression/overview.html>.

Paul A. Johnson

Diabetes

Definition

Diabetes is the Greek term for "passing through," a phrase used to describe multiple diseases characterized by excessive urination. There are multiple forms of diabetes. The most frequently described is diabetes mellitus, a chronic disorder involving the body's use of blood glucose (blood sugar) and the synthesis, or utility, of the hormone insulin. However, not all forms of diabetes involve glucose or insulin.

Description

Diabetes is a term used to describe multiple distinctive disorders that have the symptom of excessive urination in common. Although there are multiple forms of diabetes, the most common form is diabetes mellitus.

Diabetes mellitus

Diabetes mellitus is a chronic disorder of carbohydrate (sugar) metabolism. The word "mellitus" is Latin for "honey." Diabetes mellitus is characterized by abnormal, excessive levels of the sugar glucose in the blood, which is consequently passed through the urine. Most people always have some glucose in the blood to be used by cells for energy. Blood glucose originates from food ingested, the liver, and muscle cells. However, an excessive amount of glucose chronically present in the blood causes a variety of serious health complications.

Diabetics have excessive blood glucose because of a deficiency in the production or utilization of the hormone insulin. Insulin is made by the beta cells of the pancreas in response to the elevated glucose in the blood after a meal. Insulin binds to receptors on the body's cells to allow the passage of glucose into the cell as an energy source. Insulin stimulates cells to remove glucose from the blood, stimulates the liver to metabolize glucose, and thus causes the blood sugar level to return to normal. Diabetics have either a deficiency of insulin or defective insulin receptor binding. As a result, the cells of the body are unable to receive the glucose energy and are essentially starved, despite the energy source present in the blood. Because glucose is not entering the cells, it remains in the blood causing high blood sugar, or hyperglycemia. Chronic diabetes mellitus can lead to serious problems with the eyes, kidneys, nervous system, gums, and teeth. One of the most serious complications caused by diabetes is heart disease. Diabetics are more than twice as likely to develop cardiac disease or a stroke. The risk for diabetics equals that of an individual with a history of heart attacks. The use of cigarettes greatly increases the risk for vascular disease, nerve damage, and limb amputation.

Diabetes mellitus is divided into three main subtypes known as type I diabetes, type II diabetes, and gestational diabetes. Individuals can also develop a condition known as pre-diabetes that may develop into type II diabetes.

Type I diabetes was formerly called juvenile diabetes because it is usually first identified in children or young adults. It was also known as brittle diabetes and insulin-dependent diabetes mellitus (IDDM). Type I diabetes is an autoimmune condition in which the body's immune system has attacked and destroyed the beta cells of the pancreas. As a result there is a shortage of insulin, and glucose cannot enter the cells. Bodily processes involving the storage of glucose as energy and the utilization of glucose are adversely affected. The body is essentially starved of the energy it needs for normal function.

Type II diabetes was formerly called adult-onset diabetes because it usually develops in people over the age of 40 years. However, individuals can develop type II diabetes at any age. Also known as non-insulin-dependent diabetes, type II diabetes is the most common form. Type II diabetes is a condition in which the body's cells become insulin resistant and do not properly utilize the insulin being synthesized and secreted by the pancreas. In the beginning stages, the pancreas increases insulin production in response to the increased demand. However, as the disease progresses, the pancreas loses the ability to secrete sufficient insulin in response to meals.

The third subtype of diabetes mellitus is gestational diabetes. This is a form of glucose intolerance that may develop during the late stages of pregnancy. Pregnancy hormones or an insulin deficiency may cause gestational diabetes. During pregnancy, gestational diabetes requires treatment to normalize maternal blood glucose levels and avoid complications in the infant. Gestational diabetes usually disappears after the infant is born. However, females who have had gestational diabetes are more likely to develop type II diabetes in their later years.

Pre-diabetes is a condition in which blood glucose levels are abnormally elevated, but not enough for a diagnosis of diabetes. This term is used to distinguish individuals who are at increased risk of developing diabetes type II. Individuals with pre-diabetes have impaired fasting glucose (IFG), impaired glucose tolerance (IGT), or both. IFG is a condition in which the fasting blood sugar level is elevated to a level between 100 and 125 mg/dL after an overnight fast, a value that is not high enough to be classified as diabetes. IGT is a condition in which the blood sugar level is elevated to between 140 and 199 mg/dL after a two-hour oral glucose tolerance test, a value that is not high enough to be classified as diabetes. Those individuals with pre-diabetes are at increased risk for developing type II diabetes, cardiac disease, and stroke. The risk of progressing into type II diabetes can be significantly lowered with moderate weight loss and physical activity.

Diabetes insipidus

Diabetes insipidus is caused when the pituitary gland does not produce enough antidiuretic hormone (ADH), which is responsible for water reabsorption in the kidney. Without sufficient ADH, an abnormal amount of water is secreted in the urine. This results in excessive urination, thirst, weakness, and dry skin. In many cases, the cause of diabetes insipidus is unknown but may involve damage to the pituitary gland by head trauma or a tumor. In some cases, it is treatable with ADH replacement therapy.

Diabetes bronze

Diabetes bronze is a rare disease of iron metabolism that occurs in conjunction with diabetes mellitus and cardiac failure. It usually develops after 40 years. Diabetes bronze is characterized by the usual symptoms of diabetes mellitus with the addition of an enlarged liver and hyperpigmentation of the skin to a bronze color. It occurs 10 times as frequently in males than in females.

Genetic profile

Type I and type II diabetes mellitus have different causes, yet both have genetic components. A combination of inheriting a predisposition to diabetes and environmental trigger factors may make the biggest contribution to the development of the disease. A genetic predisposition contributes to, but does not automatically result, in diabetes. Studies of identical twins show that when one twin has type I diabetes mellitus, the other develops the disease about 50% of the time. When one twin has type II diabetes, the other develops the disease about 75% of the time.

Type I diabetes is an autoimmune disorder in which the immune system attacks the insulin-secreting pancreatic beta cells. The onset of type I diabetes is attributed to both inherited risk and external triggers, such as improper diet or an infection. Approximately 18 regions of the genome have been linked with risk for diabetes type I. These regions may each contain several genes that have abnormal variations in some diabetics. They are labeled IDDM1 to IDDM18.

The region, or locus, most well studied is IDDM1. IDDM1 contains genes that encode immune response proteins called the HLA genes. Variations in HLA genes are one of multiple important genetic risk factors. Normal HLA genes encode for proteins called **major histo-compatibility complex** (MHC), which assemble on the cell surface, are viewed by the immune system as "self," and therefore are not attacked. When there are variations in the HLA genes, they encode for variable MHC proteins expressed on the cell surface. The pancreatic beta cells of some diabetics have variable MHC proteins that the immune system does not recognize as self, and attacks as it would a virus or bacteria. The IDDM1 **gene** locus contains these variations in HLA genes that cause the pancreatic beta cells to be attacked and destroyed by the immune system.

The **inheritance** of particular HLA gene variations can account for more than 50% of the genetic risk of developing type I diabetes. The genes most strongly linked with diabetes are called HLA-DR, HLA-DQ, and HLA-DP. Half of the general population inherits a copy, called an allele, of the HLA-DR gene called DR3 or DR4. Less than 3% of the general population has both alleles. However, 95% of Caucasians with type I diabetes possesses at least one allele of DR3 or DR4. Individuals with both alleles are at the highest risk of developing type I diabetes mellitus. Conversely, the HLA-DR2 allele has protective effect and lowers the risk of developing diabetes.

As seen with the DR gene, specific alleles of the DQ gene are risk factors for developing type I diabetes, and specific alleles are protective. There is a tendency for individuals who inherit DR3 or DR4 to inherit a variant of DQ that increases their genetic risk of developing type I diabetes. The protective DR and DQ alleles also tend to be inherited together. These combination tendencies are not absolute, a phenomenon known as linkage disequilibrium. The IDDM1 locus contains many diabetes susceptibility genes that exhibit linkage disequilibrium, making it difficult to research the effects of any one gene on diabetes susceptibility.

The IDDM2 locus contains the insulin gene (INS) that is located on **chromosome** 11. Mutations of INS cause a rare form of diabetes that is similar to MODY. Other variations of the insulin gene may contribute to susceptibility to type I and II diabetes. The IDDM2 locus contributes about 10% toward type I diabetes susceptibility incidence. The type I diabetes risk associated area of this locus is localized to a region flanking the insulin gene that contains a short sequence of **DNA** that is repeated many times. The repeated sequences follow one behind the other (in tandem) and the number of repeats is variable between individuals, an event called a variable number tandem repeat (VNTR). There are three classes of VNTR in the insulin gene.

Class I has alleles that range 26–63 repeat units, class II has alleles with approximately 80 repeat units, and class III has alleles ranging 141–209 repeat units. In Caucasians, who have the highest rate of type I diabetes, the class-I VNTRs are most common. Class I alleles are responsible for 70% of the VNTR alleles, with nearly all the other alleles being class III. The short class I alleles are associated with a higher risk of developing type I diabetes, whereas the longer class III alleles are protective. The presence of at least one class III allele is associated with a threefold reduction in the risk of type I diabetes. Class III VNTR alleles are associated with higher levels of insulin in the thymus. The thymus gland has an important role in training the immune system to not attack the body's own cells. Immature immune cells called T cells are presented with chains of amino acids, such as insulin, to recognize as self. Any T cells that form a response to them, to attack them, are deleted to prevent autoimmunity. Because the longer VNTRs cause more insulin to be produced in the thymus, the detection and deletion of autoreactive T cells that would attack the body's cells may be more efficient. The resulting improved immune tolerance to insulin would lessen the risk of a future onset of type I diabetes caused by anti-insulin immune responses.

There is conflicting evidence for the role of INS in predisposition to type II diabetes. Certain mutations in INS can result in mutant insulin that results in rare forms of diabetes. One type of mutant insulin, called Chicago insulin, has been found in individuals who have a rare form of diabetes that resembles MODY. This form of diabetes is caused by a single gene mutation and is inherited in an autosomal dominant fashion. The INSR gene encodes the receptor for insulin. Mutations of the insulin receptor can also cause rare forms of diabetes and may play a role in susceptibility to type II diabetes. However, most diabetics have a normal sequence of the insulin receptor, indicating that if insulin receptor mutations contribute to the development of type II diabetes, they will be present only in a minor fraction of the diabetic population.

In determining the risk of developing type II diabetes mellitus, environmental factors such as diet and exercise play an important role. The majority of individuals with type II diabetes are either overweight or obese. Inherited factors are also keys to the development of type II diabetes. However, as of 2004 the multiple genes involved remained poorly defined. Genes that have been implicated may have only subtle variations that are extremely common, known as single nucleotide polymorphisms (SNPs). It is very difficult to link common gene variations with an increased risk of developing diabetes. Many of the links that have been found seem to be important in only select ethnic or geographical populations.

Calpain 10 (CAPN10) is one such gene that maps to chromosome 2. CAPN10 is a calcium-activated enzyme that breaks down proteins. SNPs in part of the CAPN10 gene are associated with a threefold increased risk of type II diabetes in Mexican Americans. It is thought that these genetic variants of CAPN10 may alter pancreatic beta cell survival, insulin production, insulin action, and liver glucose production. CAPN10 may also be involved in development of type II diabetes in Chinese populations. However, in European, Japanese, and Samoan populations, CAPN10 does not appear to play an important role.

The HFN4A gene encodes a transcription factor that is found in the liver and pancreas. HNF4A maps to a region of chromosome 20 that is linked with type II diabetes. HNF4A mutations cause a rare form of autosomal dominant diabetes. The HNF4A gene is now also being researched for involvement in predisposition to type II diabetes. It is thought that pancreatic beta cells are responsive to the amount of HNF4A present to regulate insulin production. SNPs in HNF4A have an impact on pancreatic beta cell function, increasing or decreasing insulin secretion. In the British population, individuals with SNPs that cause increased insulin secretion capacity have a reduced risk for diabetes. In the Ashkenazi Jewish population and Finnish population, four SNPs near the HNF4A gene have been identified as associated with type II diabetes via an unknown mechanism that may cause pancreatic beta cell malfunction.

In 2004, research began on various other genes that are candidates for type II diabetes predisposition in specific populations, many of which reside on various IDDM loci. The ABCC8 gene encodes the receptor for sulfonylurea. Sulfonylureas are a class of drug used to lower blood glucose levels in type II diabetics by interacting with the sulfonylurea receptor of pancreatic beta cells and stimulating insulin release. Genetic variations of ABCC8 may impair the release of insulin in some diabetics. The GCGR gene encodes the hormone glucagon, which regulates glucose levels. A mutation in GCGR has been associated with type II diabetes in the French and Sardinian population. The GCK gene encodes for the enzyme glucokinase, which speeds up glucose metabolism and acts as a glucose detector in pancreatic beta cells. Mutant glucokinase causes a rare form of diabetes and may also play a role in type II diabetes in some populations. Mutations known to activate glucokinase are all clustered in one area of the glucokinase structure that is called the allosteric activator site. These mutations cause an increase in insulin release. Research is being performed to discover pharmacological agents that act as allosteric activators to increase glucokinase activity, increase the release of insulin, and can be used in the treatment of diabetes. Because glucokinase activators also stimulate liver glucose metabolism, they would be doubly effective in reducing the blood sugar of diabetics. The GLUT2 gene encodes a glucose transporter which controls the entry of glucose into pancreatic beta cells and detects blood glucose. Mutations of GLUT2 cause a rare genetic syndrome that disturbs blood glucose control. Common variants of GLUT2 may also be linked with type II diabetes. The KCNJ11 gene encodes a potassium ion channel on the surface of pancreatic beta cells. Closure of potassium channels in these cells triggers insulin release. Pharmacological agents that close the channels are used in the treatment of diabetes.

Variations in KCNJ11 have been linked to both increased and decreased insulin release. A controlled study done in non-diabetic adults with a SNP in KCNJ11 demonstrated that the variation was associated with impaired insulin release in response to glucose and increased body mass index (BMI). Lipoprotein lipase (LPL) is an enzyme that breaks down triglycerides. LPL is functionally impaired or present at low levels in many type II diabetics. Evidence suggests that insulin may help regulate LPL synthesis. A common complication of type II diabetes is protein excreted in the urine because of chronic inflammation and kidney damage. There is a correlation between the severity of this condition and genetic variation in LPL. SNPs in the LPL gene are associated with insulin resistance in Mexican Americans. The same variation is associated with coronary artery disease, and may provide some of the link between diabetes and atherosclerosis.

An important diabetes risk factor and drug target is peroxisome proliferator activated receptor gamma (PPARc). This protein is a transcription factor that regulates fat cell development. Diabetics are prescribed drugs that activate PPARc to increase insulin sensitivity and lower blood sugar. Variations in PPARc influence the risk of developing obesity and type II diabetes. A common variation at position 12 confers a small risk of developing obesity of about 1.3% increase. For the individual, this 1.3% is a small increase of risk, but 75% of the population has this variation, which translates into a large impact on the prevalence of diabetes. The Pima Indians of Arizona, a population known for type II diabetes incidence, contain several SNPs in the gene for PPARc. There are other SNPs in the gene for PPARc that confer a degree of protection against insulin resistance and obesity. Mutations in some of these genes may also lead to a rare form of diabetes known as MODY (maturity-onset diabetes of the young). MODY is inherited in an autosomal dominant fashion. It is similar to non-insulin dependent diabetes, but develops in individuals before the age of 25.

Environmental triggers for type I diabetes are varied. Type I diabetes develops more often in cold climates than warm climates. Type I diabetes is less common in individuals who were breastfed and those whose first solid foods were at later ages. A family history of type II diabetes is only a strong risk factor for individuals living a western lifestyle of high fat diets with little exercise. Individuals who live in areas that do not have westernized lifestyles tend not to develop type II diabetes no matter how high their genetic risk. Obesity is a strong risk factor for type II diabetes; the highest environmental risk is correlated with obesity at early age or for extended periods of time. Women who develop gestational diabetes are likely to have a maternal family history of type II diabetes. The environmental factors that predispose to gestational diabetes are older age and higher weight. The ethnic group in the United States with the highest risk for type I diabetes is Caucasian. The ethnic groups in the United States with the highest risk for type II diabetes are African Americans, Mexican Americans, and Pima Indians.

Demographics

According to the American Diabetes Association, the number of individuals with diabetes in the United States in the year 2002 reached 6.3% of the population, or 18.2 million. This statistic included 210,000 individuals under the age of 20. The risk for death among individuals with diabetes is approximately two times that of non-diabetics. In 2002 research, cardiac disease and stroke were determined to be the leading cause of diabetes-related mortality, responsible for 65% of deaths. Diabetic adults have two to four times increased risk for both cardiac disease and stroke than non-diabetics. Approximately 73% of adult diabetics have elevated blood pressure or use prescription medication for hypertension. The leading cause of new cases of adult blindness from 20–74 years of age is diabetic retinopathy. Approximately 60–70% of diabetics have some degree of nervous system damage called neuropathy. Severe forms of diabetic neuropathy account for more than 60% of non-traumatic lower-limb amputations in the United States.

Preexisting diabetes that is unsuccessfully controlled before conception and during the first trimester of pregnancy can result in major birth defects in 5–10% of pregnancies and spontaneous abortions in 15–20% of pregnancies. If diabetes is unsuccessfully controlled during the second and third trimesters of pregnancy, it can cause high infant birth weight that poses a risk to both mother and child. Gestational diabetes occurs most frequently in African-American, Hispanic- or Latino-American, and Native American populations. It is most common among obese women with a family history of diabetes. Women who have gestational diabetes have a 20–50% chance of developing type II diabetes within 5–10 years.

Type II diabetes is associated with obesity, family history of diabetes, prior history of gestational diabetes, impaired glucose tolerance, physical inactivity, older age, and specific ethnicities. According to the Surgeon General, gaining between 11–18 lbs (4.9–8 kgs) above normal weight doubles the risk of developing type II diabetes. Type II diabetes is increasingly diagnosed in children and adolescents, and is most common in females. African-American, Hispanic- or Latino-American, Native American, and some Asian-American, native Hawaiian, or other Pacific Islander populations are particularly at high risk for type II diabetes.

By 2002, 8.4% of non-Hispanic Caucasians (12.5 million) over 20 years of age had diabetes. Regional studies done in 2002 indicated that type II diabetes is becoming more common among Native American, African-American, and Hispanic and Latino children and adolescents. Approximately 11.4% of non-Hispanic blacks (2.7 million) over 20 years of age had diabetes. Generally, non-Hispanic blacks are 1.6 times more likely to develop diabetes than non-Hispanic Caucasians. Approximately 8.2% of Hispanic or Latino Americans (2 million) over 20 years of age had diabetes. Generally,

Hispanic or Latino Americans are 1.5 times more likely to have diabetes than non-Hispanic Caucasians. Mexican Americans, the largest Hispanic or Latino subgroup, are more than twice as likely to have diabetes than non-Hispanic Caucasians. Correspondingly, residents of Puerto Rico are 1.8 times more likely to be diagnosed with diabetes than non-Hispanic Caucasians in the United States. Approximately 14.5% of Native Americans and Alaskan natives (107,775) who receive care from the Indian Health Service (IHS) over 20 years of age had diabetes. Within this ethnic group, diabetes is least common among Alaskan natives (6.8%) and most common among Native Americans of the southeastern United States (27%). However, Native Americans and Alaska natives generally have 2.2 times increased risk of developing diabetes than non-Hispanic Caucasians. Native Hawaiians, Japanese, and Filipino residents of Hawaii had approximately two times increased risk to be diagnosed with diabetes than Caucasian residents of Hawaii.

Type I diabetes accounts for 5–10% of diabetes cases, and affects approximately one in every 400–500 children and adolescents. Type II diabetes accounts for 90–95% of all diabetes. This form of diabetes may remain undiagnosed for many years. Increased awareness has led to a rapid rise in the number of cases diagnosed each year, in what has been described as epidemic proportions in the United States. In 1990, 4.9% of the American population was diagnosed with diabetes. In 2001, this proportion increased to 7.9%. In the year 2002, the NIH estimated that diabetes costs more than $130 billion in total health care and was the fifth leading cause of death. According to the CDC, from the year 1980 through 2002, the proportion of diabetic Americans increased from 5.8 million to 13.3 million individuals. Estimates revealed that of the children with birth year 2000, one in three will develop diabetes over their lifetime. According to the CDC, more than 1.3 million adults between 18 and 79 years of age were diagnosed as new cases of diabetes in 2003. The CDC estimates that from 1997 to the year 2003, the number of new cases of diagnosed diabetes increased by 52%. Diabetes is predicted to become one of the most common diseases in the world within decades, affecting at least half a billion individuals.

Type I diabetes may cause the sudden onset of any of the following symptoms:

- increased thirst, especially for sweet beverages
- increased urination
- weight loss, despite increased appetite
- nausea or vomiting
- abdominal pain

- fatigue

- absence of menstruation

Type II diabetes may proceed for long periods of time with no symptoms. When diabetes is present, symptoms include the following:

- increased thirst, especially for sweet beverages

- increased urination

- increased appetite

- fatigue

- blurred vision

- frequent or slow-healing infections (including urinary tract, vaginal, skin)

- dry, itchy skin

- tingling or numbness in hands or feet

- erectile dysfunction in men

Diabetes mellitus impacts many organ systems and can result in many complications. Diabetic ketoacidosis (DKA) is a complication of diabetes caused by the buildup of byproducts of fat metabolism called ketones. Ketone buildup occurs when glucose is not available as a fuel source. Diabetics have a deficiency of the insulin hormone used to metabolize glucose for energy. Because glucose is not being made available for cells to use as energy, body fat is alternatively metabolized. The byproducts of fat metabolism are ketones. The ketones accumulate in the blood and so become present in the urine. DKA develops when ketones are in high enough amounts to cause the blood to acidify. In response, the liver begins releasing glucose to use as an energy source instead of fatty acids. Because the cells cannot take in this glucose in the absence of insulin, it only further elevates the blood glucose level. DKA may be the first symptom that leads to the initial diagnosis of type I diabetes. It may also be a sign that a diagnosed type I diabetic is developing a need for increased insulin. Type I diabetics are more prone to the development of DKA than type II diabetics. In a type I diabetic, DKA can result from infection, trauma, heart attack, or surgery. Type II diabetics usually develop ketoacidosis incidentally under conditions of severe stress. Recurrent episodes of DKA in type II diabetics are usually the result of poor compliance with treatment or diet.

The symptoms of DKA may include the following:

- fruity breath odor

- fatigue

- appetite loss, nausea, or vomiting

- rapid deep breathing

- difficulty breathing, especially when lying down

- decreased consciousness

- mental stupor that may progress to coma

- muscular stiffness or aching

- headache

- low blood pressure

Diabetics may endure periods of hypoglycemia if their blood sugar is unsuccessfully controlled or if they imbibe even small amounts of alcohol. Hypoglycemia is a low level of blood glucose that occurs when the balance between insulin, food intake, and physical exertion is disturbed. Symptoms of mild hypoglycemia include hunger, sweating, anxiety, and increased heart rate. Severe hypoglycemia can lead to a confused mental state, slurred speech, weakness, lack of coordination, dizziness, drowsiness, and loss of consciousness. The loss of consciousness due to low levels of blood sugar is called a hypoglycemic coma.

Diabetics are prone to infections from even simple lacerations. Damage to the peripheral nervous system, called diabetic peripheral neuropathy, may result in decreased blood flow and loss of sensation to the limbs. When there is loss of sensation to the feet, an infection developing from a laceration may go unnoticed and therefore not be properly cared for. Diabetics also have decreased immune defenses with which to fight infection. Because of lack of peripheral sensation, deficient oxygen supply from decreased blood flow, and reduced immune defense, diabetics are prone to developing peripheral gangrene. Small cuts with infections can rapidly progress to death of the tissue, which may require amputation of the affected limb to preserve the life of the patient. Gangrene is responsible for many limb amputations in diabetics. Diabetic individuals are advised to keep their feet clean and dry, and to thoroughly inspect daily for any sign of injury or infection.

Poorly controlled blood sugar also predisposes diabetics to fungal infections of the skin, nails, female genital tract, and urinary tract. Diabetic nephropathy is kidney disease that may occur early in diabetes. Diabetics tend to have severe urinary tract infections and are prone to kidney damage as a result. Diabetics also have an increased vulnerability to kidney damage from high blood pressure. Late-stage kidney disease may display symptoms that result from excessive protein in the urine. These symptoms include swelling around the eyes in the morning, swelling of the legs, unintentional weight gain from fluid accumulation, poor appetite, fatigue, headache, and frequent hiccups.

Diabetic retinopathy develops in 80% of diabetics after 15 years with the disease. Diabetic retinopathy is damage to capillary blood vessels that nourish the retina of the eye due to the effects of poorly controlled blood

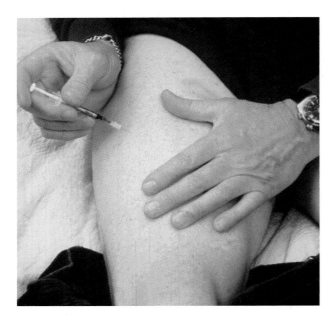

Diabetics must give themselves insulin shots to maintain proper blood sugar levels. *(Custom Medical Stock Photo, Inc.)*

sugar. Signs of diabetic retinopathy include decreased visual acuity and floating spots within the field of vision. Diabetics may also develop cataracts, which are clouding of the lens of the eye that develop slowly and painlessly with increasing visual difficulty. The signs of cataracts include cloudy vision and difficulty with night driving due to glare from bright lights. Initially, most diabetics experience only mild vision problems. However, both diabetic neuropathy and cataracts can progress into blindness. Diabetic retinopathy is a leading cause of legal blindness among adults in the United States. The best defense against severe vision loss is early detection and treatment via annual eye examinations, and steps to maintain control over blood sugar, blood pressure, and blood cholesterol.

Diagnosis

Type II diabetes is diagnosed with the following blood tests:

• Fasting blood glucose test (FGT): positive diagnosis of diabetes or pre-diabetes requires values higher than 126 mg/dL after eight hours of fasting on two separate occasions.

• Random (non-fasting) blood glucose: values higher than 200 mg/dL, accompanied by increased thirst, urination, and fatigue, cause suspicion of diabetes that must be confirmed with a fasting blood glucose test.

• Oral glucose tolerance test (OGTT): positive diagnosis of diabetes or pre-diabetes requires values higher than

200 mg/dL two hours after consuming a glucose solution.

A positive diagnosis of diabetes requires positive results on any one of the three listed tests, with confirmation from a second positive test on a different day. The fasting plasma glucose test is preferred for diagnosing type I and type II diabetes, and pre-diabetes. This convenient test is most reliably performed in the morning after eight hours of fasting, on two separate occasions. FGT values from 70–99 mg/dL are considered normal. Fasting glucose levels of 100–125 mg/dL may indicate a form of pre-diabetes called impaired fasting glucose (IFG). Individuals with IFG have an increased probability of developing type II diabetes in the future. A fasting glucose level 126 mg/dL, in conjunction with a positive OGTT on a separate testing occasion, indicates diabetes.

The random (non-fasting) glucose test can be performed at any time of day, regardless of previous food intake. Diabetes is suspected when blood glucose levels above 200 mg/dL are present in combination with classic diabetic symptoms such as increased thirst and urination, and fatigue. Diagnosis of diabetes requires a positive fasting blood glucose test or oral glucose tolerance test to be performed on a different occasion.

The oral glucose tolerance test can be used to diagnose diabetes or pre-diabetes. The patient is required to fast for eight hours and then drink a solution containing 2.6 oz (75 g) of glucose dissolved in water. Blood glucose levels are then measured at separate points over a three-hour time interval. A value less than 140 mg/dL is considered normal. Values from 140–200 mg/dL may indicate pre-diabetes. A value over 200 mg/dL, in conjunction with a positive FGT on a separate testing occasion, indicates diabetes.

Gestational diabetes is diagnosed with the OGTT. Glucose levels are normally lower during pregnancy, so the threshold values for diagnosis are proportionally lower. The presence of two plasma glucose values meeting or exceeding any of the following levels results in a diagnosis of gestational diabetes: a fasting plasma glucose level of 95 mg/dL, a one-hour level of 180 mg/dL, a two-hour level of 155 mg/dL, or a three-hour level of 140 mg/dL. Some practices deem a 1.7 oz (50 g) glucose solution with one-hour testing to be acceptable.

The hemoglobin A1c (HbA1c) test is used primarily to monitor the quality of glucose control over several weeks. Controlled blood glucose helps to minimize the development of complications caused by chronically elevated glucose levels, such as progressive damage to body organs. The HbA1c test is an overall picture of the average amount of glucose in the blood over the previous few months. HbA1c is the term for glycosylated (glu-

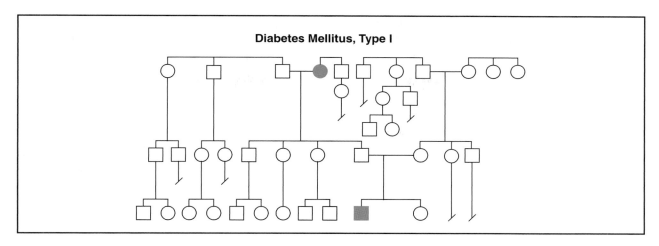

Diabetes Mellitus, Type I

(Gale Group)

cose-carrying) hemoglobin in red blood cells. It is a measurement of how successful the employed treatments are at controlling blood sugar values. The HbA1c test can determine how severe blood sugar fluctuations have been in newly diagnosed diabetics and indicate the need for treatment adjustments in the medication or diets of known diabetics. Physicians may perform HbA1c tests on a patient several times a year to verify that good control is being maintained. The HbA1c test will not reflect temporary, acute fluctuations in blood glucose. A 1% change in HbA1c reflects a fluctuation of approximately 30 mg/dL in average blood glucose. An HbA1c value of 6% corresponds to an average blood glucose value of 135 mg/dL, while an HbA1c of 9% corresponds to an average blood glucose value of 240 mg/dL. The closer the HbA1c can be kept to 5% or 6%, the better diabetic control. Risk of diabetic complications increases with increased values of HbA1c.

A urinalysis followed by a blood test for ketones and pH is used in diagnosing ketoacidosis. Type I diabetes may also require a test for insulin level to determine whether it is very low or absent. A test for C-peptide levels, a byproduct of insulin production, is also often performed.

Treatment

After a diagnosis of type I diabetes, the immediate goals of treatment are to control blood glucose levels and control diabetic ketoacidosis, if present. Type I diabetics often have a sudden onset of severe symptoms that may require hospitalization. The ongoing goals of treatment are to prolong life, reduce symptoms, and prevent diabetes-related complications. Medication, education, weight control, exercise, foot care, and self-testing of blood glucose levels are key to a good prognosis.

Insulin lowers blood sugar by allowing it to leave the blood and enter the cells to be used as energy. Type I diabetics are insulin deficient and so must take insulin every day. Insulin is either injected under the skin at set times using a syringe, or administered by an infusion pump that delivers the insulin continuously. Insulin is not available as an oral medication. There are different types of insulin that vary in how quickly they work and the duration of their effect. More than one type of insulin is sometimes mixed together in an injection. Injections are usually self-administered from one to three times daily. Type I diabetes requires that food intake is balanced by insulin intake to prevent extreme fluctuations in blood glucose.

In March of 2005, the FDA approved Symlin, the first non-insulin drug for the treatment of adult type I diabetes. Symlin is intended as an addition to insulin therapy for three hours after meals when blood glucose control is not tight enough on insulin alone. Symlin is injectable and can be used to augment treatment of both type I and type II diabetes. Appropriate use of Symlin involves close monitoring by a physician to prevent hypoglycemic attacks. However, the addition of Symlin to the therapeutic environment is hoped to result in much tighter overall control in diabetics for whom current therapies are inadequate.

After a diagnosis of type II diabetes, the immediate goals are to eliminate symptoms and stabilize blood glucose levels. The ongoing goals are to prevent complications and prolong life. The primary treatment for type II diabetes is physical activity, weight control, and diet. Non-insulin oral medication is sometimes indicated to assist in lowering blood sugar when diet and exercise are not enough. These oral medications are effective in type II diabetics, but not type I diabetics.

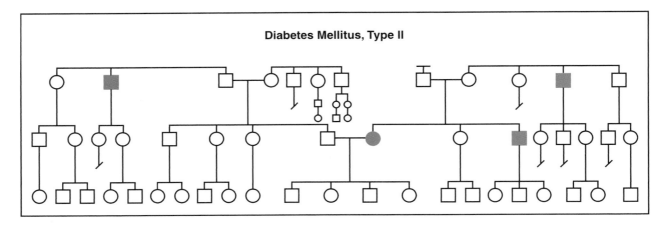

Diabetes Mellitus, Type II

(Gale Group.)

There are multiple classes of medication available for treatment of type II diabetes. Oral sulfonylureas trigger the pancreas to increase insulin production. Biguanides (metformin) cause a decrease in liver glucose production to bring down blood glucose levels, while alpha-glucosidase inhibitors (acarbose) decrease the absorption of carbohydrates from the digestive tract, thereby lowering blood glucose levels after meals. Thiazolidinediones (rosiglitazone) assist insulin functioning at the cell surface by increasing the responsiveness to insulin. Meglitinides (repaglinide and nateglinide) trigger the pancreas to increase the proportion of insulin released in response to blood glucose. Type II diabetics who continue to have poor blood glucose control despite lifestyle changes and the use of oral medicines may be prescribed insulin treatment. Type II diabetics are also sometimes prescribed insulin treatment if they cannot tolerate the oral medications. Insulin must be injected under the skin using a syringe and cannot be taken orally.

For all types of diabetes, planning balanced meals and dietary control requires education. Regular physical activity is important to help control blood glucose and weight. However, diabetics must take special precautions before engaging in intense physical activity that may alter blood glucose levels too rapidly. Blood glucose monitoring is done with specialized home kits called glucometers. A glucometer is a small device that provides an exact reading of blood glucose. A test strip is used to collect a small drop of blood obtained by pricking the finger with a small needle called a lancet. The test strip is placed in the meter and results are available within 30–45 seconds. Testing is done on a regular basis to monitor the balance between food intake, medication, and physical activity. Test results may are used to adjust meals, activity, and medications to keep blood glucose under control. Diabetes causes damage to the blood vessels and nervous system that often results in a loss of sen-

sation to the foot. Foot injuries may go unnoticed until severe infection develops due to lack of care and a depressed immune system. A daily foot care routine involves washing and inspecting the feet, and generally keeping them clean and dry.

Hypoglycemia, or low blood glucose, can occur in diabetics when they use too much insulin, drink alcohol, exercise too much, or eat too little food. Symptoms of low blood sugar typically appear when blood glucose levels fall below 70. Treatment involves eating something with sugar such as fruit juice. Sugar intake should be continued until blood glucose control is achieved. Only after blood glucose has returned to normal should more substantial food be eaten. Severe hypoglycemia may require a shot of glucagon at a hospital emergency room.

Ketones can be monitored using a simple urine test available at pharmacies. Warning signs for ketoacidosis include flushed face, dry skin and mouth, nausea or vomiting, stomach pain, deep, rapid breathing, or fruity breath odor. If left untreated, the condition can worsen and lead to death. Treatment of DKA involves lowering the blood glucose level to normal, and to replacing fluids lost through excessive urination and vomiting. It is often possible to recognize the early warning signs of DKA and make appropriate corrections at home before the condition progresses. If severe DKA develops, hospitalization is often required to control the condition.

General diabetes treatment includes regular doctor visits for an evaluation of general health and neurological function, having HbA1c measured several times a year to evaluate overall blood glucose control, regular evaluation of blood pressure, cholesterol and triglyceride levels, annual eye examinations, dental examination and cleaning every six months, daily foot inspection, and cur-

KEY TERMS

Allosteric activator site—Site at which an enzyme is regulated separate from its site of catalytic enzymatic activity.

Autosomal dominant—Inheritance apart from the sex chromosomes that only requires one copy for expression.

Body mass index (BMI)—Assessment of health related to weight and height.

Gangrene—Death of tissue due to deficient or absent blood supply.

Hemoglobin—The iron-containing pigment of red blood cells.

Maturity-onset diabetes of the young (MODY)—A rare form of diabetes inherited in an autosomal dominant fashion. It is similar to type II diabetes, but develops before the age of 25.

Transcription factor—A factor that activates the transformation of DNA to RNA (the next step is translation, where RNA is changed into protein).

rent immunizations. Diabetes education is critical to the treatment plan.

Prognosis

Diabetes is a chronic disease for which there is not yet a cure. The prognosis for diabetics is varied based on blood glucose control. Tight control of blood glucose can delay or even prevent the progression of complications and secondary illnesses caused by diabetes. However, complications may occur even when good control is achieved. Diabetics with high control of blood glucose and blood pressure significantly reduce their risk of death, stroke, and heart failure. A reduction of HbA1c by one percentage point can improve prognosis and cause a decrease in the risk for complications by 25%. Prognosis is greatly improved by a normal BMI, which uses individuals' height and weight to rate them as normal, overweight, or obese. A score of 18–24.9 is considered normal and improves the prognosis for diabetes. A score of 25–29.9 indicating overweight, or a score of 30 or more indicating obesity, results in a poorer prognosis. Diabetics have increased susceptibility to illness such as influenza. Once a diabetic has an illness, they often have a worse prognosis than non-diabetics. Smoking cigarettes drastically worsens the prognosis for diabetes, greatly increasing the risk of vascular complications, gangrene, and amputations.

Resources

BOOKS

Champe, P. C., and R. A. Harvey. *Lippincott's Illustrated Review of Biochemistry, Second Edition.* Philadelphia, PA: Lippincott, 1994.

Thompson & Thompson Genetics in Medicine, Sixth Edition. St. Louis, MO: Elsevier Science, 2004.

WEBSITES

All About Diabetes. American Diabetes Association. (April 2, 2005.) <http://www.diabetes.org/genetics.jsp>.

Diabetes. Centers for Disease Control and Prevention. (April 2, 2005.) <http://www.cdc.gov/diabetes/>.

Diabetes. MedlinePlus. (April 2, 2005.) <http://www.nlm.nih.gov/medlineplus/diabetes.html>.

Diabetes. National Diabetes Information Clearinghouse. (April 2, 2005.) <http://diabetes.niddk.nih.gov/dm/a-z.asp>.

Diabetes Data and Trends. Centers for Disease Control and Prevention. (April 2, 2005.) <http://www.cdc.gov/diabetes/statistics/index.htm>.

Diabetes Health Topics. Centers for Disease Control and Prevention. (April 2, 2005.) <http://www.cdc.gov/doc.do/id/0900f3ec802723eb>.

The Genetic Landscape of Diabetes. National Institutes of Health. (April 2, 2005.) <http://www.ncbi.nlm.nih.gov/books/bv.fcgi?call=bv.View..ShowTOC&rid=diabetes.TOC&depth=1>.

ORGANIZATIONS

American Diabetes Association. 1701 North Beauregard Street, Alexandria, VA 22311. 800-DIABETES, (800) 342-2383. (April 2, 2005.) <http://www.diabetes.org>.

National Diabetes Education Program. (800) 438-5383. (April 2, 2005.) <http://www.cdc.gov/diabetes/ndep/index.htm>.

National Diabetes Information Clearinghouse. 1 Information Way, Bethesda, MD 20892-3560. (800) 860-8747. (April 2, 2005.) <http://diabetes.niddk.nih.gov/about/index.htm>.

Maria Basile, PhD

Diastrophic dysplasia

Definition

Diastrophic **dysplasia** (DTD) is a rare genetic disorder of bone growth and formation that is evident at birth.

Description

Diastrophic dysplasia is one of the genetic osteochondrodysplasias, a group of disorders characterized by abnormal growth and formation of bone and cartilage. The main features of DTD include: malformed ears, cleft palate, short limbs, short stature, spinal and joint deformities, and abnormalities of the bones of the hands and feet. Although children with DTD may experience delays in motor development (e.g. walking at a later age than expected), they are of normal intelligence. The syndrome derives its name from the Greek word, *diastrophos*, meaning twisted or crooked. Maroteaux and Lamy first used the term diastrophic dysplasia in 1960 to describe three of their patients and eleven other cases already reported in the literature. Since then, at least 300 cases of DTD have been described. Diastrophic dysplasia is also known as diastrophic nanism or diastrophic dwarfism and is abbreviated as DTD or DD.

Genetic profile

The **gene** responsible for DTD, known as the diastrophic dysplasia sulfate transporter gene (DTDST gene), is located at the end of the long arm of **chromosome** 5, at position 5q32-33. The DTDST gene produces a protein that functions as a channel and transports sulfate across the cell membrane. DTD is inherited in an autosomal recessive manner. Affected individuals have a mutation in both copies of their DTDST gene; they inherit one mutation from each parent. Parents of affected individuals are carriers; they have a mutation in one copy of their DTDST gene and are without symptoms of the disorder.

Most bone in the body begins as cartilage and later hardens (ossifies) to form bone. In certain parts of the body such as the rib, auricle, and joints, cartilage does not ossify; it remains as cartilage and functions as load-bearing or shock-absorbing tissue. Cartilage contains sulfur-containing compounds, known as proteoglycans. It is thought that abnormal function of the DTD sulfate transporter leads to insufficient sulfate uptake by proteogycans in the cartilage. This undersulfation results in weakness and distortion of the cartilage. The exact mechanism by which this occurs is not fully understood.

Three other genetic skeletal dysplasias: recessively inherited **multiple epiphyseal dysplasia** (rMED), atelosteogenesis type 2 (AO-2), and **achondrogenesis** type IB (ACG-IB), are also due to mutations in the DTDST gene. When compared to DTD, both AO-2 and ACG-1B are more severe skeletal dysplasias, with the latter being a lethal disorder. Recessively inherited MED is a relatively mild condition. This broad range in severity, from mild to fatal, is attributed to the different types and combinations of genetic mutations within the DTDST gene that are responsible for these four related diseases.

Demographics

Diastrophic dysplasia is a rare disorder in most parts of the world except in Finland where the incidence of the disease is estimated at one in every 32,600 live births. Approximately 1–2% of Finnish people are DTD carriers. Most Finnish DTD gene carriers possess the same ancestral mutation, known as DTDST (Fin). The high frequency of this single mutation in Finland is attributed to a founder effect.

Signs and symptoms

Diastrophic dysplasia is a variable condition that tends to become more severe with age. Many manifestations of the disorder are prenatal in onset and are therefore apparent at birth.

Growth

Diastrophic dysplasia is considered a short-limbed **skeletal dysplasia** because the limbs are disproportionately short for the overall height of the individual. The newborn with DTD tends to be short with an average birth length of 16.5 in (42 cm). This growth failure continues throughout childhood and is progressive in nature. The degree of deformity caused by orthopedic complications of this disorder can influence overall height. A wide range of final adult heights has been reported with lower limits at 2 ft 10 in (86 cm) and 3 ft 5 in (104 cm) and upper limits at 4 ft 5 in (135.7 cm) and 4 ft 3 in (129 cm) for males and females respectively. On x ray, the limb bones appear short and thick with broad metaphyses and flattened, irregular epiphyses.

Craniofacial

One of the most distinct features of DTD is the so-called "cauliflower ear." In over 80% of infants with DTD, fluid-filled cysts appear on the outer ear (pinnae) during the first few weeks of life. These cysts later calcify and may eventually ossify to form bone. In as many as 75% of individuals with DTD, some form of cleft palate is present. Although individuals with DTD may have a small chin (micrognathia), the head is otherwise normal in size.

Thoracic

Occasionally there may be abnormalities of cartilage in the trachea, larynx, and bronchi, which may lead to a life-threatening complication—collapse of the airways—especially in early infancy.

Spinal

Spina bifida occulta in the neck (cervical) and upper back (thoracic) region is the most common spinal abnormality found in DTD and is present in over 50% of cases. In spina bifida occulta there is incomplete closure of bones of the spinal column. Other common spinal abnormalities include progressive curvature of the spine, either from front to back (kyphosis) or from side to side (**scoliosis**). Kyphosis in the neck region (cervical kyphosis) is present in at least 30% of affected individuals and is usually evident at birth. This type of spine curvature usually resolves over time without treatment. In severe cases however, cervical kyphosis can lead to respiratory problems. Scoliosis, which is generally not present at birth, may appear at an early age and become problematic in early adolescence. Nearly 50% of females and at least 20% of males will develop scoliosis.

Joint

Joint changes in diastrophic dysplasia are progressive in nature and can be a painful complication of this disorder. Individuals with DTD may experience limited mobility and/or permanent immobility (contractures), especially in the knees and shoulders. The joints in an individual with DTD are also prone to partial or complete dislocations in the shoulders, hips, kneecaps, and elbows.

Hands and feet

The hands of a child with diastrophic dysplasia are distinct. The fingers are short (**brachydactyly**) and there may be fusion of the joints between the bones of the fingers (symphalangism). The metacarpal bone of the thumb is short and oval-shaped; these bony deformations cause the thumb to deviate away from the hand and assume the appearance of the so-called "hitchhiker thumb," a classic feature of DTD. The bony changes in the feet are similar to those found in the hands. The great toes may deviate outward, much like the thumbs. **Clubfoot** deformity (talipes), due to abnormal formation and limited mobility of the bones of the feet, is a common birth defect found in newborns with DTD.

Diagnosis

At birth the diagnosis of diastrophic dysplasia is based on the presence of the characteristic physical and radiologic (x ray) findings. **DNA** mutation analysis may be helpful in confirmation of a suspected diagnosis. In those rarer cases where DNA mutation analysis does not detect changes, a laboratory test that measures the uptake of sulfate by fibroblasts or chondrocytes may be useful in making a diagnosis.

If there is a family history of diastrophic dysplasia and DNA is available from the affected individual, then prenatal diagnosis using DNA methods, either mutation analysis or linkage analysis, may be possible. DNA mutation analysis detects approximately 90% of DTDST mutations in suspected patients. In patients where the mutations are unknown or undetectable, another DNA method known as linkage analysis may be possible and, if so, it can usually distinguish an affected from an unaffected pregnancy with at least 95% certainty. In linkage analysis, DNA from multiple family members, including the person with DTD, is required. DNA-based testing can be performed through chorionic villus sampling or through **amniocentesis**.

If DNA-based testing is not possible, prenatal diagnosis of diastrophic dysplasia in an at-risk pregnancy may be made during the second and third trimesters through ultrasound. The ultrasound findings in an affected fetus may include: a small chin (micrognathia), abnormally short limbs, inward (ulnar) deviation of the hands, the "hitchhiker" thumb, clubfoot, joint contractures, and spinal curvature.

General population carrier screening is not available except in Finland where the frequency of a single ancestral mutation is high.

Treatment and management

There is currently no treatment that normalizes the skeletal growth and development in a child with diastrophic dysplasia. The medical management and treatment of individuals with DTD generally requires a multidisciplinary team of specialists that should include experts in orthopedics. At birth it is recommended that a neonatologist be present because of the potential for respiratory problems. Surgery may be indicated in infancy if congenital abnormalities such as open cleft palate and/ or clubfoot deformity are present. Throughout childhood and adulthood, bracing, surgery, and physical therapy are measures often used to treat the spinal and joint deformities of DTD. Such measures, however, may not fully correct these deformities.

Due to the significant short-limbed short stature associated with diastrophic dysplasia, certain modifications to home, school, and work environments are necessary in order for a person with DTD to perform daily tasks. Occupational therapy may help affected individuals, especially children, learn how to use assistive devices and to adapt to various situations.

Prognosis

In infancy there is an increased mortality rate, as high as 25%, due to respiratory complications caused

KEY TERMS

Amniocentesis—A procedure performed at 16-18 weeks of pregnancy in which a needle is inserted through a woman's abdomen into her uterus to draw out a small sample of the amniotic fluid from around the baby. Either the fluid itself or cells from the fluid can be used for a variety of tests to obtain information about genetic disorders and other medical conditions in the fetus.

Cartilage—Supportive connective tissue which cushions bone at the joints or which connects muscle to bone.

Chondrocyte—A specialized type of cell that secretes the material which surrounds the cells in cartilage.

Chorionic villus sampling (CVS)—A procedure used for prenatal diagnosis at 10-12 weeks gestation. Under ultrasound guidance a needle is inserted either through the mother's vagina or abdominal wall and a sample of cells is collected from around the fetus. These cells are then tested for chromosome abnormalities or other genetic diseases.

Chromosome—A microscopic thread-like structure found within each cell of the body and consists of a complex of proteins and DNA. Humans have 46 chromosomes arranged into 23 pairs. Changes in either the total number of chromosomes or their shape and size (structure) may lead to physical or mental abnormalities.

Cleft palate—A congenital malformation in which there is an abnormal opening in the roof of the mouth that allows the nasal passages and the mouth to be improperly connected.

Clubfoot—Abnormal permanent bending of the ankle and foot. Also called *talipes equinovarus*.

Collagen—The main supportive protein of cartilage, connective tissue, tendon, skin, and bone.

Deoxyribonucleic acid (DNA)—The genetic material in cells that holds the inherited instructions for growth, development, and cellular functioning.

DNA mutation analysis—A direct approach to the detection of a specific genetic mutation or mutations using one or more laboratory techniques.

Dysplasia—The abnormal growth or development of a tissue or organ.

Epiphyses—The growth area at the end of a bone.

Fibroblast—Cells that form connective tissue fibers like skin.

Founder effect—increased frequency of a gene mutation in a population that was founded by a small ancestral group of people, at least one of whom was a carrier of the gene mutation.

Gene—A building block of inheritance, which contains the instructions for the production of a particular protein, and is made up of a molecular sequence found on a section of DNA. Each gene is found on a precise location on a chromosome.

Linkage analysis—A method of finding mutations based on their proximity to previously identified genetic landmarks.

Metacarpal—A hand bone extending from the wrist to a finger or thumb.

Metaphyses—The growth zone of the long bones located between the epiphyses the ends (epiphyses) and the shaft (diaphysis) of the bone.

Mutation—A permanent change in the genetic material that may alter a trait or characteristic of an individual, or manifest as disease, and can be transmitted to offspring.

Nanism—Short stature.

Sulfate—A chemical compound containing sulfur and oxygen.

Vertebra—One of the 23 bones which comprise the spine. *Vertebrae* is the plural form.

---

by weakness and collapse of the cartilage of the wind pipe (trachea) and/or the voice box (larynx), conditions which may require surgical intervention. Some forms of cleft palate and micrognathia may be life threatening in early life as they can result in respiratory obstruction. Severe spinal abnormalities such as cervical kyphosis may also cause respiratory problems. After the newborn period, the life span of an individual with DTD is usually normal with the exception of those

cases where spinal cord compression occurs as a result of severe cervical kyphosis with vertebrae subluxation. Spinal cord compression is a significant medical problem that can lead to muscle weakness, paralysis, or death. In a susceptible individual, spinal cord compression may occur for the first time during surgery due to the hyperextended neck position used during intubation. Other anesthetic techniques may be indicated for such cases.

People with diastrophic dysplasia are of normal intelligence and are able to have children. Since many of the abnormalities associated with DTD are relatively resistant to surgery, many individuals with DTD will have some degree of physical handicap as they get older. They may continue to require medical management of their spinal and joint complications throughout adult life.

Resources

BOOKS

Bianchi, Diana W., et al. *Fetology: Diagnosis and Management of the Fetal Patient.* New York: McGraw-Hill, 2000.

Jones, Kenneth Lyons. *Smith's Recognizable Patterns of Human Malformation.* Philadelphia: W.B. Saunders Company, 1997.

PERIODICALS

Makitie, Outi, et al. "Growth in Diastrophic Dysplasia." *The Journal of Pediatrics* 130 (1997): 641–6.

Remes, Ville, et al. "Cervical Kyphosis in Diastrophic Dysplasia." *Spine* 24, no. 19 (1999): 1990–95.

Rossi, Antonio, et al. "Mutations in the Diastrophic Dysplasia Sulfate Transporter (DTDST) gene (SLC26A2): 22 Novel Mutations, Mutation Review, Associated Skeletal Phenotypes, and Diagnostic Relevance." *Human Mutation* 17 (2001): 159–71.

Satoh, Hideshi, et al. "Functional analysis of Diastrophic Dysplasia Sulfate Transporter." *The Journal of Biological Chemistry* 273, no. 20 (1998): 12307–15.

ORGANIZATIONS

National Organization for Rare Disorders (NORD). PO Box 8923, New Fairfield, CT 06812-8923 (203) 746-6518 or (800) 999-6673. Fax: (203) 746-6481. <http://www.rarediseases.org>.

WEBSITES

Diastrophic Help Web Site. <http://pixelscapes.com/ddhelp/>.

The Kathryn and Alan C. Greenberg Center for Skeletal Dysplasias Web Page. <http://www.med.jhu.edu/Greenberg.Center/Greenberg.htm>.

Dawn Cardeiro, MS, CGC

Distal arthrogryposis syndrome

Definition

Distal arthrogryposis syndrome is a rare genetic disorder in which affected individuals are born with a characteristic bending at the joints of the hands and feet. A contracture is the word used to describe what happens at the joints to cause this bending. In addition to contractures of the hand and feet, individuals with distal arthrogryposis are born with a tightly clenched fist and overlapping fingers.

Description

The word arthrogryposis means a flexed (bent) or curved joint. Distal means the furthest from any one point of reference or something that is remote. Therefore, distal arthrogryposis syndrome causes the joints at the most remote parts of our limbs, the hands and feet, to be flexed.

Consistent fetal movement during pregnancy is necessary for the development of the joints. Without regular motion, the joints become tight resulting in contractures. The first cases of arthrogryposis were identified in 1923. Arthrogryposis multiple congenital (AMC) is also referred to as fetal akinesia/hypokinesia sequence that is not a disorder, but describes what happens when there is no fetal movement during fetal development. The reasons for lack of fetal motion include neurologic, muscular, connective tissue, or skeletal abnormalities or intrauterine crowding. There are various disorders involving some form of arthrogryposis.

Distal arthrogryposis was identified as a separate genetic disorder in 1982. Two types of distal arthrogryposis have been identified. Type 1 or typical distal arthrogryposis, is used to describe individuals with distal contractures of the hands and feet, characteristic positioning of the hands and feet, and normal intelligence. Type 2 distal arthrogryposis is known as the atypical form. It is characterized by additional birth defects and mild intellectual delays.

There are other syndromes which include arthrogryposis, however distal arthrogryposis has been characterized as its own syndrome by its **inheritance** pattern. In addition to the inheritance pattern, there are other features that differentiate this type of arthrogryposis from other forms. Some of these features include a characteristic position of the hands at birth—the fists are clenched and the fingers are bent and overlapping. In addition, problems with the positioning of the feet, called **clubfoot** is often seen in these individuals. Another distinguishing characteristic is an extremely wide variability in the severity and number of joint contractures someone may exhibit. This variability is often noticed between two affected individuals from the same family.

Genetic profile

Distal arthrogryposis syndrome is inherited in an autosomal dominant manner. Autosomal dominant inheritance patterns only require one genetic mutation on one of the **chromosome** pairs to exhibit symptoms of the disease. Chromosomes are the structures that carry genes. Genes are the blueprints for who we are and what we look like. Humans should have 23 pairs, or 46 total chromosomes in every cell of their body. The first 22 chromosomes are numbered 1–22 and are called autosomes. The remaining (23rd) pair is assigned a letter, either an X or a Y, and are the sex determining chromosomes. A typical male is described as 46, XY. A typical female is 46, XX.

Each parent contributes one of their paired chromosomes to their children. Before fertilization occurs, the father's sperm cell divides in half and the total number of chromosomes reduces from 46 to 23. The mother's egg cell undergoes the same type of reduction as well. At the time of conception, each parent contributes 23 chromosomes, one of each pair, to their children. All of the genetic information is contained on each chromosome.

If either the father or the mother is affected with distal arthrogryposis, there is a 50% chance they will pass on the chromosome with the **gene** for this disease to each of their children. The specific gene for distal arthrogryposis is not known, however we do know that it is located on chromosome number 9.

The symptoms of distal arthrogryposis can be different between two affected relatives. For example, a mother may have contractures in all of her joints, but her child may only be affected with contractures in the hands. Because of this variability in the symptoms of this disease, it is believed there is more than one gene mutation that causes distal arthrogryposis. The only gene thought to cause this disease is on chromosome number 9. The exact location and type of genetic mutation on chromosome 9 is not known and, therefore, the only **genetic testing** available is research based.

Demographics

Distal arthrogryposis can affect individuals from all types of populations and ethnic groups. This disease can affect both males and females. There have been only a handful of individuals described with this type of arthrogryposis. The physician, Dr. Hall, who named the disorder in 1982, had initially identified 37 patients with type 1 and type 2 distal arthrogryposis syndrome. She

identified 14 individuals with type 1 and 23 individuals with type 2. Since then, numerous other individuals have been diagnosed with distal arthrogryposis. The exact incidence has not been reported in the literature.

Signs and symptoms

At birth, many individuals have been diagnosed based on their characteristic hand positioning. Virtually all individuals with distal arthrogryposis are born with their hands clenched tightly in a fist. The thumb is turned inwards lying over the palm, called abduction. The fingers are also overlapping on each other. This hand positioning is also characteristic of a more serious condition called **trisomy 18**. The majority of patients with distal arthrogryposis will also have problems with the positioning of their feet. Many patients will have some form of clubfoot, where the foot is twisted out of shape or position. Another word for clubfoot is talipes.

In addition to the hand and foot involvement, a small percentage of patients will have a dislocation or separation of the hip joint as well as difficulty bending at the hips and tendency for a slight degree of unnatural bending at the hip joints. The knees may also exhibit similar problems of being slightly bent and fixed at that point. Even fewer individuals are born with stiff shoulders.

Type 2 distal arthrogryposis syndrome includes other birth defects not seen in type 1 individuals. For example, type two distal arthrogryposis involves problems with the closure of the lip called cleft lip or an opening in the roof of the mouth called cleft palate.

Other abnormalities seen in type 2 distal arthrogryposis include a small tongue, short stature, a curvature of the spine, more serious joint contractures, and mental delays.

Diagnosis

The diagnosis of distal arthrogryposis can sometimes be made during pregnancy from an ultrasound evaluation. An ultrasound may detect the characteristic hand finding as well as the flexion deformities of both the hands and the feet. An affected fetus may have difficulty swallowing and this is exhibited on an ultrasound evaluation as extra amniotic fluid surrounding the baby called polyhydraminos. Another very important and specific diagnostic sign for distal arthrogryposis during a pregnancy is no fetal movement. Ultrasound findings have been detected as early as 17 weeks of a pregnancy.

After birth, a diagnosis is made by a physician performing a physical examination of a baby suspected of

KEY TERMS

Amniotic fluid—The fluid which surrounds a developing baby during pregnancy.

Cell—The smallest living units of the body which group together to form tissues and help the body perform specific functions.

Flexion—The act of bending or condition of being bent.

Inheritance pattern—The way in which a genetic disease is passed on in a family.

Neurologic—Pertaining the nervous system.

Trisomy 18—A chromosomal alteration where a child is born with three copies of chromosome number 18 and as a result is affected with multiple birth defects and mental retardation.

Ultrasound evaluation—A procedure which examines the tissue and bone structures of an individual or a developing baby.

having this disorder. If a baby is affected with type 2 distal arthrogryposis, they may have a difficult time eating properly. The only type of genetic testing available is research based. Because there is likely more than one gene that causes the disease, the genetic testing being performed at this time is not yet offered to affected individuals in order to confirm a diagnosis.

Treatment and management

The treatment for individuals with distal arthrogryposis is adjusted to the needs of the affected child. With therapy after birth to help loosen the joints and retrain the muscles, most individuals do remarkably well. The hands do not remain clenched an entire lifetime, but will eventually unclench. Sometimes the fingers will remain bent to some degree. Clubfoot can usually be corrected so that the feet can be positioned to be straight.

Prognosis

The prognosis depends on how severely affected an individual is and how many joints are involved. Some of the more severe cases may be associated with an early death due to sudden respiratory failure and difficulty breathing properly. The majority of individuals with distal arthrogryposis do very well after receiving the necessary therapies and sometimes surgery to correct severe joint contractions.

Resources

BOOKS

Fleischer, A., et al. *Sonography in Obstetrics and Gynecology, Principles & Practice.* Stamford, Conn.: 1996.

Jones, Kenneth. *Smith's Recognizable Patterns of Human Malformation.* 5th ed. Philadelphia: W.B. Saunders Company, 1997.

PERIODICALS

Sonoda, T. "Two brothers with distal arthrogryposis, peculiar facial appearance, cleft palate, short stature, hydronephrosis, retentio testis, and normal intelligence: a new type of distal arthrogryposis?" *American Journal of Medical Genetics.* (April 2000): 280–85.

Wong, V. "The spectrum of arthrogryposis in 33 Chinese children." *Brain Development.* (April 1997): 187–96.

WEBSITES

"Arthrogryposis Multiplex Congenita, Distal, Type 1." *Online Mendelian Inheritance in Man.* <http://www.ncbi.nlm.gov/Omim/>.

Limb Anomalies. <http://www.kumc.edu/gec/support/limb.html>.

Katherine S. Hunt, MS

DNA (deoxyribonucleic acid)

Genetics is the science of heredity that involves the study of the structure and function of genes and the methods by which genetic infomation contained in genes is passed from one generation to the next. The modern science of genetics can be traced to the research of Gregor Mendel (1823–1884), who was able to develop a series of laws that described mathematically the way hereditary characteristics pass from parents to offspring. These laws assume that hereditary characteristics are contained in discrete units of genetic material now known as genes.

The story of genetics during the twentieth century is, in one sense, an effort to discover the **gene** itself. An important breakthrough came in the early 1900s with the work of the American geneticist, Thomas Hunt Morgan (1866–1945). Working with fruit flies, Morgan was able to show that genes are somehow associated with the chromosomes that occur in the nuclei of cells. By 1912, Hunt's colleague, American geneticist A. H. Sturtevant (1891–1970) was able to construct the first **chromosome** map showing the relative positions of different genes on a chromosome. The gene then had a concrete, physical referent; it was a portion of a chromosome.

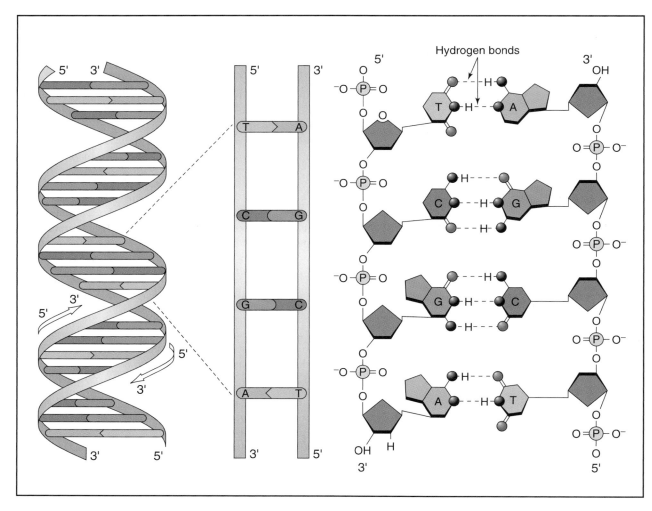

The structure of a DNA molecule. *(Gale Group.)*

During the 1920s and 1930s, a small group of scientists looked for a more specific description of the gene by focusing their research on the gene's molecular composition. Most researchers of the day assumed that genes were some kind of protein molecule. Protein molecules are large and complex. They can occur in an almost infinite variety of structures. This quality is expected for a class of molecules that must be able to carry the enormous variety of genetic traits.

A smaller group of researchers looked to a second family of compounds for potential candidates as the molecules of heredity. These were the nucleic acids. The nucleic acids were first discovered in 1869 by the Swiss physician Johann Miescher (1844–1895). Miescher originally called these compounds "nuclein" because they were first obtained from the nuclei of cells. One of Miescher's students, Richard Altmann, later suggested a new name for the compounds, a name that better reflected their chemical nature: nucleic acids.

Nucleic acids seemed unlikely candidates as molecules of heredity in the 1930s. What was then known about their structure suggested that they were too simple to carry the vast array of complex information needed in a molecule of heredity. Each nucleic acid molecule consists of a long chain of alternating sugar and phosphate fragments to which are attached some sequence of four of five different nitrogen bases: adenine, cytosine, guanine, uracil and thymine (the exact bases found in a molecule depend slightly on the type of nucleic acid).

It was not clear how this relatively simple structure could assume enough different conformations to "code" for hundreds of thousands of genetic traits. In comparison, a single protein molecule contains various arrangements of twenty fundamental units (amino acids) making it a much better candidate as a carrier of genetic information.

Yet, experimental evidence began to point to a possible role for nucleic acids in the transmission of hereditary characteristics. That evidence implicated a specific sub-family of the nucleic acids known as the deoxyribonucleic acids, or DNA. DNA is characterized by the presence of the sugar deoxyribose in the sugar-phosphate backbone of the molecule and by the presence of adenine, cytosine, guanine, and thymine, but not uracil.

As far back as the 1890s, the German geneticist Albrecht Kossel (1853–1927) obtained results that pointed to the role of DNA in heredity. In fact, historian John Gribbin has suggested that the evidence was so clear that it "ought to have been enough alone to show that the hereditary information... *must* be carried by the DNA." Yet, somehow, Kossel himself did not see this point, nor did most of his colleagues for half a century.

As more and more experiments showed the connection between DNA and genetics, a small group of researchers in the 1940s and 1950s began to ask how a DNA molecule could code for genetic information. The two who finally resolved this question were a somewhat unusual pair, James Watson, a 24-year old American trained in genetics, and Francis Crick, a 36-year old Englishman, trained in physics and self-taught in chemistry. The two met at the Cavendish Laboratories of Cambridge University in 1951, and became instant friends. They were united by a common passionate belief that the structure of DNA held the key to understanding how genetic information is stored in a cell and how it is transmitted from one cell to its daughter cells.

In one sense, the challenge facing Watson and Crick was a relatively simple one. A great deal was already known about the DNA molecule. Few new discoveries were needed, but those few discoveries were crucial to solving the DNA-heredity puzzle. Primarily the question was one of molecular architecture. How were the various parts of a DNA molecule oriented in space such that the molecule could hold genetic information?

The key to answering that question lay in a technique known as x-ray crystallography. When x rays are directed at a crystal of some material, such as DNA, they are reflected and refracted by atoms that make up the crystal. The refraction pattern thus produced consists of a collection of spots and arcs. A skilled observer can determine from the refraction pattern the arrangement of atoms in the crystal.

The technique is actually more complex than described here. For one thing, obtaining satisfactory x-ray patterns from crystals is often difficult. Also, interpreting x-ray patterns—especially for complex molecules like DNA—can be extremely difficult.

Watson and Crick were fortunate in having access to some of the best x-ray diffraction patterns that then

existed. These "photographs" were the result of work being done by Maurice Wilkins and Rosalind Elsie Franklin at King' s College in London. Although Wilkins and Franklin were also working on the structure of DNA, they did not recognize the information their photographs contained. Indeed, it was only when Watson accidentally saw one of Franklin's photographs that he suddenly saw the solution to the DNA puzzle.

Racing back to Cambridge after seeing this photograph, Watson convinced Crick to make an all-out attack on the DNA problem. They worked continuously for almost a week. Their approach was to construct tinker-toy-like models of the DNA molecule, shifting atoms around into various positions. They were looking for an arrangement that would give the kind of x-ray photograph that Watson had seen in Franklin's laboratory.

Finally, on March 7, 1953, the two scientists found the answer. They built a model consisting of two helices (corkscrew-like spirals), wrapped around each other. Each helix consisted of a backbone of alternating sugar and phosphate groups. To each sugar was attached one of the four nitrogen bases, adenine, cytosine, guanine, or thymine. The sugar-phosphate backbone formed the outside of the DNA molecule, with the nitrogen bases tucked inside. Each nitrogen base on one strand of the molecule faced another nitrogen base on the opposite strand of the molecule. The base pairs were not arranged at random, however, but in such a way that each adenine was paired with a thymine, and each cytosine with a guanine.

The Watson-Crick model was a remarkable achievement, for which the two scientists won the 1954 Nobel Prize in Chemistry. The molecule had exactly the shape and dimensions needed to produce an x-ray photograph like that of Franklin's. Furthermore, Watson and Crick immediately saw how the molecule could "carry" genetic information. The sequence of nitrogen bases along the molecule, they said, could act as a genetic code. A sequence, such as A-T-T-C-G-C-T...etc., might tell a cell to make one kind of protein (such as that for red hair), while another sequence, such as G-C-T-C-T-C-G...etc., might code for a different kind of protein (such as that for blonde hair). Watson and Crick themselves contributed to the deciphering of this genetic code, although that process was long and difficult and involved the efforts of dozens of researchers over the next decade.

Watson and Crick had also considered, even before their March 7th discovery, what the role of DNA might be in the manufacture of proteins in a cell. The sequence that they outlined was that DNA in the nucleus of a cell might act as a template for the formation of a second type of nucleic acid, **RNA (ribonucleic acid)**. RNA would then leave the nucleus, emigrate to the cytoplasm and then itself act as a template for the production of protein. That theory, now known as the Central Dogma, has since been largely confirmed and has become a critical guiding principal of much research in molecular biology.

Scientists continue to advance their understanding of DNA. Even before the Watson-Crick discovery, they knew that DNA molecules could exist in two configurations, known as the "A" form and the "B" form. After the Watson-Crick discovery, two other forms, known as the "C" and "D" configurations, were also discovered. All four of these forms of DNA are right-handed double helices that differ from each other in relatively modest ways.

In 1979, however, a fifth form of DNA known as the "Z" form was discovered by Alexander Rich and his colleagues at the Massachusetts Institute of Technology. The "Z" form was given its name partly because of its zig-zag shape and partly because it is different from the more common A and B forms. Although Z-DNA was first recognized in synthetic DNA prepared in the laboratory, it has since been found in natural cells whose environment is unusual in some respect or another. The presence of certain types of proteins in the nucleus, for example, can cause DNA to shift from the B to the Z conformation. The significance and role of this most recently discovered form of DNA remains a subject of research among molecular biologists.

Donohue syndrome

Definition

Donohue syndrome, also formerly called leprechaunism, is a genetic disorder caused by mutations in the insulin receptor **gene**. W. L. Donohue first described this rare syndrome in 1948.

Description

Donohue syndrome is a disorder that causes low birth weight, unusual facial features, and failure to thrive in infants. Donohue syndrome is associated with the over-development of the pancreas, a gland located near the stomach. It is also considered to be the most insulin resistant form of **diabetes**.

Donohue syndrome results from a mutation of the insulin receptor gene which prevents insulin in the blood from being processed. Therefore, even before birth, the fetus exhibits "insulin resistance" and has high levels of unprocessed insulin in the blood. Insulin is one of two hormones secreted by the pancreas to control blood sugar (glucose) levels. Donohue syndrome is known as a progressive endocrine disorder because it relates to the growth and functions of the endocrine system, the collection of glands and organs that deliver hormones via the bloodstream.

Hormones are chemicals released by the body to control cellular function (metabolism) and maintain equilibrium (homeostasis). These hormones are released either by the endocrine system or by the exocrine system. The endocrine system consists of ductless glands that secrete hormones into the blood stream. These hormones then travel through the blood to the parts of the body where they are required. The exocrine system consists of ducted glands that release their hormones via ducts directly to the site where they are needed. The pancreas is both an endocrine and an exocrine gland. As part of the endocrine system, the pancreas acts as the original producer of estrogen and other sex hormones in fetuses of both sexes. It also regulates blood sugar through its production of the hormones insulin and glucagon. The pancreas releases insulin in response to high levels of glucose in the blood. Glucagon is released when glucose levels in the blood are low. These two hormones act in direct opposition to each other (antagonistically) to maintain proper blood sugar levels. As an exocrine gland, the pancreas secretes digestive enzymes directly into the small intestine.

In an attempt to compensate for the high blood insulin level, the pancreas overproduces glucagon as well as the female hormone estrogen and other related (estrogenic) hormones. As excess estrogen and related hormones are produced, they affect the development of the external and internal sex organs (genitalia) of the growing baby.

Insulin mediates the baby's growth in the womb through the addition of muscle and fat. A genetic link between fetal insulin resistance and low birth weight has been suggested. Without the proper processing of insulin, the fetus will not gain weight as fast as expected. Therefore, the effects of Donohue syndrome tend to become visible during the seventh month of development when the fetus either stops growing entirely or shows a noticeable slowdown in size and weight gain. This lack of growth is further evident at birth in affected infants, who demonstrate extreme thinness (emaciation), difficulty in gaining weight, a failure to thrive, and delayed maturation of the skeletal structure.

Genetic profile

Donohue syndrome is a non-sex-linked (autosomal) recessive disorder. In 1988, Donohue syndrome was identified as the first insulin receptor gene mutation directly related to a human disease. The gene responsible for the appearance of Donohue syndrome is the insulin receptor gene located at 19p13.2. Over 40 distinct mutations of this gene have been identified. Besides Donohue syndrome, other types of non-insulin-dependent (Type II) diabetes mellitus (NIDDM) can result from mutations of this gene, including Rabson-Mendenhall syndrome and type A insulin resistance.

Demographics

Donohue syndrome occurs in approximately one out of every four million live births. As in all recessive **genetic disorders**, both parents must carry the gene mutation in order for their child to have the disorder. Therefore, Donohue syndrome has been observed in cases where the parents are related by blood (consanguineous). Parents with one child affected by Donohue syndrome have a 25% likelihood that their next child will also be affected with the disease.

Signs and symptoms

Infants born with Donohue syndrome have characteristic facial features that have been said to exhibit "elfin" or leprechaun-like qualities, such as: a smallish head with large, poorly developed and low-set ears; a flat nasal ridge with flared nostrils, thick lips, a greatly exaggerated mouth width, and widely spaced eyes. They will be very thin and have low blood sugar (hypoglycemia) due to their inability to gain nutrition through insulin processing. They will exhibit delayed bone growth and maturation, and difficulty in gaining weight and developing (failure to thrive).

Donohue syndrome patients are prone to persistent and recurrent infections. Delayed bone growth not only leads to skeletal abnormalities, it also leads to a compromised immune system. Many of the chemicals used by the body to fight infection are produced in the marrow of the bones. When bone maturation is delayed, these chemicals are not produced in sufficient quantities to fight off or prevent infection.

At birth, affected individuals can also have an enlarged chest, with possible breast development, excessive hairiness (hirsutism), as well as overdeveloped external sex organs, because of increased estrogen production caused by an overactive pancreas. As an additional side effect of the increased sex hormones released in Donohue syndrome, these individuals often have extremely large hands and feet relative to their non-affected peer group. As the result of a lack of insulin, the infant is likely to have a relatively small amount of muscle mass, very little fat, and a distended abdomen (due to malnutrition). Additional symptoms of Donohue syndrome include pachyderma, or elephant skin, in which there is excess skin production causing large, loose folds; and abnormal coloration (pigmentation) of the skin. These individuals are also quite susceptible to both umbilical and inguinal hernias.

In addition to the defect in the insulin receptor gene, Donohue syndrome is associated with problems in the epidermal growth factor receptor, which controls growth of the skin. An abnormal functioning of the epidermal growth factor receptor has been identified in three unrelated individuals affected with Donohue syndrome. This suggests that the probable cause of leprechaunism is more than just the insulin receptor. These observations may help explain the physical symptom of pachyderma in those affected with Donohue syndrome. It has also been suggested that the high concentrations of insulin close to the cell membranes lead to a lowering of growth hormone receptor activity at these locations. This lowered growth hormone activity, in turn, causes slowed cellular growth which leads to systemic growth failure in affected patients.

Diagnosis

In families with a history of the disease, diagnosis *in utero* before birth of the fetus is possible through molecular **DNA** analysis of tissue samples from the chorionic villi, which are cells found in the placenta. After birth, the diagnosis of Donohue syndrome is usually made based on the blood tests that show severe insulin resistance coupled with hypoglycemia. The presence of several of the physical symptoms listed above in addition to positive results in a test for severe insulin resistance, such as an insulin receptor defect test or a fasting hypoglycemia test, is usually sufficient for a diagnosis of Donohue syndrome. The diagnosis of Donohue syndrome may be confirmed by observed cellular (histologic) changes in the ovaries, pancreas, and breast that are not normal for the age of the patient.

Treatment and management

Genetic counseling of parents with a Donohue syndrome affected child may help prevent the conception of additional children affected with this genetic disorder. After birth, affected infants may require treatment for malnutrition as well as insulin resistant diabetes. Patients with a demonstrated residual insulin receptor function may survive past infancy. In these cases, the treatment regimen must certainly include on-going insulin resistant diabetes care and dietetic counseling to assist with weight gain. It may also be necessary to administer

KEY TERMS

Autosomal—Relating to any chromosome besides the X and Y sex chromosomes. Human cells contain 22 pairs of autosomes and one pair of sex chromosomes.

Chorionic villus sampling (CVS)—A procedure used for prenatal diagnosis at 10-12 weeks gestation. Under ultrasound guidance a needle is inserted either through the mother's vagina or abdominal wall and a sample of cells is collected from around the fetus. These cells are then tested for chromosome abnormalities or other genetic diseases.

Consanguineous—Sharing a common bloodline or ancestor.

Endocrine system—A system of ductless glands that regulate and secrete hormones directly into the bloodstream.

Fibroblast—Cells that form connective tissue fibers like skin.

Hirsutism—The presence of coarse hair on the face, chest, upper back, or abdomen in a female as a result of excessive androgen production.

Histologic—Pertaining to histology, the study of cells and tissues at the microscopic level.

Hypoglycemia—An abnormally low glucose (blood sugar) concentration in the blood.

Insulin—A hormone produced by the pancreas that is secreted into the bloodstream and regulates blood sugar levels.

Insulin receptor gene—The gene responsible for the production of insulin receptor sites on cell surfaces. Without properly functioning insulin receptor sites, cells cannot attach insulin from the blood for cellular use.

Insulin resistance—An inability to respond normally to insulin in the bloodstream.

Insulin-like growth factor I—A hormone released by the liver in response to high levels of growth hormone in the blood. This growth factor is very similar to insulin in chemical composition; and, like insulin, it is able to cause cell growth by causing cells to undergo mitosis (cell division).

Pachyderma—An abnormal skin condition in which excess skin is produced that appears similar to that of an elephant (pachyderm).

Pancreas—An organ located in the abdomen that secretes pancreatic juices for digestion and hormones for maintaining blood sugar levels.

Serological—Pertaining to serology, the science of testing blood to detect the absence or presence of antibodies (an immune response) to a particular antigen (foreign substance).

growth hormone therapy to certain patients to spur growth, but this is only indicated in those individuals who show signs of functioning growth hormone receptors and no signs of higher than normal resistance to growth hormone.

The revolutionary impact of recombinant DNA technology, whereby scientists can mass produce genetic material for use in medicine, has made possible another treatment method which involves the introduction of recombinant human insulin-like growth factor 1 (rhIGF-1) into the body. A case study has been reported of a female affected with Donohue syndrome and low levels of insulin-like growth factor 1 (IGF-1), which is indicative of a higher than normal resistance to growth hormone.

Examination of the patient's fibroblasts showed normal binding of IGF-1 and normal functioning of these fibroblasts in response to IGF-1. Fibroblasts are connective tissue cells that accomplish growth in humans by differentiating into chondroblasts, collagenoblasts, and osteoblasts, all of which are the precursor cells necessary to produce bone growth in humans. This case report indicates that if enough IGF-1 could get to the fibroblasts in the patient's body, there is every reason to believe that these fibroblasts would function normally and mature into the precursor cells needed for bone growth. This finding made the patient an ideal candidate for rhIGF-1 treatments.

In this study, the long- and short-term effects on growth patterns and glucose metabolism in the patient were studied after the treatment with recombinant human insulin-like growth factor 1 (rhIGF-1). The rhIGF-1 that was not immediately utilized by the patient was rapidly destroyed in the cellular conditions produced by Donohue syndrome. Therefore, to maintain the desired levels of rhIGF-1 in the blood, the patient received rhIGF-1 both in injection form prior to every meal and via a continuous subcutaneous infusion method similar to that used to continuously pump insulin for some patients with diabetes. Recombinant human IGF-1 was administered to this patient over a period of six years with an observation of normal blood glucose levels and a return to normal growth patterns. Moreover, the treatment did not cause negative side effects. The results of this case study offer a promising new treatment for certain individuals affected with Donohue syndrome. Other clinical studies of treatments with rhIGF-1 are in progress.

Prognosis

Individuals born with Donohue syndrome generally die in infancy from either malnutrition or recurrent and persistent infection. All individuals affected with Donohue syndrome that survive past infancy have severe mental retardation and profound motor skill impairment. Survival into childhood is thought to be due to some remaining insulin receptor function and the ability of extremely high insulin concentrations to transmit signals through alternate pathways.

Resources

PERIODICALS

Desbois-Mouthon, C., et al. "Molecular analysis of the insulin receptor gene for prenatal diagnosis of leprechaunism in two families." *Prenatal Diagnosis* (July 1997): 657–63.

Hattersley, A. "The fetal insulin hypothesis: an alternative explanation of the association of low birth weight with diabetes and vascular disease." *Lancet* (May 1999): 1789–92.

Nakae, J., et al. "Long-term effect of recombinant human insulin-like growth factor I on metabolic and growth control in a patient with leprechaunism." *Journal of Clinical Endocrinology and Metabolism* (February 1998): 542–9.

Psiachou, H., et al. "Leprechaunism and homozygous nonsense mutation in the insulin receptor gene." *Lancet* (October 1993): 924.

Reddy, S., D. Muller-Wieland, K. Kriaciunas, C. Kahn. "Molecular defects in the insulin receptor in patients with leprechaunism and in their parents." *Journal of Laboratory and Clinical Medicine* (August 1989): 1359–65.

ORGANIZATIONS

Children Living with Inherited Metabolic Diseases. The Quadrangle, Crewe Hall, Weston Rd., Crewe, Cheshire, CW1-6UR. UK 127 025 0221. Fax: 0870-7700-327. <http://www.climb.org.uk>.

National Center for Biotechnology Information. National Library of Medicine, Building 38A, Room 8N805, Bethesda, MD 20894. (301) 496-2475. <http://www.ncbi.nlm.nih.gov>.

National Organization for Rare Disorders (NORD). PO Box 8923, New Fairfield, CT 06812-8923. (203) 746-6518 or (800) 999-6673. Fax: (203) 746-6481. <http://www.rarediseases.org>.

WEBSITES

OMIM—Leprechaunism. Online Mendelian Inheritance in Man. (June 17, 2005.) <http://www.ncbi.nlm.nih.gov/entrez/dispomim.cgi?id=246200>.

Paul A. Johnson

Down syndrome

Definition

Down syndrome is the most common **chromosome** disorder and genetic cause of mental retardation. It occurs because of the presence of an extra copy of chromosome 21. For this reason, it is also called trisomy 21.

Description

When a baby is conceived, the sperm cell from the father and the egg cell from the mother undergo a reduction of the total number of chromosomes from 46 to 23. Occasionally an error occurs in this reduction process and instead of passing on 23 chromosomes to the baby, a parent will pass on 24 chromosomes. This event is called nondisjunction and it occurs in 95% of Down syndrome cases. The baby therefore receives an extra chromosome at conception. In Down syndrome, that extra chromosome is chromosome 21. Because of this extra chromosome 21, individuals affected with Down syndrome have 47 instead of 46 chromosomes.

Genetic profile

In approximately one to two percent of Down syndrome cases, the original egg and sperm cells contain the correct number of chromosomes, 23 each. The problem occurs sometime shortly after fertilization—during the phase when cells are dividing rapidly. One cell divides abnormally, creating a line of cells with an extra copy of chromosome 21. This form of genetic disorder is called mosaicism. The individual with this type of Down syndrome has two types of cells: those with 46 chromosomes (the normal number), and those with 47 chromosomes (as occurs in Down syndrome). Individuals affected with this mosaic form of Down syndrome generally have less severe signs and symptoms of the disorder.

Another relatively rare genetic accident that causes Down syndrome is called translocation. During cell division, chromosome 21 somehow breaks. The broken off piece of this chromosome then becomes attached to another chromosome. Each cell still has 46 chromosomes, but the extra piece of chromosome 21 results in the signs and symptoms of Down syndrome. Translocations occur in about 3–4% of cases of Down syndrome.

Once a couple has had one baby with Down syndrome, they are often concerned about the likelihood of future offspring also being born with the disorder. Mothers under the age of 35 with one Down syndrome-affected child have a 1% chance that a second child will also be born with Down syndrome. In mothers 35 and older, the chance of a second child being affected with Down syndrome is approximately the same as for any woman at a similar age. However, when the baby with Down syndrome has the type that results from a translocation, it is possible that one of the two parents is a carrier of a balanced translocation. A carrier has rearranged chromosomal information and can pass it on, but he or she does not have an extra chromosome and therefore is not affected with the disorder. When one parent is a carrier of a translocation, the chance of future offspring having Down syndrome is greatly increased. The specific risk will have to be assessed by a genetic counselor.

Demographics

Down syndrome occurs in about one in every 800 live births. It affects an equal number of male and female babies. The majority of cases of Down syndrome occur due to an extra chromosome 21 within the egg cell supplied by the mother (nondisjunction). As a woman's age (maternal age) increases, the risk of having a Down syndrome baby increases significantly. By the time the woman is age 35, the risk increases to one in 400; by age 40 the risk increases to one in 110; and, by age 45, the risk becomes one in 35. There is no increased risk of either mosaicism or translocation with increased maternal age.

Down syndrome occurs with equal frequency across all ethnic groups and subpopulations.

Signs and symptoms

While Down syndrome is a chromosomal disorder, a baby is usually identified at birth through observation of a set of common physical characteristics. Not all affected babies will exhibit all of the symptoms discussed. There is a large variability in the number and severity of these characteristics from one affected individual to the next. Babies with Down syndrome tend to be overly quiet, less responsive to stimuli, and have weak, floppy muscles. A number of physical signs may also be present. These include: a flat appearing face; a small head; a flat bridge of the nose; a smaller than normal, low-set nose; small mouth, which causes the tongue to stick out and to appear overly large; upward slanting eyes; bright speckles on the iris of the eye (Brushfield spots); extra folds of skin located at the inside corner of each eye near the nose (epicanthal folds); rounded cheeks; small, misshapen ears; small, wide hands; an unusual deep crease across the center of the palm (simian crease); an inwardly curved little finger; a wide space between the great and the second toes; unusual creases on the soles of the feet; overly flexible joints (sometimes referred to as being double-jointed); and shorter-than-normal stature.

Other types of defects often accompany Down syndrome. Approximately 30–50% of all children with Down syndrome are found to have heart defects. A number of different heart defects are common in Down syndrome. All of these result in abnormal patterns of blood flow within the heart. Abnormal blood flow within the heart often means that less oxygen is sent into circulation throughout the body, which can cause fatigue, a lack of energy, and poor muscle tone.

Malformations of the gastrointestinal tract are present in about 5–7% of children with Down syndrome. The most common malformation is a narrowed, obstructed duodenum (the part of the intestine into which the stomach empties). This disorder, called duodenal atresia, interferes with the baby's milk or formula leaving the stomach and entering the intestine for digestion. The baby often vomits forcibly after feeding, and cannot gain weight appropriately until the defect is repaired.

Another malformation of the gastrointestinal tract that is seen in patients with Down syndrome is an abnormal connection between the windpipe (trachea) and the digestive tube of the throat (esophagus) called a tracheoesophageal fistula (T-E fistula). This connection interferes with eating and/or breathing because it allows air to enter the digestive system and/or food to enter the airway.

Other medical conditions occurring in patients with Down syndrome include an increased chance of developing infections, especially ear infections and pneumonia; certain kidney disorders; thyroid disease (especially low or hypothyroid); hearing loss; vision impairment requiring glasses (corrective lenses); and a 20 times greater chance than the population as a whole of developing leukemia.

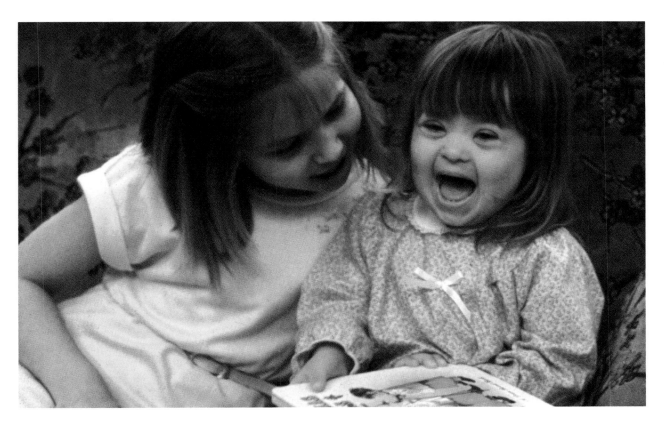

The sibling on the right has Down syndrome. *(Photo Researchers, Inc.)*

Development in a baby and child affected with Down syndrome occurs at a much slower than normal rate. Because of weak, floppy muscles (hypotonia), babies learn to sit up, crawl, and walk much later than their unaffected peers. Talking is also quite delayed. The level of mental retardation is considered to be mild-to-moderate in Down syndrome. The degree of mental retardation varies a great deal from one child to the next. While it is impossible to predict the severity of Down syndrome at birth, with proper education, children who have Down syndrome are capable of learning. Most children affected with Down syndrome can read and write and are placed in special education classes in school. The majority of individuals with Down syndrome become semi-independent adults, meaning that they can take care of their own needs with some assistance.

As people with Down syndrome age, they face an increased chance of developing the brain disease called Alzheimer's (sometimes referred to as **dementia** or senility). Most people have a 12% chance of developing Alzheimer's, but almost all people with Down syndrome will have either **Alzheimer disease** or a similar type of dementia by the age of 50. Alzheimer disease causes the brain to shrink and to break down. The number of brain cells decreases, and abnormal deposits and structural

arrangements occur. This process results in a loss of brain functioning. People with Alzheimer's have strikingly faulty memories. Over time, people with Alzheimer's disease will lapse into an increasingly unresponsive state.

As people with Down syndrome age, they also have an increased chance of developing a number of other illnesses, including cataracts, thyroid problems, **diabetes**, and seizure disorders.

Diagnosis

Diagnosis is usually suspected at birth, when the characteristic physical signs of Down syndrome are noted. Once this suspicion has been raised, **genetic testing** (chromosome analysis) can be undertaken in order to verify the presence of the disorder. This testing is usually done on a blood sample, although chromosome analysis can also be done on other types of tissue, including the skin. The cells to be studied are prepared in a laboratory. Chemical stain is added to make the characteristics of the cells and the chromosomes stand out. Chemicals are added to prompt the cells to go through normal development, up to the point where the chromosomes are most visible, prior

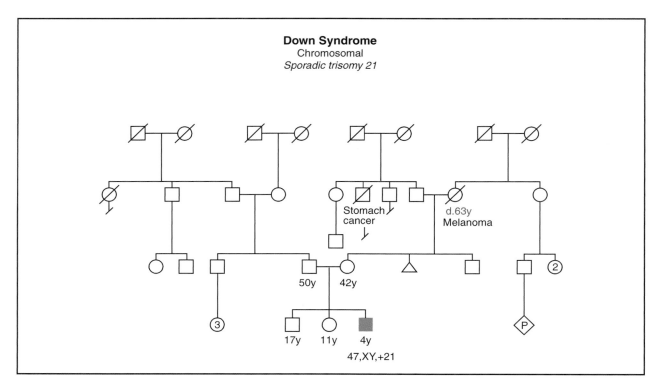

Down Syndrome
Chromosomal
Sporadic trisomy 21

(Gale Group.)

to cell division. At this point, they are examined under a microscope and photographed. The photograph is used to sort the different sizes and shapes of chromosomes into pairs. In most cases of Down syndrome, one extra chromosome 21 will be revealed. The final result of such testing, with the photographed chromosomes paired and organized by shape and size, is called the individual's **karyotype**. An individual with Down syndrome will have a 47 XX+21 karyotype if they are female and a 47 XY+21 karyotype if they are male.

Women who become pregnant after the age of 35 are offered prenatal tests to determine whether or not their developing baby is affected with Down syndrome. A genetic counselor meets with these families to inform them of the risks and to discuss the types of tests available to make a diagnosis prior to delivery. Because there is a slight risk of miscarriage following some prenatal tests, all testing is optional, and couples need to decide whether or not they desire to take this risk in order to learn the status of their unborn baby.

Screening tests are used to estimate the chance that an individual woman will have a baby with Down syndrome. A test called the maternal serum alpha-fetoprotein test (MSAFP) is offered to all pregnant women under the age of 35. If the mother decides to have this test, it is performed between 15 and 22 weeks of pregnancy. The MSAFP screen measures a protein and two hormones that are normally found in maternal blood during pregnancy. A specific pattern of these hormones and protein can indicate an increased risk for having a baby born with Down syndrome. However, this is only a risk and MSAFP cannot diagnose Down syndrome directly. Women found to have an increased risk of their babies being affected with Down syndrome are offered **amniocentesis**. The MSAFP test can detect up to 60% of all babies who will be born with Down syndrome.

Ultrasound screening for Down syndrome is also available. This is generally performed in the mid-trimester of pregnancy. Abnormal growth patterns characteristic of Down syndrome such as growth retardation, heart defects, duodenal atresia, T-E fistula, shorter than normal long-bone lengths, and extra folds of skin along the back of the neck of the developing fetus may all be observed via ultrasonic imaging.

The only way to definitively establish (with about 99% accuracy) the presence or absence of Down syndrome in a developing baby is to test tissue during the pregnancy itself. This is usually done either by amniocentesis, or chorionic villus sampling (CVS). All women under the age of 35 who show a high risk for having a

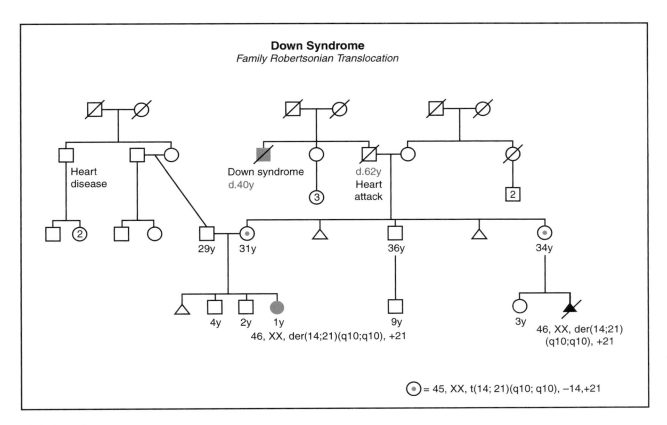

Down Syndrome
Family Robertsonian Translocation

⊙ = 45, XX, t(14; 21)(q10; q10), −14,+21

(Gale Group.)

baby affected with Down syndrome via an MSAFP screen and all mothers over the age of 35 are offered either CVS or amniocentesis. In CVS, a tiny tube is inserted into the opening of the uterus to retrieve a small sample of the placenta (the organ that attaches the growing baby to the mother via the umbilical cord, and provides oxygen and nutrition). In amniocentesis, a small amount of the fluid in which the baby is floating is withdrawn with a long, thin needle. CVS may be performed as early as 10 to 12 weeks into a pregnancy. Amniocentesis is generally not performed until at least the fifteenth week. Both CVS and amniocentesis carry small risks of miscarriage. Approximately 1% of women miscarry after undergoing CVS testing, while approximately one-half of one percent miscarry after undergoing amniocentesis. Both amniocentesis and CVS allow the baby's own karyotype to be determined.

Approximately 75% of all babies diagnosed prenatally as affected with Down syndrome do not survive to term and spontaneously miscarry. In addition, these prenatal tests can only diagnose Down syndrome, not the severity of the symptoms that the unborn child will experience. For this reason, a couple might use this information to begin to prepare for the arrival of a baby with Down syndrome, to terminate the pregnancy, or in the case of miscarriage or termination, decide whether to consider adoption as an alternative.

Treatment and management

No treatment is available to cure Down syndrome. Treatment is directed at addressing the individual concerns of a particular patient. For example, heart defects may require surgical repair, as will duodenal atresia and T-E fistula. Many Down syndrome patients will need to wear glasses to correct vision. Patients with hearing impairment benefit from hearing aids.

While some decades ago all children with Down syndrome were quickly placed into institutions for lifelong care, research shows very clearly that the best outlook for children with Down syndrome is a normal family life in their own home. This requires careful support and education of the parents and the siblings. It is a life-changing event to learn that a new baby has a permanent condition that will affect essentially all aspects of his or her development. Some community groups help families deal with the emotional effects of raising a child with Down syndrome. Schools are required to provide services to children with Down syndrome, sometimes in separate special education classrooms, and sometimes in

KEY TERMS

Chromosome—A microscopic thread-like structure found within each cell of the body and consists of a complex of proteins and DNA. Humans have 46 chromosomes arranged into 23 pairs. Changes in either the total number of chromosomes or their shape and size (structure) may lead to physical or mental abnormalities.

Karyotype—A standard arrangement of photographic or computer-generated images of chromosome pairs from a cell in ascending numerical order, from largest to smallest.

Mental retardation—Significant impairment in intellectual function and adaptation in society. Usually associated an intelligence quotient (IQ) below 70.

Mosaic—A term referring to a genetic situation in which an individual's cells do not have the exact same composition of chromosomes. In Down syndrome, this may mean that some of the individual's cells have a normal 46 chromosomes, while other cells have an abnormal 47 chromosomes.

Nondisjunction—Non-separation of a chromosome pair, during either meiosis or mitosis.

Translocation—The transfer of one part of a chromosome to another chromosome during cell division. A balanced translocation occurs when pieces from two different chromosomes exchange places without loss or gain of any chromosome material. An unbalanced translocation involves the unequal loss or gain of genetic information between two chromosomes.

Trisomy—The condition of having three identical chromosomes, instead of the normal two, in a cell.

regular classrooms (this is called mainstreaming or inclusion).

In May 2000, the genetic sequence for chromosome 21 was fully determined, which opens the door to new approaches to the treatment of Down syndrome through the development of gene-specific therapies.

Prognosis

The prognosis for an individual with Down syndrome is quite variable, depending on the types of complications (heart defects, susceptibility to infections, development of leukemia, etc.). The severity of the retardation can also vary significantly. Without the presence of heart defects, about 90% of children with Down syn-

drome live into their teens. People with Down syndrome appear to go through the normal physical changes of aging more rapidly, however. The average age of death for an individual with Down syndrome is about 50 to 55 years.

Still, the prognosis for a baby born with Down syndrome is better than ever before. Because of modern medical treatments, including antibiotics to treat infections, and surgery to treat heart defects and duodenal atresia, life expectancy has greatly increased. Community and family support allows people with Down syndrome to have rich, meaningful relationships. Because of educational programs, some people with Down syndrome are able to hold jobs.

There has only been one report of a male affected with Down syndrome becoming a father. Approximately 60% of women with Down syndrome are fully capable of having children. The risk of a woman with trisomy 21 having a child affected with Down syndrome is 50%.

Resources

BOOKS

Pueschel, Siegfried M. *A Parent's Guide to Down Syndrome: Toward a Brighter Future*. Revised ed. New York: Paul H. Brookes Publishing Co., 2000.

Selikowitz, Mark. *Down Syndrome: The Facts*. 2nd ed. London: Oxford University Press, 1997.

Stray-Gunderson, K. *Babies with Down Syndrome: A New Parents' Guide*. Kensington: Woodbine House, 1986.

PERIODICALS

Carlson, Tucker, and Jason Cowley. "When a Life is Worth Living: Down's Syndrome Children." *The Times* (29 November 1996): 18+.

Cohen, William, ed. "Health Care Guidelines for Individuals with Down Syndrome: 1999 Revision." *Down Syndrome Quarterly* (September 1999).

Hattori, M., A. Fujiyama, D. Taylor, H. Watanabe, et al. "The DNA sequence of human chromosome 21." *Nature* (18 May 2000): 311–19.

ORGANIZATIONS

National Down Syndrome Congress. 7000 Peachtree-Dunwoody Rd., Bldg 5, Suite 100, Atlanta, GA 30328-1662. (770) 604-9500 or (800) 232-6372. Fax: (770) 604-9898. ndsccenter@aol.com. <http://www.ndsccenter.org>.

National Down Syndrome Society. 666 Broadway, New York, NY 10012-2317. (212) 460-9330 or (800) 221-4602. Fax: (212) 979-2873. <http://www.ndss.org info@ndss.org>.

WEBSITES

Down Syndrome Health Issues. <http://www.ds-health.com/>. (15 February 2001).

Down Syndrome Information Network. <http://www.down-syndrome.net/>. (15 February 2001).

Down Syndrome WWW Page. <http://www.nas.com/downsyn/>. (15 February 2001).

Recommended Down Syndrome Sites on the Internet. <http://www.ds-health.com/ds_sites.htm#natl>. (15 February 2001).

Paul A. Johnson

DRPLA *see*
Dentatorubral-pallidoluysian atrophy

Duane retraction syndrome

Definition

Duane retraction syndrome is a congenital disorder that limits the movement of the eye. It may also involve other systems of the body.

Description

Duane retraction syndrome (DRS or DURS) is an inherited disorder characterized by a limited ability to move the eye to one side or the other. DRS is congenital, meaning that it is present at birth. It results from abnormal connections among the nerves that control the muscles of the eyes. About 80% of DRS cases involve one eye (unilateral) and about 20% involve both eyes (bilateral). Most unilateral DRS cases (72%) involve the left eye.

DRS was first described in 1905 by A. Duane. It also is known as: Duane syndrome (DUS)

- DR syndrome
- eye retraction syndrome
- retraction syndrome
- Stilling-Turk-Duane syndrome

DRS is one of a group of conditions known as strabismus, or misalignment of the eye. DRS is classified as an incomitant strabismus, because it is a misalignment of the eye that varies depending on the direction that the eye is gazing. It is further classified as an extraocular muscle fibrosis syndrome. This means that it is a condition associated with the muscles that move the eyes. Both the active and the passive movement of the eyeball are affected in DRS.

Physiology

DRS is believed to result from an abnormality that occurs during the development of the fetus in the womb.

It may be caused by either environmental or genetic factors, or a combination of both. The developmental abnormality is believed to occur between the third and eighth weeks of fetal development. This is the period when the ocular muscles that rotate the eye, and the cranial nerves from the brain that control the ocular muscles, are forming in the fetus.

DRS appears to result from the absence of cranial nerve VI, which is known as the abducens nerve. The nerve cells in the brain that connect to the abducens nerve are also missing. The abducens nerve controls the lateral rectus muscle of the eye. This muscle moves one eye outward toward the ear, as a person looks toward that side. This movement is called abduction. In DRS, the nerves from a branch of cranial nerve III (the oculomotor nerve) also are abnormal. The oculomotor nerve controls several eye muscles, including the medial rectus muscle. This muscle moves the eye inward toward the nose, as the person looks toward the other side. This movement is called adduction.

The majority of individuals with DRS have limited or no ability to move an eye outward toward the ear. Instead, the opening between the eyelids of that eye widens and the eyeball protrudes. In addition, individuals with DRS may have only a limited ability to move the eye inward, toward the nose. Instead, when looking inward toward the nose, the medial and lateral recti muscles contract simultaneously. This causes the eyeball to retract, or pull into the skull, and causes the opening between the eyelids to narrow, as if one were squinting. Sometimes, the eye moves up or down as the individual attempts to look in toward the nose. This is called upshoot or downshoot, respectively.

In some individuals with DRS, the eyes may cross when looking straight ahead. Gazing straight ahead is called the primary position or primary gaze. Crossed eyes may cause the person to turn the head to one side or the other, to restore binocular vision. In such individuals, this "head turn" may become habitual.

Associated syndromes

About 30-50% of individuals with DRS have associated abnormalities. These may include additional eye problems, deafness, and nervous system or skeletal abnormalities. In particular, DRS may be associated with abnormalities in the upper extremities, especially the hands. Sometimes DRS is associated with **Holt-Oram syndrome**, a hereditary heart defect.

Okihiro syndrome is DRS in association with other abnormalities that may include: flatness in the normally-fleshy region between the thumb and the wrist (the thenar eminence) of one or both hands

- inability to flex the joint in the thumb
- hearing loss or deafness in one or both ears

Okihiro syndrome also is known as:

- Duane syndrome with radial ray anomalies (as in the arms and hands)
- Duane/radial **dysplasia** syndrome (referring to abnormal tissue growth in the arms and hands)
- DR syndrome (the "D" refers to Duane anomaly and deafness; the "R" refers to radial and renal (kidney) dysplasia, or abnormal tissue growth in the arms, hands, and kidneys)
- Duane anomaly with radial ray abnormalities and deafness

Genetic profile

The genetic basis of DRS is unclear. The specific **gene** or genes that are responsible for DRS and the associated syndromes have not been identified. DRS may arise from a combination of environmental factors and defects in one or more genes.

Portions of several of the 23 pairs of human chromosomes may be associated with DRS. A gene that is involved in DRS has been localized to a region of **chromosome** 2. Deletions of portions of chromosomes 4 and 8 have also been associated with DRS. The presence of an additional small chromosome, thought to be broken off from chromosome 22, has been associated with DRS. It is possible that these chromosome rearrangements and abnormalities may account for the wide range of symptoms and syndromes that can occur with DRS.

The **inheritance** of DRS is autosomal, meaning that the trait is not carried on either the X or Y sex chromosomes. The most common type of DRS, DRS1, is inherited as an autosomal dominant trait. This means that only a single copy of a DRS gene, inherited from one parent, can result in the condition. The offspring of a parent with DRS is expected to have a 50% chance of inheriting the disorder. However, the autosomal dominant form of DRS sometimes skips a generation in the affected family; for example, a grandparent and grandchildren may have DRS, but the middle generation does not. Some forms of DRS may be recessive, requiring two copies of a gene, one inherited from each parent.

Family members may exhibit different types of DRS, indicating that the same genetic defect may be expressed by a range of symptoms. The severity of DRS also may vary among family members. Furthermore, the majority of individuals with DRS do not appear to have a family history of the disorder. There are very few reports of single families with a large number of affected individuals. However, close relatives of individuals with DRS often are affected by some of the other abnormalities that may be associated with the disorder.

Okihiro syndrome, or Duane syndrome with radial ray anomalies, and Holt-Oram syndrome both are inherited as autosomal dominant traits. However, like DRS, Okihiro syndrome may skip a generation in a family, or may be expressed by a range of symptoms within one family.

Demographics

DRS is estimated to affect 0.1% of the general population. It accounts for 1-5% of all eye movement disorders. Although it is not a sex-linked disorder, females are more likely than males to be affected by DRS (60% compared with 40%).

Signs and symptoms

Types of DRS

There are three generally-recognized types of DRS. Type 1 DRS (DRS1) accounts for about 70% of cases. With DRS1, abduction, the ability to move the eye toward the ear, is limited or absent. The eye widens and the eyeball protrudes when the eye is moved outward. In contrast, adduction, the ability to move the eye toward the nose, is normal or almost normal. However, the eye narrows and the eyeball retracts during adduction. The eyes of infants and children with DRS1 are usually straight ahead in the primary position. However, some children develop an increasing misalignment in the primary position and may compensate by turning their head.

With DRS type 2, adduction is limited or absent but abduction is normal, or only slightly limited. The eye narrows and the eyeball retracts during adduction. Type 2 accounts for approximately 7% of DRS cases.

With DRS Type 3, both abduction and adduction are limited. The eye narrows and the eyeball retracts during adduction. Type 3 accounts for about 15% of DRS cases.

Each type of DRS is subclassified, depending on the symptoms that occur when the individual is looking straight ahead (primary gaze). With subgroup A, the eye turns in toward the nose when gazing ahead. With subgroup B, the eye turns out toward the ear during a primary gaze. With subgroup C, the eyes are straight ahead in the primary position.

Associated symptoms

The majority of individuals with DRS are healthy and have no other symptoms. However, other body systems that may be affected with DRS include:

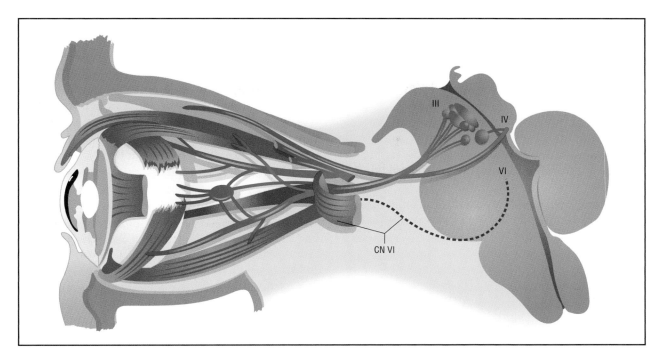

Absence of cranial nerve VI (dashed line) is indicative of Duane retraction syndrome and results in abnormal head and eye movements. *(Gale Group)*

- skeleton

- ears and hearing

- additional involvement of the eyes

- nervous system

With Okihiro syndrome, the DRS can be unilateral or bilateral. In addition to a flatness at the base of the thumb, there may be difficulty with thumb movements. There also may be abnormalities or the complete absence of the radial and ulnar bones of the forearm. In extreme cases, the thumb or forearm may be absent. Okihiro syndrome may be accompanied by hearing loss, abnormal facial appearance, and heart, kidney, and spinal abnormalities.

Sometimes Wildervanck syndrome is associated with DRS. This syndrome may include congenital deafness and a fusion of the cervical (neck) vertebrae (C2 and C3).

Diagnosis

Diagnosis of DRS usually occurs by the age of ten. The clinical evaluation includes a complete family history, an eye examination, and examinations for other eye involvement or other physical abnormalities.

Eye examinations include the following measurements:

- visual acuity or sharpness

- alignment of the eyes

- range of motion of the eyes

- retraction (pulling in) of the eyeballs

- size of the eye opening between the eyelids

- upshoots and downshoots

- head turns

Hearing tests are frequently conducted. The cervical (neck) and thoracic (chest) parts of the spine, the vertebrae, the hands, and the roof of the mouth all are included in the examination as well.

Treatment and management

Special glasses with prisms can eliminate the head turning that is associated with DRS. Vision therapy may help with secondary vision problems.

Surgery may be performed for the following cosmetic reasons: abnormalities in the primary gaze (when looking straight ahead)

- an unusual compensatory head position

- a large upshoot or downshoot

- severe retraction of the eye The goal of surgery is to reduce or eliminate the misalignment of the eye that

KEY TERMS

Abducens nerve—Cranial nerve VI; the nerve that extends from the midbrain to the lateral rectus muscle of the eye and controls movement of the eye toward the ear (abduction).

Abduction—Turning away from the body.

Adduction—Movement toward the body. In Duane retraction syndrome, turning the eye inward toward the nose.

Autosomal dominant—A pattern of genetic inheritance where only one abnormal gene is needed to display the trait or disease.

Congenital—Refers to a disorder which is present at birth.

Downshoot—Downward movement of the eye.

Dysplasia—The abnormal growth or development of a tissue or organ.

Extraocular muscle fibrosis—Abnormalities in the muscles that control eye movement.

Head turn—Habitual head position that has been adopted to compensate for abnormal eye movements.

Holt-Oram syndrome—Inherited disorder characterized by congenital heart defects and abnormalities of the arms and hands; may be associated with Duane retraction syndrome.

Lateral rectus muscle—The muscle that turns the eye outward toward the ear (abduction).

Medial rectus muscle—The muscle that turns the eye inward toward the nose (adduction).

Oculomotor nerve—Cranial nerve III; the nerve that extends from the midbrain to several of the muscles that control eye movement.

Okihiro syndrome—Inherited disorder characterized by abnormalities of the hands and arms and hearing loss; may be associated with Duane retraction syndrome.

Primary position, primary gaze—When both eyes are looking straight ahead.

Recessive—Genetic trait expressed only when present on both members of a pair of chromosomes, one inherited from each parent.

Strabismus—An improper muscle balance of the ocular muscles resulting in crossed or divergent eyes.

Upshoot—Upward movement of the eye.

---

causes abnormal head turning, as well as to reduce the retraction of the eyeball and the upshoots and downshoots. The surgery is directed at the affected muscles of the eye.

Children with DRS, as well as their siblings, require complete medical examinations to detect other abnormalities that may be associated with DRS.

Prognosis

If children with DRS go undiagnosed, a permanent loss of vision may occur. Surgical procedures may eliminate head turns and improve the misalignment of the eyes, particularly in the primary position. However, the absence of nerves for controlling the muscles of the eye cannot be corrected. Thus, no surgical procedure can completely eliminate the abnormal eye movements. However, the condition does not get worse during the course of one's life.

Resources

BOOKS

Engle, E. "The Genetics of Strabismus: Duane, Moebius, and Fibrosis Syndromes." In *Genetic Diseases of the Eye: A Textbook and Atlas.* Edited by E. Traboulsi, 477–512. New York: Oxford University Press, 1998.

PERIODICALS

Appukuttan, B., et al. "Localization of a Gene for Duane Retraction Syndrome to Chromosome 2q31." *American Journal of Human Genetics* 65 (1999): 1639–46.

Chung, M., J. T. Stout, and M. S. Borchert. "Clinical Diversity of Hereditary Duane's Retraction Syndrome." *Ophthalmology* 107 (2000): 500–03.

Evans, J.C., T. M. Frayling, S. Ellard, and N. J. Gutowski. "Confirmation of Linkage of Duane's Syndrome and Refinement of the Disease Locus to an 8.8-cM Interval on Chromosome 2q31." *Human Genetics* 106 (2000): 636–38.

ORGANIZATIONS

American Association for Pediatric Ophthalmology and Strabismus. <http://med-aapos.bu.edu/>.

Genetic Alliance. 4301 Connecticut Ave. NW, #404, Washington, DC 20008-2304. (800) 336-GENE (Helpline) or (202) 966-5557. Fax: (888) 394-3937. info@geneticalliance. <http://www.geneticalliance.org>.

March of Dimes Birth Defects Foundation. 1275 Mamaroneck Ave., White Plains, NY 10605. (888) 663-4637 or (914)

428-7100. resourcecenter@modimes.org. <http://www.modimes.org>.

National Eye Institute. National Institutes of Health. 31 Center Dr., Bldg. 31, Rm 6A32, MSC 2510, Bethesda, MD 20892-2510. (301) 496-5248. 2020@nei.nih.gov. <http://www.nei.nih.gov/>.

Schepens Eye Research Institute. 20 Staniford St., Boston, MA 02114-2500. (617) 912-0100. <http://www.eri.harvard.edu>.

WEBSITES

Cooper, Jeffrey. "Duane's Syndrome." *All About Strabismus.* Optometrists Network. 2001. (22 Apr. 2001). <http://www.strabismus.org/Duane_Syndrome.html>.

Duane's Retraction Syndrome. Yahoo! Groups. 2001. (22 Apr. 2001). <http://groups.yahoo.com/group/duanes>.

The Engle Laboratory. *Research: Duane Syndrome.* Children's Hospital Boston. (22 Apr. 2001). <http://www.tch.harvard.edu/research/engle/duane.html>.

Margaret Alic, PhD

Dubowitz syndrome

Definition

Dubowitz syndrome is a genetic disorder defined by slow growth, a characteristic facial appearance, and a small head.

Description

Dubowitz syndrome was first described in 1965 by the English physician Dr. Victor Dubowitz. This genetic disorder causes growth retardation both before and after birth. It is primarily diagnosed through the distinctive facial features of affected individuals, including a small triangular-shaped face with a high forehead and wide-set, slitted eyes. A number of other symptoms, most commonly irritation and itching of the skin (eczema), may be present in infants born with Dubowitz syndrome.

Genetic profile

Dubowitz syndrome is passed on through an autosomal recessive pattern of **inheritance**. Autosomal means that the syndrome is not carried on a sex **chromosome**, while recessive means that both parents must carry the **gene** mutation in order for their child to have the disorder. Parents with one child affected by Dubowitz syndrome have a 25% chance that their next child will also be affected with the disease.

The specific gene mutation responsible for Dubowitz syndrome had not yet been identified.

Demographics

Cases of Dubowitz syndrome have been reported from many different regions of the world with the majority coming from the United States, Germany, and Russia. There does not appear to be any clear-cut ethnic pattern to the incidence of the syndrome. Dubowitz syndrome appears to affect males and females with equal probability. The overall incidence of the disorder has not been established since it is very rare. Only about 142 cases have been reported worldwide.

Signs and symptoms

Physical characteristics

The symptoms of people diagnosed with Dubowitz syndrome vary considerably. However, the most common physical characteristics associated with Dubowitz syndrome are growth retardation, characteristic facial appearance, and a very small head (microcephaly). A wide variety of secondary physical characteristics may be present.

GROWTH RETARDATION Children born with Dubowitz syndrome usually have a low birth weight. Slower than normal growth continues after birth. Even if the infant is born in the normal range, the height and weight gradually falls toward the low end of growth curves during childhood. However, Dubowitz syndrome is not a form of dwarfism, because affected individuals have normally proportioned bodies.

FACIAL APPEARANCE The characteristic facial appearance of people with Dubowitz syndrome is the primary way in which the disorder is recognized. The face is small and often triangular in shape with a pointed, receding chin. The nose is broad with a wide or rounded tip. The eyes are set far apart and sometimes appear slitted due to a decreased distance between top and bottom eyelids or a drooping top eyelid. The forehead is high, broad, and sloping. Eyebrows and hair are thin or absent. The ears may be abnormally shaped or placed.

MICROCEPHALY Infants born with Dubowitz syndrome have primary microcephaly, or a small head size at birth. By definition, in microcephaly the circumference of the head is in the second percentile or less, meaning that 98% or more of all infants have a larger head circumference than an infant with microcephaly.

OTHER PHYSICAL CHARACTERISTICS There are many other physical characteristics that have been observed in the majority of cases of Dubowitz syndrome, although they are not present in all affected individuals. These include:

- A soft or high-pitched cry or voice
- Partial webbing of the toes
- Cleft palate or less severe palate malformations
- Genital abnormalities, including undescended testicles
- Gastroesophophageal reflux
- Inflammation and itching of the skin (eczema)

Mental and behavioral characteristics

Despite the small head size of children born with Dubowitz syndrome, developmental delay is not observed in all cases. Estimates of the incidence of developmental delay in cases of Dubowitz syndrome range from 30% to 70%, and in most cases the level of the mental retardation is rather mild.

A number of behavioral characteristics have been described by parents of children with Dubowitz syndrome as well as in the medical literature. These include:

- Extreme hyperactivity
- Temper tantrums, difficulty in self-calming
- Preference for concrete thinking rather than abstract thinking
- Language difficulties
- Shyness and aversion to crowds
- Fondness for music and rhythm

Diagnosis

Since the genetic cause is not known, there is no specific medical test that can definitively assign the diagnosis of Dubowitz syndrome. The diagnosis is usually based on the characteristic facial appearance of the affected individual as well as on other factors such as growth data and medical history. The diagnosis is easily missed if the physician is not familiar with genetic pediatric conditions.

Treatment and management

A number of chronic medical conditions are associated with Dubowitz syndrome. These include:

- Inflammation and itching of the skin (eczema)
- Susceptibility to viral infections
- Allergies

- Chronic diarrhea or constipation
- Feeding difficulties and vomiting

These conditions need to be managed individually with appropriate treatments. For example, skin creams containing corticosteroid drugs are used to treat eczema.

Other physical problems caused by Dubowitz syndrome, such as drooping eyelids (ptosis) or cardiovascular defects, can be corrected through surgery.

Prognosis

The prognosis for individuals affected by Dubowitz syndrome is good provided that management of their medical conditions is maintained. Dubowitz syndrome has not been reported to cause shortened lifespan or any degenerative conditions. People with Dubowitz syndrome can expect to survive to adulthood and lead a fairly normal lifestyle, although most have some level of mental retardation.

Resources

PERIODICALS

Tsukahara, M., and J. Opitz. "Dubowitz Syndrome: Review of 141 Cases Including 36 Previously Unreported Patients." *American Journal of Human Genetics* (1996): 277-289.

ORGANIZATIONS

Dubowitz Syndrome Nationwide Support Group Network. RR 1 Box 114, Downs, IL 61736. (309) 724-8407.

Dubowitz Syndrome Parent Support. PO Box 173, Wheatland, IN 47597. (812) 886-0575.

WEBSITES

Dubowitz Syndrome Information and Parent Support. <http://www.dubowitz.org/> (20 April 2001).

"Dubowitz Syndrome." *Online Mendelian Inheritance in Man.* <http://www.ncbi.nlm.nih.gov/htbin-post/Omim/dispmim?223370> (20 April 2001).

Paul A. Johnson

Duchenne muscular dystrophy

Definition

The group of conditions called muscular dystrophies are characterized by muscle weakness and degeneration. Duchenne is a relatively common, severe **muscular dystrophy**. Becker muscular dystrophy is less common and less severe. Becker and Duchenne muscular dystrophy were once considered to be separate conditions. In the 1990s, researchers showed that Duchenne and Becker muscular dystrophy have the same etiology (underlying cause). However, the two disorders remain distinct based on different ages on onset, rates of progression, and some distinct symptoms.

Description

Duchenne muscular dystrophy (DMD) and Becker muscular dystrophy (BMD) are both defined by progressive muscle weakness and atrophy. Both conditions are caused by a mutation in the same **gene** and usually affect only boys. Symptoms of Duchenne muscular dystrophy usually begin in childhood, and boys with DMD are often in wheelchairs by the age of 12 years. Symptoms of Becker muscular dystrophy begin later, and men with BMD typically do not require wheelchairs until their 20s.

Boys with Duchenne muscular dystrophy are usually diagnosed at a young age. Boys with Becker muscular dystrophy are diagnosed much later. Both conditions are progressive, although DMD progresses more quickly than BMD. Unfortunately, no treatments exist to slow or prevent progression of the disease. Skeletal muscles are affected initially. Eventually the muscles of the heart are also affected, and both conditions are fatal. The life expectancy of males with Duchenne and Becker is 18 years and approximately 45 years, respectively. Both conditions are caused by disorders of the muscle, not of the nerves that control the muscle.

Genetic profile

Duchenne and Becker muscular dystrophy are both caused by mutations in the DMD gene on the X **chromosome**. This is an exceptionally large gene, and control of its expression is complex.

Humans each have 46 chromosomes, of which 23 are inherited from the mother and 23 are inherited from the father. The sets of 23 chromosomes are complimentary: each contains the same set of genes. Therefore, every human has a pair of every gene. Genes are the sequences of **DNA** that encode instructions for growth,

development, and functioning. One of the 23 pairs of chromosomes may not be complimentary: the sex chromosomes. Boys have an X chromosome and a Y chromosome. Girls have two X chromosomes.

Scientists often say that every person has the same genes, and that the genes on a pair of complimentary chromosomes are the same. It is true that a specific gene at a specific place on each chromosome provides the body with a very specific instruction, i.e. plays a particular functional role. However, most genes have multiple forms. Scientists call the various forms of a gene *alleles*. A given gene may have multiple alleles that function normally and multiple alleles that lead to physical problems.

Mutations (changes) in the DMD gene cause Duchenne and Becker muscular dystrophy. The DMD gene provides instructions for a protein called dystrophin. Mutations in DMD associated with Duchenne often completely disrupt production of dystrophin, such that no dystrophin is present. Mutations in DMD associated with Becker lead to a reduced amount of dystrophin being made and/or abnormal dystrophin. Certain mutations (alleles) in the DMD gene lead to the symptoms of DMD and other mutations lead to the symptoms of BMD.

Sex linked inheritance

Because the DMD gene is on the X chromosome, Duchenne and Becker muscular dystrophy affect only boys. Most females have two X chromosomes. Thus, if a female inherits an X chromosome with a mutation in the DMD gene, she has another normal DMD gene on her other X chromosome that protects her from developing symptoms. Women who have one mutated gene and one normal gene are called *carriers*. Boys, on the other hand, have an X and a Y chromosome. The Y chromosome has a different set of genes than the X chromosome; it mostly contains genes that provide instructions for male development. If a boy has a mutation in the DMD gene on his X chromosome, he has no normal DMD gene and he has muscular dystrophy.

If a woman has one son with Duchenne or Becker and no other family history, she may or may not be a carrier. If a woman has another family member with Duchenne or Becker muscular dystrophy, *and* a son with muscular dystrophy, it is assumed that she is a carrier. The risk for a male child to inherit the mutated gene from his carrier mother is 50% with each pregnancy. Based on the family history, geneticists can determine the likelihood that a woman is or is not a carrier. Based on this estimate, risks to have a son with muscular dystrophy can be provided.

New mutations

The DMD gene is very large and new mutations are fairly common. A new mutation is a mutation that occurs for the first time, that no other members have. Approximately 1/3 of males with Duchenne who have no family history of muscular dystrophy have the condition because of a new mutation that is only present in themselves. In this case, the affected male's mother is not a carrier. Approximately 2/3 of males with Duchenne and no family history have it because of a new mutation that occurred in a relative. In other words, even if the affected male is the first in his family his mother may still be carrier. The new mutation could have happened for the first time in the affected male's mother, or the new mutation could have occurred in his maternal grandmother or grandfather (or their parents, or their parents, etc.).

Sometimes a woman or man has mutations in the DMD gene of his or her sperm or eggs, but not in the other cells of his or her body. The mutation may even be in some sperm and/or eggs but not in others. This situation is called "germline mosaicism." Germline cells are the egg and sperm cells. A woman or man with germline mosaicism may have more than one affected son even though genetic studies of his or her blood show that he or she is not a carrier. Geneticists can estimate the risk that a person has germline mosaicism, and provide information regarding the risk for a person with germline mosaicism to have a child with muscular dystrophy.

Demographics

Duchenne muscular dystrophy affects approximately one in 3,500 males. Males from every ethnicity are affected. Becker muscular dystrophy is much less common than Duchenne muscular dystrophy. The incidence of Becker muscular dystrophy is approximately one in 18,000.

Signs and symptoms

Both Becker and Duchenne muscular dystrophy initially affect skeletal muscle. Muscle weakness is the first symptom. Both conditions are progressive. Duchenne progresses more rapidly than Becker. People with Duchenne usually begin to use a wheelchair in their early teens, while people with Becker muscular dystrophy may not use a wheelchair until their twenties or later. In the late stages of both diseases, the cardiac muscles begin to be affected. Impairment of the heart and cardiac muscles leads to death. Some female carriers have mild muscle weakness.

People with muscular dystrophy often develop contractures. A contracture makes a joint difficult to move.

The joint becomes frozen in place, sometimes in a painful position. **Scoliosis** (curvature of the spine) is another common problem. Most people with Duchenne have normal intelligence, but cognition is affected in some. Cognition is not usually affected in Becker muscular dystrophy.

Dystrophin

The DMD gene contains instructions for a protein called dystrophin. Dystrophin is part of muscle cells and some nerve cells. Its function is not entirely understood. Based on its location in the muscle cell, scientists think that dystrophin may help maintain the structural integrity of muscle cells as they contract. People with Duchenne make very little or no dystrophin, and people with Becker make less than normal and/or semi-functional dystophin. When there is not enough dystrophin in the muscle, it becomes weak and starts to waste away. The muscle tissue is replaced by a fatty, fibrous tissue.

Duchenne muscular dystrophy

The first symptoms of Duchenne muscular dystrophy are usually noticed in early childhood. Delays in developmental milestones, such as sitting and standing, are common. The affected child's gait is often a characteristic waddle or toe-walk. He often stumbles, and running is difficult. While parents notice these symptoms retrospectively, and may notice them at the time, muscular dystrophy often is not suspected until additional signs are apparent. By the age of four to five years, it is difficult for the child to climb stairs or rise from a sitting position on the floor. It is around this time that the diagnosis is usually made. A particular method, called the *Gower sign* is used by the child to raise himself from sitting on the floor. These motor problems are caused by weakness in large muscles close to the center of the body (proximal).

Although some muscles, such as the calves, appear to be large and defined, the muscle is actually atrophied and weak. It appears large because deposits of fatty, fibrous tissue are replacing muscle tissue. Enlarged calves are a characteristic sign of Duchenne muscular dystrophy, and are said have pseudohypertrophy. "Pseudo" means false, "hyper" is excessive, and "trophy" is growth or nourishment. Other muscles may also have pseudohypertophy. These muscles feel firm if massaged.

The weakness begins at the center of the body (the pelvis) and progresses outward from the hips and shoulders to the large muscles of the legs, lower trunk, and arms. The weakness is symmetrical; i.e., both sides of the body are equally weak. Early signs of weakness, such as stumbling and difficulty climbing, progress to the point that the affected boy is unable to walk. Boys with Duchenne muscular dystrophy usually require wheelchairs by the age of 12 years. Eventually the muscles that support the neck are affected. The muscles of the digestive tract are affected in some males in the later stages of the disease. Contractures and scoliosis develop. Some boys also have learning disabilities or mild mental retardation.

Cardiac symptoms and life expectancy

The weakness usually affects skeletal muscles first, then cardiac muscle. Skeletal muscles are those that attach to bones and produce movement. The muscle weakness of both Duchenne and Becker muscular dystrophy progresses to affect the cardiac muscles. Weak, abnormal cardiac muscles cause breathing difficulties and heart problems. Breathing difficulties lead to lung infections, such as pneumonia. These problems are fatal in Duchenne, and often fatal in Becker. The life expectancy for a boy with Duchenne muscular dystrophy is the late teens or early twenties. The average life expectancy of males with Becker muscular dystrophy is the mid-forties.

Becker muscular dystrophy

The initial signs of Becker muscular dystrophy may be subtle. The age at which symptoms become apparent is later and more variable than that of DMD. The progression of Becker muscular dystrophy is slower than that of DMD. Like Duchenne muscular dystrophy, boys with BMD develop symmetrical weakness of proximal muscles. The calf muscles often appear especially large. Boys with Duchenne muscular dystrophy develop weakness in the muscles that support their necks, but boys with BMD do not. The incidence and severity of learning disabilities and mild mental retardation is less in Becker muscular dystrophy than in Duchenne.

The first symptoms of Becker muscular dystrophy usually appear in the twenties and may appear even later. Weakness of the quadriceps (thigh muscle) or cramping with exercise may be the first symptom. The age of onset and rate of progression are influenced by how much dystrophin is made and how well it functions. Not all males with Becker muscular dystrophy become confined to wheelchairs. If they are, the age at which they begin to use the wheelchair is later than in Duchenne. Many males with Becker muscular dystrophy are ambulatory in their twenties. However, many males with Becker eventually develop cardiac problems, even if they do not have a great deal of skeletal muscle weakness. Cardiac problems are typically fatal by the mid-40s. Some men with Becker muscular dystrophy remain ambulatory (and alive) into their sixties.

Since Duchenne and Becker muscular dystrophy are caused by a mutation (change) in the same gene, the two conditions are usually distinguished based on age of onset and rate of progression. Males with Duchenne usually require wheelchairs by the age of 12 years and males with Becker usually do not require wheelchairs until after the age of 16. However, some males with muscular dystrophy develop symptoms at an intermediate age. Similarly, some males have elevated creatine kinase and abnormal muscle biopsies but do not develop most of the symptoms typical of muscular dystrophy. Some doctors would classify these males with very mild symptoms as having "mild Becker muscular dystrophy." Some individuals who have Becker muscular dystrophy with mildly affected skeletal muscles still develop abnormalities of their cardiac muscle.

Many other forms of muscular dystrophy exist and are part of the diagnoses considered when a person develops signs of Duchenne or Becker muscular dystrophy. The symptoms of Becker muscular dystrophy, in particular, may be caused by many other conditions. However, diagnostic studies can definitively confirm whether an individual has Becker muscular dystrophy.

Affected females

It is unusual, but some females have some or all of the symptoms of muscular dystrophy. Assuming that the diagnosis is correct, this can happen for various reasons. If a woman has **Turner syndrome**, in which she has one X chromosome instead of two, she could also have Duchenne or Becker muscular dystrophy. (She has no second X chromosome with a normal DMD gene to protect her.) Alternatively, a woman may have muscular dystrophy because of random unfavorable "X inactivation," or because she has a chromosomal translocation. Rarely, she may also have inherited both X chromosomes from the same parent.

Diagnosis

The diagnosis of muscular dystrophy is based on physical symptoms, family history, muscle biopsy, measurement of creatine kinase, and **genetic testing**. Creatine kinase (CK) may also be called creatine phosphokinase or CPK. It is a protein present in skeletal muscle, cardiac muscle, and the brain.

Creatine kinase is released into the blood as muscle cells die. The level of CK in the blood is increased if a person has muscular dystrophy. The level in a male with Duchenne is often more than ten times the normal level, and the level in a male with Becker is often at least five times more than the normal level. The level of CK in the blood of female carriers is variable. Approximately 50% of Duchenne muscular dystrophy carriers have slightly to greatly elevated serum creatine kinase. Only about 30% of carriers of Becker muscular dystrophy have elevated creatine kinase. Therefore, the measurement of creatine kinase is not an accurate predictor of carrier status.

If a muscle biopsy is performed, a small piece of muscle tissue is removed from the patient. Special studies are performed on the tissue. Early in the course of the disease, the muscle shows general abnormalities. Later in the disease, the muscle tissue appears more abnormal. The fat and fibrous tissues that are replacing the muscle fibers are visible.

Another specialized test of muscle function, the electromyogram (EMG) may be performed. The EMG records the electrical activity of a muscle. This test is used to determine whether the symptoms are the result of an underlying muscle problem or a nerve problem. Nerves stimulate muscles to contract. A non-functioning muscle due to a nerve problem often causes the same symptoms as a non-functioning muscle caused by a problem with the muscle.

Genetic testing

Genetic testing is a useful diagnostic tool because the diagnosis can be made without an invasive muscle biopsy. Blood from the person suspected to have muscular dystrophy is analyzed at a specialty laboratory. Genetic testing will confirm that the DMD gene is abnormal in most males affected with muscular dystrophy (70% with DMD and 85% with BMD). The disease causing mutation will be unidentifiable in some males who have muscular dystrophy. Therefore, an abnormal test result is definitive, but a normal test result is not. In these cases, muscle biopsy may be necessary to confirm the diagnosis. Muscle biopsy may be helpful to determine whether a young person with mild symptoms has Duchenne or Becker even when the diagnosis of muscular dystrophy is established by genetic testing.

The severity of the mutation is correlated to the severity of the disease. For example, mutations that completely eliminate the dystrophin protein are associated with DMD much more often than they are associated with BMD. Particular mutations have been associated with intellectual impairment. The severity of symptoms can be somewhat predicted by the mutation present.

Even when a mutation in the DMD gene has been identified in the affected family member, genetic testing to determine whether or not the females are carriers may not be straightforward.

In some families, a special form of genetic testing called "linkage testing" may be helpful. Linkage genetic testing can be performed when the diagnosis of Duchenne or Becker muscular dystrophy is certain in more than one family member but no mutation is identified in the DMD gene. Linkage testing requires the participation of multiple family members. Unique DNA sequences within the gene and flanking the gene are analyzed to determine whether the sequences are those associated with the deleterious gene or with the normal gene. This method is not 100% accurate.

If a woman knows that she is a carrier, prenatal and preimplantation diagnosis are available. If the specific DMD or BMD mutation has been identified in a family member, genetic testing can be performed on the fetus. The procedures used to obtain fetal cells are chorionic villus sampling (CVS) and **amniocentesis**. CVS is usually performed between 10 and 12 weeks of pregnancy, and amniocentesis is usually performed after 16 weeks. Whether amniocentesis or CVS is performed, chromosomal analysis of the fetal cells will show whether the baby is male or female. Linkage testing may also be performed prenatally.

Treatment and management

There is no cure for muscular dystrophy. However, doctors are getting better at treating the symptoms. Many researchers are searching for preventative measures and for a cure. Currently, therapies focus on treating the associated symptoms.

Preventative measures

Exercise and physical therapy help to prevent joint contractures and maintain mobility. Avoiding obesity is important. Orthopedic devices may delay the age at which an affected boy begins to use a wheelchair, and are often used to treat scoliosis. Motorized wheelchairs and other devices help an affected person who has become disabled to maintain his independence as long as possible. When the cardiac muscles become affected, respiratory care may be necessary. Cardiac function should be evaluated in adult males with Becker muscular dystrophy even when skeletal muscles are mildly affected. Some women who are carriers of Duchenne muscular dystrophy develop heart disease related to changes in their cardiac muscle. Therefore, surveillance for heart disease should be a consideration for women who are carriers of DMD.

KEY TERMS

Cardiac muscle—The muscle of the heart.

Chromosome—A microscopic thread-like structure found within each cell of the body and consists of a complex of proteins and DNA. Humans have 46 chromosomes arranged into 23 pairs. Changes in either the total number of chromosomes or their shape and size (structure) may lead to physical or mental abnormalities.

Contracture—A tightening of muscles that prevents normal movement of the associated limb or other body part.

Mutation—A permanent change in the genetic material that may alter a trait or characteristic of an individual, or manifest as disease, and can be transmitted to offspring.

Scoliosis—An abnormal, side-to-side curvature of the spine.

Skeletal muscle—Muscles under voluntary control that attach to bone and control movement.

Translocation—The transfer of one part of a chromosome to another chromosome during cell division. A balanced translocation occurs when pieces from two different chromosomes exchange places without loss or gain of any chromosome material. An unbalanced translocation involves the unequal loss or gain of genetic information between two chromosomes.

X inactivation—Sometimes called "dosage compensation." A normal process in which one X chromosome in every cell of every female is permanently inactivated.

Experimental therapies

Some researchers are trying to deliver normal dystrophin protein to the muscle. If this were done by **gene therapy**, a normal copy of the DMD gene would be inserted into the muscle cells. Neither gene therapy nor dystrophin protein replacement is available, however. In fact, this research is in the early stages. But the theoretical possibility gives researchers hope that in the future there may be a cure.

Researchers have also experimentally transferred healthy muscle cells into the tissue of individuals with muscular dystrophy. This is not a standard treatment. However, it provides another hope that in the future an effective treatment will be developed.

Claims have been made that a class of medications called corticosteroids slows the progression of muscle destruction in muscular dystrophy. The use of these drugs is controversial. Corticosteroids have not been proven to have a long-term effect. Also, corticosteroids have many serious side effects. Cortisone is a corticosteroid, and prednisone is similar to cortisone.

Discovering the DMD gene allowed researchers to create animal models for muscular dystrophy. They have created mice and other animals that have Duchenne muscular dystrophy in order to more effectively study the disease and test the efficacy of treatments. This development also provides hope for the future.

Prognosis

The prognosis of Duchenne muscular dystrophy is confinement to a wheelchair by the age of 12 years, and usually death by the late teens or early twenties. The prognosis for Becker muscular dystrophy varies. Some individuals with BMD require a wheelchair after 16 years of age, but others remain ambulatory into middle adulthood. Some mildly affected individuals never require a wheelchair. The average life expectancy for Becker muscular dystrophy is the mid-forties. Both conditions are progressively debilitating.

Because Duchenne is a relatively common and severe condition, many people very actively promote further funding, research, and support of affected individuals. Associations to help families with muscular dystrophy have chapters all over the world. Families and researchers are hopeful that the genetic discoveries of the 1990s will lead to new treatments and cures in the next millennium. However, the obstacles between understanding the pathogenesis of a disease and creating an effective treatment are large. This is especially true of muscular dystrophy.

Resources

BOOKS

Bayley, Susan C. *Our Man Sam: Making the Most Out of Life with Muscular Dystrophy.* 1998.

Bergman, Thomas. *Precious Time: Children Living with Muscular Dystrophy.* Stevens, Gareth Inc., 1996.

Burnett, Gail Lemley. *Muscular Dystrophy, Health Watch Series.* Enslow Publishers, Inc., 2000.

Emery, Alan. *Muscular Dystrophy, Oxford Medical Publications.* 2nd ed. New York: Oxford University Press, Inc., 2000.

Lockshin, Michael. *Guarded Prognosis: A Doctor and His Patients Talk About Chronic Disease and How to Cope with It.* New York: Hill and Wang, 1998.

Siegal, Irwin M. *Muscular Dystrophy in Children: A Guide for Families.* Demos Medical Publishing, Inc., 1999.

PERIODICALS

Leahy, Michael. "A Powerful Swimmer, Boy with Muscular Dystrophy Relishes Competition." *The Washington Post* (29 July 1999).

ORGANIZATIONS

Muscular Dystrophy Association. 3300 East Sunrise Dr., Tucson, AZ 85718. (520) 529-2000 or (800) 572-1717. <http://www.mdausa.org>.

Muscular Dystrophy Campaign. 7-11 Prescott Place, London, SW4 6BS. UK +44(0) 7720 8055. info@muscular-dystrophy.org. <http://www.muscular-dystrophy.org>.

Muscular Dystrophy Family Foundation. 615 North Alabama St., Ste. 330, Indianapolis, IN 46204-1213. (317) 632-8255 or (800) 544-1213. mdff@prodigy.net. <http://www.mdff.org>.

Parent Project for Muscular Dystrophy Research. 1012 N. University Blvd., Middletown, OH 45042. (413) 424-0696 or (800) 714-5437. parentproject@aol.com. <http://www.parentdmd.org>.

WEBSITES

Iowa Health Book: Orthopaedics. "Treating Scoliosis in Muscular Dystrophy." <http://www.vh.org/Patients/IHB/Ortho/Peds/Scoliosis/MD/ScoliosisMD.html>.

Leiden University Medical Center, Netherlands. "Information for Non-scientists on Muscular Dystrophies." <http://dmd.nl/nonsciuk.html>.

National Center for Biotechnology Information. "Duchenne Muscular Dystrophy." <http://www.ncbi.nlm.nih.gov/disease/DMD.html>.

National Institute of Neurological Disorders and Stroke. "NINDS Muscular Dystrophy Information Page." <http://nindsiis2.ninds.nih.gov/health_and_medical/disorders/md.htm>.

OTHER

Facts About Duchenne and Becker Muscular Dystrophies (DMD and BMD). Booklet. Muscular Dystrophy Association. <http://www.mdausa.org/publications/fa-dmdbmd.html>.

Muscular Dystrophy. Videotape. Dartmouth-Hitchcock Medical Center. <http://www.dartmouth.edu/~drisin/videos/md.shtml>.

A Teacher's Guide to Duchenne Muscular Dystrophy. Booklet. Muscular Dystrophy Association. <http://www.mdausa.org/publications/tchrdmd/index.html>.

Michelle Q. Bosworth, MS, CGC

Dwarfism *see* **Pituitary dwarfism syndrome**

Dyschondrosteosis

Definition

Dyschondrosteosis (DCO) is a genetic form of dwarfism characterized by short forearms, short lower legs, normal-sized torso, normal-sized head, and a wrist and arm bone abnormality called Madelung deformity.

Description

Dyschondrosteosis (DCO) was first described by Leri and Weill in 1929. Leri and Weill described patients with dwarfism characterized by short lower legs, normal-sized torso, and a specific wrist and arm bone abnormality called Madelung's deformity. Other names for DCO include Leri-Weill dyschondrosteosis (LWD), Leri-Weill syndrome (LWS), Leri-Weill disease, Mesomelic dwarfism- Madelung deformity, Lamy-Bienefeld syndrome, Langer's syndrome, Langer's mesomelic dwarfism, and Langer's mesomelic **dysplasia**.

Genetic profile

Dyschondrosteosis (DCO) is a pseudoautosomal dominant condition caused by a change or mutation in one of two genes called SHOX and SHOY. The SHOX **gene** is located on the short arm of the X **chromosome** in the pseudoautosomal region (Xpter-p22.32). SHOY is located on the Y chromosome in the pseudoautosomal region (Ypter-p11.2). Chromosomes are the structures found in all cells that contain genes. In each cell, there are 46 chromosomes, which come in 23 pairs. One member of each pair comes from the mother, and the other from the father. The first 22 pairs are called autosomes, and are the same in males and females. The last pair of chromosomes is the sex chromosomes, X and Y. Females have two X chromosomes and males have one X chromosome and one Y chromosome. On the sex chromosomes, there are regions that contain the same genes. These regions are called the pseudoautosomal region because the genes in those regions behave as if they were on an autosomal chromosome and are the same in males and females. In 2004, it was found that 70% of families affected by DCO have a mutation in the SHOX gene. The remaining families have a mutation in the SHOY gene, or possibly another gene related to the SHOX and SHOY genes that leads to problems in bone development.

When DCO is caused by a mutated SHOX or SHOY gene, it is inherited through the family in an pseudoautosomal dominant pattern. In a pseudoautosomal dominant condition, only one nonworking copy of the gene for a particular condition is necessary for a person to experience symptoms of the condition. If a parent has a pseudoautosomal dominant condition, there is a 50% chance for each child to have the same or similar condition. DCO can also appear in an individual for the first time, and not be found in the affected individual's parents. An individual who is the first member of the family to be affected by DCO passes DCO to their children in a pseudoautosomal dominant pattern of **inheritance**. Accordingly, the individual who has *de novo* (new) DCO has the same 50% chance to have affected children.

Individuals inheriting the same nonworking gene in the same family can have very different symptoms. For example, some family members affected by DCO may be affected by proportional dwarfism with no visible arm bone deformity, while other family member may have very short (mesomelic) arms and legs and severe Madelung deformity. The difference in physical findings within the same family is known as variable penetrance, or intrafamilial variability.

Studies in 1998 and 1999 suggested that another form of severe dwarfism, called Langer mesomelic dysplasia, is the result of inheriting two copies of the mutated gene that causes DCO. Langer mesomelic dysplasia is characterized by severe short stature with underdeveloped or missing arm bones.

Demographics

Dyschondrosteosis (DCO) is a rare genetic condition. The ethnic origins of individuals affected by DCO are varied, and DCO is not more common in any specific ethnicity. There are more females than males affected by DCO, and females affected by DCO appear to be more severely affected than males.

Signs and symptoms

Most individuals affected by Dyschrondrosteosis have short stature, short lower legs and forearms (mesomelia), normal head size, normal torso size, and a specific form of arm bone abnormality called Madelung deformity. Madelung deformity occurs when one of the bones of the forearms (the radius) is short and bends toward the shortened and partially dislocated and bent ulna (subluxation), which causes the wrist to be shifted toward the thumb. Affected individuals may also exhibit abnormalities of the large bone of the upper arm (humerus), abnormal bony growths projecting outward from the surface of the shin bones (exostoses of the tibia), unusually short, broad bones in the fingers and toes, and abnormalities of the hipbones. One study in 2000 found that some males have overdeveloped muscles (or muscular hypertrophy). There is

also some evidence that conductive hearing loss may be found as a symptom in some individuals. Depending on the individual, DCO can result in severe to very mild symptoms (variable expression). Females affected by DCO tend to have more severe symptoms, including a more frequent occurrence of Madelung deformity.

Some individuals affected by DCO can also be affected by other symptoms not usually considered part of the DCO features. These features, such as mental retardation, Hodgkin's lymphoma, kidney disease, and skin disorders, are believed to be caused by errors in genes close to the mutated SHOX or SHOY gene. In 1995, based on a finding of two sisters with dyschondrosteosis who both developed Hodgkin's lymphoma in late adolescence, it was suggested that a gene that increased the risk to develop Hodgkin's lymphoma may be located very near to the SHOX and SHOY genes. Individuals affected by Hodgkin's lymphoma, or other unusual symptoms, and DCO are most likely affected by an Xp22.3 contiguous gene syndrome. The name refers to a syndrome caused by the deletion or incorrect working of several genes found side-by-side on the X chromosome.

Diagnosis

Diagnosis of dyschondrosteosis is usually made from physical examination by a medical geneticist and x rays of the legs and arms. The characteristic Madelung deformity of the arms is generally not yet present in children through physical exam, but the first signs of the Madelung deformity, like forearm bone bowing, can be identified by x rays between children aged 2–5 years. The condition's characteristic bone abnormalities become more pronounced during adolescence. Clinical **genetic testing** for dyschondrosteosis is now available to examine portions of the SHOX or SHOY genes to look for a mutation that would cause the gene not to work correctly. Although clinical testing is available, testing cannot identify all mutations causing DCO. Physical exam and x rays may diagnosis an individual without an identifiable mutation SHOX or SHOY. In families in which a mutation is identified, prenatal diagnosis through **amniocentesis** is available.

Treatment and management

Dyschondrosteosis (DCO) is a genetic disorder and does not have a specific therapy that removes, cures, or fixes all signs of the condition. Treatment and management of DCO focuses on treatment of specific symptoms of the disorder. Some progress in increasing height has been made by growth hormone (GH) supplementation in affected children. However, hormone supplementation

KEY TERMS

Madelung's deformity—A forearm bone malformation characterize by a short forearm, a arced or bow-shaped radius, and dislocation of the ulna, resulting in wrist abnormalities.

Mesomelia—Shortness of the portion of arm connecting the elbow to the wrist or forearm.

Pseudoautosomal dominant inheritance—The pattern of inheritance for a disorder caused by genes in the pseudoautosomal regions of the sex chromosomes. Individuals only require one mutated or nonworking copy of a gene to have signs and symptoms of the disorder. Affected individuals have a 50% chance to have an affected child with each pregnancy.

Pseudoautosomal region—Genes found on the sex chromosomes that contain the same genetic information whether they are on the X or Y chromosome.

causes disproportionate growth, leading to longer arms and trunk and shorter legs. The Madelung deformity found in many individuals with DCO can be treated surgically by addressing the deforming bone ligaments, correcting the abnormal position of the lower arm bones, and equalizing the length of the arm's radius and ulna bones. Operative treatment for the Madelung deformity is indicated for pain relief and appearance of the arm and wrist, but may not greatly improve the wrists' range of motion. Individuals with conductive hearing loss may wish to consider surgery or hearing aids to improve hearing.

Prognosis

The symptoms of individuals affected by DCO can be severe or mild, and prognosis depends on the severity of the symptoms. Severe Madelung deformity may cause pain in adolescence that is most often relieved through surgery. Individuals affected by DCO are of short stature and may need adjustments in their living space to optimize their living conditions. Individuals affected by DCO have an excellent prognosis.

Resources

BOOKS

Rieser, Patricia, and Heino F. L. Mayer-Bahlburg. *Short and OK: A Guide for Parents of Short Children*. Falls Church, VA: Human Growth Foundation, 1997.

PERIODICALS

Binder, G., et al. "SHOX Haploinsufficiency and Leri-Weill Dyschondrosteosis: Prevalence and Growth Failure in Relation to Mutation, Sex, and Degree of Wrist Deformity." *J Clin Endocrinol Metab*. 89, no. 9 (September 2004): 4403–08.

ORGANIZATIONS

Human Growth Foundation. 997 Glen Cove Road, Glen Head, NY 11545. (516) 671-4041 or (800) 451-6434. E-mail: hgf1@hgfound.org. (April 9, 2005.) <http://www.hgfound.org>.

Little People of America, Inc. P.O. Box 65030Lubbock, TX 79464-5030. (888) 572-2001. E-mail: lpadatabase@juno.com. (April 9, 2005.) <http://www.lpaonline.org>.

MAGIC Foundation for Children's Growth. 6645 West North Avenue, Oak Park, IL 60302. (708) 383-0808 or (800) 362-4423. E-mail: mary@magicfoundation.org. (April 9, 2005.) <http://www.magicfoundation.org>.

WEB SITES

On-line Mendelian Inheritance in Man (OMIM). (April 9, 2005.) <http://www.ncbi.nlm.nih.gov/entrez/dispomim.cgi?id=158300>.

Support group for people with dyschondrosteosis (DCS)and/or Madelung wrist deformity (MWD). (April 9, 2005.) <http://www.divdev.fsnet.co.uk/dysch.htm>.

Dawn Jacob Laney

Dysplasia

Definition

Dysplasia is a combination of two Greek words; *dys-*, which means difficult or disordered; and *plassein*, to form. In other words, dysplasia is the abnormal or disordered organization of cells into tissues. All abnormalities relating to abnormal tissue formation are classified as dysplasias.

Description

Tissues displaying abnormal cellular organization are called dysplastic. Dysplasias may occur as the result of any number of stimuli. Additionally dysplasia may occur as a localized or a generalized abnormality. In a localized dysplasia, the tissue abnormality is confined to the tissue in a single area, or body part. In a generalized dysplasia, the abnormal tissue is an original defect leading to structural consequences in different body parts.

Localized dysplasia

Localized dysplasia may occur as the result of any number of stimuli and affect virtually any organ. Stimuli leading to localized dysplasia may include viruses, chemicals, mechanical irritation, fire, or even sunlight. Sunburned skin, for example, is dysplastic. The dysplasia caused from sunburn, however, corrects itself as the sunburned skin heals.

Any source of irritation causing inflammation of an area will result in temporary dysplasia. Generally, when the source of irritation is removed the dysplasia will correct itself. Removing the irritant generally allows cell structure and organization to return to normal in a localized dysplasia.

Unfortunately, dysplasia can become permanent. This can occur when a source of irritation to a given area cannot be found and removed, or for completely unknown reasons. A continually worsening area of dysplasia can develop into an area of malignancy (**cancer**). Tendencies toward dysplasia can be genetic. They may also result from exposure to irritants or toxins, such as cigarette smoke, viruses, or chemicals.

The Pap smear, a medical procedure commonly performed on women, is a test for dysplasia of a woman's cervix. The cervix is the opening to a woman's uterus that extends into the vagina. It is a common area where cancers may develop. A Pap smear involves sampling the outer cells of a woman's cervix to look for microscopic cellular changes indicative of dysplasia, or abnormal tissue changes. Less than five percent of Pap smears indicate cervical dysplasia. Cervical dysplasia is most common in women who are 25–35 years old.

The degree of dysplasia present in cervical cells can be used as an indicator for progression to a cancerous condition. Early treatment of cervical dysplasia is very effective in halting progression of the dysplasia to cancer. Essentially, all sexual risk factors correlate with dysplasia. Exposure to the AIDS virus (HIV) or certain strains of human papilloma virus (HPV) raises a woman's risk to develop cervical dysplasia. Increased risk is also linked to having unprotected sex at an early age, having unprotected sex with many partners, or becoming pregnant before age 20. Smoking increases a woman's risk to develop cervical dysplasia. Prenatal exposure to diethylstilbestrol (DES), a hormonal drug prescribed from 1940 to 1971 to reduce miscarriages, also increases a woman's risk for cervical dysplasia. Exactly how these risk factors are connected to cervical dysplasia is not well understood.

The American Cancer Society recommends that all women begin yearly Pap tests at age 18, or when they

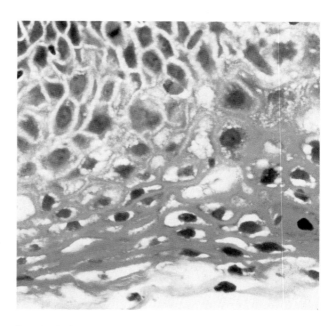

Dysplasia is characterized by abnormal cell organization in body tissues. The tissue sample above shows a variety of cell shapes and arrangements typical of this disorder. *(Photo Researchers, Inc.)*

become sexually active, whichever occurs earlier. If a woman has had three negative annual Pap tests in a row, this test may be done less often at the judgment of a woman's health care provider.

Generalized dysplasia

A generalized dysplasia often presents as multiple malformations in a variety of structures. Any structural consequences are due to the particular tissue organization defect and the spectrum of organs that utilize the dysplastic tissue. Generalized dysplasias are often genetic. They may be inherited or occur due to a new genetic change in an individual. The structural problems associated with generalized dysplasias usually begin during embryonic development.

This type of dysplasia is classified according to the specific tissue affected. Generalized dysplasias account for some important groups of inherited disorders including the skeletal dysplasias and ectodermal dysplasias.

SKELETAL DYSPLASIAS Skeletal dysplasias affect the growth, organization, and development of the bony skeleton. These conditions are always genetic. The effects of skeletal dysplasias vary. A mild **skeletal dysplasia** may cause someone to be of shortened height without any other complication. Other skeletal dysplasias may severely reduce height, causing dwarfism with disproportion and other bone deformity. The most severe

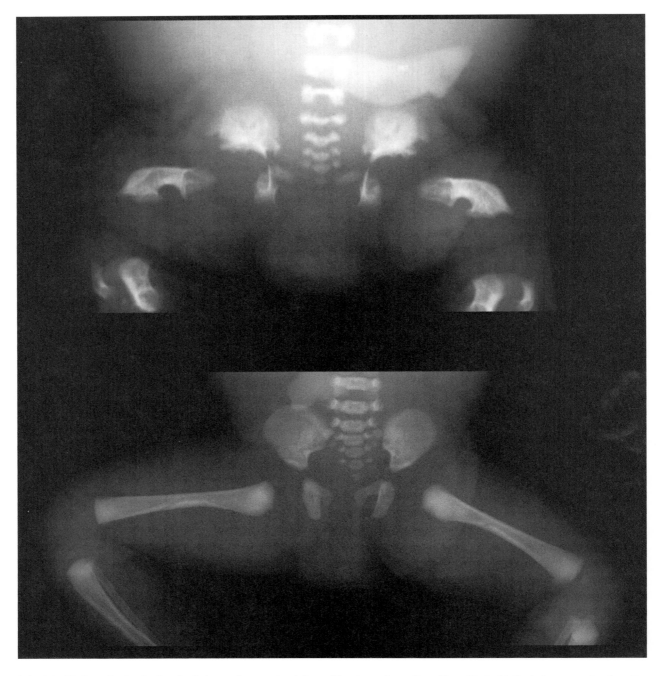

Infants with thanatophoric dysplasia have abnormal pelvic and leg bone formation. The affected infant shown on top has the characteristic "telephone receiver" shape. An infant with normal bone formation is shown on the bottom for comparison. *(Greenwood Genetic Center.)*

skeletal dysplasias are incompatible with life, causing babies to die before or soon after birth.

The skeletal dysplasias include **achondroplasia**, **hypochondroplasia**, **thanatophoric dysplasia**, **achondrogenesis**, **diastrophic dysplasia**, atelosteogenesis, **spondyloepiphyseal dysplasia**, Kniest dysplasia, **Stick-**

ler syndrome, pseudoachondoplasia, **metaphyseal dysplasia**, and several others.

Achondroplasia is a common, highly recognizable skeletal dysplasia. This disorder occurs in approximately one in 20,000 live births. Achondroplasia affects bone growth resulting in short stature, a large head, characteris-

KEY TERMS

Acondroplasia—An autosomal dominant form of dwarfism caused by a defect in the formation of cartilage at the ends of long bones. Affected individuals typically have short limbs, a large head with a prominent forehead and flattened profile, and a normal-sized trunk.

Amastia—A birth defect involving absent breast(s).

Amniocentesis—A procedure performed at 16-18 weeks of pregnancy in which a needle is inserted through a woman's abdomen into her uterus to draw out a small sample of the amniotic fluid from around the baby. Either the fluid itself or cells from the fluid can be used for a variety of tests to obtain information about genetic disorders and other medical conditions in the fetus.

Autosomal—Relating to any chromosome besides the X and Y sex chromosomes. Human cells contain 22 pairs of autosomes and one pair of sex chromosomes.

Cartilage—Supportive connective tissue which cushions bone at the joints or which connects muscle to bone.

Chondrocyte—A specialized type of cell that secretes the material which surrounds the cells in cartilage.

Chorionic villus sampling (CVS)—A procedure used for prenatal diagnosis at 10-12 weeks gestation. Under ultrasound guidance a needle is inserted either through the mother's vagina or abdominal wall and a sample of cells is collected from around the early embryo. These cells are then tested for chromosome abnormalities or other genetic diseases.

Chromosome—A microscopic thread-like structure found within each cell of the body and consists of a complex of proteins and DNA. Humans have 46 chromosomes arranged into 23 pairs. Changes in either the total number of chromosomes or their shape and size (structure) may lead to physical or mental abnormalities.

Cleft palate—A congenital malformation in which there is an abnormal opening in the roof of the mouth that allows the nasal passages and the mouth to be improperly connected.

Clubfoot—Abnormal permanent bending of the ankle and foot. Also called *talipes equinovarus*.

Collagen—The main supportive protein of cartilage, connective tissue, tendon, skin, and bone.

Corpus callosum—A thick bundle of nerve fibers deep in the center of the forebrain that provides communications between the right and left cerebral hemispheres.

***de novo* mutation**—Genetic mutations that are seen for the first time in the affected person, not inherited from the parents.

Deoxyribonucleic acid (DNA)—The genetic material in cells that holds the inherited instructions for growth, development, and cellular functioning.

DNA mutation analysis—A direct approach to the detection of a specific genetic mutation or mutations using one or more laboratory techniques.

Dysplasia—The abnormal growth or development of a tissue or organ.

Ectoderm—The outermost of the three embryonic cell layers, which later gives rise to the skin, hair, teeth, and nails.

Ectrodactyly—A birth defect involving a split or cleft appearance of the hands and/or feet, also referred to as a "lobster-claw malformation."

Epiphyses—the growth area at the end of a bone.

Fetus—The term used to describe a developing human infant from approximately the third month of pregnancy until delivery. The term embryo is used prior to the third month.

Fibroblast—Cells that form connective tissue fibers like skin.

Founder effect—Increased frequency of a gene mutation in a population that was founded by a small ancestral group of people, at least one of whom was a carrier of the gene mutation.

Gene—A building block of inheritance, which contains the instructions for the production of a particular protein, and is made up of a molecular sequence found on a section of DNA. Each gene is found on a precise location on a chromosome.

Genitals—The internal and external reproductive organs in males and females.

Gonads—The organ that will become either a testis (male reproductive organ) or ovary (female reproductive organ) during fetal development.

Hallucal polydactyly—The appearance of an extra great toe.

(continued)

KEY TERMS (CONTINUED)

Hormone—A chemical messenger produced by the body that is involved in regulating specific bodily functions such as growth, development, and reproduction.

Hypertelorism—A wider-than-normal space between the eyes.

Hyperthermia—Body temperature that is much higher than normal (i.e. higher than 98.6°F).

Hypochondroplasia—An autosomal dominant form of dwarfism whose physical features are similar to those of achondroplasia but milder. Affected individuals have mild short stature and a normal facial appearance.

Linkage analysis—A method of finding mutations based on their proximity to previously identified genetic landmarks.

Metacarpal—A hand bone extending from the wrist to a finger or thumb.

Metaphyses—The growth zone of the long bones located between the epiphyses the ends (epiphyses) and the shaft (diaphysis) of the bone.

Mutation—A permanent change in the genetic material that may alter a trait or characteristic of an individual, or manifest as disease, and can be transmitted to offspring.

Nanism—Short stature.

Ovary—The female reproductive organ that produces the reproductive cell (ovum) and female hormones.

Philtrum—The center part of the face between the nose and lips that is usually depressed.

Sulfate—A chemical compound containing sulfur and oxygen.

Testes—The male reproductive organs that produce male reproductive cells (sperm) and male hormones.

Tetralogy of Fallot—A congenital heart defect consisting of four (tetralogy) associated abnormalities: ventricular septal defect (VSD—hole in the wall separating the right and left ventricles); pulmonic stenosis (obstructed blood flow to the lungs); the aorta "overrides" the ventricular septal defect; and thickening (hypertrophy) of the right ventricle.

Tissue—Group of similar cells that work together to perform a particular function. The four basic types of tissue include muscle, nerve, epithelial, and connective tissues.

Vertebra—One of the 23 bones which comprise the spine. *Vertebrae* is the plural form.

---

tic facial features, and disproportionately short arms and legs. This disorder is caused by a mutation in a single **gene** called fibroblast growth gactor receptor three (FGFR3). Achondroplasia may be inherited like most generalized dysplasias, but more commonly it occurs due to a new mutation in a family. Over 80% of cases of achondroplasia are sporadic, or due to new mutations. The appearance of new mutations for achondroplasia is more frequently observed in children born to older fathers.

Hypochondroplasia is a common, milder skeletal dysplasia caused by different mutations in the gene responsible for achondroplasia, the FGFR3 gene. People with hypochondroplasia display varying degrees of short stature and disproportion of limbs. People with mild symptoms may never be diagnosed. The body of a person with hypochondroplasia appears short and broad with a long torso and short limbs. Life span is normal. Like achondroplasia, hypochondroplasia is inherited in an autosomal dominant manner.

ECTODERMAL DYSPLASIAS Ectodermal dysplasias affect the growth and development of tissues derived

from the early outer layer of embryonic tissue known as the ectoderm. Tissues derived from the ectoderm include hair, fingernails, skin, sweat glands, and teeth. People with ectodermal dysplasias display abnormalities in at least two derivatives of the ectoderm. **Ectodermal dysplasia** (ED) can take many different forms because so many tissues are derived from the ectoderm. Over 150 types of ectodermal dysplasias have been identified.

The effects of ectodermal dysplasias range from mild to severe. They are divided into two major groups based on the presence or absence or normal sweating. Sweat production is normal in hidrotic (sweating) types and reduced in hypohidrotic (decreased sweating) types. Types with reduced or absent sweating are generally more severe.

Christ-Siemens-Touraine syndrome (CST), a hypohidrotic (decreased sweating) ectodermal dysplasia, is a common, well-understood type of ectodermal dysplasia. People with this type of ectodermal dysplasia are not able to sweat or form tears normally. They are very sensitive to light and are not able to control their body temperature well due to their reduced sweating. Intelligence is normal. People with CST often have small or missing teeth, eyebrows, and eyelashes. Head hair is usually sparse, but fingernails are normal. CST is usually X-linked recessive, affecting only males with full symptoms of the disease. In some cases, female carriers show mild symptoms of the disease. Rarer autosomal dominant and autosomal recessive forms can affect males and females.

Clouston ectodermal dysplasia, a hidriotic (sweating) ectodermal dysplasia, also known as ectodermal Dysplasia 2 (ED2) is found more commonly in people of French Canadian descent. People with this form of ED have partial to total baldness with normal teeth, severely abnormal fingernails, and darkly pigmented areas of skin, especially over joints. They have underdeveloped eyebrows and eyelashes and may be born with teeth. They may also have thickened skin on the soles of their feet and the palms of their hands. Features including mental retardation and strabismus, or crossed eyes, may occur with this disorder, however intelligence is usually normal. This form of ED is inherited in an autosomal dominant manner. Any affected person has a 50% chance to pass the disorder to each of their children.

Resources

BOOKS

Moore, Keith L. *The Developing Human: Clinically Oriented Embryology.* Philadelphia: W.B. Saunders Company, 1998.

PERIODICALS

Wright, Michael J. "Hypochondroplasia." *Gene Map Locus* (2001): 16.

ORGANIZATIONS

American Cancer Society. 1599 Clifton Rd. NE, Atlanta, GA 30329. (800) 227-2345. <http://www.cancer.org>.

Children's Craniofacial Association. PO Box 280297, Dallas, TX 75243-4522. (972) 994-9902 or (800) 535-3643. contactcca@ccakids.com. <http://www.ccakids.com>.

FACES: The National Craniofacial Assocation. PO Box 11082, Chattanooga, TN 37401. (423) 266-1632 or (800) 332-2373. faces@faces-cranio.org. <http://www.faces-cranio.org/>.

Greenberg Center for Skeletal Dysplasias. 600 North Wolfe St., Blalock 1012C, Baltimore, MD 21287-4922. (410) 614-0977 <http://www.med.jhu.edu/Greenberg.Center/Greenbrg.htm>.

Johns Hopkins University-McKusick Nathans Institute of Genetic Medicine 600 North Wolfe St., Blalock 1008, Baltimore, MD 21287-4922. (410) 955-3071.

Little People of America, Inc. National Headquarters, PO Box 745, Lubbock, TX 79408. (806) 737-8186 or (888) LPA-2001. lpadatabase@juno.com. <http://www.lpaonline.org>.

National Foundation for Ectodermal Dysplasias. PO Box 114, 410 E Main, Mascoutah, IL 62258-0114. (618) 566-2020. Fax: (618) 566-4718. <http://www.nfed.org>.

National Organization for Rare Disorders (NORD). PO Box 8923, New Fairfield, CT 06812-8923. (203) 746-6518 or (800) 999-6673. Fax: (203) 746-6481. <http://www.rarediseases.org>.

Judy C. Hawkins, MS, CGC

Dysplasia giantism syndrome X-linked (DGSX) *see* **Simpson-Golabi-Behmel syndrome**

Dystonia

Definition

Dystonia is a group of complex neurological movement disorders. While the disorders vary in their symptoms, causes, progression, and treatment, dystonia is characterized by involuntary muscle contractions and spasms that result in abnormal postures and movements. Focal dystonias—which affect a single part of the body, such as the face, arms, or vocal chords—are the most common.

Description

Dystonia is not a single disease, but a group of disorders with a variety of symptoms. The most common characteristic of dystonia is twisting, repetitive, and sometimes painful movements that affect a specific part of the body, such as the arms, legs, trunk, neck, eyelids, face, or vocal cords. Cervical dystonia, which affects the head and neck, is the most common adult form of dystonia, followed by blepharospasm (eyelids), spasmodic dysphonia (larynx), and limb dystonias (hands).

Researchers believe that dystonia is caused by a malfunction in the basal ganglia, the part of the brain involved in regulating voluntary and involuntary movement. A Berlin neurologist, Hermann Oppenheim, first coined the term "dystonia" in 1911 after observing muscle spasm and variation in muscle tone in several of his young patients. The term was widely accepted and used by neurologists; however, the definition has changed over time.

Today dystonia is classified in several ways, based on cause, location, and age at onset.

Dystonia can be caused by many different factors. It may occur due to trauma, stroke, certain infections and diseases (e.g., **Wilson disease**, **multiple sclerosis**), reactions to certain neuroleptic or antipsychotic drugs (e.g., haloperidol or chlorpromazine), birth injury, or heavy-metal or carbon monoxide poisoning. This type of dystonia is called secondary or symptomatic dystonia. About half of dystonia cases have no connection to disease or injury and are referred to as primary dystonia. Many of these cases appear to be inherited.

The most useful classification for physicians is location, or distribution of the dystonia. Focal dystonia involves a single body part while multifocal dystonia affects multiple body parts. In generalized dystonia, symptoms begin in an arm or a leg and advance, eventually affecting the rest of the body.

The patient's age at the onset of symptoms helps physicians identify the cause and determine the probability of disease progression. Dystonia that begins in childhood is often hereditary, begins in the leg or (less commonly) the arm, and may progress to other parts of the body. Dystonia that begins in adolescence (early on-set dystonia) may be hereditary, often begins in the arm or neck, and is more likely to progress than the childhood form. Adult-onset dystonia typically begins as focal or multifocal and is sporadic in origin.

Genetic profile

The majority of primary dystonia cases are believed to be hereditary and occur as the result of a faulty **gene**. Most cases of early-onset primary dystonia are due to a mutation in the DYT-1 gene, which was first identified as a factor in the disorder in 1987.

Dystonia appears when an individual has one copy of the mutated gene and one copy of the normal gene; however, only 30–40% of individuals with the mutated genes develop symptoms.

Demographics

Dystonia affects more than 300,000 people in North America, affecting all races and ethnic groups. Early onset idiopathic torsion dystonia has a higher frequency among Ashkenazi Jews—Jews of Eastern European ancestry.

Dystonia is the third most common movement disorder, after **Parkinson disease** and tremor.

Signs and symptoms

Early symptoms of dystonia may include a deterioration in handwriting, foot cramps, tremor, voice or speech difficulties, and a tendency of one foot to pull up or drag while walking. Initially, the symptoms may be very mild and only noticeable after prolonged exertion, stress, or fatigue. Over a period of time, the symptoms may become more noticeable and widespread.

Symptoms may first occur in childhood (between the ages of 5 and 17 years) or early adulthood. In general, the earlier the onset of symptoms, the greater the chance that the disease will progress with advancing age.

Diagnosis

There is no specific diagnostic test for dystonia and the diagnosis is often based on clinical signs and symptoms. Diagnosis may be difficult because the signs are similar to those of other disorders; the involuntary muscle contractions are often incorrectly attributed to stress, stiff neck, dry eyes, tics, or psychogenic or neurological disorders. According to Mount Sinai Medical Center, 90% of dystonia patients are initially misdiagnosed.

One thing that is helpful in differentiating dystonic movements from those caused by other disorders is the timing of the movements. Dystonic movements tend to increase during activity, nervousness, and emotional stress; and usually disappear during sleep.

Treatment and management

There is no cure for dystonia. However, symptoms such as spasms and pain can usually be managed with a combination of treatments.

No one treatment has proven universally effective. A physician's approach to treatment is typically three-tiered, encompassing oral medications, injections of therapeutic agents (e.g., botulinum toxin) directly into dystonic muscle, and surgery. Surgery, which involves cutting nerves and muscles or placing a lesion in the basal ganglia to reduce movement, is usually reserved for the most severe cases. Alternative medicine, such as physical therapy, speech therapy, and biofeedback, may also have a role in treatment management.

The cause and location of a patient's dystonia will play a factor in the treatment methods chosen by the physician. In secondary dystonia, treating the underlying cause may prove effective in improving or eliminating the associated symptoms. Patients with focal dystonia often respond best to targeted methods—such as injections of botulinum toxin or surgery—while patients with

KEY TERMS

Basal ganglia—A section of the brain responsible for smooth muscular movement.

Blepharospasm—A focal dystonia marked by excessive blinking and involuntary closing of the eyes.

Cervical dystonia—A focal dystonia that causes neck muscles to contract involuntarily, leading to abnormal movements and posture of the head and neck. Also known as spasmodic torticollis.

Early on-set dystonia—Dystonia that begins in adolescence. Most common among Jewish persons of Eastern European ancestry.

Limb dystonia—Involuntary cramp or spasm that affects the hands. Also known as writer's cramp.

Primary dystonia—Dystonia that has no connection to disease or injury. Often hereditary.

Secondary dystonia—Dystonia that occurs due to disease, injury, or another non-hereditary factor. Also known as symptomatic dystonia.

Spasmodic dysphonia—A focal dystonia that causes involuntary "spasms" of the vocal cords—leading to interruptions of speech and a decrease in voice quality.

dystonia may first need to be treated with oral medications to alleviate the multiple symptoms.

Prognosis

Dystonia is not fatal; however, it is a chronic disorder and prognosis can be difficult to predict.

Resources

PERIODICALS

Adler, Charles H. "Strategies for Controlling Dystonia; Overview of Therapies That May Alleviate Symptoms." *Postgraduate Medicine* (October 2000). <http://www.postgradmed.com/issues/2000/10_00/adler.htm>.

Ozelius, Laurie J., et al. "The Early-Onset Torsion Dystonia Gene (DYT1) Encodes an ATP-Binding Protein." *Nature Genetics* 17 (September 1997): 40.

ORGANIZATIONS

Bachmann-Strauss Dystonia & Parkinson Foundation, Inc. Mount Sinai Medical Center, One Gustave L. Levy Place, Box 1490, New York, NY 10029. (212) 241-5614. <http://www.dystonia-parkinsons.org>.

Dystonia Medical Research Foundation. One East Wacker Dr., Suite 2430, Chicago, IL 60601. (312) 755-0198. <http://www.dystonia-foundation.org>.

National Institute of Neurological Disorders and Stroke. 31 Center Drive, MSC 2540, Bldg. 31, Room 8806, Bethesda, MD 20814. (301) 496-5751 or (800) 352-9424. <http://www.ninds.nih.gov>.

National Organization for Rare Disorders (NORD). PO Box 8923, New Fairfield, CT 06812-8923. (203) 746-6518 or (800) 999-6673. Fax: (203) 746-6481. <http://www.rarediseases.org>.

WE MOVE (Worldwide Education and Awareness for Movement Disorders). Mount Sinai Medical Center, One Gustave L. Levy Place, Box 1490, New York, NY 10029. (800) 437-6682. <http://www.wemove.org>.

WEBSITES

"Early Onset Primary Dystonia." *GeneClinics*. March 30, 1999. <www.geneclinics.org/profiles/dystonia>.

"Gene Sequenced for Disabling Childhood Movement Disorder: Early-Onset Torsion Dystonia Protein Found." *National Institute of Neurological Disorders and Stroke.* September 3, 1997. <www.ninds.nih.gov/news_and_events/pressrelease_disabling_childhhod_movement_090397.htm>.

Michelle L. Brandt

Dystrophia myotonica 2 *see*
Myotonic dystrophy

Ectodermal dysplasia

Definition

The ectodermal dysplasias are a group of hereditary conditions characterized by abnormal hair, teeth, fingernails and toenails, and sweat glands.

Description

All ectodermal dysplasias have a genetic etiology and involve abnormal development and growth of tissues derived from the ectoderm. The ectoderm is the outermost layer of the developing embryo, which gives rise to the hair, teeth, nails, and skin. More than 100 different ectodermal **dysplasia** conditions have been described in the medical literature. The most common of these is hypohidrotic ectodermal dysplasia, which may account for up to 80% of all ectodermal dysplasias.

Other ectodermal dysplasia conditions include ectrodactyly-ectodermal dysplasia-clefting (EEC) syndrome, hidrotic ectodermal dysplasia (Clouston syndrome), Hay-Wells syndrome, incontintentia pigmenti, Rapp-Hodgkin syndrome, tricho-dento-osseous syndrome, and tooth-nail (Witkop) syndrome. Each of these conditions appears to account for 1–4% of all ectodermal dysplasias.

Most ectodermal dysplasia conditions are associated with sparse hair that has abnormal texture. The hair may appear thin, dry and brittle. In some cases, premature balding may occur.

The teeth of those with ectodermal dysplasia are typically abnormal and reduced in number. A characteristic conical and sharply pointed tooth shape is often present. In some cases, the majority of teeth are missing.

In some ectodermal dysplasia conditions, the fingernails and toenails may be absent or abnormally formed. The nails may be thickened, thinned, brittle, or display unusual ridging or pitting.

The skin may be thin, show abnormal pigmentation, and be prone to eczema (a condition of dry skin characterized by inflammation and itching). The nasal and respiratory passages may be dry, leading to abnormal discharges and increased infections. In hypohidrotic ectodermal dysplasia, the sweat glands are reduced in number, which may lead to dangerous hyperthermia (high body temperature).

Other abnormalities that may occur in the ectodermal dysplasia conditions include amastia (absent mammary glands), cleft lip and/or palate, ectrodactyly (split hand or split foot), and abnormal bands of skin in the mouth or connecting the eyelids.

Many individuals with ectodermal dysplasia have normal cognitive function. A minority of cases may involve some degree of mental retardation. In the case of hypohidrotic ectodermal dysplasia, untreated hyperthermic episodes can lead to brain damage and cognitive impairment.

Genetic profile

Hypohidrotic ectodermal dysplasia is inherited in an X-linked recessive manner. Sixty to 75% of carrier females may show variable manifestations of the condition. The responsible **gene** has been named EDA; it has been mapped to the Xq12-q13.1 chromosomal region but has not yet been identified.

Incontinentia pigmenti is caused by chromosomal rearrangements disrupting the Xp11 region (type I incontinentia pigmenti) or by a gene mapping to Xq28 (type II or familial incontintentia pigmenti). Both forms appear to be lethal in males, as nearly all affected patients (97–98%) are female.

Most other ectodermal dysplasias are transmitted in an autosomal dominant fashion. Rarely, autosomal recessive transmission may occur.

The molecular genetics of the ectodermal dysplasia conditions are poorly understood. Investigation has been hampered by the great variability displayed by

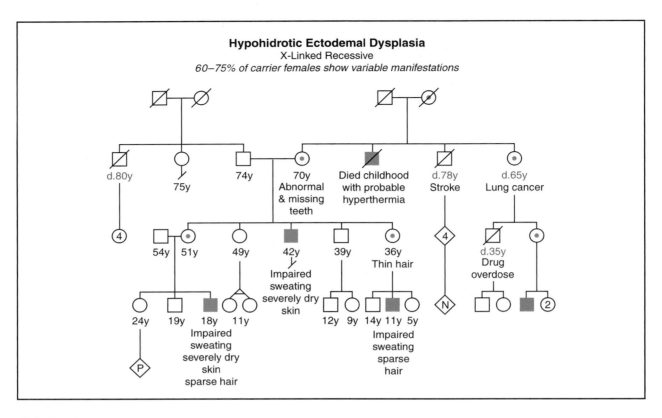

Hypohidrotic Ectodemal Dysplasia
X-Linked Recessive
60–75% of carrier females show variable manifestations

(Gale Group)

many of these conditions, similar features shown by different ectodermal dysplasias, and genetic heterogeneity (different genetic alterations producing identical physical features). As with many other human genetic conditions, mouse models are being used to identify candidate genes that may be responsible for these disorders.

Demographics

The exact incidence of ectodermal dysplasia conditions has not yet been studied accurately and is not known. One published report estimated the incidence of these conditions collectively as seven per 10,000 births. The disorders have been reported in individuals and families of diverse ethnic backgrounds. One early description of an ectodermal dysplasia came from Charles Darwin, who cited a report of an affected individual from the Indian subcontinent in an 1897 publication.

Signs and symptoms

Most ectodermal dysplasia conditions cause significant dental abnormalities. In some cases, the majority of the primary (baby) and secondary (adult) teeth are miss-

ing. Teeth that are present may show a characteristic conical, pointed shape (peg-teeth), or have abnormal enamel that is prone to cavities.

Hair is often thin with an abnormal texture. In hypohidrotic ectodermal dysplasia, the scalp hair is thin during childhood and ultimately shows premature balding. Although body hair, eyebrows, and eyelashes are also sparse in this condition, beard and mustache hair are normal. Hair is also sparse in EEC syndrome. In trichodento-osseous syndrome and Hay-Wells syndrome, the hair is sparse, coarse, and wiry. Individuals with incontinentia pigmenti may have patchy, bald areas of abnormal skin on the scalp. Frequent scalp infections occur in many of the ectodermal dysplasias.

A variety of skin abnormalities may occur in ectodermal dysplasia conditions. The skin may be dry, thin, and prone to eczema, infection, cracking, bleeding, and other problems. In hypohidrotic ectodermal dysplasia, sebaceous glands (the oil glands within the skin) are absent, causing severe dryness. Increased pigmentation may occur around the eyes (in hypohidrotic dysplasia), over the joints (in hidrotic ectodermal dysplasia), or in a linear pattern over the trunk (in incontinentia pigmenti). Hyperkeratosis, or thickened skin, occurs on the palms and soles of the feet in hidrotic ectodermal dysplasia. Reddening and blistering of the skin may occur during infancy in incontintentia pigmenti. In Hay-Wells syndrome, abnormal bands of skin may occur between the upper and lower jaws and between the eyelids.

Decreased numbers of sweat glands and associated impaired sweating ability is an important feature of hypohidrotic ectodermal dysplasia. This can lead to life-threatening hyperthermia in hot environments or with physical exertion. Sweating is normal in most other ectodermal dysplasias.

Many ectodermal dysplasias involve abnormalities of the mucous membranes. Production of tears and saliva may be deficient. In hypohidrotic ectodermal dysplasia, the mucous glands in the respiratory tract may be absent or decreased in number, leading to dryness, infections and an unusual foul-smelling secretion known as ozena. In some cases, dryness of the pharynx and larynx may affect the quality of the voice.

Finger and toenails are abnormal in many of the ectodermal dysplasias. In EEC syndrome, the nails may be thin and brittle. Nails may be absent or abnormally formed in Hay-Wells syndrome, Rapp-Hodgkin syndrome, hidrotic ectodermal dysplasia, tooth and nail syndrome, and incontintentia pigmenti. Nails are normal in hypohidrotic ectodermal dysplasia.

Some individuals with ectodermal dysplasia, particularly those with EEC syndrome, may have hearing impairment.

Structural birth defects may occur in some ectodermal dysplasias. In EEC, Hay-Wells, and Rapp-Hodgkin syndromes, **cleft lip and palate** may occur. EEC is also characterized by split hand/split foot (or "lobster claw") malformations and genitourinary anomalies. Amastia (absence of the breast) may occur in hypohidrotic ectodermal dysplasia and breasts may be underdeveloped in incontintia pigmenti and EEC syndrome. Some individuals with incontinentia pigmenti may have defects of the eye (such as congenitally crossed eyes, cataracts, or atrophy of the optic nerve) or central nervous system (such as a small head size, mental retardation, or seizures).

Diagnosis

The diagnosis of an ectodermal dysplasia condition is typically based on clinical findings (physical examination, medical and family history). With the exception of type I incontinentia pigmenti, there are no laboratory studies that are considered diagnostic. High resolution **chromosome** study may be considered diagnostic for type I incontintentia pigmenti as it can reveal the X chromosome rearrangements that appear to cause the condition.

The high degree of variability within and overlap between the different ectodermal dysplasia conditions can lead to difficulty identifying the specific syndrome. The presence or absence of nail and sweat gland involvement are important distinguishing features.

In hypohidrotic ectodermal dysplasia, determining whether or not a female relative of an affected male also carries the EDA gene may be difficult. A variety of clinical tests based on sweat pore and dental analysis have been attempted, but are considered unreliable. Linkage analysis by way of tracing the Xq12-13 gene locus through the family is considered to be the best way of determining carrier status. When linkage analysis is successful, it may also be used for prenatal diagnosis.

Treatment and management

In hypohidrotic ectodermal dysplasia, males are at risk for hyperthermia and potential central nervous system damage or death. Hot environments and fevers must be avoided or managed with cooling methods, such as misting the skin with water. Air conditioning of home, school, and work environments is considered essential. The dry nasal passages may be treated with moisturizing inhalers or other solutions. Various skin treatments may be used to prevent cracking, bleeding and infection.

Early and extensive dental work is required in most ectodermal dysplasia conditions. In childhood, successive dentures may be used, while dental implants and bridges may be used in adults. Orthodontic treatment may also be necessary.

The abnormal hair in the ectodermal dysplasias is primarily a cosmetic problem and may be managed with wigs.

In EEC, Rapp-Hodgkin syndrome, and Hay-Wells syndrome, clefting of the lip and palate requires surgical correction, with treatment of any associated speech, dental, or hearing problems.

Hand and foot malformations in EEC may require orthopedic or plastic surgery, and/or occupational therapy. The abnormal skin banding that may occur in the mouth and between the eyelids in Hay-Wells syndrome also requires surgical correction.

Prognosis

Among males with hypohidrotic ectodermal dysplasia, unrecognized episodes of hyperthermia are a dangerous complication. The mortality rate during infancy and early childhood in affected, undiagnosed males is 20% due to neurologic damage associated with hyperthermic episodes. If affected males are diagnosed and managed

KEY TERMS

Amastia—A birth defect involving absent breast(s).

Dysplasia—The abnormal growth or development of a tissue or organ.

Ectoderm—The outermost of the three embryonic cell layers, which later gives rise to the skin, hair, teeth, and nails.

Ectrodactyly—A birth defect involving a split or cleft appearance of the hands and/or feet, also referred to as a "lobster-claw malformation."

Hyperthermia—Body temperature that is much higher than normal (i.e. higher than 98.6°F).

appropriately, a normal life expectancy and normal intelligence can be expected.

Otherwise, the tissue abnormalities and birth defects that occur in the ectodermal dysplasias are usually not life-threatening.

These conditions typically do not cause mental retardation, although a minority of cases of incontinentia pigmenti and EEC syndrome may involve cognitive impairment.

Resources

PERIODICALS

Coskun, Yavuz, and Ziya Bayraktaroglu. "Ectodermal dysplasia." (Pathological Case of the Month) *Archives of Pediatrics & Adolescent Medicine* 151, no. 7 (July 1997): 741–2.

WEBSITES

National Foundation for Ectodermal Dysplasias. <www.nfed.org>.

Jennifer Ann Roggenbuck, MS, CGC

Ectrodactyly-ectodermal dysplasia-clefting syndrome

Definition

Ectrodactyly-ectodermal dysplasia-clefting (EEC) syndrome is one of more than 100 **ectodermal dysplasia** syndromes. EEC syndrome is characterized by deformities of the hands and feet (ectrodactyly), abnormalities of the skin, hair, and nails (ectodermal **dysplasia**), and

cleft lip and/or cleft palate (clefting). Other symptoms include dental, eye, skin, and kidney abnormalities.

Description

Ectodermal dysplasias (ED) are a group of inherited disorders that result from problems in early development of the ectodermal layer in the embryo. Problems with the ectoderm cause the hair, teeth, nail, and glands to develop and function abnormally. EEC syndrome is characterized by deformities of the hands and feet (ectrodactyly) that are sometimes referred to as lobster-claw deformities, abnormalities of the skin, hair, and nails (ectodermal dysplasia), and cleft lip and/or cleft palate (clefting). Other abnormalities include absence of the teeth and other dental abnormalities, decreased ability to sweat, absence of tear ducts, photophobia (increased sensitivity to light), and kidney abnormalities. Most individuals with EEC syndrome have some of these abnormalities, but very few individuals have all of these abnormalities.

EEC syndrome is genetic disorder with autosomal dominant **inheritance** with incomplete penetrance and variable expression. It can be inherited from a parent, but many individuals are the first in their family to be affected. **DNA** testing is now available and may be used to clarify the diagnosis in an individual with characteristic symptoms of the syndrome.

The cosmetic concerns of EEC can have a tremendous impact on the quality of life of an individual with EEC syndrome. The facial and limb differences can be socially isolating and physically challenging. Children and adults with EEC may be socially ostracized due to their physical appearance. Many individuals erroneously assume that people with EEC syndrome have limited abilities. It is important to increase awareness with educational programs and to take proactive steps to foster self-esteem in children with EEC syndrome.

Genetic profile

EEC syndrome has autosomal dominant inheritance with incomplete penetrance and variable expression. It is caused by mutations in the p63 **gene**, which is located on the long arm of **chromosome** 3 (3q27). The p63 gene appears to be necessary for the normal development of the skin and limbs, although its exact function is not known as of 2005.

Mutations in the p63 gene are inherited in an autosomal dominant manner. Every individual has two p63 genes: one from their father and one from their mother. In an autosomal dominant disorder, only one gene has to have a mutation for the person to have the EEC disorder. Some individuals with EEC syndrome are born to unaffected parents. Their EEC syndrome is the result of a *de novo*, or new mutation. No one knows the cause of *de novo* mutations or why they occur so frequently in EEC syndrome. Because individuals pass half of their genes onto their children, a person with EEC syndrome has a 50% chance that their child will also inherit EEC syndrome. If two unaffected people have a child with EEC syndrome, they have about a 4% risk to have another child with EEC syndrome. This increased recurrence risk is due to the possibility of germline mosaicism. Germline mosaicism is the presence of two cell lines in the reproductive cells (eggs or sperm cells) of an individual. Thus, a parent of a child with EEC syndrome may have one normal cell line and one cell that contains the mutation for EEC syndrome.

While EEC syndrome has autosomal dominant inheritance, it also shows incomplete penetrance. Incomplete penetrance is the term that is used to describe individuals with a mutation in a gene that do not have any symptoms of a particular disease. Although this is very rare, there are some large families in which this phenomenon has been documented. Because the physical findings of EEC syndrome can be so variable, it is important to carefully examine other family members to make sure that they do not have an extremely mild case of EEC syndrome.

The findings or symptoms of EEC vary from family to family and even from person to person within the same family. For example, one sibling may have cleft lip and hand abnormalities, while another sibling may have kidney and eye abnormalities. This phenomenon is referred to as variable expression. Most ectodermal dysplasias show some degree of variable expression. This can often make it very difficult for a physician to make an exact diagnosis.

Demographics

The overall incidence of ectodermal dysplasias in the United States is seven out of 10,000 people. Because the findings of EEC syndrome overlap those seen in other ectodermal dysplasia, the exact prevalence of EEC syndrome is not known. With the advent of DNA testing, it may soon be possible to get an accurate prevalence figure for EEC syndrome, but, as of 2005, this is not yet possible.

Signs and symptoms

In order to understand the signs and symptoms of EEC syndrome it is important to understand a little about early embryonic development. Very early in pregnancy, the cells that will develop into the embryo are organized as a small round ball. These cells eventually separate into three distinct layers: the endoderm, the mesoderm, and the ectoderm. The endoderm can be thought of as the inside layer. Cells from the endoderm will eventually form into

the lining of the digestive tract and the respiratory tract. The mesoderm can be thought of as the middle layer, and the cells of the mesoderm will eventually become the muscles, bones, cartilage, heart, and blood vessels. The ectoderm (involved in EEC syndrome) can be thought of as the outside layer. The cells of the ectoderm will eventually become the skin, hair, nails, brain, and nervous system. Any disruption of the development of the ectoderm will lead to disruption of the organs formed from this layer.

EEC syndrome is the result of a disruption of the ectoderm layer very early in development. This disruption causes the specific defects seen in EEC syndrome, including defects of the skin, hair, nails, and other organs. As of 2005, the exact nature of this disruption or problem in formation of the ectooderm is not known. Research in this area is ongoing.

EEC syndrome is a disorder that causes multiple congenital abnormalities. Although these anomalies appear to be diverse, they all arise from the same underlying defect, or insult, to the early embryonic ectodermal tissue. Ectodermal tissue is responsible for the formation of the limbs, nails, eyes, skin, hair, teeth, kidneys, glands, and face. All of these organs and systems are affected to some degree in EEC syndrome. Most individuals will have some of the EEC abnormalities, but it is very rare for one individual to have all of these abnormalities.

Abnormalities of the hands and feet of individuals affected with EEC may include:

- ectrodactyly (lobster-claw deformity) of the hands and feet

- syndactyly (webbed fingers or toes)

Abnormalities of the eyes of affected individuals may include:

- nasolacrimal duct obstruction (tear duct obstruction)

- excessive lacrimation (tears)

- blephariphimosis/blepharospasm

- corneal ulcers and scarring

- telecanthus

- photophobia

Skin abnormalities of individuals affected with EEC may include:

- dry skin

- lack of sweat pores

- thin skin/generalized skin atrophy

- hyperkeratosis (thickened skin)

Individuals affected with EEC may have hair abnormalities, including:

• dry, brittle hair

• generalized depigmentation of hair

• fine hair

• sparse hair, or alopecia areata

Teeth abnormalities in affected individuals may include:

• abnormalities in the tooth buds, resulting in missing or abnormally shaped teeth

• defective enamel

• small teeth

Abnormalities of the kidneys of affected individuals may include:

• dilated ureters or uretral atresia

• double ureters

• hydronephrosis

• multiple renal cysts

• renal agenesis

• renal dysplasia

Gland abnormalities of individuals affected with EEC may include:

• absent or hypoplastic thymus

• hypopituitarism

• isolated growth hormone deficiency

• pituitary **diabetes** insipidus

Facial abnormalities of affected individuals may include:

• cleft lip

• cleft palate

• malformed ears

Additionally, individuals affected with EEC can experience nail dystrophy.

There are two other ectodermal dysplasia syndromes that closely resemble EEC syndrome: Rapp-Hodgkin syndrome (RHS) and ankyloblepharon-ectodermal defects-cleft lip and palate (AEC) syndrome (also known as Hay Wells syndrome). These syndromes share some of the specific findings of EEC syndrome, but differ in important ways.

The Rapp-Hodgkin syndrome (RHS) is another type of ED associated with **cleft lip and palate**. However, RHS does not share the hand and foot defects of EEC

syndrome. People with RHS do have some sweating problems, and their hair grows slowly and is coarse. Some affected individuals have persistent scalp dermatitis. As a rule, individuals with RHS have more teeth than those with EEC. General health, intelligence, and lifespan are within normal expectations.

The Hay-Wells syndrome (HWS), also known as the anklyloblepharon-ectodermal dysplasia-cleft lip and palate syndrome, is one of several syndromes that affect both the ectoderm and structures that do not derive from the ectoderm. The scalp hair is sparse and wiry, while the eyelashes are sparse or absent. The nails may be absent or malformed, and the teeth and sweat glands may also be affected. The feature that differentiates HWS from the other ectodermal dysplasias is the fusion of the upper and lower eyelids usually by narrow bands of tissue connecting the lids (anklyloblepharon). Patients may also have inflammatory dermatitis of the scalp.

Diagnosis

The diagnosis of EEC syndrome can be complex because of the overlap of symptoms with other ectodermal dysplasia syndromes. The diagnosis of EEC syndrome is usually made through a combination of clinical exam, x rays, kidney imaging tests, skin biopsy, and DNA testing.

To make the diagnosis of EEC, a physician must evaluate which ectodermally derived structures are involved and look for physical features that do not develop from the ectoderm. By looking at the specific pattern of defects, it may be possible to make a correct diagnosis, but because of the overlap between other ectodermal dysplasias, it can often be difficult to make a definitive diagnosis based only clinical exam alone. DNA testing and other tests can help aid in the diagnosis.

X rays are often helpful in establishing the diagnosis of EEC syndrome. X rays may be taken of the jaw to look for dental abnormalities, while x rays of the limbs may be done to look for subtle abnormalities that may not be seen with a clinical exam. The presence of dental abnormalities or limb abnormalities would add to the suspicion that a person had EEC syndrome.

Because individuals with EEC syndrome can have kidney abnormalities, it is important to assess their kidney structure. This can be done using an IV pyelogram or ultrasound. The presence of a kidney abnormality would lend credence to the diagnosis of EEC syndrome, but the absence of a kidney abnormality does not rule out the diagnosis as not every person with EEC syndrome has every symptom.

A skin biopsy involves removing a small amount of several layers of skin to examine them under a microscope. In EEC syndrome, the skin cells themselves may be abnormal. In addition, the sweat glands may be abnormal in number or shape.

DNA testing can also be performed on blood samples from children or adults. The presence of a mutation in the p63 gene would confirm the diagnosis of EEC syndrome. Because scientist have not yet found all of the mutations in this gene, the absence of a detectable mutation does not completely rule out the diagnosis.

The diagnosis of EEC syndrome can also be made prenatally (during pregnancy) either by ultrasound (sonogram) or by prenatal DNA testing. Sonograms use sound waves to provide an image of a fetus. The structural abnormalities of EEC syndrome, including cleft lip, kidney abnormalities, and limb abnormalities, can be detected during the second trimester of pregnancy. Because of the overlap in the some of the structural abnormalities of the ectodermal dysplasias, it can be very difficult to definitively diagnose EEC syndrome by sonogram. Other ectodermal dysplsias can look very similar to EEC syndrome on a sonogram. DNA testing can have a role in clarifying ambiguous ultrasound findings.

Prenatal testing can also be done using DNA testing. A sample of tissue from a fetus is obtained by either chorionic villi sampling (CVS) or by **amniocentesis**. Chorionic villi sampling is generally done between 10 and 12 weeks of pregnancy, and amniocentesis is done between 14 and 18 weeks of pregnancy. Chorionic villi sampling involves removing a small amount of tissue from the developing placenta. The tissue in the placenta contains the same DNA as the fetus. Amniocentesis involves removing a small amount of fluid from around the fetus. This fluid contains some fetal skin cells. DNA can be isolated from these skin cells. The fetal DNA is then tested to determine if it contains mutations in the p63 gene that causes EEC syndrome. Because not all of the mutations causing EEC syndrome have been found, DNA testing is not always definitive and the interpretation of the test results is best done by a genetics professional.

Treatment and management

There is no cure for EEC syndrome, but there are many treatments available to address the symptoms. These treatments include surgery, dental care, prevention of complications from hypohydrosis (abnormal sweating), and other preventative treatments.

Individuals with EEC syndrome may need surgery to correct cleft lips, cleft palates, and abnormalities with their hands and feet. Correction of cleft lip is usually done in infancy, as is surgery for cleft palate. Correction of cleft palate is important for feeding and for speech.

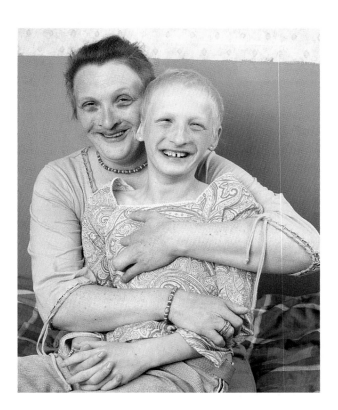

Mother and child with ectrodactyly-ectodermal dysplasia-clefting (EEC) syndrome. © *Science Photo Library / Photo Researchers, Inc.*

Surgery may be done on hand and foot abnormalities to improve the function of these limbs, to improve the appearance of these limbs, and to aid in shoe fit.

Typically patients with EEC syndrome will need extensive dental work. X rays may be taken to document the presence or absence of teeth. Abnormal teeth may be pulled or capped. Replacement dentures may be worn during childhood. After growth has ended, many individuals will receive dental implants.

Hypohydrosis, or impaired sweating, is a major complication of EEC syndrome. Without normal sweating, the body cannot regulate temperature properly. Therefore, overheating is a common problem, and can lead to seizures, coma, and death in severe cases. It is important that affected individuals with an impaired ability to sweat follow the general precautions of using air conditioning when necessary, avoiding vigorous exercise, wear light clothing, and avoid hot temperatures.

Abnormal development of the eye can result in dryness of the eye, cataracts, and vision defects. Artificial tears can be used to protect the eyes from corneal scarring, which can lead to blindness if left untreated.

KEY TERMS

Ectoderm—Embryonic cells that are affected in EEC syndrome.

Ectrodactyly—Lobster-claw deformities of the hands and feet, and missing digits on the hands and feet.

Incomplete penetrance—Absence of disease in an individual known to carry the gene for that disease.

Variable expression—Ability of the same gene to cause different symptoms in different people (with the same disorder).

Prognosis

The prognosis for most individuals with EEC syndrome is very good. Life expectancy ranges from slightly reduced to normal. The most life-threatening complications come from sweating problems. Individuals with an impaired ability to sweat are at risk to overheat, which can lead to seizures, coma, and death. The life expectancy of individuals with EEC syndrome without sweating problems is expected to be normal.

The prognosis for most people with EEC syndrome is very good. In general, they have minimal and manageable serious medical problems, normal IQ, and most achieve success and have a long life, irregardless of their disabilities. Successful social adaptation plays an important role in the ultimate success and happiness of an individual with EEC syndrome. It is very important that the career and life choices of an individual with EEC syndrome not be limited by preconceived ideas about their abilities.

Resources

ORGANIZATIONS

National Foundation for Ectodermal Dysplasias. PO Box 114. 410 East Main. Mascoutah, IL 62258-0114. (618) 566-2020. Email: info@nfed.org.

WEBSITES

American Cleft Palate-Craniofacial Association. (April 10, 2005.) <http://www.cleftline.org>.

National Foundation for Ectodermal Dysplasia. (April 10, 2005.) <http://www.nfed.org>.

Kathleen A. Fergus, MS, CGC

Edwards syndrome *see* **Trisomy 18**

Ehlers-Danlos syndrome

Definition

The Ehlers-Danlos syndromes (EDS) refer to a group of inherited disorders that affect collagen structure and function. Genetic abnormalities in the manufacturing of collagen within the body affect connective tissues, causing them to be abnormally weak.

Description

Collagen is a strong, fibrous protein that lends strength and elasticity to connective tissues such as the skin, tendons, organ walls, cartilage, and blood vessels. Each of these connective tissues requires collagen tailored to meet its specific purposes. The many roles of collagen are reflected in the number of genes dedicated to its production. There are at least 28 genes in humans that encode at least 19 different types of collagen. Mutations in these genes can affect basic construction as well as the fine-tuned processing of the collagen.

Genetic profile

There are numerous types of EDS, all caused by changes in one of several genes. The manner in which EDS is inherited depends on the specific **gene** involved. There are three patterns of **inheritance** for EDS: autosomal dominant, autosomal recessive, and X-linked (extremely rare).

Chromosomes are made up of hundreds of small units known as genes, which contain the genetic material necessary for an individual to develop and function. Humans have 46 chromosomes, which are matched into 23 pairs. Because chromosomes are inherited in pairs, each individual receives two copies of each **chromosome** and likewise two copies of each gene.

Changes or mutations in genes can cause genetic diseases in several different ways, many of which are represented within the spectrum of EDS. In autosomal dominant EDS, only one copy of a specific gene must be changed for a person to have EDS. In autosomal recessive EDS, both copies of a specific gene must be changed for a person to have EDS. If only one copy of an autosomal recessive EDS gene is changed, the person is referred to as a carrier meaning they do not have any of the signs or symptoms of the disease itself, but carry the possibility of passing on the changed gene to a future child. In X-linked EDS, a specific gene on the X chromosome must be changed. This affects males and females differently because males have one and females have two X chromosomes.

The few X-linked forms of EDS fall under the category of X-linked recessive. As with autosomal recessive, this implies that both copies of a specific gene must be changed for a person to be affected. However, because males only have one X chromosome, they are affected if an X-linked recessive EDS gene is changed on their single X chromosome. That is, they are affected even though they have only one changed copy. On the other hand, that same gene must be changed on both of the X chromosomes in a female for her to be affected.

Although there is much information regarding the changes in genes that cause EDS and their various inheritance patterns, the exact gene mutation for all types of EDS is not known.

Demographics

EDS was originally described by Dr. Van Meekeren in 1682. Dr. Ehlers and Dr. Danlos further characterized the disease in 1901 and 1908, respectively. Today, according to the Ehlers-Danlos National Foundation, one in 5,000 to one in 10,000 people are affected by some form of EDS.

Signs and symptoms

EDS is a group of **genetic disorders** that usually affects the skin, ligaments, joints, and blood vessels. Classification of EDS types was revised in 1997. The new classification involves categorizing the different forms of EDS into six major subtypes including classical, hypermobility, vascular, kyphoscoliosis, arthrochalasia, and dermatosparaxis, as well as a collection of rare or poorly defined varieties. This new classification is simpler and based more on descriptions of the actual symptoms.

Classical type

Under the old classification system, EDS classical type was divided into two separate types: type I and type II. The major symptoms involved in EDS classical type affect the skin and joints. The skin has a smooth, velvety texture and bruises easily. Affected individuals typically have extensive scarring, particularly at the knees, elbows, forehead, and chin. The joints are hyperextensible, so there is a tendency towards dislocation of the hip, shoulder, elbow, knee, or clavicle. Due to decreased muscle tone, affected infants may experience a delay in reaching motor milestones. Children may have a tendency to develop hernias or other organ shifts within the abdomen. Sprains and partial or complete joint dislocations are also common. Symptoms can range from mild to severe. EDS classical type is inherited in an autosomal dominant manner.

There are three major clinical diagnostic criteria for EDS classical type. These include skin hyperextensibil-

ity, unusually wide scars, and joint hypermobility. At this time there is no definitive test for the diagnosis of classical EDS. Both **DNA** and biochemical studies have been used to help identify affected individuals. In some cases, a skin biopsy has been found to be useful in confirming a diagnosis. Unfortunately, these tests are not sensitive enough to identify all individuals with classical EDS. If there are multiple affected individuals in a family, it may be possible to perform prenatal diagnosis using a DNA information technique known as a linkage study.

Hypermobility type

Excessively loose joints are the hallmark of this EDS type, formerly known as EDS type III. Both large joints, such as the elbows and knees, and small joints, such as toes and fingers, are affected. Partial and total joint dislocations are common, and particularly involve the jaw, knee, and shoulder. Many individuals experience chronic limb and joint pain, although x rays of these joints appear normal. The skin may also bruise easily. **Osteoarthritis** is a common occurrence in adults. EDS hypermobility type is inherited in an autosomal dominant manner.

There are two major clinical diagnostic criteria for EDS hypermobility type. These include skin involvement (either hyperextensible skin or smooth and velvety skin) and generalized joint hypermobility. At this time there is no test for this form of EDS.

Vascular type

Formerly called EDS type IV, EDS vascular type is the most severe form. The connective tissue in the intestines, arteries, uterus, and other hollow organs may be unusually weak, leading to organ or blood vessel rupture. Such ruptures are most likely between ages 20 and 40, although they can occur any time, and may be life-threatening.

There is a classic facial appearance associated with EDS vascular type. Affected individuals tend to have large eyes, a thin pinched nose, thin lips, and a slim body. The skin is thin and translucent, with veins dramatically visible, particularly across the chest.

The large joints have normal stability, but small joints in the hands and feet are loose, and hyperextensible. The skin bruises easily. Other complications may include collapsed lungs, premature aging of the skin on the hands and feet, and ruptured arteries and veins. After surgery there may be poor wound healing, a complication that tends to be frequent and severe. Pregnancy also carries the risk complications. During and after pregnancy there is an increased risk of the uterus rupturing and of arterial bleeding. Due to the severe complications associated with EDS type IV, death usually occurs before age 50. A study of 419 individuals with EDS vascular type, completed in 2000, found that the median survival rate was 48 years, with a range of 6–73 years. EDS vascular type is inherited in an autosomal dominant manner.

There are four major clinical diagnostic criteria for EDS vascular type. These include thin translucent skin, arterial/intestinal/uterine fragility or rupture, extensive bruising, and characteristic facial appearance. EDS vascular type is caused by a change in the gene COL3A1, which codes for one of the collagen chains used to build collage type III. Laboratory testing is available for this form of EDS. A skin biopsy may be used to demonstrate the structurally abnormal collagen. This type of biochemical test identifies more than 95% of individuals with EDS vascular type. Laboratory testing is recommended for individuals with two or more of the major criteria.

DNA analysis may also be used to identify the change within the COL3A1 gene. This information may be helpful for **genetic counseling** purposes. Prenatal testing is available for pregnancies in which an affected parent has been identified and the DNA mutation is known or their biochemical abnormality has been demonstrated.

Kyphoscoliosis type

The major symptom of kyphoscoliosis type, formerly called EDS type VI, is general joint looseness. At birth, muscle tone is poor and motor skill development is subsequently delayed. Also, infants with this type of EDS have an abnormal curvature of the spine (**scoliosis**). The scoliosis becomes progressively worse with age, with affected individuals usually unable to walk by age 20. The eyes and skin are fragile and easily damaged, and blood vessel involvement is a possibility. The bones may also be affected as demonstrated by a decrease in bone mass. Kyphoscoliosis type is inherited in an autosomal recessive manner.

There are four major clinical diagnostic criteria for EDS kyphoscoliosis type. These include generally loose joints, low muscle tone at birth, scoliosis at birth (which worsens with age), and fragility of the eyes, which may give the white area of the eye a blue tint or cause the eye to rupture. This form of EDS is caused by a change in the PLOD gene on chromosome 1, which encodes the enzyme lysyl hydroxylase. A laboratory test is available in which urinary hydroxylysyl pryridinoline is measured. This urine test is extremely sensitive and specific for EDS kyphoscoliosis type. Laboratory testing is recommended for infants with three or more of the major diagnostic criteria.

Prenatal testing is available if a pregnancy is known to be at risk and an identified affected family member has had positive laboratory testing. An **amniocentesis** may be performed in which fetal cells are removed from the amniotic fluid and enzyme activity is measured.

Arthrochalasia type

Dislocation of the hip joint typically accompanies arthrochalasia type EDS, formerly called EDS type VIIB. Other joints are also unusually loose, leading to recurrent partial and total dislocations. The skin has a high degree of stretchability and bruises easily. Individuals with this type of EDS may also experience mildly diminished bone mass, scoliosis, and poor muscle tone. Arthrochalasia type is inherited in an autosomal dominant manner.

There are two major clinical diagnostic criteria for EDS arthrochalasia type. These include sever generalized joint hypermobility and bilateral hip dislocation present at birth. This form of EDS is caused by a change in either of two components of Collage type I, called proa1(I) type A and proa2 (I) type B. A skin biopsy may be performed to demonstrate an abnormality in either component. Direct DNA testing is also available.

Dermatosparaxis type

Individuals with this type of EDS, once called type VIIC, have extremely fragile skin that bruises easily but does not scar excessively. The skin is soft and may sag, leading to an aged appearance even in young adults. Individuals may also experience hernias. Dermatosparaxis type is inherited in an autosomal recessive manner.

There are two major clinical diagnostic criteria for EDS dematosparaxis type. These include severe skin fragility and sagging or aged appearing skin. This form of EDS is caused by a change in the enzyme called procollagen I N-terminal peptidase. A skin biopsy may be preformed for a definitive diagnosis of dermatosparaxis type.

Other types

There are several other forms of EDS that have not been as clearly defined as the aforementioned types. Forms of EDS within this category may present with soft, mildly stretchable skin, shortened bones, chronic diarrhea, joint hypermobility and dislocation, bladder rupture, or poor wound healing. Inheritance patterns within this group include X-linked recessive, autosomal dominant, and autosomal recessive.

Diagnosis

Clinical symptoms such as extreme joint looseness and unusual skin qualities, along with family history, can lead to a diagnosis of EDS. Specific tests, such as skin biopsies are available for diagnosis of certain types of EDS, including vascular, arthrochalasia, and dermatosparaxis types. A skin biopsy involves removing a small sample of skin and examining its microscopic structure. A urine test is available for the kyphoscoliosis type.

Management of all types of EDS may include genetic counseling to help affected individuals and their families understand the disorder and its impact on other family members and future children.

If a couple has had a child diagnosed with EDS, the chance that they will have another child with the same disorder depends on with what form of EDS the child has been diagnosed and if either parent is affected by the same disease or not.

Individuals diagnosed with an autosomal dominant form of EDS have a 50% chance of passing the same disorder on to a child in each pregnancy. Individuals diagnosed with an autosomal recessive form of EDS have an extremely low risk of having a child with the same disorder.

X-linked recessive EDS is accompanied by a slightly more complicated pattern of inheritance. If a father with an X-linked recessive form of EDS passes a copy of his X chromosome to his children, his sons will be unaffected and his daughters will be carriers. If a mother is a carrier for an X-linked recessive form of EDS, she may have affected or unaffected sons, and carrier or unaffected daughters, depending on the second sex chromosome inherited from the father.

Prenatal diagnosis is available for specific forms of EDS, including kyphoscoliosis type and vascular type. However, prenatal testing is only a possibility in these types if the underlying defect has been found in another family member.

Treatment and management

Medical therapy relies on managing symptoms and trying to prevent further complications. There is no cure for EDS.

Braces may be prescribed to stabilize joints, although surgery is sometimes necessary to repair joint damage caused by repeated dislocations. Physical therapy teaches individuals how to strengthen muscles around joints and may help to prevent or limit damage. Elective surgery is discouraged due to the high possibility of complications.

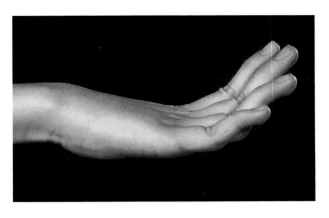

Hyperflexion of the joints, the ability to bend them beyond normal, is seen in most patients with Ehlers-Danlos syndrome. Overflexing of the hand is demonstrated by this patient. (*Custom Medical Stock Photo, Inc.*)

Alternative treatment

There are anecdotal reports that large daily doses (1–4 g) of vitamin C may help decrease bruising and aid in wound healing. Constitutional homeopathic treatment may be helpful in maintaining optimal health in persons with a diagnosis of EDS. Individuals with EDS should discuss these types of therapies with their doctor before beginning them on their own. Therapy that does not require medical consultation involves protecting the skin with sunscreen and avoiding activities that place stress on the joints.

Prognosis

The outlook for individuals with EDS depends on the type of EDS with which they have been diagnosed. Symptoms vary in severity, even within one subtype, and the frequency of complications changes on an individual basis. Some individuals have negligible symptoms while others are severely restricted in their daily life. Extreme joint instability and scoliosis may limit a person's mobility. Most individuals will have a normal life span. However, those with blood vessel involvement, particularly those with EDS vascular type, have an increased risk of fatal complications.

EDS is a lifelong condition. Affected individuals may face social obstacles related to their disease on a daily basis. Some people with EDS have reported living with fears of significant and painful skin ruptures, of becoming pregnant (especially those with EDS vascular type), of their condition worsening, of becoming unemployed due to physical and emotional burdens, and of social stigmatization in general.

Constant bruises, skin wounds, and trips to the hospital take their toll on both affected children and their parents. Prior to diagnosis, parents of children with EDS have found themselves under suspicion of child abuse.

Some people with EDS are not diagnosed until well into adulthood and, in the case of EDS vascular type, occasionally not until after death due to complications of the disorder. Not only may the diagnosis itself be devastating to the family, but in many cases other family members find out for the first time they are at risk for being affected.

Although individuals with EDS face significant challenges, it is important to remember that each person is unique with his or her own distinguished qualities and potential. Persons with EDS go on to have families, careers, and become accomplished citizens, surmounting the challenges of their disease.

Resources

PERIODICALS

"Clinical and Genetic Features of Ehlers-Danlos Syndrome Type IV, the Vascular Type." *The New England Journal of Medicine* 342, no. 10 (2000).

"Ehlers-Danlos Syndromes: Revised Nosology, Villefranche, 1997." *American Journal of Medical Genetics* 77 (1998): 31–37.

"Living a Restricted Life with Ehlers-Danlos Syndrome." *International Journal of Nursing Studies* 37 (2000): 111–118.

ORGANIZATIONS

Elhers-Danlos National Foundation. 6399 Wilshire Blvd., Ste 203, Los Angeles, CA 90048 (323) 651-3038. Fax: (323) 651-1366. <http://www.ednf.org>.

Ehlers-Danlos Support Group—UK. PO Box 335, Farnham, Surrey, GU10 1XJ. UK 01252 690 940. <http://www.atv.ndirect.co.uk>.

WEBSITES

GeneClinics. <http://www.geneclinics.org>.

Java O. Solis, MS

Elattoproteus syndrome *see* **Proteus syndrome**

Ellis-van Creveld syndrome

Definition

Ellis-van Creveld syndrome is an individually recognized genetic condition characterized by short stature and malformations of the heart, limbs, nails, and teeth. The name given to this condition originates from Richard W. B. Ellis of Scotland and Simon van Creveld of the

Netherlands. Each had a patient with this syndrome in his care when the two met by chance in an English train car on the way to a pediatric conference in the late 1930s.

Description

Ellis-van Creveld (EvC) syndrome primarily affects the skeletal system, but is also associated with congenital heart defects. EvC syndrome is one of the six short rib **polydactyly** syndromes, or SRPS. There is considerable overlap between the features of these six syndromes. Clinical, radiological, and pathological studies are being conducted to determine if there are indeed six distinct SRPS, or if each is a different mutation at the **gene** that also causes Ellis-van Creveld syndrome.

Ellis-van Creveld syndrome is alternatively known as chondroectodermal **dysplasia** or mesoectodermal dysplasia. The name chondroectodermal dysplasia is meant to indicate a dysplasia, or abnormal growth or development, of the skeleton (chondro-) and the skin (ectodermal). The name mesoectodermal dysplasia is meant to indicate an abnormal growth or development of the skin (ectodermal) and primarily the middle portion of the bone (meso-). However, neither medically descriptive term defines the syndrome completely, and Ellis-van Creveld syndrome remains the most used name for both medical and common purposes.

Ellis-van Creveld syndrome is characterized by short arms and legs; short ribs; short fingers; polydactyly, or extra fingers or toes; and dysplastic, or abnormal, teeth and nails. Limb shortening is more noticeable in the legs than in the arms. Many older children affected by EvC syndrome develop knock-knee, or genu valgum, which may have to be corrected by orthopedic surgery. The underdeveloped ribs generally cause a condition known as pectus carinatum, in which the chest is narrow and elongated. A sixth finger on both hands occurs in all patients with EvC syndrome, while extra toes are observed in approximately 20% of the EvC syndrome population. Polydactyly in affected individuals is always symmetric. That is, if the left hand possesses a sixth finger, the right hand will also possess a sixth finger.

Dysplastic, or abnormal, teeth and nails are observed in all individuals with EvC syndrome. The most common dental anomalies are: teeth present at birth; wide spaces between permanent teeth; the late eruption of, or the complete lack of, some permanent teeth; and permanent teeth that more closely resemble baby teeth than permanent teeth. The most common nail abnormalities are absent or malformed fingernails or toenails. Thin, brittle hair is also observed in a majority of patients with EvC syndrome.

Congenital heart defects occur in approximately 50-60% of affected individuals. The most common cardiac abnormality observed is a common atrium rather than the normal two-chambered atrium. This "hole in the heart" can often be surgically repaired, resulting in normal heart function.

Genetic profile

Ellis-van Creveld syndrome is an autosomal, or non-sex linked, recessive condition. The gene responsible for EvC syndrome has been identified and its locus determined on the distal short arm of **chromosome** 4p. In 2000, it was shown that the EvC gene is the same gene that causes Weyers acrofacial dysostosis.

Certain mutations in the EvC gene cause EvC syndrome. In order for EvC syndrome to appear, the affected child must inherit a mutation of this gene from each parent. The child must receive two abnormal genes.

When the child receives only a single copy of an abnormal gene that would cause EvC syndrome, that child is affected with Weyers acrofacial dysostosis. Weyers acrofacial dysostosis is an autosomal dominant condition characterized by tooth and nail abnormalities, extra fingers and toes, and milder limb anomalies than those observed in Ellis-van Creveld syndrome. As is often the case in homozygous disorders, EvC syndrome presents much more pronounced physically observable and potentially life-threatening signs than the corresponding heterozygous condition, Weyers acrofacial dysostosis.

Demographics

Ellis-van Creveld syndrome has an incidence of approximately one out of 150,000 live births. Ellis-van Creveld syndrome has a much higher occurrence among the Old Order Amish, an isolated and inbred religious community in Lancaster County, Pennsylvania.

As a homozygous condition, both parents of an affected child must carry the abnormal EvC gene. The parents of a child with EvC syndrome have a one in four chance of having additional children affected with EvC syndrome. The transmission of such homozygous **genetic disorders** is facilitated by the close association among potentially related individuals in a relatively small and isolated population such as that of the Amish. Also, a relatively high frequency of Ellis-van Creveld syndrome has been observed in the Aboriginal people of Western Australia. This high frequency has been attributed to a founder effect from Dutch castaways and genetic drift caused by the isolation and interbreeding of these peoples.

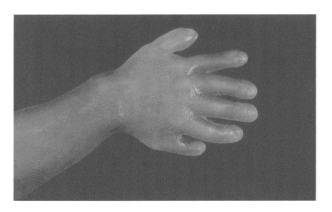

Polydactyly, having extra fingers or toes, is a common feature in patients with Ellis van Creveld syndrome. (*Greenwood Genetic Center*)

Signs and symptoms

Ellis-van Creveld syndrome is characterized by short limbs and short body length identifiable at birth. The average adult height range for those affected by EvC syndrome is 43–60 in (109–152 cm). The head and neck are generally unaffected other than possible abnormalities of the upper lip, and dental anomalies including delayed eruption of the permanent teeth, which are generally underdeveloped and more similar to a child's teeth than to those of an adult. EvC syndrome is further characterized by congenital heart defects, usually a single upper chamber (atrium) rather than the normal two upper chambers. Affected individuals have short, poorly developed ribs, which leads to a narrow chest; this is termed pectus carinatum.

Males affected by EvC syndrome may present abnormalities of the penis in which the urethral opening occurs on the underside of the penis rather than at the tip of the glans (**hypospadias**); they may also have one or both testicles undescended (cryptorchidism). Further skeletal anomalies associated with EvC syndrome include: low hips; a spur-like projection at the acetabula, the socket in the hipbone that accepts the head of the thighbone; a fusion of the capitate and hamate bones; two carpal bones, the fusion of which makes the formation of a fist difficult or impossible; knock-knee; clubfeet that turn down and in; and postaxial polydactyly, or extra fingers/toes that arise outside the normal fifth digit. Fingernails and toenails are generally malformed. Neurologically, mental retardation has been observed in patients with EvC syndrome, but it is not the norm. A brain abnormality of one of the normal cavities of the brain (Dandy-Walker syndrome) is also occasionally associated with EvC syndrome.

Diagnosis

Ultrasound imaging of developing fetuses can reveal the limb shortening and underdeveloped ribs that are characteristic of the short rib polydactyly syndromes (SRPS), which includes Ellis-van Creveld syndrome. An ultrasound scan is now available after the sixteenth week of gestation that may identify extra digits in the developing fetus.

Ellis-van Creveld syndrome is generally differentially diagnosed from the other SRPS by the additional presence of atrial abnormalities. However, it is often difficult to distinguish Ellis-van Creveld syndrome from two other forms of **skeletal dysplasia**. These are asphyxiating thoracic dysplasia (ATD), also known as Jeune syndrome; and short rib polydactyly syndrome (SRPS) type III, or Verma-Naumoff type SRPS. Individuals with Jeune syndrome often die of respiratory distress shortly after birth, whereas individuals diagnosed with EvC syndrome are more likely to die from congenital heart failure. Individuals with Jeune syndrome often have extra fingers or toes; but, unlike those with EvC syndrome, this polydactyly is often not symmetric. Individuals with Jeune syndrome do not show the nail and hair abnormalities observed in EvC syndrome. Older children can often be differentially diagnosed with Jeune syndrome rather than EvC syndrome if they develop kidney problems, which may also later lead to kidney failure as adults. Kidney dysfunction is not associated with Ellis-van Creveld syndrome.

Verma-Naumoff type SRPS is virtually indistinguishable from EvC syndrome prior to birth. However, individuals with Verma-Naumoff type SRPS also exhibit heart, kidney, and intestinal malformations that are not present in the Ellis-van Creveld population. Verma-Naumoff type SRPS has an essentially 100% mortality rate within hours of birth, as those affected die from respiratory distress. All three of these conditions arise from autosomal recessive **inheritance**. The genetic evidence is beginning to further the hypothesis that these three conditions are the result of mutations of the same gene on chromosome 4p that has been identified as the cause of Ellis-van Creveld syndrome.

Treatment and management

Genetic counseling of individuals affected with either Ellis-van Creveld syndrome or the allelic disorder, Weyers acrofacial dysostosis, may prevent the conception of EvC syndrome-affected children. Congenital heart defects associated with Ellis-van Creveld syndrome may be surgically corrected. The potential outcome of such a procedure is normal heart function. Extra fingers or toes (polydactyly) can be surgically removed shortly after birth. This is more a cosmetic treatment than a necessary one in the case of fully developed extra digits. If person affected with EvC syndrome develops

KEY TERMS

Autosomal—Relating to any chromosome besides the X and Y sex chromosomes. Human cells contain 22 pairs of autosomes and one pair of sex chromosomes.

Dysplasia—The abnormal growth or development of a tissue or organ.

Heterozygous—Having two different versions of the same gene.

Homozygous—Having two identical copies of a gene or chromosome.

Postaxial polydactyly—A condition in which an extra finger or toe is present outside of the normal fifth digit.

Primary atrial septation—An improper division of the atria of the heart, or a "hole in the heart," which results in the formation of a common atrium rather than the normal two-chambered atrium.

Short rib polydactyly syndromes—A collection of genetic disorders characterized by abnormally short ribs and extra fingers or toes. Research is ongoing to determine if these disorders are the result of mutations in a common gene.

Weyers acrofacial dysostosis—The condition resulting from a mutation of the same gene that shows mutation in Ellis-van Creveld syndrome. As is usually the case when comparing expressions of the same gene mutation, the single dose Weyers acrofacial dysostosis presents milder symptoms than the double dose Ellis-van Creveld syndrome.

---

genu valgum (knock-knee), he or she may require orthopedic surgery to straighten the legs at the knee. Dental treatment also has an important role in management of Ellis-van Creveld syndrome.

Many people of extremely short stature adapt their surroundings to their size. Others choose to undergo one of the bone lengthening procedures that have increasingly become available. These bone lengthening procedures are generally performed only on the limbs. They often do not offer complete relief to the EvC syndrome patient who may also have a smaller than normal thoracic cavity caused by undersized ribs.

Prognosis

Ellis-van Creveld syndrome is generally non-lethal with approximately two-thirds of those affected surviving to adulthood. Mortality is higher when the congenital

heart defects associated with EvC syndrome are also present. Approximately half of those affected with Ellis-van Creveld syndrome with heart abnormalities die in childhood due to cardiorespiratory problems associated with these congenital heart defects or associated with pressure on the chest, primarily the lungs, caused by an underdeveloped rib cage. Of these, approximately one-half die within the first six months of life.

Resources

PERIODICALS

Polymeropoulos, M., et al. "The gene for the Ellis-van Creveld syndrome is located on chromosome 4p16." *Genomics* (July 1996): 1–5.

Ruiz-Perez, V., et al. "Mutations in a new gene in Ellis-Van Creveld syndrome and Weyers acrodental dysostosis." *Nature Genetics* (March 2000): 283–86.

ORGANIZATIONS

Ellis-Van Creveld Foundation. Farthingdale Farm, Hackmans Lane, Purleigh, Chelmsford, CM3 6RW. UK 01-621-829675. <http://www.cafamily.org.uk/Direct/e24.html>.

Genetic Alliance. 4301 Connecticut Ave. NW, #404, Washington, DC 20008-2304. (800) 336-GENE (Helpline) or (202) 966-5557. Fax: (888) 394-3937 info@geneticalliance. <http://www.geneticalliance.org>.

WEBSITES

Johns Hopkins Hospital Greenberg Center for Skeletal Dysplasias. <http://www.med.jhu.edu/Greenberg.Center/evc.htm>. (February 7, 2001).

OMIM—Online Mendelian Inheritance in Man. <http://www.ncbi.nlm.nih.gov/htbin-post/Omim/dispmim?225500>. (February 7, 2001).

WebMD—Ellis-van Creveld syndrome. <http://webmd.lycos.com/content/asset/adam_disease_ellis-van_creveld_syndrome>. (February 7, 2001).

Paul A. Johnson

Emery-Dreifuss muscular dystrophy

Definition

Emery-Dreifuss **muscular dystrophy** (EDMD) is a rare childhood-onset degenerative muscle disease seen almost exclusively in males. Emery-Dreifuss muscular dystrophy is characterized by a classic triad of symptoms. These include early-onset contractures, very slow progressive muscle weakness and degeneration involving the upper arms and lower legs, and cardiac (heart) muscle disease.

Description

Emery-Dreifuss muscular dystrophy affects the arms, legs, spine, face, neck, and heart. This disease is characterized by contractures of the elbows and the Achilles tendons at an early age, slowly progressive muscle wasting and weakness, and life potentially life-threatening heart muscle disease. Intelligence is normal, however physical problems may be severe.

Symptoms and disease severity may vary between individuals. Three modes of **inheritance** exist: X-linked, autosomal dominant, and autosomal recessive. The symptoms of the autosomal dominant and X-linked forms of the disease are identical, however the autosomal dominant form appears to have a later onset of symptoms.

Genetic profile

Emery Dreifuss muscular dystrophy is inherited in different ways in different families. Most commonly EDMD is inherited in an X-linked recessive manner. Autosomal dominant inheritance of EDMD is also well characterized. Only one case of autosomal recessive inheritance of EDMD has been reported.

Rarely a new mutation causing EDMD can also occur, causing disease in a person with no family history. This is called a sporadic occurrence and is the ressult of a new change in a **gene** (new mutation) in that individual. New mutations account for approximately 10% of cases of EDMD.

X-linked recessive form

Emery-Dreifuss muscular dystrophy is usually inherited in an X-linked recessive manner. EDMD is the third most common type of X-linked muscular dystrophy. Symptoms begin in the first decade of life. A tendency to walk on the toes is often one of the first signs of EDMD. Muscle weakness first affects the lower extremities usually at age four or five.

X-linked diseases map to the human X **chromosome**, a sex chromosome. Females have two X chromosomes, whereas males have one X chromosome and one Y chromosome. Because males only have one X chromosome, they only require one X-linked disease gene to display disease. Since females have two X chromosomes, the effect of one X-linked recessive disease gene is masked by the disease gene's normal counterpart on her other X chromosome.

In classic X-linked inheritance males are affected, presenting full clinical symptoms of the disease. Females are usually not affected. Affected fathers can never pass X-linked diseases to their sons. However, affected fathers always pass X-linked disease genes to their daughters. Females who inherit the faulty gene but do not show the disease are known as carriers. Female carriers of X-linked EDMD have a 50% chance to pass the disease-causing gene to each of their children.

It is unusual for female carriers of an X-linked disease to show symptoms of the disease. In X-linked EDMD, carrier females can exhibit certain symptoms of the disease. Females have two X chromosomes in each of their body cells. Very early on in fetal development, one X chromosome in each cell of a female is inactivated. The pattern of inactivation is random, so carrier females may express the disease-causing gene in some of their cells. An estimated 10–20% of female carriers of X-linked EDMD display varying symptoms of the disease. Female carriers can display the dangerous heart symptoms of EDMD. Less commonly, carrier females may show late-onset muscle weakness.

In 1994 it was recognized that the X-linked recessive form of Emery-Dreifuss muscular dystrophy is caused by changes, or mutations, in a gene now known as EMD or STA. This gene is located on the long arm of the human X chromosome at a location designated as Xq28. The STA gene is approximately 2,100 base pairs in length. This gene codes for emerin, an amino acid protein.

Emerin is an important protein normally found on the inner nuclear membrane of skeletal, cardiac, and smooth muscle cells as well as in other tissues. Emerin is missing from the nuclear membranes of males affected with X-linked EDMD. Emerin is not altered in other neuromuscular disorders.

Autosomal dominant form

In some families, Emery-Dreifuss muscular dystrophy may be inherited in an autosomal dominant pattern. Autosomal dominant EDMD is known as Emery-Dreifuss muscular dystrophy 2 (EDMD2), Hauptmann-Thannhauser muscular dystrophy, and Scapuloilioperoneal atrophy with cardiopathy. Autosomal dominant disorders affect both sexes equally. In autosomal dominant conditions a person, male or female, requires only one faulty gene to produce disease. There are no unaffected carriers of EDMD2. In families with EDMD2, both males and females can be affected and father to son inheritance of the disease can occur. Every child of a person affected with EDMD2 has a 50% chance of inheriting the disease.

In families with EDMD2, affected members exhibit a later onset of the same symptoms as someone affected with X-linked EDMD. Symptoms begin between the ages of 17 and 42. EDMD2 and X-linked EDMD are caused by changes in different genes on different chromosomes.

Muscle biopsy of people with EDMD2 are found to have normal emerin levels. In families with EDMD2, the disease is caused by changes, or mutations, in a gene known as Lamin A/C, or LMNA. Lamin A/C is located in a specific area on the long arm of chromosome 1 known as 1q21.2.

Lamin A/C codes for two proteins, lamins A and C. Like emerin, these lamins are associated with the nuclear membrane. People with autosomal dominant EDMD2 have normal levels of emerin and low levels of these lamin proteins. Emerin and these lamins form an important protein complex in a cell's nuclear membrane. The exact role of this complex is unclear. Scientists theorize that this important complex of proteins stabilizes the nuclear membrane and plays a role in regeneration of muscle fibers.

Autosomal recessive form

As of early 2001 a single case of autosomal recessively inherited EDMD has been documented. EDMD of autosomal recessive inheritance has been named Emery-Dreifuss muscular dystrophy 3 (EDMD3). For someone to be affected with an autosomal recessive disease they must inherit two copies of a disease-causing gene, one from each parent. A parent who has only one gene associated with autosomal recessive EDMD is not affected by the disease and is known as a carrier of the disease. Two carriers of autosomal recessive EDMD have a 25% chance to have a child affected with the disorder in each pregnancy.

Like EDMD2, EDMD3 is caused by mutations in the Lamin A/C gene located on the long arm of chromosome 1 at an area designated as 1q21.2. The single known mutation associated with EDMD3 has not been found to also lead to EDMD2.

The single known patient with autosomal recessively inherited EDMD (EDMD3) displayed symptoms similar to those of X-linked and autosomal dominant EDMD without any heart involvement. He had difficulties when he started walking at 14 months of age. At five years of age, his contractures were so severe that he could not stand. At age 40, he was confined to a wheelchair and exhibited severe widespread muscle wasting. He displayed normal intelligence and did not have any heart problems. His carrier parents had no heart, skeletal, or muscle abnormalities.

Demographics

X-linked EDMD is estimated to occur in one in 100,000 births. EDMD2 and EDMD3 are far less common. Only one case of EDMD3 has been documented.

Only males exhibit full symptoms of X-linked EDMD. EDMD2 and EDMD3 may occur in males and females. X-linked EDMD and EDMD2 have been documented in many countries. There does not appear to be a single founder of these diseases, as many families have distinctly different backgrounds and different disease-causing mutations.

Signs and symptoms

Emery-Dreifuss muscular dystrophy is recognized by a classic triad of symptoms: contractures at a young age, progressive muscle weakness and degeneration involving the upper arms and lower legs, and cardiac (heart) muscle disease.

Contractures

Contractures, or frozen joints, are a hallmark of all forms of EDMD. A contracture is the abnormal shortening of a body part, usually a muscle or a tendon. This shortening creates joint deformity. Contractures usually begin in childhood or adolescence before any muscle weakness is evident. In most cases, contractures are recognized before patients reach 10 years of age.

Contractures may display as flexion or extension deformities. In a flexion contracture a muscle or tendon remains abnormally flexed, permanently bending a body part at a joint. In an extension contracture a muscle or tendon remains abnormally extended, not allowing a body part to bend at a joint. Affected persons cannot control these contractures and cannot release them at will. Contractures are treated with stretching, physical therapy, bracing, and surgery.

People affected with EDMD often have flexion contractures of the elbows and ankles. Elbow contractures force the elbow to remain bent at an angle. Contractures of the Achilles tendons, or heel cords, force the feet to remain in a pointed toe position. Children with EDMD often walk on their toes due to heel cord contractures. Neck and trunk contractures may also occur, restricting movement of the neck or the entire spine. **Scoliosis** is commonly found in patients with EDMD.

Muscle weakness and degeneration

Muscle weakness and degeneration are slowly progressive, affecting a distinct pattern of muscles. This pattern includes the muscles of the upper arms and the muscles of the lower legs. The biceps (inner upper arm), triceps (outer upper arm), tibialis anterior (inner lower leg), and peroneal (outer lower leg) muscles are commonly involved. Later, the muscles of the shoulder girdle and pelvic girdle, the shoulder and hip area muscles that stabilize and support the attachment of the arms and legs, may also be affected. Additionally, the highly specialized muscle of the heart is at risk for weakness and degeneration.

Heart disorders

Heart disease associated with EDMD may be life threatening. It is, however, potentially treatable. Not all patients with EDMD develop heart involvement. Any heart involvement often becomes apparent in the second to third decade of life. In rare cases heart problems may be the first symptom of EDMD. Early recognition of heart involvement is of utmost importance as surgical placement of a pacemaker may be life saving.

EDMD is associated with cardiac conduction defects (electrical impulse problems), heart muscle degeneration, and unusual tissues (abnormal fatty and fibrous tissues) growing into the heart. Conduction defects can manifest as heart rhythm disturbances known as arrhythmias or, more seriously, heart block. Heart block is a dangerous situation where the heart is unable to respond correctly to its own electrical system. Arrhythmias and heart block can lead to fainting or even sudden death.

One uncommon type of heart conduction problem, total permanent auricular paralysis (TPAP), is relatively specific to EDMD. Scientists have found that 33% of 109 published cases of TPAP were due to EDMD.

The level of skeletal involvement in a patient with EDMD is not indicative of their level of heart involvement. Heart problems can be unpredictable, occasionally leading to sudden death without any prior symptom. In a review of 73 cases of X-linked EDMD, scientists found that 30 patients died suddenly between ages 25 and 39. Frequent careful checkups with a cardiologist (heart specialist) are necessary. Preventive surgical implantation of a pacemaker is often considered.

Female carriers of X-linked EDMD

Female carriers of X-linked EDMD may display some symptoms of disease. They can have the dangerous heart problems or, less commonly, muscle weakness. One case of sudden death of a female carrier of X-linked EDMD has been reported. It is recommended that female carriers of X-linked EDMD have regular examinations by a cardiologist.

Diagnosis

Diagnosis of EDMD is based on the classic triad of distinctive clinical symptoms seen in this disease. A diagnosis based on careful neuromuscular examination may be confirmed with muscle biopsy or **DNA** testing.

Other special laboratory tests and neuromuscular tests may help physicians to confirm or rule out EDMD.

Creatine kinase (CK), a muscle enzyme, is often measured when symptoms of muscular dystrophy are present. CK levels are only mildly elevated in EDMD. Muscle biopsy can show microscopic changes in muscle fibers. Muscle biopsy also allows for a very practical test for X-linked EDMD where muscle tissue is stained with a chemical that binds specifically to emerin. If emerin is present, X-linked EDMD can be ruled out. If emerin is reduced or absent, X-linked EDMD is diagnosed.

Genetic testing and prenatal diagnosis for X-linked Emery-Dreifuss muscular dystrophy is available on a clinical basis. To perform DNA testing for X-linked EDMD a blood sample is required. This method of testing can diagnose female carriers of X-linked EDMD. Prenatal testing requires fetal cells obtained via **amniocentesis** or chorionic villus sampling. Once the specific alteration in the gene is identified in an affected family member, female relatives at risk to be carriers can be tested and prenatal diagnosis can be offered. Prenatal testing is performed on DNA extracted from fetal cells obtained by amniocentesis or chorionic villus sampling.

Treatment and management

The muscle and skeletal symptoms of EDMD are treated as they appear. People with EDMD should see a neurologist at least once a year. Stretching and working with a physical therapist is useful in preventing or delaying contractures. Occupational therapy can help patients adapt their activities and environment to their own particular needs. Ankle and foot braces are used to prevent leg deformity. Surgery may be necessary to release contractures. Exercise can help maintain muscle use and overall good health. Affected individuals may eventually require a wheelchair or other adaptive equipment.

Persons affected with EDMD require frequent, at least yearly, heart checkups with a cardiologist. Heart symptoms can appear suddenly with disastrous consequences, so patients often have a pacemaker implanted before they have had any serious heart problem. Anti-arrhythmia drugs, diuretics, ACE inhibitors, and blood thinners may help with some of the cardiovascular symptoms associated with EDMD. Heart transplant has been successful. Relatives of patients with EDMD, especially female carriers of X-linked EDMD, should also be offered yearly screening for heart involvement via electrocardiography and echocardiography.

Scientists are currently researching **gene therapy** as a possible treatment for EDMD. STA, the gene known to be involved in the X-linked form of EDMD, is a

KEY TERMS

Amniocentesis—A procedure performed at 16-18 weeks of pregnancy in which a needle is inserted through a woman's abdomen into her uterus to draw out a small sample of the amniotic fluid from around the baby. Either the fluid itself or cells from the fluid can be used for a variety of tests to obtain information about genetic disorders and other medical conditions in the fetus.

Autosomal—Relating to any chromosome besides the X and Y sex chromosomes. Human cells contain 22 pairs of autosomes and one pair of sex chromosomes.

Chorionic villus sampling (CVS)—A procedure used for prenatal diagnosis at 10-12 weeks gestation. Under ultrasound guidance a needle is inserted either through the mother's vagina or abdominal wall and a sample of cells is collected from around the fetus. These cells are then tested for chromosome abnormalities or other genetic diseases.

Contracture—A tightening of muscles that prevents normal movement of the associated limb or other body part.

Sporadic—Isolated or appearing occasionally with no apparent pattern.

relatively small, less complicated gene. A small gene with a widespread product, such as STA, shows great promise for gene therapy.

Prognosis

Without serious heart involvement, most people with EDMD are expected to survive at least into middle age. Slow progression of muscle involvement allows most patients to walk and work until middle age or late adult life. Intellect is not affected.

Resources

BOOKS

Emery, Alan E. H. *Muscular Dystrophy: The Facts.* New York: Oxford University Press, Inc., 2000.

ORGANIZATIONS

Muscular Dystrophy Association. 3300 East Sunrise Dr., Tucson, AZ 85718. (520) 529-2000 or (800) 572-1717. <http://www.mdausa.org>.

WEBSITES

Gene Clinics. <http://www.geneclinics.org>.

Online Mendelian Inheritance in Man. <http://www3.ncbi.nlm.nih.gov/Omim>.

Judy C. Hawkins, MS

Emery-Dreifuss syndrome *see*
Emery-Dreifuss muscular dystrophy

Encephalocele

Definition

An encephalocele is a defect characterized by the herniation of brain tissue and membranes through an opening in the cranium.

Description

Encephlaoceles are classified as **neural tube defects**, which are a group of disorders occurring due to the failure of closure of the neural tube at about week four of fetal development.

Other neural tube defects include **anencephaly** and **spina bifida**. Anencephaly results from failure of closure of the cranial end of the neural tube. This is a lethal condition. Spina bifida results from failure of neural tube closure in the spine. Spina bifida is a variable condition that is usually not lethal, but causes problems with bladder and bowel control and ambulation. It is usually associated with **hydrocephalus** (water on the brain) which can be treated with a shunt to drain the fluid into the body cavity. Encephalocele is the most rare neural tube defect.

Encephaloceles are classified according to their location. Occipital (arising at the back of the head where the head meets the neck) encephaloceles occur in 75% of cases, parietal encephaloceles in 10%, and anterior encephaloceles (arising from the base of the nose) in 15%. Anterioposterior encephaloceles have a poorer prognosis.

Genetic profile

The genetics of neural tube defects, including encephalocele, are not well understood.

Most encephaloceles are sporadic, following a multifactorial pattern (genetic and environmental factors involved) of **inheritance**. It is known that there is a genetic basis to encephaloceles and other neural tube defects, and it is believed that neural tube defects may be caused by different genetic factors in different subsets of families. Proof that genetic factors contribute to encephaloceles is that it is

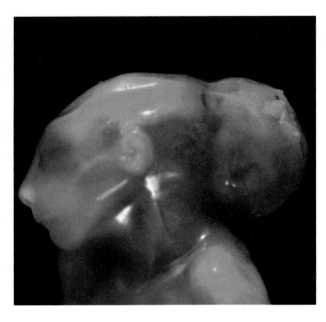

This 16 week old fetus has developed an encephalocele. The formation of the brain outside of the skull is visible. (*Custom Medical Stock Photo, Inc.*)

known to run in families, and it has been seen in association with some **chromosome** abnormalities. The number of genes and their location is still not known.

Occipital encephaloceles are associated with several single **gene** syndromes, including Meckle syndrome, dyssegmental dwarfism, Knobloch syndrome, Warburg syndrome, cryptophthalmos, and Voss syndrome. Anterior encephalocele may occur with **frontonasal dysplasia**. Encephalocele can also be seen in the amniotic band syndrome.

Demographics

The frequency of encephalocele has been reported to be between one in 2,000 to one in 5,000 live births. Anterior encephalocele is more common in Africa, Thailand and India. Females outnumber males for occipital encephalocele but not other types.

The incidence of all neural tube defects is different in different parts of the world. It is highest in northern Europe, specifically the British Isles and especially South Wales. In the United States, it is higher on the East Coast than the West Coast.

The rate of sporadic neural tube defects in the general population is about one in 1,000. The rate is higher in areas with higher incidence. The chance for a recurrence of a neural tube defect after having an affected child is 2%. After two affected children the risk is 10%.

The chance for an affected person to have an affected child is 4%. The chance for a second degree relative to have an affected child is 0.5%. Third degree relatives do not have an increased risk. Recurrence risks are given for neural tube defects as a group. A family with a previous child with anencephaly could have a child with spina bifida or encephalocele (the types do not "breed true" in families).

Care must be taken to be sure that the neural tube defect in the family was sporadic and not associated with a genetic syndrome, which would have a higher risk of recurrence.

Signs and symptoms

Symptoms of encephalocele may include hydrocephalus, spastic quadriplegia (paralysis of all four limbs), developmental delay, mental and growth retardation, uneven gait (ataxia), or seizures.

The size of the cerebral and skull abnormalities associated with encephaloceles are variable. Large encephaloceles are usually associated with microcephaly (abnormally small head). Microcephaly is usually associated with mental retardation.

Occipital encephalocele may be asymptomatic. If the ventricles are involved, hydrocephalus may occur. Anterior encephalocele may progress in size and may be solid, cystic, or both. There may be microcephaly and/or hydrocephaly, ocular hypertelorism (widespaced eyes), and cleft palate. There may be problems with vision, breathing, and feeding in patients with anterior encephaloceles. Many patients have mental retardation.

Diagnosis

Encephalocele can be diagnosed by ultrasound examination. Ultrasound examination is a screening test, the quality of which is affected by many factors including the machine used, skill of the operator, size and location of the lesion, and position of the fetus.

It is not likely that maternal serum alpha-fetoprotein testing (AFP) or **amniocentesis** would detect encephalocele. Alpha fetoprotein is a normal serum protein produced by the fetal liver. The AFP normally stays within the fetus, with a small amount present in the amniotic fluid from the fetal urine. When there is an "open" neural tube defect, there is a high amount of AFP in the amniotic fluid and the maternal serum. Although encephalocele is a neural tube defect, AFP testing on maternal blood or amniotic fluid only detects open neural tube defects. Encephaloceles are closed neural tube defects, meaning they are covered by a thick covering. This covering does not allow the AFP to leak into the maternal blood or the amniotic fluid in increased amounts that would be detected by the aforementioned tests. Pregnancies in which an encephalocele is diagnosed should be offered an amniocentesis and amniotic fluid biochemistry to better understand the cause of the disorder.

CT scan can be used to determine the contents of the encephalocele once the baby is born. Some centers offer fetal MRI to attempt to classify the encephalocele prior to deliver. This is usually done at 22 weeks gestation.

Treatment and management

Nutrition, specifically deficiency of folic acid, has been implicated as causing an increased risk for neural tube defects. All women of childbearing age should take 0.4 mg of folic acid to reduce the risk of birth defects. Women with a previous child with a neural tube defect should take 4.0 mg of folic acid. This amount has been shown to reduce the recurrence risk for neural tube defects by 50%.

Prognosis

Size, location, and contents of the encephalocele determine the outcome for the child. Anterior encephaloceles have a much better prognosis than posterior. Mortality due to occipital encephalocele is reported as about 30% if hydrocephalus is present, and 2% if it is not. For all types of encephalocele with hydrocephalus, the mortality rate is 60%. Most patients with parietal encephalocele have associated brain malformations, and mental retardation occurs in 40%. Massive occipital encephalocele with microcephaly have a mortality rate of nearly 100%. Patients with encephaloceles that contain a single frontal lobe are more likely to have normal intelligence without hydrocephalus. Posterior have a poorer prognosis if they contain large amounts of the contents of the posterior fossa (an area of the brain at the back of the head), especially the brain stem. Complications such as hemorrhage or air embolism (stroke) can occur.

Resources

BOOKS

Goodman, Richard M., and Robert J. Gorlin. *Encephalocele.* New York: Oxford University Press, 1983.

ORGANIZATIONS

Association of Birth Defects in Children. 930 Woodcock Rd., Suite 225, Orlando, FL 32803. (407) 895-0802. <http://www.biethdefects.org>.

March of Dimes Birth Defects Foundation. 1275 Mamaroneck Ave., White Plains, NY 10605. (888) 663-4637. resourcecenter@modimes.org. <http://www.modimes.org>.

WEBSITES

National Institute of Neurological Disorders and Stroke. <http://www.ninds.nih.gov/health_and_medical/disorders/encephaloceles>.

Online Mendelian Inheritance in Man. <http://www.ncbi.nlm.nih.gov/htbin-post/OMIM>.

Amy Vance, MS, CGC

Engelmann disease

Definition

Engelmann disease is a rare genetic condition that causes the long bones in the legs to become abnormally wide and may change the structure of other bones in the body. Its effects include bone pain (especially in the legs), skeletal disorders, and weak, underdeveloped leg muscles.

Description

Despite their strength and durability, human bones are living organisms. Throughout the life span, bones are constantly being broken down and rebuilt again without losing their proper size and shape. Diseases that interfere with this delicately orchestrated process (called bone remodeling) can produce pain and restrict our freedom of movement. In Engelmann disease, which was first described in 1920, the shafts of the long bones in the legs become thicker than normal. The femur (thigh bone) and tibia (shin bone) are primarily affected. These changes often cause severe bone pain and weak muscles in the legs. The weak, aching muscles associated with Engelmann disease may result in an unusual walk that resembles a "waddle." People with Engelmann may be bow-legged and have thin, elongated legs that look as if they are "wasting away."

Aside from bones in the leg, Engelmann disease can cause abnormal changes in other bones. People with Engelmann may develop **scoliosis** (in which the spine curves to the left or right side) or lumbar lordosis (a forward curvature of the spine). Engelmann disease can also cause bones to become abnormally hardened (a process referred to as sclerosis). This hardening can affect the bones at the base of the skull as well as those in the hands and feet. In rare cases, sclerosis may affect the jaw. Bone pain and aching, weak muscles may occur in parts of the body affected by the disease.

Engelmann can also affect internal organs and sight. The liver and spleen may become enlarged. Loss of vision may occur if bones near the eye sockets are affected. Some people with Engelmann report headaches, fatigue, and lack of appetite.

The underlying cause of Engelmann disease is unknown. It is often referred to in the medical literature as Camurati-Engelmann disease or progressive diaphyseal **dysplasia** (PDD). Less common names for the condition include osteopathia hyperostotica scleroticans and multiplex infantalis. Engelmann disease was sometimes referred to as ribbing disease in the past but this name is no longer used.

Genetic profile

Engelmann is considered an inherited disease, though occasionally mutations may produce sporadic cases. It is passed from parent to child as an autosomal dominant trait. This means that a person may develop the condition after receiving just one copy of the abnormal **gene** (associated with Engelmann disease) from either the mother or father.

While the gene (or genes) responsible for Engelmann disease is still unknown, medical researchers have narrowed their search to a specific region of human **DNA**, which may eventually lead to identification. This chromosomal region is known as 19q13. A gene known as TGFB1 (transforming growth factor-beta 1), which plays a role in regulating bone growth, is located in this region and is therefore considered a possible candidate.

Demographics

Engelmann, which affects men and women equally, is a very rare disease that develops during childhood or young adulthood. It usually develops between ages four and ten, but may affect children as young as three months old. Other people may develop Engelmann disease anytime before age 30.

Signs and symptoms

The main symptoms of Engelmann disease are severe pain in the legs, weak and underdeveloped leg muscles, and a "waddling" walk. Other symptoms include bowed legs, unusually long limbs, spine problems such as scoliosis or lumbar lordosis, and flat feet. People with the disease may complain of headaches, lack of energy or appetite, vision problems, and an aching feeling in their hands and feet and, less often, in the jaw. Infants with Engelmann disease may experience feeding problems or a failure to thrive, and have a "malnourished" appearance.

In simple terms, Engelmann disease causes telltale changes in the structure of the femur and tibia, around the mid-shaft areas. Certain bone regions (specifically, the endosteal and periosteal surfaces) become abnormally thickened and hardened, which in turn narrows the

---

medullary canal. Engelmann disease also causes the long bones to become "fusiform," a technical term indicating a tapered, spindle-like shape. In addition to these changes, Engelmann may cause abnormal hardening of other bones: in the hands and feet, at the base of the skull, and in the jaw. Engelmann may also involve liver and spleen enlargement, compression of the optic nerves, and increased intracranial pressure.

Diagnosis

Classic symptoms such as severe leg pain, underdeveloped leg muscles, and a "waddling" gait are often the first indication of the disease. An infant may initially experience feeding problems or failure to thrive (though these are more often the result of other, less serious problems). Imaging procedures such as a CT scan are used to detect the bone abnormalities associated with the condition, which mainly involve the thickening and sclerosis of the long bones of the legs. In some cases, x-ray studies of the skull are necessary. Blood tests and a biopsy of muscle tissue may be recommended.

In diagnosing Engelmann disease, a doctor must distinguish it from other conditions that produce similar symptoms, such as Paget disease and certain types of **muscular dystrophy**.

Treatment and management

The treatment of Engelmann disease focuses on alleviating symptoms. While the changes in bone associated with the condition cannot be reversed, the use of steroid drugs such as cortisone or prednisone can ease bone pain and strengthen muscle. Surgery to repair muscles or bones is rarely necessary, while procedures to repair nerves in the eye are generally considered ineffective.

Prognosis

While Engelmann disease does not affect life expectancy, the prognosis for the condition varies. Some people affected by the disease are virtually free of symptoms; others are severely disabled. In some cases, the muscle weakness associated with Engelmann diminishes or goes away completely with the passage of time. In other people, the effects of the disease seem to remain the same or slowly worsen during adulthood.

Resources

BOOKS

Jones, Kenneth L., ed. *Smith's Recognizable Patterns of Human Malformation.* 5th ed. Philadelphia: W.B. Saunders, 1997.

PERIODICALS

Janssens, K., et al. "Localisation of the gene causing diaphyseal dysplasia Camurati-Engelmann to chromosome 19q13." *Journal of Medical Genetics* 37, no. 4 (2000): 245–9.

Kinoshita, A., T. Saito, H. Tomita, et al. "Domain-specific mutations in TGFB1 result in Camurati-Engelmann disease." *Nature Genetics* 26, no. 1 (2000): 19–20.

ORGANIZATIONS

National Arthritis and Musculoskeletal and Skin Diseases Information Clearinghouse. One AMS Circle, Bethesda, MD 20892-3675. (301) 495-4484.

National Organization for Rare Disorders (NORD). PO Box 8923, New Fairfield, CT 06812-8923. (203) 746-6518 or (800) 999-6673. Fax: (203) 746-6481. <http://www.rarediseases.org>.

WEBSITES

Genetic Alliance. <http://www.geneticalliance.org>.

National Organization for Rare Disorders (NORD). <http://www.rarediseases.org>.

Greg Annussek

▌Epidermolysis bullosa

Definition

Epidermolysis bullosa (EB) is a group of rare inherited skin diseases that are characterized by the development of blisters following minimal pressure to the skin. Blistering often appears in infancy in response to simply being held or handled. In rarer forms of the disorder, EB can be life-threatening. There is no cure for the disorder. Treatment focuses on preventing and treating wounds and infection.

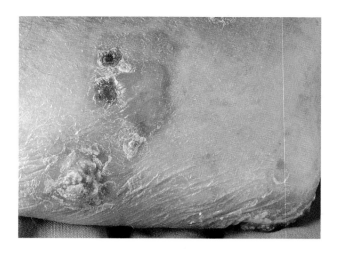

Hemorragic blisters such as those seen on this patients arm form as a result of even slight trauma to the body for patients with epidermolysis bullosa. *(Custom Medical Stock Photo, Inc.)*

Description

Epidermolysis bullosa has three major forms and at least 16 subtypes. The three major forms are EB simplex, junctional EB, and dystrophic EB. These can range in severity from mild blistering to more disfiguring and life-threatening disease. Physicians diagnose the form of the disease based on where the blister forms in relation to the epidermis (the skin's outermost layer) and the deeper dermis layer.

Genetic profile

EB can be inherited as the result of a dominant genetic abnormality (only one parent carries the abnormal **gene**) or a recessive genetic abnormality (both parents carry the abnormal gene).

EB simplex results from mutations in genes responsible for keratin 5 and 14, which are proteins that give cells of the epidermis its structure. EB simplex is transmitted in an autosomal dominant fashion.

Dystrophic EB is caused by mutations in genes for type VII collagen, the protein contained in the fibers anchoring the epidermis to the deeper layers of the skin. The genetic mutations for junctional EB are found in the genes responsible for producing the protein Laminin-5. Dystrophic EB is an autosomal disorder and will only result if both parents transmit an abnormal gene during conception.

Demographics

The prevalence of epidermolysis varies among different populations. A study in Scotland estimated the

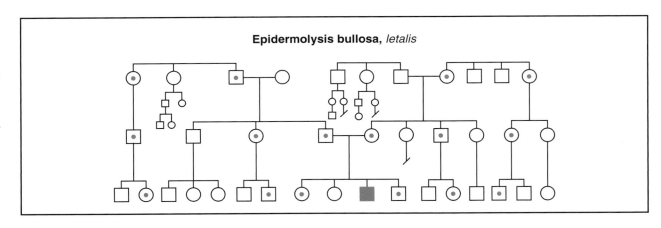

Epidermolysis bullosa, *letalis*

(*Gale Group*)

prevalence to be one in 20,400. Researchers in other parts of the world estimate the prevalence to be one in 100,000. This variance is due to the variability of expression. Many cases of epidermolysis bullosa are often not accurately diagnosed and thus, are not reported.

Signs and symptoms

EB simplex, the most common form of EB, is the least serious form of the disease. In most affected individuals, the blisters are mild and do not scar after they heal. Some forms of EB simplex affect just the hands and feet. Other forms of EB simplex can lead to more widespread blistering, as well as hair loss and missing teeth. Recurrent blistering is annoying but not life threatening.

The second, or junctional, form of EB does not lead to scarring. However, skin on the areas prone to blistering, such as elbows and knees, often shrinks. In one variation of junctional EB, called gravis junctional EB of

Herlitz, the blistering can be so severe that affected infants may not survive due to massive infection and dehydration.

The third form of EB, dystrophic EB, varies greatly in terms of severity, but more typically affects the arms and legs. In one variation, called Hallopeau-Siemens EB, repeated blistering and scarring of the hands and feet causes the fingers and toes to fuse, leaving them dysfunctional and with a mitten-like appearance.

Diagnosis

Physicians and researchers distinguish between the three major subtypes of EB based on which layer of the epidermis separates from the deeper dermis layer of the skin below. Patients suspected of having EB should have a fresh blister biopsied for review. This sample of tissue is examined under an electron microscope or under a conventional microscope using a technique called immunofluorescence, which helps to map the underlying structure.

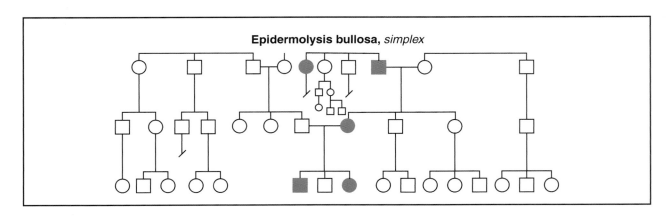

Epidermolysis bullosa, *simplex*

(*Gale Group*)

KEY TERMS

Collagen—The main supportive protein of cartilage, connective tissue, tendon, skin, and bone.

Dermis—The layer of skin beneath the epidermis.

Epidermis—The outermost layer of the skin.

Keratin—A tough, nonwater-soluble protein found in the nails, hair, and the outermost layer of skin. Human hair is made up largely of keratin.

Knowing that a family member has EB can help establish the diagnosis, but it is possible that parents or siblings will show no sign of the disease, either because it is caused by a new genetic mutation, or because the parents are carriers of the recessive trait and do not display the disease.

Treatment and management

The most important treatment for EB is daily wound care. Because the skin is very fragile, care must be taken to be certain that dressing changes do not cause further damage. Tape should not be applied directly to skin and bandages should be soaked off. Infection is a major concern, so a topical antibiotic, such as bacitracin, mupirocin, or sulfadiazine, should be routinely applied. Among persons with recessive dystrophic EB, the anticonvulsant phenytoin is sometimes effective because it decreases production of an enzyme that breaks down collagen.

Prognosis

The prognosis of EB varies depending on the subtype of the disease. Individuals with EB simplex can live long, fulfilling lives. The severity of the junctional and dystrophic forms of EB can vary greatly. Infants affected with some forms of the disease often do not survive infancy; other forms can lead to severe scarring and disfigurement.

Resources

BOOKS

Fine, Jo-David, et al. *Epidermolysis Bullosa: Clinical, Epidemiologic, and Laboratory Advances, and the Findings of the National Epidermolysis Bullosa Registry.* Baltimore: Johns Hopkins Univ Press, 1999.

Fitzpatrick, Thomas B., Richard A. Johnson, Wolff Klaus, and Dick Suurmond. *Color Atlas and Synopsis of Clinical Dermatology.* 4th ed. New York: McGraw-Hill, 2000.

Lin, Andrew N., and D. Martin Carter. *Epidermolysis Bullosa: Basic and Clinical Aspects.* New York: Springer Verlag, 1992.

Mallory, S. B. *Atlas of Pediatric Dermatology.* Pearl River, NY: Parthenon, 2001.

PERIODICALS

Brust, Mary D., and Andrew N. Lin. "Epidermolysis Bullosa: Practical Management and Clinical Update." *Dermatology Nursing* 8 (April 1996): 81–9.

Cotell, S., N. D. Robinson, and L. S. Chan. "Autoimmune blistering skin diseases." *American Journal of Emerging Medicine.* 18, no. 3 (2000): 288–99.

Eichenfield, L. F., and P. J. Honig. "Blistering disorders in childhood." *Pediatric Clinics of North America* 38, no. 4 (1991): 959–76.

Horn, H. M., G. C. Priestley, R. A. Eady, and M. J. Tidman. "The prevalence of epidermolysis bullosa in Scotland." *British Journal of Dermatology* 136, no. 4 (1997): 560–64.

Lin, Andrew N. "Management of Patients with Epidermolysis Bullosa." *Dermatologic Clinics* 14 (April 1996): 381–87.

McKenna, K. E., M.Y. Walsh, and E. A. Bingham. "Epidermolysis bullosa in Northern Ireland." *British Journal of Dermatology* 127, no. 4 (1992): 318–21.

ORGANIZATIONS

American Academy of Dermatology. PO Box 4014, 930 N. Meacham Rd., Schaumburg, IL 60168-4014. (847) 330-0230. Fax: (847) 330-0050. <http://www.aad.org>.

Dystrophic Epidermolysis Bullosa Research Association of America (DebRA). 40 Rector St., Suite 1403, New York, NY 10006. (212) 513-4090. Fax: (212) 513-4099. staff.debra@exario.net. <http://www.debra.org>.

Dystrophic Epidermolysis Bullosa Research Association of United Kingdom, (DebRA). 13 Wellington Bus. Park, Dukes Ride, Crowthorne, Berkshire, RG45 6LS. UK 011-01344 771961. admin@debra.org.uk. <http://www.debra.org.uk>.

National Epidermolysis Bullosa Registry. University of North Carolina at Chapel Hill, Bolin Heights Bldg. #1, CB# 3369, Chapel Hill, NC 27514-3369. (919) 966-2007. Fax: (919) 966-7080. eb_registry@med.unc.edu. <http://www.med.unc.edu/derm/nebr_site>.

WEBSITES

Dermatology Online Atlas. <http://www.dermis.net/doia/diagnose.asp?zugr=d&lang=e&diagnr=757320&topic=t>.

Dystrophic Epidermolysis Bullosa Research Association International. <http://debra-international.org/index1.htm>.

Epidermolysis Bullosa Medical Research Foundation. <http://www.med.stanford.edu/school/dermatology/ebmrf/>.

Oregon Health Sciences University. <http://www.ohsu.edu/cliniweb/C17/C17.800.865.410.html>.

University of Iowa College of Medicine. <http://tray.dermatology.uiowa.edu/EBA-001.htm>.

L. Fleming Fallon, Jr., MD, PhD, DrPH

Epidermolysis bullosa junctionalis-disentis type *see* **Epidermolysis bullosa**

Epilepsy

Definition

Epilepsy is a chronic (persistent) disorder of the nervous system. The primary symptoms of this disease are periodic or recurring seizures that are triggered by sudden episodes of abnormal electrical activity in the brain. The term "seizure" refers to any unusual body functions or activities that are under the control of the nervous system.

Description

The word epilepsy is derived from the Greek term for seizure. Seizures can involve a combination of sensations, muscle contractions, and other abnormal body functions. Seizures may appear spontaneously—without any apparent cause—or can be triggered by a specific type of stimulus such as a flashing light. Specific cases of epilepsy may result from known causes, such as brain injury, or may have no apparent cause (referred to as *ideopathic epilepsy*). Ideopathic epilepsy may be initiated by a combination of genetic and environmental factors.

An epileptic seizure involves a transient (temporary) episode of abnormal electrical activity in the brain. During a seizure, many nerve cells within a specific region of the brain may begin to fire at the same time. This activity may then spread out over other parts of the brain. In addition to abnormal physical symptoms, seizures can bring on emotions ranging from fear, anger, and rage, to joy or happiness. During a seizure, patients may experience disorientation, spontaneous sensations of sounds, smells, visions, and distorted visual perception—such as misshapen objects and places.

Epilepsy can be caused by some event or condition that results in damage to the brain such as strokes, tumors, abscesses, trauma (physical injury), or infections such as meningitis. Epilepsy can also be triggered by inherited (genetic) factors or some form of injury or trauma at birth. Epilepsy cases that seem to have no read-ily identifiable cause are referred to as "idiopathic" cases in medical terminology. Symptoms of this disease can appear at any age. Seizures can damage and destroy brain cells and scar tissue can develop in the section of brain tissue where seizures originate.

There are many forms of epileptic seizures. The parts of the body that are affected by a seizure and the distinctive characteristics, duration and severity of the symptoms can distinguish each type of epilepsy. Patients can experience more than one type of seizure. The nature of the symptoms depends on where in the brain the seizure originated and how much of the brain is involved. Seizures can be classified as either "generalized" or "partial." Partial seizures involve abnormal activity in a specific region of the brain.

Generalized (also called tonic-clonic) seizures last about two minutes and are the result of abnormal electrical activity that spreads out over both sides or hemispheres of the brain. They were formerly referred to as grand mal seizures. The patient will usually lose consciousness and fall during the episode. The term "tonic" refers to the first phase of a generalized seizure in which the body muscles become taunt or stiff. This is followed by strong, rhythmic muscular contractions (convulsions) of the "clonic" phase. Sometimes a patient's breathing may be hampered by a brief stoppage of the respiratory muscles, causing the skin to develop a bluish tinge due to lack of oxygen.

Epileptic seizures can also be classified as "complex" or "simple." Complex seizures generally involve a loss of consciousness, whereas simple seizures do not. Simple partial seizures can begin as a localized (focal) seizure and then evolve into a secondary generalized episode in which the initial abnormal electrical activity spreads to involve other parts of the brain. Patients may actually remember the physical and psychological events that occur during a simple seizure, such as the types of movement, emotions, and sensations, but frequently are completely unaware of the event. Partial seizures are more common in adults.

An absence seizure (once called *petit mal*) typically results in brief periods of "lack of awareness" and some abnormal muscle movement. The patient generally remains conscious during the seizure episode, but may become absent-minded and unresponsive. They may also appear to be starring. Absence seizures last about 5–10 seconds.

How seizures affect a person's memory depends where in the brain seizures occur. Seizures can interfere with learning, storage, and retrieval of new information. For example, a form of epilepsy that produces seizures in the temporal lobe of the brain can cause a serious deterioration (loss) of memory function. Early treatment can help prevent or reduce memory loss.

In some forms of epilepsy, seizures can be triggered by a particular mental—or cognitive—activity. For example, the simple activity of reading aloud can trigger a seizure in patients with reading epilepsy. Symptoms include face muscle spasms. In medical terms, this type of epilepsy is referred to as idiopathic localization-related epilepsy. This means that seizures occur in one part of the brain (in this case, the temporal lobes) and that there is no apparent cause that brought on the disease.

Genetic profile

Genetic factors contribute to about 40% of all epilepsy cases. Most of the generalized epilepsy syndromes and some of the partial epilepsy syndromes have an inherited component. Medical researchers suggest that at least 500 genes may somehow be involved in the development of various forms of epilepsy. It is believed that some of these genes can make people with epilepsy more susceptible or sensitive to environmental factors that initiate or start seizures. Only a few types of epilepsy are thought to be caused by just one type of **gene**.

Gene mutations can cause a variety of nervous system abnormalities that are associated with epilepsy. Different mutations may lead to abnormal brain development or progressive degeneration of brain tissue. Some gene mutations make nerve cells hyperexcitable. These abnormal nerve cells can trigger outbursts of abnormal patterns of electrical activity that can initiate an epileptic seizure.

Specific gene locations (called gene markers) have been linked to various forms of the disease, such as juvenile myoclonic epilepsy. However, researchers have discovered that some individuals who possess this gene do not develop symptoms of this disease. In some pairs of identical twins with this gene, one twin may appear normal while the other develops typical symptoms of epilepsy. Thus, genetic **inheritance** seems to be just one of many factors that influence the possibility of developing epilepsy symptoms.

Some genetic mutations may also reduce the effectiveness of antiepileptic medication. One of the major goals of epilepsy research is to determine how a patient's genetic makeup can influence their drug therapy.

Demographics

Epilepsy affects about one percent of the population. Approximately 2.3 million Americans and 40 million people throughout the world have epilepsy. It is the second-most common neurological disorder. The highest incidence is in children under 10 and elderly over 70.

Signs and symptoms

Patients have little warning that they are about to experience an epileptic seizure. Some unusual feeling or "aura" which can act as a warning that an episode is about to start generally precedes actual seizures. An "aura" may take the form of an unusual sensation such as a fearful feeling, a mental image, or an unusual taste, smell, or sound. Some patients who do not experience seizures during the day or who have prolonged "auras" or warnings of an impending seizure can be permitted to drive. Getting a good night's sleep is a common problem for young children with epilepsy. Lack of sleep can then lead to behavior problems and constant drowsiness during the daytime. A stupor may follow a seizure.

Diagnosis

Early symptoms of epilepsy include excessive staring, easy distraction, and difficulty maintaining attention. To confirm the diagnosis, doctors look for neurological (nervous system) abnormalities such as speech or vision defects, defects in brain structure or other parts of the nervous system. The goal of the diagnositic testing is to identify where the seizures are originating. EEGs (electroencephalographs) are used to monitor electric activity—patterns of nerve impulses in the brain. A type of brain scan called MRI is also used extensively to try to pinpoint the location and type of abnormalities (referred to as lesions) in brain structure, which cause episodes of epileptic seizures. Idiopathic epilepsy—those cases for which no specific cause can be identified—are presumed to have a genetic basis.

Treatment and management

Currently, no cure exists for epilepsy. However, a wide range of treatment programs are available that provide varying degrees of success in controlling the symptoms of epilepsy.

Medication is the most effective and widely used treatment for the symptoms of epilepsy. Most medications work by interfering with or stopping the abnormal electrical activity in nerve cells that cause seizures. This form of treatment is generally referred to as anticonvulsant therapy. Medication is considered effective if the patient is free of seizures for at least one year.

Anticonvulsants are powerful drugs that can produce a variety of side effects, including nausea, fatigue, dizziness, and weight change. They can also increase the risk of birth defects, especially involving the early stages of embryonic development of the nervous system if taken during pregnancy.

Doctors prefer to put their patients on just one type of anticonvulsant drug. Some patients, however, experience more effective relief from their epilepsy symptoms by taking a combination of two different but complementary forms of medication. The choice of medication depends on the type of seizure that affects a patient, the patient's medical history—including response to other drug therapies, their age, and gender. For example, the drug Carbamazepine is one of the most effective medications and has little impact on important cognitive functions such as thinking, memory and learning.

Newer medications generally produce fewer side effects than their predecessors. Research into **gene therapy** may ultimately be the most effective form of epilepsy treatment, but is still in the very early stages.

Unfortunately, medication is ineffective for more than one third of known cases of epilepsy. More than 30% of patients with epilepsy cannot maintain adequate control of their seizures. Some genetic mutations may reduce the effectiveness of antiepileptic medications.

Surgery is recommended for some patients for whom medication cannot effectively control the frequency or severity of their seizures. Surgery is a treatment option only in extreme cases where doctors can identify the specific site in the brain where seizures originate. The most promising candidates for surgery are those with a single lesion on the temporal, frontal, or occipital lobes of the brain.

Prior to surgery, the patient must complete extensive testing to determine the precise patterns of seizures and to locate their point of origin in the brain. Patients spend extended stays in hospital during which their seizures are recorded on video and with the aid of EEGs. This machine records patterns of electrical activity in the brain using sensors (referred to as "electrodes") attached to various parts of the body.

The surgical procedure involves the removal of a small part of brain tissue in the "suspected" region. The anterior temporal lobe and hippocampus are the most common areas in which tissue is removed. In some studies, more than 83% of patients become free of seizures following surgery. Ninety-seven percent show significant improvement in their condition.

Vagus Nerve Stimulation (VNS) is another form of treatment for some cases of epilepsy that are unresponsive (referred to as refractory epilepsy) to other forms of medi-

cal therapy. VNS may also be recommended for patients who cannot tolerate the side effects of medication. This procedure involves implanting a device that stimulates the Vagus nerve, located in the left side of the neck. In one study, this treatment reduced seizures by 78%.

A special dietary program is another treatment option for patients who are not good candidates for surgery or who have had little success with anticonvulsant medication. This form of treatment called the Ketogenic Diet can be effective for many types of epilepsy. It is most appropriate for young children whose parents can follow the rigid requirements of the diet. Older children and adults tend to have greater difficulty in sticking to the dietary rules for an extended period of time. The Ketogenic Diet is a stringent diet that is very high in fat, but low in proteins, carbohydrates, and calories. The excessive fat produces high levels of a substance called ketones (which the body makes when it breaks down fat for energy). Somehow these ketones help reduce the incidence of epileptic seizures. The success of this form of treatment varies. For some patients, the high fat diet is the best form of treatment. For others, the diet is less effective.

Resources

PERIODICALS

Berkovic, S. F., and I. E. Scheffer. "Genetics of the epilepsies." *Current Opinion in Neurobiology* 12, no. 2 (April 1999): 177–82.

Farooqui S., W. Boswell, J. M. Hemphill, and E. Pearlman. "Vagus nerve stimulation in pediatric patients with intractable epilepsy: case series and operative technique." *The American Surgeon* 67, no. 2 (February 2001): 119–21.

Hirose S., M. Okada, S. Kaneko, and A. Mitsudome. "Are some idiopathic epilepsies disorders of ion channels?: A working hypothesis." *Epilepsy Research* 41, no. 3 (Oct 2000): 191–204.

Kwan, Patrick, and Martin J. Brodie. "Early Identification of Refractory Epilepsy." *The New England Journal of Medicine* 342, no. 5 (February 3, 2000).

ORGANIZATIONS

American Epilepsy Society, 342 North Main Street, West Hartford, Connecticut 06117, (860) 586-7505. <http://www.aesnet.org.>

Epilepsy and Brain Mapping Program: Huntington Memorial Hospital. 10 Congress Street, Suite 505, Pasadena, California 91105. (800) 621-2102. e-mail: info@epipro.com, <http://www.epipro.com/meds.html>.

Epilepsy Foundation. 4351 Garden City Drive, Landover, Maryland 20785. (800) 332-1000. <http://www.epilepsyfoundation.org.>

WEBSITES

"Seizures." MayoClinic.com. <http://www.mayohealth.org/home?id=SP3.1.4.7>.

Surgical Treatment of Epilepsy. G. Rees Cosgrove, M.D., F.R.C.S.(C) and Andrew J. Cole M.D., FRCP(C). Department of Neurosurgery, Massachusetts General Hospital. 15 Parkman St., ACC Suite # 331, Boston, MA 02114. (617) 724-0357. Fax: (617) 726-5546. cosgrove@helix.mgh.harvard.edu. <http://neurosurgery.mgh.harvard.edu/ep-sxtre.htm>.

Marshall G. Letcher, MA

Essential hypertension

Definition

Essential or primary hypertension, the most common form of hypertension, is elevated blood pressure that develops without apparent cause. Genetic factors, however, appear to play role in increasing the risk of developing the disorder.

Normal blood pressure refers to a range of values rather than a specific set of numbers and varies with factors such as age, race, and gender. However, a blood pressure reading greater than 140/90 mm Hg (millimeters of mercury pressure) is generally considered to be elevated. In this measurement, 140 refers to the systolic pressure (the maximum pressure in the arteries when the heart contracts). The 90 refers to the diastolic pressure (the lowest pressure in the arteries when the heart is between contractions).

Description

More than 95% of all elevated blood pressure can be classified as essential hypertension. When a disease, other physical problems, medications, or even temporary physical exertion or stress cause high blood pressure, the condition is called secondary hypertension.

Blood pressure refers to the force exerted by blood against the interior walls of the body's blood vessels. There are three categories of blood pressure, corresponding to the three types of blood vessels: arterial, capillary, and venous. In individuals with hypertension, arterial pressure (recorded as two numbers: systolic and diastolic pressure) is the most important measurement to obtain. The reason is that because of their relative proximity to blood flowing forcefully from the heart, arteries must withstand the highest pressures of all the body's blood vessels.

The body requires a relatively constant blood pressure level to ensure adequate passage of nutrients and oxygen to organs and tissues. To maintain a constant level of pressure, the body must balance and react to a number of factors such as these:

• volume of blood in the circulatory system

• amount of blood ejected by the heart (stroke volume)

• heart rate

• thickness of the blood (viscosity)

• elasticity of the arteries

When the systolic or diastolic pressure is elevated for an extended period of time, such as months or years, the heart has to work harder and may become damaged, along with the blood vessels. If it remains untreated, high blood pressure can lead to a variety of serious health problems, including heart disease, stroke, and kidney failure.

Genetic profile

Studies suggest that some people with essential hypertension may inherit abnormalities of the sympathetic nervous system—the part of the nervous system that controls heart rate, blood pressure, and the diameter of blood vessels. It is estimated that the risk of developing essential hypertension is increased two- to four-fold if one or both parents are diagnosed with the disorder.

Researchers have identified the chromosomes (11 and 18) that house the genes responsible for blood pressure regulation, although narrowing down the range of specific genes involved in hypertension is more difficult.

Genes under intense study are those that regulate a group of hormones known as the angiotensin-renin-aldosterone system. This system influences all aspects of blood pressure control, including blood vessel contraction, sodium and water balance, and cell development in the heart.

When blood pressure drops, the kidneys release an enzyme called renin, which initiates a chain reaction to bring blood pressure back up. Renin acts on angiotensinogen (a plasma protein) to produce the hormone, angiotensin I (an inactive form), which is then converted to angiotensin II (an active form of the hormone) by the angiotensin-converting enzyme (ACE). Angiotensin II then stimulates the adrenal glands to release the hormone aldosterone, which decreases kidney sodium excretion, thereby causing blood vessels to constrict. When blood vessels constrict, blood pressure goes up.

Researchers believe that this angiotensin-renin-aldosterone system evolved millions of years ago to protect humans. By retaining salt and water and narrowing blood vessels, the body was ensured an adequate blood flow and the ability to repair injured tissue. Over time, however, this system outlived its original protective function and led to serious health complications.

Demographics

It is estimated that one in four Americans have high blood pressure; it is also estimated that one in three people who have high blood pressure are unaware of the problem. Also, hypertension is much more common among African-Americans and Mexican-Americans than in Caucasian populations. Low levels of nitric oxide, which have been observed in individuals—particularly African-Americans—with elevated blood pressure, may be an important factor in the development of essential hypertension.

The prevalence of essential hypertension increases with age until at least the age of 80. Statistics indicate that more than half of all Americans over the age of 65 have hypertension. In those under the age of 55, essential hypertension is more common in males than females. Over age 55, there is an equal distribution among males and females.

Signs and symptoms

Essential hypertension may cause no symptoms for years. For this reason, high blood pressure is often called the "silent killer." The first symptom may be a heart attack or stroke. However, many people with hypertension may experience one or more of the following symptoms:

- headache
- dizziness
- blurred vision
- irregular or rapid heartbeat
- nosebleeds
- fatigue

Diagnosis

Although genetic studies hold hope for detecting, evaluating, and treating hypertension in the future, there are no reliable genetic screening tests for the disorder yet. Thus, essential hypertension is a condition that cannot be diagnosed until it has developed; it is often diagnosed during a routine physical or medical examination.

Blood pressure is measured by an instrument called a sphygmomanometer. A cloth-covered rubber cuff is wrapped around the upper arm and inflated. When the cuff is inflated, an artery in the arm is squeezed to momentarily stop the flow of blood. Then the air is let out of the cuff, while a stethoscope placed over the artery is used to detect the sound of the blood spurting back through the artery. This first sound is the systolic pressure. The last sound heard as the rest of the air is released is the diastolic pressure. Both sounds are recorded on the mercury gauge of the sphygmomanometer.

Because a number of factors such as pain, stress, or anxiety can cause a temporary increase in blood pressure, hypertension is not diagnosed on the basis of one elevated reading. Also, blood pressure results may be different depending on which arm is used. Thus, if a blood pressure reading is 140/90 or higher for the first time, the physician will have the individual return for another blood pressure check. Diagnosis of essential hypertension is usually made based on two or more readings after the first visit.

A typical physical examination to evaluate hypertension includes:

- medical and family history (especially important to determine a genetic contribution)
- physical examination
- examination of the blood vessels in the eye
- chest x ray
- electrocardiograph (EKG)
- blood and urine tests

Treatment and management

There is no complete cure for essential hypertension because unlike secondary hypertension, there is no single cause of the problem; it is a complex disorder only determined, in part, by genes. Environmental (lifestyle) factors interact with genetic factors to produce hypertension.

However, essential hypertension can be treated and managed effectively, even if an individual has a genetic predisposition to the disorder. If essential hypertension is mildly or even moderately high, it may be possible to bring it down to a normal level without medication. Weight loss, changes in diet, and exercise may be the only treatment necessary. General nonpharmacologic recommendations include:

- reducing the amount of salt (sodium) and fat in the diet
- exercising regularly
- maintaining a healthy weight
- limiting alcohol and caffeine consumption
- quitting smoking
- reducing stress through stress management techniques, relaxation exercises, or counseling

If lifestyle changes are not effective in lowering blood pressure to a normal level, medication may be prescribed. There are many types of drugs available to treat essential hypertension. The main categories of drugs include:

- diuretics (help kidneys eliminate excess salt and water from the body's tissues and blood, thereby reducing swelling and lowering blood pressure)
- beta-blockers, alpha-blockers, and alpha/beta blockers (act on nervous system to slow heart rate and reduce the force of the heart's contractions
- angiotensin-converting enzyme (ACE) inhibitors (block the production of substances that constrict blood vessels and reduce salt and water build-up in the tissues)
- calcium channel blockers (block the entry of calcium into muscle cells in artery walls, making arteries more relaxed)
- vasodilators (relax artery walls and lower blood pressure rapidly)
- peripheral acting adrenergic antagonists (act of nervous system to relax arteries and reduce the force of the heart's contractions)
- Centrally acting agonists (act on nervous system to relax arteries)

When a blood pressure medication is prescribed, it is important to:

- take the medication regularly, exactly as prescribed
- report any side effects immediately
- have regular follow-up visits with a physician

It may take weeks or even months to find the most effective pharmacologic treatment. Once an effective drug or combination of drugs is found, individuals with high blood pressure may require treatment for the rest of their lives.

KEY TERMS

Angiotensinogen—A plasma globulin (protein) formed in the liver and directly involved in the regulation of blood pressure.

Diastolic blood pressure—Blood pressure when the heart is resting between beats.

Renin—An enzyme produced by the kidneys.

Sphygmomanometer—An inflatable cuff used to measure blood pressure.

Systolic blood pressure—Blood pressure when the heart contracts (beats).

Vasodilator—A drug that relaxes blood vessel walls.

Prognosis

The higher the blood pressure, the worse the prognosis. However, most serious complications of essential hypertension can be delayed or even avoided by getting regular blood pressure checks and by treating the disorder as soon as it is diagnosed.

Resources

BOOKS

Appel, Lawrence, Robert McNamara, and Jerilyn Allen, eds. *High Blood Pressure: What You Need to Know.* New York: Time Life, 1999.

Whitaker, Julian. *Hypertension: A Vital New Program to Prevent, Treat, and Reduce High Blood Pressure.* New York: Warner Books, 2000.

PERIODICALS

Ambler, S. Kelly, and R. Dale Brown. "Genetic Determinants of Blood Pressure Regulation." *Journal of Cardiovascular Nursing* 13, no. 4 (July 1999): 59–72.

Lifton, Richard P. "Molecular genetics of human blood pressure variation." *Science* 272, no. 5262 (May 3, 1996): 676–80.

Phillips, Robert A. "Hypertension: What's new in diagnosis?" *Consultant* 39, no. 8 (August 1999): 2337–41.

Rowe, Paul M. "Identification of Hypertension Genes Comes Closer." *Lancet* 355, no. 9214 (April 29, 2000): 1525–28.

Seppa, N. "Male hypertension may have genetic link." *Science News* 153, no. 20 (May 16, 1998): 310–12.

ORGANIZATIONS

American Heart Association. 7272 Greenville Ave., Dallas, TX 75231-4596. (214) 373-6300 or (800) 242-8721. inquire@heart.org. <http://www.americanheart.org>.

American Society of Hypertension. 515 Madison Ave., Suite 1212, New York, 10022. (212) 644-0600. <http://www.ash-us.org>.

WEBSITES

Heart Information Network. <http://www.heartinfo.org>.

Genevieve T. Slomski, PhD

Essential tremor

Definition

Tremor is derived from the Latin "to shake." It is an involuntary, rhythmic, back and forth oscillation or shaking of a part of the body, resulting from alternating or irregularly synchronous contractions of antagonist muscles. Essential tremor (ET) is the most common movement disorder. It is a syndrome characterized by a slowly progressive postural and/or kinetic tremor of certain body parts, most commonly the arms, hands, and head when the respective body part is maintained in a constant position.

Description

James Parkinson in 1817 was the first to describe and differentiate ET from the tremor seen in **Parkinson's disease**. ET is also called benign essential tremor or familial tremor. ET is called benign as it does not increase an individual's risk of mortality, and is called essential as the cause was initially unknown. Two genes for ET were discovered in 1997. ET is caused by abnormal communication between certain areas of the brain, including the cerebellum, thalamus, and brainstem. In most cases, the tremor is mild and non-progressive, whereas a minority of people has a slowly progressive condition with the tremor eventually involving the voice box, tongue, legs, and trunk. There can be several periods when the symptoms do not worsen and remain stable. ET can be quite disabling if the tremor is severe and widespread and can substantially affect a person's quality of life.

Demographics

ET is probably the most common neurologic movement disorder of adults and affects about 10 million people in the United States alone. Various estimates indicate that about 5% of patients older than 60 years of age have ET and that it is more prevalent than Parkinson's disease or **Alzheimer's disease**. The incidence is bimodal with the first peak occurring in an individual's early 20s and the second peak in the 60s. It can even occur in children, although onset is rare before age 10. Sometimes, ET appears in adolescence and can go into remission, only to surface later in life. There is no major ethnic or gender differences, although males tend to have more severe extremity tremor and females have more severe head tremor. The actress Katherine Hepburn is one of the well-known personalities who had ET involving the head and voice.

Genetic profile

ET can occur either as a truly sporadic form or more commonly as an autosomal dominant **inheritance** with variable penetrance. Some cases appear to be sporadic, but this could be due to decreased penetrance in certain families, which means that all persons who inherit the **gene** need not express symptoms. In familial ET, 50% of patients develop symptoms by 40 years of age and this differentiates it from truly sporadic ET, which has a later age of onset. Most studies indicate that 50–70% of ET is familial and first-degree relatives are five times more likely to develop ET than a person without an affected relative. Children of affected individuals have a 50% risk of inheriting the gene and expression of this is nearly complete by 70 years of age.

Two susceptibility genes have been identified in ET. One is a familial essential tremor gene (FET1 or ETM1), found on the long arm of **chromosome** 3. The second one is ETM2 on the short arm of chromosome 2. It is not clear if the phenomenon of anticipation occurs in ET, whereby symptoms occur earlier with each successive generation. A third mutation in chromosome 4p may also cause postural tremor.

No structural lesions in the brain have been detected using sophisticated brain imaging techniques like computerized tomography (CT) or magnetic resonance imaging (MRI). Positron emission tomography (PET), which examines the biochemistry in various parts of the brain, and functional MRI (fMRI) scans have shown increased activity in the cerebellum and olivo-cerebellar pathways. It is postulated that certain circuits in the brain may become unstable and drive muscle contractions. These are called central oscillators, and one such oscillating generator/pacemaker is a part of the brainstem near the inferior olivary nucleus, which becomes unmasked in ET. Other possible generators include the red nucleus, globus pallidus, and cerebellum. Disturbances in neural transmission involving the amino acid gamma amino butyric acid (GABA) are thought to be important in ET.

Signs and symptoms

Tremor is usually the only symptom seen in ET. There are three types of tremor that can be observed in ET.

The most common is postural tremor is seen when the patient is voluntarily maintaining a fixed anti-gravity position of a limb (e.g., outstretched hands). This resembles a physiologic tremor that is present in everyone, but is more severe in an affected individual. The postural tremor appears as a fine to moderate tremor with a frequency of 4–12 Hertz (Hz). This usually begins in both hands simultaneously, but 10–15% patients notice tremor onset in the dominant hand. A mild degree of asymmetry in tremor severity is not unusual. Tremor usually moves from the hands to the arms over time. Initially the tremor may be noticeable only during periods of fatigue or anxiety, but it becomes more constant over time. The severity of tremor varies considerably even from day to day. Tremor amplitude worsens with emotion, cold, hunger, and fatigue, and tends to increase with age. Changing the angle of the limb position can significantly alter the magnitude of the tremor. Handwriting becomes shaky and rounded letters take on a sharp angularity. There is a component of the tremor that can be voluntarily suppressed. The tremors can range from being mild and a minor annoyance in one individual to severe and disabling in another family member.

Some patients have worsening of tremor while performing goal-directed tasks, such as writing, buttoning a shirt, or drinking from a cup, and this is called intention tremor, or kinetic tremor. This type of tremor is higher in amplitude than positional tremor and is the major cause of disability. The third type of tremor is a feeling of general shakiness or a sensation of vibration inside the body referred as internal tremor.

In about 30% of patients, the tremor involves the head region. Head tremor (titubation) is the second most common body part to be affected and can occur either in isolation or with hand tremors. Head tremor is mostly a horizontal sideways pattern, as if indicating no. Voice and tongue tremor causes dysarthria (difficulty in articulating words) and causes quavering or shaky speech and is usually seen with advancing age above 65.

Tremor generally disappears during sleep and is minimal during periods of rest. Although the typical picture is that of gradually increasing postural and kinetic tremor of the hands and forearms, there exists considerable variation among patients. Muscle tone and strength are usually not affected. Memory, intellect, strength, and muscle tone remain intact. Some associated symptoms like ataxia (unsteady and uncoordinated gait) and **dystonia** can also be seen. It is still controversial if there is a higher-than-chance incidence of Parkinson's disease among people with ET.

Diagnosis

Although ET is a common condition seen in general medical practice, diagnosis may be difficult and treatment challenging. Correct diagnosis is crucial to implement early treatment and to avoid unnecessary anxiety about a misdiagnosis of more severe neurological conditions like Parkinson's disease or other neurodegenerative disorders. It is best diagnosed and treated by a neurologist or a physician trained in movement disorders. No biomarkers, blood tests, or imaging tools is available to assist in diagnosis. Thyroid disease, excess caffeine consumption, and medication side effects should be excluded as these can mimic ET. MRI scans are used only to exclude other causes of tremor, such as **multiple sclerosis**.

Diagnosis is mainly clinical and depends on recognizing the postural tremor, absence of rest tremor that is seen in Parkinson's disease, presence of tremor for more than three years, a decrease in tremor with alcohol consumption, and a family history of similar tremor. Clinical tremor questionnaires and rating scales can be helpful in the diagnosis and in assessing response to treatment. During the neurological assessment, the physician may use simple tests like spiral or line drawing, handwriting, tasks such as taking a water-filled cup to the mouth, articulating vowels, etc., to determine the extent and severity of ET. Accelerometer is a simple device attached to the fingers that measures tremor frequency.

Diagnostic criteria

Inclusion criteria include the following symptoms:

- Bilateral, largely symmetrical postural, or kinetic tremor in hands/forearms that is visible and persistent.
- Isolated head tremor may occur, but without abnormal posturing.

Exclusion criteria include the following symptoms:

- Prominent dystonia
- Known causes of enhanced physiologic tremor
- Psychogenic origin of tremor
- Primary orthostatic tremor
- Isolated voice tremor
- Isolated position or task-specific tremor
- Isolated tongue or chin tremor
- Isolated leg tremor

Treatment and management

Various population-based studies have found that only about 15% of patients with ET seek treatment, mostly because of lack of awareness of the disease and treatment options. Treatment is based on how disabling the symptoms are to the patient, as early treatment has not been shown to stop or delay the disease progression.

There is a 50% chance that the tremor will respond to currently available medications without undue side effects. Sometimes, trials with multiple medications may have to be done before the tremor responds. Depending on coexisting medical conditions and neurological diseases, treatment must be individualized.

Lifestyle changes, including elimination of caffeinated foods like sodas, coffee, and chocolates, and other stimulants like cigarettes, are the first step in treatment. Biofeedback, acupuncture, yoga, tai-chi, and guided imagery are techniques that can be used in patients in whom the tremor worsens with stress and anxiety. In 50% of patients, alcohol may reduce tremor for up to two hours, but this is not to be considered as therapy. Excessive alcohol consumption can worsen tremor as a rebound phenomenon. Adaptive devices like wrist weights and plate guards can help to minimize tremor and interference with daily activities. Specially designed utensils (such as rocker knives and utensils with large handles) and electrical appliances (such as can openers and toothbrushes) can make daily activities easier. Certain simple precautions can enable many people to continue their normal daily activities. For example, objects should be grasped firmly but comfortably and held close to the body. Cylinders of foam can be placed around handles to make them easier to hold. Other helpful measures include using straws, button hooks, Velcro fasteners, zipper pulls, and shoe horns. Counseling may be needed to help patients deal with social isolation resulting from severe tremor.

The most commonly used medication to treat ET is propranolol, which is a beta blocker. It prevents the action of adrenaline and reduces tremor amplitude. It is available in a short- and long-acting form. The effect of the short-acting form lasts for 3–4 hours and is suitable for taking prior to a specific task, such as giving a speech, attending a social gathering, etc. It is rare for the tremor to completely disappear with treatment, but about 60% of patients respond to it. The medication works best for hand tremor. Side effects include lowering of blood pressure and heart rate, aggravation of **asthma** and **depression**, fatigue, and impotence. Primidone is a barbiturate and is the second most commonly used medication. It was originally developed as an anti-seizure medication and is taken once a day at night in order to minimize the side effects of drowsiness and fatigue. It can be used for long periods of time with minimal side effects. Other medications include gabapentin and benzodiazepines like Valium and clonazepam. A combination of propranolol and primidone can be used in resistant cases. Newer therapeutic approaches include botulinum toxin injection into the muscles, such as neck muscles to treat head tremor. Transient weakness may be experienced, but the therapeutic effect lasts for 3–6 months.

Invasive surgical intervention is usually reserved for patients with severe disabling unilateral tremor, bilateral tremor, head and voice tremor, functional disability that interferes with the activities of daily living, or tremor that is unresponsive to the highest tolerated doses of medications.

The thalamus is a paired structure deep inside the brain and its ventral intermediate nucleus (VIM) is intimately involved in movement regulation. In thalamotomy, a small pea-sized hole is made in the thalamus on the side opposite to the tremor to disrupt faulty circuits. As the thalamus is close to vital brainstem structures, the surgery has to be done only by an experienced neurosurgeon. Postoperatively, some temporary side effects like confusion, weakness, and speech difficulty may occur. Bilateral thalamotomy is not advised as it may cause loss of speech and other permanent neurologic problems. Thalamotomy is especially helpful in patients with severe unilateral hand, arm, and leg tremor and is effective in up to 80% of patients with either decrease or cessation of medications. In a similar method using gamma knife, a small burn is made in the thalamus without a hole or operation being necessary.

Thalamic stimulation, or deep brain stimulation (DBS), is an alternative to thalamotomy. Unilateral DBS for tremor was approved by the Food and Drug Administration (FDA) in 1997. It involves implanting an electrode (a fine wire) deep in the VIM nucleus of the thalamus. The electrode is connected to a stimulation device (implantation pulse generator), similar to a pacemaker, which is placed under the skin below the collarbone. By sending painless, high-frequency electrical currents through the electrode, it interrupts communication between tremor cells and helps the thalamus rebalance the tremor control messages. Patients may turn the pulse generator off and on by passing a hand-held magnet over the device. The batteries that power the pulse generator need to be surgically replaced every 3–5 years. Tremor reduction occurs within seconds of activation and can be quite dramatic. Significant or complete tremor reduction occurs in approximately 80% of people with this procedure and, thus far, efficacy has continued for 6–7 years. The main advantages of this procedure are that implantation on both sides of the brain is possible, the device can be adjusted for optimal effect, and it may be removed if desired. Other potential targets for DBS in ET include globus pallidus and sub-thalamic nucleus.

There are two ongoing clinical trials sponsored by the National Institute of Neurological Diseases and Stroke (NINDS). One of these measures the reduction of tremor by a substance called Octanol. The other looks at

KEY TERMS

Acupuncture—An alternative health procedure based on ancient Chinese methods, involving insertion of thin needles at specific pressure points in the body.

Alzheimer's disease—A neurodegenerative disease marked by the loss of cognitive ability, generally over a period of 10–15 years, associated with the development of abnormal tissues and protein deposits in the brain.

Anticipation—The apparent tendency of certain diseases to appear at earlier ages and with increasing severity in successive generations.

Ataxia—A condition of bodily incoordination and unsteadiness that is most often caused by disease activity in the cerebellum.

Autosomal dominant—A type of genetic inheritance where a trait (or a disease) is produced even when only one copy of an abnormal gene is present.

Biofeedback—A technique in which patients are trained to gain some voluntary control over certain physiological conditions, such as blood pressure and muscle tension, and to promote relaxation.

Cerebellum—The lower back part of the brain responsible for functions such as maintaining balance, and coordinating and controlling voluntary muscle movement.

Computed tomography(CT)—A special radiographic technique to visualize internal organs using a computer to combine multiple x-ray images into a two-dimensional cross-sectional image.

Dysarthria—Refers to a group of speech disorders caused by disturbances in the strength or coordination of the muscles of the speech mechanism as a result of damage to the brain or nerves.

Dystonia—A movement disorder involving prolonged muscle contractions that cause twisting and repetitive movements or abnormal posture.

Functional magnetic resonance imaging (fMRI)—A form of imaging of the brain that registers blood flow to functioning areas of the brain.

Gamma knife—Equipment that precisely delivers a concentrated dose of radiation to a predetermined target using gamma rays.

Gamma amino butyric acid (GABA)—An amino acid that functions as the major inhibitory neurotransmitter in the nervous system.

Globus pallidus—A small paired structure present in the deep portion of the brain, in front of the brain-

stem, that is considered a part of the basal ganglia and helps in movement control.

Inferior olivary nucleus—A small collection of cells seen in the lower part of the brainstem, which has connections to the cerebellum and is involved in control of movements.

Magnetic resonance imaging (MRI)—An imaging technique that uses the properties of magnetism to create nondestructive, three-dimensional, internal images of the soft tissues of the body, including the brain, spinal cord, and muscle.

Multiple sclerosis—A progressive autoimmune disease in which the body attacks its own central nervous system, gradually destroying the white fatty substance that surrounds nerve fibers, thereby damaging sites in the brain and spinal cord.

Orthostatic—Posture that is maintained while standing.

Parkinson's disease—A progressive disease occurring most often after the age of 50, associated with the destruction of brain cells that produce dopamine and characterized by tremor, slowing of movement, and gait difficulty.

Penetrance—The extent to which a disease expresses itself in individuals that have the mutation; for example, if all individuals with the abnormal gene exhibit the disease, the disease is said to have complete penetrance.

Positron emission tomography (PET)—A form of nuclear medicine scanning that measures brain activity using low doses of a radioactive substance.

Red nucleus—A small structure present in the brainstem that is involved in the control of movement.

Sporadic—Disease that is apparently not hereditary.

Tai-chi—A Chinese system of physical exercises that uses slow, smooth body movements to help with posture control and relaxation.

Thalamus—A pair of large egg-shaped structures near the brainstem that act as the main sensory relay station and help with control of movement.

Titubation—Tremor of the head.

Yoga—An exercise that combines relaxation and breathing techniques to combat stress and help circulation and movement of the joints; yoga has its origin in ancient Indian medicine.

tremor reduction by Botox (botulinum toxin). The Essential Tremor Organization is also conducting a trial looking at the efficacy of a medication called topiramate. Fetal neural implant (or nigral implant) is an experimental technique that involves transplanting fetal tissue into the brain to replace degenerated nerves. Many issues are still unresolved, such as the source of embryonic tissue, the amount of tissue required, the number of brain penetrations needed, and rejection of transplanted tissue.

Prognosis

ET does not increase a person's risk of mortality, but can result in varying levels of functional difficulty and disability depending on how severe the tremor is. With advancing age, the amplitude of the tremor worsens and it is this feature that results in major disability. The patient with ET is disabled either due to physical limitations or from the resulting social embarrassment, which can lead to social withdrawal and depression. Everyday tasks that need fine motor skills and manipulation become difficult, such as writing, using utensils, drinking from a glass, applying makeup, etc. Several patients even opt for early retirement or change jobs due to the severity of tremor. Patients should be educated about the disease and emphasized that it is not life-threatening or a forerunner of a neurodegenerative disorder like Parkinson's disease.

RESOURCES

BOOKS

Bradley, Walter G., Robert B. Daroff, Gerald M. Fenichel, and Joseph Jankovic. *Neurology in Clinical Practice*, 4th ed. Philadelphia: Butterworth Heinemann, 2004.

PERIODICALS

Louis, Elan D. "Essential Tremor". *Lancet Neurology* 4 (February 2005): 100–110.

Sullivan, Kelly L., Robert A. Hauser, and Theresa A. Zesiewicz. "Essential Tremor". *The Neurologist* 10 (September 2004): 250–258.

ORGANIZATIONS

International Essential Tremor Foundation. P.O.Box 14005, Lenexa, Kansas 66285-4005. (888) 387 3667. (April 4, 2005.) <http://www.essentialtremor.org>.

National Institutes of Health/National Institute of Neurological Disorders and Stroke Brain Resources and Information Network. PO Box 5801, Bethesda, MD 20824. (301) 496 5751. (April 4, 2005.) <http://www.ninds.nih.gov>.

Worldwide Education and Awareness for Movement Disorders (WE MOVE). 204 West 84th Street, New York, NY 10024. (April 4, 2005.) <http://www.wemove.org>.

OTHER

Medtronic Neurological Patient Services. LN 360, 710 Medtronic Parkway NE, Minneapolis, MN 55432-5604. (800) 325-2518. (April 4, 2005.) <http://www.medtronic.com>.

National Institute of Neurological Disorders and Stroke, Patient Recruitment and Public Liaison Office. 9000 Rockville Pike, Bethesda, MD 20892. (800) 411-1222. (April 4, 2005.) <http://www.clinicaltrials.gov>.

Tremor Action Network. PO Box 5013, Pleasanton, CA 94566-0513. (952) 462-0111. (April 4, 2005.) <http://www.tremoraction.org>.

Chitra Venkatasubramanian, MBBS, MD

F

Fabry disease

Definition

Fabry disease is a genetic condition that typically affects males. It is caused by deficiency of an enzyme, a chemical that speeds up another chemical reaction. Fabry disease can affect many parts of the body including the kidneys, eyes, brain, and heart. Pain in the hands and feet and a characteristic rash are classic features of this disease.

Description

The symptoms of Fabry disease were first described by Dr. Johann Fabry and Dr. William Anderson in 1898. The enzyme deficiency that leads to the disease was identified in the 1960s. Fabry disease is caused by a change (mutation) in the GLA **gene**. This gene is responsible for the production of the enzyme alpha-galactosidase A. Alpha-galactosidase A normally breaks down globotriaosylceramide. Globotriaosylceramide is a natural substance in the body, made of sugar and fat. A mutation in the GLA gene leads to a decrease in alpha-galactosidase A activity which, in turn, leads to an excess of globotriaosylceramide. The excess globotriaosylceramide builds up in blood vessels (veins, arteries, and capillaries) and obstructs normal blood flow. It also builds up in parts of the skin, kidneys, heart, and brain. It is this build-up that inhibits normal function and leads to the symptoms associated with the disease.

The symptoms of Fabry disease are variable. Some individuals with Fabry disease have severe complications, while others have very mild symptoms. The first sign of the disease may be a painful burning sensation in the hands and feet (acroparesthesias). A red rash, most commonly between the belly button and the knees (angiokeratoma) is also common. The outer portion of the eye (cornea) may also become clouded in individuals with Fabry disease. The progressive build up of globotriaosylceramide can also lead to kidney problems and heart disease in adulthood.

Genetic profile

The gene that produces alpha-galactosidase A is located on the X **chromosome**. It is called the GLA gene. Since the GLA gene is located on the X chromosome, Fabry disease is considered to be X-linked. This means that it generally affects males.

A person's sex is determined by his or her chromosomes. Males have one X chromosome and one Y chromosome. Females, on the other hand, have two X chromosomes. Males who possess a mutation or change in their GLA gene will develop Fabry disease. Females who possess a mutation in one of their GLA genes typically do not develop many of the symptoms associated with Fabry disease. This is because a female's other X chromosome does not have the mutation, and the normal chromosome can take over the function of the abnormal chromosome and keep her from getting the disease. These women are considered to be carriers. If a woman is a carrier, she has a 50% risk with any pregnancy to pass on her X chromosome with the mutation. Therefore, with every male pregnancy she has a 50% risk of having an affected son, and with every female pregnancy she has a 50% risk of having a daughter who is a carrier.

Demographics

Fabry disease affects approximately one in 40,000 live births. It occurs evenly among all ethnic groups. Almost always, only male children are affected. Although female carriers of the disease occasionally develop symptoms of the disease, it is rare for a female carrier to be severely affected.

Signs and symptoms

The signs and symptoms of Fabry disease vary. Some individuals with Fabry disease have many severe symptoms, while other individuals' symptoms may be few and mild. The symptoms typically increase or intensify over time. This progression is caused by the slow buildup of globotriaosylceramide as the person ages.

A painful burning sensation in the hands and feet (acroparesthesias) is one of the first symptoms of Fabry disease. This pain can be severe and may grow worse with exercise, stress, illness, extreme heat, or extreme cold. Another symptom of Fabry disease typically present during childhood is a red rash (angiokeratoma). This rash typically develops between the navel and the knees. Children with Fabry disease may also have a clouding of the outer most portion of the eye (cornea). This symptom is usually diagnosed by an eye doctor (ophthalmologist). The cloudiness may increase with time. A decreased ability to sweat is another common symptom of Fabry disease.

Due to the progressive nature of Fabry disease, most affected individuals develop additional symptoms by age 40. The buildup of globotriaosylceramide in the heart can lead to heart problems. These heart problems can include changes in the size of the heart (left ventricular enlargement), differences in the heart beat, and leaky heart valves. Mitral valve prolapse is a particular type of leaky heart valve that is common in Fabry disease, even in childhood. The excess globotriaosylceramide can also disrupt normal blood flow in the brain. In some cases this can cause dizziness, seizures, and stroke. The kidneys are other organs affected by Fabry disease. Kidney problems can lead to an abnormal amount of protein in the urine (proteinuria). Severe kidney problems can lead to kidney failure.

Although the symptoms of Fabry disease usually occur in males, female carriers may occasionally exhibit symptoms of the disease. Some carriers experience pain in their hands and feet. Carrier females may also have proteinuria and clouding of their cornea. It is rare for a female to experience all of the symptoms associated with Fabry disease.

Diagnosis

Initially, the diagnosis of Fabry disease is based on the presence of the symptoms. It should also be suspected if there is a family history of the disorder. The diagnosis of Fabry disease is definitively made by measuring the activity of the alpha-galactosidase enzyme. When the activity is very low, it is diagnostic of Fabry disease. This enzyme analysis can be performed through a blood test. Measuring the activity of the enzyme can also detect if female carrier. Women who are carriers of Fabry disease have enzyme activity that is lower than normal.

Prenatal diagnosis is possible by measuring the alpha-galactosidase A activity in fetal tissue drawn by **amniocentesis** or chorionic villus sampling (CVS). Fetuses should be tested if the mother is a carrier. A

KEY TERMS

Acroparesthesias—Painful burning sensation in hands and feet.

Amniocentesis—A procedure performed at 16-18 weeks of pregnancy in which a needle is inserted through a woman's abdomen into her uterus to draw out a small sample of the amniotic fluid from around the baby. Either the fluid itself or cells from the fluid can be used for a variety of tests to obtain information about genetic disorders and other medical conditions in the fetus.

Angiokeratoma—Skin rash comprised of red bumps. Rash most commonly occurs between the navel and the knees.

Blood vessels—General term for arteries, veins, and capillaries that transport blood throughout the body.

Chorionic villus sampling (CVS)—A procedure used for prenatal diagnosis at 10-12 weeks gestation. Under ultrasound guidance a needle is inserted either through the mother's vagina or abdominal wall and a sample of cells is collected from around the fetus. These cells are then tested for chromosome abnormalities or other genetic diseases.

Cornea—The transparent structure of the eye over the lens that is continuous with the sclera in forming the outermost protective layer of the eye.

Dialysis—Process by which special equipment purifies the blood of a patient whose kidneys have failed.

Enzyme replacement therapy—Giving an enzyme to a person who needs it for normal body function. It is given through a needle that is inserted into the body.

Left ventricular enlargement—Abnormal enlargement of the left lower chamber of the heart.

Mitral valve prolapse—A heart defect in which one of the valves of the heart (which normally controls blood flow) becomes floppy. Mitral valve prolapse may be detected as a heart murmur, but there are usually no symptoms.

Mutation—A permanent change in the genetic material that may alter a trait or characteristic of an individual, or manifest as disease, and can be transmitted to offspring.

Proteinuria—Excess protein in the urine.

woman is at risk of being a carrier if she has a son with Fabry disease or someone in her family has Fabry disease.

Treatment and management

There is currently no cure for Fabry disease. However, there are clinical trials underway in which individuals with Fabry disease are being given the alpha-galactosidase A enzyme as a form of enzyme replacement therapy. If successful, this enzyme replacement therapy may reduce or eliminate the symptoms associated with Fabry disease.

Until the enzyme replacement therapy is proven to be safe and effective, individuals with Fabry disease must rely on traditional treatments. Individuals with Fabry disease are recommended to have routine evaluations of the their heart and kidneys. Some individuals with kidney disease require a special diet that is low in sodium and protein. Dialysis and kidney transplantation may be necessary for patients with severe kidney disease. Certain medications may reduce the risk of stroke. Finally, individuals with Fabry disease are recommended to avoid the situations that cause the pain in their hands and feet to grow worse. In some situations medication may be required to reduce the pain.

Prognosis

The prognosis for individuals with Fabry disease is good, especially with the arrival of enzyme replacement therapy. Currently, affected individuals survive into adulthood with the symptoms increasing over time.

Resources

BOOKS

Desnick, Robert J., Yiannis Ioannou, and Christine Eng. Galactosidase A Deficiency: Fabry Disease.'' In *The Molecular Bases of Inherited Disease*. 8th ed. New York: McGraw Hill, 2001.

ORGANIZATIONS

Alliance of Genetic Support Groups. 4301 Connecticut Ave. NW, Suite 404, Washington, DC 20008. (202) 966-5557. Fax: (202) 966-8553. <http://www.geneticalliance.org>.

Deptartment of Human Genetics, International Center for Fabry Disease. Box 1497, Fifth Ave. at 100th St., New York, NY 10029. (866) 322-7963. <http://www.mssm.edu/genetics/fabry>.

Fabry Support and Information Group. PO Box 510, 108 NE 2nd St., Suite C, Concordia, MO 64020. (660) 463-1355. <http://www.cpgnet.com/fsig.nsf>.

National Institute of Neurological Disorders and Stroke. 31 Center Drive, MSC 2540, Bldg. 31, Room 8806, Bethesda, MD 20814. (301) 496-5751 or (800) 352-9424. <http://www.ninds.nih.gov>.

National Organization for Rare Disorders (NORD). PO Box 8923, New Fairfield, CT 06812-8923. (203) 746-6518 or (800) 999-6673. Fax: (203) 746-6481. <http://www.rarediseases.org>.

WEBSITES

Fabry Disease Home Page. <http://www.sci.ccny.cuny.edu/~fabry/>.

Online Mendelian Inheritance in Man(OMIM). <http://www.ncbi.nlm.nih.gov/htbin-post/Omim/dispmim?301500>.

Holly Ann Ishmael, MS, CGC

Facioauriculovertebral sequence (FAVS) *see* **Hemifacial microsomia**

Faciopalatoosseous syndrome *see* **Otopalatodigital syndrome**

Facioscapulohumeral muscular dystrophy

Definition

The term **muscular dystrophy** refers to a group of conditions characterized by progressive muscle weakness and atrophy (deterioration). Many different types of muscular dystrophy have been described, each of which have unique features and usually a unique underlying genetic cause. Facioscapulohumeral (FSH) muscular dystrophy affects the muscles of the face and shoulders first. Usually the first signs of weakness appear before the age of 20 years. The symptoms of FSH muscular dystrophy are variable and are not fatal. One in five people who are affected require a wheelchair after the age of 40 years.

Description

Facio refers to the face, *scapulo* to the shoulder blades, and *humeral* to the bone of the upper arm. The symptoms of FSH muscular dystrophy are quite variable, even within the same family. Some individuals who have the altered **DNA** sequence never develop noticeable symptoms. Most people with the condition first notice weakness in their teenage years. Muscles of the shoulders and face are usually the first to be affected. These may remain the only parts of the body that are affected, or the weakness may progress to include the pelvic muscles, the lower limbs, and the hands. Intelligence and life expectancy are not affected.

Genetic profile

FSH muscular dystrophy has autosomal dominant **inheritance**. This means that an affected person has a 50% chance, with each pregnancy, to pass the altered **gene** on to the child. Every person has two copies of every DNA sequence, one inherited maternally and the other inherited paternally. The altered DNA sequence that causes FSH muscular dystrophy is on **chromosome** 4. If a person has one normal sequence and one altered sequence, he or she will probably develop FSH muscular dystrophy.

When an autosomal dominant condition is present in multiple generations of a family, usually someone from each generation is affected. If a person is the first in his or her family to have an autosomal dominant condition, doctors often assume that the gene mutated for the first time in the egg or sperm that came together to make that person. (This is called a new mutation.) However, when the physical symptoms associated with an altered gene are highly variable, the distinction between these two scenarios is less obvious.

The term nonpenetrance refers to altered genes that do not always cause a person to have the typical associated symptoms. FSH muscular dystrophy is nonpenetrant in some individuals. Therefore, an individual who appears to be the first person affected in his or her family may have actually inherited the mutated DNA sequence from his or her mother or father. If so, his or her siblings would be at a 50% risk to also have inherited the altered sequence. Similarly, a mildly affected individual may have a child who is severely affected. Occasionally, two affected siblings are born to unaffected parents because of a genetic process called germline mosaicism.

Describing the genetics of FSH muscular dystrophy is slightly complicated by an interesting phenomenon. Genes are the DNA sequences that give the body instructions for growth, development, and functioning. Usually a mutation that causes a disease occurs in the gene associated with that disease. The above description refers to the mutation in FSH muscular dystrophy as an altered DNA sequence because it does not appear that this sequence is actually part of a gene. The mutated sequence affects the gene for FSH muscular dystrophy, but probably is not part of the gene itself.

Demographics

The incidence of FSH muscular dystrophy is approximately one in 20,000. Some references report a lower incidence. Individuals from all ethnic groups are affected.

Signs and symptoms

The severity of the symptoms of FSH muscular dystrophy is highly variable. Some people are debilitated while others are minimally affected. Symptoms of progressive muscle weakness are usually first noticed in the teenage years, but may be noticed much later. For unknown reasons, more males than females with FSH muscular dystrophy develop symptoms by the age of 30 years. Specific muscle groups are affected. FSH muscular dystrophy does not lead to reduced sensation, nor does it affect intelligence.

Progressive muscle weakness of the shoulders/upper arms and face muscles are usually noticed first. The facial muscle weakness may be noticed as difficulty puckering the lips, smiling, sucking a straw, and closing the eyes while sleeping. Weakness may be asymmetrical, i.e. one shoulder may be weaker than the other shoulder. As the condition progresses, the muscles of the lower legs, abdomen, and hips may also become weak. The muscle weakness leads to abnormal positioning such as forward-sloping shoulders and exaggerated curvature of the spine. Although the weakness progresses continuously, the affected individual may perceive it as progressing rapidly at times and slowly at other times. This is because he or she notices the weakness when it results in loss of function. Reflexes are often weaker than normal. Twenty percent of affected individuals eventually require wheelchairs.

Describing the weakness as shoulder weakness or facial weakness is an oversimplification. In FSH muscular dystrophy, very specific muscles are affected. Not all of the facial muscles are affected, and not all of the muscles of the shoulder are affected. For example, the biceps and triceps of the upper arm are affected before the deltoids, and the forearm is relatively unaffected.

Some researchers report that more males than females with FSH muscular dystrophy develop symptoms by the age of 30 years. The reasons for this are unknown. Other researchers report that men and women are equally affected. Autosomal dominant conditions such as FSH muscular dystrophy usually affect men and women equally.

Many individuals with early–onset FSH muscular dystrophy develop hearing loss of the high tones. Some individuals have more significant hearing loss. Slight changes of the retina are also a symptom of FSH muscular dystrophy. These changes usually do not affect vision.

A subset of FSH muscular dystrophy patients are severely affected. Individuals with severe infantile FSH muscular dystrophy are symptomatic at birth.

Diagnosis

The diagnosis of FSH muscular dystrophy is based on clinical history (symptoms), family history, and **genetic testing**. Many evaluations may be necessary to confirm the diagnosis. A thorough physical examination will be performed. Additional testing may include measuring the level of creatine kinase (CK) in the blood, special analysis of tissue obtained by muscle biopsy, and electromyogram (EMG). Sometimes it is difficult to rule out other possible causes of the muscle weakness.

Genetic testing is available for FSH muscular dystrophy, but it is complicated. Not everyone who is shown to have the associated abnormality of chromosome 4 develops symptoms of FSH muscular dystrophy. Alternately, not everyone who has FSH muscular dystrophy shows the typical genetic abnormality. Therefore, the test is helpful, but it must be interpreted in the context of the individual's medical history. A small subset of people tested will have inconclusive results. This is not due to lab error; some people have a genetic change that is midway between normal and abnormal.

Genetic testing can be performed on fetal cells that are obtained by **amniocentesis**, performed after the sixteenth week of pregnancy, or chorionic villus sampling (CVS). CVS is usually performed between 10 and 12 weeks of pregnancy.

Researchers have shown some correlation between the type of mutation in the FSH region of chromosome 4 and the severity of the disease. Abnormal genetic results fall into a range from nearly normal or far from normal. People with certain abnormal genetic testing results tend to have earlier onset of symptoms and more rapidly progressive muscle weakness. Although many researchers have observed this correlation, the cause and effect relationship is not clear.

Because of the variable severity of symptoms, assumptions should not be made about the family history. A thorough clinical examination by an experienced physician may show that a person believed to be unaffected actually has mild symptoms.

Treatment and management

There is no effective treatment, prevention, or cure for FSH muscular dystrophy. Available treatments help affected persons with the effects of the disease but do not treat the disease itself. Supportive therapies include orthodic devices such as splints and braces, and sometimes surgery. Physical and occupational therapy may be helpful to ease discomfort and adjust to physical changes. Researchers continue to study various medica-

---

KEY TERMS

Gene—A building block of inheritance, which contains the instructions for the production of a particular protein, and is made up of a molecular sequence found on a section of DNA. Each gene is found on a precise location on a chromosome.

Genome—All of the DNA in one cell.

Germ line mosaicism—A rare event that occurs when one parent carries an altered gene mutation that affects his or her germ line cells (either the egg or sperm cells) but is not found in the somatic (body) cells.

Retina—The light-sensitive layer of tissue in the back of the eye that receives and transmits visual signals to the brain through the optic nerve.

---

tions. Previous studies indicated that prednisone may improve muscle strength. However, this was not confirmed in more recent studies. Another medication, albuterol, was shown to be beneficial in early studies.

Prognosis

The prognosis for FSH muscular dystrophy is extremely variable. Prognosis cannot be predicted based on family history. Most people remain ambulatory, but some do not. Progression is usually slow. One third of affected individuals over 40 years of age have mild symptoms. A few people with FSH muscular dystrophy never develop muscle weakness. The typical course is weakness that becomes noticeable before the age of 20 years and progresses slowly but continuously throughout life.

Although FSH muscular dystrophy is rare in the general population, it is a relatively common neuromuscular disorder. Identification of the altered DNA sequence associated with FSH muscular dystrophy has stimulated research efforts. If the mechanism underlying the disease practice is discovered, researchers can better study possible treatments.

Resources

ORGANIZATIONS

FacioScapuloHumeral Society, Inc. 3 Westwood Rd., Lexington, MA 02420. (781) 860-0501. carol.perez@fshsociety.org. <http://www.fshsociety.org>.

Muscular Dystrophy Association. 3300 East Sunrise Dr., Tucson, AZ 85718. (520) 529-2000 or (800) 572-1717. <http://www.mdausa.org>.

Muscular Dystrophy Campaign. 7-11 Prescott Place, London, SW4 6BS. UK +44(0) 7720 8055. info@muscular-dystrophy.org. <http://www.muscular-dystrophy.org>.

WEBSITES

"Facioscapulohumeral Muscular Dystrophy." *Gene Clinics.* <http://www.geneclinics.org/profiles/fsh/details.html>.

National Institute of Neurological Disorders and Stroke. Summary of "Conference on the Cause and Treatment of Facioscapulohumeral Muscular Dystrophy," held May 2000. <http://nindsiis2.ninds.nih.gov/news_and_events/fshmdconference.htm>.

OTHER

Facioscapulohumeral Muscular Dystrophy. Fact Sheet. Yale Neuromuscular MDA/ALS Program. http://pandora.med.yale.edu/neurol/Cneruophysiol/FSH.html.

Facts About Muscular Dystrophy (MD). Booklet. Muscular Dystrophy Association. <http://www.mdausa.org/publications/fa-md.html>.

FSH Muscular Dystrophy. Fact Sheet. Disability Information & Resources Center Inc. http://www.dircsa.org.au/pub/docs/fsh.htm.

Michelle Q. Bosworth, MS, CGC

Factor V deficiency *see* **Factor V leiden thrombophilia**

Factor V Leiden thrombophilia

Definition

Factor V Leiden thrombophilia is a common genetic disorder that leads to a predisposition or increased chance to develop blood clots in the veins (venous thrombosis).

Description

Factor V Leiden thrombophilia is a disorder caused by an inherited change or mutation in the genetic instructions for making a substance called factor V. The factor V change leads to an increased chance to develop blood clots in blood vessels.

Blood clots form in two steps. In the first step, the body produces platelets that are "sticky" and can form initial plugs or clots when needed. However, the first platelets only form the first temporary plugs. To form a more lasting plug or clot the platelets release chemicals to attract more platelets and other substances called clotting factors (or clotting proteins). In the second step, the platelets come together with the clotting proteins and form fibers. The fibers weave together and make the clot stronger and longer lasting.

Individuals affected by factor V Leiden thrombophilia have a genetic mutation that makes a longer lasting, "stickier" form of the clotting factor or protein called factor V. This different form of factor V is called factor V Leiden. The factor V Leiden clotting protein lasts longer in the blood because a chemical produced by the body called Activated Protein C (or APC), which is supposed to help "break-down" the factor V clotting protein, cannot break down the factor V Leiden clotting protein as easily and quickly as it breaks down normal factor V. The factor V Leiden clotting protein breaks down ten times slower than an average clotting factor V and accordingly stays in the blood longer.

Since there is longer lasting, extra sticky Factor V Leiden in the blood, individuals affected by factor V Leiden thrombophilia have an increased chance to have free-floating blood clots (thrombosis) that can get stuck in the veins and other blood vessels. An alternative name used to describe this condition is Hereditary Resistance to Activated Protein C.

Genetic profile

Factor V Leiden thrombophilia occurs when a specific **gene** on the long arm of **chromosome** one is changed or mutated. This gene is called *F5*. Every person has approximately 30,000-35,000 genes that tell our bodies how to form and function. Each gene is present in pairs, since one is inherited from the mother, and one is inherited from the father. Depending on the **inheritance** of the changed or mutated *F5* gene, factor V Leiden thrombophilia runs in families in a more severe and less severe form.

The less severe form of factor V Leiden thrombophilia is called "heterozygous" and occurs when an individual inherits only one copy of the altered or mutated gene that causes factor V Leiden. The more severe form of factor V is called "homozygous" and is caused by the inheritance of two non-working or mutated copies of the gene that causes factor V Leiden thrombophilia.

Heterozygous factor V Leiden is inherited in an autosomal dominant pattern. In an autosomal dominant condition, only one changed or mutated copy of the gene for a particular condition is necessary for a person to experience symptoms of the condition. If a parent has an autosomal dominant condition, there is a 50% chance for each child to have the same or similar condition. In heterozygous factor V Leiden thrombophilia, the chance of being affected by venous blood clots is four to eight times greater than the general population.

Homozygous factor V Leiden thrombophilia is inherited in an autosomal recessive pattern. An autosomal recessive condition is caused by the inheritance of two changed or mutated copies of a gene. Individuals who are affected by heterozygous factor V Leiden thrombophilia have only one copy of the altered gene. However, when two people with heterozygous factor V Leiden thrombophilia have children together, there is a 25% chance, with each pregnancy, for the child to inherit two copies, one from each parent. That child then has two altered copies of the gene and therefore, has homozygous factor V Leiden thrombophilia. When an individual inherits two non-working copies of the gene that lead to homozygous factor V Leiden thrombophilia, there is an up to 80 times increased risk to be affected by blood clots stuck in the veins (venous thrombosis). Additionally, most individuals affected by homozygous factor V Leiden thrombophilia develop blood clots at a younger age than individuals affected by heterozygous factor V Leiden thrombophilia.

Demographics

Factor V Leiden thrombophilia is the most common inherited form of increased blood clotting in the general population. Factor V Leiden thrombophilia is more common in the Caucasian population. In the general U.S. and European population, heterozygous factor V Leiden thrombophilia occurs in approximately three to eight individuals per 100. In the same general U.S. and European population, homozygous factor V Leiden thrombophilia affects approximately one in 5,000 individuals. The frequency in African Americans, Asian Americans, Hispanic Americans and Native Americans is smaller than that of Caucasian Americans, but is still present at approximately 0.45-2% of individuals tested. Factor V Leiden thrombophilia is very rare in individuals who have only Asian, African, and indigenous Australian descent.

Signs and symptoms

The symptoms of factor V Leiden thrombophilia vary. Some affected individuals have no physical problems. Other individuals will have complications including blood clots blocking blood vessels (thromboembolism), deep vein thrombosis, unexplained multiple miscarriages and stillborn infants, gall bladder dysfunction, strokes, and heart attacks. The most common physical sign of factor V Leiden thrombophilia is thromboembolism (a blockage in the veins caused by a free floating clot [embolus]). Venous thromboembolism is most common in the deep veins of the legs (deep venous thrombosis or DVT of the legs). Since non-specific and common factor V Leiden thrombophilia are

suspected in individuals who have had multiple blood clots in the veins (venous thrombosis), more than three unexplained miscarriages, or a family history of individuals with multiple blood clots in the blood vessels.

Diagnosis

Diagnosis of factor V Leiden thrombophilia can be done through a blood coagulation screening test or **DNA** analysis of the gene that codes for factor V.

The blood coagulation screening test uses the breakdown protein APC in a resistance study to see how quickly the factor V is broken down as compared to other blood clotting factors. An individual with factor V Leiden thrombophilia has factor V that is resistant or much slower to being broken down by the APC protein. At this time there are two types of APC resistance screening tests for factor V Leiden thrombophilia. The preferred test is the "modified second generation" APC resistance study because an extra step in the testing (dilution by plasma without factor V) makes it almost 100% accurate even in pregnant women and patients being treated by medications such as heparin and warfarin.

The DNA or molecular analysis examines the *F5* gene to learn if the gene is altered or mutated.

Prenatal diagnosis is not offered routinely because the disorder is fairly mild and effective treatment is available.

Treatment and management

The treatment and management of individuals affected by factor V Leiden thrombophilia is focused on prevention of floating blood clots (thrombosis) and thromboembolism. The management of affected individuals should be overseen by a hematologist who specialized in blood clotting disorders and a general practitioner or internist who can work closely with the hematologist.

At different times of life, different specialists may need to be added. For example, when pregnant, a perinatologist or high-risk obstetrician should work with the hematologist during pregnancy. Additionally, individuals who have had a deep vein clot or stroke may need to consult a vascular specialist and/or neurologist.

The physicians managing an affected individual's care should discuss with them the timing, risks, and benefits of taking birth control pills and taking "blood thinning" anticoagulant medications like warfarin, aspirin, and heparin. Individuals affected by factor V Leiden

KEY TERMS

Deep vein thrombosis—A blood clot in one of the systemic veins deep in the body.

Heterozygous—Having two different versions of the same gene.

Homozygous—Having two identical copies of a gene or chromosome.

Thromboembolism—A condition in which a blood vessel is blocked by a free-floating blood clot carried in the blood stream.

Venous thrombosis—A condition caused by the presence of a clot in the vein.

thrombophilia should also be examined to make sure they do not have other blood clotting disorders in addition to factor V Leiden thrombophilia.

Prognosis

Individuals affected by factor V Leiden thrombophilia have a wide range of symptoms and signs. Some individuals affected by factor V Leiden thrombophilia will never develop physical signs and symptoms of the disorder. Other individuals will be more severely affected. Most affected individuals will not experience their first clotting event until adulthood. However, individuals with homozygous factor V Leiden thrombophilia have a significantly increased risk to have symptoms of the disease at a younger age. Treatment and close management of the disorder can reduce the risk of thromboembolism significantly.

Resources

PERIODICALS

Major, D. A., et al. "Cardiovascular Implications of the Factor V Leiden Mutation." *American Heart Journal* (August 2000): 189-195.

ORGANIZATIONS

Thrombophilia Support. <http://www.fvleiden.org>.

WEBSITES

"Factor V Leiden Thrombophilia." *GeneClinics.* <http://www.geneclinics.org/profiles/factor-v-leiden/index.html>.

Thrombophilia Support Page. <http://www.fvleiden.org>.

"Venous Thrombosis and Factor V (Leiden) Mutation." *Genetic Drift Newletter* 14 (Spring 1997). <http://www.mostgene.org>.

Dawn A. Jacob, MS, CGC

Fahr disease

Definition

Fahr disease is a rare, progressive neurological disorder that is often hereditary. Characterized by deposits of calcium in the basal ganglia and other parts of the brain, Fahr disease causes worsening **dementia** and the loss of routine motor skills, among other symptoms.

Description

Though calcium is important for good health, this mineral can have harmful effects when it appears in parts of the body where it does not belong. In Fahr disease, abnormal deposits of calcium build up in a region of the brain called the basal ganglia (mainly in a section called the globus pallidus), as well as in other parts of the brain. The basal ganglia is the technical name given to clusters of nerve cells that help to initiate and control movements of the body—for example, reaching for a cup of coffee or taking a step forward while walking. The presence of these calcium deposits (referred to as calcifications) interferes with the working of the brain, causing a variety of debilitating mental and physical symptoms that worsen over time. Aside from the basal ganglia, the calcium deposits associated with Fahr disease often appear in other areas of the brain such as the cerebral cortex.

Two important effects of the disease are dementia and the loss of learned motor skills. People affected by Fahr disease may become overly forgetful and easily confused or disoriented. They have trouble performing relatively simple tasks that require basic hand-eye coordination. Most people with the disease experience slurred speech and problems involving involuntary movements or poor coordination. In addition, personality changes and disorders of mood may develop. In one study of 18 people with Fahr disease, half of the participants had symptoms of obsessive-compulsive disorder, major **depression**, or **bipolar disorder**. People with Fahr disease may have psychotic symptoms, including hallucinations (visual and auditory), a distorted perception of reality, and paranoid delusions.

As the disease progresses, it causes an increasing degree of paralysis. Muscles become stiff and physical movement is restricted. Aside from these symptoms, people with Fahr disease may experience specific movement disorders: slow, twisting movements of the hands and feet (athetosis) and jerky, rapid movements that resemble spasms (chorea). Vision may also be affected. Because the disease can weaken nerves that carry signals from the eyes to the brain, people with Fahr disease may experience partial or almost complete vision loss. Ear infections have also been reported.

The underlying cause of Fahr disease is unknown. For this reason, it is described as an idiopathic disorder. Fahr disease is often referred to in the medical literature as idiopathic basal ganglia calcification (IBGC). Less common names for the disease include cerebrovascular ferrocalcinosis, non-arteriosclerotic cerebral calcifications, and striopallidodentate calcinosis.

Genetic profile

Fahr disease often runs in families and is believed to be inherited either as a recessive or dominant trait. In the recessive version of Fahr, a person must inherit the same abnormal **gene** (associated with Fahr) from both parents in order to develop the disease. Therefore, a child who receives only one recessive gene for the disease can become a carrier but will not usually develop symptoms. In the dominant version of Fahr disease, a person may develop the condition after receiving just one copy of the abnormal gene from either the mother or father.

Researchers studying a particular family affected by Fahr disease over several generations discovered a pattern regarding the age at which the condition strikes. The results of this medical study, indicated that each generation with Fahr developed symptoms at an earlier age than previous generations, a phenomenon described as "genetic anticipation." The family (referred to as a "kindred") being analyzed in this study was affected by the dominantly inherited version of the disease.

While studying this kindred, researchers located a gene believed to play a role in the disorder. The gene was named IBGC1 ("IBGC" is short for "idiopathic basal ganglia calcification," another name for Fahr disease). The gene location was identified as 14q, situated on the long arm (called q) of **chromosome** 14. Despite this finding, more research is necessary to determine the identity and nature of the gene or genes associated with Fahr disease.

Aside from inherited forms, Fahr disease can occur sporadically for reasons that are not well understood. Some medical studies suggest that sporadic cases of Fahr disease may result from an as-yet unidentified infection that affects the fetus in the womb.

Demographics

Fahr disease, which appears to affect men and women equally, can appear at any stage of life, from infancy to adulthood. Some people diagnosed with the disease have no family history of the condition, while in many cases Fahr disease runs in families and affects members of several generations. In people with dominantly inherited Fahr disease, symptoms usually appear anywhere between the ages of 30 and 60. The recessive form of Fahr disease emerges at a younger age, between infancy and young adulthood.

Signs and symptoms

People with Fahr disease have abnormal calcium deposits in the basal ganglia, primarily in the globus pallidus region, and often in other parts of the brain. Loss of brain cells in these areas also occurs. The results of electrocardiogram (ECG) studies, which monitor heartbeats, are often abnormal in people with Fahr disease. Other signs include malfunctioning parathyroid glands and low blood calcium levels.

The disease causes a variety of physical and psychological symptoms. The head of a person with Fahr disease is often smaller and rounder than normal. The condition causes worsening dementia and loss of routine motor skills. Muscle stiffness, movement disorders, and paralysis may occur. Speech often becomes slurred. In some cases, Fahr disease causes vision problems and ear infections. Symptoms of **Parkinson's disease** may develop as well.

Diagnosis

In simple terms, Fahr disease is diagnosed when calcifications in the basal ganglia are associated with slurred speech, movement disorders, and other specific symptoms. Special imaging procedures such as a CT scan can detect the presence of calcium deposits. Symptoms can be determined by physical and psychological examinations. Friends or family members with relevant observations of the patient's behavior can also be helpful. Blood tests may be recommended to evaluate blood calcium levels and the parathyroid glands. The appearance of Parkinson-like symptoms is not essential to a diagnosis of Fahr disease.

In the absence of other factors, calcium deposits in the basal ganglia do not necessarily indicate the presence of Fahr disease. Such calcifications may be due to a metabolism disorder, infectious disease, or a genetic disorder other than Fahr. In fact, sometimes these calcifications may be present without producing any symptoms or harmful effects, especially in people older than age 60.

Treatment and management

There is no cure for Fahr disease, which worsens over time. The process of calcification cannot be stopped or reversed. Where possible, clinicians focus on alleviating its various mental and physical effects. These may vary to some degree depending on the individual, even

KEY TERMS

Calcification—A process in which tissue becomes hardened due to calcium deposits.

Cerebral cortex—The outer surface of the cerebrum made up of gray matter and involved in higher thought processes.

Cerebrum—The largest section of the brain, which is responsible for such higher functions as speech, thought, vision, and memory.

Computed tomography (CT) scan—An imaging procedure that produces a three-dimensional picture of organs or structures inside the body, such as the brain.

Dementia—A condition of deteriorated mental ability characterized by a marked decline of intellect and often by emotional apathy.

Idiopathic—Of unknown origin.

Neurological—Relating to the brain and central nervous system.

Parathyroid glands—A pair of glands adjacent to the thyroid gland that primarily regulate blood calcium levels.

among members of the same family. Lithium carbonate, for example, may be recommended to control psychotic symptoms, while antidepressant medications are often used to combat depression. Ear infections associated with Fahr disease can be treated with antibiotics and pain medication.

Prognosis

Due to its damaging effects on the brain and nervous system, Fahr disease is eventually fatal.

Resources

BOOKS

Victor, Maurice, et al. *Principles of Neurology.* 7th ed. New York: McGraw-Hill, 2001.

PERIODICALS

Geschwind, D. H., et al. "Identification of a Locus on Chromosome 14q for Idiopathic Basal Ganglia Calcification (Fahr Disease)." *American Journal of Human Genetics* 65 (1999): 764-772.

Lauterbach, E. C., et al. "Neuropsychiatric Correlates and Treatment of Lenticulostriatal Diseases: A Review of the Literature and Overview of Research Opportunities in Huntington's, Wilson's, and Fahr's Diseases. A report of the ANPA Committee on Research. American

Neuropsychiatric Association." *Journal of Neuropsychiatry and Clinical Neurosciences* 10 (1998): 249-66.

Rosenblatt, A., and I. Leroi. "Neuropsychiatry of Huntington's Disease and Other Basal Ganglia Disorders." *Psychosomatics* 41(2000): 24-30.

ORGANIZATIONS

National Institute of Neurological Disorders and Stroke. 31 Center Drive, MSC 2540, Bldg. 31, Room 8806, Bethesda, MD 20814. (301) 496-5751 or (800) 352-9424. <http://www.ninds.nih.gov>.

National Organization for Rare Disorders (NORD). PO Box 8923, New Fairfield, CT 06812-8923. (203) 746-6518 or (800) 999-6673. Fax: (203) 746-6481. <http://www.rarediseases.org>.

WEBSITES

Association of Birth Defect Children, Inc. <http://www.birthdefects.org>.l

Greg Annussek

Familial adenomatous polyposis

Definition

Familial adenomatous polyposis is an inherited condition that typically presents with extensive adenomatous polyps of the colon. These polyps often develop into colorectal **cancer** in early adult life. Other symptoms are often present as well. These signs include polyps in the upper gastrointestinal tract, malignancies in the brain or thyroid, pigmented retinal lesions, and osteomas.

Description

Familial adenomatous polyposis (FAP) was first clearly described as a dominantly inherited colorectal cancer susceptibility by Lockhart-Mummery in an article published in 1925. FAP has since served as a paradigm for hereditary cancer and has taught much about the diagnosis, surveillance, and management of colon cancer. It is one of the most clearly defined and well understood of the inherited colon cancer syndromes. FAP is thought to account for approximately 1% of all cases of colorectal cancer.

FAP is a disorder that is characterized by the development of hundreds to thousands of glandular colorectal tumors called adenomas or adenomatous polyps, meaning that they are benign growths made of the tissue that lines the inside of the colon. They are described as polyps because they protrude from mucous membranes. In FAP, these tumors generally develop by the second or third decade of life. They are found in the internal lining of the colon and the rectum, with a particular affinity for the left side of the colon or the rectosigmoid. By themselves, these polyps are benign but they have the ability to become malignant, leading to colorectal cancer. If the polyps are not treated properly, it is almost certain that a person affected with FAP will develop colorectal cancer by the age of 40.

Other clinical findings that may be associated with FAP include polyps in the upper gastrointestinal tract, extraintestinal manifestations such as osteomas and epidermoid cysts, desmoid formation, retinal lesions, and malignant changes in other organs. Symptoms are thought to manifest anywhere between the ages of 16 and 50 years.

FAP is also known as familial polyposis coli (FPC) and adenomatous polyposis coli (APC). Gardner syndrome and Turcot syndrome are variants of FAP. Gardner syndrome is used to describe patients with FAP and the extracolonic symptoms of osteomas, soft tissue tumors, desmoids, and dental abnormalities. Turcot syndrome is used when FAP is seen in conjunction with tumors of the central nervous system called medulloblastomas (cerebral tumors that occur in childhood). Attenuated FAP (AFAP) is another variant of FAP. In this condition, individuals present with fewer polyps, usually fewer than 100 in number and often in the right colon. Patients with AFAP may have a later onset of cancer than those with classic FAP.

Genetic profile

FAP is inherited in an autosomal dominant pattern; thus, an affected person has a 50% chance of passing the disease on to each of his or her children. It is almost 100% penetrant, meaning that nearly everyone who carries the **gene** mutation will show signs of the disorder. The majority of patients with FAP inherit the mutation from one of their parents. However, in approximately 25% of cases, there is no family history of the disorder and FAP occurs because of a new mutation in the affected individual.

The majority of cases of FAP are due to mutations of the *APC* gene, located on the long arm (or "q" arm) of **chromosome** 5. This gene encodes a protein that is important in cell adhesion and signal transduction. More than 300 different APC mutations have been described in FAP patients. Most APC mutations seen in individuals with FAP result in translation of a protein that is shorter than normal. This shortened protein cannot function properly.

Studies have shown that the type and location of the *APC* mutation seems to correlate to the clinical symptoms that a person manifests. For example, if the mutation is located near the center of the gene, colonic polyps tend to be more dense and numerous. A mutation towards the ends of the gene often leads to polyps that are fewer and more sparse, as in attenuated FAP. Additionally, mutations at one particular end (the 3′ end) of the APC gene seem to be associated with a higher risk of desmoid formation. However, it is known that family members who carry identical mutations often have different clinical features. This suggests that modifying genes and/or environmental factors also influence the expression of the APC gene mutation.

The APC gene is a tumor suppressor gene, meaning that its function is to control cell growth. When APC is mutated, it does not function correctly and allows cells to grow out of control. This results in tumors that may lead to cancer. Carriers of mutations in APC inherit a germline mutation in one allele of the gene. Thus, in every one of their cells, one gene does not make the APC protein but the corresponding gene on the other chromosome continues to produce the functional protein. Thus, tumor suppression continues. However, if a somatic mutation occurs in the remaining functional gene, no APC protein is made, tumor suppression fails, and tumors develop. These somatic mutations occur in various parts of the body at various times, leading to multiple tumors forming in distinct parts of the body over a period of time. In the case of FAP, many of these tumors are confined to the colon but can occur in other organs as well.

Demographics

Approximately one of 8,000 people are affected with FAP. It is seen in all racial and ethnic groups. Both sexes are affected equally.

Signs and symptoms

Colorectal

FAP is characterized by multiple (more than 100) adenomatous polyps of the colon and rectum. These generally develop after the first decade of life but the age of onset of adenomas is variable. Fifteen percent of individuals with FAP will show these polyps by age 10, 75% by age 20, and 90% by the age of 30. More than 95% of affected individuals will have adenomatous polyps by the age of 35. Although these polyps are benign, it is inevitable that, if left untreated, at least one of the hundreds of polyps will eventually progress to cancer. The majority of cancers appear by the age of 40 and over 90% appear by the age of 45. Symptoms of polyps and/ or colorectal cancer may include rectal bleeding, change in bowel habits, iron deficiency anemia, or abdominal pain.

Upper gastrointestinal tract

Many individuals with FAP will develop adenomas in the upper gastrointestinal tract as well. The second portion of the duodenum is particularly prone to these polyps. These adenomas are benign, as they are in the colon, but about 5–8% of patients with FAP will eventually develop cancer in this area. Duodenal cancer seems to cluster in certain FAP families while being absent in others. Adenomas of other portions of the small bowel may also occur but with lesser frequency.

In people affected with FAP, benign adenomas can also be seen in the stomach. Gastric cystic fundic gland polyps are also common. These are benign polyps that occur in the fundic gland of the stomach, an organ that secretes enzymes and mucus. It is rare for these polyps to become cancerous in individuals of Western origin. However, in Japanese and Korean families with FAP, the risk of **gastric cancer** is reported to be increased three- to four-fold over the general population.

Ocular, skeletal, and cutaneous

Approximately two thirds of individuals with FAP will have congenital hypertrophy of the retinal pigment epithelium (CHRPE). These lesions are typically flat, oval, and pigmented. They can be detected by an ophthalmology examination. In FAP patients, these lesions are usually multiple, bilateral, or large. CHRPE does not affect vision nor does it have the potential to become malignant. However, CHRPE is a very important finding for families with a history of FAP. If CHRPE runs in a family with FAP, all or nearly all affected individuals in the family will have this finding. It can be detected at birth and can thus identify susceptible family members at a young age.

Other manifestations of FAP include dental abnormalities, such as impacted teeth, supernumerary teeth, and congenitally missing teeth. Osteomas can occur, often in the jaw area or on the forehead. Soft tissue tumors, such as lipomas, epidermoid cysts, and fibromas, are observed in some patients with FAP as well.

Other tumors and malignancies

Abdominal desmoid tumors occur in approximately 15% of individuals with FAP. Desmoids are tumors made of connective tissue. Although they are not cancerous, approximately 10% grow very aggressively and can become life threatening. They may lead to obstruction of blood vessels, the intestine, or ureters. They may also result in abdominal distention and associated pain and discomfort. Over 70% of these tumors develop in women aged 20–40 years, suggesting a hormonal role in their development. Additionally, they occur more commonly in those who have had prior abdominal surgery. Desmoids may occur as part of classical FAP, as part of Gardner syndrome, or sporadically, without the colonic findings of FAP.

Additionally, patients with FAP are at an increased risk for cancers in organs outside of the gastrointestinal tract. These include brain tumors, thyroid tumors, and hepatoblastoma. Hepatoblastoma is a malignant tumor of the liver and occurs in approximately 1.6% of patients with FAP in the first five years of life. Tumors of the adrenal cortex, biliary tract, and pancreas have also been reported.

Diagnosis

FAP can be diagnosed clinically in any individual with greater than 100 polyps in the colon or rectum. The diagnosis is usually made via flexible sigmoidoscopy. This procedure may be done on a routine basis or to investigate possible symptoms of colon polyps and/or colorectal cancer. Flexible sigmoidoscopy involves inspecting the interior of the rectum and the sigmoid colon, or the terminal part of the colon that leads to the rectum. Once polyposis has been established, complete colonoscopy may be necessary to further evaluate the extent of the polyps. Colonoscopy is a more invasive procedure that examines the interior of the entire colon and rectum, rather than only the terminal part.

In regards to a diagnosis in someone who does not yet have colon polyps, retinoscopy, or examination of the retina, can be useful in a family where CHRPE has been associated with FAP. In these families, CHRPE is almost 100% predictive of FAP; thus, if someone shows CHRPE on an ophthalmology exam, it is very likely that he or she is affected with FAP. Although **genetic testing** yields more certain predictive information, retinoscopy is a relatively inexpensive and noninvasive alternative diagnostic screening measure in families with a history of FAP associated with CHRPE.

Polyps may be first detected by the passage of occult (non-visible) blood in the stool by means of fecal occult blood testing. This testing is also inexpensive and noninvasive, and if positive, could indicate that additional testing is needed.

FAP can also be diagnosed by genetic testing. This type of testing may be used to identify someone who is affected but does not yet show any symptoms of FAP. It can also confirm the diagnosis of FAP in someone who has polyposis discovered via flexible sigmoidoscopy. APC gene testing is most commonly performed by using a protein truncation test, which looks for the presence of shortened proteins caused by a mutation in the gene. This test identifies approximately 80% of those affected with FAP. The other 20% of patients likely have mutations that do not lead to a shortened protein. It is important to test an affected family member first to determine whether or not a detectable mutation is present. If a mutation is identified in this affected person, other at-risk family members can be tested for this particular mutation. However, if a mutation is not identified in the affected individual, it is likely that the mutation does not produce a shortened protein. In this case, protein truncation testing would not be informative for the rest of the family.

FAP can also be diagnosed by linkage analysis. This testing identifies approximately 95% of affected individuals, however, blood samples are required from numerous family members, including at least one affected individual. Thus, logistically, this procedure is more complicated than the protein truncation testing mentioned above.

Treatment and management

There is no treatment for FAP because the genetic abnormality cannot be fixed. Management focuses on routine surveillance of at-risk and affected individuals for early detection and treatment of colonic polyps and other manifestations.

For individuals diagnosed with FAP, either clinically or via linkage analysis or protein truncation testing, an annual sigmoidoscopy must be performed beginning around the age of 10 years. Sigmoidoscopy is preferred because it is less invasive, safer, and will generally detect the polyps in FAP, since they are numerous and located throughout the colon. Colonoscopy may be the screening tool of choice if attenuated FAP is suspected since, in this case, the adenomas are fewer in number and may be confined to the proximal region of the colon.

If polyposis is established, complete colonoscopy may be necessary to determine the extent of the polyposis and the timing of surgery. As for surgical intervention, total proctocolectomy (removal of the colon and rectum) is generally favored. In some cases, however, other options may be explored, such as total colectomy (removal of the colon only) with ileorectal anastomosis (the small intestine is attached to the upper portion of the rectum). Another option, a total colectomy with rectal mucosal protectomy and ileoanal anastomosis, involves removing the entire colon and mucosal lining of the rectum. The ileum then attaches to the anus. Fecal continence is preserved since the muscular wall and the sensory functions of the rectum are preserved.

All FAP patients require an annual medical examination with palpation of the thyroid and review of systems. Children with FAP should be screened for hepatoblastoma with liver palpation. In some cases, hepatic ultrasonography and determination of serum alpha-fetoprotein levels can be helpful as well. Upper endoscopy (visual examination of the upper GI tract) should be completed every one to four years to evaluate for gastric and duodenal polyps. Duodenal polyps that increase in size or number or show signs of becoming cancerous may require treatment. This treatment may include evaluation by computed tomography or ultrasonography. If necessary, the polyps may be removed by laser or other procedures.

For at-risk relatives of affected individuals, regular screening should begin between the ages of 10 and 12 years. This screening can be accomplished by protein truncation testing. If the test result is a true negative (i.e., negative result in a person whose affected relative had a positive result), further screening is debatable. This test result should theoretically eliminate the risk of FAP but, in very few cases, laboratory errors or other circumstances may lead to an inaccurate test result. Thus, some experts suggest that flexible sigmoidoscopy should be performed at ages 18, 25, and 35 years in these individuals, with standard screening thereafter.

After colectomy, continued surveillance of patients with FAP is advised. Ileoscopy is recommended every three to five years. This procedure examines the ileum, or lowest third of the small intestine, and serves to rule out polyps, which may become cancerous with time. Surgical removal of desmoid tumors is invasive but often necessary to prevent reoccurrence. Various nonoperative treatments have been attempted, such as medication and radiation, none of which have yielded consistent results. Additionally, the examination of any remaining rectal tissue by proctoscopy is necessary every six months to assess for signs of rectal cancer.

As with any abdominal surgeries in people affected with FAP, there is a risk of developing desmoid tumors after the colectomy. If desmoids are suspected, computed tomography is the recommended imaging study. MRI may also be used in certain cases.

Surveillance of the upper GI tract, even after total proctocoloectomy, is appropriate due to the incidence of tumors in this area previously discussed.

Prognosis

Without colectomy, the prognosis for individuals with FAP is very poor. Patients who have not undergone colectomy develop colorectal cancer at an average age of 39 years. The majority of untreated people die from colorectal cancer by the age of 42 years. For those who do

KEY TERMS

Benign—A non-cancerous tumor that does not spread and is not life-threatening.

Duodenum—Portion of the small intestine nearest the stomach; the first of three parts of the small intestine.

Epidermoid cyst—Benign, cystic tumor derived from epithelial cells.

Fibroma—A non-malignant tumor of connective tissue.

Hypertrophy—Increase in the size of a tissue or organ brought on by the enlargement of its cells rather than cell multiplication.

Lipoma—A benign tumor composed of well-differentiated fat cells.

Malignant—A tumor growth that spreads to another part of the body, usually cancerous.

Osteoma—A benign bone tumor.

Somatic—Relating to the nonreproductive parts of the body.

undergo a colectomy, prognosis is variable, depending on development and progression of other tumors. For example, desmoids can also be detrimental to those affected with FAP, accounting for 11–31% of all mortality in these individuals.

Resources

PERIODICALS

King, John E., Roger R. Dozois, Noralane M. Lindor, and David A. Ahlquist. "Care of Patients and Their Families With Familal Adenomatous Polyposis." *Mayo Clinic Proceedings* 75, no. 1 (January 2000): 57–67.

Lynch, Henry T., and Thomas C. Smyrk. "Hereditary Colorectal Cancer." *Seminars in Oncology* 26, no. 5 (October 1999): 478–484.

Olson, Sharon J., and Kristin Zawacki. "Hereditary Colorectal Cancer." *Clinical Genetics* 35, no. 3 (September 2000): 671–685.

ORGANIZATIONS

Colon Cancer Alliance. 175 Ninth Ave. New York, NY 10011. (212) 627-7451. <http://ccalliance.org>.

Colorectal Cancer Network. PO Box 182, Kensington, MD 20895-0182. (301) 879-1500. <http://www.colorectal-cancer.net>.

Hereditary Colon Cancer Association (HCCA). 3601 N 4th Ave., Suite 201, Sioux Falls, SD 57104. (800) 264-6783. <http://hereditarycc.org>.

WEBSITES

"Familial Adenomatous Polyposis." *Gene Clinics.* <http://www.geneclinics.org>.

Johns Hopkins Medical Institutions. "FAP. Hereditary Colorectal Cancer." <http://www.hopkins-coloncancer.org/subspecialties/heredicolor_cancer/overview.htm>.

National Cancer Institute. "Genetics of Colorectal Cancer (PDQ)." *CancerNet.* <http://cancernet.nci.nih.gov>.

Mary E. Freivogel, MS

Familial dysautonomia

Definition

Familial dysautonomia (FD) is a rare inherited disorder in which affected individuals experience multiple malfunctions of the autonomic nervous system (the part of the nervous system that regulates heart muscle, smooth muscle, and glands) as well as the sensory, motor, and central components of the nervous system. The disorder is progressive with a continual loss of nerve cells of the sensory and autonomic nervous systems.

Description

Familial dysautonomia is an inherited disorder that occurs almost exclusively in people of Eastern European (Ashkenazi) Jewish descent. FD is one of a larger group of at least five hereditary sensory and autonomic neuropathies (HSANs), meaning conditions that stem from abnormalities of the nervous system. FD was first described in 1949 by pediatricians Conrad Riley and Richard Day. They reported five children, all Jewish, who had an unusual set of reactions to mild anxiety, attributed to a disturbance of the autonomic nervous system. FD is also known as HSAN type III or Riley-Day syndrome. Decades of studies have determined the cause to be a genetic abnormality that causes poor development of nerve cells in the fetus, leading to a progressive loss of nerve cells of the autonomic and sensory nervous systems. The depletion of nerve cells in the autonomic system causes problems with unstable heart rate, blood pressure, and body temperature, as well as gastrointestinal dysfunction, poor motor coordination, and emotional instability. Abnormal development of the sensory nervous system results in poor perception of pain, heat, and cold. This causes affected individuals to injure themselves without being aware of it. This deterioration of the nervous system worsens throughout life and causes multiple health problems that lead to the death of 50% of those affected by adulthood.

Genetic profile

FD is caused by mutations (genetic errors) in the IKBKAP **gene** that is found on human **chromosome** 9, specifically located at region 9q31. The disease is inherited as an autosomal recessive trait. This means that both parents have one copy of the mutant gene but do not have the disease. For these parents, there is a 25% chance with each pregnancy that the child will have the disease.

The IKBKAP gene has two known mutations, which together account for 100% of the Ashkenazi Jewish (AJ) cases of FD. There is also a third mutation causing FD that is rarely seen in the non-AJ population. This mutation's gene location has not yet been determined.

Demographics

The abnormal gene causing FD is rare in the general population but has a fairly high incidence in the Ashkenazi Jewish population, originating from Eastern Europe. Both males and females are affected. In the at-risk group, one in 30 people is thought to be a carrier of the abnormal gene, with a disease frequency of one in 3,600 live births. Rare non-Jewish individuals affected with FD have been reported.

Signs and symptoms

Sensory and autonomic nervous systems fail to develop properly in the fetus. Newborn babies with FD have poor or decreased muscle tone and have poor sucking and swallowing reflexes that make feeding difficult. Affected babies are prone to periods of abnormally low body temperature and are unable to produce adequate tears when crying.

Although symptoms vary markedly, by adolescence affected children have a 90% likelihood of spinal curvature and experience weakness and leg cramping. They have difficulty concentrating and undergo personality changes including negativism, **depression**, irritability, and insomnia. Forty percent of affected people have regular vomiting crises in response to either emotional or physical stress. A crisis typically involves one to three days of compulsive vomiting, rapid heart rate, high blood pressure, profuse sweating, and red, blotchy skin.

Between crises, affected individuals may experience low blood pressure when rising to a standing position. They often have unexplained fevers and may have convulsions in response to even mild infections. Uncoordinated swallowing, reflux of stomach contents, and a poor gag reflex result in food or fluids being misdirected into the trachea and lungs. Aspiration pneumonia (lung infections) often follows. Kidney function may deteriorate with age. Affected people have an abnormal response to low oxygen or high carbon dioxide in their blood. They do not experience the expected "air hunger," or urge to breathe, and may faint or have a seizure. Lack of tears, decreased blink frequency, and insensitivity of the eye to pain from foreign objects can cause inflammation and ulcers of the cornea.

A characteristic sign in those affected with familial dysautonomia is a lack of the sense of taste. This is due to the absence of taste buds on the tongue. Other sensory problems include an inability to feel pain or distinguish between hot and cold temperatures; sensory loss increases with age. Deep tendon reflexes in affected individuals are decreased. Poor speech and motor coordination result in abnormal gait, unsteadiness, tongue thrusting, and abnormal rhythmic facial movements. Growth is stunted, with an average adult height of 5 ft (1.5 m). Puberty is delayed in both sexes. However, fertility and offspring of affected individuals are normal.

Diagnosis

The presentation of FD varies between affected people. However, of the many manifestations of the disease, five signs are key to the diagnosis:

- flat, smooth tongue due to lack of taste buds,
- lack of red flare following histamine injection under the skin,
- decreased or absent deep tendon reflexes,
- absence of overflow tears with emotional crying,
- parents of Ashkenazi Jewish background.

Other frequent signs are decreased response to pain and temperature, decreased corneal reflexes, unstable blood pressure, low blood pressure when standing erect, red blotching of the skin, and increased sweating. Further supportive evidence of the FD diagnosis are feeding difficulties, repeated aspiration pneumonia, episodes of low body temperature, breath holding spells, poor muscle tone, delayed motor development, repeated vomiting, spinal curvature, and poor growth. Prenatal diagnosis, screenings for carrier status, and **genetic counseling** are available.

Treatment and management

The identification of the FD gene as IKBKAP was reported in March 2001, and is expected to lead to new treatment approaches as the function of the gene is better understood. Until that time, treatment is preventive and supportive. Management of vomiting crises is attempted with drugs, replacement of body fluids, prevention of aspiration of stomach contents into lungs, control of

KEY TERMS

Aspiration pneumonia—Lung infection due to food or liquids accidentally getting into lungs.

Autonomic nervous system—The part of the nervous system that regulates heart muscle, smooth muscle, and glands.

Autosomal—Relating to any chromosome besides the X and Y sex chromosomes. Human cells contain 22 pairs of autosomes and one pair of sex chromosomes.

Carrier—A person who possesses a gene for an abnormal trait without showing signs of the disorder. The person may pass the abnormal gene on to offspring.

Mutation—A permanent change in the genetic material that may alter a trait or characteristic of an individual, or manifest as disease, and can be transmitted to offspring.

Recessive—Genetic trait expressed only when present on both members of a pair of chromosomes, one inherited from each parent.

blood pressure, and promotion of sleep. Care of the eyes includes artificial tears, eyewashes, and topical antibiotics to avoid ulcers of the cornea. Early and adequate treatment of even mild infections is important to avoid triggering vomiting crises. Children should be protected from injury and watched for any unusual swellings or skin discolorations as a way of coping with decreased pain and temperature perception.

Physical and occupational therapy, braces, and other orthopedic aids are used for spinal curvature and poor motor coordination. Speech therapy, special feeding techniques, and respiratory care enhance quality of life. It is important to maintain adequate fluid intake and avoid situations such as high elevations, air travel, and diving underwater where oxygen concentration is decreased. Psychological intervention is helpful to alleviate emotional instability and mood swings in children and depression, anxiety, and phobias in adults.

Prognosis

The disease process of familial dysautonomia can not be prevented at present but 80% of affected individuals survive beyond childhood and 50% reach age 30. With the 2001 determination of the exact location of the gene abnormality, prospects for new treatments and possible **gene therapy** are on the horizon.

Resources

BOOKS

Gilbert, Patricia. *Riley-Day Syndrome. The A-Z Reference Book of Syndromes and Inherited Disorders.* 2nd ed. San Diego: Singular Publishing Group, Inc., 1996.

PERIODICALS

Axelrod, Felicia B. "Familial Dysautonomia: A 47-year Perspective." *Journal of Pediatrics* 132, no.3 (March 1998): S2-5.

Gelbart, Marsh. "In Our Parents' Shadow. Riley-Day Syndrome." *Nursing Times* 95, no. 6 (February 10-16, 1999): 33.

ORGANIZATIONS

Dysautonomia Foundation, Inc. 633 Third Ave., 12th Floor, New York, NY 10017-6706. (212) 949-6644. <www.med.nyu.edu/fd/fdcenter.html>.

Marianne O'Connor, MT (ASCP), MPH

Familial endocrine adenomatosis *see* **Multiple endocrine neoplasia**

Familial fatal insomnia *see* **Prion diseases**

Familial infiltrative fibromatosis *see* **Hereditary desmoid disease**

Familial Mediterranean fever

Definition

Familial Mediterranean fever (FMF) is an inherited disorder of the inflammatory response characterized by recurring attacks of fever, accompanied by intense pain in the abdomen, chest, or joints. Attacks usually last 12–72 hours, and can occasionally involve a skin rash. Kidney disease is a serious concern if the disorder is not treated. FMF is most prevalent in people of Armenian, Sephardic-Jewish, Arabic, and Turkish ancestry.

Description

FMF could be described as a disorder of "inappropriate" inflammation. That is, an event that in a normal situation causes a mild or unnoticeable inflammation might cause a severe inflammatory response in someone with FMF. Certain areas of the body are at risk for FMF-related symptoms. A serosa is a serous (fluid-producing) membrane that can be found inside the abdominal cavity (peritoneum), around the lungs (pleura), around the heart (pericardium), and inside the joints (synovium). The symptoms of FMF are due to inflammation of one or more of the serosal membranes (serositis). Thus, FMF is also sometimes called recurrent polyserositis.

During an attack, large numbers of neutrophils, a type of white blood cell, move into the affected areas causing painful inflammation and fever. These episodes may be accompanied by a skin rash or joint pain. In a few cases, chronic arthritis is a problem. Amyloidosis is a potentially serious condition in which proteins called amyloids are mistakenly produced and deposited in organs and tissues throughout the body. Left untreated, amyloidosis often leads to kidney failure, which is the major long-term health risk in FMF.

In most cases, the attacks of fever and pain are first noticed in childhood or adolescence. The interval between these episodes may be days or months, and is not predictable. However, during these intervals people with FMF typically lead normal lives. It is not entirely clear what brings on an attack, but people with FMF often report mild physical trauma, physical exertion, or emotional stress just prior to the onset of symptoms. Treatment for FMF involves an oral medication called colchicine, which is highly effective for the episodes of fever and pain, as well as for amyloidosis and the kidney disease that can result from it.

FMF is most common in certain ethnic groups from the eastern Mediterranean region, but cases in other ethnic groups in other parts of the world are increasingly being reported. FMF is also known by many other names. They include: recurrent hereditary polyserositis, benign paroxysmal peritonitis, familial paroxysmal polyserositis, paroxysmal polyserositis, familial recurrent polyserositis, periodic fever, periodic amyloid syndrome, periodic peritonitis syndrome, Reimann periodic disease, Reimann syndrome, Siegel-Cattan-Mamou syndrome, and Armenian syndrome.

Genetic profile

FMF is a genetic condition inherited in an autosomal recessive fashion. Mutations in the MEFV **gene** (short for Mediterranean Fever) on **chromosome** number 16 are the underlying cause of FMF. Autosomal recessive **inheritance** implies that a person with FMF has mutations in both copies of the MEFV gene. All genes come in pairs, and one copy of each pair is inherited from each parent. If neither parent of a child with FMF has the condition, it means they carry one mutated copy of the MEFV gene, but also one normal copy, which is enough to protect them from disease. If both parents carry the same autosomal recessive gene, there is a one in four chance in each pregnancy that the child will inherit both recessive genes, and thus have the condition.

The MEFV gene carries the instructions for production of a protein called pyrin, named for pyrexia, a medical term for fever. The research group in France that co-discovered the protein named it marenostrin, after ancient Latin words that referred to the Mediterranean Sea. The movement of neutrophils into an area of the body where trauma or infection has occurred is the major cause of inflammation, which is a normal process. Research has shown that pyrin has some function in controlling neutrophils. In a situation where minor trauma or stress occurs, some initial inflammation may follow, but a functional pyrin protein is responsible for shutting-down the response of neutrophils once they are no longer needed. An abnormal pyrin protein associated with FMF may be partly functional, but unstable. In some instances, the abnormal pyrin itself seems to be "stressed," and loses its ability to regulate neutrophils and inflammation. Left unregulated, a normal, mild inflammation spirals out of control. Exactly what causes pyrin in FMF to lose its ability to control neutrophils in some situations is not known.

Demographics

Estimates of the incidence of FMF in specific eastern Mediterranean populations range from one in 2,000 to one in 100, depending on the population studied. Specific mutations in the MEFV gene are more common in certain ethnic groups, and may cause a somewhat different course of the disease. A few mutations in the MEFV gene likely became common in a small population in the eastern Mediterranean several thousand years ago. It is postulated that carrying a single copy of a mutated gene produced a modified (but not abnormal) inflammatory response that may have been protective against some infectious agent at that time. Those who carried a single "beneficial" mutation in the MEFV gene were more likely to survive and reproduce, which may explain the high carrier frequency (up to one in five) in some populations. People of Armenian, Sephardic-Jewish, Arabic, and Turkish ancestry are at greatest risk for FMF. However, a better understanding and recognition of the symptoms of FMF in recent years has resulted in more reports of the condition in other ethnic groups, such as Italians and Armenian-Americans.

Signs and symptoms

The recurrent acute attacks of FMF typically begin in childhood or adolescence. Episodes of fever and painful inflammation usually last 12–72 hours. About 90% of people with FMF have their first attack by age 20. The group of symptoms that characterizes FMF includes the following:

Fever

An FMF attack is nearly always accompanied by a fever, but it may not be noticed in every case. Fevers are typically 100–104°F (38–40°C). Some people experience chills prior to the onset of fever.

Abdominal pain

Nearly all people with FMF experience abdominal pain at one point or another, and for most it is the most common complaint. The pain can range from mild to severe, and can be diffuse or localized. It can mimic appendicitis, and many people with undiagnosed FMF have had appendectomies or exploratory surgery of the abdomen done, only to have the fever and abdominal pain return.

Chest pain

Pleuritis, also called pleurisy, occurs in up to half of the affected individuals in certain ethnic groups. The pain is usually on one side of the chest. Pericarditis would also be felt as chest pain.

Joint pain

About 50% of people with FMF experience joint pain during attacks. The pain is usually confined to one joint at a time, and often involves the hip, knee, or ankle. For some people, however, the recurrent joint pain becomes chronic arthritis.

Myalgia

Up to 20% of individuals report muscle pain. These episodes typically last less than two days, and tend to occur in the evening or after physical exertion. Rare cases of muscle pain and fever lasting up to one month have been reported.

Skin rash

A rash, described as erysipelas-like erythema, accompanies attacks in a minority of people, and most often occurs on the front of the lower leg or top of the foot. The rash appears as a red, warm, swollen area about 4–6 in (10–15 cm) in diameter.

Amyloidosis

FMF is associated with high levels in the blood of a protein called serum amyloid A (SAA). Over time, excess SAA tends to be deposited in tissues and organs throughout the body. The presence and deposition of excess SAA is known as amyloidosis. Amyloidosis may affect the gastrointestinal tract, liver, spleen, heart, and testes, but effects on the kidneys are of greatest concern.

The frequency of amyloidosis varies among the different ethnic groups, and its overall incidence is difficult to determine because of the use of colchicine to avert the problem. Left untreated, however, those individuals who do develop amyloidosis of the kidneys may require a renal transplant, or may even die of renal failure. The frequency and severity of a person's attacks of fever and serositis seem to have no relation to whether they will develop amyloidosis. In fact, a few people with FMF have been described who have had amyloidosis but apparently no other FMF-related symptoms.

Other symptoms

A small percentage of boys with FMF develop painful inflammation around the testes. Headaches are a common occurrence during attacks, and certain types of vasculitis (inflammation of the blood vessels) seem to be more common in FMF.

Diagnosis

Individually, the symptoms that define FMF are common. Fevers occur for many reasons, and nonspecific pains in the abdomen, chest, and joints are also frequent ailments. Several infections can result in symptoms similar to FMF (Mallaret meningitis, for instance), and many people with FMF undergo exploratory abdominal surgery and ineffective treatments before they are finally diagnosed. Membership in a less commonly affected ethnic group may delay or hinder the correct diagnosis.

In general, symptoms involving one or more of the following broad groups should lead to suspicion of FMF: Unexplained recurrent fevers, polyserositis, skin rash, and/or joint pain; abnormal blood studies (see below); and renal or other disease associated with amyloidosis. A family history of FMF or its symptoms would obviously be an important clue, but the recessive nature of FMF means there usually is no family history. The diagnosis may be confirmed when a person with unexplained fever and pain responds to treatment with colchicine since colchicine is not known to have a beneficial effect on any other condition similar to FMF. Abnormal results on a blood test typically include leukocytosis (elevated number of neutrophils in the blood), an increased erythrocyte sedimentation rate (rate at which red blood cells form a sediment in a blood sample), and increased levels of proteins associated with inflammation (called acute phase reactants) such as SAA.

Direct analysis of the MEFV gene for FMF mutations is the only method to be certain of the diagnosis. However, it is not yet possible to detect all MEFV **gene mutations** that might cause FMF. Thus, if **DNA** analysis is negative, clinical methods must be relied upon. If both members of a couple were proven to be FMF carriers through **genetic testing**, highly accurate prenatal diagnosis would be available in any subsequent pregnancy.

Similar syndromes of periodic fever and inflammation include familial Hibernian fever and hyperimmunoglobulinemia D syndrome, but both are more rare than FMF.

Treatment and management

Colchicine is a chemical compound that can be used as a medication, and is frequently prescribed for gout. Some years ago, colchicine was discovered to also be effective in reducing the frequency and severity of attacks in FMF. Treatment for FMF at this point consists of taking colchicine daily. Studies have shown that about 75% of FMF patients achieve complete remission of their symptoms, and about 95% show marked improvement when taking colchicine. Lower effectiveness has been reported, but there is some question about the number of FMF patients who choose not to take their colchicine between attacks when they are feeling well, and thus lose some of the ability to prevent attacks. Compliance with taking colchicine every day may be hampered by its side effects, which include diarrhea, nausea, abdominal bloating, and gas. There is a theoretical risk that colchicine use could damage chromosomes in sperms and eggs, or in an embryo during pregnancy, or that it might reduce fertility. However, studies looking at reproduction in men and women who have used colchicine have so far not shown any increased risks. Colchicine is also effective in preventing, delaying, or reversing renal disease associated with amyloidosis.

Other medications may be used as needed to deal with the pain and fever associated with FMF attacks. Dialysis and/or renal transplant might become necessary in someone with advanced kidney disease. Given its genetic nature, there is no cure for FMF, nor is there likely to be in the near future. Any couple that has a child diagnosed with FMF, or anyone with a family history of the condition (especially those in high-risk ethnic groups), should be offered **genetic counseling** to obtain the most up-to-date information on FMF and testing options.

Prognosis

For those individuals who are diagnosed early enough and take colchicine consistently, the prognosis is excellent. Most will have very few, if any, attacks of fever and polyserositis, and will likely not develop serious complications of amyloidosis. The problem of misdiagnosing FMF continues, but education attempts directed at both the public and medical care providers should improve the situation. Future research should

provide a better understanding of the inflammation process, focusing on how neutrophils are genetically regulated. That information could then be used to develop treatments for FMF with fewer side effects, and might also assist in developing therapies for other diseases in which abnormal inflammation and immune response are a problem.

Resources

BOOKS

Kastner, Daniel L. "Intermittent and Periodic Arthritic Syndromes." In *Arthritis and Allied Conditions: A*

KEY TERMS

Acute phase reactants—Blood proteins whose concentrations increase or decrease in reaction to the inflammation process.

Amyloid—A waxy translucent substance composed mostly of protein, that forms plaques (abnormal deposits) in the brain.

Amyloidosis—Accumulation of amyloid deposits in various organs and tissues in the body such that normal functioning of an organ is compromised.

Colchicine—A compound that blocks the assembly of microtubules, which are protein fibers necessary for cell division and some kinds of cell movements, including neutrophil migration. Side effects may include diarrhea, abdominal bloating, and gas.

Leukocyte—A white blood cell. The neutrophils are a type of leukocyte.

Leukocytosis—An increase in the number of leukocytes in the blood.

Neutrophil—The primary type of white blood cell involved in inflammation. Neutrophils are a type of granulocyte, also known as a polymorphonuclear leukocyte.

Pericarditis—Inflammation of the pericardium, the membrane surrounding the heart.

Peritonitis—Inflammation of the peritoneum, the membrane surrounding the abdominal contents.

Pleuritis—Inflammation of the pleura, the membrane surrounding the lungs.

Pyrexia—A medical term denoting fevers.

Serositis—Inflammation of a serosal membrane. Polyserositis refers to the inflammation of two or more serosal membranes.

Synovitis—Inflammation of the synovium, a membrane found inside joints.

Textbook of Rheumatology, edited by William J. Koopman. 13th ed. Baltimore: Williams & Wilkins, 1996.

Sha'ar, Khuzama H., and Haroutone K. Armenian. "Familial Paroxysmal Polyserositis (Familial Mediterranean Fever)." In *Genetic Disorders Among Arab Populations,* edited by Ahmad S. Teebi, and Talaat I. Faraq. New York: Oxford University Press, 1997.

PERIODICALS

Ben-Chetrit, Eldad, and Micha Levy. "Familial Mediterranean Fever." *The Lancet* 351 (February 28, 1998): 659-64.

Kastner, Daniel L. "Familial Mediterranean Fever: The Genetics of Inflammation." *Hospital Practice* 33 (April 15, 1998):131-146.

Samuels, Jonathan, et al. "Familial Mediterranean fever at the millennium: clinical spectrum, ancient mutations, and a survey of 100 American referrals to the National Institutes of Health." *Medicine* 77, (July 1998):268-97.

ORGANIZATIONS

National Institute of Arthritis and Musculoskeletal and Skin Diseases. National Institutes of Health, One AMS Circle, Bethesda, MD 20892. <http://www.nih.gov/niams>.

National Organization for Rare Disorders (NORD). PO Box 8923, New Fairfield, CT 06812-8923. (203) 746-6518 or (800) 999-6673. Fax: (203) 746-6481. <http://www.rarediseases.org>.

National Society of Genetic Counselors. 233 Canterbury Dr., Wallingford, PA 19086-6617. (610) 872-1192. <http://www.nsgc.org/GeneticCounselingYou.asp>.

Scott J. Polzin, MS, CGC

Familial nephritis

Definition

Familial nephritis is an inheritable form of kidney disease. There are multiple distinct forms of kidney disease that are **genetic disorders**. The main inheritable types are Alport's syndrome, autosomal recessive **polycystic kidney disease**, and autosomal dominant polycystic kidney disease. These are all forms of kidney disease in which the nephrons, the basic functional units of the kidney, are diseased or damaged.

Description

Kidneys perform many important bodily functions. Having at least one kidney is necessary for life. Kidneys filter waste and extra fluid from the blood, keep a healthy blood level of electrolytes and minerals such as sodium, phosphorus, calcium, and potassium, help to maintain healthy blood pressure, and release hormones that are important for bodily functions. Normally, there are two fist-sized kidneys present, one on each side of the spinal column of the back just below the rib cage. Each kidney contains microscopic filter lobules called nephrons that transfer bodily waste products from the bloodstream to the urinary system. Healthy nephrons are critical for maintaining bodily functions, and the buildup of waste products can be life-threatening.

Hereditary nephritis (Alport's syndrome) is a genetic disease in which there is significant damage to the nephrons of the kidney. The disease is characterized by the onset of bloody urine in early childhood, which later leads to renal failure. The onset is typically in males before six years of age. After years of recurrent or persistent bloody urine, the kidneys begin to malfunction. Renal dysfunction typically occurs in the third or fourth decade of life, but occasionally before 20 years of age. Alport's syndrome also involves the complication of high-frequency hearing loss and eye complications.

Polycystic kidney disease (PKD) involves the development of renal cysts on the nephrons. A renal cyst is defined as an enclosed sac, or nephron segment, that is dilated to more than 200 micrometers. A cystic kidney is defined as a kidney with three or more cysts. PKD occurs in two forms. The first form is the dominant form (denoting form of **inheritance**), known as autosomal dominant PKD (ADPKD). ADPKD is an adult-onset genetic disorder that is a common cause of chronic renal failure. Early in life, the kidneys are a normal size with normal functional capacities. The disease may remain undetected, until in the fourth or fifth decade. At onset, the kidneys become enlarged by cysts that appear along the nephron. The cysts cause pain, damage, and renal failure. Some cases also include cysts on the liver, pancreas, and spleen.

The second form of PKD is the recessive form (denoting form of inheritance), known as autosomal recessive PKD (ARPKD). This form most often has an onset in the first few days of life (neonatal), but may also onset in infants or in juveniles. In younger patients, most complications involve the kidneys, whereas in older patients, most complications involve the liver. With neonatal onset, the kidneys are greatly enlarged and cause the abdomen to protrude. The kidneys may have taken up so much space during fetal development, that the lungs may be underdeveloped (pulmonary hypoplasia). There are many cysts that may contain fluid or blood covering the nephrons. When the onset occurs in the neonatal period, renal failure usually causes fatality within the first two years of life. When the onset is infantile (three to six months of age), the primary symptoms are renal cysts, with an enlarged and damaged liver.

When onset is juvenile (between three and 10 years of life), the most prominent symptom is liver disease and the associated high blood pressure (portal hypertension). In this form, there may only be a few cysts on the nephrons. It is speculated that **cancer** may also occur with higher prevalence in association with cysts in all forms of ARPKD.

Genetic profile

Mendelian genetics demonstrates that an individual inherits two functional copies (alleles) of every non-sex linked **gene**. One copy is paternally inherited, and the other is maternally inherited. When genes follow the Mendelian inheritance pattern, both the paternal and maternal copies are functionally expressed, regardless of which parent they came from.

There are different modes of inheritance for genetic disorders. An autosomal dominant mode of inheritance means that one gene in the pair needs to have a mutation in order for an individual to become affected with the disease. Since a parent only passes one copy of each gene on to their offspring, there is a 50%, or one in two, chance that a person who has autosomal dominant disorder will pass it on to each of their offspring. Males and females are equally likely to be affected in this mode of inheritance.

Autosomal recessive diseases are caused by the inheritance of two defective copies of a gene. Each parent may contribute one copy of autosomal genes to their offspring. In autosomal recessive inheritance, only if both copies are mutated does disease occur. If only one defective copy is present, the disease does not occur, but the mutated gene can still be passed on to subsequent generations. If both parents are carrying a mutated gene, then each offspring has a 25% chance of inheriting the disease. Populations with a high frequency of healthy individuals carrying defective genes will also have higher prevalence of offspring with the disease.

The sex-linked genes are denoted XX in females and XY in males. A female receives an X gene from each parent. A male receives the X gene maternally and the Y gene paternally. Some genetic disorders display X-linked recessive inheritance. In this mode of inheritance, mothers carrying defective X-linked genes can pass one copy to each offspring. However, because female offspring also receive a normal X-linked gene from the father, female offspring do not actually develop the disease. But since male offspring receive their only X **chromosome** from the mother, if their mother has the mutated X gene, the males can develop the disease. In this case, the mother is known as a carrier.

Alport's syndrome is a genetic disorder that can be inherited in different ways. The mode of inheritance is X-linked in 85% of cases and autosomal recessive in 15% of cases. Rare cases of autosomal dominant mode of inheritance have also been reported. Alport's syndrome frequently affects the ears and eyes in addition to the kidneys. The inherited defect involves the basement membranes of the affected organs, as a result of mutations in type IV collagen genes. The basement membrane is a sheet-like structure made up of type IV collagen that supports the kidney cells. Type IV collagen is made up of six segments called chains designated A1 through A6. Each chain is encoded for by a distinct gene. These genes are distributed in pairs on three chromosomes. The A1 and A2 chains are encoded by the genes COL4A1 and COL4A2 on chromosome 13; the A3 and A4 chains are encoded by COL4A3 and COL4A4 on chromosome 2; and the A5 and A6 chains are encoded by COL4A5 and COL4A6 on the X chromosome. Alport's syndrome involves mutations in the COL4A3, COL4A4, or COL4A5 genes. All of the A chains encoded for by these genes are present in the basement membranes of the glomerulus (portion of the kidney that filters the blood), cochlea (portion of the ear involved with hearing), and the eye. Consequently, there are abnormalities in the basement membranes causing the symptoms associated with Alport's syndrome.

The gene responsible for ADPKD was first localized to chromosome 16, in the region designated PKD1. A mutation at this locus occurs in 85–90% of ADPKD cases. The remaining 10–15% of cases is linked to chromosome 4 at the locus designated PKD2. An additional unidentified locus may exist, as some cases have been reported with no linkage to either of these loci. The abnormal gene for ARPKD has been localized to chromosome 6.

Demographics

In the United States, the frequency of Alport's syndrome is estimated at one in 5,000 individuals. There is no distinction between ethnic populations. The X-linked form of Alport's syndrome is the most common and predominantly affects males. However, there are cases of symptoms reported in females carrying the X-linked form of the disease. In a process known as breakthrough expression, some female patients with X-linked Alport's syndrome have mild disease with a normal lifespan. The autosomal recessive form of Alport's syndrome is uncommon and affects both sexes equally.

ADPKD frequency is one in 1,250 live births, and is discovered in every 500–800 autopsies in the world. In the United States, ADPKD frequency is one per every 200–1,000 individuals. ADPKD is responsible for 0.6–1%

of end-stage renal disease cases in the United States and Europe. ARPKD has a frequency of one per 10,000 live births. ARPKD is twice as common in females as in males. The onset of ARPKD generally occurs in neonates and children, while the onset of ADPKD is in adults usually between 20 and 40 years of age.

Signs and symptoms

Alport's syndrome usually has an onset of persistent microscopic bloody urine (hematuria). The amount of blood in the urine is too small to be detected visually, but can be detected in a laboratory test. The onset is usually in males before six years of age, and is sometimes exacerbated by upper respiratory illness into visibly bloody urine. The hematuria may last for many years, eventually resulting in renal dysfunction between 20 and 40 years of age. Hearing loss is variable. A high-frequency hearing loss is the most common complication, but may progress as far as complete deafness. Hearing complications are usually present by early adolescence, and may require a hearing aid. Other associated complications may include abnormalities of the cornea or lens of the eye, near-sightedness, degeneration of the retina, and blood platelet abnormalities. Hypertension usually begins by the second decade of life. With the onset of renal insufficiency, anemia and bone degeneration may occur. Females with Alport's disease usually have only a mild version of the disorder with only microscopic hematuria that does not progress to renal failure.

When ARPKD presents in the neonatal period, it is often detected by ultrasound imaging techniques that show the formation of cysts. Other signs that a fetus may have ARPKD are a low level of amniotic fluid or underdevelopment of the lungs. When ARPKD presents in childhood, the symptoms often include a painless abnormal mass detectable in the abdomen that is caused by an enlarged liver and enlarged kidneys. Other initial symptoms often include hypertension, an enlarged spleen, and blood in the urine detectable by laboratory tests or visually. Adolescents may also present with liver disease from ARPKD. ADPKD mostly has signs in a young adult of an abdominal mass with or without abdominal pain. ADPKD also often has initial symptoms of blood in the urine detectable by laboratory tests, or visually, and hypertension.

Diagnosis

Alport's syndrome is investigated through multiple tests. Urinalysis in individuals with Alport's syndrome presents with microscopic or visible hematuria. The presence of high protein levels in the urine (proteinuria) is indicative of kidney disease. Proteinuria eventually develops in males with X-linked Alport's syndrome, and in both sexes with the autosomal recessive form of the disease. Proteinuria usually becomes worse as kidney disease progresses. Blood tests are also performed to look for standard protein markers of kidney dysfunction. If kidney disease has progressed, there may also be high cholesterol in the blood. Some cases of autosomal dominant Alport's syndrome also have defects in platelets of the blood.

All children with a medical history that suggests Alport's syndrome are tested for high-frequency hearing loss. To confirm a diagnosis of high-frequency hearing loss, a special tool called an audiometer is used. Eye complications can be diagnosed through an ophthalmologic examination.

Ultrasound imaging studies of the kidneys may be normal in the early stages of Alport's disease. In the later stages of the disease, the kidneys may progressively decrease in size. A renal biopsy is performed to confirm the diagnosis. Physicians search for abnormalities in collagen indicative of Alport's syndrome. The **gene mutations** that cause collagen abnormalities in the kidneys in Alport's syndrome also cause similar collagen abnormalities in skin. For this reason, a skin biopsy may also be used. Skin biopsies are preferred if the patient has end-stage renal disease, in which case a renal biopsy may be unsafe. Genetic analysis is the only method by which to diagnose asymptomatic carrier females that carry an X-linked Alport's syndrome gene. Genetic analysis is also the only method by which to make a prenatal diagnosis.

PKD can be investigated through a variety of laboratory tests. A basic set of urine and blood tests is performed to assist with diagnosis and subsequent monitoring of the disease. The ability of the kidneys to remove waste from the bloodstream is initially tested. The portion of the kidney that acts as a filter is the glomerulus. A reduced ability to filter the blood is known as a reduced glomerular filtration rate (GFR). Complications of PKD may include proteinuria and reduced GFR. A diagnosis of proteinuria is made through urinalysis. In a primary urinalysis test, a strip of testing paper is dipped into a urine sample to provide an immediate, rough indication of whether or not there is protein in the urine. High levels of protein in the urine indicate kidney damage.

Highly sensitive urinalysis tests are also performed to diagnose proteinuria. These tests calculate the protein-to-creatinine ratio. A high protein-to-creatinine ratio in urine indicates that the kidney is leaking protein that should be kept in the blood, which indicates kidney damage. The GFR can be measured by injecting a measurable substance (a contrast medium) into the bloodstream. The injection is followed by a 24-hour urine collection to determine how much of the medium was filtered through the kidney. A more recent method of determining GFR is to measure blood creatinine levels and perform calculations that involve weight, age, and values assigned for sex and race. If GFR remains consistently below 60, a diagnosis of chronic kidney disease is made.

If PKD is present, blood tests will show altered levels of electrolytes and minerals that the kidney normally filters and normalizes. Such altered levels include low sodium and high potassium blood levels seen in PKD. PKD also alters vitamin D metabolism, which is indicated by blood calcium levels. Urinalysis commonly reveals blood in the urine, and blood tests reveal abnormalities in various blood cell types. Liver function tests are also performed. In the early stages of PKD, liver function may be normal, but as the disease progresses, liver disease becomes a more prominent symptom. Even with successful dialysis and kidney transplantation, liver disease may persist and worsen. Abnormalities of lipid metabolism are also commonly seen with chronic renal failure, occur early in the course of PKD, and progressively worsen as well as renal function.

Ultrasound imaging is an important part of diagnosis for PKD. Prenatal diagnosis of ARPKD using ultrasound imaging is sometimes possible based on enlarged kidneys, a small bladder, and oligohydramnios. No cysts are observed during **prenatal ultrasound**. These findings may be the same in the dominant form of PKD. Imaging done on infants with ARPKD may reveal small cysts and kidney enlargement. In the diagnosis of ARPKD in older children, ultrasound imaging usually reveals enlarged kidneys with many very small cysts. The presence of large cysts may occur in later stages, and increase in number over time. Ultrasound imaging varies with the age of onset. Older children may also present with an enlarged, cystic liver and a cystic pancreas.

Diagnosis of ADPKD also involves ultrasound imaging, and was the main method prior to genetic linkage studies. Since PKD1 and PKD2 were identified as the genes involved in ADPKD, **DNA** linkage analysis has been the standard form of diagnosis. Genetic linkage studies have also verified that the ultrasound imaging criteria are accurate in the detection of previously undiagnosed disease. Currently, the criteria for diagnosis include the presence of bilateral cysts with at least two cysts in one kidney. This criterion is most reliable for individuals 30 years of age and older. Sometimes a less stringent criterion is applied to establish a diagnosis for ADPKD between 15 and 29 years of age. The less stringent criteria include the presence of at least two renal cysts total. An individual greater than 60 years of age requires at least four cysts in each kidney for a diagnosis of PKD. Individuals who are

considered at risk may be periodically screened with ultrasound imaging. Computer tomography (CA) scan imaging can be used to diagnose the volume of kidney enlargement and cystic hemorrhaging involved in ADPKD.

Treatment and management

For Alport's syndrome, there is no treatment that prevents the progression to end-stage renal disease. However, there is some initial evidence that suggests that cyclosporine therapy or angiotensin-converting enzyme (ACE) inhibitors may slow the rate of progression. Cyclosporine is an immune-suppressing agent that may reduce some of the inflammatory process involved in Alport's syndrome. ACE inhibitors decrease hypertension and pressure on the kidneys. Other therapy treats the complications that arise as a result of Alport's syndrome. Therapy includes erythropoietin for chronic anemia, medications that affect phosphate and vitamin D levels to combat bone loss, bicarbonate to correct acidic blood conditions, and antihypertensive therapy.

Kidney transplantation is also the main treatment to combat end-stage renal disease in individuals with Alport's syndrome. Unfortunately, 3–5% of males develop immune complications after kidney transplant. Those at risk are individuals with early-onset Alport's syndrome, significant hearing loss, and end-stage renal disease by the time they are 20 years of age. The onset of immune complications after kidney transplant usually happens within the first year. Severe complications result, and 75% of the kidney transplants fail within a few weeks of onset. These immune complications are recurrent in patients who receive more than one transplant regardless of time intervals between transplants and experience an absence of immune complications prior to retransplantation. All other subtypes of Alport's syndrome are at very low risk for this complication and usually have successful transplants. Because of the rarity of transplant complications, donor organs are generally recommended. Generally, there is no restriction of activity for individuals with Alport's syndrome.

The hypertension associated with ARPKD requires extensive treatment with antihypertensive agents, particularly the ACE inhibitors, calcium channel blockers, beta-blockers, and sometimes diuretic agents. Antibiotics may be used to treat urinary tract infections. For children with ARPKD and chronic renal dysfunction, the complication of bone loss is treated with calcium and vitamin D supplements and medications that affect phosphate usage. Erythropoietin is used to increase blood levels. Human growth hormone may be used to improve growth. Sodium bicarbonate may be used to treat metabolic acidosis. If severe dehydration occurs as a result of kidney dysfunction and diarrhea or fever, increased water and salt may be used as treatment.

Drug therapy is not a component of the standard treatment for ARPKD or ADPKD. Drug development of compounds that inhibit cystic growth factors is under research. In the meantime, dialysis is an important part of treatment, along with kidney transplantation. Successful kidney transplantation prolongs survival, and may improve growth and development. Individuals with primarily liver complications may also require a liver transplant, depending on the stage of renal disease.

Prognosis

The prognosis for males with X-linked Alport's syndrome and for all patients with autosomal recessive disease is poor. Most patients develop hypertension and end-stage renal disease. Deafness and visual loss may also be components of the poor prognosis. Many patients with a family history of juvenile-onset Alport's syndrome or early-onset deafness usually develop end-stage renal disease by 20–30 years of age. The prognosis is predicted by the amount of proteinuria present.

In contrast, the prognosis for females with X-linked Alport's syndrome is generally good, with most having normal life spans and clinically mild renal disease.

The prognosis of prenatal ARPKD is very poor. Fetuses develop oligohydramnios and pulmonary hypoplasia. Most infants die from respiratory complications shortly after birth. In fetuses with less severe renal disease who survive the neonatal period, end-stage renal failure may still develop and cause death. The prognosis for children with ARPKD is improved if kidney transplantation is successful, but liver disease may still result. ADPKD is a significant cause of chronic renal failure in adults. The prognosis for ADPKD depends to some extent on the age of onset. If the disease is diagnosed before symptoms develop (through ultrasound imaging) and the patient is less than 40 years of age, the risk of developing end-stage renal failure is 2%. The percentage increases to approximately 50% risk by the seventh decade of life. Prognosis is also dependent on the degree of disease progression. Continued improvements in medical management of end-stage renal disease provide hope for improved prognosis in the future.

Resources

BOOKS

Moore, Keith L., and T. V. N. Persaud. *The Developing Human, Clinically Oriented Embryology, Seventh Edition.* St. Louis, MO: Elsevier Science, 2003.

Thompson & Thompson Genetics in Medicine, Sixth Edition. St. Louis, MO: Elsevier Science, 2004.

KEY TERMS

Amniotic fluid—The protective fluid surrounding a fetus in the womb.

Anemia—Condition in which there are low levels of red blood cells.

Asymptomatic—Without symptoms.

Computerized axial tomography (CAT) scan—An imaging technique that visualizes organs or tissues.

Cornea—The transparent, curved, fibrous coat of the front of the eye.

Creatinine—A normal component of blood kept in low levels in urine by functioning kidneys.

Dialysis—Filtering of blood to remove waste products that the kidneys would normally remove if they were present and functioning.

DNA—Deoxyribonucleic acid, inheritable material that constitutes the building blocks of life.

Locus (plural: loci)—Position occupied by a gene on a chromosome.

Mendelian genetics—A set of parameters describing the traditional method of the transmission of genes from one generation to the next.

Neonate—A newborn infant up to six weeks of age.

Nephron—Basic functional filtration unit of the kidney.

Oligohydramnios—An abnormally small amount of amniotic fluid.

Platelet—An important component of blood that forms clots to close wounds.

Pulmonary hypoplasia—Underdevelopment of the lungs.

Retina—The light-sensitive layer of tissue in the back of the eye that receives and transmits visual signals to the brain through the optic nerve.

WEBSITES

"Alport Syndrome." E-medicine. (April 18, 2005.) <http://www.emedicine.com/ped/topic74.htm>.

"Polycystic Kidney Disease." E-medicine. (April 18, 2005.) <http://www.emedicine.com/ped/topic1846.htm>.

ORGANIZATIONS

National Kidney and Urologic Diseases Information Clearinghouse. 3 Information Way Bethesda, MD 20892-3580. (800) 891-5390. E-mail:

Maria Basile, PhD

Familial polyposis coli (FPC) *see* **Familial adenomatous polyposis**

Familial somatotrophinoma *see* **Acromegaly**

Familial spastic parapelegia *see* **Hereditary spastic paraplegia**

Fanconi anemia

Definition

Fanconi anemia is an inherited disorder characterized by a severe form of anemia and various other physical malformations. Patients with Fanconi anemia are susceptible to various types of **cancer**.

Description

Fanconi anemia (FA) was first described in 1927 by a Swiss pediatrician named Guido Fanconi. It is a rare, inherited form of aplastic anemia. Aplastic anemia is a life-threatening condition in which a person is unable to produce adequate amounts of red blood cells, white blood cells, or platelets. Red blood cells serve to carry oxygen to all areas of the body. White blood cells help to fight infection and disease. Platelets are responsible for clotting to help to heal wounds and control bleeding. Without adequate amounts of these important blood cells, patients affected with aplastic anemia are easily fatigued and susceptible to infections. Most cases of aplastic anemia develop throughout the course of a person's lifetime. However, in FA, the aplastic anemia is inherited, or present from birth.

FA is also associated with various other findings. These include short stature, skeletal abnormalities, kidney problems, and heart defects. Additionally, people with FA experience a high incidence of leukemia and an increased incidence of other types of cancer.

The chromosomes in the cells of FA patients break and rearrange easily. Chromosomes are the information manuals of our cells. Genes are arranged on chromosomes in a linear fashion, like beads are arranged on a string. Genes tell our cells how to make proteins. These proteins perform many vital functions in the body. When chromosomes break, genes are disrupted and they do not function correctly. This leads to abnormal proteins and various health problems. The **chromosome** breakage in FA can be seen in the laboratory and is used to diagnose the disorder.

Genetic profile

It has been determined that at least eight different genes are associated with FA. A change in any one of these genes causes the disorder. The proteins made by these genes are not yet known and their role in FA is not yet understood.

For someone to be affected with FA, each of their parents must have a defect in the same **gene**. Parents that carry the defective gene do not show symptoms of FA because they have a corresponding gene on the other chromosome that produces an adequate amount of protein. Thus, they often do not know they are carriers until they have an affected child. If both parents carry the same defective gene, each pregnancy has a 25% chance of inheriting both abnormal genes and being affected with FA. Likewise, each pregnancy has a 25% chance of inheriting two functional copies of the gene and being unaffected. This leaves a 50% chance that the pregnancy will have one functional gene and one defective gene and will be an unaffected carrier of the disorder. This pattern is known as autosomal recessive **inheritance**.

The FA genes are designated by a letter of the alphabet. Defects in the FA-A gene account for approximately 65% of FA cases. Defects in the FA-C gene account for about 15% of FA cases. In the Ashkenazi Jewish population, however, defects in this particular gene are responsible for nearly all cases of FA.

Demographics

FA occurs equally in males and females. The total number of FA patients has not been documented. It has been estimated, however, that between one in 100 and one in 600 people carry one of the defective genes. FA is found in all ethnic groups but is more frequent in the Ashkenazi Jewish population. One in every 89 people in this population carry a mutation in the FA-C gene.

Signs and symptoms

The signs and symptoms of FA generally appear between the ages of three and 12. In rare cases, symptoms do not present until adulthood. These symptoms vary in severity from case-to-case. Even within a family, siblings who are both affected may show very different signs of the disorder.

Aplastic anemia is the first sign of FA in many patients. In some cases, it may be the only sign of the

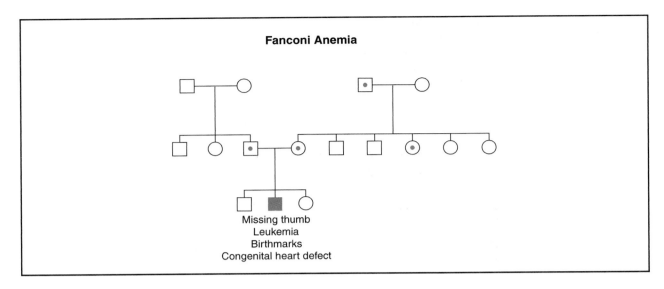

Fanconi Anemia

Missing thumb
Leukemia
Birthmarks
Congenital heart defect

(Gale Group)

disorder. In aplastic anemia, the bone marrow does not produce an adequate amount of red cells, white cells, or platelets. This can lead to several conditions. Anemia can result due to the deficiency in red blood cells, leading to weakness, fatigue, and a pale appearance. Without enough white blood cells, the patient may be vulnerable to common germs and infections. The deficiency in platelets can cause easy bruising, nosebleeds, and possible internal bleeding.

Ten to fifteen percent of patients with FA develop leukemia, specifically acute myelogenous leukemia (AML). Leukemia is a cancer of the blood system in which abnormal white blood cells grow rapidly in number and suppress the development of healthy blood cells. AML is a particularly aggressive type of leukemia and is difficult to treat successfully. Individuals with FA are very sensitive to the toxic drugs used to fight leukemia, which makes treatment even more difficult.

Among the physical defects associated with FA, short stature is very common. Additionally, an affected child may be born with missing, misshapen, or extra thumbs, or an underdeveloped or missing bone in the arm. Approximately one-fifth of patients with FA exhibit other skeletal abnormalities, such as those of the hip, spine, or rib. About 25% of individuals with FA are born with abnormalities of the kidneys. Some are born with defects of the heart, stomach, esophagus, or intestinal tract. These problems may require immediate surgery at birth.

FA is also associated with hyperpigmentation, or a darkening of the skin, in approximately 65% of patients. This darkening may be present in the form of spots or it may be more diffuse over a larger portion of the body. Additionally, the head or eyes might be smaller than average and some patients may not grow properly. Learn-

ing disabilities are thought to be fairly common in FA as well. Hearing loss has been reported in 10% of patients.

As these individuals become older, other problems may result. In males, it is common to see underdeveloped male organs and infertility. Females often have a delay in the start of their menstrual periods and a decrease in fertility. Menopause may occur as early as age 30.

People with FA, especially those over the age of 20, are at a high risk to develop cancerous tumors in the head, neck, intestines, urinary tract, liver, and esophagus. Women are also at an increased risk for cancers of the reproductive tract.

Diagnosis

The most common test for FA is called a chromosome breakage test. White blood cells are isolated from a patient's blood sample and destructive chemicals are added to these cells. The chromosomes are then viewed under a microscope. If the person is not affected with FA, the chromosomes will appear normal. If the person is affected with FA, the chromosomes will be broken and rearranged. Skin cells can be tested in a similar fashion and will often show this chromosome breakage as well. This particular test can be completed prenatally if a family desires to know whether or not a child is affected before he or she is born. Cells obtained from the mother's placenta or cells floating in the amniotic fluid that surrounds the fetus in the womb can be used to detect chromosome breakage.

For families who have a defect in the FA-C gene, it is possible to look directly at the gene to determine whether or not a defect is present. This can detect those who carry the gene defect as well as those who are affected. Carrier testing is offered routinely to those in the Ashkenazi Jewish population since the frequency of carriers is so high.

Treatment and management

Once the diagnosis of FA has been made, several initial tests should be completed, including liver and kidney function studies, a formal hearing evaluation, a developmental assessment, and an ultrasound examination of the kidneys and urinary system.

People affected with FA should be followed closely by a physician. Their blood cell and platelet counts should be monitored frequently. Symptoms caused by anemia and low platelets, such as bleeding, fatigue, chest pain, and dizziness, can be treated with transfusions as needed. Antibiotics are often given to fight infections. At times, hospitalization may be necessary to adequately tend to these complications. As patients get older, they should be monitored for any signs of solid tumor cancers.

Due to either aplastic anemia or leukemia, many individuals with FA will eventually require a bone marrow transplant. The donor must be carefully matched to the patient. The prognosis for transplant is best for young patients who have an sibling donor with a matching tissue type.

Between 50 and 75% of individuals with FA will respond to androgens. These are artificial male hormones that can stimulate production of one or more types of blood cells. They are most effective in increasing the number of red blood cells but can increase platelets and white cells as well. These drugs prolong the lives of individuals with FA but are not a cure.

Various hematopoietic growth factors have been studied in relation to FA. These substances are already present in the body and serve to stimulate the production of blood cells and platelets. Scientists have developed a way to manufacture these substances. They have been given to patients with FA and show promise in increasing the counts of blood cells and platelets.

Prognosis

FA is an unpredictable illness. The average life expectancy for an affected individual is 22 years, but any one individual can have a life span that is quite different from this average. Research discoveries have led to life-extending treatments and improved bone marrow transplant outcome. However, as patients live longer, they become at an increased risk to develop other types of tumors.

KEY TERMS

Androgens—A group of steroid hormones that stimulate the development of male sex organs and male secondary sex characteristics.

Anemia—A blood condition in which the level of hemoglobin or the number of red blood cells falls below normal values. Common symptoms include paleness, fatigue, and shortness of breath.

Aplastic anemia—A form of anemia characterized by a greatly decreased formation of red and white blood cells as a result of abnormal bone marrow.

Hematopoietic growth factors—Substances that assist in the formation of blood cells.

Hyperpigmentation—An abnormal condition characterized by an excess of melanin in localized areas of the skin, which produces areas that are much darker than the surrounding unaffected skin.

Leukemia—Cancer of the blood forming organs which results in an overproduction of white blood cells.

Platelets—Small disc-shaped structures that circulate in the blood stream and participate in blood clotting.

Red blood cells—Hemoglobin-containing blood cells that transport oxygen from the lungs to tissues. In the tissues, the red blood cells exchange their oxygen for carbon dioxide, which is brought back to the lungs to be exhaled.

White blood cell—A cell in the blood that helps fight infections.

Resources

BOOKS

Frohnmayer, Lynn and Dave. *Fanconi Anemia: A Handbook for Families and Their Physicians.* Fanconi Anemia Research Fund, Inc., 2000.

PERIODICALS

Auerbach, A. D. "Fanconi Anemia." *Dermatologic Clinics* 13 (January 1995): 41-49.

ORGANIZATIONS

Aplastic Anemia Foundation. PO Box 613, Annapolis, MD 21404-0613. (800) 747-2820. <http://www.aplastic.org>.

Fanconi Anemia Research Fund. 1801 Willamette St., Suite 200, Eugene, OR 97401-4030. (800) 828-4891. <http://www.fanconi.org>.

Leukaemia Research Fund. 43 Great Ormond St., London, WC1N 3JJ. 020-7405-3139. <http://dspace.dial.pipex.com/lrf>.

WEBSITES

"Fanconi Anemia." *Leukaemia Research Fund.* <http://dspace.dial.pipex.com/lrf-/diseases/fanconi_book.htm>.

Fanconi Anemia Research Fund. <http://www.fanconi.org>.

Mary E. Freivogel, MS

Fanconi-Bickel syndrome

Definition

Fanconi-Bickel syndrome (FBS) is a rare inherited disorder of carbohydrate metabolism caused by mutations in the **gene** known as GLUT2.

Description

Also known as glycogen storage disease type XI, the disease was first described by scientists G. Fanconi and Horst Bickel in 1949. Since then, only a few dozen cases of FBS have been studied, most in the United States, Europe, and Japan.

Onset of FBS is within the first year of life, with the overt symptom being a failure to thrive. At age two, an enlarged liver and kidneys are present and the child has rickets. The incidence of FBS has not been determined but it is believed to occur in less than one in one million births.

Genetic profile

Fanconi-Bickel syndrome is believed to be an autosomal recessive disorder. This means that an individual with FBS would have to inherit an abnormal copy of the gene from both parents in order to show symptoms of FBS. People with only one abnormal gene are carriers and do not have the disorder. When both parents have the abnormal gene, there is a 25% chance with each birth that their child will inherit both abnormal genes and have the disease. There is a 50% chance each birth that the child will inherit one abnormal gene and become a carrier of the disorder but not have the disease itself. There is a 25% chance each child will inherit neither abnormal gene and not have the disease nor be a carrier. The specific genetic defect of FBS has not been identified.

Demographics

Since there is so little research on Fanconi-Bickel syndrome, no clear pattern of demographics has been established. However, the disorder is known to affect both males and females. One common thread in some of the cases that have been studied has been consanguinity, meaning that FBS is found in the children of two persons of the same blood relation. In several of these cases the consanguinity is between two first cousins.

Signs and symptoms

In a 1987 study by researchers at the Research Institute for Child Nutrition in Dortmund, Germany, nine cases of Fanconi-Bickel syndrome were compared for clinical symptoms, behavior symptoms, and physical appearance. The initial symptoms reported were fever, vomiting, growth failure, and rickets between the ages of between three and ten months. Later, these same patients showed signs of dwarfism, a protruding abdomen, enlarged liver, moon-shaped face, and abnormal fat deposits around the shoulders and abdomen. Also, cutting of teeth and puberty were delayed. Complications present included fractures and pancreatitis (an enlarged pancreas). Later in life, rickets and **osteoporosis** were constant features.

The German study, whose researchers included H. Bickel, co-discoverer of the syndrome, also used ultrasound to determine increased kidney size and growth in relation to body height. The most prominent finding was glucosuria (glucose, or sugar, in the urine). Polyuria (increased urination) was also a constant finding. The study noted that liver size was normal or slightly increased at birth in all nine cases but became greatly enlarged during infancy. The liver size and glycogen (a glucose storage molecule) content were reduced when the patients were placed on an antiketogenic (high carbohydrate) diet.

Other laboratory findings included fasting hypoglycemia (low levels of sugar in the blood), ketonuria (high levels of ketones in the urine), high hypercholesterolemia (high cholesterol), **hypophosphatemia** (high phosphate levels in the blood), and high levels of amino acids and protein in the urine. In a 1995 study at Children's Hospital in Philadelphia of an eight-year-old with Fanconi-Bickel syndrome, doctors reported additional symptoms of overworked kidneys, very small amounts of albumin (a class of water soluble proteins) in the urine, and an increase in the number of cells in the inner part of the kidney that filters blood.

Diagnosis

Fanconi-Bickel syndrome can usually be identified in patients by neonatal screening for galactose, a type of sugar. Patients with FBS are intolerant to galactose. Other diagnostic factors include an impaired glucose

KEY TERMS

Carbohydrate—Any of various natural compounds of carbon, hydrogen, and oxygen (as in sugars and starches) that are burned by the body for energy.

Diabetes mellitus—The clinical name for common diabetes. It is a chronic disease characterized by inadequate production or use of insulin.

Hyperlordosis—An exaggerated curve in the lower (lumbar) portion of the back.

Osteoporosis—Loss of bone density that can increase the risk of fractures.

Pancreas—An organ located in the abdomen that secretes pancreatic juices for digestion and hormones for maintaining blood sugar levels.

Pancreatitis—Inflammation of the pancreas.

Rickets—A childhood disease caused by vitamin D deficiency, resulting in soft and malformed bones.

tolerance test, x ray to determine the pattern of rickets, urine tests to measure levels of glycose, phosphates, amino acids, and bicarbonate, and a liver biopsy to detect abnormal galactose oxidation.

Treatment and management

There is no effective treatment for Fanconi-Bickel syndrome. However, some of the symptoms can be treated with adequate supplementation of water, electrolytes, and vitamin D, restriction of galactose, and a **diabetes** mellitus-like diet (low sugar and low carbohydrate) presented in frequent small meals. These treatments can improve growth and give the patient a general sense of well-being.

Prognosis

The long-term prognosis has not been determined. It may depend on the severity of symptoms and early diagnosis and treatment of symptoms. The first person diagnosed with the disorder in 1949 was a four-year-old Swiss boy with consanguineous parents. At six months, the boy had excessive thirst, constipation, and was not thriving. He was treated with vitamin D and calcium supplements. At about age four, the boy had short stature, a protruding abdomen, an enlarged liver, facial obesity, osteopenia, and hyperlordosis. At age 12, the boy was found to be resistant to glycogen. In 1997 at age 52, the patient, without any treatment other than vitamin D and calcium supplements, was of short stature (4 ft 8 in, 140

cm), weighed about 95 lbs (43 kg), had a moderately protruding abdomen, and a smaller than normal liver. Other than arthritis, he had no medical complaints. However, other people diagnosed as children with FBS had much shorter life spans. Long-term follow-up studies of nine persons with FBS showed severely retarded growth, partly compensated for by late onset of puberty.

Resources

PERIODICALS

Manz, F., et al. "Fanconi-Bickel Syndrome." *Pediatric Nephrology* (July 1987): 509-518.

Muller, D., et al. "Fanconi-Bickel Syndrome Presenting in Neonatal Screening for Galactosaemia." *Journal of Inherited Metabolic Disease* (August 1997): 20-24.

Sahin, Figen, et al. "Glycogen Storage Disease with Renal Tubular Dysfunction (Type XI, Fanconi-Bickel Syndrome)." *Archives of Pediatrics and Adolescent Medicine* (November 2000): 1165.

ORGANIZATIONS

American Association of Kidney Patients. 100 S. Ashley Dr., Suite 280, Tampa, FL 33602. (800) 749-2257. <http://www.aakp.org>.

National Kidney Foundation. 30 East 33rd St., New York, NY 10016. (800) 622-9010. <http://www.kidney.org>.

National Organization for Rare Disorders (NORD). PO Box 8923, New Fairfield, CT 06812. (203) 746-6518 or (800) 999-6673. Fax: (203) 746-6481. <http://www.rarediseases.org>.

WEBSITES

"Fanconi-Bickel Syndrome; FBS." (Entry No. 227810). National Center for Biotechnology Information, *Online Mendelian Inheritance in Man (OMIM)*. <http://www3.ncbi.nlm.nih.gov/>.

Ken R. Wells

Fatty aldehyde dehydrogenase deficiency (FALDH10 deficiency) *see* **Sjögren Larsson syndrome**

Feingold syndrome *see* **Oculo-digito-esophago-duodenal syndrome**

Fetal alcohol syndrome

Definition

Fetal alcohol syndrome (FAS) is a pattern of birth defects, learning, and behavioral problems affecting individuals whose mothers consumed alcohol during pregnancy.

Description

FAS is the most common preventable cause of mental retardation. This condition was first recognized and reported in the medical literature in 1968 in France and in 1973 in the United States. Alcohol is a **teratogen**, the term used for any drug, chemical, maternal disease or other environmental exposure that can cause birth defects or functional impairment in a developing fetus. Some features may be present at birth including low birth weight, prematurity, and microcephaly. Characteristic facial features may be present at birth, or may become more obvious over time. Signs of brain damage include delays in development, behavioral abnormalities, and mental retardation, but affected individuals exhibit a wide range of abilities and disabilities. It has only been since 1991 that the long-term outcome of FAS has been known. Learning, behavioral, and emotional problems are common in adolescents and adults with FAS. Fetal Alcohol Effect (FAE), a term no longer favored, is sometimes used to describe individuals with some, but not all, of the features of FAS. In 1996, the Institute of Medicine suggested a five-level system to describe the birth defects, learning and behavioral difficulties in offspring of women who drank alcohol during pregnancy. This system contains criteria including confirmation of maternal alcohol exposure, characteristic facial features, growth problems, learning and behavioral problems, and birth defects known to be associated with prenatal alcohol exposure.

The incidence of FAS varies among different populations studied, and ranges from approximately one in 200 to one in 2,000 at birth. However, a recent study reported in 1997, utilizing the Institute of Medicine criteria, estimated the prevalence in Seattle, Washington from 1975-1981 at nearly one in 100 live births. Avoiding alcohol during pregnancy, including the earliest weeks of the pregnancy, can prevent FAS. There is no amount of alcohol use during pregnancy that has been proven completely safe.

Genetic profile

FAS is not a genetic or inherited disorder. It is a pattern of birth defects, learning, and behavioral problems that are the result of maternal alcohol use during the pregnancy. The alcohol freely crosses the placenta and causes damage to the developing embryo or fetus. Alcohol use by the father cannot cause FAS. If a woman who has FAS drinks alcohol during pregnancy, then she may also have a child with FAS. Not all individuals from alcohol exposed pregnancies have obvious signs or symptoms of FAS; individuals of different genetic backgrounds may be more or less susceptible to the damage that alcohol can cause. The dose of alcohol, the time during pregnancy that alcohol is used, and the pattern of alcohol use all contribute to the different signs and symptoms that are found.

Demographics

There is no racial or ethnic predilection for FAS. Individuals from different genetic backgrounds exposed to similar amounts of alcohol during pregnancy may exhibit different signs or symptoms of FAS. Several studies have estimated that 25-45% of chronic alcoholic women will give birth to a child with FAS if they continue to drink during pregnancy. The risk of FAS appears to increase as a chronic alcoholic woman progresses in her childbearing years and continues to drink. That is, a child with FAS will often be one of the last born to a chronic alcoholic woman, although older siblings may exhibit milder features of FAS. Binge drinking, defined as sporadic use of five or more standard alcoholic drinks per occasion, and "moderate" daily drinking (two to four 12 oz bottles of beer, eight to 16 ounces of wine, two to four ounces of liquor) can also result in offspring with features of FAS.

Signs and symptoms

Classic features of FAS include short stature, low birth weight and poor weight gain, microcephaly, and a characteristic pattern of facial features. These facial features in infants and children may include small eye openings (measured from inner corner to outer corner), epicanthal folds (folds of tissue at the inner corner of the eye), small or short nose, low or flat nasal bridge, smooth or poorly developed philtrum (the area of the upper lip above the colored part of the lip and below the nose), thin upper lip, and small chin. Some of these features are nonspecific, meaning they can occur in other conditions, or be appropriate for age, racial, or family background. Other major and minor birth defects that have been reported include cleft palate, congenital heart defects, strabismus, hearing loss, defects of the spine and joints, alteration of the hand creases and small fingernails, and toenails. Since FAS was first described in infants and children, the diagnosis is sometimes more difficult to recognize in older adolescents and adults. Short stature and microcephaly remain common features, but weight may normalize, and the individual may actually become overweight for his/her height. The chin and nose grow proportionately more than the middle part of the face and dental crowding may become a problem. The small eye openings and the appearance of the upper lip and philtrum may continue to be characteristic. Pubertal changes typically occur at the normal time.

Newborns with FAS may have difficulties with feeding due to a sucking difficulties, have irregular sleep-wake cycles, decreased or increased muscle tone, or seizures or tremors. Delays in achieving developmental milestones such as rolling over, crawling, walking and talking may become apparent in infancy. Behavior and learning difficulties typical in the preschool or early school years include poor attention span, hyperactivity, poor motor skills, and slow language development. Attention deficit-hyperactivity disorder is a common associated diagnosis. Learning disabilities or mental retardation may be diagnosed during this time. Arithmetic is often the most difficult subject for a child with FAS. During middle school and high school years the behavioral difficulties and learning difficulties can be significant. Memory problems, poor judgment, difficulties with daily living skills, difficulties with abstract reasoning skills, and poor social skills are often apparent by this time. It is important to note that animal and human studies have shown that neurologic and behavioral abnormalities can be present without characteristic facial features. These individuals may not be identified as having FAS, but may fulfill criteria for alcohol-related diagnoses, as set forth by the Institute of Medicine.

In 1991, Streissguth and others reported some of the first long-term follow-up studies of adolescents and adults with FAS. In the approximately 60 individuals they studied, the average IQ was 68, with 70 being the lower limit of the normal range. However, the range of IQ was quite large, as low as 20 (severely retarded) to as high as 105 (normal). The average achievement levels for reading, spelling, and arithmetic were fourth grade, third grade and second grade, respectively. The Vineland Adaptive Behavior Scale was used to measure adaptive functioning in these individuals. The composite score for this group showed functioning at the level of a seven-year-old. Daily living skills were at a level of nine years, and social skills were at the level of a six-year-old.

In 1996, Streissguth and others published further data regarding the disabilities in children, adolescents and adults with FAS. Secondary disabilities, that is, those disabilities not present at birth and that might be preventable with proper diagnosis, treatment, and intervention, were described. These secondary disabilities include: mental health problems; disrupted school experiences; trouble with the law; incarceration for mental health problems, drug abuse, or a crime; inappropriate sexual behavior; alcohol and drug abuse; problems with employment; dependent living; and difficulties parenting their own children. In that study, only seven out of 90 adults were living and working independently and successfully. In addition to the studies by Streissguth, several other authors in different countries have now reported on long term outcome of individuals diagnosed with FAS. In general, the neurologic, behavioral and

emotional disorders become the most problematic for the individuals. The physical features change over time, sometimes making the correct diagnosis more difficult in older individuals, without old photographs and other historical data to review. Mental health problems including attention deficit, **depression**, panic attacks, psychosis, and suicide threats and attempts were present in over 90% of the individuals studied by Streissguth. A 1996 study in Germany reported more than 70% of the adolescents they studied had persistent and severe developmental disabilities and many had psychiatric disorders, the most common of which were emotional disorders, repetitive habits, speech disorders, and hyperactivity disorders.

Diagnosis

FAS is a clinical diagnosis, which means that there is no blood, x ray or psychological test that can be performed to confirm the suspected diagnosis. The diagnosis is made based on the history of maternal alcohol use, and detailed physical examination for the characteristic major and minor birth defects and characteristic facial features. It is often helpful to examine siblings and parents of an individual suspected of having FAS, either in person or by photographs, to determine whether findings on the examination might be familial, of if other siblings may also be affected. Sometimes, genetic tests are performed to rule out other conditions that may present with developmental delay or birth defects. Individuals with developmental delay, birth defects or other unusual features are often referred to a clinical geneticist, developmental pediatrician, or neurologist for evaluation and diagnosis of FAS. Psychoeducational testing to determine IQ and/or the presence of learning disabilities may also be part of the evaluation process.

Treatment and management

There is no treatment for FAS that will reverse or change the physical features or brain damage associated with maternal alcohol use during the pregnancy. Most of the birth defects associated with prenatal alcohol exposure are correctable with surgery. Children should have psychoeducational evaluation to help plan appropriate educational interventions. Common associated diagnoses such as attention deficit-hyperactivity disorder, depression, or anxiety should be recognized and treated appropriately. The disabilities that present during childhood persist into adult life. However, some of the secondary disabilities mentioned above may be avoided or lessened by early and correct diagnosis, better understanding of the life-long complications of FAS, and intervention. Streissguth has described a model in which an individual affected by FAS has one or more advocates to help provide guidance, structure, and support as the

KEY TERMS

Cleft palate—A congenital malformation in which there is an abnormal opening in the roof of the mouth that allows the nasal passages and the mouth to be improperly connected.

Congenital—Refers to a disorder which is present at birth.

IQ—Abbreviation for Intelligence Quotient. Compares an individual's mental age to his/her true or chronological age and multiplies that ratio by 100.

Microcephaly—An abnormally small head.

Miscarriage—Spontaneous pregnancy loss.

Placenta—The organ responsible for oxygen and nutrition exchange between a pregnant mother and her developing baby.

Strabismus—An improper muscle balance of the ocular muscles resulting in crossed or divergent eyes.

Teratogen—Any drug, chemical, maternal disease, or exposure that can cause physical or functional defects in an exposed embryo or fetus.

individual seeks to become independent, successful in school or employment, and develop satisfying social relationships.

Prognosis

The prognosis for FAS depends on the severity of birth defects and the brain damage present at birth. Miscarriage, stillbirth or death in the first few weeks of life may occur in very severe cases. Major birth defects associated with FAS are usually treatable with surgery. Some of the factors that have been found to reduce the risk of secondary disabilities in FAS individuals include diagnosis before the age of six years, stable and nurturing home environments, never having experienced personal violence, and referral and eligibility for disability services. The long-term data helps in understanding the difficulties that individuals with FAS encounter throughout their lifetime and can help families, caregivers, and professionals provide the care, supervision, education and treatment geared toward their special needs.

Prevention of FAS is the key. Prevention efforts must include public education efforts aimed at the entire population, not just women of child-bearing age, appropriate treatment for women with high-risk drinking habits, and increased recognition and knowledge about FAS by professionals, parents, and caregivers.

Resources

BOOKS

Jones, Kenneth Lyons. *Smith's Recognizable Patterns of Human Malformation.* 5th ed. Philadelphia: W.B. Saunders Company, 1997.

Streissguth, Ann. *Fetal Alcohol Syndrome: A Guide for Families and Communities.* Baltimore, MD: Paul H. Brookes Publishing Company, 1997.

PERIODICALS

Committee of Substance Abuse and Committee on Children with Disabilities. "Fetal Alcohol Syndrome and Alcohol-Related Neurodevelopmental Disorders." *Pediatrics* 106 (August 2000): 358-361.

Cramer, C., and F. Davidhizar. "FAS/FAE: Impact on Children." *Journal of Child Health Care* 3 (Autumn 1999): 31-34.

Gladstone, J., et al. "Reproductive Risks of Binge Drinking During Pregnancy." *Reproductive Toxicology* 10 (Jan-Feb 1996): 3-13.

Hannigan, J.H., and D.R. Armant. "Alcohol in Pregnancy and Neonatal Outcome." *Seminars in Neonatology* 5 (August 2000): 243-54.

Olson, Heather Carmichael, et al. "Association of Prenatal Alcohol Exposure with Behavioral and Learning Problems in Early Adolescence." *Journal of the American Academy of Child and Adolescent Psychiatry* 36 (September 1997): 1187-1194.

"Prenatal Exposure to Alcohol." *Alcohol Research and Health* 24 (2000): 32-41.

Sampson, Paul D., et al. "Incidence of Fetal Alcohol Syndrome and Prevalence of Alcohol-Related Neurodevelopmental Disorder." *Teratology* 56 (Nov 1997): 317-326.

Streissguth, Ann Pytkowicz, et al. "Fetal Alcohol Syndrome in Adolescents and Adults." *JAMA* 265 (April 1991): 1961-1967.

ORGANIZATIONS

Arc's Fetal Alcohol Syndrome Resource Guide. The Arc's Publication Desk, 3300 Pleasant Valley Lane, Suite C, Arlington, TX 76015. (888) 368-8009. <http://www.thearc.org/misc/faslist.html>.

Fetal Alcohol Syndrome Family Resource Institute. PO Box 2525, Lynnwood, WA 98036. (253) 531-2878 or (800) 999-3429. <http://www.fetalalcoholsyndrome.org>.

Institute of Medicine. National Academy Press, Washington, DC <http://www.come-over.to/FAS/IOMsummary.htm>.

March of Dimes Birth Defects Foundation. 1275 Mamaroneck Ave., White Plains, NY 10605. (888) 663-4637. resourcecenter@modimes.org. <http://www.modimes.org>.

Nofas. 216 G St. NE, Washington, DC 20002. (202) 785-4585. <http://www.nofas.org>.

Laurie Heron Seaver, MD

Fetal facies syndrome *see* **Robinow syndrome**

FG syndrome

Definition

FG syndrome (FGS) is a genetic disorder characterized by mental retardation, low muscle tone (hypotonia), large head, constipation, and anal abnormalities.

Description

FGS refers to a rare genetic condition that has a variety of physical and mental symptoms. Most individuals affected by FGS have symptoms including mental retardation, low muscle tone, brain abnormalities (partial agenesis of the corpus callosum), seizures, large head, characteristic facial features, large intestinal and anal abnormalities, constipation, short stature, joints that tend to stay in one place (fixed), broad big toes, and light and dark skin streaking. The syndrome was first described by Opitz and Kaveggia in 1974 based on physical findings and family history. All of these features appear to be caused by mutated or changed genes on the X **chromosome**. Although the full effect of the mutation or change in the **gene** is not fully understood, the mutations are believed to interrupt the genes' normal functions in the brain, digestive tract, and muscle tissue.

Other names for FG syndrome include Opitz-Kaveggia Syndrome and Keller syndrome.

Genetic profile

FG syndrome (FGS) is caused by mutations on the long arm of the X-chromosome. Studies in 1998 and 2000 found that individuals affected by FGS can have a mutation on the X-chromosome in two different locations on the long arm (q) of the X-chromosome: Xq12-Xq21 [called FGS1] and Xq28 [called FGS2]. When a set of symptoms are caused by **gene mutations** at different locations, the disorder is called heterogeneous. Although a gene mutation causing FGS can appear in an individual for the first time and is not found in the affected individual's parents, most cases of FGS are inherited.

Since both possible gene mutations are found on the X chromosome, FGS is inherited in an X-linked recessive pattern. Every individual has approximately 30,000–35,000 genes that tell their bodies how to form and function. Each gene is present in pairs, since one is inherited from their mother and one is inherited from their father. Females have two X chromosomes, while males have a single X chromosome and Y chromosome. In other words, females receive two copies of the genetic information stored on the X chromosome. When a female inherits the gene for an X-linked recessive condi-

tion, she is known as a "carrier." She usually has no problems related to that condition, because the gene on her other X chromosome continues to function properly and "masks" the abnormal gene. However, males only inherit one copy of the information stored on the X chromosome. When a male inherits the gene for an X-linked recessive condition, he will experience the symptoms associated with that condition. The mutated or changed genes which cause FGS are located on the X chromosome and thus the full-blown disorder primarily affects males carrying the mutated or changed gene on their one X chromosome. When a condition is X-linked, the gene for the condition travels through the family on the X chromosome. In X-linked genetic conditions, the risk for a carrier female to have an affected son is 50%, while the risk to have a carrier daughter is also 50%. An affected male has a 100% chance of having carrier daughters and no chance to have an affected son.

Individuals inheriting the same mutated gene in the same family can have very different symptoms. For example, approximately 38% of individuals affected by FGS have anal anomalies, like a missing anal opening (imperforate anus), while mental retardation is present in 97% of individuals affected by FGS. The difference in physical findings within the same family is known as variable penetrance or intrafamilial variability.

Demographics

FG syndrome can appear in any ethnic population. FGS has been described in individuals of Japanese, American, European, African, and other ethnic background. FGS is not believed to be more common in one specific population.

Signs and symptoms

Individuals affected by FG syndrome can be affected by a variety of symptoms. Most affected individuals have signs of FGS such as mental retardation, low muscle tone and physical development, seizures, large heads, big foreheads, a front cowlick of hair, wide-spaced eyes, extra eye folds (short, palpebral fissures), constipation, and an outgoing, talkative personality. Other fairly common signs of FGS include anal abnormalities (imperforate anus), brain abnormalities (partial agenesis of the corpus callosum, hearing impairments, broad thumbs and big toes, small ears, fine/thinning hair, fused fingers, minor back bone abnormalities, **cleft lip and palate**, heart defects, and fetal fingertip pads.

Diagnosis

Diagnosis of FGS is usually made from physical examination by a medical geneticist. The physical

KEY TERMS

Heterogeneous—A set of symptoms or a disorder caused by several different gene mutations.

Imperforate anus—Also known as anal atresia. A birth defect in which the opening of the anus is absent or obstructed.

Variable penetrance—A term describing the way in which the same mutated gene can cause symptoms of different severity and type within the same family.

examination looks for the combined characteristic features, low muscle tone, mental retardation, etc., of FGS.

Although mutations in specific genes that cause FGS have been found, molecular **genetic testing** (prenatal or diagnostic) is not yet available.

Treatment and management

FG syndrome (FGS) is a genetic disorder and does not have a specific therapy that removes, cures, or fixes all signs of the disorder.

Management and treatment for FGS mainly focuses on the treatment of specific symptoms. More specifically, individuals with incompletely formed anal openings and serious heart defects would need surgery to try to correct the problems. Individuals affected by FGS who have mental retardation benefit from special school and early intervention programs.

Prognosis

The prognosis of an individual affected by FG syndrome depends on the severity of the symptoms by which they are affected. For example, approximately one-third of individuals affected by FGS will die before two years of age due to the severity of heart defects and anal abnormalities.

Most individuals affected by FGS who do not have severe physical problems, such as serious heart defects and anal abnormalities, are still affected by mental retardation. Individuals affected by FGS who have mental retardation benefit from special schools and early intervention programs.

Resources

BOOKS

Smith, Raomayne, and Eunice Kennedy Shriver, eds. *Children with Mental Retardation, A Parents' Guide*. Bethesda, MD: Woodbine House, 1993.

Trainer, Marilyn, and Helen Featherstone. *Differences in Common: Straight Talk on Mental Retardation, Down Syndrome, and Your Life*. Bethesda, MD: Woodbine House, 1991.

PERIODICALS

FG Syndrome Family Alliance Print Newsletter FG Syndrome Family Alliance, subscribe by sending email to : FGSNewsl@aol.com.

ORGANIZATIONS

Arc (a National Organization on Mental Retardation). 1010 Wayne Ave., Suite 650, Silver Spring, MD 20910. (800) 433-5255. <http://www.thearclink.org>.

WEBSITES

The Family Village. <http://www.familyvillage.wisc.edu>.

FG Syndrome Family Alliance. FG Syndrome Homepage. <http://www.geocities.com/HotSprings/Spa/3687/>.

On-line Mendelian Inheritance of Man. <http://www3.ncbi.nlm.nih.gov/Omim/>.

Dawn A. Jacob, MS, CGC

Fibroblast growth factor receptor mutations

Definition

Fibroblast growth factor receptors (FGFRs) are a family of proteins specialized in growth inhibition. Mutations in these molecules lead to various **genetic disorders** involving short stature and/or premature fusion of the bones of the skull. There are at least four known FGFRs (FGFR1, FGFR2, FGFR3, FGFR4).

Description

As a group, FGFRs are very similar to each other in their structure and function. All are transmembrane proteins composed of three distinct parts. A binding site on the exterior of the cell membrane, an active site on the interior of the cell membrane, and a connecting section spanning the cell membrane and joining the inner and outer components.

Fibroblast growth factors (FGFs) attach to the binding site of extracellular portion of the FGFR protein. There are at least 17 known FGFs that bind and interact with FGFRs. Two FGFs must first bind with each other and, as a pair, are able to fit into the FGFR binding site forming an FGF/FGFR complex. FGF pairing and FGF/FGFR binding is non-specific, with any two FGFs coupling and binding any FGFR.

When the binding site is empty and no FGF is bound, the FGFR is inactive and cellular growth continues unchecked. When an FGF pair binds, the FGF/FGFR

TABLE 1

FGFR Genes

Gene	Chromosome	Protein product
FGFR1	8p11	FGFR1
FGFR2	10q26	FGFR2
FGFR3	4p16	FGFR3
FGFR4	5q35	FGFR4

complex sends a signal that travels the length of the FGFR protein, resulting in the stimulation of the active site on the inside of the cell membrane.

The active site of the FGFR stimulates molecules within the cell through the biochemical process of phosphorylation. Each activated molecule goes on to affect another molecule, thereby propagating the original signal and, much like the domino effect, a cascade of events is triggered. The process continues, molecule by molecule, until the signal reaches the nucleus of the cell, ultimately resulting in the inhibition of cell growth.

Although highly recognized in the process of growth restriction, FGFRs are also thought to be involved in a wide variety of biological processes including migration of cells during embryo development, blood vessel growth, wound healing, cell death, and **cancer**.

Genes

A different **gene** codes for each of the four types of FGFR proteins (Table 1). Genes are the genetic material passed down from generation to generation that tell a person's body how to work and how to grow. Genes are packaged into chromosomes, with hundreds of genes on each **chromosome**. Individual cells contain 46 chromosomes, which may be matched into 23 pairs. One of each pair is inherited from the egg of the mother and one of each pair is inherited from the sperm of the father.

A mutation, a change in an FGFR gene, also changes the structure of the FGFR protein, which then affects the protein's function. Most FGFR **gene mutations** are thought to cause the protein receptors to become overly active. These defective receptors continuously start the activation cascade independent of FGF binding. This causes a strong slowing-down effect on growth, which is readily observed in the symptoms of affected individuals. Common features of the disease include abnormalities of the limbs, skin, head, and face.

Inheritance

Approximately ten genetic disorders have been linked to abnormal FGFRs. All FGFR-related syndromes are autosomal dominant. That is, although individuals

inherit two copies of each gene FGFR gene, only one copy must be mutated for a person to be affected with a disorder. Some individuals with an FGFR-related disorder have a parent affected by the same disease, in which case the disease is said to be familial. Other individuals are the first person in their family to be affected. These cases are considered sporadic, meaning they arose from a new mutation in the affected person's **DNA**.

Whether familial or sporadic, all affected individuals have a 50% chance of passing on the disease to a child in any future pregnancy. The overall risk for a pregnancy can change if an affected person has a child with an individual affected by the same disease.

Prenatal testing

Prenatal testing is available for all of the FGFR-associated syndromes. Some cases are diagnosed based on clinical presentation, while others are diagnosed by DNA mutation analysis. Chorionic villus sampling (CVS) or **amniocentesis** may be used when there is a known familial mutation. If there is no family history of FGFR-related disease, but prenatal examination by ultrasound gives rise to concern, prognosis and diagnosis are traditionally based on clinical findings after birth.

Disease causing mutations

Syndromes involving FGFR gene mutations fall into two categories. The first category includes four disorders of short stature, all caused by mutations in the FGFR3 gene. The second category includes six syndromes involving skull malformations (**craniosynostosis**), all caused by mutations in the FGFR1, FGFR2, or FGFR3 genes. There have been no disease-causing mutations reported in the FGFR4 gene.

Dwarfism

FGFR-related dwarfism disorders are all due to abnormal FGFR3 function (Table 2). Mutations in the FGFR3 gene are among the most common mutations in the human genome.

Achondroplasia was the first disease associated with FGFRs. It is the most common form of inherited disproportionate short stature with an incidence of one in 15,000 to one in 40,000 live births. Over 80% of cases of achondroplasia are sporadic, with a strong link to advanced paternal age.

Achondroplasia is characterized by abnormal bone growth that results in short stature with disproportionately short arms and legs, a large head, and characteristic facial features. Intelligence and life span are usually normal, although there is an increased risk of death in

TABLE 2

FGFR-related dwarfism syndromes

Syndrome*	Incidence	Gene	Common mutations≈
Achondroplasia (ACH)	1/15,00 — 1/40,000	FGFR3	Gly380Arg
Hypochondroplaisa (HCH)	Unknown	FGFR3	Asn540Lys
Thanatophoric dysplasia Type I (TD1)	1/60,000 (TD1 and TD2)	FGFR3	Arg248Cys
Thanatophoric dysplasia type II (TD2)	See above	FGFR3	Lys650Glu
Severe achondroplasia with developmental delay and acanthosis nigricans (SADDAN)	3 reported cases	FGFR3	Lys650Met

*Please see the entry of the specific disease for further information and an exact description of the disorder.
≈This represents common mutations and is not a complete list of mutations.

TABLE 3

FGFR-related Craniosynostosis Syndromes

Syndrome*	Incidence	Gene	Common Mutations≈
Muenke syndrome	Unknown	FGFR3	Pro250Arg
Crouzon syndrome	1.6/100,000	FGFR2	25 mutations
Crouzon with Acanthosis Nigricans	Unknown	FGFR3	Ala391Glu
Jackson-Wiess syndrome	Unknown	FGFR2	Cys342Arg, Ala344Gly
Apert syndrome	1/100,000	FGFR2	Pro250Arg, Ser252Trp
Pfeiffer types 1–3	1/100,000 (collective)	FGFR1, FGFR2	Pro250Arg
Beare-Stevenson cutis gyrata	<10 cases reported	FGFR2	Ser372Cys, Tyr375Cys

*Please see the entry of the specific disease for further information and an exact description of the disorder.
≈This represents common mutations and is not a complete list of mutations.

infancy from compression of the spinal cord and/or upper airway obstruction.

Hypochondroplasia is a form of short-limbed dwarfism also caused by a mutation in the FGFR3 gene. Although it appears clinically as a mild form of dwarfism, hypochondroplasia is caused by unique mutations in the FGFR3 gene, different than those that cause achondroplasia.

Thanatophoric dysplasia types I and II and severe achondroplasia with developmental delay and acanthosis nigricans (SADDAN) **dysplasia** are the most severe forms of FGFR-related dwarfism. Both types of thanatophoric dysplasia are fatal with death occurring before birth or during early infancy. There have been only three reported cases of SADDAN dysplasia. Although it is much like thanatophoric dysplasia in its presentation, affected individuals survive past infancy. Affected individuals are severely affected both mentally and physically. Both SADDAN dysplasia and thanatophoric dysplasia Types I and II have their own distinct FGFR3 gene mutations.

Craniosynostosis

Craniosynostosis is the hallmark feature of the second subset of disorders caused by FGFR gene mutations (Table 3). Craniosynostosis is the premature fusion of some or all of the bones of the skull. During normal development the bones of the skull do not completely fuse until the first to second year of life. This allows for passage through the narrow birth canal at delivery and for maximum brain growth during early developmental years.

There are over 150 genetic disorders that involve craniosynostosis that are not related to FGFR mutations. The collective incidence of all forms of craniosynostosis is one in 2,000 to one in 2,500 live births.

There are six craniosynostosis syndromes thought to be FGFR-related. All six display some form of craniosynostosis, distinctive facial features, and hand and foot deformations. Syndromes range from severe (neonatal death) to mild (no clinical manifestations). The characteristic facial features observed include underdevelopment of the midface, protruding eyes, down-slanting eyes, small beaked nose, protruding jaw (prognathism), and eyes that are unusually far apart (hypertelorism). Hand and foot anomalies are distinct for each syndrome and are sometimes used to distinguish between the disorders.

Future

Although the FGFR-related syndromes have been well-characterized, scientists continue to face some puzzling questions. It has been observed that identical FGFR

KEY TERMS

Amniocentesis—A procedure performed at 16–18 weeks of pregnancy in which a needle is inserted through a woman's abdomen into her uterus to draw out a small sample of the amniotic fluid from around the baby. Either the fluid itself or cells from the fluid can be used for a variety of tests to obtain information about genetic disorders and other medical conditions in the fetus.

Chorionic villus sampling (CVS)—A procedure used for prenatal diagnosis at 10–12 weeks gestation. Under ultrasound guidance, a needle is inserted either through the mother's vagina or abdominal wall and a sample of cells is collected from around the fetus. These cells are then tested for chromosome abnormalities or other genetic diseases.

Deoxyribonucleic acid (DNA)—The genetic material in cells that holds the inherited instructions for growth, development, and cellular functioning.

Genome—A term used to describe a complete representation of all of the genes in a species.

Phosphorylation—The addition of phosphoric acid to another compound.

Transmembrane—Anything that spans the width of a membrane.

gene mutations may result in two or more clinically distinct disorders, meaning with different symptoms. For example, a single mutation in the FGFR1 gene has been shown to result in **Pfeiffer syndrome**. The same mutation in the FGFR2 gene leads to **Apert syndrome**, while the equivalent mutation in the FGFR3 gene produces Muenke craniosynostosis. Likewise, a single mutation in the FGFR2 gene may lead to any of the Crouzon, Pfeiffer, or Jackson-Weiss syndromes. The mechanism by which a particular mutation may lead to multiple different genetic disorders is not clearly understood.

Resources

BOOKS

Jorde, Lynne B., et al. *Medical Genetics.* St. Louis: Mosby, 1999.

PERIODICALS

Burke, David, et al. "Fibroblast Grown Factor Receptors: Lessons From the Genes." *Trends in Biochemical Science* (February 1998): 59-62.

Vajo, Z., et al. "The Molecular and Genetic Basis of Fibroblast Growth Factor Receptor 3 Disorders: The Achondroplasia Family of Skeletal Dysplasias, Muenke Craniosynostosis, and Crouzon Syndrome with Acanthosis Nigricans." *Endocrine Reviews* (February 2000): 23-39.

Webster, M. K., and D. J. Donoghue. "FGFR Activation in Skeletal Disorders: Too Much of a Good Thing." *Trends in Genetics* (May 1997): 178-182.

WEBSITES

GeneClinics. <http://www.geneclinics.org>.

Little People Online. <http://www.lpaonline.org>.

Online Inheritance of Man. <http://www3.ncbi.nlm.nih.gov/Omim>.

Java O. Solis, MS

Fifth digit syndrome *see* **Coffin-Siris syndrome**

FISH *see* **Fluorescent in situ hybridization**

▌Fluorescent in situ hybridization

Definition

Fluorescent in situ hybridization (FISH) is a powerful technique used to identify the presence of specific chromosomes or parts of chromosomes through the attachment (hybridization) of fluorescent **DNA** probes to available chromosomal DNA. The fluorescent DNA sequence used to attach to the cellular DNA is called the probe and is created in the experimental laboratory. Sometimes an **RNA** sequence is used as the probe instead of DNA. Examining the labeled cellular DNA under special lighting reveals the presence or absence of a fluorescent signal that indicates specific genes. FISH can be used on tissue preparations, blood or bone marrow smears, directly on cells, or on nuclear isolates.

Description

In situ is Latin for "in the original place," which, in the case of FISH, means inside a human cell or tissue. To hybridize with something means to attach to it in a very selective, specific manner. In situ hybridization (ISH) is the attachment of a very specifically designed DNA probe to cellular DNA (the original place). FISH uses a DNA probe that can be labeled with a fluorescent compound, and emit colored light when it is exposed to specific light wavelengths under a microscope. FISH can detect specific DNA or RNA sequences that are present in a human cell, by taking advantage of DNA's double stranded nature.

FISH and DNA structure

In a normal human cell, DNA is compartmentalized in an area known as the cell's nucleus. Within this nucleus, the preferred conformation of DNA is two strands wrapped around each other and twisted. This twisted structure is known as the DNA helix. DNA is made up of chemical bases that are represented by the letters C, T, G, and A. This is the DNA alphabet that makes up each strand of DNA. The letters of each strand pair up in a specific manner when twisting to form the helix. All the T bases pair with A bases, and all the G bases pair with C bases. Different combinations of these bases are put together in three-letter "words." The arrangement of the words is what determines what a **gene** will encode for, give the gene its meaning, and therefore tell the body how to grow and develop. DNA is transcribed into RNA, the beginning of expression of DNA in a cell. To express the product that the gene is encoding, RNA is translated into proteins that function in many capacities for life.

FISH takes advantage of the tendency of DNA to form base pairs with its corresponding letters. The DNA inside a cell can be experimentally exposed and temporarily unraveled from its helical structure. To denature DNA means to take the unraveling a step farther and undo or the bonds between the bases from the two strands. Once the single stranded bases are exposed, carefully designed DNA sequences that can be fluorescently labeled can be used to probe the cell's set of DNA or RNA. At specific temperatures and under standardized laboratory conditions, the probe is able to hybridize with (pair up with) and therefore label the cellular DNA. This technique can be used to search for specific gene sequences in human tissue that would cause clinical complications. FISH can also reveal the actual location of a DNA sequence on a **chromosome**.

The FISH technique

The general procedure for FISH involves fixing samples of chromosomes or human tissue onto a piece of glass known as a slide (it slides into place on the viewing platform of a microscope when the sample is ready to examine). To prepare the tissue on the slide for hybridization, it is treated with chemicals to permeabilize (open up) the cells and expose the DNA. The chemicals also denature the DNA so that it is single stranded and ready for the probe. A specific chemical hybridization solution containing the probe is applied to the slide so that the probe can hybridize with cellular DNA. This hybridization solution controls the degree of specificity to which the probe hybridizes to the target sequence. Factors such as the temperature, pH, and salt concentration can be changed to control the specificity of the hybridization. When the probe is made of RNA or is being hybridized to RNA, special precautions must be taken because single stranded RNA is less stable than DNA and easily degraded. Any excess probe is washed away.

Probes can be labeled directly with an attached fluorescent molecule, or indirectly, where a specific fluorescent-labeled antibody or labeled binding protein is used to detect a tag attached to the probe sequence. Using the indirect method, the probe itself only contains an attachment point for the fluorescent antibody or binding protein. With this method, the probe by itself is not fluorescent. Once the fluorescent binding molecules are applied, the slide can be viewed on a special microscope designed for fluorescence. The microscope applies a beam of light, set at a specific light wavelength to the DNA on the slide. The fluorescent tags on the DNA emit colored light in response to specific wavelengths. The fluorescent molecules do not fluoresce under sunlight.

Fluorescent labeling

Fluorescent compounds are known as fluorochromes. An example of a fluorochrome that may be used is fluorescein isothiocyanate (FITC). FITC can be attached, or conjugated, to an antibody for the tag on the DNA probe. FITC can only fluoresce under specific narrow wavelengths of light, and does not fluoresce in sunlight. Sunlight contains many wavelengths of light measured in nanometers (nm). Short wavelengths less than 400 nm are types of ultraviolet light that have very high energy. The visible spectrum of light ranges from 400–760 nm. The infrared, long wavelengths of light lie between 760–3,000 nm. FITC compounds are designed to only fluoresce when specific narrow ranges of wavelengths are shining on them. The wavelength required varies from compound to compound. A dark room and a special microscope equipped with such lighting are used for this purpose. Fluorescent labeling can allow two or more different probes to be visualized at the same time because they fluoresce with different colors and can be distinctly visualized. Special filters have been developed to allow simultaneous visualization of several fluorescent molecules at once. When many gene loci (locations) on a chromosome are being labeled, the process is referred to as a chromosome paint. Fluorescent dyes are subject to photobleaching (fading) and so are not permanent preparations. Digital imaging systems can store the fluorescent images permanently and make quantitative measurements.

Once the DNA has been visualized, many types of information can be revealed. FISH is an extremely powerful technique used for many applications in medical

KEY TERMS

Aneuploidy—Having too many or too few copies of a specific chromosome; the most common forms are trisomy (three) and monosomy (one); two copies of a chromosome is normal.

Chromosome—A thread-like structure of DNA and associated proteins called chromatin that carries multiple genes.

DNA—Deoxyribonucleic acid, inheritable material that constitutes the building blocks of life.

Fluorochrome—A fluorescent compound used for visualization in FISH.

Gene—A sequence of chromosomal DNA that functions as a hereditary unit and encodes for the production of a functional product.

Locus (plural: loci)—Position occupied by a gene on a chromosome.

Nuclear isolate—An isolated preparation of the contents of the nucleus of a cell, which contains the DNA.

RNA—Ribonucleic acid, the intermediate step between DNA and its final expression product. DNA is transcribed into RNA and RNA is translated into protein.

Transcription—The process by which DNA is changed into RNA.

Translation—The process by which RNA is changed into protein.

research and diagnosis. FISH can be used to determine chromosome structure, chromosome deletions, chromosomal gene mapping, detect the expression of genes when probing RNA, to localize viral DNA sequences, diagnose viral diseases based on the presence of viral DNA sequences, localize genes involved in **cancer** formation, in forensics, and in sex determination. There are so many uses and different approaches to FISH that it impacts many different types of medicine and research fields.

FISH applications in medicine

There are specific types of **genetic disorders** whose detection and diagnosis have been revolutionized by the FISH technique in accuracy, time, and cost. FISH findings have been determined as so important, that the standing committee for the International System on Cytogenetic Nomenclature (ISCN) established a specific genetic nomenclature just to describe FISH findings. Deletion syndromes, such as **Prader-Willi syndrome**,

were first characterized by high-resolution analysis of chromosomes. Because the deletions in some of these disorders are small and difficult to detect, they are referred to as microdeletion syndromes. The FISH technique has revolutionized the detection and diagnosis of microdeletion syndromes. In some cases, the prevalence of these diseases had not been realized before FISH.

FISH has had a great impact on the characterization of chromosome structural abnormalities that are difficult to diagnose. Given a patient with a genetic disease that has multiple possible **gene mutations**, FISH, with multiple fluorochromes, can be used to determine the precise nature of the chromosomal rearrangements. FISH can be used to literally map out the exact chromosomal structure in DNA samples from such patients, to a level of accuracy previously unknown. This kind of diagnosis would not have been confirmed prior to the advent of FISH. FISH studies can also be used to screen for fetal aneuploidies (too many or too few of one type of chromosome), such as **Down syndrome**.

FISH is used in cancer analysis. Exploration of the acquired **chromosomal abnormalities** found in cancer cells is an important area of research. Techniques other than FISH usually require growing sample cells in laboratories for study, a task that can prove very difficult. Because FISH can be used on non-dividing cells, it can greatly augment standard research techniques. FISH studies are also being used to look for early relapse and residual disease in cancer patient bone marrow transplants from opposite sex donors. The success of transplant engraftments is monitored by dual fluorochrome FISH studies that can label and differentiate between the proportions of female XX and male XY cells in bone marrow and blood.

FISH is used in gene mapping of specific chromosomes and chromosomal regions. The DNA sequences within a chromosome can be determined by labeling FISH probes with multiple different fluorochromes and distinguishing their hybridization color patterns. Chromosomes are composed of DNA and associated proteins. The combination of DNA and protein found in chromosomes is called chromatin. In a new technique called fiber FISH, chromosome-specific chromatin fibers are stretched out on a glass slide and hybridized with gene locus-specific probes. Fiber FISH achieves higher levels of fine resolution mapping of DNA sequences than normal FISH.

FISH is a powerful technique. Because of its high accuracy, time efficiency, and relative low cost, it is quickly becoming the preferred method by which to accomplish many clinical and research applications.

Resources

BOOKS

Thompson & Thompson Genetics in Medicine, Sixth Edition. St. Louis, MO: Elsevier Science, 2004.

PERIODICALS

Heiskanen, M., O. Kallioniemi, and A. Palotie. "Fiber-FISH: Experiences and A Refined Protocol." *Genet Anal.* 12, nos. 5–6 (March 1996): 179–84.

Maria Basile, PhD

Focal dermal hypoplasia (DHOF) *see* **Goltz syndrome**

Fragile site (FRAXE) *see* **Fragile X syndrome**

Fragile site mental retardation 1 (FMR1) *see* **Fragile X syndrome**

Fragile X syndrome

Definition

Fragile X syndrome is the most common form of inherited mental retardation. Individuals with this condition have developmental delay, variable levels of mental retardation, and behavioral and emotional difficulties. They may also have characteristic physical traits. Generally, males are affected with moderate mental retardation and females with mild mental retardation.

Description

Fragile X syndrome is also known as Martin-Bell syndrome, Marker X syndrome, and FRAXA syndrome. It is the most common form of inherited mental retardation. Fragile X syndrome is caused by a mutation in the FMR-1 **gene**, located on the X **chromosome**. The role of the gene is unclear, but it is probably important in early development.

Genetic profile

In order to understand fragile X syndrome it is important to understand how human genes and chromosomes influence this condition. Normally, each cell in the body contains 46 (23 pairs of) chromosomes. These chromosomes consist of genetic material (**DNA**) needed for the production of proteins, which lead to growth, development, and physical/intellectual characteristics. The first 22 pairs of chromosomes are the same in males and females. The remaining two chromosomes are called the sex chromosomes (X and Y). The sex chromosomes

determine whether a person is male or female. Males have only one X chromosome, which is inherited from the mother at conception, and they receive a Y chromosome from the father. Females inherit two X chromosomes, one from each parent. Fragile X syndrome is caused by a mutation in a gene called FMR-1. This gene is located on the X chromosome. The FMR-1 gene is thought to play an important role in the development of the brain, but the exact way that the gene acts in the body is not fully understood.

The mutation involves a short sequence of DNA in the FMR-1 gene. This sequence is designated CGG. Normally, the CGG sequence is repeated between six and 54 times. People who have repeats in this range do not have fragile X syndrome and are not at increased risk to have children with fragile X syndrome. Those affected by fragile X syndrome have expanded CGG repeats (over 200) in the first exon of the FMR1 gene (the full mutation)

For reasons not fully understood, the CGG sequence in the FMR-1 gene can expand to contain between 54 and 230 repeats. This stage of expansion is called a premutation. People who carry a premutation do not usually have symptoms of fragile X syndrome; although there have been reports of individuals with a premutation and subtle intellectual or behavioral symptoms. Individuals who carry a fragile X premutation are at risk to have children or grandchildren with the condition. Female premutation carriers may also be at increased risk for earlier onset of menopause; however, premutation carriers may exist through several generations of a family and no symptoms of fragile X syndrome will appear.

The size of the premutation can expand over succeeding generations. Once the size of the premutation exceeds 230 repeats, it becomes a full mutation and the FMR-1 gene is disabled. Individuals who carry the full mutation may have fragile X syndrome. Since the FMR-1 gene is located on the X chromosome, males are more likely to develop symptoms than females. This is because males have only one copy of the X chromosome. Males who inherit the full mutation are expected to have mental impairment. A female's normal X chromosome may compensate for her chromosome with the fragile X gene mutation. Females who inherit the full mutation have an approximately 50% risk of mental impairment. The phenomenon of an expanding trinucleotide repeat in successive generations is called anticipation. Another unique aspect fragile X syndrome is that mosaicism is present in 15-20% those affected by the condition. Mosaicism is when there is the presence of cells of two different genetic materials in the same individual.

Fragile X syndrome is inherited in an X-linked dominant manner (characters are transmitted by genes on the

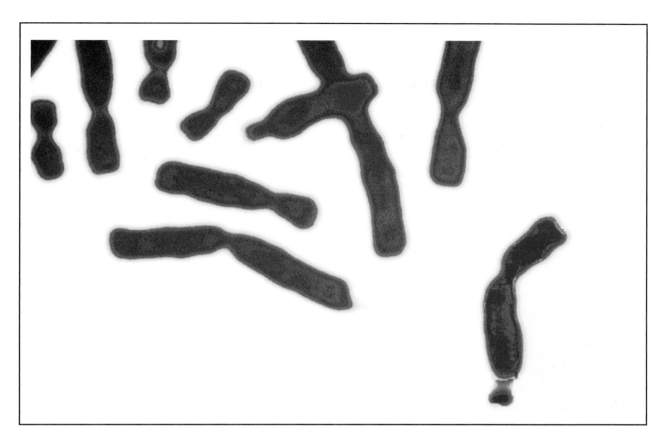

A fragile X chromosome is identified as purple. *(Custom Medical Stock Photo, Inc.)*

X chromosome). When a man carries a premutation on his X chromosome, it tends to be stable and usually will not expand if he passes it on to his daughters (he passes his Y chromosome to his sons). Thus, all of his daughters will be premutation carriers like he is. When his daughter, who carries a premutation, has children, the premutation becomes unstable and can expand as she passes it on. Therefore, a man's grandchildren are at greater risk of developing the syndrome. There is a 50% risk for a premutation carrier female to transmit an abnormal mutation with each pregnancy. The likelihood for the premutation to expand is related to the number of repeats present; the higher the number of repeats, the greater the chance that the premutation will expand to a full mutation in the next generation. All mothers of a child with a full mutation are carriers of an FMR-1 gene expansion. Ninety-nine percent of patients with fragile X syndrome have a CGG expansion, and less than one percent have a point mutation or deletion on the FMR-gene.

Demographics

Fragile X syndrome affects males and females of all ethnic groups. It is estimated that there are about one in 4,000 to one in 6,250 males affected with fragile X syn-

drome. There are approximately half as many females with fragile X syndrome as there are males. The carrier frequency in unaffected females is one in 100 to one in 600, with one study finding a carrier frequency of one in 250.

Signs and symptoms

Individuals with fragile X syndrome appear normal at birth but their development is delayed. Most boys with fragile X syndrome have mental impairment. The severity of mental impairment ranges from learning disabilities to severe mental retardation. Behavioral problems include attention deficit and hyperactivity at a young age. Some may show aggressive behavior in adulthood. Short attention span, poor eye contact, delayed and disordered speech and language, emotional instability, and unusual hand mannerisms (hand flapping or hand biting) are also seen frequently. Characteristic physical traits appear later in childhood. These traits include a long and narrow face, prominent jaw, large ears, and enlarged testes. In females who carry a full mutation, the physical and behavioral features and mental retardation tend to be less severe. About 50% of females who have a full mutation are mentally retarded. Other behavioral characteristics include whirling, spinning, and occasionally **autism**.

KEY TERMS

Amniocentesis—A procedure performed at 16-18 weeks of pregnancy in which a needle is inserted through a woman's abdomen into her uterus to draw out a small sample of the amniotic fluid from around the baby. Either the fluid itself or cells from the fluid can be used for a variety of tests to obtain information about genetic disorders and other medical conditions in the fetus.

CGG or CGG sequence—Shorthand for the DNA sequence: cytosine-guanine-guanine. Cytosine and guanine are two of the four molecules, otherwise called nucleic acids, that make up DNA.

Chorionic villus sampling (CVS)—A procedure used for prenatal diagnosis at 10-12 weeks gestation. Under ultrasound guidance a needle is inserted either through the mother's vagina or abdominal wall and a sample of cells is collected from around the fetus. These cells are then tested for chromosome abnormalities or other genetic diseases.

Chromosome—A microscopic thread-like structure found within each cell of the body and consists of a complex of proteins and DNA. Humans have 46 chromosomes arranged into 23 pairs. Changes in either the total number of chromosomes or their shape and size (structure) may lead to physical or mental abnormalities.

FMR-1 gene—A gene found on the X chromosome. Its exact purpose is unknown, but it is suspected that the gene plays a role in brain development.

Mitral valve prolapse—A heart defect in which one of the valves of the heart (which normally controls blood flow) becomes floppy. Mitral valve prolapse may be detected as a heart murmur but there are usually no symptoms.

Premutation—A change in a gene that precedes a mutation; this change does not alter the function of the gene.

X chromosome—One of the two sex chromosomes (the other is Y) containing genetic material that, among other things, determine a person's gender.

Children with fragile X syndrome often have frequent ear and sinus infections. Near-sightedness and lazy eye are also common. Many babies with fragile X syndrome may have trouble with sucking and some experience digestive disorders that cause frequent gagging and vomiting. A small percentage of children with fragile X syndrome may experience seizures. Children with fragile X syndrome also tend to have loose joints which may result in joint dislocations. Some children develop a curvature in the spine, flat feet, and a heart condition known as mitral valve prolapse.

Diagnosis

Any child with signs of developmental delay of speech, language, or motor development with no known cause should be considered for fragile X testing, especially if there is a family history of the condition. Behavioral and developmental problems may indicate fragile X syndrome, particularly if there is a family history of mental retardation. Definitive identification of the fragile X syndrome is made by means of a genetic test to assess the number of CGG sequence repeats in the FMR-1 gene. Individuals with the premutation or full mutation may be identified through **genetic testing**. Genetic testing for the fragile X mutation can be done on the developing baby before birth through **amniocentesis** or chorionic villus sampling (CVS), and is 99% effective in detecting the condition due to trinucleotide repeat expansion. Prenatal testing should only be undertaken after the fragile X carrier status of the parents has been confirmed and the couple has been counseled regarding the risks of recurrence. While prenatal testing is possible to do with CVS, the results can be difficult to interpret and additional testing may be required.

Treatment and management

Presently there is no cure for fragile X syndrome. Management includes such approaches as speech therapy, occupational therapy, and physical therapy. The expertise of psychologists, special education teachers, and genetic counselors may also be beneficial. Drugs may be used to treat hyperactivity, seizures, and other problems. Establishing a regular routine, avoiding over stimulation, and using calming techniques may also help in the management of behavioral problems. Children with a troubled heart valve may need to see a heart specialist and take medications before surgery or dental procedures. Children with frequent ear and sinus infections may need to take medications or have special tubes placed in their ears to drain excess fluid. Mainstreaming of children with fragile X syndrome into regular classrooms is encouraged because they do well imitating behavior. Peer tutoring and positive reinforcement are also encouraged.

Prognosis

Early diagnosis and intensive intervention offer the best prognosis for individuals with fragile X syndrome.

Adults with fragile X syndrome may benefit from vocational training and may need to live in a supervised setting. Life span is typically normal.

Resources

BOOK

Sutherland, Grant R., and John C. Mulley. "Fragile X Syndrome." In *Emery and Rimoin's Principles and Practice of Medical Genetics*. Edited by David L. Rimoin, J. Michael Connor, and Reed E. Pyeritz. New York: Churchill Livingstone, 1997, pp. 1745–66.

PERIODICALS

de Vries, B. B. A., et al. "The Fragile X Syndrome." *Journal of Medical Genetics* 35 (1998): 579–89.

Kaufmann, Walter E., and Allan L. Reiss. "Molecular and Cellular Genetics of Fragile X Syndrome." *American Journal of Medical Genetics* 88 (1999): 11–24.

ORGANIZATIONS

Arc of the United States (formerly Association for Retarded Citizens of the US). 500 East Border St., Suite 300, Arlington, TX 76010. (817) 261-6003. <http://thearc.org>.

National Fragile X Foundation. PO Box 190488, San Francisco, CA 94119-0988. (800) 688-8765 or (510) 763-6030. Fax: (510) 763-6223. natlfx@sprintmail.com. <http://nfxf.org>.

National Fragile X Syndrome Support Group. 206 Sherman Rd., Glenview, IL 60025. (708) 724-8626.

WEBSITES

"Fragile X Site Mental Retardation 1;FMR1." *Online Mendelian Inheritance in Man* <http://www3.ncbi.nlm.nih.gov/Omim/>. (March 6, 2001).

Tarleton, Jack, and Robert A. Saul. "Fragile X Syndrome." *GeneClinics* <http://www.geneclinics.org>. (March 6, 2001).

Nada Quercia, MS, CCGC, CGC

Francois dyscephalic syndrome *see* Hallermann-Streiff syndrome

Fraser syndrome

Definition

Fraser syndrome, also called cryptophthalmos with other malformations, is a rare non-sex linked (autosomal) recessive genetic disorder that primarily affects the eyes.

Description

Fraser syndrome is named for Canadian geneticist C. R. Fraser, who first described the syndrome in 1962.

The syndrome is also referred to as cryptophthalmos with other malformations because over 90% of the people born with this syndrome have hidden (crypto-) eyes (ophthalmos). It is alternately called cryptophthalmos-syndactyly syndrome since most affected individuals also have partial fusion or webbing of their fingers or toes (syndactyly).

Individuals affected with Fraser syndrome appear to have hidden eyes (cryptophthalmos) because the skin of their eyelids is partially or fully sealed shut. Cryptophthalmos is classified into three types: complete, in which the eyelid is completely fused over an existing eye; incomplete, in which the eyelid is only partially fused over the underlying eye; and abortive, in which the eyelid is completely fused and the underlying eye does not form.

Approximately half of all individuals affected with Fraser syndrome have abnormalities of the genitals, while 37% have kidney (renal) problems, including the lack of one or both kidneys. Some individuals also have abnormalities of the voice box (larynx) and of the middle and outer ear.

Genetic profile

The **gene** responsible for Fraser syndrome has not yet been identified, but it is known to be transmitted as a non-sex linked (autosomal) recessive trait. It seems likely that the gene responsible for Fraser syndrome alters the normally programmed cell death process (apoptosis) in affected individuals. This is suggested by the fact that several of the symptoms of Fraser syndrome result from a failure of apoptosis.

Cells are normally programmed to die when certain conditions have been met. These cells are then replaced by new cells in an ongoing process. **Cancer** cells do not have the ability to undergo this natural cell death process. It is for this reason that many cancers are associated with tumor growth. Tumors are made up of cells that do not undergo apoptosis. The cells in individuals with Fraser syndrome that do not seem to undergo apoptosis are those cells that cause the overgrowth of certain tissues, such as the eyelids in the case of cryptophthalmos or the tissues of the fingers and toes in the case of syndactyly.

Demographics

Fraser syndrome is very rare, occurring in fewer than one of every 100,000 births. It has been reported that the frequency of the syndrome is over 100 times higher in the Roma (gypsy) population as in the non-Roma population. As in all recessive **genetic disorders**, both parents must carry the gene mutation in order for their child to have the disorder. Approximately 15% of individuals diagnosed with Fraser syndrome have been observed in cases where the parents are related by blood (consanguineous). Parents with one child affected by Fraser syndrome have a 25% likelihood that their next child will also be affected with the disease. The specific **gene mutations** responsible for Fraser syndrome have not been identified.

Signs and symptoms

Fraser syndrome is characterized by hidden eyes (cryptophthalmos) resulting from either partial or complete fusion of the eyelids. This condition may be observed on only one side (unilaterally), but it is generally observed in both eyes of affected individuals (bilateral cryptophthalmos). In most cases the underlying eyes are not fully formed which causes small eyes (microphthalmia). In some cases of Fraser syndrome the underlying eyes are completely absent (abortive cryptophthalmos).

Individuals with Fraser syndrome have abnormal or absent tear ducts and widely spaced eyes (hypertelorism). Blindness from birth is quite common in affected individuals. However, in cases where there is a functioning visual pathway to the inner, light-sensitive layer of the eye (retina), partial vision has been observed.

Approximately half of those individuals affected with Fraser syndrome have partial or complete fusion of the fingers or toes (syndactyly). In cases of Fraser syndrome, the observed syndactyly is most often of the third and fourth digits of the hands or feet. An extra finger or toe situated outside the normal fifth digit (postaxial **polydactyly**) and webbing of the fingers or toes (cutaneous syndactyly) are also symptoms seen in individuals with Fraser syndrome. The only other bone abnormality seen with any high frequency is a greater than normal width of the cartilaginous joint between the pubic bones in the front of the pelvis (symphysis pubis).

Abnormalities of the middle and/or outer ear occur in approximately 50% of affected individuals. These symptoms range from malformations and closures of the outer ear (called the pinna or the auricle) to an absence of the auditory canal (Eustachian tube). In cases where the Eustachian tube is absent, connective tissue fills the space where the auditory canal should be and bone covers what would be the opening of the auditory canal to the outer ear. As a result of these abnormalities, some individuals may be deaf or suffer from hearing problems.

Approximately 85% of those affected with Fraser syndrome have abnormalities of the nose. The most common nasal abnormalities are blockage or narrowing of the nasal cavities that open into the mouth and throat (the internal nares or choanae) by either excess bone or by membranous tissue. Forking of the tongue and cleavage of the internal nasal passage are also seen.

Blockage and narrowing of the voice box (larynx) are also commonly associated with Fraser syndrome. Occasionally an abnormal web-like structure is seen in the vocal apparatus of the larynx (glottis) that causes an inability of speech if not corrected.

Abnormalities of the digestive system, otherwise known as the gastrointestinal, or GI, tract are also common. These abnormalities include an incomplete development of the membrane (mesentery) that connects the small intestine to the back wall of the abdominal cavity; malrotation of the small intestine; a protrusion of parts of the large intestine through an abnormal opening in the abdominal wall near the navel (umbilical hernia); and, defects of the muscle beneath the lungs (diaphragm) that is responsible for the flow of air into and out of the lungs.

Approximately 50-80% of all individuals with Fraser syndrome have abnormalities of the genitalia. Affected females may have partial or complete fusion of the folds of skin on either side of the vagina (labia), an abnormally large clitoris, a malformation of the paired tubes that connect the ovaries to the uterus (fallopian tubes), and/or an abnormally shaped uterus (bicornate uterus). Affected females beyond puberty also may not have a menstrual cycle. In affected males, one or both testicles may fail to descend into the scrotum, the urinary opening may occur on the underside of the penis rather than at the tip of the penis (**hypospadias**), the penis may be abnormally small, and/or the urinary opening of the penis may be fused shut (anterior urethral atresia).

Another complication of Fraser syndrome is malformations of one or both kidneys. These malformations may include improper development (renal **dysplasia**), underdevelopment (renal hypoplasia), or the complete absence of one or both kidneys (unilateral or bilateral **renal agenesis**).

Both the navel and the nipples may develop in irregular locations. The navel can be located lower than normal and the nipples are generally wider set. A hairline that extends forward over the temples is an additional cosmetic symptom of Fraser syndrome.

Many infants with Fraser syndrome suffer from water on the brain (hydrocephaly) and some cases have been found in which one of the normal cavities within the brain (the left ventricle) is not present. **Dandy-Walker** syndrome, a brain malformation of the fourth ventricle of the brain, has also been associated with Fraser syndrome. These brain abnormalities can all cause mental retardation.

Diagnosis

The symptoms of Fraser syndrome have been classified into four major and eight minor characteristics.

A patient is diagnosed with Fraser syndrome rather than another genetic syndrome by the presence of at least two of the four major characteristics of the syndrome accompanied by at least one of the eight minor characteristics of the syndrome, or by the presence of one major characteristic and at least four minor characteristics.

The four major characteristics of Fraser syndrome are hidden eyes (cryptophthalmos), fused or partially fused fingers and/or toes (syndactyly), abnormalities of the genitals, and the existence of an affected sibling.

The eight minor characteristics of Fraser syndrome are malformations of the nose, malformations of the ears, malformations of the voice box, a protrusion of parts of the large intestine through an abnormal opening in the abdominal wall near the navel (umbilical hernia), the absence or the incomplete development of one or both kidneys (renal agenesis), abnormalities of the bones other than syndactyly, cleavage of the tongue or other oral clefts, and mental retardation.

Prenatal diagnosis of Fraser syndrome is possible as early as 18 weeks into the pregnancy and is accomplished by the observance via ultrasound of a combination of some or all of the following conditions: blockage of urine flow out of the bladder; small eyes; fused or partially fused fingers and/or toes; blockage of the lungs (pulmonary obstruction) resulting from an absence or closure of the voice box (laryngeal atresia); the accumulation of thin, watery fluid (serous fluid) in the abdominal cavity (ascites); a blood disorder (fetal hydrops) that prevents proper formation of the oxygen-carrying molecule of blood (hemoglobin); a presence of an abnormally high amount of fluid in the tissues comprising the nape of the neck (nuchal edema), and an absence of amniotic fluid due to an incomplete development of the kidney (oligohydramnios).

Treatment and management

Genetic counseling is particularly important in the prenatal treatment and management of Fraser syndrome. This is because the severity of symptoms and appearance of an infant with this syndrome is likely to be very similar in a sibling also born with the disease.

Surgery is almost always necessary to correct the improperly fused tissues of the eyelids, ears, nose, and genitals. Most affected individuals are blind at birth, however, if some visual function is observed to be present, such as a wincing reaction to strong light, partial vision is possible after surgery to repair the damaged eyelids. Recently, corneal transplant surgery has been used to achieve improvements in vision. In cases of a missing eye (anophthalmia) reshaping of the eye socket may be necessary and a glass eye will need to be fitted

for cosmetic purposes. Many infants diagnosed with Fraser syndrome are also deaf or partially deaf at birth. Special programs for the hearing and vision impaired will be necessary for these affected persons.

The most serious and life-threatening abnormalities associated with Fraser syndrome are those of the kidneys and the larynx. In some cases, the laryngeal malformations cannot be repaired, which leads to either stillbirth or death shortly after birth. This is particularly true of blockage of the larynx (laryngeal atresia). Corrective surgery is often possible in cases of narrowing of the larynx (laryngeal stenosis).

If both kidneys are absent (bilateral renal agenesis), the affected individual is usually stillborn. If only one kidney is present (unilateral renal agenesis), the kidney or kidneys are improperly developed (renal dysplasia), or underdeveloped (renal hypoplasia) the affected individual may require kidney dialysis or a kidney transplant. The abnormalities of the small intestine that are associated with Fraser syndrome are generally correctable through surgery.

Prognosis

The type and severity of the kidney and voice box malformations that may result in Fraser syndrome usually determine the prognosis. Overall, 25% of all babies born with Fraser syndrome are stillborn. Another 20% die within the first year of infancy, often in the first few weeks of life. The cause of death is usually lack of kidney function or blockage of the larynx. Kidney and larynx defects tend to be either very slight or absent in the surviving 55% of Fraser syndrome affected individuals, but developmental delay is observed in most patients.

Resources

PERIODICALS

"Craniofacial Clinic: Correction of Ptosis in Children." *Pediatrics & Medical Genetics News of the Cedars-Sinai Medical Center* (Summer 1997): 6-7.

Martinez-Frias, M., et al. "Fraser Syndrome: Frequency in our Environment and Clinical-Epidemiological Aspects of a Consecutive Series of Cases." *Anales Espanoles de Pediatria* (June 1998): 634-8.

Thomas, I., et al. "Isolated and Syndromic Cryptophthalmos." *American Journal of Medical Genetics* (September 1996): 85-98.

ORGANIZATIONS

Children's Craniofacial Association. PO Box 280297, Dallas, TX 75243-4522. (972) 994-9902 or (800) 535-3643. contactcca@ccakids.com. <http://www.ccakids.com>.

National Kidney Foundation. 30 East 33rd St., New York, NY 10016. (800) 622-9010. <http://www.kidney.org>.

National Organization for Rare Disorders (NORD). PO Box 8923, New Fairfield, CT 06812-8923. (203) 746-6518 or (800) 999-6673. Fax: (203) 746-6481. <http://www.rarediseases.org>.

WEBSITES

"Fraser Syndrome." *OMIM—Online Mendelian Inheritance in Man.* <http://www.ncbi.nlm.nih.gov/htbin-post/Omim/dispmim?219000>. (06 February 2001).

Jeanty, Philippe, MD, PhD, and Sandra R. Silva, MD. "Fraser Syndrome." (May 13, 1999) *TheFetus.Net.* <http://www.thefetus.net/sections/articles/Syndromes/Fraser_syndrome.html#_ednref10>. (February 6, 2001).

"Multiple Congenital Anomaly/Mental Retardation (MCA/MR) Syndromes: Fraser Syndrome." *Jablonski's Multiple Congenital Anomaly/Mental Retardation (MCA/MR) Syndromes Database.* <http://www.nlm.nih.gov/cgi/jablonski/syndrome_cgi?index=302>. (February 6, 2001)

Paul A. Johnson

FRDA-1 *see* **Friedreich ataxia**

Freeman-Sheldon syndrome

Definition

Freeman-Sheldon syndrome (FSS) is a very rare genetic disorder characterized by a small, puckered mouth, which gives the appearance of a person whistling. For this reason, Freeman-Sheldon syndrome is also known as whistling face syndrome. FSS may also be referred to as windmill vane hand syndrome or craniocarpotarsal dystrophy.

Description

Ernest Freeman and Joseph Sheldon, two British physicians, first described this distinct disorder in 1938. The syndrome is characterized by skeletal malformations in the hands and feet and facial abnormalities.

In addition to the small mouth, characteristics of FSS include a flat, mask-like face, underdeveloped nose cartilage, contracted muscles of the joints of fingers and hand, and clubbed feet. Most of the features of FSS are caused by muscle weakness. In addition to those characteristics noted above, individuals with FSS may also have crossed eyes, drooping upper eyelids, **scoliosis**, hearing loss, and walking difficulties. Intelligence is usually normal, health is generally good, and life expectancy is normal.

Genetic profile

Usually, FSS follows an autosomal dominant **inheritance** pattern. With this pattern of inheritance, the syndrome appears when a child inherits one defective **gene** from one parent. In some families, FSS follows an autosomal recessive inheritance pattern. In these cases, the condition only appears when a child receives the same defective gene from each parent. This syndrome can also occur sporadically, that is, neither parent passes on the gene responsible for FSS.

The gene responsible for FSS has not been located. Current genetic research is focusing on **chromosome** 11. Some experts consider FSS a form of distal arthrogryposis, which has been mapped to chromosome 11, specifically to location 11p15.5.

Demographics

Freeman-Sheldon syndrome is extremely rare. It affects males and females in equal numbers.

Signs and symptoms

Doctors can recognize Freeman-Sheldon syndrome at birth. Babies born with FSS usually have distinct abnormalities of the head, face, hands, and feet.

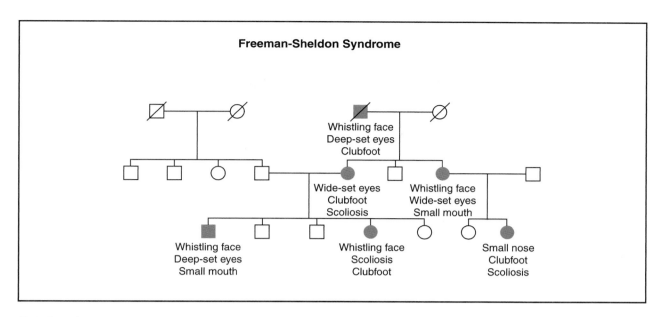

Freeman-Sheldon Syndrome

Whistling face
Deep-set eyes
Clubfoot

Wide-set eyes
Clubfoot
Scoliosis

Whistling face
Wide-set eyes
Small mouth

Whistling face
Deep-set eyes
Small mouth

Whistling face
Scoliosis
Clubfoot

Small nose
Clubfoot
Scoliosis

(Gale Group)

Facial abnormalities usually include an extremely small and puckered mouth, a full forehead, prominent cheeks, and thin, pursed lips. The middle part of the face may be flat, giving the baby a mask-like appearance. There may be a high palate, unusually small jaw, abnormally small tongue, and a raised mark or dimpling in the shape of an "H" or "V" on the chin. Other common facial abnormalities associated with FSS include widely-spaced, deep-set eyes, crossed eyes, and down-slanting eye openings.

Infants born with FSS may have malformations of the hands or feet, including clubbed feet. The muscles in the joints of the fingers and hands may be contracted.

Characteristics of FSS are often linked with other problems such as impaired speech, swallowing and eating difficulties, and vomiting. Children may fail to grow and gain weight at the expected rate, and there may be respiratory problems. Although most of the characteristics of FSS will be discovered fairly early in life, scoliosis (curvature of the spine) may be diagnosed later in childhood or adolescence as the child grows.

Diagnosis

There is no laboratory test to diagnose Freeman-Sheldon syndrome. Because many of the characteristics of FSS are present at birth, doctors can recognize and diagnose FSS following birth based on these characteristics. FSS has also been diagnosed prenatally using ultrasound imaging. Since the gene responsible for FSS has not yet been identified, chromosomal tests are not used in diagnosis.

Because FSS can run in families, parents of children with FSS may wish to seek **genetic counseling**.

Treatment and management

Most children with Freeman-Sheldon syndrome will require orthopedic or plastic surgery to correct their hand problems, clubbed feet, and tight mouth. Plastic surgery can improve the function and appearance of the mouth and nose. Craniofacial surgery can reshape the frontal bone and increase eyelid openings. A potential surgical complication in FSS patients is **malignant hyperthermia** (a serious problem with inhaled anesthetic agents). A muscle biopsy prior to surgery can rule out this risk. The thumb may be repositioned to improve hand function.

Prognosis

Life expectancy for infants diagnosed with Freeman-Sheldon syndrome is normal. Infants and children with

FSS may be referred to physical and speech therapists. Physical therapy may help children improve the use of their hands, and it also can improve ambulation (walking). Speech therapy may improve tongue movement, which helps speech and swallowing. Sometimes, adaptive devices are recommended to aid muscular function.

Resources

PERIODICALS

Bamshad, M., L. B. Jorde, and J. C. Carey. "A Revised and Extended Classification of Distal Arthrogryposis." *American Journal of Medical Genetics* 65 (1996): 277-281.

Lev, D., et al. "Progressive Neurological Deterioration in a Child with Distal Arthogryposis and Whistling Face." *Journal of Medical Genetics* 37 (2000): 231-233.

Ohyama, K., et al. "Freeman-Sheldon Syndrome: Case Management from Age 6 to 16 Years." *Cleft Palate Craniofacial Journal* 34 (1997): 151-153.

ORGANIZATIONS

Freeman-Sheldon Parent Support Group. 509 East Northmont Way, Salt Lake City, UT 84103-3324. (801) 364-7060.

Lisa Ann Fratt

Friedreich ataxia

Definition

Friedreich ataxia (FA) is an inherited, progressive nervous system disorder causing loss of balance and coordination.

Description

Ataxia is a condition marked by impaired coordination. Friedreich ataxia is the most common inherited ataxia, affecting between 3,000–5,000 people in the United States.

Genetic profile

FA is an autosomal recessive disease, which means that two defective **gene** copies must be inherited to develop symptoms, one from each parent. A person with only one defective gene copy is called a carrier and will not show signs of FA, but has a 50% chance of passing along the gene to offspring with each pregnancy. Couples in which both parents are carriers of FA have a 25% chance with each pregnancy of conceiving an affected child. The gene for FA is on **chromosome** 9 and codes for a protein called frataxin. Normal frataxin is found in the cellular energy structures known as mitochondria, where it is involved in regulating the transport of iron.

In approximately 96% of patients with FA, both copies of the frataxin gene are expanded with nonsense information known as a "triple repeat" of a particular sequence of **DNA** bases called "GAA." Normally, the GAA sequence is repeated between six and 34 times, but those with FA have between 67 and 1,700 copies. About 4% of patients have been found to have the triple repeat in only one copy of the frataxin gene and a different gene change in the other. Longer GAA repeats are associated with more severe disease, but the severity of disease in a particular individual cannot be predicted from the repeat length. The extra DNA or other gene change interferes with normal production of frataxin, thereby impairing iron transport. FA is thought to develop at least in part because defects in iron transport prevent efficient use of cellular energy supplies. Extra iron builds up in the mitochondria, leading to the accumulation of damaging chemicals called free-radicals.

The nerve cells most affected by FA are those in the spinal cord involved in relaying information between muscles and the brain. Tight control of movement requires complex feedback between the muscles promoting a movement, those restraining it, and the brain. Without this control, movements become uncoordinated, jerky, and inappropriate for the desired action.

Demographics

The prevalence of FA in the Caucasian population is approximately one in 50,000 to one in 25,000. Prevalence appears to be highest in Italy. Approximately 1% of Caucasian individuals carry one defective copy of the gene for frataxin. Friedreich ataxia is very rare in people of Asian or African descent

Signs and symptoms

Symptoms of FA usually first appear between the ages of eight and 15, although onset as early as 18 months or as late as age 25 is possible. The first symptom is usually gait incoordination. For instance, a child with FA may graze doorways when passing through or trip over low obstacles. Unsteadiness when standing still and deterioration of position sense is common. Foot deformities and walking up off the heels often results from uneven muscle weakness in the legs. Muscle spasms and cramps may occur, especially at night.

Ataxia in the arms usually follows within several years, leading to decreased hand-eye coordination. Arm weakness does not usually occur until much later. Speech and swallowing difficulties are common. The loss of reflexes in the lower legs is common. **Diabetes** mellitus, a condition characterized by elevated blood sugar, may also occur. One study suggested that carriers of one FAA gene with an "intermediate" sized GAA region (10 to 36 copies of GAA) are also at increased risk for diabetes, but other similar studies did not show this finding. Nystagmus, or eye tremor, is common in FA, along with some loss of visual acuity. Hearing loss may also occur. A side-to-side curvature of the spine (**scoliosis**) occurs in many cases and may become severe.

Heart muscle enlargement with or without heartbeat abnormality occurs in about two thirds of FA patients, leading to shortness of breath after exertion, swelling in the lower limbs, and frequent complaints of cold feet.

There are some atypical forms of FA. For example, the Acadian population that descended from Northern France and now live in Louisiana, have a very slow progressing disease and rarely have heart problems, leading them to live longer than most patients with FA. Other forms include late onset Friedreich ataxia (LOFA), in which symptoms begin after the age of 25 years, and Friedreich ataxia with retained reflexes (FARR). All three of these forms have been shown to result from changes in the same gene as the "classic" form. There have been a few patients with classic FA described in which the frataxin gene on chromosome 9 has been shown not to be the cause. A form of ataxia caused by a gene change resulting in vitamin E deficiency, but having similar symptoms to FA, has been identified with changes in a different gene on chromosome 8.

In 1988, a Spanish family was reported in which several members had FA along with congenital **glaucoma**, a disease caused by increased pressure inside the eye. Glaucoma is not normally seen in patients with Friedreich ataxia or other types of inherited ataxia. Most of the affected family members had parents who were closely related to each other, which placed children at increased risk for autosomal recessive conditions in general. Therefore, the glaucoma and FA may have been caused by two distinct genes inherited in an autosomal recessive manner. It is not known if their unusual disease was caused by a gene other than the since-identified frataxin gene or if the glaucoma and the FA were caused by two different genes.

Diagnosis

Diagnosis of FA involves a careful medical history and thorough neurological exam. Lab tests include electromyography, an electrical test of muscle, and a nerve conduction velocity test. An electrocardiogram may be performed to diagnose heart arrhythmia.

Direct DNA testing is available, allowing FA to be more easily distinguished from other types of ataxia. Testing is accomplished by counting the number of GAA repeats in the frataxin gene to see if there is an expansion (67 or more sets of the DNA bases GAA) and by looking

for other gene changes in patients who only show a GAA expansion in one copy of the frataxin gene. As of 2001, no patient with FA has been reported to have non-GAA changes in both copies of the frataxin gene. Many of these non-GAA changes completely prevent the frataxin protein from being made, so having two copies may not be compatible with life. The same genetic test may be used to determine the presence of the genetic defect in the carrier state (i.e., one normal copy and one defective copy of the frataxin gene) in unaffected individuals, such as adult siblings, who would like to learn their chances of producing an affected child. During pregnancy, the DNA of a fetus can be tested using cells obtained from procedures called chorionic villi sampling (CVS), in which cells from the placenta are studied, and **amniocentesis**, in which skin cells from the amniotic fluid surrounding the baby are tested.

Treatment

There is no prevention or cure for FA, nor any proven treatment that can slow its progress. One recent (1999) study in three patients has suggested that a drug called idebenone can reduce heart problems. Idebenone is an antioxidant—a drug that captures free-radicals, the toxic chemicals generated by increased iron. Amantadine may provide some limited improvement in ataxic symptoms, but is not recommended in patients with cardiac abnormalities. Physical and occupational therapy are used to maintain range of motion in weakened muscles, and to design adaptive techniques and devices to compensate for loss of coordination and strength. Some patients find that using weights on the arms can help dampen the worst of the uncoordinated arm movements.

Heart problems and diabetes are treated with drugs specific to those conditions.

Prognosis

The rate of progression of FA is highly variable. Most patients lose the ability to walk within 15 years of symptom onset, and 95% require a wheelchair for mobility by age 45. Reduction in life span from FA complications, usually cardiac, is also quite variable. Average age at death, usually from heart problems, is in the mid-30s, but may be as late as the mid-60s. The particular length of the triple repeat has not been correlated strongly enough with disease progression to allow prediction of the course of the disease on this basis.

Resources

BOOKS

Isselbacher, Kurt J., et al., eds. "Spinocerebellar Degeneration (Friedreich's Ataxia)." In *Harrison's Principles of Internal Medicine.* New York: McGraw-Hill, 1994, p. 2285.

PERIODICALS

Delatycki, Martin B., Robert Williamson, and Susan M. Forrest. "Friedreich Ataxia: An Overview." *Journal of Medical Genetics* 37 (2000): 1-8.

ORGANIZATIONS

Friedreich's Ataxia Research Alliance. 2001 Jefferson Davis Highway #209, Arlington, VA 22202. (703) 413-4468. <http://www.frda.org>.

Muscular Dystrophy Association. 3300 East Sunrise Dr., Tucson, AZ 85718. (520) 529-2000 or (800) 572-1717. <http://www.mdausa.org>.

National Ataxia Foundation. 2600 Fernbrook Lane, Suite 119, Minneapolis, MN 55447. (763) 553-0020. Fax: (763) 553-0167. naf@ataxia.org. <http://www.ataxia.org>.

National Institute of Neurological Disorders and Stroke. 31 Center Drive, MSC 2540, Bldg. 31, Room 8806, Bethesda, MD 20814. (301) 496-5751 or (800) 352-9424. <http://www.ninds.nih.gov>.

Toni I. Pollin, MS, CGC

Frontonasal dysplasia

Definition

Frontonasal **dysplasia**, also called median cleft syndrome, is a rare disorder affecting primarily the face and head. The causes of frontonasal dysplasia are unknown. Most cases appear to occur randomly (sporadically), but it is suspected that some cases are genetically inherited. The term frontonasal dysplasia was first used in 1970 to describe this disorder.

Description

Frontonasal dysplasia is characterized by malformations of the central portion of the face, especially of the forehead, the nose, and the philtrum (the area between the nose and upper lip). A cleft, or divided area, that traverses one or more of the upper lip, philtrum, nose, and forehead is a hallmark of the disease. Occasionally, affected individuals also experience abnormalities of the brain, heart, and certain bones. In the most severe cases, mild to moderate mental retardation has been observed.

Genetic profile

Most cases of frontonasal dysplasia do not seem to show any genetic linkage. However, a case of an affected male with a spontaneous **chromosome** rearrangement, in which the abnormality was not inherited from either parent (a *de novo* rearrangement), involving chromosomes 3, 7, and 11 has been reported in the medical literature. From this case report, it is suggested that the search for the genetic mutation, or mutations, responsible for the appearance of frontonasal dysplasia should focus on locations 3q23, 3q27, 7q22.1, and 11q21. Other researchers have suggested an X-linked dominant trait or a non-sex linked (autosomal) recessive trait is responsible for genetic cases of frontonasal dysplasia. Further research into the genetic origin of this disorder is still needed.

Demographics

Frontonasal dysplasia is rare and statistical data on its occurrence has not been reported. It has not been associated with any particular ethnic or social group. Some reports show frontonasal dysplasia occurs twice as often in males as in females, and that it is associated with increased parental age, which points to chromosome mutation being a possible cause.

Signs and symptoms

Individuals affected with frontonasal dysplasia most often have widely spaced eyes (hypertelorism), a broadening of the nose (nasal root), absence of the skin that forms the tip of the nose, and a hairline that extends farther than normal and comes to a point in the center of the forehead (widow's peak). A cleft lip along the centerline (median cleft lip) of the skin between the nose and the upper lip (philtrum) is also generally seen in individuals affected with the condition.

In some cases, an individual diagnosed with frontonasal dysplasia may also have a vertical groove down the middle of the face; which, in the most extreme instances, may cause the nose to vertically separate into two parts (median cleft nose). Additionally, in some cases of frontonasal dysplasia, a skin-covered gap may be present in the bones of the forehead (anterior cranium bifidum occultum). In cases where the bone deformations of the nose and forehead are quite severe, there may be a malformation of the bony structures (orbits) that hold the eyeballs. Eye defects and even blindness may be present.

In a few cases of frontonasal dysplasia, the group of heart abnormalities known as the tetralogy of Fallot have been observed. This is a combination of four disorders of the heart: an abnormal narrowing of the valve that opens from the right ventricle of the heart into the pulmonary artery (pulmonary stenosis); a hole or perforation in the wall between the left and right ventricles of the heart that allows blood to flow directly from the higher pressure left ventricle to the lower pressure right ventricle (ventricular septal defect); abnormal positioning of the aorta on the right, rather than the left, side of the heart (dextroposition of the aorta), which means that blood flows out of the right ventricle into the aorta so that deoxygenated blood rather than oxygenated blood is being delivered to the body; and finally, an abnormally large right ventricle (hypertrophy of the right ventricle), which is generally associated with the three other anomalies since each of these over-burdens the right ventricle. This set of conditions leads to an improper oxygenation of the blood causing "blue baby" at birth. When these defects are observed, surgery is required.

Skeletal deformities have also been observed in some cases of frontonasal dysplasia. These include the presence of an extra toe arising from the great toe (hallucal **polydactyly**) and a severe under-development of the major bone of the shin (tibial aplasia).

Brain anomalies are also associated with frontonasal dysplasia. These include the absence of the connection between the left and right hemispheres of the brain (corpus callosum) and swelling or hernias of the brain (basal **encephalocele**). In extreme cases of frontonasal dysplasia, mental retardation may be seen. The extent of retardation appears linked with the degree of hypertelorism, which is an abnormal increase of the distance between the eye sockets. The greater the observed distance between the eyes, the greater the likelihood of mental retardation or developmental delays.

Diagnosis

Frontonasal dysplasia is generally diagnosed at birth based on the observed facial abnormalities. A presence of two or more of the following symptoms is considered a positive diagnosis for frontonasal dysplasia: a skin-covered gap in the bones of the forehead (anterior cranium bifidum occultum); hypertelorism; median cleft lip; median cleft nose; and/or any abnormal development of the center (median cleft) of the face.

Because the genetic cause of frontonasal dysplasia remains unclear and because the majority of cases are sporadic, the only way to diagnose frontonasal dysplasia before birth (prenatally) is via ultrasound observation of craniofacial deformations (**holoprosencephaly**). This is a technique that produces pictures of the fetus.

Treatment and management

Cosmetic surgery to correct the facial defects associated with frontonasal dysplasia is recommended for all affected individuals. In severe cases, additional facial surgeries may be required after the initial surgery. These include reformation of the eyelids (canthoplasty), reformation of the orbits (orbitoplasty), surgical positioning of the eyebrows, and plastic surgery of the nose (rhinoplasty).

In cases of congenital heart defects, surgery to correct the defects is required shortly after birth.

Surgery is available to remove the extra toe seen in some affected individuals. Surgeries to correct under-development of the tibia, or shin bone, may also be required. The tibia supports five-sixths of the body weight when a person is standing, with the smaller fibula supporting the remaining one-sixth. If surgery is not performed to correct the shin bone defects seen in some cases of frontonasal dysplasia, the affected individual may never be able to stand or walk.

In the rare instance of mental retardation associated with frontonasal dysplasia, early and continuing intervention programs may be necessary to assist the affected individual.

Prognosis

Individuals diagnosed with frontonasal dysplasia usually are of average intelligence and can expect a normal life span. In the rare cases of associated heart abnormalities, the affected individual may die shortly after birth if corrective surgery is not performed as soon as possible.

Resources

PERIODICALS

Guion-Almeida, M., et al. "Frontonasal Dysplasia: Analysis of 21 Cases and Literature Review." *International Journal of Oral and Maxillofacial Surgery* (April 1996): 91-7.

Stevens, C., and M. Qumsiyeh. "Syndromal Frontonasal Dysostosis in a Child with a Complex Translocation Involving Chromosomes 3, 7, and 11." *American Journal of Medical Genetics* (February 1995): 494-7.

Trifiletti, R., et al. "Aicardi Syndrome with Multiple Tumors: A Case Report with Literature Review." *Brain Development* (July-August 1995): 283-5.

ORGANIZATIONS

Children's Craniofacial Association. PO Box 280297, Dallas, TX 75243-4522. (972) 994-9902 or (800) 535-3643. contactcca@ccakids.com. <http://www.ccakids.com>.

FACES: The National Craniofacial Assocation. PO Box 11082, Chattanooga, TN 37401. (423) 266-1632 or (800) 332-2373. faces@faces-cranio.org. <http://www.faces-cranio.org/>.

National Organization for Rare Disorders (NORD). PO Box 8923, New Fairfield, CT 06812-8923. (203) 746-6518 or (800) 999-6673. Fax: (203) 746-6481. <http://www.rarediseases.org>.

WEBSITES

OMIM—Online Mendelian Inheritance in Man. <http://www.ncbi.nlm.nih.gov/htbin-post/Omim/dispmim?136760> (14 February 2001).

Reader's Digest Health—Frontonasal Dysplasia. <http://rdhealth.com/kbase/nord/nord809.htm> (14 February 2001).

Paul A. Johnson

Frontonasal malformation *see* **Frontonasal dysplasia**

▌Frontotemporal dementia

Definition

Frontotemporal **dementia** (FTD) is one of a group of conditions that cause progressive degeneration of the anterior temporal lobe (the decision-making and behavior control center) and frontal lobe (the language and emotion control center) of the brain. Dementia is not a disease in itself, but is a general term used to describe the loss of the ability to think, reason, and remember, all symptoms that may accompany a wide variety of conditions and diseases.

Description

Although less common than **Alzheimer's disease,** the most common of the dementias, FTD is a relatively new category and is the third most common dementia. The second more common is dementia with Lewy bodies, a condition in which brain cells abnormally accumulate a protein called alphasynuclein in structures called Lewy bodies, which are deposits in the brain containing damaged nerve cells.

Arnold Pick, a neuropsychiatrist, identified the first type of FTD in the early 1890s, when he noticed the dramatic shrinkage in frontal and temporal brain regions during the autopsies of some people with a dementia. This shrinkage seriously disrupted the ability of these individuals to use language.

In later examinations of Pick's tissue samples, the pioneer neuropathologist, Alois Alzheimer, the first to identify Alzheimer's disease, observed that the shrunken brain regions showed similar microscopic changes. Some nerve cells appeared swollen; others contained spherical abnormalities. Later, the swollen cells became known as Pick's cells; the tiny spheres were called Pick's bodies; and the disorder itself became known as Pick's disease.

As scientists acquired more knowledge of brain pathology, they observed that in some cases of FTD degeneration, Pick's cells or bodies were not present. And during the 1970s and 1980s, new diagnostic imaging techniques revealed that frontotemporal degeneration comprised a wide variety of symptoms aside from language difficulties. Imaging studies also suggested that frontotemporal disease is more common than was originally believed, representing up to 20% of dementia cases.

A combination of all of these factors, including reduced emphasis on Pick's abnormalities, varied symptoms, and newly recognized frequency, contributed to an expanding list of names for frontotemporal disorders. To help clarify the situation, researchers adopted the term frontotemporal dementia to encompass all the disorders resulting from gradual deterioration of the frontal and temporal regions of the brain. Sometimes, however, the terms Pick's disease, FTD, and frontotemporal lobar degeneration (FTLD) are used interchangeably.

A variety of pathologic findings has been identified in the brains of patients with FTD. Although some findings are specific to one or two of the FTD subtypes, there is a general profile of FTD brain pathology that emerges.

In general terms, damage to cells in the temporal lobe appears to produce language and emotional dysfunction. Patients with the most severe damage to the frontal lobe experience more severe problems with decision-making function and behavior. Initially, the damage may occur on just one side of the brain. In most cases, however, as the disease progresses, both sides of the brain are affected.

Scientists have recently demonstrated that in some FTD subtypes, these damaged cells contain deposits of an abnormal form of a protein called tau. Tau is present in all neurons and plays an important role in the structure and function, that is, the metabolism, of normal neuron function. In the brain cells of patients with FTD, however, pathologists are finding a variety of combinations: excessive deposits of tau, abnormal versions of tau, or an absence of tau. This evidence is providing increasing support for the scientific theory that different forms of FTD are caused by abnormalities in the tau protein. In most cases, however, the cause of these tau abnormalities is unknown.

Frontotemporal dementia most commonly refers to a group of specific disorders. These include:

- Pick's disease: A rare brain disease that is characterized by shrinkage of the tissues of the brain's frontal and temporal lobes and the presence of small deposits (Pick's bodies) in the nerve cells of the affected area. Pick's bodies are not always present in FTD. The disease resembles Alzheimer's disease in the personality changes and disorientation that may precede memory loss.

- Corticobasal degeneration: A progressive neurologic disorder that is characterized by nerve cell loss and shrinkage of multiple areas of the brain, including the cerebral cortex and basal ganglia. Symptoms, such as rigidity and loss of muscle coordination, resemble those symptoms found in **Parkinson's disease.**

- Progressive aphasia: A rare neurologic disorder that is characterized by progressively impaired language abilities, although other mental functions and activities of daily living are preserved.

- Semantic dementia: Also known as fluent progressive aphasia, semantic dementia is a language disorder in which patients exhibit a progressive deterioration of the understanding and recognition of words, although impairment in other cognitive faculties is not present.

- Frontotemporal dementia with Parkinsonism-17 (FTDP-17): A type of progressively worsening dementia that involves the frontal and temporal areas of the brain and is characterized by behavioral and cognitive changes, psychiatric symptoms, language difficulties, and Parkinsonian symptoms, such as tremor and muscle rigidity. This form of FTD is linked to **chromosome** 17.

- Frontotemporal dementia with motor neuron disease (FTD-MND): A disorder in which FTD coexists with MND and primarily affects the temporal lobe of the brain; also known as **amyotrophic lateral sclerosis** (ALS, or Lou Gehrig's disease) with dementia. ALS is a neuromuscular disease that progressively weakens and destroys motor neurons, the cells in the nervous system that send messages from the brain to the rest of the body.

Genetic profile

Frontotemporal dementia may be sporadic (occurring in one family member), familial (involving two or more family members), or hereditary. In most cases (about 60%), FTD is sporadic. When FTD is diagnosed in a person with no family history of FTD or dementia, the isolated, or sporadic, case appears to pose no increased risk to family members.

About 40% of FTD cases are believed to have a genetic component, such as a positive family history for FTD or a related neurodegenerative condition or dementia. Of those, about 10% have mutations in the microtubule-associated protein tau (MAPT) **gene**, which is located on chromosome 17. The children of a person with a mutation in this gene have a 50% chance of inheriting that same disease-causing mutation. Researchers have found some linkage to chromosome 9 and some to chromosome 3, and other FTD genes are likely to be found in the future.

About 5–10% of patients have a family history that suggests a hereditary condition with an autosomal dominant patter of **inheritance**, meaning that there is a clear pattern of FTD-type diagnoses being passed from parent to child, with virtually every patient having an affected parent, and each child of an affected person having a 50% chance of inheriting the disorder. Only one of the subtypes, FTDP-17, is exclusively hereditary.

Demographics

It is estimated that as many as seven million Americans may be affected with some form of dementia, and FTD may account for about 25% of those dementias. Frontotemporal dementia occurs most frequently between the ages of 35 and 75, and was believed to affect men and women equally. Recent studies, however, have indicated that FTD appears to be more common in men and is a more common cause of early-onset dementia than previously recognized.

Signs and symptoms

Frontotemporal dementia comprises a wide variety of symptoms that vary widely from person to person, depending on the degree of involvement of the frontal and temporal lobes and the side of the brain affected.

Although two major symptom patterns emerge in all forms of FTS, namely gradual and progressive changes in behavior and language, some symptoms are more closely associated with one subtype of FTD than another. In general, the range of symptoms associated with FTD includes behavioral, linguistic, cognitive, emotional, neurologic, and psychiatric.

A progressive deterioration in the ability to control or adjust behavior appropriately in different social contexts is the characteristic feature of all the behavioral changes. This results in embarrassing, inappropriate social situations that can be one of the most disturbing aspects of FTD. Patients with FTD often present two seemingly opposite behavioral profiles in the early and middle stages of the disease. Some people are hyperactive, restless, distracted, and uninhibited. Others are apathetic, lack spontaneity, and are emotionally blunted.

Behavioral symptoms include:

- compulsive behaviors involving, for example, eating, drinking, or dressing
- repetitive behaviors, such as turning the television on and off
- deteriorating personal hygiene habits, such as bathing, grooming, and dressing
- hyperactive behaviors, such as pacing, agitation, aggression
- impulsive or inappropriate behaviors involving, for example, sexuality
- changes in sleep patterns, including prolonged sleepiness, especially in those with more apathetic behaviors

Linguistic symptoms include:

- decreasing speech to the point of total silence in some patients, and conversation is not spontaneous but, rather, mechanical
- weak-sounding, imprecise, or incoherent speech
- difficulties remembering grammar rules
- repetition of a word or phrase uttered by another
- repetition of a word or phrase uttered by the person themselves
- loss of the ability to speak

Cognitive symptoms include:

- distractibility and impatience
- rigid and inflexible thinking and impaired judgment
- abstract reasoning difficulty
- poor financial judgment

As opposed to those affected by Alzheimer's disease, patients with FTD tend to have normal results on intelligence tests until that point in the disease process at which apathy results in lower scores.

Emotional symptoms include:

- apathy or indifference to people and events
- lack of understanding of self and others
- lack of empathy toward and understanding of others, including family members and close friends
- frequent and abrupt mood changes

Neurologic symptoms include:

- movement dysfunction, including decreased facial expression, slow movements, rigidity, difficulties with posture, and sometimes abnormal eye movements
- muscle dysfunction, such as weakness, muscle jerking, or atrophy

Psychiatric symptoms include:

- **depression**
- manic behavior
- paranoia
- visual or auditory hallucinations

Diagnosis

Although medical knowledge of FTD is still evolving and a broad range of subtypes is involved, current technology is providing the first evidence of the pathologic changes that occur in specific areas of the brain that cause FTD's varied symptoms. For example, loss of function in an individual's temporal lobe produces language changes, and loss of function in the frontal lobe appears to lead to behavioral symptoms, including aggressive, antisocial, and other socially unacceptable behaviors.

Because of its symptoms, FTD is often initially misdiagnosed as a psychiatric problem, Alzheimer's disease, or Parkinson's disease. However, there are features that rule out other diagnoses and identify features that pinpoint FTD.

Medical history

The presentation of the disorder within families can vary. Some people may have FTD alone, and others may develop parkinsonism or psychiatric symptoms. Because of this variability, a careful analysis of family medical and social history can help clarify whether an affected person has a sporadic or a hereditary form of the disorder.

It is important to interview another source, such as a spouse, partner, or adult child, regarding changes in the patient's cognitive performance or behavior that are having a negative impact on the patient's activities of daily living. This source is important in establishing information about past performance and behavior, as well as the progression of symptoms that the patient may not be able to provide reliably. The additional source may also provide information that can be used to test the patient's recent and long-term memory. Significant functional changes in memory and other cognitive domains that interfere with everyday activities (such as driving, functioning at work, and/or interactions with family and friends) signal a disease state and are not part of the typical aging process.

It is essential to determine the potential for medication-induced confusion or dementia by studying the patient's drug inventory and looking for compounds that may cause or exacerbate any loss of mental capacity.

Physical examination

A targeted physical examination should be performed in all patients with dementia. Signs of systemic disorders, such as vasculitis, systemic lupus erythematosus (SLE, a chronic inflammatory condition), tuberculosis, and hypothyroidism, suggest that further evaluation is necessary. Physical problems, such as profound hearing or visual loss, may exacerbate FTD.

Laboratory studies

The American Academy of Neurology practice parameters suggest that routine evaluation of a patient with dementia should include: complete blood count (CBC); serum electrolytes, including calcium; glucose; blood urea nitrogen (BUN) and creatinine; liver function tests; thyroid tests; vitamin B12 level; and syphilis serology.

Neurologic examination

Neurologic examination may reveal signs that vary according to which part of the brain is affected, either the temporal or the frontal lobe, with associated behavioral and language changes. Careful neurologic examination should include observation of gait and posture, cranial nerves, motor strength, sensation, and reflexes. In more advanced stages of FTD, neurologic examination often reveals motor dysfunction and reflex abnormalities.

Neuropsychological examination

This examination assesses, for example, language, behavior, abstraction, memory, executive, motor skills, and visual-spatial functioning. There are many tools available for cognitive testing. The goal of testing is to demonstrate a decline in intellectual function, to assess whether depression is a contributing factor, to make predictions about future functioning, and to plan care. The Mini-Mental State Examination (MMSE) and the Geriatric Depression Scale may be administered by primary caregivers and should be performed on all patients with dementia. More detailed evaluation, such as the Wechsler Adult Intelligence Scale (WAIS), the Blessed Information-Memory-Concentration Test, visuospatial testing, and the Boston Diagnostic Aphasia Evaluation, also may be helpful in making a diagnosis.

Neuroimaging studies

These studies include magnetic resonance imaging (MRI), computed tomography (CT), positron emission tomography (PET), and single-photon computed tomography (SPECT). They help to determine the exact location and extent of atrophy in the brain as well as areas of decreased blood flow. Electroencephalogram (EEG), or brain scan, results are usually normal, however, even in advanced stages of the disease.

Although differentiating FTD from dementias, such as Alzheimer's disease, has been difficult, with more sophisticated brain imaging, such as SPECT, some researchers have claimed that they can diagnose Alzheimer's disease with an accuracy rate of nearly 100%. Differentiating among the various subtypes of FTD, however, still remains a challenge. Sometimes definitive diagnosis of these conditions can be made only by brain autopsy.

Treatment and management

There is no cure for FTD, and in most cases, disease progression cannot be slowed. Although no medications have been proven effective specifically for FTD, many physicians look to the medications and treatment approaches used in other, similar disorders to develop a therapeutic approach. For example, some patients with FTD benefit from selective serotonin reuptake inhibitors (SSRIs), which are used in treating depression, and acetylcholinesterase inhibitors, which are used in treating Alzheimer's disease, to help prolong the activity of neurotransmitters in the brain. Physicians may also use antioxidants, such as vitamin E or coenzyme Q10, which are known to slow the progression of damage to brain cells in general.

Over time, FTD is progressive, and after a few years, a patient's ability to live and function

Acetylcholine—A neurotransmitter (chemical messenger) used to certain nerve cells to send messages to adjacent cells.

Aphasia—Impairment of ability to comprehend or communicate through speech, writing, or signs due to brain dysfunctions.

Autosomal dominant—A gene on one of the non-sex chromosomes that is always expressed, even if only one copy is present.

Cholinesterase—Enzyme whose role is to break down released acetylcholine in the gap between nerve cells.

Familial—A trait observed with higher frequency within the same family, whether the origin is genetic, environmental, or a combination of both.

independently are decreased, leaving them dependent on others for activities of daily living.

Care of patients with FTD focuses on maximizing quality of life, treating neuropsychiatric complications, ensuring patient safety, and supporting and educating caregivers. It is important for caregivers and families to consider long-term management issues and identify a team of experts who can help with difficult medical, financial, and emotional challenges. Also, it is important to have a physician who is knowledgeable about FTD and comprehensive approaches to treatment. In addition, speech therapists, occupational and physical therapists, neuropsychologists, nurses, and genetic counselors may be helpful.

Prognosis

Prognosis varies, but studies have shown that a person with FTD may live with the disease an average of eight years, with a range of 3–17 years. A more slowly progressive form of FTD occurs in the small percentage of people with familial tau-positive disease. People with FTD-MND have the shortest life expectancy, both before and after diagnosis.

Resources

BOOKS

Radin, Lisa, and Gary Radin, eds. *What If It's Not Alzheimer's? A Caregiver's Guide to Dementia.* Amherst, NY: Prometheus Books, 2003.

Weiner, Myron F., and Anne M. Lipton, eds. *The Dementias: Diagnosis, Treatment, Research, 3rd Edition.* Arlington, VA: American Psychiatric Publishing, 2003.

PERIODICALS

Wilhelmsen, Kirk C., et al. "17q-Linked Frontotemporal Dementia–Amyotrophic Lateral Sclerosis without Tau Mutations with Tau and alfa-Synuclein Inclusions." *Archives of Neurology* Vol. 61 (3) March 2004: 398–406.

WEBSITES

Kirshner, Howard. "Frontal and Temporal Lobe Dementia." Emedicine. (March 29, 2005 [April 19, 2005].) <http://www.emedicine.com/NEURO/topic140.htm>.

Rabheru, Kiran. "Depression in Dementia: Diagnosis and Treatment." Psychiatric Times (November 2004 [April 20, 2005].) Available online: <http://www.psychiatrictimes.com/p041139.html>.

ORGANIZATIONS

Alzheimer's Association. 919 North Michigan Avenue, Suite 1100, Chicago, IL. 60611-1676. (800) 272-3900. (April 20, 2005.) <http:www.alz.org>.

Alzheimer's Disease Education and Research (ADEAR), National Institute on Aging. P.O. Box 8250, Silver Spring, MD. 20907-8250 (800) 4388-4380). (April 20, 2005.) <http:www.alzheimers.org/>.

Association for Frontotemporal Dementias (AFTD). P.O. Box 7191, St. David's, PA 19087-7191. (April 20, 2005.) <http://www.ftd-picks.org>.

The Genetic Alliance. 4301 Connecticut Ave., NW, Suite 404, Washington, DC 20008-2369. (202) 966-5557). (April 20, 2005.) <http:www.geneticalliance.org>.

National Organization for Rare Disorders (NORD), Inc. P.O. Box 8923, New Fairfield, CT 06812-8923. (203) 746-6518. (April 20, 2005.) <http:www.rarediseases.org>.

Genevieve T. Slomski, PhD

Fryns syndrome

Definition

Fryns syndrome is a multiple congenital anomaly syndrome usually resulting in neonatal death.

Description

Fryns syndrome is a genetic condition involving abnormalities in many organ systems that usually results in neonatal death. The condition was first reported in 1979 by J. P. Fryns.

Typical anomalies include a characteristic facial appearance, including a broad nasal bridge (part of the nose between the eyes), small jaw, abnormal ears, cleft palate, abnormal fingers, underdevelopment of the lungs, and abnormalities of the urogenital system (kidneys and genitals). Diaphragmatic hernia (opening in the diaphragm muscle that can allow contents of the lower abdomen like the liver or intestine or stomach to move up into the chest cavity through the hole) can also be seen in some cases. Some researchers believe that there may be a distinct subset of patients without diaphragmatic hernia who are more mildly affected.

Genetic profile

Fryns syndrome is inherited in an autosomal recessive manner. This means that two defective **gene** copies must be inherited, one from each parent, for the disease to manifest itself. Persons with only one gene mutation are carriers for the disorder. A person who is a carrier for Fryns syndrome does not have any symptoms and does not know he/she is a carrier unless he/she has had a child with Fryns syndrome. Carrier testing is not available since the gene location is not known at this time. The likelihood that each member of a couple would be a carrier for a mutation in the same gene is higher in people who are related (called consanguineous). When both parents are carriers for Fryns syndrome, there is a one in four chance (25%) in each pregnancy for a child to have the disease. There is a two in three chance that a healthy sibling of an affected child is a carrier.

There have been several different **chromosome** abnormalities reported with a Fryns syndrome–like appearance. Investigation for a candidate gene causing Fryns syndrome has not yet identified the causative gene.

Demographics

The number of affected individuals is reported as seven in 100,000. There does not appear to be any ethnic difference in prevalence. There are more than 50 documented cases of Fryns syndrome in the literature.

Signs and symptoms

The most frequent anomalies have been described as diaphragmatic defects, underdeveloped lungs, **cleft lip and palate** (usually on both sides, called bilateral), heart defects, cysts in the kidneys, urinary tract abnormalities, and limb underdevelopment.

Most patients also have underdeveloped external genitals, abnormal internal reproductive structures, abnormalities in the digestive tract, and abnormalities in the structure of the brain. Fewer patients have eye abnormalities.

Other reported anomalies include fetal hydops (fluid surrounding the fetus prenatally, usually fatal), prematurity, **scoliosis** (curvature of the spine), extra vertebrae or ribs, abnormal bone formation, and small chest cavity.

Diagnosis

Prenatal diagnosis has been possible in several fetuses by use of ultrasound to identify in one fetus fetal hydrops, diaphragmatic hernia, and dilation of the cerebral ventricles and in another with cystic hygroma and diaphragmatic hernia. These anomalies themselves can be isolated or as a part of another genetic syndrome; it is the specific combination of anomalies that would lead one to suspect Fryns syndrome. Definitive diagnosis is not possible until after birth or autopsy.

Treatment and management

Since Fryns syndrome is a genetic disease, caused by mutations in specific genes, there is no cure at this time. Some of the anomalies may be amenable to surgery, such as diaphragmatic hernia or cleft palate, but the entire prognosis for the baby must be considered.

Special education for mentally retarded individuals is indicated if the child survives.

Prognosis

Unfortunately, the prognosis for babies with Fryns syndrome is poor, with usual neonatal death occurring due to the lung hyperplasia and respiratory distress or other anomalies. Approximately 14% of infants survive the neonatal period. Survivors typically do not have complex heart malformations and less frequently have diaphragmatic hernias, milder lung hypoplasia, and neurologic impairment (usually severe to profound mental retardation with serious brain malformations).

Resources

PERIODICALS

Ramsing, M., et al. "Variability in the Phenotypic Expression of Fryns Syndrome: A Report of Two Sibships." *American Journal of Medical Genetics* 95 (2000): 415.

ORGANIZATIONS

Genetic Alliance. 4301 Connecticut Ave. NW, #404, Washington, DC 20008-2304. (800) 336-GENE (Helpline) or (202) 966-5557. Fax: (888) 394-3937 info@geneticalliance. <http://www.geneticalliance.org>.

SHARE-Pregnancy and Infant Loss Support, Inc. St Joseph Health Center, 300 First Capital Dr., St. Charles, MO 63301. (800) 821-6819.

WEBSITES

Online Mendelian inheritance in Man (OMIM). <http://www.ncbi.nlm.nig.gov>.

Amy Vance, MS, CGC

FSH muscular dystrophy *see* **Facioscapulohumeral muscular dystrophy**

G

Galacktokinase deficiency

Definition

Galactokinase deficiency is a one of a set of three distinct autosomal recessive-inherited disorders that causes **galactosemia**, or build up of the dietary sugar galactose in the body as a result of inborn errors of metabolism. This relatively rare form of the galactosemia disorder can lead to toxic injury to the eyes unless all forms of galactose, found chiefly in dairy products, are eliminated from the diet early in life.

Description

Lactose, the principle carbohydrate of human milk, commercial infant formulas, and other dairy products, is broken down in the human intestine into its component sugars: glucose and galactose. After absorption by the intestine, galactose is sequentially metabolized by three separate enzymes (galactokinase, galactose-1-phosphate uridyl transferase, and galactose-4-epimerase) to convert it to glucose, a usable form of fuel for individual cells.

The term, galactosemia, denotes the abnormally elevated level of galactose in the blood and body tissues that results when any of these three enzymes are missing or defective. Thus, inherited defects in any one of these three enzymes will result in galactosemia.

Classic galactosemia, the most common form of galactosemia, is due to the deficiency of the second enzyme in the pathway, galactose-1-phosphate uridyl transferase (GALT), and is typically associated with cataract formation, mental retardation, and liver damage. Galactokinase deficiency (also known as GALK deficiency, or Galactosemia Type II) is a rarer form of galactosemia caused by the absence of the enzyme, galactokinase, which is responsible for the first step of the conversion of galactose to glucose. However, unlike the more serious form of classic galactosemia, galactokinase deficiency mainly manifests as injury to the eyes without damage to other organ systems. The third and final form of galactosemia, uridine-diphosphate galactose-4-epimerase deficiency, is the rarest of the group; few cases have been described, and the symptoms of this form of galactosemia are variable, but usually mild.

Galactosemia may have been described in German medical publications as early as 1908, and in 1917, F. Goeppert noted symptoms of galactosemia in an infant and sibling, suggesting that the disorder could be inherited. In 1935, the American scientists H. H. Mason and M. F. Turner described a patient with a group of symptoms that could be prevented by removal of milk from the diet. In 1954, the individual steps in the metabolic pathway for the conversion of galactose to glucose was described by L. F. Leloir, who was later awarded a Nobel Prize in Chemistry for his efforts. Leloir's work made it possible for scientists, such as V. Schwatz and K. J. Isselbacher to demonstrate that defects in this metabolic pathway were responsible for galactosemia and its associated symptoms.

Genetic profile

Galactokinase deficiency, like other causes of galactosemia, is transmitted as an autosomal recessive trait. Individuals that are heterozygous for the defective allele have half the normal enzyme levels, which is still sufficient to convert all of their dietary galactose to glucose. Thus, heterozygotes experience neither galactosemia nor its symptoms.

Using advanced scientific techniques, the location of a **gene** that encodes for the galactokinase enzyme (GALK1) was localized to the human **chromosome** 17 (17p24) by D. Stambolian in 1995. At least 13 different types of mutations in the GALK1 gene have been identified that result in a nonfunctional galactokinase enzyme. A second human galactokinase gene (GK2), located on human chromosome 15, was also identified in 1992 by R. T. Lee. However, it is unclear whether this second gene plays an active role in galactose metabolism.

Demographics

Galactokinase deficiency has an estimated incidence ranging from one in 500,000 to one in one million births and is much more rare than classic galactosemia. However, there is evidence that this trait may be unevenly distributed between various ethic and geographical groups. In 1967, R. Gitzelman characterized galactokinase deficiency in two related Romani (Gypsy) individuals. Later, in 1999, L. Kalaydijeva studied six Gypsy families from Bulgaria with galactokinase deficiency and found the same specific mutation in all cases. It was estimated that the carrier rate of the mutation in this population was as high as 5%, and Kalaydijeva suggested that this same mutation was likely responsible for the cases originally described by Gitzelman in 1967. As a result of the widespread prevalence of this mutation, incidence of galactokinase deficiency in Bulgaria has been reported to be one in 50,000 and among the Gypsy population, even higher, at one in 2,000.

The mutant galactokinase gene also shows higher prevalence in several other groups. In 1982, M. Magnani estimated the heterozygote frequency in Italy to be one in 310. In 1972, T. A. Tedesco presented evidence that African-Americans have an allele in high frequency that causes a decrease in red cell galactokinase activity that is likely different from the mutant allele that causes galactokinase deficiency. This finding was confirmed in 1988, when T. Soni found the same mutation in a group of African-Americans living in Philadelphia.

Signs and symptoms

Galactokinase deficiency is associated with galactosemia and cataracts (clouding of the lens of the eyes resulting in blurred vision), but without the systemic manifestations of liver disease and severe mental retardation that are commonly found in classic galactosemia. The cause of the cataract is an accumulation of galactitol (sugar alcohol derivative of galactose) within the lens of the eye. This galactitol accumulation attracts water, resulting in swelling and damage of the lens fiber.

There are infrequent reports of mild mental retardation in people with galactokinase deficiency, but the overwhelming majority of people have been shown to have normal intelligence. The rare finding of pseudotumor cerebri (a syndrome of raised pressure within the skull) has also been reported. Several investigators have reported premature development of cataracts (between the ages of 20 and 40 years old), even in individuals who are heterozygous for the galactokinase deficiency mutation.

Diagnosis

Newborn screening is the act of testing all infants for a specific disease shortly after birth for the purpose of preventing disease progression through prompt medical treatment. When newborn screening for the inherited disease **phenylketonuria** (PKU) began in 1962, it quickly became clear that many infants with PKU were being identified for early treatment and that the mental retardation caused by the disease was being prevented.

This success encouraged R. Guthrie and others to consider additional metabolic disorders that might benefit from newborn screening. Since restricting dietary galactose early in life would prevent the development of irreversible symptoms, galactosemia appeared to be an ideal candidate for newborn screening. In 1963, Guthrie and his colleague, K. Paigen, developed a method to detect galactosemia that could be applied to the newborn blood specimen, and screening for galactosemia in the newborn became practical.

When trying to establish a diagnosis of galactokinase deficiency, an initial test is performed to detect galactosuria, or high levels of galactose in the urine that is seen with galactosemia. If that test proves positive, the next step is to determine which of the three enzymes needed to convert galactose to glucose is defective. When looking for galactokinase deficiency, blood samples are taken, and galactokinase activity is measured from red blood cells. If galactokinase activity is low, then the person has galactokinase deficiency. Thus, the diagnosis is made by demonstrating the deficiency of galactokinase in red blood cells and can be further confirmed by showing normal levels of the other two enzymes involved in this pathway using other tests. The disease can also be diagnosed before birth by testing fluid surrounding the unborn fetus for high levels of galactose, but this is rarely done.

Before widespread institution of newborn screening, these diagnostic tests were performed in infants with symptoms consistent with any form of galactosemia. As of the year 2000, newborn screening was mandated by law in every U.S. state except Louisiana, Pennsylvania, and Washington state.

Treatment and management

The galactosemia syndromes are effectively treated by rigid dietary exclusion of all lactose and galactose, primarily involving the elimination of milk and its products. A galactose-free diet should be initiated as early as possible, particularly because cataract formation may be reversed in early stages. Non-lactose milk substitutes are often used. Although soybean preparations contain

KEY TERMS

Allele—One of two or more alternate forms of a gene.

Cataract—A clouding of the eye lens or its surrounding membrane that obstructs the passage of light resulting in blurry vision. Surgery may be performed to remove the cataract.

Enzyme—A protein that catalyzes a biochemical reaction or change without changing its own structure or function.

Galactitol—An alcohol derivative of galactose that builds up in the lens and causes cataracts.

Galactose—One of the two simple sugars, together with glucose, that makes up the protein, lactose, found in milk. Galactose can be toxic in high levels.

Galactosemia—Abnormally high levels of galactose in the blood due to an inherited defect in the conversion of galactose to glucose.

Galactosuria—High levels of galactose found in the urine that is seen with galactosemia.

Glucose—One of the two simple sugars, together with galactose, that makes up the protein, lactose, found in milk. Glucose is the form of sugar that is usable by the body to generate energy.

Heterozygous—Having two different versions of the same gene.

Lactose—A sugar made up of glucose and galactose. It is the primary sugar in milk.

Mutation—A permanent change in the genetic material that may alter a trait or characteristic of an individual, or manifest as disease, and can be transmitted to offspring.

Newborn screening—The act of testing all infants for a specific disease shortly after birth for the purpose of preventing disease progression through prompt medical treatment.

Phenylketornuria (PKU)—An inborn error of metabolism that causes buildup of the amino acid, phenylalanine, in the body. The first disease to be used for newborn screening.

Pseudotumor cerebri—A syndrome of raised pressure within the skull that may cause vomiting, headache, and double vision.

This galactose-free diet must be followed for life and requires close supervision, normally overseen by a team of health care professionals including a primary care provider, specialist physician, and a nutritionist. Periodic blood or urine measurements of galactose can be performed to monitor compliance with the restricted diet. Even with early diagnosis and strict dietary restrictions, people with galactosemia are at increased risk for cataract development in adulthood and should have regular eye examinations.

One detrimental effect of eliminating milk and milk products from the diet is the loss of adequate intake of vital nutrients such as protein, calcium, phosphorus, and riboflavin. As a result, nutritional deficiencies may develop, resulting in poor growth. Great care must be taken to achieve adequate daily supplementation with these nutrients after an infant is weaned from the enriched non-dairy formula. However, studies have demonstrated that children, adolescents, and adults often fail to routinely take prescribed supplements.

It also should be noted that exclusion of milk and milk products alone does not constitute a galactose-restricted diet, as galactose is found in other foods as well. Some fruits and vegetables with higher galactose content must also be avoided. Education of parents and children regarding galactose content of specific foods is important, and lists of foods can be obtained from nutritionists that prove useful in management.

Prognosis

Abundant experience with early treatment supports the concept that effective treatment instituted in the initial weeks of life can prevent all symptoms of the disease. In the rare event that some degree of mild retardation results, it is likely irreversible. Cataracts appear to be reversible if treatment is started within the initial three months of life.

Resources

BOOKS

Chen, Y. "Defects in Metabolism of Carbohydrates." In *Nelson Textbook of Pediatrics,* edited by R.E. Behrman. Philadelphia: W.B. Saunders, 2000, pp. 413-414.

Isselbacher, K. J. "Galactosemia, Galactokinase Deficiency, and Other Rare Disorders of Carbohydrate Metabolism." In *Harrison's Principles of Internal Medicine,* edited by A. S. Fauci. New York: McGraw-Hill, 1998, pp.2131-2132.

Naviaux, R. K. "Galactosemia." In *Cecil Textbook of Medicine,* edited by R. E. Behrman, Philadelphia: W.B. Saunders, 2000, pp, 413-414.

bound galactose, they appear to be well-tolerated because the bound galactose is not readily absorbed by the intestine.

Nyhan, W.E. "Galactosemia." In *Atlas of Metabolic Disease*. London: Chapman & Hall, 1998, pp. 322-329.

ORGANIZATIONS

National Newborn Screening and Genetics Resource Center. 1912 W. Anderson Lane, Suite 210, Austin, TX 78757. Fax: (512) 454-6419. <http://www.genes-r-us.uthscsa.edu>.

Parents of Galactosemic Children, Inc. 1100 West 49th St., Austin, TX 78756-3199. (512) 458-7111. <http://www.tdh.state.tx.us/newborn/galac_1.htm>.

OTHER

Roberts, R. and Meyer, B. *Living with Galactosemia: A Handbook for Families*. 1993. University School of Medicine Department of Pediatrics, 702 Barnhill Dr., Indianapolis, Indiana 46202-5225.

Oren Traub, MD, PhD

Galactose-1-phosphate uridyl transferase deficiency *see* **Galactosemia**

Galactosemia

Definition

Galactosemia is an inherited disease in which the transformation of galactose to glucose is blocked, allowing galactose to increase to toxic levels in the body. If galactosemia is untreated, high levels of galactose cause vomiting, diarrhea, lethargy, low blood sugar, brain damage, jaundice, liver enlargement, cataracts, susceptibility to infection, and death.

Description

Galactosemia is a rare but potentially life-threatening disease that results from the inability to metabolize galactose. Serious consequences from galactosemia can be prevented by screening newborns at birth with a simple blood test.

Galactosemia is an inborn error of metabolism. "Metabolism" refers to all chemical reactions that take place in living organisms. A metabolic pathway is a series of reactions where the product of each step in the series is the starting material for the next step. Enzymes are the chemicals that help the reactions occur. Their ability to function depends on their structure, and their structure is determined by the **deoxyribonucleic acid**

(**DNA**) sequence of the genes that encode them. Inborn errors of metabolism are caused by mutations in these genes which do not allow the enzymes to function properly.

Sugars are sometimes called "the energy molecules," and galactose and glucose are both sugars. For galactose to be utilized for energy, it must be transformed into something that can enter the metabolic pathway that converts glucose into energy (plus water and carbon dioxide). This is important for infants because they typically get most of their nutrient energy from milk, which contains a high level of galactose. Each molecule of lactose, the major sugar constituent of milk, is made up of a molecule of galactose and a molecule of glucose, and so galactose makes up 20% of the energy source of a typical infant's diet.

Three enzymes are required to convert galactose into glucose-1-phosphate (a phosphorylated glucose that can enter the metabolic pathway that turns glucose into energy). Each of these three enzymes is encoded by a separate **gene**. If any of these enzymes fail to function, galactose build-up and galactosemia result. Thus, there are three types of galactosemia with a different gene responsible for each.

Genetic profile

Every cell in a person's body has two copies of each gene. Each of the forms of galactosemia is inherited as a recessive trait, which means that galactosemia is only present in individuals with two mutated copies of one of the three genes. This also means that carriers (who only one copy of a gene mutation) will not be aware that they are carrying a mutation (unless they have had a genetic test), because it is masked by the normal gene on the second **chromosome** they also carry and the fact that they have no symptoms of the disease. For each step in the conversion of galactose to glucose, if only one of the two copies of the gene controlling that step is normal (i.e., for carriers), enough functional enzyme is made so that the pathway is not blocked at that step. If a person has galactosemia, both copies of the gene coding for one of the enzymes required to convert glucose to galactose are defective and the pathway becomes blocked. If two carriers of the same defective gene have children, the chance of any of their children getting galactosemia (the chance of a child getting two copies of the defective gene) is 25% (one in four) for each pregnancy.

Demographics

Classic galactosemia occurs in the United States about one in every 50,000–70,000 live births.

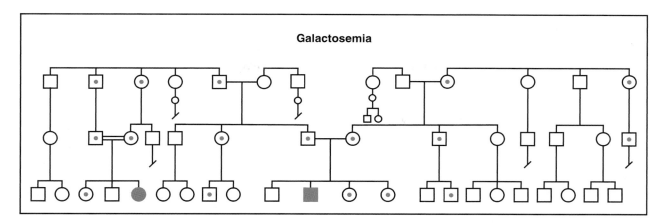

Galactosemia

(*Gale Group.*)

Signs and symptoms

Galactosemia I

Galactosemia I (also called classic galactosemia), the first form to be discovered, is caused by abnormalities in both copies of the gene that codes for an enzyme called galactose-1-phosphate uridyl transferase (GALT). There are 30 known different mutations in this gene that cause GALT to malfunction.

Newborns with galactosemia I appear normal at birth, but begin to develop symptoms after they are given milk for the first time. Symptoms include vomiting, diarrhea, lethargy (sluggishness or fatigue), low blood glucose, jaundice (a yellowing of the skin and eyes), enlarged liver, protein and amino acids in the urine, and susceptibility to infection, especially from gram negative bacteria. Cataracts (a grayish white film on the eye lens) can appear within a few days after birth. People with galactosemia frequently have symptoms as they grow older even though they have been given a galactose-free diet. These symptoms include speech disorders, cataracts, ovarian atrophy and infertility in females, learning disabilities, and behavioral problems.

Galactosemia II

Galactosemia II is caused by changes in both copies of the gene that codes for an enzyme called galactokinase (GALK). The frequency of occurrence of galactosemia II is about one in 100,000–155,000 births.

Galactosemia II is less harmful than galactosemia I. Babies born with galactosemia II will develop cataracts at an early age unless they are given a galactose-free diet. They do not generally have liver damage or neurologic disturbances.

Galactosemia III

Galactosemia III is caused by changes in the gene that codes for an enzyme called uridyl diphosphogalactose-4-epimerase (GALE). This form of galactosemia is very rare.

There are two forms of galactosemia III, a severe form, which is exceedingly rare, and a benign form. The benign form has no symptoms and requires no special diet. However, newborns with galactosemia III: including the benign form, have high levels of galactose-1-phosphate that show up on the initial screenings for elevated galactose and galactose-1-phosphate. This situation illustrates one aspect of the importance of follow-up enzyme function tests. Tests showing normal levels of GALT and GALK allow people affected by the benign form of galactosemia III to enjoy a normal diet.

The severe form has symptoms similar to those of galactosemia I, but with more severe neurological problems, including seizures. Only a few cases of this rare form have been reported.

Diagnosis

The newborn screening test for classic galactosemia is quick and straightforward; all but three states require testing on all newborns. Blood from a baby who is two to three days old is usually screened for high levels of galactose and galactose-1-phosphate. If either of these compounds is elevated, further tests are performed to find out which enzymes (GALT, GALK, or GALE) are present or missing. DNA testing may also be performed to confirm the diagnosis.

If there is a strong suspicion that a baby has galactosemia, galactose is removed from their diet right away. In this case, an initial screen for galactose or galactose-1-phosphate will be meaningless. In the absence of galactose in the diet, this test will be negative whether the baby has galactosemia or not. In this case, tests to measure enzyme levels must be given to find out if the suspected baby is indeed galactosemic.

In addition, galactosemic babies who are refusing milk or vomiting will not have elevated levels of galactose or galactose phosphate, and their condition will not be detected by the initial screen. Any baby with symptoms of galactosemia (for example, vomiting) should be given enzyme tests.

Treatment and management

Galactosemia I and II are treated by removing galactose from the diet. Since galactose is a break-down product of lactose, the primary sugar constituent of milk, this means all milk and foods containing milk products must be totally eliminated. Other foods like legumes, organ meats, and processed meats also contain considerable galactose and must be avoided. Pills that use lactose as a filler must also be avoided. Soy-based and casein hydrolysate-based formulas are recommended for infants with galactosemia.

Treatment of the severe form of galactosemia III with a galactose-restricted diet has been tried, but this disorder is so rare that the long-term effects of this treatment are unknown.

Prognosis

Early detection in the newborn period is the key to controlling symptoms. Long-term effects in untreated babies include severe mental retardation, cirrhosis of the liver, and death. About 75% of the untreated babies die within the first two weeks of life. On the other hand, with treatment, a significant proportion of people with galactosemia I can lead nearly normal lives, although speech defects, learning disabilities, and behavioral problems are common. In addition, cataracts due to galactosemia II can be completely prevented by a galactose-free diet.

Prevention

Since most people are unaware that they are carriers of a gene mutation causing galactosemia, the disease is usually detected on a newborn screening test. For couples with a previous child with galactosemia, prenatal diagnosis is available to determine whether a pregnancy is similarly affected. Families who have a child diagnosed with galactosemia can have DNA testing, which would enable other relatives to determine their carrier status. Prospective parents can then use that information

---

KEY TERMS

Casein hydrolysate—A preparation made from the milk protein casein, which is hydrolyzed to break it down into its constituent amino acids. Amino acids are the building blocks of proteins.

Catalyst—A substance that changes the rate of a chemical reaction, but is not physically changed by the process.

Enzyme—A protein that catalyzes a biochemical reaction or change without changing its own structure or function.

Galactose—One of the two simple sugars, together with glucose, that makes up the protein, lactose, found in milk. Galactose can be toxic in high levels.

Glucose—One of the two simple sugars, together with galactose, that makes up the protein, lactose, found in milk. Glucose is the form of sugar that is usable by the body to generate energy.

Lactose—A sugar made up of glucose and galactose. It is the primary sugar in milk.

Metabolic pathway—A sequence of chemical reactions that lead from some precursor to a product, where the product of each step in the series is the starting material for the next step.

Metabolism—The total combination of all of the chemical processes that occur within cells and tissues of a living body.

Recessive trait—An inherited trait or characteristic that is outwardly obvious only when two copies of the gene for that trait are present.

---

to conduct family planning or to prepare for a child with special circumstances. Children born with galactosemia should be put on a special diet right away to reduce the symptoms and complications of the disease.

Resources

BOOKS

Ng, Won G., Thomas F. Roe, and George N. Donnell. "Carbohydrate Metabolism." In *Emery and Rimoin's Principles and Practice of Medical Genetics,* edited by David L. Rimoin, J. Michael Connor, and Reed E. Pyeritz. 3rd. ed. New York: Churchill Livingstone, 1998.

ORGANIZATIONS

Association for Neuro-Metabolic Disorders. 5223 Brookfield Lane, Sylvania, OH 43560. (419) 885-1497.

Metabolic Information Network. PO Box 670847, Dallas, TX 75367-0847. (214) 696-2188 or (800) 945-2188.

Parents of Galactosemic Children, Inc. 2148 Bryton Dr., Powell OH 43065. <http://www.galactosemia.org/index.htm>.

OTHER

"GeneCards: Human Genes, Proteins and Diseases." <http://bioinfo.weizmann.ac.il/cards/>.

"Vermont Newborn Screening Program: Galactosemia." <http://www.vtmednet.org/~m145037/vhgi_mem/nbsman/galacto.htm>.

Amy Vance, MS, CGC

GALK deficiency *see* **Galactokinase deficiency**

Gangliosidosis-GM1 *see* **GM1 gangliosidosis**

Gardner syndrome *see* **Familial adenomatous polyposis**

Gastric cancer

Definition

Gastric **cancer** (also known as stomach cancer) is a disease in which the cells forming the inner lining of the stomach become abnormal and start to divide uncontrollably, forming a mass or a tumor.

Description

The stomach is a J-shaped organ that lies in the abdomen, on the left side. The esophagus (or the food pipe) carries the food from the mouth to the stomach. The stomach produces many digestive juices and acids that mix with the food and aid in the process of digestion. The stomach is divided into five sections. The first three are together referred to as the proximal stomach, and produce acids and digestive juices, such as pepsin. The fourth section of the stomach is where the food is mixed with the gastric juices. The fifth section of the stomach acts as a valve and controls the emptying of the stomach contents into the small intestine. The fourth and the fifth sections together are referred to as the distal stomach. Cancer can develop in any of the five sections of the stomach. The symptoms and the outcomes of the disease may vary depending on the location of the cancer.

In many cases, the cause of the gastric cancer is unknown. Several environmental factors have been linked to gastric cancer. Consuming large amounts of smoked, salted, or pickled foods has been linked to increased gastric cancer risk. Nitrates and nitrites, chemicals found in some foods such as cured meats may be linked to gastric cancer as well.

Infection by the *Helicobacter pylori* (*H. pylori*) bacterium has been found more often in people with gastric cancer. *H. pylori* can cause irritation of the stomach lining (chronic atrophic gastritis), which may lead to precancerous changes of the stomach cells.

People who have had previous stomach surgery for ulcers or other conditions may have a higher likelihood of developing gastric cancers, although this is not certain. Another risk factor is developing polyps, benign growths in the lining of the stomach. Although polyps are not cancerous, some may have the potential to turn cancerous.

While no particular **gene** for gastric cancer has yet been identified, people with blood relatives who have been diagnosed with gastric cancer are more likely to develop the disease. In addition, people who have inherited disorders such as familial adenomatous polyps (FAP) and Lynch syndrome have an increased risk for gastric cancer. For unknown reasons, gastric cancers occur more frequently in people with the blood group A.

Genetic profile

Although environmental or health factors may explain frequent occurrences of gastric cancer in families, it is known that inherited risk factors also exist. Some studies show close relatives having an increased risk of gastric cancer two to three times that of the general population. Interestingly, an earlier age at the time of gastric cancer diagnosis may be more strongly linked to familial gastric cancer. Two Italian studies estimated that about 8% of gastric cancer is due to inherited factors. Some of these hereditary factors are known genetic conditions while in other instances, the factors are unknown.

Familial cancer syndromes are hereditary conditions in which specific types of cancer, and perhaps other features, are consistently occurring in affected individuals. Familial adenomatosis (FAP) and hereditary nonpolyposis colon cancer (HNPCC) are familial cancer syndromes that increase the risk of colon cancer.

FAP is due to changes in the *APC* gene. Individuals with FAP typically have more than 100 polyps, mushroom-like growths, in the digestive system as well as other effects. Polyps are noncancerous growths that have the potential to become cancerous if not removed. At least one study estimated that the risk of gastric cancer was seven times greater for individuals with FAP than the general population.

The number of polyps present is an important distinction between FAP and HNPCC. Polyps do not form at such a high rate in HNPCC but individuals with this condition are still at increased risk of colon, gastric, and other cancers. At least five genes are known to cause HNPCC, but alterations in the *hMSH2* or *hMLH1* genes have been found in the majority of HNPCC families.

Other inherited conditions such as **Peutz-Jeghers,** Cowden and **Li-Fraumeni syndromes** and other syndromes have been associated with gastric cancer. All of these syndromes have distinct features beyond gastric cancer that aid in identifying the specific syndrome. The **inheritance** pattern for most of these syndromes is dominant, meaning only one copy of the gene needs to be inherited for the syndrome to be present.

In 1999, the First Workshop of the International Gastric Cancer Linkage Consortium developed criteria for defining hereditary gastric cancer not due to known genetic conditions, such as those listed above. In areas with low rates of gastric cancer, hereditary gastric cancer was defined according to the Consortium as: (1) families with two or more cases of gastric cancer in first or second degree relatives (siblings, parents, children, grandparents, nieces/nephews or aunts/uncles) with at least one case diagnosed before age 50 or (2) three or more cases at any age. In countries with higher rates of gastric cancer, such as Japan, the suggested criteria are: (1) at least three affected first degree relatives (sibling, children or parents) and one should be the first degree relative of the other two; (2) at least two generations (without a break) should be affected; and (3) at least one cancer should have occurred before age 50.

Inherited changes in the *E-Cadherin/CDH1* gene first were reported in three families of native New Zealander (Maori) descent with gastric cancer and later were found in families of other ancestry. The E-Cadherin/CDH1 gene, which plays a role in cell to cell connection, is located on the **chromosome** 16 at 16q22. The percentage of hereditary gastric cancer that is due to E-Cadherin/CDH1 gene alterations is uncertain. In summary, most gastric cancer is due to environmental or other non-genetic causes. A small portion of cancer of the stomach, about 8%, is due to inherited factors one of which is E-Cadherin/CDH1 gene alterations.

Demographics

The American Cancer Society estimated, based on previous data from the National Cancer Institute and the United States Census, that 21,700 Americans were diagnosed with gastric cancer during 2001. In some areas, nearly twice as many men are affected by gastric cancer than women. Most cases of gastric cancer are diagnosed between the ages of 50 and 70 but in families with a hereditary risk of gastric cancer, younger cases are more frequently seen. Gastric cancer is one of the leading causes of cancer deaths in many areas of the world, most notably Japan, but the number of new gastric cancer cases is decreasing in some areas, especially in developed countries. In the United States, the use of refrigerated foods and increased consumption of fresh fruits and vegetables, instead of preserved foods, may be a reason for the decline in gastric cancer.

Signs and symptoms

Gastric cancer can be difficult to detect at early stages since symptoms are uncommon and frequently unspecific. The following can be symptoms of gastric cancer:

- poor appetite or weight loss
- fullness even after a small meal
- abdominal pain
- heart burn, belching, indigestion or nausea
- vomiting, with or without blood
- swelling or problems with the abdomen
- anemia or blood on stool (feces) examination

Diagnosis

In addition to a physical examination and fecal occult blood testing (checking for blood in the stool), special procedures are done to evaluate the digestive system including the esophagus, stomach, and upper intestine. Procedures used to diagnose gastric cancer include: barium upper gastrointestinal (GI) x rays, upper endoscopy, and endoscopic ultrasound. **Genetic testing** can also be used to determine an individuals predisposition to gastric cancer.

Upper GI x rays

The first step in evaluation for gastric cancer may be x ray studies of the esophagus, stomach, and upper intestine. This type of study requires drinking a solution with barium to coat the stomach and other structures for easier viewing. Air is sometimes pumped into the stomach to help identify early tumors.

Upper endoscopy

Endoscopy allows a diagnosis in about 95% of cases. In upper endoscopy, a small tube, an endoscope, is

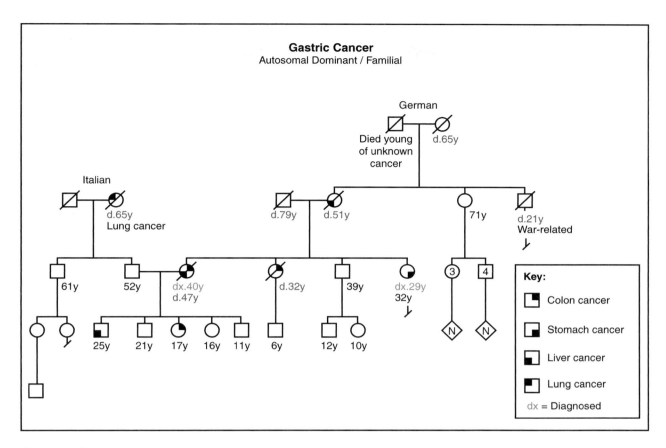

Gastric Cancer
Autosomal Dominant / Familial

German

Died young of unknown cancer

d.65y

Italian

d.65y
Lung cancer

d.79y

d.51y

71y

d.21y
War-related

61y

52y

dx.40y
d.47y

d.32y

39y

dx.29y
32y

3

4

25y

21y

17y

16y

11y

6y

12y

10y

N

N

Key:

Colon cancer

Stomach cancer

Liver cancer

Lung cancer

dx = Diagnosed

(*Gale Group*)

placed down the throat so that the esophagus, stomach and upper small intestine can be viewed. If a suspicious area is seen, a small sample of tissue, a biopsy, is taken. The tissue from these samples can be examined for evidence of cancer.

Endoscopic ultrasound

Endoscopic ultrasound allows several layers to be seen and so it is useful in determining where cancer may have spread. With this test, an endoscope is placed into the stomach and sound waves are emitted. A machine analyzes the sound waves to see differences in the tissues in order to identify tumors.

Genetic testing

If a certain genetic syndrome such as FAP or HNPCC is suspected, genetic testing may be available either through a clinical laboratory or through a research study. Testing for E-cadherin/CDH1 gene alterations is mainly available through research studies. Once an E-cadherin/CDH1 gene change is identified through research, the results can be confirmed through a certified laboratory.

When a gene change is identified, genetic testing may be available for other family members. For most genetic tests, it is helpful to test the affected individual first, since they are most likely to have a gene change. Genetic testing is usually recommended for consenting adults, however, for syndromes in which gastric cancer is a common feature, testing of children may be reasonable for possible prevention of health problems.

The detection rate and usefulness of genetic testing depends on the genetic syndrome. If genetic testing is under consideration, a detailed discussion with a knowledgeable physician, genetic counselor, or other practitioner is helpful in understanding the advantages and disadvantages of the genetic test. It is also important to realize that testing positive for the E-cadherin/CDH1 gene does not necessarily mean the individual will be affected with cancer. However, they may have an increased risk compared to an individual without the gene.

Treatment and management

Regular mass screening for gastric cancer has not been found useful in areas, such as the United States,

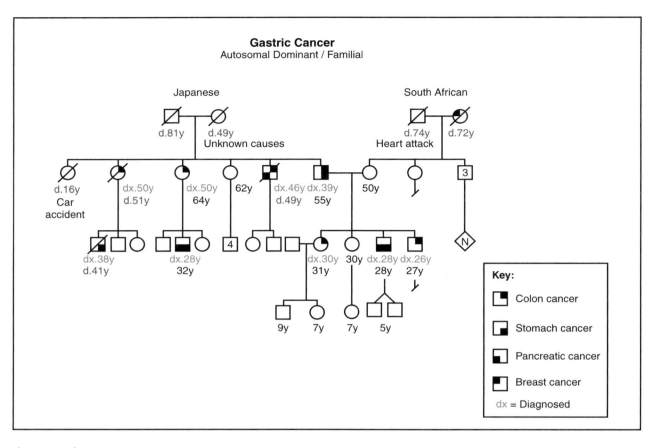

Gastric Cancer
Autosomal Dominant / Familial

Japanese

South African

Key:
- Colon cancer
- Stomach cancer
- Pancreatic cancer
- Breast cancer
- dx = Diagnosed

(*Gale Group*)

where gastric cancer is less common. When gastric cancer is diagnosed in the United States, it is usually discovered at later, less curable stages. However, individuals with an increased risk of gastric cancer, including those with a known genetic syndrome or with a family history of the disease, may consider regular screening before the development of cancer. If a known hereditary cancer syndrome is suspected, screening should follow the generally accepted guidelines for these conditions.

In 1999, the First Workshop of the International Gastric Cancer Linkage Consortium recommended that regular detailed upper endocopy and biopsy be done in families with hereditary gastric cancer, including screening every six to 12 months for individuals with known E-cadherin gene alterations, if no other treatment has been done. Some individuals with a known hereditary gastric cancer risk have surgery to remove the stomach prior to development of any gastric cancer, but the effectiveness of this prevention strategy is uncertain. Several other less drastic prevention measures have been considered including changes in diet, use of vitamins, and antibiotic treatment of *H. pylori*.

The American Cancer Society recommends limiting use of alcohol and tobacco.

Treatment of gastric cancer, in nearly all cases, involves some surgery. The amount of the stomach or surrounding organs that is removed depends on the size and location of the cancer. Sometimes, surgery is performed to try to remove all of the cancer in hopes of a cure while other times, surgery is done to relieve symptoms. Possible side effects of stomach surgery include leaking, bleeding, changes in diet, vitamin deficiencies, and other complications.

Chemotherapy involves administering anti-cancer drugs either intravenously (through a vein in the arm) or orally (in the form of pills). This can either be used as the primary mode of treatment or after surgery to destroy any cancerous cells that may have migrated to distant sites. Side effects (usually temporary) of chemotherapy may include low blood counts, hair loss, vomiting, and other symptoms.

Radiation therapy is often used after surgery to destroy the cancer cells that may not have been completely removed during surgery. Generally, to treat

Adenocarcinoma—A type of cancer which is in a gland-like form.

Barium—A chemical put into a solution and swallowed to help with outlining the gastrointestinal system during an x ray study.

Biopsy—The surgical removal and microscopic examination of living tissue for diagnostic purposes.

Cancer—A disease caused by uncontrolled growth of the body's cells.

Chemotherapy—Treatment of cancer with synthetic drugs that destroy the tumor either by inhibiting the growth of the cancerous cells or by killing the cancer cells.

Chronic atrophic gastritis—Irritation and break down of the stomach wall over a period of time.

Dominant inheritance—A type of genetic inheritance pattern results in one form of a gene being dominant over other forms. Therefore, the dominant allele can express itself and cause disease, even if only one copy is present.

Duodenum—Portion of the small intestine nearest the stomach; the first of three parts of the small intestine.

E-Cadherin/CDH1—A gene involved in cell-to-cell connection. Alterations in this gene have been found in several families with increased rates of gastric cancer.

Endoscopy—A slender, tubular optical instrument used as a viewing system for examining an inner part of the body and, with an attached instrument, for biopsy or surgery.

Esophagus—The part of the digestive tract which connects the mouth and stomach; the foodpipe.

Familial adenomatous polyposis (FAP)—Inherited syndrome causing large numbers of polyps and increased risk of colon cancer and other cancers.

Familial gastric cancer—Gastric cancer that occurs at a higher rate in some families.

Fecal occult blood test—Study of stool (feces) to identify loss of blood in the gastrointestinal system.

Gastric—Associated with the stomach.

Gastrointestinal (GI) system—Body system involved in digestion, the breaking down and use of food.

Gene—A building block of inheritance, which contains the instructions for the production of a particular protein, and is made up of a molecular sequence found on a section of DNA. Each gene is found on a precise location on a chromosome.

Genetic counselor—A health professional with advanced training in genetics and psychology who educates people about genetic conditions and testing.

Helicobacter pylori (*H. pylori*)—Bacterium that infects humans and may be associated with an increased risk of gastric cancer.

Hereditary non-polyposis colon cancer (HNPCC)—A genetic syndrome causing increased cancer risks, most notably colon cancer. Also called Lynch syndrome.

Li-Fraumeni syndrome—Inherited syndrome known to cause increased risk of different cancers, most notably sarcomas.

Lymph node—A bean-sized mass of tissue that is part of the immune system and is found in different areas of the body.

Maori—A native New Zealand ethnic group.

Nitrates/nitrites—Chemical compounds found in certain foods and water that, when consumed, may increase the risk of gastric cancer.

Pernicious anemia—A blood condition with decreased numbers of red blood cells related to poor vitamin B12 absorption.

Peutz-Jeghers syndrome (PJS)—Inherited syndrome causing polyps of the digestive tract and spots on the mouth as well as increased risk of cancer.

Polyp—A mass of tissue bulging out from the normal surface of a mucous membrane.

Radiation—High energy rays used in cancer treatment to kill or shrink cancer cells.

Staging—A method of describing the degree and location of cancer.

Stomach—An organ that holds and begins digestion of food.

Ultrasound—An imaging technique that uses sound waves to help visualize internal structures in the body.

X ray—An image of the body made by the passing of radiation through the body.

gastric cancer, external beam radiation therapy is used. In this procedure, high-energy rays from a machine that is outside of the body are concentrated on the area of the tumor. In the advanced stages of gastric cancer, radiation therapy is used to ease the symptoms such as pain and bleeding.

Prognosis

"Staging" is a method of describing cancer development. There are five stages in gastric cancer with stage 0 being the earliest cancer that has not spread while stage IV includes cancer that has spread to other organs. Expected survival rate can be roughly estimated based on the stage of cancer at the time of diagnosis.

The prognosis for patients with early stage cancer depends on the location of the cancer. When cancer is in the proximal part of the stomach, only 10-15% of people survive five years or more, even if they have been diagnosed with early stage cancer. For cancer that is in the distal part of the stomach, if it is detected at an early stage, the outlook is somewhat better. About 50% of the people survive for at least five years or more after initial diagnosis. However, only 20% of the patients are diagnosed at an early stage. Chance of survival depends on many factors and it is difficult to predict survival for a particular individual.

Resources

BOOKS

Flanders, Tamar, et al. "Cancers of the Digestive System." In *Inherited Susceptibility: Clinical, Predictive and Ethical Perspectives,* edited by William D. Foulkes and Shirley V. Hodgson. Cambridge University Press, 1998. pp.158-165.

Lawrence, Walter, Jr. "Gastric Cancer." In *Clinical Oncology Textbook,* edited by Raymond E. Lenhard, Jr., et al. American Cancer Society, 2000, pp.345-360.

ORGANIZATIONS

American Cancer Society. 1599 Clifton Road NE, Atlanta, Georgia 30329. (800) 227-2345. <http://www.cancer.org>.

National Cancer Institute. Office of Communications, 31 Center Dr. MSC 2580, Bldg. 1 Room 10A16, Bethesda MD 20892-2580. (800) 422-6237. <http://www.nci.nih.gov>.

WEBSITES

CancerBACUP. <http://www.cancerbacup.org.uk>.

Oncolink. University of Pennsylvania Cancer Center. <http://cancer.med.upenn.edu>.

STOMACH-ONC. <http://www.listserv.acor.org/archives/stomach-org.html>.

Kristin Baker Niendorf, MS, CGC

Gastroschisis

Definition

Gastroschisis, which literally means "split abdomen," is a hernia (open fissure) in the muscle and skin of the abdominal wall that allows the contents of the abdominal cavity to be exposed to the outside of the body. The opening is usually 2–5 in (5–12.7 cm) long and located in the median plane of the abdomen to the right of the umbilical cord.

Gastroschisis appears during the fetal period and causes the fetal intestines to be exposed to the amniotic fluid with no covering sac. Because amniotic fluid contains the urine of the fetus, this exposure may irritate the fetal intestines, causing swelling and shortening during development. As fetal development progresses, the opening becomes smaller relative to the size of the intestines. Consequently, the bowel may either become strangulated or malrotated. After the infant is born, the intestines are placed back inside the abdominal cavity and the opening is closed surgically. However the intestines may still pose long-term functional problems because of the previous irritation and formation of adhesions.

Description

Gastroschisis is caused by a defect in the normal fetal developmental pattern. In fetal development, the midgut (intestines) loops out of the abdominal cavity in a normal process known as physiological umbilical herniation. This process begins in the sixth week of fetal development because there is not enough room in the abdominal cavity for the growing liver, kidneys, and intestines. By the tenth week of fetal development, the liver and kidneys have decreased in size and the abdominal cavity has grown. In a normal fetus the intestines return to the abdominal cavity at this time, and the abdominal wall forms around them. In a fetus with gastroschisis, the return of the intestine to the abdominal cavity fails to occur. The pancreas, stomach, liver, spleen, bladder, uterus, ovaries, or fallopian tubes are rarely also herniated. The cause of the failure of the intestines to return to the abdominal cavity is unknown. The attachment of the umbilical cord is normal.

Genetic profile

The cause of gastroschisis is unknown; no definite genetic association has been determined. **Chromosomal abnormalities** are rarely associated with gastroschisis, and familial occurrence is exceptionally rare. Most genetic centers do not recommend the testing of infants with isolated gastroschisis. The familial cases that have been reported include occurrence in twins. Gastroschisis is not usually seen in association with other types of birth defects. Deformations of the fetal urinary tract can develop because of gastroschisis. These do not represent separate malformations, and **genetic testing** is not indicated.

A genetically associated issue that may arise is the misdiagnosis of gastroschisis for the distinct condition known as **omphalocele**. This misdiagnosis occurs in 5% of patients with omphalocele and has serious implications because omphalocele is often associated with chromosomal abnormalities and additional non-gastrointestinal malformations.

Demographics

Gastroschisis is not a common birth defect. It occurs in approximately two infants per 10,000 live births in the United States and internationally. Most cases of gastroschisis are sporadic with no familial association. Abnormalities of the intestines as a direct consequence of gastroschisis are seen in 5% of patients. Gastroschisis occurs slightly more often in males than in females. Young maternal age, maternal drug usage, and origination from a socially or economically disadvantaged background all increase the risk of gastroschisis. Very low maternal weight is associated with three times increased risk for gastroschisis. High maternal intake of nitrosamines found in preserved meat and beer doubles the risk of gastroschisis. High maternal weight reduces risk. A low maternal intake of chemicals called carotenoids found in many fruit and vegetables or glutathione from animal protein causes three to four times increased risk for gastroschisis. Carotenoids and glutathione are antioxidants that have a protective effect on the fetus and decrease oxygen stress or oxygen deprivation. Any factor that reduces blood flow to the fetus, thereby causing oxygen stress, can be a factor in the development of gastroschisis. Maternal intake of aspirin or ibuprofen (found in Advil) causes four to five times increased risk for gastroschisis. Both medications are inhibitors of the cyclooxygenase enzyme and influence blood flow to the fetus. Acetaminophen (found in Tylenol) has no demonstrated association with gastroschisis. Decongestants, especially pseudoephedrine and phenylpropanolamine, more than double the risk because they cause constriction of blood vessels and decrease blood flow to the fetus. Illness and fever have no association with the development of gastroschisis.

Signs and symptoms

A mother carrying a fetus with gastroschisis will not experience any unusual signs or symptoms in early preg-

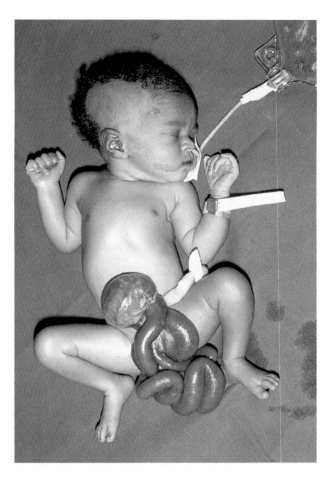

Gastroschisis is an opening in the muscle and skin of the abdominal wall that exposes the contents of the abdominal cavity. It appears during the fetal period and causes the fetal intestines to be exposed to the amniotic fluid. After the infant is born, the intestines are placed back inside the abdominal cavity and the opening is closed surgically. (© Ansary / Custom Medical Stock Photo.)

nancy. Gastroschisis may be suspected when maternal serum screening, which is typically performed at 15-20 weeks of gestation, reveals an elevated alpha-fetoprotein level (AFP). Gastroschisis is an open defect in the fetal abdominal wall which allows the leakage of AFP from the fetal tissues into the amniotic fluid. The increased amount of amniotic fluid AFP is absorbed into the maternal circulation and can be easily measured in a maternal serum screening test. An elevated AFP level detected in maternal serum is not indicative of gastroschisis specifically, but this does alert the obstetrician that a detailed ultrasound of the fetus is indicated. An elevated maternal serum AFP level is present in approximately 75 to 80% of cases of gastroschisis. Gastroschisis may also be incidentally detected in the second trimester during routine ultrasonography.

Diagnosis

Ultrasonogram is the primary method of diagnosis for gastroschisis because it is noninvasive, rapid, and allows for real-time fetal monitoring. Gastroschisis is often diagnosed before 20 weeks of gestation by an ultrasonogram that may show some or all of the following: loops of fetal intestines floating exposed to amniotic fluid with or without other organs, signs of intestinal obstruction, or a defect in the middle of the abdominal wall to the right of a normal umbilical cord.

With a transvaginal sonogram, the diagnosis has been made as early as 12 weeks of gestation. The diagnosis may be made difficult by flexed fetal limbs. The detection rate in the United States is approximately 75% with the use of ultrasonogram. Frequent ultrasonograms may be necessary to monitor potential injury to the fetal intestines as the pregnancy progresses. A blood clot around the umbilicus as a result of a traumatic **amniocentesis** or premature detachment of the placenta may mimic gastroschisis on an ultrasonogram.

Once the infant is born and has received corrective surgery, radiographs and bowel contrast studies may be necessary to diagnose intestinal complications. While these procedures are noninvasive, they expose the infant to a degree of radiation. A computed axial tomography (CAT) scan is not considered a medically suitable method by which to diagnose gastroschisis. Magnetic resonance imaging (MRI) is not usually used for diagnosis due to high expense and limited availability.

Treatment and management

In cases of gastroschisis, the infant is usually delivered in a hospital with a neonatal intensive care unit. If the infant's other organs are mature enough, the child is often delivered at 36, often using a Caesarian section. At birth, infants with gastroschisis die without immediate corrective surgery and intensive hospital care. The infant is given intravenous fluids, and the intact intestinal contents are temporarily placed in a surgical plastic clinging film attached to the infant's stomach. The plastic film helps to prevent infection, heat loss, and dehydration.

If the fissure and intestinal spillage is small to medium, the intestines are re-inserted into the abdominal cavity and the fissure is surgically closed within 12–24 hours after birth. If the fissure is large or complicated then the procedure may occur in stages over several days. A silastic bag (silicone plastic called a silo) is used to gradually return the intestines to the abdominal cavity at each stage. Finally the silo is removed and the skin is surgically closed.

Approximately 48% of infants with gastroschisis are small for gestational age. During the recovery period the infants receive nutrition and fluids intravenously. Once the intestines are able to receive food, infants may begin breast- or bottle-feeding. Normal feedings usually begin by the fourth week from delivery date. However, some infants with gastroschisis have associated complications that require months of intravenous feeding. Infants are discharged from the hospital once they are attaining sufficient weight gain and are followed closely over several months.

Prognosis

The overall prognosis for an infant with gastroschisis without extensive complications is very good. Most deaths occur as a result of premature delivery, infection, and bowel necrosis. The clinical outcome is not correlated with the size of the hernia as estimated using ultrasonography or with the known time of exposure to amniotic fluid. Although the survival rate is high, the postoperative hospitalization is often lengthy with complications. If the intestines sustained damage from exposure to amniotic fluid or from twisting, then the prognosis is of poorer quality. Complications that negatively influence prognosis include intestinal damage, prematurity, fetal growth restriction, and shortening of the gut secondary to irritation. Gastroschisis diagnosed prenatally may resolve in utero, causing the death of portions of the intestines. This may result in a condition known as chronic short gut syndrome with a poor prognosis, including problems with diarrhea, slow weight gain, vitamin or mineral deficiencies, and increased mortality. Spontaneous resolution of gastroschisis and closure of the abdominal hernia have been reported. Gastroschisis may also cause deformations of the fetal urinary tract, resulting in a poor prognosis.

Resources

BOOKS

Moore, Keith L., and T. V. N. Persaud. *The Developing Human, Clinically Oriented Embryology, Seventh Edition.* New York: Elsevier Science, 2003.

ORGANIZATIONS

Office of Rare Diseases National Institutes of Health 6100 Executive Boulevard, 3B-01 Bethesda, Maryland 20892-7518. (301) 402-4336. Patient Support Groups. <http://ord.aspensys.com/asp/resources/pat_supgrp.asp>.

WEB SITES

California Birth Defects Monitoring Program. California State Health Department and March of Dimes (March 22, 2005). <http://www.cbdmp.org/index.htm>.

Children's Hospital of Philadelphia Center for Fetal Diagnosis and Treatment. (March 22, 2005.) <http://fetalsurgery.chop.edu/gastroschisis.shtml>.

Gastroschisis. Children's Hospital of Boston (March 22, 2005). <http://www.childrenshospital.org/cfapps/A2ZtopicDisplay.cfm?Topic=Gastroschisis>.

Gastroschisis. E Medicine (March 22, 2005). <http://www.emedicine.com>.

Gastroschisis. Medline Plus (March 22, 2005). <http://www.nlm.nih.gov/medlineplus/ency/article/000992.htm>.

National Center for Birth Defects and Developmental Disabilities Conference. Centers of Disease Control and Prevention 2004 (March 22, 2005). <http://www.cdc.gov/ncbddd/conference/NCBDDD%20Program%20Book.pdf>.

Omphalocele and Gastroschisis E Medicine (March 22, 2005). <http://www.emedicine.com>.

Surgeon General's Report 2004—Health Consequences of Smoking. (March 22, 2005.) <http://www.cdc.gov/tobacco/sgr/sgr_2004/pdf/chapter5.pdf>.

University of California San Francisco Fetal Treatment Services. (March 22, 2005.) <http://www.ucsfhealth.org/childrens/medical_services/fetal_treatment/index.html>.

Maria Basile, PhD

Gaucher disease

Definition

Gaucher disease is a rare genetic disorder that results in accumulation of fatty molecules called cerebrosides. It can have serious effects on numerous body organs including the liver, spleen, bones and central nervous system. Treatments based on molecular biology are becoming available, but are very expensive.

Description

Gaucher disease was first described by the French physician Philippe Gaucher in 1882. It is the most common of a class of diseases called lysosomal storage diseases, each of which is characterized by the accumulation of a specific chemical substance (a different substance depending on the exact disease). Gaucher disease is characterized by a wide array of different symptoms and the severity of the disease ranges from undetectable to lethal.

Three forms of the disease are recognized: Types I, II, and III. Type I is by far the most common and shows the mildest symptoms. It is non-neuronopathic, meaning that the nervous system is not attacked. The onset of Type I can occur at any age in childhood or adult life, with the average age of onset at about 21 years. Some affected individuals have no symptoms throughout adult life. Type II, the infantile form, accounts for less than 1% of patients with Gaucher disease. It is neuronopathic (attacks the nervous system); nervous system effects are severe, and victims often die within the first year of life. Type III most often has its onset during childhood and has some of the features of both the adult and infantile forms. This affects less than 5% of persons with Gaucher disease.

Gaucher disease is caused by the absence, or near absence, of activity of an enzyme called glucocerebrosidase (GC). The normal action of GC is to break down a common molecule called glucocerebroside. If not broken down, glucocerebroside accumulates in certain cells to levels that can cause damage, especially in the spleen, liver, and bone. The common link among these organs is that they house a cell type called a macrophage. A macrophage is a large cell that surrounds and consumes a foreign substance (such as bacteria) in the body. The cellular structures in which glucocerebroside accumulates are called lysosomes.

Genetic profile

Lack of the GC enzyme is caused by a mutation in the glucocerebrosidase **gene**. The gene is located on **chromosome** 1. There have been over 100 mutations described in this gene that causes Gaucher disease. Gaucher disease is inherited in an autosomal recessive pattern. This means that two defective gene copies must be inherited, one from each parent, for the disease to manifest itself. Persons with only one gene mutation are carriers for the disorder. A person who is a carrier for Gaucher disease does not have any symptoms and does not know he or she is a carrier unless he or she has had specific testing. When both parents are carriers for Gaucher disease, there is a one in four chance (25%) in each pregnancy for a child to have Gaucher disease. There is a two in three chance that a healthy sibling of an affected child is a carrier.

Demographics

The three forms of Gaucher disease also differ in their population genetics. Type I is most common in persons of eastern European (Ashkenazi) Jewish descent. Among this population, the disease occurs at a rate of one in 450 live births and about one in 10 to 15 persons are carriers, making it the most common genetic disease affecting Jewish people. The other two types are equally frequent in all ethnic groups. Type II occurs at a rate of one in 100,000 live births, while Type III is estimated to occur in one in 50,000 live births.

Signs and symptoms

The results of Gaucher disease are widespread in the body and include excessive growth of the liver and spleen (hepatosplenomegaly), weakening of bones, and, in acute cases, severe nervous system damage. Many patients experience "bone crises," which are episodes of extreme pain in their bones.

There is a wide array of other problems that occur with Gaucher disease, such as anemia (fewer than normal red blood cells). Just how these other symptoms are caused is not known, nor is it known why some patients have very mild disease and others have much more significant problems. Even identical twins with the disease can have differing symptoms.

Diagnosis

Diagnosis of Gaucher disease, based initially on the symptoms described above, can be confirmed by microscopic, enzymatic, and molecular tests. Biopsy (surgical removal of tissue from a problem area) of tissue is helpful for microscopic diagnosis. When biopsy tissue is examined under the microscope, cells will appear swollen and will show characteristic features of the cytoplasm (part of the cell body along with the nucleus) and nucleus. Enzyme tests will show deficiency (<30% of normal levels) of the enzyme GC. Molecular analysis of **DNA** samples looking at four of the more common mutations will show defects in the gene for GC in 95% of Ashkenazi Jewish individuals and in 75% of non-Jewish people. Diagnosis can be performed prenatally (before birth) if the parents' mutations are known using **amniocentesis** or chorionic villus sampling.

Diagnosis as to which of the three types of Gaucher disease an individual has is based on the symptoms, rather than on test results.

Treatment and management

Until the 1990s, only supportive therapy could be offered. Analgesics are used to control pain. Orthopedic treatment is used for bone fractures. In some cases, surgical removal of the spleen may be necessary. Several treatments for anemia have been used, including vitamin and iron supplements, blood transfusions, and bone marrow transplants.

The newest form of treatment for Gaucher disease is enzyme replacement therapy, in which GC can be administered intravenously. The enzyme can be prepared either by purification from placentas (alglucerase) or by recombinant DNA manufacturing techniques (imiglucerase). Either way, the cost of treatment ranges from $100,000 to $400,000 per year, which can prevent many from obtaining treatment.

Enzyme replacement is effective at reducing most Gaucher symptoms. The notable exception is neurologic damage in Type II disease, which remains unimproved by this treatment. This treatment is not recommended for individuals who are asymptomatic. The efficacy for the treatment of Type III Gaucher disease is not known. Many questions remain about enzyme replacement therapy in regard to dosage, and method and frequency of administration. The treatment program should be individualized for each patient.

Prognosis

A patient's expected life span varies greatly with the type of Gaucher disease. Infants with Type II disease have a life span of one to four years. Patients with Types I and III of the disease have highly variable outcomes, with some patients dying in childhood and others living full lives. Little is known about the reasons for this variability.

Prevention

Genetic counseling is advised for individuals with Gaucher disease and for their relatives to accurately assess risk and discuss testing options. For couples who previously had a child with Gaucher or in situations where both parents are carriers for known Gaucher mutations, prenatal diagnosis is available to determine whether a pregnancy is affected. Families in which a person has been diagnosed with Gaucher disease can have DNA testing, which enables other relatives to determine their carrier status. Prospective parents can then use that information to conduct family planning or to prepare for a child who may have special circumstances.

Families in which both parents are known to be a carrier of a mutation for Gaucher disease could consider preimplantation genetic diagnosis. This relatively new procedure can select an embryo without both Gaucher

KEY TERMS

Cerebrosides—Fatty carbohydrates that occur in the brain and nervous system.

Enzymatic replacement therapy—A treatment method used to replace missing enzymes. It is possible to synthesize enzymes and then inject them intravenously into patients.

Glucocerebroside—A cerebroside that contains glucose in the molecule.

disease mutations prior to implantation of the embryo into the uterus. This technique is only available at selected genetics centers.

Population screening for Gaucher disease is not standard care.

Resources

PERIODICALS

Beutler, E. "Gaucher Disease." *Archives of Internal Medicine* 159 (1999): 881-2.

Charrow, J., et al. "Gaucher Disease: Recommendations on Diagnosis, Evaluation, and Monitoring." *Archives of Internal Medicine* 158 (1998): 1754-1760.

Grabowski, Gregory A. "Current Issues in Enzyme Therapy for Gaucher Disease." *Drugs* 52 (August 1996): 159-167.

NIH Technology Assessment Conference. "Gaucher Disease: Current Issues in Diagnosis and Treatment." *JAMA* 275 (February 12, 1996): 548-553.

ORGANIZATIONS

Alliance of Genetic Support Groups. 4301 Connecticut Ave. NW, Suite 404, Washington, DC 20008. (202) 966-5557. Fax: (202) 966-8553. <http://www.geneticalliance.org>.

Children's Gaucher Research Fund. PO Box 2123, Granite Bay, CA 95746-2123. (916) 797-3700. Fax: (916) 797-3707. <http://www.childrensgaucher.org>.

National Gaucher Foundation. 11140 Rockville Pike, Suite 350, Rockville, MD 20852-3106. (800) 925-8885. <http://www.gaucherdisease.org>.

National Organization for Rare Disorders (NORD). PO Box 8923, New Fairfield, CT 06812-8923. (203) 746-6518 or (800) 999-6673. Fax: (203) 746-6481. <http://www.rarediseases.org>.

WEBSITES

"Cerezyme." *Genzyme Therapeutics.* <http://www.cerezyme.com>.

"Gaucher Disease: Current Issues in Diagnosis and Treatment." <http://text.nlm.nih.gov/nih/ta/www/16.html>.

"Living with Gaucher Disease: A Guide for Patients, Parents, Relatives, and Friends." <http://neuro-www3.mgh.harvard.edu/gaucher/living.html>.

National Foundation for Jewish Genetic Diseases (NFJGD). <http://www.nfjgd.org/>.

Amy Vance, MS, CGC

Gene

A gene is the fundamental physical and functional unit of heredity. It is an individual element of an organism's genome and determines a trait or characteristic by regulating biochemical structure or metabolic process.

Genes are segments of nucleic acid, consisting of a specific sequence and number of the chemical units of nucleic acids, the nucleotides. In most organisms the nucleic acid is **deoxyribonucleic acid (DNA)** although in retroviruses the genetic material is composed of **ribonucleic acid (RNA)**. Some genes in a cell are active more or less all the time, which means that they are continuously transcribed and provide a constant supply of their protein product. These are the "housekeeping" genes that are always needed for basic cellular reactions. Others may be rendered active or inactive depending on the needs and functions of the organism under particular conditions. The signal that masks or unmasks a gene can come from outside the cell, for example, from a steroid hormone or a nutrient, or it can come from within the cell itself as a result of the activity of other genes. In both cases, regulatory substances can bind to the specific DNA sequences of the target genes to control the synthesis of transcripts.

In a paper published in 1865, Gregor Mendel (1823–1884) advanced a theory of **inheritance** dependent on material elements that segregate independently from each other in sex cells. Before Mendel's findings, inherited traits were thought to be passed on through a blending of the mother and father's characteristics, much like a blending of two liquids. The term "gene" was coined later by the Danish botanist Wilhelm Johannsen (1857–1927), to replace the variety of terms used up until then to describe hereditary factors. His definition of the gene led him to distinguish between **genotype** (an organism's genetic makeup) and **phenotype** (an organism's appearance). Before the chemical and physical nature of genes were discovered they were defined on the basis of phenotypic expression and algebraic symbols were used to record their distribution and segregation.

Because sexually reproducing, eukaryotic organisms possess two copies of an inherited factor (or gene), one acquired from each parent, the genotype of an individual for a particular trait is expressed by a pair of letters or symbols. Each of the alternative forms of a gene is also known as alleles. Dominant and recessive alleles are denoted by the use of higher and lower case letters. It can be predicted mathematically, for example, that a single allele pair will always segregate to give a genotype ratio 1AA:2Aa:1aa, and the phenotype ratio 2A:1aa (where A represents both AA and Aa since these cannot be distinguished phenotypically if dominance is complete).

The molecular structure and activity of genes can be modified by mutations and the smallest mutational unit is now known to be a single pair of nucleotides, also known as a muton. To indicate that a gene is functionally normal it is assigned a plus (+) sign, whereas a damaged or mutated gene is indicated by a minus (−) sign. A wild type *Escherichia coli* able to synthesize its own arginine would thus be symbolized as *arg+* and strains that have lost this ability by mutation of one of the genes for arginine utilization would be *arg-*. Such strains, known as arginine auxotrophs, would not be able to grow without a supplement of arginine. At this level of definition, the plus or minus actually refer to an operon rather than a single gene and finer genetic analysis can be used to reveal the exact location of the mutated gene.

The use of mutations in studying genes is well illustrated in a traditional genetic test called the "cis-trans test" which also gave the gene the alternative name, cistron. This is a complementation test that can be used to determine whether two different mutations (m1 and m2) occur in the same functional unit, i.e., within the same gene or cistron. It demonstrates well how genes can be defined phenomenologically and has been performed successfully in microorganisms such as yeasts. It works on the principle that pairs of homologous chromosomes containing similar genes can complement their action. Two types of heterozygotes of the test organism are prepared. Heterozygotes are organisms with different alleles in the two homologous chromosomes each of which was inherited from one parent. One heterozygote contains the mutations under investigation within the same **chromosome**, that is in the cis-configuration, which is symbolically designated ++/m1m2 (m1 and m2 are the two mutations under investigation and the symbol "+" indicates the same position on the homologous chromosome in the unmutated, wild type state). The second mutant is constructed to contain the mutations in such a way that one appears on each of the homologous chromosomes. This is called the trans-configuration and is designated, for example, by m2+/+m1. If two recessive mutations are present in the same cistron, the heterozygous trans-configuration displays the mutant phenotype, whereas the cis-configuration displays the normal, wild type, phenotype. This is because in the cis-configuration, there is one completely functional, unmutated, cistron (++) within the system which masks the two mutations on the other chromosome and allows for the expression of the wild type phenotype. If one or both mutations are dominant, and the cis- and trans-heterozygotes are phenotypically different, then both mutations must be present in the same cistron. Conversely, if the cis- and trans-heterozygotes are phenotypically identical, this is taken as evidence that the mutations are present in different cistrons.

In 1910, the American geneticist Thomas Hunt Morgan (1866–1945) began to uncover the relationship between genes and chromosomes. He discovered that genes were located on chromosomes and that they were arranged linearly and associated in linkage groups, with all the genes on one chromosome being linked. For example, the genes on the X and Y chromosomes are said to be sex-linked because the X and Y chromosomes determine the sex of the organisms (in humans X determining femaleness and Y determining maleness). Nonhomologous chromosomes possess different linkage groups whereas homologous chromosomes have identical linkage groups in identical sequences. The distance between two genes of the same linkage group is the sum of the distances between all the intervening genes. A schematic representation of the linear arrangement of linked genes, with their relative distances of separation, is known as a genetic map. In the construction of such maps the frequency of recombination during crossing over is used as an index of the distance between two linked genes.

Advances in molecular genetics have allowed analysis of the structure and biochemistry of genes in greater detail. They are no longer the nebulous units described by Mendel purely in terms of their visible expression (phenotypic expression). It is now possible to understand their molecular structure and function in considerable detail. The biological role of genes is to carry, encode, or control information on the composition of proteins. The proteins, together with their timing of expression and amount of production, are possibly the most important determinants of the structure and physiology of organisms. Each structural gene is responsible for one specific protein or part of a protein and codes for a single polypeptide chain via messenger RNA (mRNA). Some genes code specifically for transfer RNA (tRNA) or ribosomal RNA (rRNA) and some are merely sequences that are recognized by regulatory proteins. The latter are termed regulator genes. In higher organisms, or eukaryotes, genes are organized in such a way that at one end there is a region to which various regulatory proteins can bind, for example, RNA polymerase during transcription, and at the opposite end there are sequences encoding the termination of transcription. In between lies the protein encoding sequence. In the genes of many eukaryotes this sequence may be interrupted by intervening non-coding sequence segments called introns, which can range in number from one to many. Transcription of eukaryotic DNA produces pre-mRNA containing complementary sequences of both introns and the information carrying sections of the gene called exons. The pre-mRNA then undergoes post-transcriptional modification or processing in which the introns are excised and exons are spliced together, leaving the complete coding transcript of connected exons ready to code directly for the protein. When the central dogma of genetics was first established, a "one gene-one enzyme" hypothesis was proposed, but today it is more accurate to restate this as a one-to-one correspondence between a gene and the polypeptide for which it codes. This is because a number of proteins are now known to be constituted of multiple polypeptide subunits coded by different genes.

Judyth Sassoon, ARCS, PhD

Gene mutations

In a strict sense, mutations are changes in genes not caused by genetic recombination. A change in the base sequence of **DNA**, for example, represents a mutational change. Spontaneous mutations are mutations that occur at a given frequency without the need for an inducing agent of change (mutagenic agent). The term mutation is also used in a less technical sense to describe changes in the human genome (i.e., evolution) that result from a broad spectrum of processes that act to increase or decrease genetic variation within a population.

By definition, a **gene** is a hereditary unit that carries information used to construct proteins via the processes of transcription and translation. The human **gene pool** is the set of all genes carried within the human population. Genetic changes, including mutations, can be beneficial, neutral or deleterious. In general, mutations, along with recombination and gene flow, act to increase genetic variation (i.e., the number of types of genes or alleles) within the human species.

The term mutation was originally used by Dutch botanist Hugo De Vries (1848–1935) to describe rapid changes in **phenotype** from one generation to the next.

Subsequently, scientists used the term mutation to describe long-term, multi-generational, and heritable physical changes to genes.

Mutations generally occur via chromosomal mutations, point mutations, frame shifts, and breakdowns in DNA repair mechanisms. Chromosomal mutations include translocations, inversions, deletions and **chromosome** non-disjunction. Essentially there are five types of genetic rearrangements: deletions, duplications, inversions, translocations, and transposition.

Mutational deletions physically remove portions of genes (e.g., a portion of the DNA comprising the gene). Deletional mutations range from the single base point mutations to mutations that can span many functional genes. Chemical and radioactive agents account for the majority of induced point mutations. Scientists currently argue that most cancers and other degenerative diseases result from acquired genetic mutations due to environmental exposure, and not as an outcome of inherited traits. Chemicals capable of inducing genetic mutation (i.e., chemical mutagenesis or genotoxic compounds) are present a wide variety of natural and man-made products.

Point mutations may be nonsense mutations leading to the early termination of protein synthesis, missense mutations (a mutation that results an a substitution of one amino acid for another in a protein), or silent mutations that cause no detectable change. Accordingly, the effects of point mutational changes range from 100% lethality (all individuals die, usually early in fetal development) to no observable (phenotypic) change.

Duplications result in multiple copies of genes, and can occur as a result of unequal crossover or chromosome breaks. In addition, because some alteration of DNA is inevitable in the replication process, any mutation that hinders DNA repair mechanism will also increase the chance that a mutation will go uncorrected. Duplications also manifest a range of deleterious effects.

Inversions (changes in the orientation of gene bearing chromosomal regions) may cause deleterious effects if the inversion breaks through a gene critical for a particular protein or enzyme.

Translocations occur when one a portion of one chromosome becomes linked to a non-homologous chromosome (a chromosome outside its normal pairing) or when portions of non-homologous chromosomes make a reciprocal exchange. Once again, the effect of such genetic change is a result of whether such translocations physically or functionally alter vital genes.

Recombination involves the reassortment of genes through new chromosome combinations. Recombination occurs via an exchange of DNA between homologous chromosomes (crossing over) during meiosis. Recombination also includes linkage disequilibrium. With linkage disequilibrium, variations of the same gene (alleles) occur in different combinations in the gametes (sexual reproductive cells) than should occur according to the rules of probability.

Gene flow occurs when individuals change their local genetic group by moving from one place to another. These migrations allow the introduction of new variations of the same gene (alleles) when they mate and produce offspring with members of their new group. In effect, gene flow acts to increase the gene pool in the new group. Because genes are usually carried by many members of a large population that has undergone random mating for several generations, random migrations of individuals away from the population or group usually do not significantly decrease the gene pool of the group left behind.

In contrast to mechanisms that operate to increase genetic variation, there are fewer mechanisms that operate to decrease genetic variation. Mechanisms that decrease genetic variation include genetic drift and natural selection.

Genetic drift results form the changes in the numbers of different forms of a gene (allelic frequency) that result from sexual reproduction. Genetic drift can occur as a result of random mating (random genetic drift) or be profoundly affected by geographical barriers, catastrophic events (e.g., natural disasters or wars that significantly affect the reproductive availability of selected members of a population), and other political-social factors.

Natural selection is based upon the differences in the viability and reproductive success of different genotypes with a population (differential reproductive success). Natural selection can only act on those differences in **genotype** that appear as visible (phenotypic) differences that affect the ability to attract a mate and produce viable offspring that are, in turn, able to live, mate and continue the species. The term evolutionary fitness describes the success of an entity in reproducing (i.e., contributing alleles to the next generation).

There are three basic types of natural selection. With directional selection, an extreme phenotype is favored (high or low body fat). Stabilizing selection occurs when an intermediate phenotype is fittest (e.g., body fat content is neither too high nor low) and for this reason, it is often referred to a normalizing selection. Disruptive selection occurs when two extreme phenotypes are more fit than an intermediate phenotype. In studying changes in the human genome, the operation of natural evolutionary mechanisms is complicated by geographic, ethnic, religious, and social groups and customs.

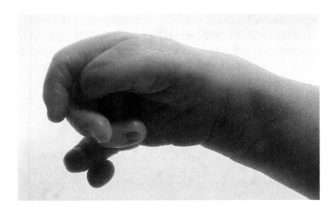

Polydactyly, which results in extra fingers or toes, is one type of genetic mutation. (*Custom Medical Stock Photo, Inc.*)

Accordingly, the effects of various evolution mechanisms on human populations are not as easy to predict. Increasingly sophisticated statistical studies are carried out by population geneticists to characterize changes in the human genome.

K. Lee Lerner

Gene pool

Definition

The term **gene** pool refers to the total sum of genetic information present in a population at any given time. A gene pool can be assigned to any set group or population. This is true for plants, animals, and humans alike. Each gene pool contains all of the inherited information for all of the traits of the members of the population.

Genetic information

Genetic information, in the form of **deoxyribonucleic acid (DNA)**, is passed down from generation to generation. DNA tells a person's body how to work and how to grow. It provides instructions that assign features to each individual, such as giving one person brown hair and another person blonde hair, and one person brown eyes and another person green eyes.

DNA is much like a linear string, with individual segments along the string known as genes. Genes provide the specific directions for the body. Each gene is a segment of DNA, and sequencing of the four base molecules of DNA create the gene. Variations in the sequence account for variations in genes. A gene is the equivalent of an allele, and each particular gene is found on the same **chromosome** in each individual. The long, linear strings of DNA are arranged into smaller packages known as chromosomes. In general, there are 46 chromosomes in each cell of a person's body. The 46 chromosomes can be matched into 23 pairs. One of each pair is inherited from the mother's egg and one of each pair is inherited from the father's sperm. Most animals, including humans, contain two copies of each chromosome and likewise two copies of each gene. Each individual receives one allele from each parent because they receive one of each of the 23 chromosomes from each parent.

Although each person has 46 chromosomes, the DNA that makes up those chromosomes is slightly different from individual to individual. It is this variation within specific genes that gives the diversity observed throughout populations around the world.

Alleles

Different versions of the same gene are referred to as alleles. Blood types are examples of alleles. In humans there are several different blood types, including A, B, O, and AB. These arise by various combinations of the three blood-type alleles; the A-allele, the B-allele, and the O-allele. The specific blood type a person has depends on the exact blood type alleles they inherited from their parents. For example, a person may inherit two O-alleles, in which case they would have type O blood, or they may inherit an A- and a B-allele, in which case they would have type AB blood, and so on.

Population genetics

Population genetics is the study of genetic variation within a population. This includes the subtle changes in DNA sequences and the frequencies of these different forms. Changes within the DNA sequences may arise through several pathways. Mechanisms commonly studied by population geneticists include mutation, natural selection, and genetic drift.

Mutations are changes within the DNA sequence that alter the original directions encoded within DNA. Mutation may result from damage to DNA, or a mistake in the replication of DNA resulting in a sequence change. The majority of mutations arise by chance, although some may be caused by environmental factors, such as toxins that penetrate the cells of the body and attack the DNA. Natural selection is the difference in mortality (death rates) and fertility (birth rates) between different genetic types. The interplay of the

expressed **phenotype** and the environment influences natural selection. If the phenotype is favorable, the individual survives and perpetuates his or her genetic profile in the gene pool. Genetic drift is a process by which the frequencies of specific alleles change, by chance, within a population.

Each gene pool accounts for all of the alleles for all of the traits of the members of a population. Within a population, different alleles will occur at different frequencies. For instance, approximately 44% of the population has type O blood, 42% of the population has type A blood, 10% of the population has type B blood, and 4% of the population has type AB blood. The percentages of each blood type are directly related to the frequency of each blood type allele. The more frequent the A-allele, the more frequent type A blood would be seen in the population.

The gene frequency of an allele is equal to the number of times the allele occurs compared to the total number of alleles for that trait.

Gene frequency equals the number of a specific type of allele, or the total number of alleles in the gene pool

DNA changes and genetic disorders

Genetic disorders are caused by changes in the DNA sequence. In general, there is a non-disease causing allele and a disease-causing allele. Some genetic disorders arise by sporadic mutations in the DNA sequence. Others are inherited from one or both of the parents.

There are several different **inheritance** patterns associated with genetic disorders. Autosomal dominant and autosomal recessive are two of the most common. Chromosomes come in pairs, one from the egg and one from the sperm. Autosomal dominant disorders require that a person inherit only one disease-causing allele in order to be affected. Even though the corresponding gene on the other chromosome in the pair may be the non-disease-causing allele, having one disease-causing allele is enough to cause the disorder to be present. Autosomal recessive disorders require that a person inherit two disease-causing alleles, one on each chromosome of the pair, for the individual to be affected. If a person inherits only one disease-causing allele of a recessive disorder they are called a carrier. Carriers are not affected by disease; however, they carry the possibility of passing that disease on to a future child.

Hardy-Weinberg equilibrium

The frequency of disease-causing and non-disease-causing alleles along with the frequency of affected individuals, carriers, and unaffected individuals are related

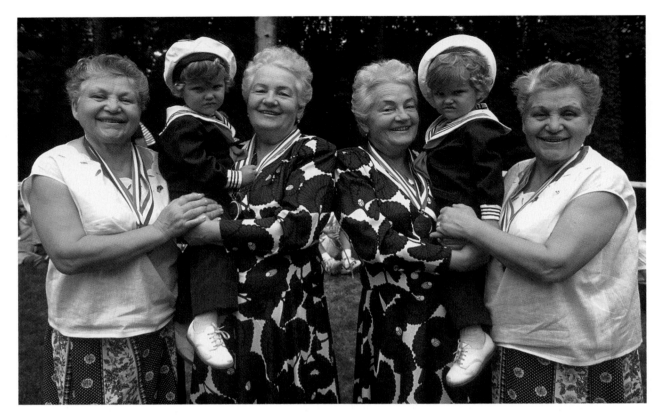

Three generations of female twins. (*Phototake*)

within a mathematical equation known as the Hardy-Weinberg equation.

The equation itself is written as p2+2pq+q2 = 1. For autosomal recessive disorders, p2 represents the people within the population that have two non-disease-causing alleles (unaffected), 2pq represents the people within the population with one disease-causing allele and one non-disease-causing allele (carriers), and q2 represents the people within the population that have two disease-causing alleles (affected). Because the Hardy-Weinberg equation deals with allele frequencies, the equation p + q = 1 may also be used. In this case, p represents the frequency of the non-disease-causing allele within the population and q represents the frequency of the disease-causing allele within the population.

The Hardy-Weinberg equation is based on the work of Drs. Hardy and Weinberg. Independently, they suggested that there should exist an equilibrium, or balance, between different allele frequencies. They devised a list of conditions that must be true for this balance, known as the Hardy-Weinberg equilibrium, to occur. These include:

• no evolutionary forces acting upon the population

• the population is "infinitely" large (meaning it is so large that it may be assumed to be infinitely large)

• individuals have two copies of each gene

• there is random mating between individuals within the group

• the frequencies of the alleles are the same in both males and females

• generations are non-overlapping

The Hardy-Weinberg equation has several applications including use by population geneticists to study the characteristics of certain populations and use by genetic counselors to calculate recurrence risks for individual families affected by genetic disease.

The future

There are several projects underway at this time in an effort to further understand the gene pool, population genetics, and the human genome. The Human Genome Diversity Project (HGDP) is an international project that seeks to understand the diversity and unity of the entire human species.

KEY TERMS

Allele—One of two or more alternate forms of a gene.

Chromosome—A microscopic thread-like structure found within each cell of the body and consists of a complex of proteins and DNA. Humans have 46 chromosomes arranged into 23 pairs. Changes in either the total number of chromosomes or their shape and size (structure) may lead to physical or mental abnormalities.

Deoxyribonucleic acid (DNA)—The genetic material in cells that holds the inherited instructions for growth, development, and cellular functioning.

Gene—A building block of inheritance, which contains the instructions for the production of a particular protein, and is made up of a molecular sequence found on a section of DNA. Each gene is found on a precise location on a chromosome.

Genome—A term used to describe a complete representation of all of the genes in a species.

The **Human Genome Project**, a separate venture from HGDP, made the news in 2000 when scientists announced they had elucidated a working draft of the human genome sequence.

Resources

WEBSITES

Bioethics and Human Population Genetics Research. <http://www.biol.tsukuba.ac.jp/~macer/PG.html>.

Biology Website References for Students and Teachers. <http://www.hoflink.com/~house/evolution.html#anchor25392>.

Evolution—Population Genetics. <http://www.nearctica.com/evolve/popgen.htm>.

Human Genome Diversity Project. <http://www.standford.edu/group/morrinst/hgdp.html>.

Human Genome Project. <http://www.ornl.gov/hgmis>.

Talk Origins. <http://www.talkorigins.org>.

Java O. Solis, MS

Gene therapy

Gene therapy is a rapidly growing field of medicine in which genes are introduced into the body to treat diseases. Genes control heredity and provide the basic biological code for determining a cell's specific functions. Gene therapy seeks to provide genes that correct or supplant the disease-controlling functions of cells that are not, in essence, doing their job. Somatic gene therapy introduces therapeutic genes at the tissue or cellular level to treat a specific individual. Germ-line gene therapy inserts genes into reproductive cells or possibly into embryos to correct genetic defects that could be passed on to future generations. Initially conceived as an approach for treating inherited diseases, like **cystic fibrosis** and Huntington's disease, the scope of potential gene therapies has grown to include treatments for cancers, arthritis, and infectious diseases. Although gene therapy testing in humans has advanced rapidly, many questions surround its use. For example, some scientists are concerned that the therapeutic genes themselves may cause disease. Others fear that germ-line gene therapy may be used to control human development in ways not connected with disease, like intelligence or appearance.

The biological basis of gene therapy

Gene therapy has grown out of the science of genetics or how heredity works. Scientists know that life begins in a cell, the basic building block of all multicellular organisms. Humans, for instance, are made up of trillions of cells, each performing a specific function. Within the cell's nucleus (the center part of a cell that regulates its chemical functions) are pairs of chromosomes. These threadlike structures are made up of a single molecule of **DNA (deoxyribonucleic acid)**, which carries the blueprint of life in the form of codes, or genes, that determine inherited characteristics.

A **DNA** molecule looks like two ladders with one of the sides taken off both and then twisted around each other. The rungs of these ladders meet (resulting in a spiral staircase-like structure) and are called base pairs. Base pairs are made up of nitrogen molecules and arranged in specific sequences. Millions of these base pairs, or sequences, can make up a single gene, specifically defined as a segment of the **chromosome** and DNA that contains certain hereditary information. The gene, or combination of genes formed by these base pairs ultimately direct an organism's growth and characteristics through the production of certain chemicals, primarily proteins, which carry out most of the body's chemical functions and biological reactions.

Scientists have long known that alterations in genes present within cells can cause inherited diseases like cystic fibrosis, sickle-cell anemia, and **hemophilia**. Similarly, errors in the total number of chromosomes can cause conditions such as **Down syndrome** or **Turner syndrome**. As the study of genetics advanced, however, scientists learned that an altered genetic sequence can also make people more susceptible to diseases, like atherosclerosis, **cancer**, and even **schizophrenia**. These diseases have a genetic component, but are also influenced by environmental factors (such as diet and lifestyle). The objective of gene therapy is to treat diseases by introducing functional genes into the body to alter the cells involved in the disease process by either replacing missing genes or providing copies of functioning genes to replace nonfunctioning ones. The inserted genes can be naturally occurring genes that produce the desired effect or may be genetically engineered (or altered) genes.

Scientists have known how to manipulate a gene's structure in the laboratory since the early 1970s through a process called gene splicing. The process involves removing a fragment of DNA containing the specific genetic sequence desired then inserting it into the DNA of another gene. The resultant product is called recombinant DNA and the process is genetic engineering.

There are basically two types of gene therapy. Germ-line gene therapy introduces genes into reproductive cells (sperm and eggs) or someday possibly into embryos in hopes of correcting genetic abnormalities that could be passed on to future generations. Most of the current work in applying gene therapy, however, has been in the realm of somatic gene therapy. In this type of gene therapy, therapeutic genes are inserted into tissue or cells to produce a naturally occurring protein or substance that is lacking or not functioning correctly in an individual patient.

Viral vectors

In both types of therapy, scientists need something to transport either the entire gene or a recombinant DNA to the cell's nucleus, where the chromosomes and DNA reside. In essence, vectors are molecular delivery trucks. One of the first and most popular vectors developed were viruses because they invade cells as part of the natural infection process. Viruses have the potential to be excellent vectors because they have a specific relationship with the host in that they colonize certain cell types and tissues in specific organs. As a result, vectors are chosen according to their attraction to certain cells and areas of the body.

One of the first vectors used was the retrovirus. Because these viruses are easily cloned (artificially reproduced) in the laboratory, scientists have studied them extensively and learned a great deal about their biological action. They have also learned how to remove the genetic information which governs viral replication, thus reducing the chances of infection.

Retroviruses work best in actively dividing cells, but cells in the body are relatively stable and do not divide often. As a result, these cells are used primarily for *ex vivo* (outside the body) manipulation. First, the cells are removed from the patient's body, and the virus, or vector, carrying the gene is inserted into them. Next, the cells are placed into a nutrient culture where they grow and replicate. Once enough cells are gathered, they are returned to the body, usually by injection into the blood stream. Theoretically, as long as these cells survive, they will provide the desired therapy.

Another class of viruses, called the adenoviruses, may also prove to be good gene vectors. These viruses can effectively infect nondividing cells in the body, where the desired gene product is then expressed naturally. In addition to being a more efficient approach to gene transportation, these viruses, which cause respiratory infections, are more easily purified and made stable than retroviruses, resulting in less chance of an unwanted viral infection. However, these viruses live for several days in the body, and some concern surrounds the possibility of infecting others with the viruses through sneezing or coughing. Other viral vectors include influenza viruses, Sindbis virus, and a herpes virus that infects nerve cells.

Scientists have also delved into nonviral vectors. These vectors rely on the natural biological process in which cells uptake (or gather) macromolecules. One approach is to use liposomes, globules of fat produced by the body and taken up by cells. Scientists are also investigating the introduction of raw recombinant DNA by injecting it into the bloodstream or placing it on microscopic beads of gold shot into the skin with a "gene-gun." Another possible vector under development is based on dendrimer molecules. A class of polymers (naturally occurring or artificial substances that have a high molecular weight and formed by smaller molecules of the same or similar substances), is "constructed" in the laboratory by combining these smaller molecules. They have been used in manufacturing Styrofoam, polyethylene cartons, and Plexiglass. In the laboratory, dendrimers have shown the ability to transport genetic material into human cells. They can also be designed to form an affinity for particular cell membranes by attaching to certain sugars and protein groups.

The history of gene therapy

In the early 1970s, scientists proposed "gene surgery" for treating inherited diseases caused by faulty genes. The idea was to take out the disease-causing gene and surgically implant a gene that functioned properly. Although sound in theory, scientists, then and now, lack the biological knowledge or technical expertise needed to perform such a precise surgery in the human body.

However, in 1983, a group of scientists from Baylor College of Medicine in Houston, Texas, proposed that gene therapy could one day be a viable approach for treating Lesch-Nyhan disease, a rare neurological disorder. The scientists conducted experiments in which an enzyme-producing gene (a specific type of protein) for correcting the disease was injected into a group of cells for replication. The scientists theorized the cells could then be injected into people with Lesch-Nyhan disease, thus correcting the genetic defect that caused the disease.

As the science of genetics advanced throughout the 1980s, gene therapy gained an established foothold in the minds of medical scientists as a promising approach to treatments for specific diseases. One of the major reasons for the growth of gene therapy was scientists' increasing ability to identify the specific genetic malfunctions that caused inherited diseases. Interest grew as further studies of DNA and chromosomes (where genes reside) showed that specific genetic abnormalities in one or more genes occurred in successive generations of certain family members who suffered from diseases like intestinal cancer, manic-depression, Alzheimer's disease, heart disease, **diabetes**, and many more. Although the genes may not be the only cause of the disease in all cases, they may make certain individuals more susceptible to developing the disease because of environmental influences, like smoking, pollution, and stress. In fact, some scientists theorize that all diseases may have a genetic component.

On September 14, 1990, a four-year-old girl with a genetic disorder that prevented her body from producing a crucial enzyme became the first person to undergo gene therapy in the United States. Because her body could not produce adenosine deaminase (ADA), she had a weakened immune system, making her extremely susceptible to severe, life-threatening infections. W. French Anderson and colleagues at the National Institutes of Health's Clinical Center in Bethesda, Maryland, took white blood cells (which are crucial to proper immune system functioning) from the girl, inserted ADA producing genes into them, and then transfused the cells back into the patient. Although the young girl continued to show an increased ability to produce ADA, debate arose as to whether the improvement resulted from the gene therapy or from an additional drug treatment she received.

Nevertheless, a new era of gene therapy began as more and more scientists sought to conduct clinical trial (testing in humans) research in this area. In that same year, gene therapy was tested on patients with melanoma (skin cancer). The goal was to help them produce antibodies (disease fighting substances in the immune system) to battle the cancer.

These experiments have spawned an ever-growing number of attempts at gene therapies designed to perform a variety of functions in the body. For example, a gene therapy for cystic fibrosis aims to supply a gene that alters cells, enabling them to produce a specific protein to battle the disease. Another approach was used for brain cancer patients, in which the inserted gene was designed to make the cancer cells more likely to respond to drug treatment. Gene therapy for patients who have artery blockage, which can lead to strokes, induces the growth of new blood vessels near clogged arteries, thus ensuring normal blood circulation.

Currently, there are a host of new gene therapy agents in clinical trials. In the United States, both nucleic acid-based (*in vivo*) treatments and cell-based (*ex vivo*) treatments are being investigated. Nucleic acid-based gene therapy uses vectors (like viruses) to deliver modified genes to target cells. Cell-based gene therapy techniques remove cells from the patient in order to genetically alter them then reintroduce them to the patient's body. Presently, gene therapies for the following diseases are being developed: cystic fibrosis (using adenoviral vector), HIV infection (cell-based), malignant melanoma (cell-based), **Duchenne muscular dystrophy** (cell-based), hemophilia B (cell-based), kidney cancer (cell-based), **Gaucher disease** (retroviral vector), **breast cancer** (retroviral vector), and lung cancer (retroviral vector). When a cell or individual is treated using gene therapy and successful incorporation of engineered genes has occurred, the cell or individual is said to be *transgenic*.

The medical establishment's contribution to transgenic research has been supported by increased government funding. In 1991, the U.S. government provided $58 million for gene therapy research, with increases in funding of $15–40 million dollars a year over the following four years. With fierce competition over the promise of societal benefit in addition to huge profits, large pharmaceutical corporations have moved to the forefront of transgenic research. In an effort to be first in developing new therapies, and armed with billions of dollars of research funds, such corporations are making impressive strides toward making gene therapy a viable reality in the treatment of once elusive diseases.

Diseases targeted for treatment by gene therapy

The potential scope of gene therapy is enormous. More than 4,200 diseases have been identified as resulting directly from abnormal genes, and countless others that may be partially influenced by a person's genetic makeup. Initial research has concentrated on developing gene therapies for diseases whose genetic origins have been established and for other diseases that can be cured or ameliorated by substances genes produce.

The following are examples of potential gene therapies. People suffering from cystic fibrosis lack a gene needed to produce a salt-regulating protein. This protein regulates the flow of chloride into epithelial cells, (the cells that line the inner and outer skin layers) which cover the air passages of the nose and lungs. Without this regulation, patients with cystic fibrosis build up a thick mucus that makes them prone to lung infections. A gene therapy technique to correct this abnormality might employ an adenovirus to transfer a normal copy of what scientists call the cystic fibrosis transmembrane conductance regulator, or CTRF, gene. The gene is introduced into the patient by spraying it into the nose or lungs.

Familial hypercholesterolemia (FH) is also an inherited disease, resulting in the inability to process cholesterol properly, which leads to high levels of artery-clogging fat in the blood stream. Patients with FH often suffer heart attacks and strokes because of blocked arteries. A gene therapy approach used to battle FH is much more intricate than most gene therapies because it involves partial surgical removal of patients' livers (*ex vivo* transgene therapy). Corrected copies of a gene that serve to reduce cholesterol build-up are inserted into the liver sections, which are then transplanted back into the patients.

Gene therapy has also been tested on patients with AIDS. AIDS is caused by the human immunodeficiency virus (HIV), which weakens the body's immune system to the point that sufferers are unable to fight off diseases like pneumonias and cancer. In one approach, genes that produce specific HIV proteins have been altered to stimulate immune system functioning without causing the negative effects that a complete HIV molecule has on the immune system. These genes are then injected in the patient's blood stream. Another approach to treating AIDS is to insert, via white blood cells, genes that have been genetically engineered to produce a receptor that would attract HIV and reduce its chances of replicating.

Several cancers also have the potential to be treated with gene therapy. A therapy tested for melanoma, or skin cancer, involves introducing a gene with an anticancer protein called tumor necrosis factor (TNF) into test tube samples of the patient's own cancer cells, which are then reintroduced into the patient. In brain cancer, the approach is to insert a specific gene that increases the cancer cells' susceptibility to a common drug used in fighting the disease.

Gaucher disease is an inherited disease caused by a mutant gene that inhibits the production of an enzyme called glucocerebrosidase. Patients with Gaucher disease have enlarged livers and spleens and eventually their bones deteriorate. Clinical gene therapy trials focus on inserting the gene for producing this enzyme.

Gene therapy is also being considered as an approach to solving a problem associated with a surgical procedure known as balloon angioplasty. In this procedure, a stent (in this case, a type of tubular scaffolding) is used to open the clogged artery. However, in response to the trauma of the stent insertion, the body initiates a natural healing process that produces too many cells in the artery and results in restenosis, or reclosing of the artery. The gene therapy approach to preventing this unwanted side effect is to cover the outside of the stents with a soluble gel. This gel contains vectors for genes that reduce this overactive healing response.

The Human Genome Project

Although great strides have been made in gene therapy in a relatively short time, its potential usefulness has been limited by lack of scientific data concerning the multitude of functions that genes control in the human body. For instance, it is now known that the vast majority of genetic material does not store information for the creation of proteins, rather, it is involved in the control and regulation of gene expression, and is therefore much more difficult to interpret. Even so, each individual cell in the body carries thousands of genes coding for proteins, with some estimates as high as 150,000 genes. For gene therapy to advance to its full potential, scientists must discover the biological role of each of these individual genes and where the base pairs that make them up are located on DNA.

To address this issue, the National Institutes of Health initiated the **Human Genome Project** in 1990. Led by James D. Watson (one of the co-discoverers of the chemical makeup of DNA), the project's 15-year goal is to map the entire human genome (a combination of the words gene and chromosomes). A genome map would clearly identify the location of all genes as well as the more than three billion base pairs that make them up. With a precise knowledge of gene locations and functions, scientists may one day be able to conquer or control diseases that have plagued humanity for centuries.

Scientists participating in the Human Genome Project have identified an average of one new gene a day, but many expect this rate of discovery to increase. Their goal is to determine the exact location of all the genes on human DNA and the exact sequence of the base pairs that make them up (see the "Human Genome Project" entry for updated information). Some of the genes

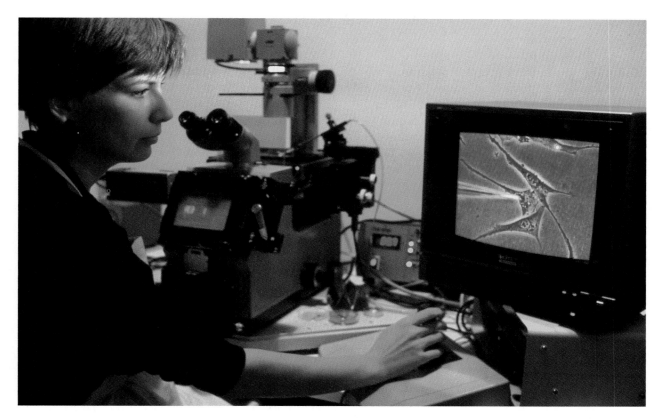

Geneticist performing DNA microinjection technique. The monitor shows the micropipette injecting DNA into a cell. (*Photo Researchers, Inc.*)

identified through this project include a gene that predisposes people to obesity, one associated with programmed cell death (apoptosis), a gene that guides HIV viral reproduction, and the genes of inherited disorders like **Huntington disease**, Lou Gehrig's disease, and some colon and breast cancers. With fewer than the anticipated number of genes found, between 30,000 and 40,000, the consequences of this announcement are enormous. Scientists caution however, that the initial publication is only a draft of the human genome and much more work is still ahead for the completion of the project. As the human genome is completed, there will be more information available for gene therapy research and implementation.

The future of gene therapy

Gene therapy seems elegantly simple in its concept: supply the human body with a gene that can correct a biological malfunction that causes a disease. However, there are many obstacles and some distinct questions concerning the viability of gene therapy. For example, viral vectors must be carefully controlled lest they infect the patient with a viral disease. Some vectors, like retro-

viruses, can also enter cells functioning properly and interfere with the natural biological processes, possibly leading to other diseases. Other viral vectors, like the adenoviruses, are often recognized and destroyed by the immune system so their therapeutic effects are short-lived. Maintaining gene expression so it performs its role properly after vector delivery is difficult. As a result, some therapies need to be repeated often to provide long-lasting benefits.

One of the most pressing issues, however, is gene regulation. Genes work in concert to regulate their functioning. In other words, several genes may play a part in turning other genes on and off. For example, certain genes work together to stimulate cell division and growth, but if these are not regulated, the inserted genes could cause tumor formation and cancer. Another difficulty is learning how to make the gene go into action only when needed. For the best and safest therapeutic effort, a specific gene should turn on, for example, when certain levels of a protein or enzyme are low and must be replaced. But the gene should also remain dormant when not needed to ensure it does not oversupply a substance and disturb the body's delicate chemical makeup.

Cell—The smallest living units of the body which group together to form tissues and help the body perform specific functions.

Chromosome—A microscopic thread-like structure found within each cell of the body and consists of a complex of proteins and DNA. Humans have 46 chromosomes arranged into 23 pairs. Changes in either the total number of chromosomes or their shape and size (structure) may lead to physical or mental abnormalities.

Clinical trial—The testing of a drug or some other type of therapy in a specific population of patients.

Clone—A cell or organism derived through asexual (without sex) reproduction containing the identical genetic information of the parent cell or organism.

Deoxyribonucleic acid (DNA)—The genetic material in cells that holds the inherited instructions for growth, development, and cellular functioning.

Embryo—The earliest stage of development of a human infant, usually used to refer to the first eight weeks of pregnancy. The term *fetus* is used from roughly the third month of pregnancy until delivery.

Enzyme—A protein that catalyzes a biochemical reaction or change without changing its own structure or function.

Eugenics—A social movement in which the population of a society, country, or the world is to be improved by controlling the passing on of hereditary information through mating.

Gene—A building block of inheritance, which contains the instructions for the production of a particu-

lar protein, and is made up of a molecular sequence found on a section of DNA. Each gene is found on a precise location on a chromosome.

Gene transcription—The process by which genetic information is copied from DNA to RNA, resulting in a specific protein formation.

Genetic engineering—The manipulation of genetic material to produce specific results in an organism.

Genetics—The study of hereditary traits passed on through the genes.

Germ-line gene therapy—The introduction of genes into reproductive cells or embryos to correct inherited genetic defects that can cause disease.

Liposome—Fat molecule made up of layers of lipids.

Macromolecules—A large molecule composed of thousands of atoms.

Nitrogen—A gaseous element that makes up the base pairs in DNA.

Nucleus—The central part of a cell that contains most of its genetic material, including chromosomes and DNA.

Protein—Important building blocks of the body, composed of amino acids, involved in the formation of body structures and controlling the basic functions of the human body.

Somatic gene therapy—The introduction of genes into tissue or cells to treat a genetic related disease in an individual.

Vectors—Something used to transport genetic information to a cell.

One approach to gene regulation is to attach other genes that detect certain biological activities and then react as a type of automatic off-and-on switch that regulates the activity of the other genes according to biological cues. Although still in the rudimentary stages, researchers are making headway in inhibiting some gene functioning by using a synthetic DNA to block gene transcriptions (the copying of genetic information). This approach may have implications for gene therapy.

The ethics of gene therapy

While gene therapy holds promise as a revolutionary approach to treating disease, ethical concerns over its use and ramifications have been expressed by scientists and lay people alike. For example, since much needs to

be learned about how these genes actually work and their long-term effect, is it ethical to test these therapies on humans, where they could have a disastrous result? As with most clinical trials concerning new therapies, including many drugs, the patients participating in these studies have usually not responded to more established therapies and are often so ill the novel therapy is their only hope for long-term survival.

Another questionable outgrowth of gene therapy is that scientists could possibly manipulate genes to genetically control traits in human offspring that are not health related. For example, perhaps a gene could be inserted to ensure that a child would not be bald, a seemingly harmless goal. However, what if genetic manipulation was used to alter skin color, prevent homosexuality, or ensure good looks? If a gene is found that can enhance intelligence of children who are not yet born, will everyone in society, the rich and the poor, have access to the technology or will it be so expensive only the elite can afford it?

The Human Genome Project, which plays such an integral role for the future of gene therapy, also has social repercussions. If individual genetic codes can be determined, will such information be used against people? For example, will someone more susceptible to a disease have to pay higher insurance premiums or be denied health insurance altogether? Will employers discriminate between two potential employees, one with a "healthy" genome and the other with genetic abnormalities?

Some of these concerns can be traced back to the eugenics movement popular in the first half of the twentieth century. This genetic "philosophy" was a societal movement that encouraged people with "positive" traits to reproduce while those with less desirable traits were sanctioned from having children. Eugenics was used to pass strict immigration laws in the United States, barring less suitable people from entering the country lest they reduce the quality of the country's collective **gene pool**. Probably the most notorious example of eugenics in action was the rise of Nazism in Germany, which resulted in the Eugenic Sterilization Law of 1933. The law required sterilization for those suffering from certain disabilities and even for some who were simply deemed "ugly." To ensure that this novel science is not abused, many governments have established organizations specifically for overseeing the development of gene therapy. In the United States, the Food and Drug Administration and the National Institutes of Health requires scientists to take a precise series of steps and meet stringent requirements before approving clinical trials.

In fact, gene therapy has been immersed in more controversy and surrounded by more scrutiny in both the health and ethical arena than most other technologies (except, perhaps, for cloning) that promise to substantially change society. Despite the health and ethical questions surrounding gene therapy, the field will continue to grow and is likely to change medicine faster than any previous medical advancement.

Resources

BOOKS

Hyde, Margaret O., and Lawrence E. Hyde. *Cloning and the New Genetics.* Springfield, NJ: Enslow Publishers, Inc., 1984.

Stwertka, Eve, and Albert Stwertka. *Genetic Engineering.* New York: Franklin Watts, 1989.

Thompson, Larry. *Correcting the Code: Inventing the Genetic Cure for the Human Body.* New York: Simon & Schuster, 1994.

PERIODICALS

Christensen R. "Cutaneous Gene Therapy—An Update." *Histochemical Cell Biology* (January 2001): 73-82.

"Initial Sequencing and Analysis of the Human Genome." *Nature* (February 15, 2001): 860-921.

Nevin, Norman. "What Has Happened to Gene Therapy?" *European Journal of Pediatrics* (2000): S240-S242.

Pekkanen, John. "Genetics: Medicine's Amazing Leap." *Readers Digest* (September 1991): 23-32.

Schemck, Harold M., Jr. "A New Era of Gene Therapy." *FDA Consumer* (December 1991): 14-19.

Weiss, Rick. "Gene Therapy at a Crossroads." *Washington Post* (October 19, 1994): 12-15.

ORGANIZATIONS

The National Human Genome Research Institute. The National Institutes of Health. 9000 Rockville Pike, Bethesda, MD 20892. (301) 496-2433. <http://www.nhgri.nih.gov>.

WEBSITES

Online Mendelian Inheritance in Man. Online genetic testing information sponsored by National Center for Biotechnology Information. <http://www.ncbi.nlm.nih.gov/Omim/>.

Katherine Hunt, MS

Genetic counseling

Definition

Genetic counseling is a communication process by which personal genetic risk information is translated into practical information for families. Genetic counselors are health care professionals with specialized training and experience in the areas of medical genetics and counseling. Genetic counselors are able to assist families by:

- Helping families understand information about birth defects or **genetic disorders**. This includes explaining patterns of **inheritance**, recurrence risks, natural history of diseases, and **genetic testing** options.

- Providing nondirective supportive counseling regarding emotional issues related to a diagnosis or testing options.

- Helping individuals or families make decisions that they are comfortable with based on their personal ethical and religious standards.

• Connecting families with appropriate resources, such as support groups or specific types of medical clinics, locally and nationally.

Types of genetic counseling

Genetic counselors work with people concerned about the risk of an inherited disease. These patients represent several different patient populations. Prenatal genetic counseling is provided to couples that have an increased risk for birth defects or inherited conditions and are expecting a child or planning a pregnancy. Pediatric genetic counseling is provided to families with children suspected of having a genetic disorder or with children previously diagnosed with a genetic disorder. Adult genetic counseling is provided to adults with clinical features of an inherited disease or a family history of an inherited disease. **Cancer** genetic counseling is provided to those with a strong family history of certain types of cancer.

Prenatal genetic counseling

There are several different reasons a person or couple may seek prenatal genetic counseling. If a woman is age 35 or older and pregnant, there is an increased chance that the fetus may have a change in the number of chromosomes present. Changes in **chromosome** number may lead to mental retardation and birth defects. **Down syndrome** is the most common change in chromosome number that occurs more often in the fetuses of older women. Couples may seek prenatal genetic counseling because of abnormal results of screening tests performed during pregnancy. A blood test called the alpha fetal protein (AFP) test is offered to all pregnant women. This blood test screens for Down syndrome, open spine defects (**spina bifida**) and another type of mental retardation caused by a change in chromosome number called **Trisomy 18**. When this test is abnormal, further tests are offered to get more information about the chance of these conditions in the fetus. Another reason that people seek prenatal genetic counseling is a family history of birth defects or inherited diseases. In some cases, blood tests on the parents may be available to indicate if their children would be at risk of being affected. Genetic counselors assess risk in each case, help patients understand their risks and explore how patients feel about or cope with these risks.

Prenatal tests that are offered during genetic counseling include level II ultrasounds, maternal serum AFP screening, chorionic villus sampling (CVS), and **amniocentesis**. Level II ultrasound is a detailed ultrasound surveying fetal anatomy for birth defects. Ultrasound is limited to detection of structural changes in anatomy and cannot detect changes in chromosome number. The maternal serum AFP screening is used to indicate if a pregnant woman has a higher or lower chance of certain birth defects. This test can only change the chances for a birth defect. The screening cannot diagnose a birth defect. CVS is a way of learning how many chromosomes is present in a fetus. A small piece of placental tissue is obtained for these studies during the tenth to twelfth weeks of pregnancy. Amniocentesis is also a way of learning how many chromosomes are present in a fetus. Amniotic fluid is obtained for these studies, usually between 16 and 18 weeks of pregnancy. There is a small risk for miscarriage with both of these tests. Genetic counseling regarding these procedures involves the careful explanation of benefits and limitations of each testing option. The counselor also tries to explore how patients feel about prenatal testing and the impact of such testing on the pregnancy. Genetic counselors are supportive of any decision a patient makes about whether or not to have prenatal tests performed.

Pediatric genetic counseling

Families or pediatricians seek genetic counseling when a child has features of an inherited condition. Any child who is born with more than one birth defect, mental retardation, or dysmorphic features has an increased chance of having a genetic syndrome. A common type of mental retardation in males for which genetic testing is available is **fragile X syndrome**. Genetic testing is also available for many other childhood illnesses such as **hemophilia** and **muscular dystrophy**. Genetic counselors work with medical geneticists to determine if a genetic syndrome is present. This process includes a careful examination of family history, medical history of the child, review of pertinent medical records in the family, a physical examination of the child, and sometimes blood work or other diagnostic tests. If a diagnosis is made, then the medical geneticist and genetic counselor review what is known about the inheritance of the condition, the natural history of the condition, treatment options, further examinations that may be needed for health problems common in the diagnosed syndrome and resources for helping the family. The genetic counselor also helps the family adjust to the diagnosis by emotional support and counseling. Many families are devastated by receiving a diagnosis, learning of the likely outcome for the child, and by the loss of the hoped-for healthy child. There would also be a discussion about recurrence risks in the family and who else in the family may be at risk.

Adult genetic counseling

Adults seek genetic counseling when a person in the family decides to be tested for a known genetic

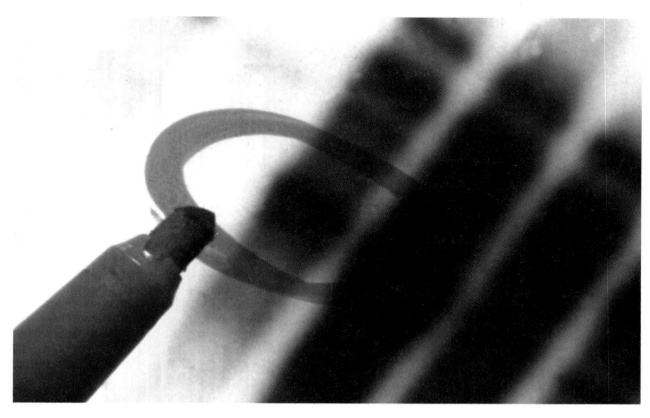

DNA sequencing is used to detect similarities and differences between gene sequences of family members. (*Custom Medical Stock Photo, Inc.*)

condition in the family, when an adult begins exhibiting symptoms of an inherited condition or when there is a new diagnosis of someone with an adult onset disorder in the family. In addition, sometimes the birth of a child with obvious features of a genetic disease leads to diagnosis of a parent who is affected more mildly. Genetic counseling for adults may lead to the consideration of presymptomatic genetic testing. Testing a person to determine if they will be symptomatic for a condition before the symptoms occur is an area of controversy. **Huntington disease** is an example of a genetic disease for which presymptomatic testing is available. Huntington disease is a neurological disease resulting in **dementia**. Onset of the condition is between 30 to 50 years of age. Huntington disease is inherited in an autosomal dominant pattern. If a person has a parent with the disease, their risk of being affected is 50%. Would presymptomatic testing relieve or create anxiety? Would a person benefit from removal of doubt about being affected? Would knowing help a person with life planning? Genetic counselors help patients sort through their feelings about such testing and whether or not the results would be helpful to them.

Cancer genetic counseling

A family history of early onset breast, ovarian, or colon cancer in multiple generations of a family is a common reason a person would seek a genetic counselor that works with cancer patients. While most cancer is not inherited, there are some families in which a dominant **gene** is present and causing the disease. The genetic counselor is able to discuss with a patient the chance that the cancer in the family is related to a dominantly inherited gene. The counselor can also discuss the option of testing for the breast and **ovarian cancer** genes, BRCA1 and BRCA2. In some cases the person seeking testing has already had cancer, and in others they have not. Therefore, presymptomatic testing is also an issue in cancer genetics. Emotional support is important for these patients as they have often lost close relatives from cancer and are fearful of their own risks. For families in which a dominant form of cancer is detected through genetic testing, a plan for increased surveillance for the disease can be made.

The pedigree

In all types of genetic counseling, an important aspect of the genetic counseling session is information

KEY TERMS

Canavan disease—A serious genetic disease more common in the Eastern European Jewish population that causes mental retardation and early death. Canavan disease is caused by the lack of an enzyme called aspartoacylase.

Cystic fibrosis—A respiratory disease characterized by chronic lung disease, pancreatic insufficiency and an average age of survival of 20 years. Cystic fibrosis is caused by mutations in a gene on chromosome 7 that encode a transmembrane receptor.

Dysmorphic feature—A subtle change in appearance such as low set ears or a flattened nasal bridge that suggests a genetic syndrome may be present.

Fragile X syndrome—A condition caused by an abnormality of a region on the X chromosome which may be expressed in males or females, and may increase in severity when inherited from the mother.

Human Genome Project—An international collaborative project among scientists to map the genetic sequence of all the chromosomes. This project is funded by the National Institute of Health in the United States.

Informed consent—Provision of complete information to a competent individual regarding a treatment or test. Part of informed consent is to ensure a patient's understanding of the pros and cons of a procedure and to get their voluntary authorization to perform the procedure.

Sickle cell anemia—A chronic, inherited blood disorder characterized by sickle-shaped red blood cells. It occurs primarily in people of African descent, and produces symptoms including episodic pain in the joints, fever, leg ulcers, and jaundice.

Tay-Sachs disease—An inherited biochemical disease caused by lack of a specific enzyme in the body. In classical Tay-Sachs disease, previously normal children become blind and mentally handicapped, develop seizures, and decline rapidly. Death often occurs between the ages of three to five years. Tay-Sachs disease is common among individuals of eastern European Jewish background but has been reported in other ethnic groups.

Thalassemia—An inherited group of anemias occurring primarily among people of Mediterranean descent. It is caused by defective formation of part of the hemoglobin molecule.

gathering about family and medical history. Information gathering is performed by drawing a chart called a pedigree. A pedigree is made of symbols and lines that represent the family history. To accurately assess the risk of inherited diseases, information about three generations of the family, including health status and/or cause of death, is usually needed. If the family history is complicated, information from more distant relatives may be helpful, and medical records may be requested for any family members who have had a genetic disorder. Through an examination of the family history a counselor may be able to discuss the probability of future occurrence of genetic disorders.

Ethnicity

In taking a family history, a genetic counselor asks the patient's ethnicity or ancestral origin. There are some ethnic groups that have a higher chance of being carriers of some genetic diseases. For instance, the chance that an African American is a carrier of a gene for **sickle cell disease** is 1/10. People of Jewish ancestry are more likely to be carriers of several conditions including **Tay-Sachs disease**, **Canavan disease** and

cystic fibrosis. People of Mediterranean ancestry are more likely to be carriers of a type of anemia called **thalassemia**. Genetic counselors discuss inheritance patterns of these diseases, carrier risks, and genetic screening or testing options.

Consangunity

Another question a genetic counselor asks in taking a family history is if the couple is related to one another by blood. The practice of marrying or having children with relatives is infrequent in the United States, but is more common in some countries. When two people are related by blood, there is an increased chance for their children to be affected with conditions inherited in a recessive pattern. In recessive inheritance, each parent of a child affected with a disease carries a single gene for the disease. The child gets two copies, one from each parent, and is affected. People who have a common ancestor are more likely than unrelated people to be carriers of genes for the same recessively inherited genes. Depending on family history and ethnic background, blood tests can be offered to couples to get more information about the chance for these conditions to occur.

Exposures during pregnancy

During prenatal genetic counseling, the counselor will ask about pregnancy history. If the patient has taken a medication or has had a harmful exposure (like radiation), the genetic counselor can discuss the possibility of harmful affects. Ultrasound is often a useful tool to look for some affects of exposures.

Ethical issues in genetic counseling

Prenatal diagnosis of anomalies or **chromosomal abnormalities** leads to a decision about whether or not a couple wishes to continue a pregnancy. Some couples chose to continue a pregnancy. Prenatal diagnosis gives them additional time to emotionally prepare for the birth of the child and to gather resources. Others choose not to continue a pregnancy in which problems have been diagnosed. These couples have unique emotional needs. Often the child is very much a desired addition to the family and parents are devastated that the child is not healthy. Presymptomatic testing for adult onset disorders and cancer raise difficult issues regarding the need to know and the reality of dealing with abnormal results before symptoms. The National Society of Genetic Counselors has created a Code of Ethics to guide genetic counselors in caring for patients. The Code of Ethics consists of four ethical principles:

- Beneficience is the promotion of personal well being in others. The genetic counselor is an advocate for the patient.
- Nonmaleficience is the idea of doing no harm to a patient.
- Autonomy is recognizing the value of the individual, the person's abilities and their point of view. Important aspects of autonomy are truthfulness with patients, respecting confidentiality, and practicing informed consent.
- Justice is providing equal care for all, freedom of choice, and providing a high quality of care.

Perhaps the main ethical principle of genetic counseling is the attempt to provide nondirective counseling. This principle again points to a patient centered approach to care by focusing on the thoughts and feelings of the patient. Five percent of the **Human Genome Project** budget is designated to research involving the best way to deal with ethical issues that arise as new genetic tests become available. Genetic counselors can help patients navigate through the unfamiliar territory of genetic testing.

Resources

BOOKS

Baker, Diane. *A Guide to Genetic Counseling.* New York: John Wiley and Sons, Inc., 1998.

Harper, Peter S. *Practical Genetic Counseling.* Oxford: Butterworth Heinmann, 1998.

ORGANIZATIONS

American Society of Human Genetics. 9650 Rockville Pike, Bethesda, MD 20814-3998. (301) 571-1825. <http://www.faseb.org/genetics/ashg/ashgmenu.htm>.

March of Dimes Birth Defects Foundation. 1275 Mamaroneck Ave., White Plains, NY 10605. (888) 663-4637. resourcecenter@modimes.org. <http://www.modimes.org>.

National Society of Genetic Counselors. 233 Canterbury Dr., Wallingford, PA 19086-6617. (610) 872-1192. <http://www.nsgc.org/GeneticCounselingYou.asp>.

Sonja Rene Eubanks, MS, CGC

Genetic disorders

Variations within the **DNA** sequence of a particular **gene** affect its function, and may cause or predispose an individual a particular disease. Alterations in the genome may increase the frequency of disorder and disease with entire populations.

Although there are many types of genetic disorders, a specific disorder does not have to be inheritable to have a genetic basis. For example, non-heritable disorders can also arise from mutations in somatic cells resulting from exposure to mutagenic factors in the environment. Mutations, whether inherited mutations that appear in every cell of the body, or random mutations affecting a particular cell, can cause groups of cells to grow out of control, or inhibit the processes (contact inhibition processes) that normally prevent this from happening.

Some diseases and disorders are traced to the presence of a single form of a gene, to a mutation in a specific normal gene. Other common conditions, including not only some cancers but also some forms of heart disease and **diabetes**, are polygenic. Variations in a number of genes, in combination with environmental conditions that determine the extent to which these genes are expressed, affect the risk that an individual will develop such conditions. The risk calculations associated with many of the disorders commonly regarded as genetic diseases are often predictable as functions of relatively simple Mendelian **inheritance**.

There are many types of genetic diseases and disorders result from a few well-established mechanisms. Autosomal dominant disorders, in which one deleterious gene or allele expresses itself over a normal complementary allele is normal is the mechanism underlying

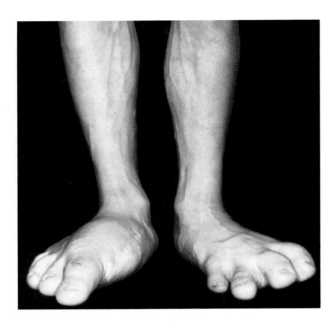

Abnormal formation of body systems and parts, for instance the gigantism of feet, often assists with diagnosis of specific inherited disorders. (*Custom Medical Stock Photos, Inc.*)

Crouzon disease. In contrast, **phenylketonuria**, is an autosomal recessive disorder, in which both deleterious alleles must be present. There are also sex-linked diseases and disorders wherein the deleterious gene or genes lie on sex chromosomes (X and Y chromosomes). There are X-linked dominant disorders (e.g., hypoplastic amelogenesis imperfecta), X-linked recessive disorders (Menkes' syndrome), and Y-linked disorders, in which the only mechanism of transmission is from father to son.

Not all genetic disorders depend on alterations to nuclear DNA. There are disorders, such as mitochondrial myopathy, that can result from alterations to mitochondrial DNA.

Genetic counseling deals with the problems associated with the diagnosis of a genetic disorder, the probable disease course, and possible treatments and management. **Genetic testing** used to assess the risks of genetic disorders and the risks of recurrence. Options for dealing with the risk of a genetic disorder and its recurrence sometimes involve methods of contraception, adoption, insemination by donor sperm, and prenatal diagnosis.

Bayes' theorem is used in genetic epidemiology in order to obtain the probability of disease in a group of people with some characteristic. In addition, Bayes' theorem is able to calculate unknown conditional probabilities (PVP) from known conditional probabilities (detection rate or sensitivity). For example, biochemical and ultrasound marker-based screening use a derivation of Bayes' theorem to select patients for whom further testing for a particular disease or disorder may be appropriate.

A variation of Bayes' theorem, termed the Bart's test, is very popular in the prenatal screening projects. Bart's test allows an adjustment of the probability of the disease (expressed as 1/total) for an appropriate factor named likelihood ratio, that is the ratio between the detection rate and the false positive rate.

Except for genes appearing on the X or Y chromosomes in males, there are usually two copies of each gene in humans. This redundancy provides a buffer to genetic diseases and disorders. In many cases, only one correctly functioning copy of a gene is necessary. Only when an individual has obtained two copies of an abnormal recessive gene will the corresponding disease manifest itself. Inheritance of this type is called homozygous recessive.

A heterozygous individual with one allele for such a condition may be completely unaffected. In other cases, the individual may even be at an advantage, which provides a clue as to why the mutation remains in the population. **Sickle cell disease**, relatively common among people of African descent, is an often-fatal condition in which red blood cells become sickle-shaped when the oxygen content of the blood decreases, as it does during physical exertion. The deformed blood cells block small blood vessels, causing tissue death (necrosis) in affected areas. Although only an individual with two alleles for sickle cell will have the disease, individuals with one sickle cell allele (type pf gene) have sickle cell trait. Trait carriers only experience disease-like symptoms at extreme low-oxygen conditions such as those found at very high altitudes. On the other hand, such an individual actually gains a significant advantage relative to malarial resistance. Malaria is endemic in Africa, and the evolutionary benefit of having a large population of people who are heterozygous for the trait overcomes the disadvantage of a fatal condition affecting homozygotes with two copies of the allele. Therefore this type of genetic disease may persist at a relatively high frequency in a population over a long period of time even if the actual disorder is serious or potentially fatal.

With dominant alleles, one copy of a defective gene is enough to produce a disease or disorder. Genetic disorders with dominant inheritance that are lethal at an early age do not remain in the population, because they kill the affected individual before he or she can reproduce. However, nonlethal dominant genetic disorders, such as the hand and foot malformation called camptobrachydactyly, do persist over time. Likewise, a lethal genetic disorder such as Huntington's disease that strikes after the individual has reached reproductive maturity can also be passed along to future generations.

If the gene associated with a disorder is found on the X **chromosome**, typically males are afflicted more often and/or more severely than females. That is because in females who are heterozygous for such an X-linked trait, there is a normal version of the gene to compensate. Males have only one X chromosome, so if a X-linked gene is mutated, it usually has a severe effect. X-linked genetic disorders include **hemophilia** and red-green **color blindness**.

Chromosome abnormalities, such as the addition or deletion of a chromosome, may result from errors that occur when gametes (sperm and egg) are formed, during fertilization, or during the early development of the **zygote**. Most chromosome aberrations are lethal, resulting in spontaneous abortion (miscarriage), or death in infancy. Only a few, including the extra copy of chromosome 21 that results in **Down syndrome**, produces individuals who, although affected by mental and physical abnormalities, can survive into adulthood.

Abdel Hakim Ben Nasr, PhD

Genetic mapping

The aim of genetic mapping is to determine the linear sequence of genes in genetic material. The mapping can be performed at several levels of detail (resolution) that fall into two broad types: traditional genetic or linkage mapping and more detailed physical mapping.

Linkage mapping shows the relative rather than absolute positions of genes along a **chromosome** and is a technique that has been used since the early 1900s. Early geneticists determined that genes were found on chromosomes. They also reasoned that because the various forms of genes, or alleles, could be precisely exchanged during meiosis through crossovers between homologous chromosomes, the genes for specific characteristics must lie at precise points along each chromosome. It followed that the mapping of chromosomes could, therefore, be made from the observation of crossovers. Between 1912 and 1915, the American scientist Thomas Hunt Morgan (1866–1945) hypothesized that if genes were arranged linearly along chromosomes, then those genes lying closer together would be separated by crossovers less often than those lying further apart. Genes lying closer together would thus have a greater

probability of being passed along as a unit. It follows that the percentage of crossovers would be proportional to the distance between two genes on a chromosome. The percentage crossover can be expressed as the number of crossovers between two genes in meiosis. One genetic map unit (m.u.) is defined as the distance between **gene** pairs for which one product out of 100 is recombinant (a product of crossover). S recombinant frequency (R.F.) of 0.01 (1%) is defined as 1 m.u., and a map unit is sometimes referred to as a centimorgan (cM) in honor of Thomas Hunt Morgan.

As an example of how linkage mapping might work, suppose two characteristics, A and B, show a 26% crossover. Assign 26 crossover units to the distance between these two genes. If a characteristic C turns out in breeding experiments to have 9% crossover with B and 17% crossover with A, it would then be located between A and B at a point 9 units from B and 17 units from A. Compiling the information from many such breeding experiments creates a chromosome map that indicates the relative positions of the genes that code for certain characteristics. Accordingly, the further apart any two genes are on the same chromosome, the greater the incidence of crossing over between them.

A linkage map is limited because recombination frequencies can be distorted relative to the physical distance between sites. As a result, the linkage map is not always the best possible representation of genetic material.

While linkage maps only indicate relative positions of genes, physical maps are more accurate and aim to show the actual number of nucleotides between each gene. Restriction maps are constructed by cleaving **DNA** into fragments with restriction enzymes. These enzymes recognize specific short DNA sequences and cut the duplex. The distances between the sites of cleavage are then measured. The positions of the target restriction sites for these enzymes along the chromosome can be used as DNA markers. Restriction sites generally exist in the same positions on homologous chromosomes so the positions of these target sites can be used rather like milestones along a road and can act as reference points for locating significant features in the chromosome.

A map of the positions of restriction sites can be made for a localized region of a chromosome. It is made by comparing the sizes of single enzyme breakages (digests) of the region of interest with double digests of the same region. This means that two different restriction enzymes are applied, one to each of two separate chromosome extracts of the region of interest, and subsequently the two enzymes are used together in a third digestion with the chromosome extract. The chromosome fragments resulting from the three digestions are then subjected to a biochemical procedure known as gel electrophoresis, which separates them and gives an estimation of their size. Comparison of the sizes of the chromosome fragments resulting from single and double restriction enzyme digestions allows for an approximate location of the target restriction sites. Thus, such maps represent linear sequences of restriction sites. As this procedure determines the sizes of digested chromosome fragments, the distances between sites in terms of the length of DNA can be calculated, because the size of a fragment estimated from an electrophoresis experiment is proportional to the number of base pairs in that fragment.

A restriction map does not intrinsically identify sites of genetic interest. For it to be of practical use, mutations have to be characterized in terms of their effects upon the restriction sites. In the 1980s, it was shown how restriction fragment length polymorphisms (RFLPs) could be used to map human disease genes. RFLPs are inherited by Mendelian segregation and are distributed in populations as classical examples of common genetic polymorphisms. If such a DNA variant is located close to a defective gene (which cannot be tested directly), the DNA variant can be used as a marker to detect the presence of the disease-causing gene. The prenatal examination of DNA for particular enzyme sites associated with certain hereditary diseases has proved to be an important method of diagnosis. Clinically useful polymorphic restriction enzyme sites have been detected within the Beta-like globin gene cluster. For example, the absence of a recognition site for the restriction enzyme HpaI is frequently associated with the allele for sickle-cell anemia, and this association has been useful in prenatal diagnosis of this disease.

The ultimate genetic map is the complete nucleotide sequence of the DNA in the whole chromosome complement, or genome, of an organism. Today, several completed genome maps already exist. Simple prokaryotic organisms, e.g., bacteria, with their relatively small chromosomes of one to two million base pairs were the first to be mapped. Later, eukaryotic organisms such as the yeast, *Saccharomyces cerevisiae*, and the nematode worm, *Caenorhabditis elegans*, were mapped. In 2000, the **Human Genome Project** produced the first draft of the human genome. The project adopted two methods for mapping the three billion nucleotides. The earlier approach was a "clone by clone" method. In this, the entire genome was cut into fragments up to several thousand base pairs long, and inserted into synthetic chromosomes known as bacterial artificial chromosomes (BACs). The subsequent mapping step involved positioning the BACs on the genome's chromosomes by looking for distinctive marker sequences called sequence tagged sites (STSs), whose location had already been

pinpointed. Clones of the BACs are then broken into smaller fragments in a process known as shotgun cloning. Each small fragment was then sequenced and computer algorithms, that recognize matching sequence information from overlapping fragments, were used to reconstruct the complete sequence inserted into each BAC. It was later argued that the first mapping step was unnecessary and that the algorithms used to reassemble the shotgunned DNA fragments could be applied to cloned random fragments taken directly from the whole genome. In this whole genome shotgun strategy, fragments were first assembled by algorithms into larger scaffolds and the correct position of these scaffolds on the genome was worked out by STSs. The latter method speeded up the whole procedure considerably and is currently being used to sequence genomes from other organisms.

Judyth Sassoon, ARCS, PhD

Genetic screening *see* **Genetic testing**

Genetic testing

Definition

A genetic test examines the genetic information contained inside a person's cells, called **DNA**, to determine if that person has or will develop a certain disease or could pass a disease to his or her offspring. Genetic tests also determine whether or not couples are at a higher risk than the general population for having a child affected with a genetic disorder.

Purpose

Some families or ethnic groups have a higher incidence of a certain disease than does the population as a whole. For example, individuals from Eastern European, Ashkenazi Jewish descent are at higher risk for carrying genes for rare conditions that occur much less frequently in populations from other parts of the world. Before having a child, a couple from such a family or ethnic group may want to know if their child would be at risk of having that disease. Genetic testing for this type of purpose is called genetic screening.

During pregnancy, the baby's cells can be studied for certain **genetic disorders** or chromosomal problems such as **Down syndrome**. **Chromosome** testing is most commonly offered when the mother is 35 years or older at the time of delivery. When there is a family medical history of a genetic disease or there are individuals in a family affected with developmental and physical delays, genetic testing may also be offered during pregnancy. Genetic testing during pregnancy is called prenatal diagnosis.

Prior to becoming pregnant, couples who are having difficulty conceiving a child or who have suffered multiple miscarriages may be tested to see if a genetic cause can be identified.

A genetic disease may be diagnosed at birth by doing a physical evaluation of the baby and observing characteristics of the disorder. Genetic testing can help to confirm the diagnosis made by the physical evaluation. In addition, genetic testing is used routinely on all newborns to screen for certain genetic diseases which can affect a newborn baby's health shortly after birth.

There are several genetic diseases and conditions in which the symptoms do not occur until adulthood. One such example is **Huntington's disease.** This is a serious disorder affecting the way in which individuals walk, talk and function on a daily basis. Genetic testing may be able to determine if someone at risk for the disease will in fact develop the disease.

Some genetic defects may make a person more susceptible to certain types of **cancer.** Testing for these defects can help predict a person's risk. Other types of genetic tests help diagnose and predict and monitor the course of certain kinds of cancer, particularly leukemia and lymphoma.

Precautions

Because genetic testing is not always accurate and because there are many concerns surrounding insurance and employment discrimination for the individual receiving a genetic test, **genetic counseling** should always be performed prior to genetic testing. A genetic counselor is an individual with a master's degree in genetic counseling. A medical geneticist is a physician specializing and board certified in genetics.

A genetic counselor reviews the person's family history and medical records and the reason for the test. The counselor explains the likelihood that the test will detect all possible causes of the disease in question (known as the sensitivity of the test), and the likelihood that the disease will develop if the test is positive (known as the positive predictive value of the test).

Learning about the disease in question, the benefits and risks of both a positive and a negative result, and what treatment choices are available if the result is positive, will help prepare the person undergoing testing. During the genetic counseling session, the individual interested in genetic testing will be asked to consider

how the test results will affect his or her life, family, and future decisions.

After this discussion, the person should have the opportunity to indicate in writing that he or she gave informed consent to have the test performed, verifying that the counselor provided complete and understandable information.

Background

Genes and chromosomes

Deoxyribonucleic acid (DNA) is a long molecule made up of two strands of genetic material coiled around each other in a unique double helix structure. This structure was discovered in 1953 by Francis Crick and James Watson.

DNA is found in the nucleus, or center, of most cells (Some cells, such as a red blood cell, don't have a nucleus). Each person's DNA is a unique blueprint, giving instructions for a person's physical traits, such as eye color, hair texture, height, and susceptibility to disease. DNA is organized into structures called chromosomes.

The instructions are contained in DNA's long strands as a code spelled out by pairs of bases, which are four chemicals that make up DNA. The bases occur as pairs because a base on one strand lines up with and is bound to a corresponding base on the other strand. The order of these bases form DNA's code. The order of the bases on a DNA strand is important to ensuring a person is not affected with any genetic disorders. When the bases are out of order or missing, cells may often not produce important proteins; this can lead to a genetic disorder. While genes are found in every cell of the body, not every **gene** is functioning all of the time. Some genes are turned on during critical points in development and then remain silent for the rest of an individual's life. Other genes always remain active so that cells can produce important proteins such as those that help digest food properly or fight off the common cold.

The specific order of the base pairs on a strand of DNA is important in order for the correct protein to be produced. A grouping of three base pairs on the DNA strand is called a codon. Each codon, or three base pairs, comes together to spell a word. A string of many codons together can be thought of as a series of words all coming together to make a sentence. This sentence is what instructs cells to make a protein that helps bodies function properly.

DNA strands containing a hundred to several thousand copies of genes are found on structures called chromosomes. Each cell typically has 46 chromosomes arranged into 23 pairs. Each parent contributes one chromosome to each pair. The first 22 pairs are called autosomal chromosomes, or non-sex chromosomes and are assigned a number from 1–22. The last pair are the sex chromosomes and include the X and the Y chromosomes. If a child receives an X chromosome from each parent, the child is female. If a child receives an X from the mother, and a Y from the father, the child is male.

Just as each parent contributes one chromosome to each pair, so each parent contributes one gene from each chromosome. The pair of genes produces a specific trait in the child. In autosomal dominant conditions, it takes only one copy of a gene to influence a specific trait. The stronger gene is called dominant; the weaker gene is called recessive. Two copies of a recessive gene are needed to control a trait, while only one copy of a dominant gene is needed. Our sex chromosomes, the X and the Y, also contain important genes. Some genetic diseases are caused by missing or altered genes on one of the sex chromosomes. Males are most often affected by sex chromosome diseases when they inherit an X chromosome with missing or mutated genes from their mother.

Types of genetic mutations

Genetic disease results from a change, or mutation, in a chromosome or in one or several base pairs on a gene. Some of us inherit these mutations from our parents, called hereditary or germline mutations, while other mutations can occur spontaneously, or for the first time in an affected child. For many of the adult on-set diseases, genetic mutations can occur over the lifetime of the individual. This is called acquired or somatic mutations, and these occur while the cells are making copies of themselves or dividing in two. There may be some environmental effects, such as radiation or other chemicals, that can contribute to these types of mutations as well.

There are a variety of different types of mutations that can occur in the genetic code to cause a disease. And for each genetic disease, there may be more than one type of mutation to cause the disease. For some genetic diseases, the same mutation occurs in every individual affected with the disease. For example, the most common form of dwarfism, called **achondroplasia**, occurs because of a single base pair substitution. This same mutation occurs in all individuals affected with the disease. Other genetic diseases are caused by different types of genetic mutations that may occur anywhere along the length of a gene. For example, **cystic fibrosis**, the most common genetic disease in the caucasian population, is caused by hundreds of different mutations along the

gene. Individual families may carry the same mutation as each other, but not as the rest of the population affected with the same genetic disease.

Some genetic diseases occur as a result of a larger mutation that can occur when the chromosome itself is either rearranged or altered or when a baby is born with more than the expected number of chromosomes. There are only a few types of chromosome rearrangements that are possibly hereditary, or passed on from the mother or the father. The majority of chromosome alterations occur sporadically or for the first time with a new baby.

The type of mutation that causes a genetic disease will determine the type of genetic test to be performed. In some situations, more than one type of genetic test will be performed to arrive at a diagnosis. The cost of genetic tests vary: chromosome studies can cost hundreds of dollars and certain gene studies can cost thousands. Insurance coverage also varies with the company and the policy. It may take several days or several weeks to complete a test. Research testing where the exact location of a gene has not yet been identified, can take several months or years for results.

Types of Genetic Testing

Direct DNA mutation analysis

Direct DNA sequencing examines the direct base pair sequence of a gene for specific **gene mutations**. Some genes contain more than 100,000 bases; a mutation of any one base can make the gene nonfunctional and cause disease. The more mutations possible, the less likely it is for a test to detect all of them. This test is usually done on white blood cells from a person's blood, but can also be performed on other tissues. There are different ways in which to perform direct DNA mutation analysis. When the specific genetic mutation is known, it is possible to perform a complete analysis of the genetic code, also called direct sequencing. There are several different lab techniques used to test for a direct mutation. One common approach begins by using chemicals to separate DNA from the rest of the cell. Next, the two strands of DNA are separated by heating. Special enzymes (called restriction enzymes) are added to the single strands of DNA; they then act like scissors and cut the strands in specific places. The DNA fragments are then sorted by size through a process called electrophoresis. A special piece of DNA, called a probe, is added to the fragments. The probe is designed to bind to specific mutated portions of the gene. When bound to the probe, the mutated portions appear on x-ray film with a distinct banding pattern.

Indirect DNA testing

Family linkage studies are done to study a disease when the exact type and location of the genetic alteration is not known, but the general location on the chromosome has been identified. These studies are possible when a chromosome marker has been found associated with a disease. Chromosomes contain certain regions that vary in appearance between individuals. These regions are called polymorphisms and do not cause a genetic disease to occur. If a polymorphism is always present in family members with the same genetic disease, and absent in family members without the disease, it is likely that the gene responsible for the disease is near that polymorphism. The gene mutation can be indirectly detected in family members by looking for the polymorphism.

To look for the polymorphism, DNA is isolated from cells in the same way it is for direct DNA mutation analysis. A probe is added that will detect the large polymorphism on the chromosome. When bound to the probe, this region will appear on x-ray film with a distinct banding pattern. The pattern of banding of a person being tested for the disease is compared to the pattern from a family member affected by the disease.

Linkage studies have disadvantages not found in direct DNA mutation analysis. These studies require multiple family members to participate in the testing. If key family members choose not to participate, the incomplete family history may make testing other members useless. The indirect method of detecting a mutated gene also causes more opportunity for error.

Chromosome analysis

Various genetic syndromes are caused by structural chromosome abnormalities. To analyze a person's chromosomes, his or her cells are allowed to grow and multiply in the laboratory until they reach a certain stage of growth. The length of growing time varies with the type of cells. Cells from blood and bone marrow take one to two days; fetal cells from amniotic fluid take 7–10 days.

When the cells are ready, they are placed on a microscope slide using a technique to make them burst open, spreading their chromosomes. The slides are stained: the stain creates a banding pattern unique to each chromosome. Under a microscope, the chromosomes are counted, identified, and analyzed based on their size, shape, and stained appearance.

A **karyotype** is the final step in the chromosome analysis. After the chromosomes are counted, a photograph is taken of the chromosomes from one or more cells as seen through the microscope. Then the chromo-

somes are cut out and arranged side-by-side with their partner in ascending numerical order, from largest to smallest. The karyotype is done either manually or using a computer attached to the microscope. Chromosome analysis is also called cytogenetics.

Applications for genetic testing

Newborn screening

Genetic testing is used most often for newborn screening. Every year, millions of newborn babies have their blood samples tested for potentially serious genetic diseases.

Carrier testing

An individual who has a gene associated with a disease but never exhibits any symptoms of the disease is called a carrier. A carrier is a person who is not affected by the mutated gene he or she possesses, but can pass the gene to an offspring. Genetic tests have been developed that tell prospective parents whether or not they are carriers of certain diseases. If one or both parents are a carrier, the risk of passing the disease to a child can be predicted.

To predict the risk, it is necessary to know if the gene in question is autosomal or sex-linked. If the gene is carried on any one of chromosomes 1–22, the resulting disease is called an autosomal disease. If the gene is carried on the X or Y chromosome, it is called a sex-linked disease.

Sex-linked diseases, such as the bleeding condition **hemophilia**, are usually carried on the X chromosome. A woman who carries a disease-associated gene on one of her X chromosomes has a 50% chance of passing that gene to her son. A son who inherits that gene will develop the disease because he does not have another normal copy of the gene on a second X chromosome to compensate for the abnormal copy. A daughter who inherits the disease-associated gene from her mother will be at risk for having a son affected with the disease.

The risk of passing an autosomal disease to a child depends on whether the gene is dominant or recessive. A prospective parent carrying a dominant gene has a 50% chance of passing the gene to a child. A child needs to receive only one copy of the mutated gene to be affected by the disease.

If the gene is recessive, a child needs to receive two copies of the mutated gene, one from each parent, to be affected by the disease. When both parents are carriers, their child has a 25% chance of inheriting two copies of the mutated gene and being affected by the disease; a 50% chance of inheriting one copy of the mutated gene, and being a carrier of the disease but not affected; and a 25% chance of inheriting two normal genes. When only one parent is a carrier, a child has a 50% chance of inheriting one mutated gene and being an unaffected carrier of the disease, and a 50% chance of inheriting two normal genes.

Cystic fibrosis is a disease that affects the lungs and pancreas and is discovered in early childhood. It is the most common autosomal recessive genetic disease found in the caucasian population: one in 25 people of Northern European ancestry are carriers of a mutated cystic fibrosis gene. The gene, located on chromosome 7, was identified in 1989.

The gene mutation for cystic fibrosis is detected by a direct DNA test. Over 600 mutations of the cystic fibrosis gene have been found; each of these mutations cause the same disease. Tests are available for the most common mutations. Tests that check for the 86 of the most common mutations in the Caucasian population will detect 90% of carriers for cystic fibrosis. (The percentage of mutations detected varies according to the individual's ethnic background). If a person tests negative, it is likely, but not guaranteed that he or she does not have the gene. Both parents must be carriers of the gene to have a child with cystic fibrosis.

Tay-Sachs disease, also autosomal recessive, affects children primarily of Ashkenazi Jewish descent. Children with this disease die between the ages of two and five. This disease was previously detected by looking for a missing enzyme. The mutated gene has now been identified and can be detected using direct DNA mutation analysis.

Presymptomatic testing

Not all genetic diseases show their effect immediately at birth or early in childhood. Although the gene mutation is present at birth, some diseases do not appear until adulthood. If a specific mutated gene responsible for a late-onset disease has been identified, a person from an affected family can be tested before symptoms appear.

Huntington disease is one example of a late-onset autosomal dominant disease. Its symptoms of mental confusion and abnormal body movements do not appear until middle to late adulthood. The chromosome location of the gene responsible for Huntington chorea was located in 1983 after studying the DNA from a large Venezuelan family affected by the disease. Ten years later the gene was identified. A test is now available to detect the presence of the expanded base pair sequence responsible for causing the disease. The presence of this expanded sequence means the person will develop the disease.

Another late onset disease, Alzheimer's, does not have as well a understood genetic cause as Huntington disease. The specific genetic cause of **Alzheimer disease** is not as clear. Although many cases appear to be inherited in an autosomal dominant pattern, many cases exist as single incidents in a family. Like Huntington, symptoms of mental deterioration first appear in adulthood. Genetic research has found an association between this disease and genes on four different chromosomes. The validity of looking for these genes in a person without symptoms or without family history of the disease is still being studied.

CANCER SUSCEPTIBILITY TESTING Cancer can result from an inherited (germline) mutated gene or a gene that mutated sometime during a person's lifetime (acquired mutation). Some genes, called tumor suppressor genes, produce proteins that protect the body from cancer. If one of these genes develops a mutation, it is unable to produce the protective protein. If the second copy of the gene is normal, its action may be sufficient to continue production, but if that gene later also develops a mutation, the person is vulnerable to cancer. Other genes, called oncogenes, are involved in the normal growth of cells. A mutation in an **oncogene** can cause too much growth, which is the beginning of cancer.

Direct DNA tests are currently available to look for gene mutations identified and linked to several kinds of cancer. People with a family history of these cancers are those most likely to be tested. If one of these mutated genes is found, the person is more susceptible to developing the cancer. The likelihood that the person will develop the cancer, even with the mutated gene, is not always known because other genetic and environmental factors are also involved in the development of cancer.

Cancer susceptibility tests are most useful when a positive test result can be followed with clear treatment options. In families with familial polyposis of the colon, testing a child for a mutated APC gene can reveal whether or not the child needs frequent monitoring for the disease. In families with potentially fatal familial medullary thyroid cancer or multiple endocrine neoplasia type 2, finding a mutated RET gene in a child provides the opportunity for that child to have preventive removal of the thyroid gland. In the same way, MSH1 and MSH2 mutations can reveal which members in an affected family are vulnerable to familiar colorectal cancer and would benefit from aggressive monitoring.

In 1994, a mutation linked to early-onset familial breast and **ovarian cancer** was identified. BRCA1 is located on chromosome 17. Women with a mutated form of this gene have an increased risk of developing breast and ovarian cancer. A second related gene, BRCA2, was later discovered. Located on chromosome 13, it also carries increased risk of breast and ovarian cancer. Although both genes are rare in the general population, they are slightly more common in women of Ashkenazi Jewish descent.

When a woman is found to have a mutation in one of these genes, the likelihood that she will get breast or ovarian cancer increases, but not to 100%. Other genetic and environmental factors influence the outcome.

Testing for these genes is most valuable in families where a mutation has already been found. BRCA1 and BRCA2 are large genes; BRCA1 includes 100,000 bases. More than 120 mutations to this gene have been discovered, but a mutation could occur in any one of the bases. Studies show tests for these genes may miss 30% of existing mutations. The rate of missed mutations, the unknown disease likelihood in spite of a positive result and the lack of a clear preventive response to a positive result, make the value of this test for the general population uncertain.

Prenatal and postnatal chromosome analysis

Chromosome analysis is performed on fetal cells primarily when the mother is age 35 or older at the time of delivery, has experienced multiple miscarriages, or reports a family history of a genetic abnormality. Prenatal testing is done on the fetal cells from a chorionic villus sampling (from the baby's developing placenta) at 10–12 weeks or from the amniotic fluid (the fluid surrounding the baby) at 16–18 weeks of pregnancy. Cells from amniotic fluid grow for 7–10 days before they are ready to be analyzed. Chorionic villi cells have the potential to grow faster and can be analyzed sooner.

Chromosome analysis using blood cells is done on a child who is born with or later develops signs of mental retardation or physical malformation. In the older child, chromosome analysis may be done to investigate developmental delays.

Extra or missing chromosomes cause mental and physical abnormalities. A child born with an extra chromosome 21 (trisomy 21) has Down syndrome. An extra chromosome 13 or 18 also produce well known syndromes. A missing X chromosome causes **Turner syndrome** and an extra X in a male causes **Klinefelter syndrome**. Other abnormalities are caused by extra or missing pieces of chromosomes. **Fragile X syndrome** is a sex-linked disease that causes mental retardation in males.

Chromosome material may also be rearranged, such as the end of chromosome 1 moving to the end of chromosome 3. This is called a chromosomal translocation. If no material is added or deleted in the exchange, the person may not be affected. Such an exchange, however, can cause infertility or abnormalities if passed to children.

Evaluation of a man and woman's infertility or repeated miscarriages will include blood studies of both to check for a chromosome translocation. Many chromosome abnormalities are incompatible with life; babies with these abnormalities often miscarry during the first trimester. Cells from a baby that died before birth can be studied to look for chromosome abnormalities that may have caused the death.

Cancer diagnosis and prognosis

Certain cancers, particularly leukemia and lymphoma, are associated with changes in chromosomes: extra or missing complete chromosomes, extra or missing portions of chromosomes, or exchanges of material (translocations) between chromosomes. Studies show that the locations of the chromosome breaks are at locations of tumor suppressor genes or oncogenes.

Chromosome analysis on cells from blood, bone marrow, or solid tumor helps diagnose certain kinds of leukemia and lymphoma and often helps predict how well the person will respond to treatment. After treatment has begun, periodic monitoring of these chromosome changes in the blood and bone marrow gives the physician information as to the effectiveness of the treatment.

A well-known chromosome rearrangement is found in chronic myelogenous leukemia. This leukemia is associated with an exchange of material between chromosomes 9 and 22. The resulting smaller chromosome 22 is called the Philadelphia chromosome.

Preparation

Most tests for genetic diseases of children and adults are done on blood. To collect the 5–10 mL of blood needed, a healthcare worker draws blood from a vein in the inner elbow region. Collection of the sample takes only a few minutes.

Prenatal testing is done either on amniotic fluid or a chorionic villus sampling. To collect amniotic fluid, a physician performs a procedure called **amniocentesis**. An ultrasound is done to find the baby's position and an area filled with amniotic fluid. The physician inserts a needle through the woman's skin and the wall of her uterus and withdraws 5–10 mL of amniotic fluid. Placental tissue for a chorionic villus sampling is taken through the cervix. Each procedure takes approximately 30 minutes.

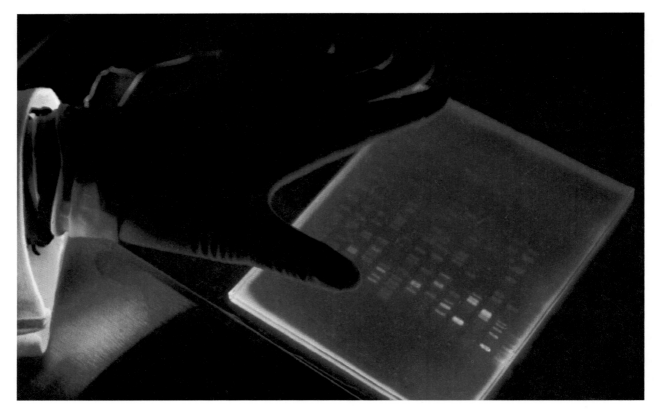

Scientist showing results of gel electrophoresis, a technique used to separate DNA molecules based on their size. (*Photo Researchers, Inc.*)

Bone marrow is used for chromosome analysis in a person with leukemia or lymphoma. The person is given local anesthesia. Then the physician inserts a needle through the skin and into the bone (usually the sternum or hip bone). One-half to 2 mL of bone marrow is withdrawn. This procedure takes approximately 30 minutes.

Aftercare

After blood collection the person can feel discomfort or bruising at the puncture site or may become dizzy or faint. Pressure to the puncture site until the bleeding stops reduces bruising. Warm packs to the puncture site relieve discomfort.

The chorionic villus sampling, amniocentesis and bone marrow procedures are all done under a physician's supervision. The person is asked to rest after the procedure and is watched for weakness and signs of bleeding.

Risks

Collection of amniotic fluid and chorionic villus sampling, have the risk of miscarriage, infection, and bleeding; the risks are higher for the chorionic villus sampling. Because of the potential risks for miscarriage,

0.5% following the amniocentesis and 1% following the chorionic villus sampling procedure, both of these prenatal tests are offered to couples, but not required. A woman should tell her physician immediately if she has cramping, bleeding, fluid loss, an increased temperature, or a change in the baby's movement following either of these procedures.

After bone marrow collection, the puncture site may become tender and the person's temperature may rise. These are signs of a possible infection.

Genetic testing involves other nonphysical risks. Many people fear the possible loss of privacy about personal health information. Results of genetic tests may be reported to insurance companies and affect a person's insurability. Some people pay out-of-pocket for genetic tests to avoid this possibility. Laws have been proposed to deal with this problem. Other family members may be affected by the results of a person's genetic test. Privacy of the person tested and the family members affected is a consideration when deciding to have a test and to share the results.

A positive result carries a psychological burden, especially if the test indicates the person will develop a

KEY TERMS

Autosomal disease—A disease caused by a gene located on an autosomal chromosome.

Carrier—A person who possesses a gene for an abnormal trait without showing signs of the disorder. The person may pass the abnormal gene on to offspring.

Chromosome—A microscopic thread-like structure found within each cell of the body and consists of a complex of proteins and DNA. Humans have 46 chromosomes arranged into 23 pairs. Changes in either the total number of chromosomes or their shape and size (structure) may lead to physical or mental abnormalities.

Deoxyribonucleic acid (DNA)—The genetic material in cells that holds the inherited instructions for growth, development, and cellular functioning.

Dominant gene—A gene, whose presence as a single copy, controls the expression of a trait.

Enzyme—A protein that catalyzes a biochemical reaction or change without changing its own structure or function.

Gene—A building block of inheritance containing the instructions for the production of a particular protein that is made up of a molecular sequence found on a section of DNA. Each gene is found on a precise location on a chromosome.

Karyotype—A standard arrangement of photographic or computer-generated images of chromosome pairs from a cell in ascending numerical order, from largest to smallest.

Mutation—A permanent change in the genetic material that may alter a trait or characteristic of an individual, or manifest as disease, and can be transmitted to offspring.

Positive predictive value (PPV)—The probability that a person with a positive test result has, or will get, the disease.

Recessive gene—A type of gene that is not expressed as a trait unless inherited by both parents.

Sensitivity—The proportion of people with a disease who are correctly diagnosed (test positive based on diagnostic criteria). The higher the sensitivity of a test or diagnostic criteria, the lower the rate of "false negatives"—people who have a disease but are not identified through the test.

Sex-linked disorder—A disorder caused by a gene located on a sex chromosome, usually the X chromosome.

disease, such as Huntington's chorea. The news that a person may be susceptible to a specific kind of cancer, while it may encourage positive preventive measures, may also negatively shadow many decisions and activities.

A genetic test result may also be inconclusive meaning no definitive result can be given to the individual or family. This may cause the individual to feel more anxious and frustrated and experience psychological difficulties.

Prior to undergoing genetic testing, individuals need to learn from the genetic counselor the likelihood that the test could miss a mutation or abnormality.

Normal results

A normal result for chromosome analysis is 46, XX or 46, XY. This means there are 46 chromosomes (including two X chromosomes for a female or one X and one Y for a male) with no structural abnormalities. A normal result for a direct DNA mutation analysis or linkage study is no gene mutation found.

There can be some benefits from genetic testing when the individual tested is not found to carry a genetic mutation. Those who learn with great certainty they are no longer at risk for a genetic disease may choose not to undergo prophylactic therapies and may feel less anxious and relieved.

Abnormal results

An abnormal chromosome analysis report will include the total number of chromosomes and will identify the abnormality found. Tests for gene mutations will report the mutations found.

There are many ethical issues to consider with an abnormal prenatal test result. Many of the diseases tested for during a pregnancy, cannot be treated or cured. In addition, some diseases tested for during pregnancy, may have a late-onset of symptoms or have minimal effects on the affected individual.

Before making decisions based on an abnormal test result, the person should meet again with a genetic counselor to fully understand the meaning of the results, learn what options are available based on the test result, and what are the risks and benefits of each of those options.

Resources

BOOKS

Berg, Paul, and Maxine Singer. *Dealing with Genes: The Language of Heredity.* Mill Valley, CA: University Science Books, 1992.

Farkas, Daniel H. *DNA Simplified: The Hitchhiker's Guide to DNA.* Washington, DC: American Association of Clinical Chemistry Press, 1996.

Gelehrter, Thomas D., Francis S. Collins, and David Ginsburg. *Principles of Medical Genetics.* 2nd ed. Baltimore: Williams and Wilkins, 1998.

Grody, Wayne W., and Walter W. Noll. "Molecular Diagnosis of Genetic Diseases." In *Clinical Diagnosis and Management by Laboratory Methods,* edited by John B. Henry. 19th ed. Philadelphia: W. B. Saunders Company, 1996, pp. 1374-1389.

Holtzman, Neil A., and Michael S. Watson, eds. *Promoting Safe and Effective Genetic Testing in the United States. Final Report of the Task Force on Genetic Testing.* National Institutes of Health-Department of Energy Working Group on Ethical, Legal, and Social Implications of Human Genome Research, 1997.

Motulsky, Arno G., Richard A. King, and Jerome I. Rotter. *The Genetic Basis of Common Diseases.* New York: Oxford University Press, 1992.

Mueller, Robert F., and Ian D. Young. *Emery's Elements of Medical Genetics.* 9th ed. New York and Edinburgh: Churchill Livingstone, 1995.

Watson, James D. *The Double Helix.* New York: Atheneum, 1968.

PERIODICALS

Auxter, Sue. "Genetic Information—What Should be Regulated?" *Clinical Laboratory News* (December 1997): 9-11.

Biesecker, Barbara Bowles. "Genetic Susceptibility Testing for Breast and Ovarian Cancer: A Progress Report." *Journal of the American Medical Women's Association* (Winter 1997): 22-27.

Fink, Leslie, and Francis S. Collins. "The Human Genome Project: View From the National Institutes of Health." *Journal of the American Medical Women's Association* (Winter 1997): 4-7, 15.

Holtzman, Neil A., et al. "Predictive Genetic Testing: From Basic Research to Clinical Practice." *Science* (October 24, 1997): 602-605.

Karnes, Pamela S. "Ordering and Interpreting DNA Tests." *Mayo Clinical Proceedings* (December 1996): 1192-1195.

Malone, Kathleen E, et al. "BRCA1 Mutations and Breast Cancer in the General Population." *Journal of the American Medical Association* (March 25, 1998): 922-929.

McKinnon, Wendy C., et al. "Predisposition Genetic Testing for Late-Onset Disorders in Adults: A Position Paper of the National Society of Genetic Counselors." *Journal of the American Medical Association* (October 15, 1997): 1217-1221.

Newman, Beth, et al. "Frequency of Breast Cancer Attributable to BRCA1 in a Population-Based Series of American Women." *Journal of the American Medical Association* (March 25, 1998): 915-921.

Ponder, Bruce. "Genetic Testing for Cancer Risk." *Science* (November 7, 1997): 1050-1054.

Roses, Allen. "Genetic Testing for Alzheimer Disease. Practical and Ethical Issues." *Archives of Neurology* (October 1997): 1226-1229.

Whittaker, Lori. "Clinical Applications of Genetic Testing: Implications for the Family Physician." *American Family Physician* (May 1996): 2077-2084.

Wisecarver, James. "The ABCs of DNA." *Laboratory Medicine* (January 1997): 48-52.

Yablonsky, Terri. "Genetic Testing Helps Patients and Researchers Predict the Future." *Laboratory Medicine* (May 1997): 316-321.

Yablonsky, Terri. "Unlocking the Secrets to Disease. Genetic Tests Usher in a New Era in Medicine." *Laboratory Medicine* (April 1997): 252-256.

Yan, Hai. "Genetic Testing-Present and Future." *Science* (September 15, 2000): 1890-1892.

ORGANIZATIONS

Alliance of Genetic Support Groups. 4301 Connecticut Ave. NW, Suite 404, Washington, DC 20008. (202) 966-5557. Fax: (202) 966-8553. <http://www.geneticalliance.org>.

American College of Medical Genetics. 9650 Rockville Pike, Bethesda, MD 20814-3998. (301) 571-1825. <http://www.faseb.org/genetics/acmg/acmgmenu.htm>

American Society of Human Genetics. 9650 Rockville Pike, Bethesda, MD 20814-3998. (301) 571-1825. <http://www.faseb.org/genetics/ashg/ashgmenu.htm>.

Centers for Disease Control. GDP Office, 4770 Buford Highway NE, Atlanta, GA 30341-3724. (770) 488-3235. <http://www.cdc.gov/genetics>.

March of Dimes Birth Defects Foundation. 1275 Manaroneck Ave., White Plains, NY 10605. (888) 663-4637. resourcecenter@modimes.org. <http://www.modimes.org>.

National Human Genome Research Institute. The National Institutes of Health, 9000 Rockville Pike, Bethesda, MD 20892. (301) 496-2433. <http://www.nhgri.nih.gov>.

National Society of Genetic Counselors. 233 Canterbury Dr., Wallingford, PA 19086-6617. (610) 872-1192. <http://www.nsgc.org/GeneticCounselingYou.asp>.

OTHER

Blazing a Genetic Trail. Online genetic tutorial. <http://www.hhmi.org/GeneticTrail/>.

The Gene Letter. Online newsletter. <http://www.geneletter.org>.

Online Mendelian Inheritance in Man. Online genetic testing information sponsored by National Center for Biotechnology Information. <http://www.ncbi.nlm.nih.gov/Omim/>.

Understanding Gene Testing. Online brochure produced by the U.S. Department of Health and Human Services. <http://www.gene.com/ae/AE/AEPC/NIH/index.html>.

Katherine S. Hunt, MS

Genetics and congenital anomalies

Definition

Any unusual variation or abnormality in the shape, structure, and/or function of an organ, body part, or tissue is commonly referred to as a birth defect. However, congenital anomaly is the more accurate and preferred term, since birth defect can be misinterpreted to mean a defect produced by the birthing process. Congenital anomalies may be external or internal, single (isolated) or multiple, major or minor, and by definition are present at (and almost always before) birth, although in some cases detection/diagnosis occurs well after birth. As a group, congenital anomalies are common, have a wide range of clinical severity, and can develop, in one form or another, in any anatomical structure or location. There are many different causes of congenital anomalies, known and unknown, but in terms of how they develop, there are four major types: malformations, deformations, disruptions, and dysplasias.

Description

Variation among individuals in physical characteristics, both external and internal, is an essential attribute of any organism that reproduces sexually, including humans. Although less obvious, but no less important, people also differ in their metabolism and other cellular/chemical processes that help form and maintain the body. The process of normal development in the body is called morphogenesis, while abnormal development is known as dysmorphogenesis. Dysmorphology, then, is the study of congenital anomalies, including their formation, causes, and patterns of occurrence.

An important task, in both medical and sociocultural contexts, lies in determining what constitutes a congenital anomaly, and what qualifies as an accepted morphological variant. Further, what distinguishes a major anomaly from a minor one? In other words, what is normal, and what is abnormal? In some cases, the distinction is obvious, in others it is not. Terms such as normal and abnormal are generally agreed to be subjective, and thus not applicable when applied to individuals in a broad context. The same can be said of terms such as defective, anomalous, deformed, malformed, aberrant, irregular,

and the like. Even though some terms and phrases are perceived as subjective, negative, and offensive when misapplied as generalities, they are nonetheless necessary in a medical context. With due sensitivity and care, these same terms can be used clinically in an objective and instructive manner.

Compared with the complex and evolving social issues of perception and acceptance, the medical approach to distinguishing normal variants from minor and major anomalies is more objective and direct. Regardless of the anatomical structure or process, the primary criterion involves evaluating whether its function, shape, structure, and/or size fall within or outside the normal (expected) range. To help answer that question, measurements of every conceivable type have been taken and catalogued over the years on countless individuals. Statistical formulas are applied to the data for a given characteristic or function (e.g., height, weight, blood pressure, serum enzyme levels, etc.) to determine its normal range. If needed, adjustments for age, gender, race, ethnicity, and many other variables can also be made. The results are often graphed and, for most human characteristics, a line drawn through the data points on the graph produces the famous bell curve, a name derived from its shape. Calculations based on such factors as the total number of individuals studied and the range of measurements obtained, among others, are used to mark off a section in the middle of the curve, such that most individuals (usually between 80% and 95%) fall within that range. Therefore, any values above or below (i.e., outside) that range are considered anomalous or abnormal. Measured values for minor anomalies might fall several percentage points on either side of the upper and lower boundaries of the normal range, while major anomalies lie at the ends of the curve.

Among other new challenges, parents and families of children with congenital anomalies are exposed to a bewildering array of new medical terms and phrases, and asked to understand, process, and remember these while likely under a great deal of stress. The practice of medical genetics consists primarily of communicating with individuals and families about difficult and complex issues. Geneticists and genetics counselors are especially sensitive to the psychosocial impact terminology can have on perception and understanding of congenital anomalies/genetic disorders. Parents of a newly diagnosed child inevitably want to know how the anomaly or genetic syndrome occurred. An understanding of the different types of anomalies is the basis for answering that question.

Malformations

A malformation is an abnormality in the shape or structure of an organ, body part, or larger section of the body resulting from an intrinsically dysfunctional developmental process. In other words, the genetic instructions for development are faulty, interfered with, or both.

All cells in the body carry the same set of genes, copied from the original set provided by the sperm and the egg at conception. Some genes are primarily responsible for directing a portion of embryonic/fetal development, and their influence may be anywhere from general (entire body or entire tissue) to specific (small component of one organ). This is why many single-gene (inherited) and most chromosomal disorders are characterized by multiple major and minor malformations in various anatomic locations. Any disorder, including most with a genetic basis, that can be uniquely characterized by a specific group of anomalies that occur more frequently together in that condition than would be expected by chance is defined as a syndrome. Multiple malformation patterns that have no discernible or consistent genetic pattern or teratogenic cause are known as associations (e.g., CHARGE association and **VATER association**).

Most isolated malformations follow a **multifactorial inheritance** pattern, and often involve incomplete morphogenesis of a midline organ or structure (e.g., septal defects (holes) in the heart, cleft lip/palate, diaphragmatic hernia, or **spina bifida**). These same types of malformations occur in some syndromes, in combination with a wide variety of other malformation types. Organs, body parts, or other structures may be extra/missing, abnormally positioned, over developed (hyperplastic), under developed (hypoplastic), or any of a number of minor variations.

Deformations

A deformation is an anomaly in the form, shape, or position of a body part or section that results from mechanical forces on the embryo/fetus. Deformations can have extrinsic (outside the fetus) or intrinsic (internal) causes. Examples of possible extrinsic causes include small maternal stature, oligohydramnios (decreased amniotic fluid volume), breech presentation, uterine malformation, and multiple pregnancy (i.e., twins, triplets, etc.). Some intrinsic (fetal) factors capable of producing deformations include neuromuscular disease, connective tissue defects, central nervous system disorders, and kidney malformations.

Joint contractures, such as talipes equinovarus (clubfeet), are the most common type of deformation, and have both extrinsic and intrinsic causes. As the fetus develops and grows, it must be able to move (flex and extend) the joints or they can become locked in position (contracted). Chronic oligohydramnios produces intrauterine constraint

(IUC), which compresses and immobilizes the fetus, causing joint contractures. Oligohydramnios itself may be caused by leakage of fluid from the amniotic sac (extrinsic cause), or result from decreased fluid production secondary to malformation or absence (agenesis) of the fetal kidneys. (Amniotic fluid is comprised mostly of fetal urine in the later stages of pregnancy.)

Agenesis of the fetal kidneys also exemplifies a malformation/deformation sequence. Specifically, an original, isolated malformation (**renal agenesis**) produces a sequence of events (oligohydramnios plus IUC plus fetal compression) that results in deformations, such as joint contractures and a characteristic facial pattern, which is sometimes referred to as the Potter sequence. A neuromuscular disease that causes partial or total prenatal paralysis of the limbs (decreased mobility) is another example of an intrinsic cause of joint contractures.

Disruptions

A disruption is an anomaly of an organ or body structure resulting from an extrinsic factor that interferes with, or disrupts, an originally normal developmental process. For example, certain types of maternal infection or drug use at a critical time in pregnancy have the potential to arrest the developmental process in specific fetal tissues. Another type of disruption can occur when a strip of the amniotic membrane surrounding the fetus detaches and wraps around one of the developing limbs or a section of the body. Known as an amniotic band, it acts somewhat like a tourniquet, restricting blood flow and inhibiting further growth.

Dysplasias

Dysplasia refers to an abnormal organization of cells in a particular tissue type, and any resulting abnormal morphological development. Dysplasias usually have a genetic basis, and examples include skeletal dysplasias (e.g., fragile, short, and/or abnormally curved bones), ectodermal dysplasias (skin, hair, nails, and associated tissues), and renal dysplasias (multiple cysts or tumors in the kidneys).

Genetic profile

Of all major congenital malformations, 60% have an undetermined cause, and 20% are attributed to multifactorial **inheritance**. The remaining 20% are divided roughly equally between single-gene disorders, chromosomal syndromes, and teratogenic causes. Considering that inclusion in the multifactorial group does not imply a specifically determined cause in any particular case, about 80% of all major malformations have no readily identifiable cause. The most frequently malformed organs are the brain, heart, and urinary tract (kidneys, ureters, bladder, and urethra). Deformations and disruptions most often affect the extremities (hands and feet), limbs (arms and legs), skull, and face.

Multifactorial inheritance is assumed for most isolated congenital anomalies, with a risk for recurrence in subsequent pregnancies of 3–5%. Single-gene (e.g., autosomal dominant, autosomal recessive, sex-linked, etc.) and chromosomal syndromes present a broad range of recurrence risks, but most often are 1–3% for chromosomal syndromes, and 25% or 50% for single-gene disorders.

Demographics

Considered individually, most anomalies and genetic syndromes are uncommon, and some are quite rare. As a group, however, they are quite common. Major congenital anomalies are the leading cause of death for children less than one year old, and the second and third most frequent cause for those less than five and 15 years old, respectively. Approximately 40% of all pediatric hospital admissions are related to congenital anomalies.

As already noted, malformations may be isolated or multiple, with minor or major clinical significance. Of all newborns, about 14% have a single minor malformation, 3% have a single major malformation, and up to 0.7% have multiple major malformations. The frequency of major malformations is even higher at conception, estimated at 10–15%, but most of these result in spontaneous pregnancy loss. About 2% of newborns are found to have a disruption of some type. In the presence of a major congenital malformation, especially if it affects the central nervous system or urinary tract, there is an 8% risk that a deformation will also occur. Skeletal dysplasias have an overall incidence of about 0.5%, with diagnosis of some of the milder forms often delayed until childhood. Ectodermal dysplasias occur in about 0.7% of individuals, but only several types associated with major malformations are usually diagnosed at birth. Other forms of congenital dysplasias are rare.

Diagnosis

Many anomalies are now detected/diagnosed prenatally, either through testing chosen because of a known or suspected risk factor, as a coincidental finding during testing chosen for another purpose, or as a chance finding by routine prenatal evaluations. Prenatal testing is done either through imaging studies, most often routine (level I) or detailed (level II) obstetric ultrasound, or through direct biochemical or **genetic testing** of the fetus using chorionic villus sampling (CVS) or **amniocentesis**.

Fetal echocardiography is sometimes used to confirm heart defects, and some rare conditions might require x rays or magnetic resonance imaging (MRI) of the fetus (via the mother), while a few others can only be diagnosed by a fetal skin biopsy. Some tests are designed only to screen for certain anomalies or syndromes (increase or decrease the likelihood).

Evaluating congenital anomalies postnatally usually involves attempts to confirm the suspected or most likely diagnosis, while at the same time excluding other possible diagnoses. Major external anomalies are easily detected, but those affecting internal organs require recognition of the signs and symptoms they produce (e.g., a baby with breathing difficulty who turns blue (cyanotic) while crying may have a heart defect), which could be subtle and/or not appear until well after birth.

Any child with an apparently isolated congenital anomaly should have this confirmed (i.e., exclude subtle or hidden signs of an association or syndrome). Multiple congenital anomalies are best evaluated by a geneticist, if possible, even in cases involving an obvious diagnosis, such as a common condition like **Down syndrome**. The family may wish to have a consultation in a genetics clinic, where a comprehensive approach helps to ensure that a thorough evaluation and explanation of the condition are provided. In addition, psychosocial issues are addressed, appropriate referrals can be made (e.g., other specialists, support groups, or more extensive psychological assistance as needed), and the most complete and current information on testing and other options are available. In cases with an unusual presentation of symptoms, or rare syndromes, geneticists have the best chance of establishing a diagnosis, often in consultation with colleagues who specialize in a particular syndrome or class of disorders. In other situations, a geneticist might suggest periodic revaluations if a diagnosis is unclear initially, since some children grow into a syndrome (i.e., the defining characteristics only become apparent as the child grows). Unfortunately, all too often a diagnosis is never established, regardless of effort expended or specialists consulted. Even in these cases, a geneticist may be able to offer a reasonable estimation as to a cause and recurrence risk, based on a process of eliminating some factors, making others more likely, and applying any available empirical data from similar cases.

Regardless of situation, a genetics evaluation includes as many of the following as possible:

- a complete physical examination of the affected child
- a review of medical records
- evaluation of the pregnancy history
- a consultation to obtain and evaluate the medical history of the immediate and extended family

KEY TERMS

Association—A non-random occurrence in two or more individuals of the same group of anomalies that are not otherwise known to be a sequence or syndrome.

Congenital—Present at birth.

Deformation—Abnormal shape or function in otherwise normal tissue produced by unusual mechanical forces on the embryo/fetus.

Disruption—A type of anomaly formation in which a breakdown or inhibition of normal tissue development occurs.

Dysmorphic—Literally meaning misshapen, it is most often used as a general descriptive term for individuals with one or more anomalous physical characteristics.

Dysplasia—The structural and functional results of the abnormal organization of cells into tissues, affecting one or more of the derivatives of a primary tissue type (endoderm, mesoderm, or ectoderm).

Etiology—The cause of a disease, syndrome, or anomaly.

Idiopathic—One or more anomalies of unknown cause in an individual.

Malformation—An abnormality in an organ or body structure caused by a dysfunctional developmental process.

Morphogenesis—The normal developmental process of the body's structure and form.

Sequence—The combination of both a primary structural or functional anomaly, and the secondary anomalies produced by any abnormal forces or processes it generates.

Syndrome—A pattern of multiple major and minor anomalies that occur as a group more often than would be expected by chance alone, implying the same underlying cause or mechanism in all affected individuals.

Based on these evaluations, one or more of a wide variety of possible medical tests could be suggested. If a hereditary syndrome is suspected, physical examination, medical record review, and testing might also be requested of one or more family members to help establish a diagnosis. The importance of making a diagnosis rests in the ability it provides to answer other questions

parents inevitably have. The diagnostic process also attempts to determining how a malformation, deformation, disruption, dysplasia, or some combination, occurred.

Treatment and management

Deformations are typically more amenable to successful treatment and correction than other types of anomalies. For instance, infants with dislocated hips or clubfeet can usually achieve normal function after a regimen of bracing, casting, and movement therapy, although in some cases minor surgery is also necessary. Many malformations can also be successfully repaired, especially those that are isolated. However, invasive and complex surgery is often needed, with only partial improvement in some cases. Certain malformations, such as cleft lip/palate, require multiple surgeries performed in stages as the child grows. For the most part, disruptions and dysplasias are minimally treatable, if at all. However, an exception could be the use of a prosthetic device for a limb amputation anomaly caused by a disruption such as an amniotic band.

Prognosis

The prognosis for any particular congenital anomaly, whether isolated or part of a sequence or syndrome, can vary greatly. Medical complications from one anomaly may also adversely affect the prognosis of another, or affect the course of an entire syndrome. In general, however, children with extrinsically caused deformations tend to fare better than those with other types of anomalies. Likewise, isolated malformations usually carry a better prognosis than multiple malformations/deformations, intrinsically derived deformations, and most types of tissue dysplasia. Disruption anomalies have widely varying prognoses based on various factors, such as the organ or body parts affected, the degree of disruption, and the timing during morphogenesis at which the disruption began.

Resources

BOOKS
Moore, Keith L., and T. V. N. Persaud. *Before We Are Born: Essentials of Embryology and Birth Defects*, 5th edition. Philadelphia: W. B. Saunders Company, 1998.

PERIODICALS
Riddle, Robert D., and Clifford J. Tabin. "How Limbs Develop." *Scientific American*. 280 (February 1999): 74–79.

ORGANIZATIONS
Alliance of Genetic Support Groups. 4301 Connecticut Ave. NW, Suite 404, Washington, DC 20008. (202) 966-5557.

March of Dimes Birth Defects Foundation. 1275 Mamaroneck Ave., White Plains, NY 10605. (888) 663-4637. (April 19, 2005.) <http://www.marchofdimes.com>.

National Society of Genetic Counselors. 233 Canterbury Dr., Wallingford, PA 19086-6617. (610) 872-1192. (April 19, 2005.) <http://www.nsgc.org/>.

WEBSITES

Cho, Mike, Mike Cohen, and Seeta Sistla. *What Is a "Normal" Phenotype? A Paper Written as Background to Discussion.* Developmental Biology Online. April 15, 2003 (April 18, 2005). <http://www.devbio.com/article.php?ch=21&id=169>.

View Dysmorphic Syndrome Features. Institute of Child Health, University College, London. (April 18, 2004.) <http://www.hgmp.mrc.ac.uk/DHMHD/view_human.html>.

Scott J. Polzin, MS

Genitalia, ambiguous

Definition

Ambiguous genitalia is a congenital anomaly in which the genital organs do not appear to be male or female.

Description

Ambiguous genitalia, also called indeterminate sex and intersexuality, is a condition present at birth in which an individual has what appears to be both male and female external sex organs. This diagnosis is usually preliminary, based on an initial physical examination. After further evaluation and diagnostic procedures, specific genital anomalies are usually diagnosed and the underlying syndrome or condition that caused them identified.

When the genitals are abnormal, a genetic screening is usually performed to determine the genetic sex of the infant and to rule out **chromosomal abnormalities**.

In a genetic female with ambiguous genitalia, the clitoris may be enlarged, having the appearance of a small penis, the labia may be fused, resembling a scrotum, and the opening to the urinary tract may be located anywhere along the clitoris.

In a genetic male with ambiguous genitalia, the penis may be small, measuring less than .78 in (2 cm); it can be mistaken for an enlarged clitoris. The clitoris often appears enlarged in newborns. The testicles may be undescended, a condition in which they remain inside the body, and they may have a groove or cleft resembling labia. The urinary tract opening may be located any-where from the tip of the penis to any point along the underside, an anomaly known as **hypospadias**.

Ambiguous genitalia is not a medically threatening anomaly, but it can be an extremely emotional issue for parents. Often parents must decide in which gender the child will be raised. This is a complex and difficult decision. There are health care professionals who can help inform and support parents. Counselors, doctors, and surgeons should be consulted before this decision is made.

The assignment of gender is not always based solely on the genetic sex of the child. When surgical treatment is necessary, parents may choose to raise a genetic male as a female because it is easier to surgically create functional female genitalia than male genitalia.

Children with ambiguous genitalia generally have one of the following conditions that cause the external genitalia to be abnormal:

- **Congenital adrenal hyperplasia**: This is the most common cause of ambiguous genitalia in infants. It is a condition affecting only females, in which the fetus cannot process an enzyme called 21-hydroxylase, causing an inability to process steroids in the body. It is characterized by a genetic female with internal female sex organs and ambiguous or masculine external genitalia.

- True **hermaphroditism**: In this extremely rare condition, an individual has both ovarian and testicular tissue, the internal sex organs of both genders, external genitalia that are ambiguous or of both genders, and abnormalities of the X or Y **chromosome**.

- Pseudohermaphroditism: In this condition, the individual has ambiguous external genitalia, but the internal sex organs of only one gender.

- Gonadal dysgenesis: In this condition, an individual has the internal sex organs of a female, external genitalia that have characteristics of both genders, but are predominantly female, abnormalities of the X or Y chromosome, and poorly developed ovaries or testicles.

- Klinefelter's syndrome: This is a chromosomal abnormality in which males have an extra X chromosome. It is characterized by small testicles, infertility, and, in some cases, mental retardation.

Genetic profile

The development of normal genitalia is a complex sequential process, beginning with the information stored on the X and Y chromosomes. Gonadal development in the fetus is first regulated by genetic information found on the short arm of the Y chromosome. Testis-determining factor (TDF) is a genetic sequence on the 11.3 subband of the Y chromosome. In the presence of TDF, testes develop. If TDF is absent, either because of a mutation of the Y chromosome or because the fetus is a female and therefore has no Y chromosome, then ovaries develop.

Testicular tissue produces two hormones essential for the development of normal male external genitalia: testosterone and mulerian-inhibiting substance (MIS). If these hormones are present, the internal male sex organs develop. These hormones work in two ways. Testosterone promotes development of male genitalia, both external and internal, and MIS prevents the development of female internal sex organs. In the absence of these two hormones, female genitalia develop.

Until these hormones are produced, all external fetal genitalia are identical and resemble female genitalia. In males, around week eight of fetal development, testosterone and another hormone, dihydrotestosterone (DHT), cause the external sex organs to become those of a normal male.

Ambiguous genitalia as a condition is caused by an interruption in some part of this process. Such interruptions may be caused by genetic mutations, exposure to substances in utero, such as steroids, or, in very rare cases, maternal endocrine abnormalities.

The exact genetic or metabolic cause of ambiguous genitalia is determined by the underlying condition that leads to the anomaly. The following are the most common syndromes causing ambiguous genitalia:

- In cases of congenital adrenal hyperplasia, the most common cause of abnormal external genital formation is defect in production of the 21-hydroxylation enzyme. This is an autosomal recessive trait thought to be linked to the human leukocyte antigen (HLA) locus on chromosome 6.

- True hermaphroditism is extremely rare and involves development of both male and female internal and external genitalia. The most common **karyotype** of individual with this condition is 46, XX. Researchers suspect that mosaicism is present and that a translocation of one antigen from a Y chromosome to one X chromosome or to an autosome may explain the development of male sex organs. True hermaphroditism does occur in individuals with a 46, XY karyotype. Explaining the development of ovarian tissue in this individual is difficult since two X chromosomes must be present for this to occur. Researchers theorize that there may be an undetected XX cell line within these individuals.

- Pseudohermaphroditism is generally caused by a failure in the production or absorption of the hormones testosterone and DHT. There are several different types of this condition, but they all appear to be passed on to the individual via either X-linked or autosomal recessive transmission. The anomalies are caused by a failure to produce sufficient levels of testosterone or a deficiency of enzymes, namely 5-alpha-reductase, necessary for DHT production.

- Individuals with gonadal dysgenesis have an abnormality of the sex chromosomes. Karyotypes often seen in these individuals are 46, XO/XY mosaicism, and 46, XO.

Demographics

Ambiguous genitalia is a very rare condition. Researchers estimate that the most common cause, congenital adrenal hyperplasia, may occur in one of every 15,000 live births worldwide. Other conditions that affect the formation of external genitalia are even rarer.

Signs and symptoms

Primarily, ambiguous genitalia is a physical condition characterized by an abnormal appearance of the external genitals; however, the internal sex organs are typically malformed as well. There may be partially formed testes, ovaries, or both, or a complete absence of internal sex organs. Typically, individuals with ambiguous genitalia are infertile.

In some cases of pseudohermphroditism, the genitalia may appear to be slightly abnormal female at birth, but at puberty, the genitals may become more masculine as testosterone levels rise. What appeared to be an enlarged clitoris may develop into a penis of up to 2.7 in (7 cm) in length.

The long-term health risks of this condition include an increased risk of tumors. Abnormal testicular tissue is vulnerable to tumor formation. As many as 40% of genetic males with ambiguous genitalia develop tumors within this tissue by the time they reach the age of 50. For this reason, regular screening is important.

Diagnosis

Ambiguous genitalia is usually diagnosed initially during a newborn's physical exam or during subsequent well-baby check-ups. Once it is suspected that the infant has abnormal genitalia, diagnostic tests may be performed to identify the child's genetic gender; the presence of a chromosomal abnormality; the presence, absence, and type of internal sex organs; and the potential for production of sex hormones.

Diagnostic test that may be performed include:

- Chromosomal analysis to determine which sex chromosomes are present and if there are any abnormalities.

KEY TERMS

Ambiguous—Unclear or open to more than one interpretation.

Autosome—One of the 22 chromosomes that are not involved in determining gender (chromosomes 1 through 22 and not the X or Y chromosome).

Clitoris—A small mass of erectile tissue in the female genitalia.

Congenital anomaly—An abnormality that is present at birth.

Genitalia—The organs of reproduction.

Genetic sex—The gender determined by the sex chromosomes; XX is female, XY is male.

Hypospadias—A birth defect in which the opening to the urinary tract, called the urethra, is located away from the tip of the penis.

Infertile—Incapable of reproduction.

Karyotype—A photographic representation of the full set of chromosomes numbered and arranged in pairs.

Labia—The two parts of the vulva (the external female genitalia).

Mosaicism—The presence of more than one cell line in a single individual.

Recessive—A genetic trait that is only expressed when another identical recessive gene is present.

Translocation—An exchange of genetic material in which a segment is moved from one location to another along the same chromosome or a different chromosome.

X-linked—A genetic trait that is carried on the X chromosome.

• Abdominal ultrasound to assess internal sex organs, if present, and to view the adrenal gland that is enlarged in females with congenital adrenal hyperplasia.

• Tests to assess the levels of male and female hormones present and the child's ability to process them; to determine if the infant can process enzymes; and to screen for other metabolic conditions that may accompany ambiguous genitalia.

Treatment and management

Treatment of ambiguous genitalia will depend on the extent of the abnormalities present, the underlying cause, and associated conditions. Treatment options include hormone replacement therapy (HRT) and surgical correction.

In some cases, gender assignment may be necessary. This can be a difficult and emotional decision for parents. Complicating the situation is the fact that when surgery is required to reconstruct external genitalia, the genetic sex of the child may not be the primary determining factor. It is far more difficult for surgeons to create functional male genitalia than female. For many years, it was thought that, in children for whom gender assignment surgery was considered the best treatment, a gender assignment should be made in the first few days of life. It was believed that environment or the influence of being raised as a girl or boy was enough to ensure gender identity. Recent data about individuals who were "assigned" a gender different from their genetic gender contradict this theory. Some individuals, who were assigned a gender different from their genetic gender as infants and were raised as the reassigned gender, chose to assume the gender identity of their genetic gender as adults. Currently, many doctors believe that gender assignment involving surgical reconstruction of the external genitalia should be delayed until the individual has an established gender identity and can be involved in the decision.

Other factors that must be considered are issues of fertility, the ability of the internal sex organs to produce gender-appropriate sex hormones, the effects of sex hormone exposure on the fetus while in the womb, and the risk of additional health problems that may develop later in life either from HRT or internal sex organs.

Prognosis

If gender assignment is successful, the prognosis for children diagnosed with ambiguous genitalia is excellent. Depending on the underlying diagnosis and associated conditions, some additional medical management may be necessary. In children with congenital adrenal hyperplasia, steroid treatment is necessary for survival. Despite the complications from long-term steroid use, if the condition is properly diagnosed and treated, children with congenital adrenal hyperplasia can have healthy and normal lives.

Resources

PERIODICALS

Committee on Genetics. "Evaluation of the Newborn with Developmental Anomalies of the External Genitalia." *Pediatrics* 106, no 1 (July 2000): 138–142.

Phornphutkul, Chanika. "Experience and Reason: Gender Self-Reassignment in an XY Adolescent Female Born with Ambiguous Genitalia." *Pediatrics* 106, no 1 (July 2000): 135–137.

ORGANIZATIONS

Ambiguous Genitalia Support Network. P. O. Box 313, Clements, CA 95227-0313.

Intersex Society of North America (ISNA). P. O. Box 31791, San Francisco, CA 94131. (April 10, 2005.) <http://www.isna.org>.

National Adrenal Diseases Foundation. 505 Northern Blvd., Great Neck, NY 11021. (April 10, 2005.) <http://www.nlm.nih.gov/medlineplus/ency/article/003269.htm>.

WEBSITES

Hutchenson, Joel, and Howard M. Snyder, III. "Ambiguous Genitalia and Intersexuality." eMedicine. (Accessed April 1, 2005; April 10, 2005.) <http://www.emedicine.com/PED/topic1492.htm>.

Deborah L. Nurmi, MS

Genotype *see* **Genotypes and phenotypes**

Genotype and phenotype

The term genotype describes the actual set (complement) of genes carried by an organism. In contrast, phenotype refers to the observable expression of characters and traits coded for by those genes. Although phenotypes are based upon the content of the underlying genes comprising the genotype, the expression of those genes in observable traits (phenotypic expression) is also, to varying degrees, influenced by environmental factors.

The term genotype was first used by Danish geneticist Wilhelm Johannsen (1857–1927) to describe the entire genetic or hereditary constitution of an organism, In contrast, Johannsen described displayed characters or traits (e.g., anatomical traits, biochemical traits, physiological traits, etc.) as an organism's phenotype.

Genotype and phenotype represent very real differences between genetic composition and expressed form. The genotype is a group of genetic markers that describes the particular forms or variations of genes (alleles) carried by an individual. Accordingly, an individual's genotype includes all the alleles carried by that individual. An individual's genotype, because it includes all of the various alleles carried, determines the range of traits possible (e.g., a individual's potential to be afflicted with a particular disease). In contrast to the possibilities contained within the genotype, the phenotype reflects the manifest expression of those possibilities

(potentialities). Phenotypic traits include obvious observable traits as height, weight, eye color, hair color, etc. The presence or absence of a disease, or symptoms related to a particular disease state, is also a phenotypic trait.

A clear example of the relationship between genotype and phenotype exists in cases where there are dominant and recessive alleles for a particular trait. Using an simplified monogenetic (one **gene**, one trait) example, a capital "T" might be used to represent a dominant allele at a particular locus coding for tallness in a particular plant, and the lowercase "t" used to represent the recessive allele coding for shorter plants. Using this notation, a diploid plant will possess one of three genotypes: TT, Tt, or tt (the variation tT is identical to Tt). Although there are three different genotypes, because of the laws governing dominance, the plants will be either be tall or short (two phenotypes). Those plants with a TT or Tt genotype are observed to be tall (phenotypically tall). Only those plants that carry the tt genotype will be observed to be short (phenotypically short).

In humans, there is genotypic sex determination. The genotypic variation in sex chromosomes, XX or XY decisively determines whether an individual is female (XX) or male (XY) and this genotypic differentiation results in considerable phenotypic differentiation.

Although the relationships between genetic and environmental influences vary (i.e., the degree to which genes specify phenotype differs from trait to trait), in general, the more complex the biological process or trait, the greater the influence of environmental factors. The genotype almost completely directs certain biological processes. Genotype, for example, strongly determines when a particular tooth develops. How long an individual retains a particular tooth, is to a much greater extent, determined by environmental factors such diet, dental hygiene, etc.

Because it is easier to determine observable phenotypic traits that it is to make an accurate determination of the relevant genotype associated with those traits, scientists and physicians place increasing emphasis on relating (correlating) phenotype with certain genetic markers or genotypes.

There are, of course, variable ranges in the nature of the genotype-environment association. In many cases, genotype-environment interactions do not result in easily predictable phenotypes. In rare cases, the situation can be complicated by a process termed phenocopy where environmental factors produce a particular phenotype that resembles a set of traits coded for by a known genotype not actually carried by the individual. Genotypic

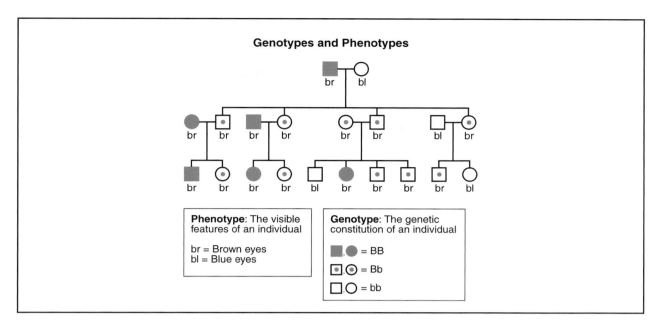

Genotypes and Phenotypes

Phenotype: The visible features of an individual

br = Brown eyes
bl = Blue eyes

Genotype: The genetic constitution of an individual

■,● = BB
▣,◉ = Bb
□,○ = bb

(*Gale Group*)

frequencies reflect the percentage of various genotypes found within a given group (population) and phenotypic frequencies reflect the percentage of observed expression. Mathematical measures of phenotypic variance reflect the variability of expression of a trait within a population.

The exact relationship between genotype and disease is an area of intense interest to geneticists and physicians and many scientific and clinical studies focus on the relationship between the effects of a genetic changes (e.g., changes caused by mutations) and disease processes. These attempts at genotype/phenotype correlations often require extensive and refined use of statistical analysis.

Antonio Farina, MD, PhD
K. Lee Lerner

Gerstmann-Straussler-Scheinker disease *see* **Prion diseases**

Gestational diabetes *see* **Diabetes mellitus**

Gilles de la Tourette syndrome *see* **Tourette syndrome**

Glanzmann thrombasthemia *see* **Thrombasthenia of Glanzmann and Naegeli**

Glaucoma

Definition

Glaucoma is a group of eye disorders that results in vision loss due to a failure to maintain the normal fluid balance within the eye. If fluid pressure builds up, then damage to the optic nerve occurs, leading to vision loss. If detected in its early stages, vision loss can be prevented through the use of medications or surgical procedures that restore the proper fluid drainage of the eye.

Description

Vision is an important and complex special sense by which the qualities of an object, such as color, shape, and size, are perceived through the detection of light. Light that bounces off an object first passes through the cornea (outer layer) of the eye and then through the pupil and the lens to project onto a layer of cells on the back of the eye called the retina. When the retina is stimulated by light, signals pass through the optic nerve to the brain, resulting in a visual image of an object.

The front chamber of the eye is bathed in a liquid called the aqueous humor. This liquid is produced by a nearby structure called the ciliary body and is moved out of the eye into the bloodstream by a system of drainage canals known as the trabecular meshwork. The proper amount of fluid within the chamber is maintained by a balance between fluid production by the ciliary body and

Types of glaucoma and related genetic information

Disorder	Alternative names	Inheritance	Abnormal protein	Abnormal gene	Gene location
Glaucoma 1, open angle, A (GLC1A)	Juvenile onset primary open-angle glaucoma; Hereditary juvenile glaucoma	Autosomal dominant	Trabecular meshwork-induced glucocorti-coid response protein (myocilin)	MYOC, (also known as TIGR, GLC1A, JOAG, GPOA)	1q24.3–q25.2;
			Unknown	Unknown	9q34.1
Glaucoma 1, open angle, B (GLC1B)	Adult onset primary open-angle glaucoma; Hereditary adult glaucoma	Autosomal dominant	Unknown	Unknown	2qcen-q13; (additional loci under investigation)
Glaucoma 1, open angle, C (GLC1C)	Adult onset primary open-angle glaucoma; Hereditary adult glaucoma	Autosomal dominant	Unknown	Unknown	3q21–q24
Glaucoma 1, open angle, D (GLC1D)	Adult onset primary open-angle glaucoma; Hereditary adult glaucoma	Autosomal dominant	Unknown	Unknown	8q23
Glaucoma 1, open angle, E (GLC1E)	Adult onset primary open-angle glaucoma; Hereditary adult glaucoma	Autosomal dominant	Unknown	Unknown	10p15–p14
Glaucoma 1, open angle, F (GLC1F)	Adult onset primary open-angle glaucoma; Hereditary adult glaucoma	Autosomal dominant	Unknown	Unknown	7q35–36
Glaucoma 3, primary infantile, A (GLC3A)	Congenital glaucoma; Buphthalmos	Autosomal recessive	CytochromeP4501B1	CYP1B1	2p22–p21
Glaucoma 3, primary infantile, B (GLC3B)	Congenital glaucoma	Autosomal recessive	Unknown	Unknown	1p36.2– 36.1
Iridogoniodysgenesis, type 1 (IRID1)	Iridogoniodysgenesis anomaly; familial glaucomaIridogonio-dysplasia	Autosomal dominant	Forkhead Transcription factor	FKHL7	6P25
Iridogoniodysgenesis, type 2 (IRID1)	Iridogoniodysgenesis anomaly; Iris hypoplasia with early-onset glaucoma	Autosomal dominant	Paired-like homeodomain transcription factor-2	PITX2 (also known as; IDG2,RIEG1, RGS, IGDS2)	4q25–q26
Rieger syndrome, type 1 (RIEG1)	Iridogoniodysgenesis with Somatic anomalies	Autosomal dominant	Paired-like homeodomain transcription factor-2	PITX2 (also known as; IDG2,RIEG1, RGS, IGDS2)	4q25–q26
Rieger syndrome, type 2 (RIEG2)	Iridogoniodysgenesis with Somatic anomalies	Autosomal dominant	Unknown	Unknown	13q14
Glaucoma-related pigment dispersion syndrome (GPDS1)	Pigment dispersion syndrome and pigmentary glaucoma	Autosomal dominant	Unknown	Unknown	7q35–q36

fluid drainage through the trabecular meshwork. When fluid accumulates in the front chamber, either because of an overproduction of fluid or because of a failure of the normal drainage routes, fluid pressure builds up within the eye. Over time, this increased fluid pressure causes damage to the optic nerve, resulting in progressive visual impairment. The condition of increased eye fluid pressure leading to vision loss is known as glaucoma.

Glaucoma is actually a group of many different eye disorders and can manifest alone or as a sign of more than 60 different diseases, or even in a healthy person who has experienced an injury to the eye. Physicians classify glaucoma by the type of abnormality in the drainage system. When the drainage passage is narrowed, but still open, it is termed open-angle glaucoma.

If the drainage passage is completely blocked, it is termed closed-angle glaucoma. Glaucoma can also be classified by the age of the affected individual: infantile or congenital glaucoma affects infants at birth or children up to three years old, juvenile glaucoma affects individuals from 3–30 years old, and adult glaucoma affects people greater than 30 years old.

Genetic profile

There are different forms of glaucoma that either occur alone or as the result of a genetic abnormality. In some cases, specific genetic abnormalities have been identified, while in other forms, the cause is unknown. The known types of glaucoma and the corresponding

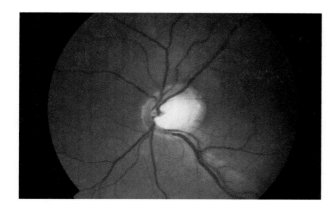

Retinal photographs, like the one shown here, can be used to check for signs of glaucoma, such as increased fluid and damage to the optic nerve. (*Custom Medical Stock Photo, Inc.*)

genetic defect include forms of glaucoma are not inherited and thus are not represented in the table.

Glaucoma can be inherited in either an autosomal recessive or an autosomal dominant fashion. In autosomal recessive inheritance, two abnormal genes are needed to display the disease. A person who carries one abnormal gene does not display the disease, and is called a carrier. A carrier has a 50% chance of transmitting the gene to a child, who must inherit one abnormal gene from each parent to display the disease. Alternatively, in autosomal dominant inheritance, only one abnormal gene is needed to display the disease, and the chance of passing the gene and the disease to offspring is 50%.

Research is ongoing concerning the heritability of genetic risk factors for primary open-angle glaucoma. This type of glaucoma is particularly troublesome since it is common, progressive, and one of the leading causes of blindness around the world. A major study done in Wisconsin, the Beaver Dam Eye Study investigated the family aggregation and heritability of risk factors of primary open-angle glaucoma among 5,924 participants. The researchers found that there are strong genetic familial effects on risk factors for open-angle glaucoma. The researchers noted that there was a strong and consistent relationship between intraocular pressure and optic cup measurements in siblings, parents, and children, with a lack of correlation of those measurements in spouses.

The genetics of juvenile open-angle glaucoma have been widely studied. Research done in the late 1990s identified a trabecular meshwork-induced glucocorticoid TIGR gene strongly associated with juvenile open-angle glaucoma. Further research identified a protein associated with the cytoskeleton of the retina that was coded for by the myocilin gene. While the exact function of the protein coded for the myocilin gene is unknown, studies have shown a high rate of mutations in this gene in patients with juvenile open-angle glaucoma.

Demographics

Glaucoma is the leading cause of preventable blindness in the United States, affecting more than two million Americans, and is the third leading cause of blindness worldwide. The prevalence of glaucoma increases with age, but the eye condition can also be present in infants and young children. The adult types of open-angle glaucoma account for the majority (70%) of glaucoma cases, while the infantile and juvenile types of glaucoma are relatively uncommon.

The types and rates of glaucoma are not distributed equally among different ethnic groups. For example, the prevalence of glaucoma in Caucasians over 70 years old is 3.5%, while the prevalence in African Americans is 12%. Also, the primary closed-angle type of glaucoma is much more common in people of Asian or Inuit descent. Apart from ethnicity, risk factors for the development of glaucoma include elevated eye pressure, increasing age, **diabetes**, and presence of glaucoma in a family member.

Signs and symptoms

In the adult and juvenile forms of open-angle glaucoma, vision loss begins at the periphery (outer edges) of the visual field, resulting in tunnel vision. Because the visual loss in not in the individual's central vision, they may not notice this change. However, if the glaucoma is left untreated, loss of vision progresses and the central vision is often affected, sometimes resulting in blindness. The average time from development of high eye fluid pressures to the appearance of visual loss is 18 years in the adult form, but much shorter in the juvenile form.

In contrast to the adult and juvenile forms, congenital or infantile open-angle glaucoma is noted at birth or within the first three years of life. Symptoms include cloudy corneas, excessive tearing, and sensitivity to light. Because the eye is very flexible in infants, increased fluid pressure may cause bulging of the eye (buphthalmos, or ox eye). Children with glaucoma in only one eye are usually diagnosed earlier because a difference in eye size can be noticed. When the disorder affects both eyes, many parents view the large eyes as attractive and do not seek help until other symptoms develop, delaying the diagnosis.

With closed-angle glaucoma, symptoms come on suddenly. People may experience blurred vision, severe pain, headache, sensitivity to light, and nausea. The development of this type of glaucoma is an emergency and requires immediate treatment.

KEY TERMS

Aqueous humor—A fluid produced by the ciliary body and contained within the front chamber of the eye.

Autosomal dominant—A pattern of genetic inheritance where only one abnormal gene is needed to display the trait or disease.

Autosomal recessive—A pattern of genetic inheritance where two abnormal genes are needed to display the trait or disease.

Buphthalmos—A characteristic enlargement of one or both eyes associated with infantile glaucoma.

Ciliary body—A structure within the eye that produces aqueous humor.

Closed-angle glaucoma—An increase in the fluid pressure within the eye due to a complete, and sometimes sudden, blockage of the fluid drainage passages.

Cornea—The transparent structure of the eye over the lens that is continuous with the sclera in forming the outermost, protective, layer of the eye.

Glaucoma—An increase in the fluid eye pressure, eventually leading to damage of the optic nerve and ongoing visual loss.

Gonioscope—An instrument used to examine the

trabecular meshwork; consists of a magnifier and a lens equipped with mirrors.

Ophthalmologist—A physician specializing in the medical and surgical treatment of eye disorders.

Ophthalmoscope—An instrument, with special lighting, designed to view structures in the back of the eye.

Optic disc—The region where the optic nerve joins the eye, also referred to as the blind spot.

Optic nerve—A bundle of nerve fibers that carries visual messages from the retina in the form of electrical signals to the brain.

Optometrist—A medical professional who examines and tests the eyes for disease and treats visual disorders by prescribing corrective lenses and/or vision therapy. In many states, optometrists are licensed to use diagnostic and therapeutic drugs to treat certain ocular diseases.

Retina—The light-sensitive layer of tissue in the back of the eye that receives and transmits visual signals to the brain through the optic nerve.

Tonometer—A device used to measure fluid pressures of the eye.

Trabecular meshwork—A sponge-like tissue that drains the aqueous humor from the eye.

Diagnosis

The diagnosis of glaucoma may be suggested by certain physical findings, especially in infants, but is confirmed by tests with special instruments. Parents may bring their young infant to a physician if they notice changes in the eye shape and size, signs of infantile glaucoma. In adults, who do not show obvious signs of glaucoma, the condition is frequently detected by routine screening eye exams and other tests.

Using an ophthalmoscope (a hand-held or machine-mounted instrument with a light source), a physician or optometrist will look through the pupil to the back of the eye. There, they may detect characteristic changes in the region where the optic nerve meets the eye, called the optic disk.

In another portion of a routine eye exam, an ophthalmologist or optometrist will measure the fluid pressure of the eye through the use of a special instrument called a tonometer. The test is painless and involves brief contact of a small probe with the surface of the eye. Presence

of elevated pressure (more than 21 mm Hg) means that a person is at risk for glaucoma.

Once high pressures or changes in the optic disk are noted, an ophthalmologist can also use a gonioscope (small lens with a reflecting mirror) to inspect the drainage passageways of the eye and determine if they are blocked. Visual field tests (in which individuals indicate whether they can see small flashing lights that are directed in different spots of their visual field) are used as a final indicator for the presence of glaucoma or a measurement of how far glaucoma-related visual loss has progressed.

Treatment and management

Although there is no treatment for the optic nerve injury and vision loss caused by glaucoma, it is possible to prevent further visual loss by lowering eye fluid pressure. In the adult, this is primarily achieved through medications. Medications can reduce eye fluid pressure by either decreasing fluid production or by increasing fluid drainage from the eye, and can be taken orally (by mouth) or applied to the eye through drops. The names of different classes of medications used to treat glaucoma include beta-blockers, alpha agonists, carbonic anhydrase inhibitors, and prostaglandin analogues.

For infantile glaucoma, the treatment is primarily surgical. Laser surgery or microsurgery to open the drainage canals can be effective in increasing drainage of eye fluid. Other types of surgery can be performed to reduce the amount of fluid production. Many children require several operations to lower or maintain their eye fluid pressures adequately, and long-term treatment with medications may be necessary. For closed-angle glaucoma, immediate hospitalization and treatment with medication is required. Once the person's condition has been stabilized, laser surgery is used to create a passageway for fluid drainage.

All individuals with glaucoma should see an ophthalmologist regularly to evaluate progress of the condition and whether it is being adequately treated. Beginning at the age of 40, all people should receive regular screening exams to detect early signs of glaucoma. People with a family history of glaucoma or with diabetes should receive these screening tests beginning in young adulthood.

Prognosis

Since even small amounts of vision loss due to glaucoma cannot be reversed, early detection of the condition through regular eye examinations is critical. If glaucoma is detected early, lifelong medical treatment can halt the progress of the disease and result in relatively normal vision. If left undiagnosed or untreated, many people with glaucoma will progress to blindness.

Closed-angle glaucoma is an emergency and the prognosis depends on how quickly medical attention is obtained and the severity of the attack. If left untreated, the condition can quickly lead to total vision loss in the affected eye.

Resources

BOOKS

Marks, E., and R. Mountauredes. *Coping With Glaucoma.* Garden City Park, NY: Avery Publishing Group, 1997.

Trope, G. E. *Glaucoma: A Patient's Guide to the Disease.* Toronto: University of Toronto Press, 1996.

PERIODICALS

Coleman, A. L. "Glaucoma." *Lancet* 354 (November 1999): 1803–1810.

Klein, B. E. K., R. Klein, and K. E. Lee. "Heritability of Risk Factors for Primary Open-angle Glaucoma: The Beaver Eye Dam Study." *Investigative*

Ophthalmology and Visual Science 45 (January 2004): 59–62.

Migdal, C. "Glaucoma Medical Treatment: Philosophy, Principles and Management." *Eye* 14 (June 2000): 515–518.

Satoko, S., P. R. Lichiter, A. T. Johnson, et al. "Age-dependent Prevalence of Mutations at the GLCIA Locus in Primary Open-angle Glaucoma." *American Journal of Opthalmology* 130 (2000): 165–177.

ORGANIZATIONS

Glaucoma Foundation. 33 Maiden Lane, New York, NY 10038. (800) 452-8266. (April 19, 2005.) <http://www.glaucoma-foundation.org>.

Glaucoma Research Foundation. 200 Pine St., Suite 200, San Francisco, CA 94104. (800) 826-6693.

WEBSITES

"Glaucoma." *Online Mendelian Inheritance in Man.* National Center for Biotechnology Information, National Library of Medicine. Building 38A, Room 8N805, Bethesda, MD 20894. (April 19, 2005.) <http://www.ncbi.nlm.nih.gov/entrez/query.fcgi?db=OMIM&cmd=search&term=glaucoma>.

Glaucoma Resources on the Internet. (April 19, 2005.) <http://www.healthcyclopedia.com/glaucoma.html>.

Oren Traub, MD, PhD
Edward R. Rosick, DO, MPH, MS

GLB1 deficiency *see* **GM1 gangliosidosis**

Globoid cell leukodystrophy (GCL) *see* **Krabbe disease**

Glucocerebrosidase deficiency *see* **Gaucher disease**

Glycogen storage disease II *see* **Glycogen storage diseases; Pompe disease**

Glycogen storage diseases

Definition

Glycogen is a form of stored glucose that the body uses as an energy source. Glycogen storage disease (GSD) involves defects that cause an abnormal accumulation of glycogen, usually found in the liver, muscle, or both. When accumulation occurs in the liver, glycogen storage diseases result in liver enlargement and in conditions ranging from mild hypoglycemia to liver failure. When the accumulation occurs in muscle, glycogen storage diseases result in conditions ranging from difficulty exercising to cardiac and respiratory failure.

Description

Glucose is a simple sugar that functions as a critical energy source for most bodily functions. Glucose can be acquired through the diet or formed within the bodily cells. Levels of glucose in the blood are maintained in a very narrow range, before and after the ingestion of food. Eating a meal supplies a high level of dietary glucose. Hormones, such as insulin, assist in the removal of glucose from the blood and into cells to be used as energy. Excess glucose is accumulated in the form of glycogen as a type of easily mobilized energy storage for use when food is not plentiful. Even while sleeping, glycogen stores are available to maintain blood glucose levels and energy for life.

The process of the formation of glycogen sheets is termed glycogenesis, and is stimulated by hormones, such as insulin. The process of the breakdown of sheets of glycogen into usable glucose is termed glycogenolysis, and is also under tight control. Hormones that stimulate glycogenolysis control enzymes to remove only the necessary amount of glucose from glycogen stores. With an average daily food intake, glycogen stores are constantly being built up and broken down based on the needs of the body. Average glycogen stores serve as a short-term supply of glucose, and need to be replenished daily. Glycogen serves as energy storage in every organ, but the liver and skeletal muscles are the main sites of glycogen deposition. The brain is dependent upon glucose for energy, and so requires a certain level of blood glucose to be available at all times. Because the brain has only minimal glycogen stores, it is mainly dependent on glycogen from other organs, such as the liver.

Glycogen has separate functions in liver and muscle. Muscle uses glycogen as a fuel source with which to produce energy during activity. As muscle is being used, glycogen stores are being broken down into glucose, turned into cellular energy called ATP, and depleted. In the liver, glycogen is mainly used as a maintenance energy source for the entire body, and is responsible for keeping blood glucose levels in a stable range. After ingestion of dietary glucose, the liver takes up many food breakdown products from the bloodstream, converts them into glucose, and stores them as glycogen. Some time after a meal, when blood glucose levels naturally fall, the liver uses its glycogen stores to replenish the blood with glucose. Organs that cannot create enough glycogen of their own are thus supplied.

Glycogen storage diseases may involve defects in glycogen breakdown or formation in muscle, liver, or both muscle and liver. Some classic features of GSDs that primarily involve muscle are muscle cramps, exercise intolerance, and easy fatigability. Some classic features of GSDs that primarily involve liver are liver enlargement, liver function defects, and hypoglycemia. Most GSDs can have subtypes with onset at different stages of life. There are many types of GSD that involve different defects in glycogen utilization. The types of GSD that are best described are types I through VIII, each with a distinct name and profile.

Von Gierke's disease

GSD type I is also known as von Gierke's disease, which has two subtypes, GSDIa and GSDIb. GSDIa is caused by a defect in an enzyme involved in the release of precursor components from liver glycogen stores; GSDIb is caused by a defect in a protein transporter used to transport the necessary precursor components of the pathway to the location of the enzyme. Without dietary glucose, the body is unable to access needed energy from the liver.

In times of fasting, which is essentially any time dietary glucose is not being ingested, severe hypoglycemia can result. Normal mechanisms are in effect in the body to sense a decrease in blood sugar, and respond by increasing rates of glycogen breakdown to maintain blood glucose. Because of the defect in glycogen breakdown, this does not occur and precursor molecules from the pathway accumulate. This causes liver enlargement and the protruding abdomen that is associated with the disease. In von Gierke's disease, the defects in glycogenolysis occur at a point in the pathway that causes accumulation of glucose-6-phosphate. When glucose-6-phosphate accumulates, it diverts into other metabolic pathways that form lactic acid and uric acid. The lactic acid can acidify the blood and cause a dangerous condition known as acidosis. Uric acid accumulation can cause kidney stones and kidney dysfunction. There are also alterations in blood-clotting factors that cause these individuals to bleed very easily and for prolonged periods of time. These alterations can be dangerous. Frequent nosebleeds are associated with von Gierke's disease as a result. Von Gierke's disease type Ib has other defects in blood immune system components that create susceptibility to some types of bacterial infections.

Pompe's disease

GSD type II is also known as **Pompe's disease.** There are three main subtypes of Pompe's disease categorized as infantile, juvenile, and adult-onset. The infantile form primarily involves defects in utilization of cardiac muscle, skeletal muscle, and respiratory muscle. This form usually presents by the age of six months and is rapidly fatal, usually due to respiratory and cardiac failure. The adult form involves muscle glycogen stores other than cardiac muscle. The adult form is a progressive disease, but there are no heart defects. However, muscle weakness often results in respiratory failure. The juvenile form includes infants and children older than six months and involves muscle weakness without cardiac defects. In general, the older a person is at the age of onset, the less the likelihood of cardiac involvement. Pompe's disease is caused by defects in an enzyme involved in a side pathway of glycogenolysis that is not critical for most glycogen degradation. The main pathway for glycogen degradation is not defective in Pompe's disease, so there is no hypoglycemia. The defect does cause an accumulation of glycogen that causes enlargement and dysfunction of the organs involved. In the infantile form of Pompe's disease, this is the cause of heart disease, respiratory deficiency, and overall muscle weakness.

Cori's disease

GSD type III is also known as Cori's disease. Cori's disease is caused by a defect in a debranching enzyme that is responsible for breaking down the highly branched structure of glycogen in the liver, skeletal muscle, and cardiac muscle. This defect results in hypoglycemia that occurs a relatively short time after food intake. It is unknown why the defect in Cori's disease may lead to liver damage and cancers not seen in von Gierke's disease. It is known that the hypoglycemia that develops in Cori's disease is directly involved and that the liver defects improve with age. Chronic hypoglycemia also contributes to skeletal and cardiac muscle damage in Cori's disease not seen in von Gierke's disease. The enzymatic defect in Cori's disease also contributes to an increase in fat breakdown. Excessive breakdown of fatty acids leads to higher than normal levels of ketone acids, fat breakdown products, in the blood. A dangerous condition known as ketoacidosis may result in organ damage. Growth retardation is associated with Cori's disease.

Andersen's disease

GSD type IV is also known as Andersen's disease, which usually causes symptoms within the first few years of life. Andersen's disease is caused by a defect in a branching enzyme, responsible for the highly branched structure of normal glycogen. In Andersen's disease, glycogen has an abnormal, unbranched structure that cannot be properly broken down into glucose molecules, and

accumulates. Most forms of Andersen's disease involve the liver. Multiple bodily organs or systems may be impacted, including the heart, gastrointestinal tract, skin, intestine, brain, blood formation, and nervous system. Andersen's disease is characterized by liver enlargement, liver-induced hypertension (portal hypertension), liver cirrhosis and failure, and often death by five years of age. Some Andersen's patients have a mild disease variant with later onset associated with a non-progressive form of liver disease. This subtype may have onset even in adulthood. Some forms of Andersen's disease have primarily muscle involvement that may include cardiac muscle. The abnormal glycogen in skeletal muscle results in weakness, exercise intolerance, and muscle wasting. Abnormal glycogen in cardiac muscle can lead to cardiac failure. The abnormal glycogen formed in Andersen's disease can also affect the nervous system by impairing mental function.

McArdle's disease

GSD type V is also known as McArdle's disease. McArdle's disease is caused by a defect in an enzyme myophosphorylase involved in initiating glycogen breakdown, specifically in skeletal muscle. As a result, glycogen is not broken down into glucose in skeletal muscle, which causes a deficit in cellular energy (ATP). Normal energy utilization in skeletal muscle involves breaking down glycogen fuel stores into glucose, and converting glucose into ATP for energy. During exercise, the amount of ATP required for performance is greatly increased. When muscle glycogen is depleted, muscle begins to use blood glucose and fat breakdown products for energy. Individuals with McArdle's disease often experience a "second wind" phenomenon in energy levels during exercise because of these secondary fuel sources. However, McArdle's disease still causes muscle cramps during exercise and exercise intolerance.

Hers' disease

GSD type VI is also known as Hers' disease. Similar to McArdle's disease, the classic form of Hers' disease is caused by a partial defect in the phosphorylase enzyme. This form of Hers' disease involves a partial defect in liver phosphorylase, which initiates glycogen breakdown, specifically in the liver. Other forms exist that are caused by similar defects. Hers' disease includes a heterogeneous group of subtypes with mild clinical consequences. Hers' disease typically involves liver enlargement, muscle weakness, growth retardation, mild fasting hypoglycemia, and mildly elevated ketone levels during childhood that resolve by puberty. Most patients have only partial impairment of glycogenolysis, due to the incomplete deficiencies of the enzymes involved.

Genetic profile

The GSDs are autosomal recessive diseases, which are caused by the **inheritance** of two defective copies of a **gene**. Each parent contributes one copy of the gene for the enzymes or transporters involved in GSDs. If both copies are defective, the result is disease. If only one defective copy is present, the disease does not occur, but the defective gene can still be passed on to subsequent generations. If both parents are carrying a defective gene, then each offspring has a one in four, or 25%, chance of inheriting the disease. Populations with a high frequency of healthy individuals carrying defective genes will also have higher prevalence of offspring with the disease.

Von Gierke's disease GSDIa and GSDIb are caused by mutations on chromosomes 17 and 11, respectively. GSDIa is caused by deficient activity of the enzyme glucose-6-phosphatase, both negatively impacting glycogenolysis. Pompe's disease is caused by mutations on **chromosome** 17 that result in different types of dysfunction of the enzyme glucosidase. Mutations in Pompe's disease may cause the complete absence of the enzyme, a normal amount of enzyme with reduced activity, or a reduced amount of enzyme with normal activity. The infantile subtype usually displays an absence of enzyme activity, whereas the other forms involve enzyme levels or functionality. Cori's disease may involve many different mutations in chromosome one, and any combination of defective genes may lead to the disease. There may be a generalized debrancher enzyme deficiency in Cori's disease, or genetic mutations in only some of the tissue-specific enzyme types.

All forms of Andersen's disease result from mutations on chromosome 3 in the genes for glycogen-branching enzymes. The branched structure of glycogen is necessary for compaction and breakdown. The mutations seen in Andersen's disease cause an abnormal, unbranched form of glycogen. Mutations may be generalized for all types of branching enzyme or tissue-specific. McArdle's disease can be caused by multiple types of mutations on chromosome 11 for the muscle-specific form of the phosphorylase enzyme. Most cases involve the functional absence of the enzyme. Hers' disease is due to mutations in multiple genes on multiple chromosomes that cause defects in liver phosphorylase enzyme pathways. Some types of the Hers' form are autosomal recessive, like other GSDs. Some subtypes have been reported that display X-linked recessive inheritance. In this mode of inheritance, mothers carrying defective X-linked genes can pass one copy to each offspring. However, because female offspring also receive a normal X-linked gene from the father, female offspring do not actually develop the disease. Male offspring who

receive their only X chromosome from the mother can develop the disease.

Demographics

GSDs are autosomal recessive inheritance and so occur with equal frequency in both sexes. GSDs as a group have a frequency of one per 20,000–25,000 births internationally. Approximately 80% of all GSD cases are a combination of von Gierke's, Cori's, and Hers' diseases, with each contributing equally. All three subtypes of Pompe's disease combined are estimated to occur at a rate of one per 40,000 individuals in the United States, and account for approximately 15% of GSD cases worldwide. Cori's disease is prevalent among Sephardic Jews of North African descent. In this population, the frequency is approximately one per 5,400 individuals. Even within the same mutation type, the physical effects of Cori's disease in this population are variable. Andersen's disease is uncommon, responsible for only 3% of all GSD cases. Andersen's disease is prevalent among the Ashkenazi Jews. McArdle's disease is also rare, with only a few hundred cases reported in the United States. McArdle's disease may be underdiagnosed because of its mild disease course. Only a few cases of early-onset McArdle's disease have been reported. Classic McArdle's disease has an adolescent onset. However, cases have been reported with onset in the sixth decade of life. Hers' disease is responsible for approximately 30% of GSD cases, while approximately 75% of Hers' disease are the X-linked form. Hers' disease is prevalent in the Mennonite population, with a frequency of 0.1%. X-linked recessive forms of Hers' disease are expressed primarily in affected males. Some breakthrough expression has still been reported in carrier females with mild symptoms.

Signs and symptoms

Von Gierke's disease

Infants born with von Gierke's disease display initial symptoms of hypoglycemia immediately following birth. These symptoms may include tremors, cyanosis (bluish tint from lack of oxygen), and seizures. Some infants are born with enlarged livers and abdomens. Onset of von Gierke's disease in an older infant may also include symptoms of fatigue, difficulty waking from long periods of sleep, tremors, extreme hunger, poor growth, short stature, and a protruding abdomen with thin limbs from liver enlargement. A doll-like facial appearance is often caused by fat deposits in the cheeks. Young children with von Gierke's disease may additionally have fat deposits called xanthomas on the elbows and knees, frequent nosebleeds, gingivitis (inflammation of the gums), and skin boils. Symptoms of severe hypoglycemia at all ages are likely to follow any illness or circumstance that causes a decrease in food intake. In later years, children may have rickets and anemia. Enlarged kidneys may be discovered by ultrasound imaging techniques. Complications that may arise from von Gierke's disease are severe hypoglycemia, liver **cancer**, kidney damage, fluid retention in the brain, coma, and death. In GSDIb, severe recurrent infections from immune compromise may also be a complication.

Pompe's disease

Infants born with Pompe's disease display initial symptoms of protruding abdomen due to liver enlargement, muscle enlargement, muscle weakness, and respiratory and feeding difficulty. Pneumonia is a complication. A heart murmur may be audible upon physical examination. Enlargement of the left ventricle of the heart may cause obstruction of blood flow and cardiac failure. The juvenile subtype of Pompe's disease displays symptoms of delayed motor development, weakness, and poor muscle tone. The adult subtype has symptoms of muscle weakness, especially when performing tasks such as climbing stairs or exercising. Approximately one third of cases involve respiratory complications.

Cori's disease

Infants born with Cori's disease may be healthy for the first few months of life, then present with initial symptoms of tremors, sweating, irritability, difficulty feeding, respiratory complications, seizures, coma, and sudden death. Older infants may also present with difficulty waking from sleep, poor growth, increased appetite, and dizziness. The level of hypoglycemia associated with this disease ranges from mild to severe. An enlarged liver may or may not be present. Some patients with Cori's disease have improvement in the liver complications as they get older, but others develop liver cirrhosis, liver failure, and liver cancer after puberty. Approximately 85% of patients with Cori's disease have significant involvement of both the liver and skeletal muscles. During childhood, complications with muscle are often minimal, but progressively get worse with age to the point of disability. Some patients may develop an enlarged heart but, otherwise, cardiac defects are rare. Often, Cori's disease causes poor growth with a short stature in children. If blood glucose levels are appropriately maintained, the attainment of normal growth is possible.

Andersen's disease

Infants born with Andersen's disease usually fail to thrive during the first year of life. In some cases, liver enlargement may lead to a protruding abdomen, liver cirrhosis, jaundice, hypertension, fatigue, bruising or bleeding easily, and liver failure. In other cases, the muscles may primarily be affected, causing weakness, fatigue, and muscle wasting. Muscle complications may extend to cardiac muscle and cause defects in function. If damage to the nervous system occurs in addition to muscular deficits, there may be decreased reflexes, sensory loss, and gait disturbances. Mild mental impairment may occur.

McArdle's disease

McArdle's disease usually has a primary symptom of exercise intolerance, with muscle weakness and fatigue. The symptoms occur during strenuous or sustained exercise and usually resolve with rest. Often there is a "second wind" of energy from glucose and fat breakdown products supplied by the blood. Symptoms may range from mild fatigue to temporarily incapacitating fatigue with muscle cramping. Late-onset cases may begin showing symptoms of progressive muscle weakness at 60–70 years of age. Other cases may present symptoms in the first year of life and become severely progressive. Even in the absence of exercise, one third of patients experience weakness. This symptom is especially common in older age. One half of cases filter blood in the urine after intense exercise, which may be indicative of impending kidney failure. A small percentage of McArdle's cases have seizures.

Hers' disease

Hers' disease usually has onset between the first and fifth year of life. Classic symptoms include a protruding abdomen due to enlarged liver, delay in growth with childhood short stature, and delayed motor development. Mild hypoglycemia may also be present, but many patients develop no other symptoms. Normal growth may be eventually achieved, along with a complete resolution in liver size to normal. Muscle strength in adults is usually normal.

Diagnosis

Von Gierke's disease

Von Gierke's disease is diagnosed through various types of testing. Characteristically, blood tests will reveal low blood sugar and the presence of lactic acid. Tests may also be performed to assess blood glucose levels after various challenges, such as administration of hormones that normally cause glycogen breakdown into glucose. Tests are done to assess for the presence of uric acid in the blood, kidney function, and liver function. GSDIa has a normal white blood cell (immune cells) level in the blood because the immune system is unaffected in this subtype. However, in subtype GSDIb, the immune system is impaired and has lower than normal blood levels of white blood cells. Most cases also involve a defect in blood coagulation, and tests are performed to assess bleeding times in a controlled setting. Ultrasound imaging of the abdomen is performed to assess liver and kidney size. To confirm a diagnosis, a biopsy of liver tissue is used to assess the function of the glucose-6-phosphatase enzyme that presents as defective in von Gierke's disease.

Pompe's disease

Blood tests are performed that can assess whether muscle disease is present by assessing for various factors, such as the enzyme creatine kinase, that are normally present inside muscle cells but not in the blood. The release of high levels of these factors into the bloodstream indicates a complication. Tests for the function of the enzyme alpha-glucosidase are performed to attain a definite diagnosis. This test may be done on white blood cells, but in infants it requires an amount of blood drawn that might not be practical. Instead, a skin biopsy is usually performed to test for the enzyme. Ultrasound imaging and tests that assess the heart's response to electrical stimulation are performed to diagnose the presence or extent of cardiac muscle defects.

Cori's disease

Blood tests are done to assess blood glucose and uric acid levels. Liver function studies are performed to determine the presence or extent of liver damage. Tests may also be performed to assess blood glucose levels after various challenges such as administration of hormones that normally cause glycogen breakdown into glucose. Both blood and urine are tested for the presence of ketone bodies, products of fat breakdown that can lead to dangerously acidic blood. Ultrasound imaging can assess for heart and liver enlargement or the presence of disease. Ultrasound imaging is also used to assess for polycystic ovaries in females, a common occurrence in Cori's disease that does not seem to affect fertility. A definite diagnosis involves tests that demonstrate abnormal, unbranched glycogen along with a debrancher enzyme deficiency in liver and muscle tissues.

Andersen's disease

To assess for liver complications, blood tests are performed to check for the presence of enzymes that are normally present in healthy liver cells and not in significant quantities in the blood. Distinct signs of liver cirrhosis or dysfunction may also be found in the blood. Ultrasound imaging can assess for liver enlargement, liver cirrhosis, and cardiac abnormalities. Cases in which there are primarily muscle, nervous system, or cardiac defects may have no sign of liver dysfunction. Blood glucose levels are tested to assess for hypoglycemia. To confirm a diagnosis of Andersen's disease, a defect in glycogen-branching enzyme activity must be demonstrated from tissue samples. Most cases can be assessed from a variety of different tissue types. A biopsy of the liver or other affected organs, such as the heart, may be taken for microscopic examination and to assess enzyme activity. In Ashkenazi Jews, deficient glycogen-branching enzyme activity is only seen in white blood cells and nerve cells. Prenatal enzyme testing can be done from amniotic samples.

McArdle's disease

Blood tests in McArdle's cases show elevated levels of enzymes, such as creatine kinase, that are normally present inside muscle cells but not in the blood. The release of high levels of these factors into the bloodstream indicates a complication. Exercise does not produce an increase in blood lactic acid in McArdle's disease. An electromyogram (EMG) is a graphic record of a muscle contraction in response to electrical stimulation. Half of all McArdle's cases have abnormalities in EMG. A muscle tissue biopsy may be assayed for muscle glycogen phosphorylase enzyme activity.

Hers' disease

The extent of abnormal blood testing results are variable and usually mild in Hers' disease. There may be some hypoglycemia, ketone bodies in blood and urine, elevated blood triglycerides, or enzyme levels that indicate liver complications. Ultrasound imaging may be used to assess liver enlargement. Tests may also be performed to assess blood glucose levels after various challenges, such as administration of hormones that normally cause glycogen breakdown into glucose. To confirm a diagnosis of Hers' disease, a liver biopsy is taken to assess to liver glycogen phosphorylase activity.

Treatment

Drug therapy and enzyme supplementation are not standard parts of treatment for the GSDs. Treatment focuses on maintaining blood glucose levels and treating the symptoms of complications that may arise from the disease. In most cases, this may involve frequent daytime feedings and, for infants, overnight use of a specialized nasogastric feeding tube equipped with an alarm. In most GSDs, children two years of age and older can be switched to cornstarch feeding at bedtime. Raw cornstarch, but not other types of starch, can sustain blood glucose for 4–6 hours if mixed with water at room temperature. Hot water significantly reduces the timeframe in which cornstarch can sustain blood glucose levels. Any illness or condition that reduces the amount of food intake requires supplemental injections of simple sugars, such as dextrose, or intravenous administration of glucose. Caregivers need to be educated in inserting feeding tubes, dietary control, and recognizing and managing hypoglycemia.

Diet is a critical component of treatment for most GSDs, and must be closely monitored by highly specialized nutritionists. Von Gierke's disease requires dietary avoidance of excessive carbohydrates, fat, or calories. All contact sports should be avoided because of the potential for excessive bleeding and liver damage. Iron supplementation is advised because of liver deficiencies. In GSDIb, an immune cell booster called granulocyte colony-stimulating factor (GCSF) is administered because of the depressed immune system. Dental and oral health needs to be actively maintained in GSDIb, to prevent infections. Cori's disease does not involve the same carbohydrate restrictions, but avoiding excessive fat intake is advised. Cori's disease is also treated with a high protein diet to supplement muscle function. Cori's disease does not involve sports restrictions past the personal limits of the individual's energy and blood glucose levels. Rupture of the liver from contact sports has not been reported in Cori's disease. The infantile subtype of Pompe's disease may not improve with dietary changes and may become fatal. A high protein diet may assist with muscle functioning in people affected with McArdle's disease and with adults with Pompe's disease. Supplementation with B vitamins may make muscles less prone to fatigue in McArdle's disease. McArdle's cases are advised to avoid sustained, strenuous, or weight-bearing exercise to prevent kidney damage. While Hers' disease requires avoiding long periods of fasting, most cases do not require significant dietary intervention or exercise reduction unless there is significant liver enlargement.

Blood glucose monitoring is done with specialized home kits called glucometers, which provides an exact reading of blood glucose. A test strip is used to collect a small drop of blood obtained by pricking the finger with a small needle called a lancet. The test strip is placed in the meter and results are available within 30–45 seconds. Testing is done on a regular basis to monitor the balance between food intake and blood sugar levels. If hypoglycemic episodes occur, drinking fruit juice or taking a few teaspoons of sugar may bring blood glucose levels back to normal. If 15 minutes have passed and blood sugar has not returned to normal, a second dose is administered.

Specialists are frequently consulted to monitor liver complications that arise in some GSDs. Andersen's disease often requires liver transplantation for effective treatment. However, some cases of Andersen's disease still result in a poor outcome after liver transplant. Specialists also monitor and provide symptom-specific management of cardiac and nervous system complications that arise from GSDs. Parents of children with GSDs are given **genetic counseling** regarding the risk of GSD to future pregnancies. There is a 25% recurrence risk for each subsequent pregnancy in most GSDs. There is a 50% of male offspring having X-linked forms of Hers' disease.

Prognosis

The prognosis of GSD is highly varied. Overall, the long-term prognosis depends on the extent, severity, and progression of the disease. GSDs are generally multisystem diseases, with many potential complications. With von Gierke's disease and Cori's disease, many patients receiving proper treatment do not encounter life-threatening hypoglycemia and have a reasonable lifespan. However, some patients may develop liver cirrhosis, liver cancer, or liver failure. Pompe's disease is also variable in prognosis. The infantile form is usually fatal within the first year of life. Death results from cardiac and respiratory failure. The juvenile (intermediate) form progresses more slowly, but is generally fatal by the second or third decade of life. Most deaths are from respiratory failure. The adult form may afford survival for several decades after onset. However, muscle weakness may interfere with normal daily activities, and death may result from respiratory failure.

Andersen's disease has a very poor prognosis, with the classic infantile form causing progressive liver cirrhosis and death by five years of age in the absence of a liver transplant. Liver transplantation still does not guarantee improvement. Cases involving non-progressive liver disease do not require liver transplantation, but are still at increased risk of liver cancer. Cases involving cardiac complications often lead to heart failure, despite medical intervention. Andersen's disease involving nervous system and skeletal muscle complications may not be life-threatening, but may be progressive and debilitating.

The prognosis of McArdle's disease is comparatively better than many other forms of GSDs. The primary complications are muscle weakness, cramping, and fatigue, which can interfere with normal daily activities. Some patients are able to adapt exercise to take advantage of the second wind phenomenon, as long as it is not too strenuous. Prognosis remains good as long as sustained, strenuous, and weight-bearing exercises are avoided, which can lead to acute renal failure. The infantile form of McArdle's disease has a poor prognosis, with death caused severe and rapidly progressive muscle weakness that leads to respiratory failure. The best

KEY TERMS

Amniotic sample—Sample of amniotic fluid, the protective fluid surrounding a fetus in the womb.

Anemia—Condition in which there are low levels of red blood cells.

Boils—Painful areas of inflammation.

Branching enzyme—Enzyme responsible for building the branched structure of glycogen stores.

Cirrhosis—Chronic disease of the liver that involves degeneration.

Coagulation—The solidification or change from a fluid state to a semisolid mass; blood coagulation helps to close open wounds.

Cyanosis—Lack of blood oxygen causing a bluish tint in the skin.

Debranching enzyme— Enzyme responsible for breaking down the branched structure of glycogen stores to release glucose into the bloodstream.

Gait disturbances—Disturbances that affect the manner of walking.

Gastrointestinal tract—The food intake and waste export system that runs from the mouth, through the esophagus, stomach, and intestines, to the rectum and anus.

Gingivitis—Inflammation of the gums of the mouth,

characterized by redness, swelling, and a tendency to bleed.

Glycogen—The storage form of many molecules of glucose, reserved for energy needs outside of dietary consumption.

Glycogenesis—The metabolic process responsible for the formation of glycogen from many glucose molecules.

Glycogenolysis—The metabolic process responsible for the break down of glycogen to mobilize glucose.

Hypoglycemia—Low blood sugar.

Jaundice—A condition that may be caused by liver disturbances characterized by yellowness of the skin.

Ketone bodies—Fat breakdown products that can make the blood acidic when present in high levels.

Left ventricle—Portion of the heart from which blood is pumped into the system.

Precursor components—Components in an enzymatic pathway that are formed by previous cellular events.

Rickets—Condition in which bone is not properly formed.

Xanthoma—Small, localized areas of fat deposition.

---

prognosis of the GSDs described is with Hers' disease. Hers' disease has a mild course with risk of growth retardation, mild fasting hypoglycemia, and delayed motor development in early childhood. However, these clinical features usually normalize by the time of puberty, along with liver enlargement and muscle weakness. Adult patients usually have normal stature and motor functions. Hers' disease may have an excellent prognosis, even without childhood dietary management.

Resources

BOOKS

Champe, P. C., and R. A. Harvey. *Lippincott's Illustrated Review of Biochemistry, Second Edition.* Philadelphia: J.B. Lippincott Company, 1994.

Thompson & Thompson Genetics in Medicine, Sixth Edition. St. Louis, MO: Elsevier Science, 2004.

WEBSITES

Anderson, W. E. *Glycogen Storage Disease, Type II.* (April 20, 2005.) <http://www.emedicine.com/med/topic908.htm>.

Ibrahim, J., and M. McGovern. *Glycogen-Storage Disease, Type II.* (April 20, 2005.) <http://www.emedicine.com/PED/topic1866.htm>.

Lerardi-Curto, L. *Glycogen-Storage Disease, Type IV.* (April 20, 2005.) <http://www.emedicine.com/PED/topic97.htm>.

Lerardi-Curto, L. *Glycogen-Storage Disease, Type VI.* (April 20, 2005.) <http://www.emedicine.com/PED/topic2564.htm>.

Roth, K.S. *Glycogen-Storage Disease, Type I.* (April 20, 2005.) <http://www.emedicine.com/ped/topic2416.htm>.

Sloan, H.R. *Glycogen-Storage Disease, Type III.* (April 20, 2005.) <http://www.emedicine.com/PED/topic479.htm>.

Wasserstein, M. *Glycogen-Storage Disease, Type V.* (April 20, 2005.) <http://www.emedicine.com/PED/topic1385.htm>.

Maria Basile, PhD

GM1-gangliosidosis

Definition

GM1-gangliosidosis is a lysosomal storage condition caused by a reduction or the absence in the amount of the enzyme, beta-galactosidase, in cells. This condition has been referred to by other names such as Norman-Landing disease, Gangliosidosis-GM1 beta-galactosidase-1 deficiency, Hurler-variant, pseudo-Hurler disease, **Tay-Sachs disease** with visceral involvement, and GLB1 deficiency.

Description

Lysosomes are structures found inside cells that contain specific proteins and enzymes that help digest or breakdown many of the complex biological substances found within the cells. After the lysosomes digest these substances, the remnants are then released from the cell. The role of the lysosome is to keep the inside of the cell clean and to help the cell function normally.

One of the lysosomal enzymes, beta-galactosidase, is necessary to digest a substance called GM1-ganglioside. When there is not enough beta-galactosidase within the lysosomes, GM1-ganglioside breaks down at a slower rate or not at all. Since GM1-ganglioside is not being digested as fast as it is being produced, GM1-ganglioside accumulates within the lysosomes. When too much GM1-ganglioside accumulates, the lysosomes stop functioning effectively, thereby causing the cell not to function properly.

When there are enough cells in an organ or organ system that stop functioning normally, the entire organ or organ system begins to experience problems. One of the first areas where GM1-ganglioside accumulates and causes problems is within the central nervous system. Other organs and systems in the body can also accumulate GM1-ganglioside; however, signs of the excessive accumulation are sometimes not immediately apparent.

There are three types of GM1-gangliosidoses; they are grouped according to the amount of beta-galactosidase detected in the individual's leukocytes (white blood cells) or skin cells, the individual's age when they start to show symptoms (called age of onset), and the specific symptoms that the individual exhibits. These types are labeled Type I, Type II, and Type III.

Genetic profile

All three types of GM1-gangliosidosis are inherited in an autosomal recessive manner. Symptoms of GM1-gangliosidosis occur when the pair of genes that produce beta-galactosidase (called GLB1) both contain a change, causing them not to work properly. When the GLB1 genes do not work properly, less or no beta-galactosidase is produced. Individuals with GM1-gangliosidosis inherit one of their non-working GLB1 genes from their mother and the other non-working GLB1 **gene** from their father. These parents are called carriers of GM1-gangliosidosis. When two people are known carriers for an autosomal recessive condition, like GM1-gangliosidosis, they have a 25% chance with each pregnancy to have a child affected with the disease.

The GLB1 gene is located on the short arm of **chromosome** 3, called 3p, in the region 21.33. This is written as 3p21.33. There have been over 20 mutations identified in the GLB1 gene that can cause the gene not to work properly. The most common type of mutation detected is a missense mutation. Typically, a gene is made up of **DNA** that codes for specific amino acids. It is the amino acids, when combined, that make a protein. When there is a missense mutation in a gene, the DNA code for a particular amino acid has been changed, often coding for a different amino acid. Changing the amino acid often changes the protein that is made. A change in the structure or production of a protein often alters its ability to function properly.

Most individuals with GM1-gangliosidosis are compound heterozygotes. This means that an individual with GM1-gangliosidosis has one GLB1 gene containing one mutation and his or her other GLB1 gene has a different mutation. Researchers do not believe that there is any correlation between specific mutations in the GLB1 gene and the severity of GM1-gangliosidosis. An exception to this is the discovery of mutations in the GLB1 gene that, instead of causing an individual to have GM1-gangliosidosis, cause the individual to have another condition called Morquio syndrome type B.

Demographics

GM1-gangliosidosis is a rare condition. It is estimated that approximately one in 100,000–200,000 live births is affected with this condition. Type I GM1-gangliosidosis is considered to occur more often than the other two types. There has also been an increased number of individuals living in Japan, Brazil, and Maltese Island diagnosed with all types of GM1-gangliosidosis. However, many researchers state that this condition is not more common in individuals of certain ethnic groups, although many of the individuals with Type III GM1-gangliosidosis are Japanese. Additionally, GM1-gangliosidosis occurs with equal frequency in males and females.

Signs and symptoms

GM1-gangliosidosis Type I

Type I GM1-gangliosidosis is also called infantile GM1-gangliosidosis or infantile type, and it is considered the most severe form of GM1-gangliosidosis. Infants with GM1-gangliosidosis Type I tend to have less than 1% of the normal amount of beta-galactosidase in their cells.

Some of the symptoms seen with Type I can be apparent at birth, but all infants with Type I will show characteristics of the condition before six months of age. All infants with Type I will reach a point where they fail to gain new skills and begin to regress and lose the skills they have learned.

Several of the initial symptoms seen in infants with Type I are caused by the storage of GM1-ganglioside in the cells of the infant's central nervous system. One sign of a problem with the central nervous system seen in some infants with Type I is the infant's inability to eat much food or formula because of a poor appetite and/or difficulties with sucking on a bottle or nipple. As a result, they tend to gain very little weight. Another sign of GM1-ganglioside storage in the central nervous system is muscle problems. Most of these infants will have low muscle tone, called hypotonia. These babies appear "floppy" or "loose." As the disease progresses, the infant presents with other central nervous system problems, such as an exaggerated reaction to sound, atrophy of the optic nerves, their bodies becoming rigid and stiff, developing tight joints (joint contractures), and experiencing seizures. Infants with Type I can also develop brain atrophy and/or areas of decreased amount of white matter in the brain.

In GM1-gangliosidosis Type I, GM1-ganglioside is also stored in the skeleton, causing visible changes on radiographs. Some of the more common bone changes are: differences with their vertebrae causing spine curvature, thicker skull, wider bones and hands, and wide, short fingers. Also, the growth of the bones tends to slow down or stop, causing infants with GM1-gangliosidosis Type I to appear smaller than expected for their age.

Additionally, infants with Type I usually develop certain characteristic facial features. The facial features typically seen in infants with Type I include frontal bossing, ears that are set lower on the head than normal, thicker skin, hair on forehead and neck, an elongated space between the nose and mouth, and an enlarged tongue. Children with these facial changes are often described as appearing "coarse." Coarse facial features can also be seen in infants and children who have other types of storage disorders.

Other characteristics of GM1-gangliosidosis Type 1 include an enlarged spleen and liver (called hepatosplenomegaly), cardiomyopathy (which has only been described in caucasian patients), and an enlargement of the cells in the bone marrow. Additionally, infants with Type I have cherry-red spots in the macula of their retinas, and several develop corneal clouding.

GM1-gangliosidosis Type II

GM1-gangliosidosis Type II is also referred to as the juvenile type. In children with Type II, the amount of beta-galactosidase in the cells is approximately 1–5% of normal.

There are no symptoms that are specific to GM1-Gangliosidosis Type II. Signs of Type II often appear late in infancy or in early childhood. Although each individual with Type II may present differently, several children with Type II have been reported to have difficulty walking and/or developed seizures. The bone changes seen in Type I may or may not occur in children with Type II. Furthermore, children with Type II do not have macular cherry-red spots, enlarged spleen or liver, or the facial changes.

GM1-gangliosidosis Type III

Individuals with GM1-gangliosidosis Type III are also labeled as having the adult or chronic type of this condition. Individuals with Type III tend to have approximately 10% of the normal amount of beta-galactosidase in their cells. The age when symptoms begin to appear in individuals with Type III is extremely variable. There have been reports of individuals with Type III exhibiting symptoms as early as three years of age to as late as 30 years old. The symptoms slowly worsen over many years.

Individuals with GM1-gangliosidosis Type III tend to experience some symptoms related to the storage of GM1-ganglioside in their central nervous system; however, these symptoms are not as severe as those seen in infants with Type I. The signs of GM1-ganglioside storage can be different in each person affected with the GM1-gangliosidosis Type III, but many individuals with Type III have been reported to have signs of **dystonia**. Other neurological symptoms in Type III can include difficulty or unusual method of walking (ataxia), mild mental delays, and slurred speech. Often the ataxia and slurred speech are some of the first symptoms to appear.

Individuals with Type III also have GM1-ganglioside storage in bone cells, but bone changes are considered milder than those seen in Type I. Often the vertebrae of individuals with Type III tend to have a flattened appearance and/or the presence of other mild vertebral

KEY TERMS

Amino acid—Organic compounds that form the building blocks of protein. There are 20 types of amino acids (eight are "essential amino acids" which the body cannot make and must therefore be obtained from food).

Ataxia—A deficiency of muscular coordination, especially when voluntary movements are attempted, such as grasping or walking.

Atrophy—Wasting away of normal tissue or an organ due to degeneration of the cells.

Basal ganglia—A section of the brain responsible for smooth muscular movement.

Cardiomyopathy—A thickening of the heart muscle.

Cytoplasm—The substance within a cell including the organelles and the fluid surrounding the nucleus.

Deoxyribonucleic acid (DNA)—The genetic material in cells that holds the inherited instructions for growth, development, and cellular functioning.

Dystonia—Painful involuntary muscle cramps or spasms.

Enzyme—A protein that catalyzes a biochemical reaction or change without changing its own structure or function.

Frontal bossing—A term used to describe a rounded forehead with a receded hairline.

Gray matter—Areas of the brain and spinal cord that are comprised mostly of unmyelinated nerves.

Lysosome—Membrane-enclosed compartment in cells, containing many hydrolytic enzymes; where large molecules and cellular components are broken down.

Mutation—A permanent change in the genetic material that may alter a trait or characteristic of an individual, or manifest as disease, and can be transmitted to offspring.

Myelin—A fatty sheath surrounding nerves in the peripheral nervous system, which help them conduct impulses more quickly.

Organelle—Small, sub-cellular structures that carry out different functions necessary for cellular survival and proper cellular functioning.

White matter—A substance found in the brain and nervous system that protects nerves and allows messages to be sent to and from to brain to the various parts of the body.

---

changes. On CT or MRI examinations, mild brain atrophy with signs of storage in the basal ganglia can be present in some individuals with Type III. Also, some individuals with Type III have experienced corneal clouding. However, the macular cherry-red spots, facial changes, and differences in the bones are not seen in individuals with GM1-gangliosidosis Type III.

Diagnosis

The diagnosis of GM1-gangliosidosis in an individual can be made by measuring the amount of beta-galactosidase in either skin cells or in leukocytes. Additionally, prenatal testing to determine if a fetus is affected with GM1-gangliosidosis prior to its delivery can be accomplished by measuring the amount of beta-galactosidase on cultured cells from an **amniocentesis** or chorionic villus sampling (CVS). Amniocentesis is a procedure used to remove some of the fluid, which contains fetal cells, from around the fetus. CVS is used to obtain cells from the placenta. With both of these procedures, the cells collected are stimulated to multiply so that there are enough cells to perform certain analyses, in this case measuring the amount of beta-galactosidase.

Both of these procedures have their own risks, benefits, and limitations.

X rays can detect bone changes and organ enlargement. However, in early stages of the condition, bone differences may not have developed or the organs may not yet be enlarged. Also, a CT scan and/or MRI can identify brain changes, such as cerebral atrophy or a loss of myelin in the white matter of the brain. An eye examination can detect any macular cherry-red spots or other changes.

Analysis of the amount of beta-galactosidase in an individual's cells cannot be used to determine if the person is a carrier of GM1-gangliosidosis. This is because the range for the amount of beta-galactosidase seen in carriers of this condition overlaps with the range of the amount of beta-galactosidase seen in individuals who are not carriers.

Treatment and management

There is no cure for GM1-gangliosidosis. Most of the treatments revolve around trying to alleviate some of the symptoms, such as helping infants with Type I to eat and devices that can help with problems walking in individuals with Type III. Additionally, there is ongoing research into **gene therapy** for GM1-gangliosidosis to infuse genes that produce beta-galactosidase into the body.

Prognosis

In Type I GM1-gangliosidosis, the child dies within a few years after the symptoms begin, typically by age two. In Type II GM1-gangliosidosis, the prognosis is variable. Some individuals have died during childhood and others have lived many years after symptoms began. In Type III GM1-gangliosidosis, no decrease in life span has been reported.

Resources

BOOKS

Suzuki, Yoshiyuki, Hitoshi Sakuraba, and Akihiro Oshima. "Beta-Galatosidase Deficiency (Beta-Galactosidosis): GM1 Gangliosidosis and Morquio B Disease." In *The Metabolic and Molecular Bases of Inherited Disease*, edited by Charles R. Scriver, et al. New York: McGraw Hill, 1995, pp. 2785-2823.

ORGANIZATIONS

Association for Neuro-Metabolic Disorders. 5223 Brookfield Lane, Sylvania, OH 43560-1809. (419) 885-1497.

WEBSITES

Lysosomal Storage Disease: A Family Source Book. <http://mcrcr2.med.nyu.edu/murphp01/lysosome/hgd.htm>.

Online Mendelian Inheritance in Man. National Center for Biotechnology Information. <http://www.ncbi.nlm.nih.gov/Omim/>.

Sharon A. Aufox, MS, CGC

Goiter-sensorineural deafness syndrome *see* **Pendred syndrome**

Golabi-Rosen syndrome *see* **Simpson-Golabi-Behmel syndrome**

Goldberg syndrome *see* **Neuraminidase deficiency with beta-galactosidase deficiency**

Goldenhar syndrome *see* **Hemifacial microsomia**

Goltz syndrome

Definition

Goltz syndrome, also known as focal dermal hypoplasia or Goltz-Gorlin syndrome, is a rare form of an abnormal skin condition that is believed to be a dominant, X-linked trait. It is named after R. W. Goltz, who first described this syndrome in 1962.

Description

Goltz syndrome is a genetic condition primarily found in females that affects the appearance and function of the skin. An unrelated syndrome, **nevoid basal cell carcinoma** syndrome (NBCCS), is also known as Gorlin-Goltz syndrome. NBCCS is a non-sex linked dominant disorder characterized by a predisposition to **cancer**, particularly of the basal cells. Care should be taken not to confuse Gorlin-Goltz syndrome with Goltz, or Goltz-Gorlin, syndrome.

Goltz syndrome has many other synonyms, but it is most often referred to as focal dermal hypoplasia (which can be found in the medical literature abbreviated as FDH, FODH or DHOF) because of the characteristic, localized (focal) skin (dermal) patches that are thin or absent (hypoplasia). Other synonyms include: combined mesoectodermal **dysplasia**, congenital ectodermal and mesodermal dysplasia, ectodermal and mesodermal dysplasia with osseous involvement, focal dermal hypoplasia syndrome, and focal dermatophalangeal dysplasia.

Goltz syndrome is part of a larger family of diseases known as the ectodermal dysplasias, or abnormalities of the skin, hair, teeth, and nails. In Goltz syndrome, the skin abnormalities take the form of areas of thin skin (lesions) where the skin is completely absent or discolored, itchy, or blistered. Hair may also be missing in patches, and the teeth are usually poorly formed. Nails may also be unusual in appearance. In addition to these characteristics of the skin and related organs, Goltz syndrome affected individuals can also have skeletal malformations and eye problems.

The obvious bodily symptoms of Goltz syndrome are the result of improper functioning of the skin, an organ whose multiple functions are often overlooked. The skin consists of two layers, the outer skin (epidermis) and the lower skin (dermis). The epidermis layer protects the body from environmental threats such as temperature variations, bacterial infections, and toxic chemicals. In Goltz syndrome, the epidermis is deformed or completely absent. The dermis layer contains cells, which manufacture the protein collagen. Collagen makes up about one-fourth of all the body's protein and plays a vital role in wound healing, skin and muscle support, and bone formation. In Goltz syndrome, abnormal formation of type IV collagen has been found in the dermis including loose collagen bundles and fibers with loss of regular bands. The importance of collagen for many of the body's tissues explains the varied symptoms of Goltz syndrome, which is observed in parts of the body as different as the bones, skin, hair, and fingernails.

Genetic profile

The locus of the **gene** responsible for Goltz syndrome has been localized to the short arm of the X **chromosome** at locus Xp22.3. At or near this same locus is the gene responsible for **microphthalmia with linear skin defects (MLS)** and the gene responsible for **Aicardi syndrome**. Because of the relatively low number of males diagnosed with this condition, it is assumed that Goltz syndrome is dominant and X-linked with close to 100% fetal mortality in males. Nearly all of the cases of Goltz syndrome are believed to result from *de novo* mutations (new mutations which occur after conception) since parents of affected individuals have normal chromosomes.

Demographics

Roughly 150 cases of Goltz syndrome in females and only 11 cases in males have been reported in the medical literature. Goltz syndrome is not linked to any particular sub-populations. It appears with equal frequency in all races and across all geographies. Because it is an X-linked dominant condition, it is observed with a much higher frequency in surviving females than it is in surviving males.

Signs and symptoms

Goltz syndrome is characterized by localized areas of malformed skin (skin lesions) that appear underdeveloped, streaked, or absent. The skin of an individual with Goltz syndrome may lack color (pigmentation) in the affected areas or the skin may look streaked with lines (linear pigmentation). The affected areas may look and feel inflamed or irritated in various ways such as by exhibiting itching, blistering, reddening and swelling, and even crusting and bleeding. Fatty deposits (papillomas) are usually present in areas of typically sensitive skin, such as the gums, lips, tongue, armpits, vaginal opening, and the anus. Nodules of yellowish fatty tissue can grow on the affected skin, particularly in skin folds.

People with Goltz syndrome often experience excessive skin growth in the palms of the hands and on the soles of the feet. Because of this overgrowth of skin layers, increased sweating (hyperhidrosis) is often noticed in these areas. Similarly, because of an undergrowth of skin in other parts of the body, many affected

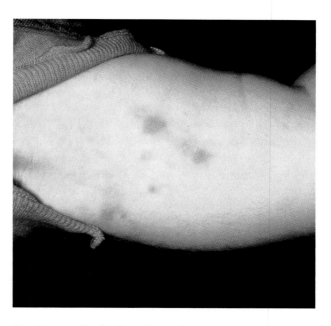

Papules, small raised sections of skin, such as that shown on this patients arm are characteristic of Goltz syndrome. (*Custom Medical Stock Photo, Inc.*)

individuals do not sweat normally (hypohidrosis) throughout the rest of their bodies.

Additionally, individuals with Goltz syndrome may present patches of hair loss on both their scalps and in their pubic regions. The teeth of Goltz syndrome patients are often malformed, mispositioned, or absent and cavities are commonplace because of missing or incomplete tooth enamel.

Unusual bone formations are also associated with Goltz syndrome. Missing or extra fingers or toes, webbed fingers or toes, permanently bent fingers or toes, and fusion of bones in the fingers or toes have all been observed in Goltz syndrome. Other skeletal abnormalities such as curvature of the spine, underdevelopment or a protrusion of the lower jaw, and fused vertebrae may also be present.

Individuals diagnosed with Goltz syndrome are likely to exhibit facial asymmetry, underdeveloped ears, wide-set eyes, and a pointed chin. Hearing loss, either developed or from birth, is frequently experienced by these individuals as well, due to the underdevelopment of the ears. Many eye abnormalities have been seen in those affected with Goltz syndrome. These range from missing eyes (anophthalmia) and incomplete formation of the eye (**coloboma**) to clouding of the cornea, drooping eyelids, and crossed eyes. The mucous membranes of the nose and throat may also be affected.

KEY TERMS

Anopthalmia—A medical condition in which one eye is missing.

Collagen—The main supportive protein of cartilage, connective tissue, tendon, skin, and bone.

Coloboma—A birth defect in which part of the eye does not form completely.

de novo **mutation**—Genetic mutations that are seen for the first time in the affected person, not inherited from the parents.

Dermis—The layer of skin beneath the epidermis.

Ectodermal dysplasia—A hereditary condition that results in the malformation of the skin, teeth, and hair. It is often associated with malfunctioning or absent sweat glands and/or tear ducts.

Epidermis—The outermost layer of the skin.

Hyperhidrosis—Excessive perspiration that may be either general or localized to a specific area.

Hypohidrosis—Insufficient perspiration or absent perspiration which may be either general or localized to a specific area.

Hypoplasia—Incomplete or underdevelopment of a tissue or organ.

Oligodactyly—The absence of one or more fingers or toes.

Papilloma—Any benign localized growth of the skin and the linings of the respiratory and digestive tracts. The most common papilloma is the wart.

Mental retardation has been observed in some, but not all, cases.

Diagnosis

Goltz syndrome is generally diagnosed by the presence of the characteristic skin abnormalities coupled with the characteristic fatty deposits in the gums, lips, armpits, vagina, or anus. It is distinguished from the other possible ectodermal dysplasias by the lack of pigmentation of the skin in some of the affected areas, the abnormal sweating experienced by those individuals affected, the lack of cysts in the eyes, and the presence of tear ducts. The papillomas in the genital areas are often misdiagnosed as genital warts, but Goltz syndrome patients will test negative for human papillomavirus (HPV), the cause of the common genital wart.

Prenatal diagnosis is not yet available, but connection to the Xp22.3 locus makes **genetic testing** for this dominant condition potentially possible. In families with a child affected by Goltz syndrome, a skin test on the parents should be conducted to evaluate the potential risk of a second child being born with this syndrome.

Treatment and management

The treatment and management of Goltz syndrome varies according to symptoms observed. Dermatological treatments such as skin creams and more targeted treatments are usually indicated. Some affected individuals will require dental work or surgery. Others will need respiratory therapies to keep the nose and throat clear. Certain skeletal deformations seen in patients with Goltz syndrome may be corrected by orthopedic surgery. Because of the associated abnormal sweating patterns, affected individuals should not be exposed to heat and should avoid heavy exercise.

Prognosis

Goltz syndrome is thought to be almost always lethal in males. Even so, a male patient as old as 68 has been reported in the medical literature. In females, a full life expectancy is possible if medical treatment is followed.

Resources

PERIODICALS

Buchner, S., and P. Itin. "Focal Dermal Hypoplasia in a Male Patient: Report of a Case and Histologic and Immunohistochemical Studies." *Archives of Dermatology* (August 1992): 1078-82.

Lee, I., et al. "Electronmicroscopic Observation of the Basement Membrane Zone in Focal Dermal Hypoplasia." *Pediatric Dermatology* (January-February 1996): 5-9.

Mendez, P., M. Vega, and A. Mosqueda. "Mucosal Lesions in Focal Dermal Hypoplasia Syndrome." *Medecina Oral* (April 1999): 366-71.

ORGANIZATIONS

Ectodermal Dyplasia Society. 108 Charlton Lane, Cheltenham, GlosGL53 9EA. UK <http://www.ectodermaldysplasia.org>.

National Foundation for Ectodermal Dysplasias. PO Box 114, 410 E Main, Mascoutah, IL 62258-0114. (618) 566-2020. Fax: (618) 566-4718. <http://www.nfed.org>.

National Organization for Rare Disorders (NORD). PO Box 8923, New Fairfield, CT 06812-8923. (203) 746-6518 or (800) 999-6673. Fax: (203) 746-6481. <http://www.rarediseases.org>.

WEBSITES

"Focal Dermal Hypoplasia." *Online Mendelian Inheritance in Man.* <http://www.ncbi.nlm.nih.gov/entrez/dispomim.cgi?id=305600> (05 February 2001).

"Focal Dermal Hypoplasia." *Reader's Digest Health.* <http://rdhealth.com/kbase/nord/nord926.htm> (February 5, 2001).

Paul A. Johnson

Goltz-Gorlin syndrome *see* Goltz syndrome

Goniodysgenesis hypodontia, iridogoniodysgenesis with somatic anomalies *see* Rieger syndrome

Goodman syndrome *see* Carpenter syndrome

Gordon syndrome *see* Distal arthrogryposis syndrome

Gorlin syndrome *see* Nevoid basal cell carcinoma

▌Greig cephalopolysyndactyly

Definition

Greig cephalopolysyndactyly is a very rare autosomal dominant disorder. The syndrome is characterized by physical abnormalities of the head, face, fingers and toes. Distinct features include extra fingers and/or toes; a large and unusual shape of the skull; a high, prominent forehead; and widely spaced eyes. The range and severity of symptoms may vary greatly between individuals. Some individuals with Greig cephalopolysyndactyly require medical or surgical intervention to manage these problems. The syndrome is familial and in most cases is transmitted as an autosomal dominant trait.

Description

The disorder is named for D. M. Greig (pronounced Gregg), a Scottish physician, who first described the features of this syndrome in 1926. He saw a mother and her daughter who had a peculiar shape of the skull (cephalus) and polysyndactyly of the hands and feet. Polysyndactyly means both extra digits (toes, fingers) as well as webbing (syndactyly) between the digits. Dr. Greig described them as having a high forehead and widely spaced eyes. Thus, the syndrome was termed Greig cephalopolysyndactyly.

Genetic profile

Greig cephalopolysyndactyly (GCPS) can be found in several generations of a family. It is an autosomal dominant disorder and can be inherited, and passed on, by men as well as women. Almost all genes come in pairs. Cells work best when both copies of the **gene** pairs are intact and do not have mutations. One copy of each pair of genes is inherited from the father, and the other copy of each pair of genes is inherited from the mother. Therefore, if a parent carries a gene mutation for GCPS, each of his/her children has a 50% chance of inheriting the gene mutation. Each child also has a 50% chance of inheriting the working copy of the gene, in which case they would not have GCPS.

The search to find the causative gene took a number of years. The first clue came in 1989, when an 11-month old infant was found to have a deletion of genetic material on **chromosome** 7. The infant had a large head and polysyndactyly of the hands and feet. Other reports soon followed, with small deletions and translocations of chromosome 7. Then, in 1991, investigators began to study a gene called GLI-3 as the candidate gene. This gene was found in the region of chromosome 7p13, which was missing in these individuals. The GLI-3 gene was also suspect because of previous studies done in mice.

The mouse gene GLI-3 normally functions in the design of the skeleton and limbs in the embryo. The GLI-3 gene also works in the developing brain. Mice lacking both copies of the gene die before birth. Many have severe birth defects of the brain, skeleton and central nervous system. However, mice with just one non-working copy of the GLI-3 gene do not die. They have minor birth defects, most notably extra digits, often of the hind feet. The mice also have a duplicated bone in their front feet, and an enlarged bone in the front portion of the skull. This combination of birth defects is unusual, but common to both Xt mice and individuals with Greig cephalopolysyndactyly.

With this in mind, the GLI3 gene was scanned for alterations (mutations) in individuals with GCPS. Of interest, both small and large mutations were found throughout the coding gene regions of the gene. As none of these mutations was found in unaffected individuals, this proved that the GLI3 gene was the cause of the condition.

In addition to GSPC, **Pallister-Hall syndrome** and post-axial **polydactyly** type A (PAP-A), two other disorders of human development, are caused by alterations in the GLI3 gene. The common feature of each disorder is polydactyly of the hands and feet. However, individuals with Pallister-Hall syndrome have additional growth problems and severe mental retardation. Extra fingers and toes are the primary feature of PAP-A, and thus, the most mild in expression of the three conditions.

Scientists have used animal models and the fruit fly *Drosophila* to study the function of the GLI3 gene. The normal function of the GLI3 protein is to bind to the **DNA** helix at specific places. By doing so, it helps to regulate which genes are activated or "turned on." Many of the mutations identified so far seem to interfere with the protein binding function. In effect, other genes that would normally be activated during development of the embryo may in fact not be turned on.

It is known that the limbs (arms, legs, fingers, toes) develop between the fourth and eighth week of pregnancy. The limb defects seen in GCPS must occur during this crucial period of development.

Demographics

Greig cephalopolysyndactyly affects both males and females equally. It most likely occurs in every race and ethnic group. In all, less than 100 individuals have been described worldwide. Therefore, it is a rare condition.

Signs and symptoms

Most individuals with Greig cephalopolysyndactyly have a large head circumference (the distance as measured around the cranium). The forehead is high and wide, and slightly rounded in front (frontal bossing). This is due to the cranial sutures closing later than normal, causing the bones of the forehead to remain apart. The widening of the forehead appears to dip down into the space between the eyes, setting the eyes farther apart than normal. The bridge of the nose is broad and flat. This adds to the impression of distance between the eyes. Many times, the rest of the face will also look broad, almost box-like. The chin is small in comparison. The mouth is wide, and the corners of the mouth may be turned downward. The ears are usually normal. Individuals with GCPS can have a short neck, making it look as if the head rests on the shoulders. Intelligence is usually normal, although a few individuals have had mild learning disabilities.

The hands are quite distinctive in appearance. Most individuals with GCPS have extra fingers, on each hand. The extra finger is rarely on the thumb side (pre-axial polydactyly). It is most often on the pinky finger side (post-axial polydactyly). Some individuals have an extra finger on each side of the hand, and thus, the possibility of 14 fingers. However, the extra finger may or may not include bone, and could just be a skin tag. The thumbs

are frequently quite wide in appearance. Sometimes the bones of the thumb are duplicated or split at the tip. There may also be duplication or fusion in some of the bones that make up the hand, which can be seen on x ray. Their hands are still quite functional, although surgery may be necessary.

Many of these patients will have extra toes. What is unusual is that the extra toe is most often on the great toe side, opposite to what is found in the hands. The toes may also be short. Syndactyly (extensive webbing of the skin) is a constant finding in these patients. The webbing is usually between the toes, but may involve the hands. The webbing can vary from being mild, to complete joining of the digits, with skin up to the nail. Sometimes, just a few of the digits are fused together; in others, all of the toes are webbed. The webbing may also be present alone, without extra toes, although this is uncommon. The syndactyly may also occur on just one foot, and can be quite variable. Foot mobility and walking is usually not a problem.

There are other occasional problems seen in GCPS. These include **craniosynostosis** (premature fusion of the skull bones), mild mental retardation, hernia of the abdominal (stomach) muscles, and lesser birth defects of the urinary tract system, such as **hypospadias**.

Diagnosis

Each individual with Greig cephalopolysyndactyly is affected somewhat differently. The features are usually quite variable, even within the same family. The facial features can be mild with most individuals only having a high and broad forehead.

Therefore, the polysyndactyly of the hands and feet remains the most distinctive feature of the syndrome. With the use of x rays, changes in the bones of the hands and feet can be seen. The diagnosis of GCPS is suspected when the physician identifies the extra digits on the outside of the hands and on the inside of the foot, along with the broad forehead. This is usually seen at birth.

The availability of direct gene testing allows for a definitive diagnosis for these patients. Using a blood sample, a direct gene test looking for alterations (mutations) in the GLI3 gene can be done. An identifiable gene mutation would confirm the diagnosis in sporadic (non-inherited) patients as well.

Treatment and management

Very often, the physical characteristics of the face do not require surgical treatment. Sometimes, the facial appearance even improves as the child grows.

KEY TERMS

Abdominal hernia—Bulging of an organ or tissue through the muscle of the stomach wall.

Chromosome deletion—A missing sequence of DNA or part of a chromosome.

Chromosome translocation—The exchange of genetic material between chromosomes, which can lead to extra or missing genetic material.

Hypospadias—An abnormality of the penis in which the urethral opening is located on the underside of the penis rather than at its tip.

Polysyndactyly—Having both extra digits (toes, fingers) as well as webbing (syndactyly) between the digits.

Post-axial polydactyly—An extra finger or toe on the outside of the hand or foot.

Pre-axial polydactyly—An extra finger or toe on the inside of the hand or foot.

Syndactyly—Webbing or fusion between the fingers or toes.

However, if the cranial sutures in the forehead close either very early or very late, there may be fairly severe disfigurement to the face. This would require surgery from a specialized craniofacial medical team. Craniofacial surgery rearranges or reconstructs the bones of the face to correct the abnormal fusion of the cranial bones.

Some degree of surgery will also be needed for the polydactyly of the hands and feet. The extra digits that are just skin tags (no bone within) are tied off at the base, and allowed to self-amputate. This is usually done at birth. For those digits that include bone, most surgeons would save the digit that would have the best use. The other digit (or digits) would then be surgically removed, usually around one year of age. Surgery is often done to release the webbing of the fingers and toes, and can be quite extensive.

Prognosis

Most individuals with Greig cephalopolysyndactyly appear to have a normal life span.

Resources

ORGANIZATIONS

AboutFace International. 123 Edwards St., Suite 1003, Toronto, ONT M5G 1E2. Canada

FACES: The National Craniofacial Association. PO Box 11082, Chattanooga, TN 37401. (423) 266-1632 or (800) 332-2373. faces@faces-cranio.org. <http://www.faces-cranio.org/>.

WEBSITES

About Face. <http://www.aboutface2000.org>.

Alliance of Genetic Support Groups. <http://www.geneticalliance.org.htm>.

Let's Face It. <http://www.faceit.org>.

Kevin M. Sweet, MS, CGC

Griscelli syndrome

Definition

Griscelli syndrome is a rare, sometimes fatal disorder that associates partial **albinism** with immunodeficiency. Partial albinism is characterized by a partial lack of melanin (pigment) in the eyes, hair, and skin. The partial albinism found in patients with Griscelli syndrome is caused by an abnormal melanosome distribution. Immunodeficiency refers to an immune system in which resistance to infection is lowered.

Description

In addition to having silvery hair, most people with Griscelli syndrome develop hemophagocytic syndrome, which causes some blood cells in the body to engulf and destroy other blood cells. Hemophagocytic syndrome leads to death unless the patient undergoes a bone marrow transplant.

Some people with Griscelli syndrome are severely impaired neurologically but have no apparent immune abnormalities. Neurologic problems may be spasticity (in which a patient has uncontrolled muscular contractions), rigidity (in which a patient is inflexible or stiff), and convulsions. Through 1994 only 19 patients were reported in the medical literature as having the disorder.

Genetic profile

Griscelli syndrome is an autosomal recessive disorder that sometimes occurs in children with parents who are related by blood. There is evidence that the disorder is caused by mutations in the **gene** that encodes myosin VA, a protein in muscle tissue. (The gene encoding myosin VA is MYO5A.) The gene associated with Griscelli syndrome has been mapped to the long end of

KEY TERMS

Autosomal recessive—A pattern of genetic inheritance where two abnormal genes are needed to display the trait or disease.

Melanin—Pigments normally produced by the body that give color to the skin and hair.

Melanocytes—A cell that can produce melanin.

Melanosomes—Granules of pigment within melanocytes that synthesize melanin.

Peptide—A molecular compound made of two or more amino acids.

Protease—An enzyme that acts as a catalyst in the breakdown of peptide bonds.

chromosome 15 at location 15q21. A second gene, RAB27A, maps very close to the same region (15q21) as MYO5A.

Demographics

Both males and females are born with Griscelli syndrome.

Signs and symptoms

Griscelli syndrome causes pigmentary dilution of the skin and hair, and clumps of pigment in hair shafts. Griscelli syndrome also causes an accumulation of melanosomes in melanocytes.

People with Griscelli syndrome may also have frequent infections in which pus is present, fever, an abnormal decrease in the number of white blood cells, and a reduction in the number of platelets in the blood.

Diagnosis

Griscelli syndrome can be diagnosed in fetuses in the womb by microscopically examining the hair shaft. After birth, patients are diagnosed with Griscelli syndrome based on the signs and symptoms.

Griscelli syndrome is similar to **Chediak-Higashi syndrome**. For example, both are autosomal recessive disorders in which partial albinism and immunodeficiency are associated. And patients with either disorder are likely to have frequent infections.

However, patients with Chediak-Higashi syndrome are likely to have giant granules in their leukocytes, a type of white blood cell. And leukocyte-specific protease activity is typically low in patients with Chediak-Higashi syndrome, and typically normal in patients with Griscelli syndrome.

Treatment and management

In patients who have hemophagocytic syndrome associated with Griscelli syndrome, treatment may be in the form of bone marrow transplantation.

Prognosis

The prognosis for babies with Griscelli syndrome is poor without bone marrow transplantation.

Resources

PERIODICALS

Bahadoran, P., et al. "Rab27a. A Key to Melanosome Transport in Human Melanocytes." *Journal of Cell Biology* 152 (February 19, 2001): 843-50.

Durandy, A., et al. "Prenatal Diagnosis of Syndromes Associating Albinism and Immune Deficiencies (Chediak-Higashi Syndrome and Variant)." *Prenatal Diagnosis* 13 (1993): 13-20.

Gogus, S., et al. "Griscelli Syndrome: Report of Three Cases." *Pediatric Pathology and Laboratory Medicine* 15 (1995): 309-319.

Griscelli, C., et al. "A Syndrome Associating Partial Albinism and Immunodeficiency." *American Journal of Medicine* 65 (1978): 691-702.

Hurvitz, H., et al. "A Kindred with Griscelli Disease: Spectrum of Neurological Involvement." *European Journal of Pediatrics* 152 (1993): 402-405.

Klein, C., et al. "Partial Albinism with Immunodeficiency (Griscelli Syndrome)." *Journal of Pediatrics* 125 (1994): 886-895.

Mancini, A. J., L. S. Chan, and A. S. Paller. "Partial Albinism with Immunodeficiency: Griscelli Syndrome: Report of a Case and Review of the Literature." *Journal of the American Academy of Dermatology* 38 (1998): 295-300.

Menasche, G. E., et al. "Mutations in RAB27A Cause Griscelli Syndrome Associated with Haemophagocytic Syndrome." *Nature Genetics* 25 (2000): 173-176.

Pastural, E., et al. "Griscelli Disease Maps to Chromosome 15q21 and Is Associated with Mutations in the Myosin-Va Gene." *Nature Genetics* 16 (1997): 289-292.

Pastural, E., et al. "Two Genes Are Responsible for Griscelli Syndrome at the Same 15q21 Locus." *Genomics* 63 (2000): 299-306.

ORGANIZATIONS

Genetic Alliance. 4301 Connecticut Ave.NW, #404, Washington, DC 20008-2304. (800) 336-GENE

(Helpline) or (202) 966-5557. Fax: (888) 394-3937
info@geneticalliance. <http://www.geneticalliance.org>.

WEBSITES

"Griscelli Syndrome." *Online Mendelian Inheritance in Man.*
<www.ncbi.nlm.nih.gov/entrez/
dispomim.cgi?id=214450>.

Sonya Kunkle

Gronblad-Strandberg-Touraine syndrome
see **Pseudoxanthoma elasticum**

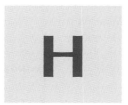

H

Haim-Munk syndrome

Definition

Haim-Munk syndrome is an extremely rare genetic disorder similar to Papillion-Lefevre syndrome. Features include callous patches of skin on the palms of the hands and the soles of the feet, long pointy fingers, and degeneration of the tissues that surround and support the teeth.

Description

Haim-Munk syndrome is characterized by red, scaly thick patches of skin on the palms of the hands and soles of the feet (palmoplantar hyperkeratosis) that are apparent at birth along with frequent pus-producing (pyogenic) skin infections, overgrowth of the fingernails and toenails (onychogryphosis), and degeneration of the gums and bone surrounding the teeth (periodontosis) beginning in childhood. The severe and ongoing periodontosis usually causes the baby teeth to fall out prematurely, and often results in the loss of the permanent adult teeth as well.

In 1965, researchers Haim and Munk reported findings similar to Papillion-Lefevre syndrome in four siblings from an inbred Jewish family that originated from Cochin, India, on the Malabar Coast and later migrated to Israel. Features that are alike in both Papillion-Lefevre syndrome and Haim-Munk syndrome include skin abnormalities and severe periodontitis. These disorders are considered alternate forms of the same genetic mutation. There are a number of additional features reported in Haim-Munk syndrome that include long, thin, pointed fingers (arachnodactyly), bone loss in the fingers or toes (acroosteolysis), abnormal changes of the nails, and a claw-like deformity of the hands.

Haim-Munk syndrome is also known as Cochin Jewish disorder or congenital keratosis palmoplantaris.

Genetic profile

Haim-Munk syndrome is a homozygous expression of an autosomal recessive trait. Among palmoplantar keratoderma disorders, only Papillion-Lefevre syndrome and Haim-Munk syndrome are associated with the premature loss of teeth. It is suspected that Haim-Munk syndrome could be genetically different from common forms of palmoplantar keratoderma that are linked to the cytokeratin **gene** families.

Preliminary findings suggest that **DNA** markers other than keratin genes are responsible for the Haim-Munk syndrome. In 1997, **genotype** data in affected individuals found that the **gene mutations** in Haim-Munk syndrome were not due to a gene defect in either type I or type II keratin gene clusters on chromosomes 12 and 17, markers common to other palmoplantar keratoderma conditions.

Because Papillion-Lefevre syndrome and Haim-Munk syndrome present different symptoms than palmoplantar keratoderma disorders, both genetic syndromes are thought to be related to specific bacterial infections in those with palmoplantar keratoderma.

The cause of Papillion-Lefevre syndrome is a mutation in the cathepsin C gene resulting in periodontal disease and palmoplantar keratosis. Haim-Munk syndrome is thought to be a variant clinical expression of Papillion-Lefevre syndrome that is caused by defects in the cathepsin C gene as well.

A study in 2000 reported a mutation of cathepsin C (exon 6, 2127A→G) that changes a highly conserved amino acid in the cathepsin C peptide. This suggests that Haim-Munk syndrome and Papillion-Lefevre syndrome are alternate forms of defects in the cathepsin C gene. The study also notes that the basis for the difference in clinical expression (symptoms) of these two syndromes caused by the mutated cathepsin C gene is not known.

Demographics

The estimated occurrence of Papillion-Lefevre syndrome, of which Haim-Munk is an extremely rare variant, is considered one to two persons per million. There appears to be no variance by gender. While

Papillion-Lefevre syndrome cases have been identified throughout the world, Haim-Munk syndrome has only been described among descendants of an inbred Jewish family originally from Cochin, India, who migrated to Israel.

Signs and symptoms

The two major manifestations of Haim-Munk syndrome are dermatological abnormalities and juvenile periodontitis.

Individuals identified with the Haim-Munk syndrome show more severe skin abnormalities than groups with Papillion-Lefevre syndrome. Extensive palmoplantar hyperkeratosis typically begins within the first two to three years of life. At birth the palms and soles are bright red in color and then progress to a callused and scaly appearance. As the patient gets older the disease often involves thick scaly patches on the entire front and back area of the hands and feet, as well as the elbows and knees.

A typical pattern of periodontis with Haim-Munk syndrome is as follows: initially the deciduous (baby) teeth appear at the normal time but the gums proceed to swell and bleed. Usually all the deciduous teeth fall out by age four, the mouth then heals and the secondary teeth begin to appear, severe gingival inflammation develops and the majority, or all, of the permanent teeth often fall out by age 15.

Individuals with Haim-Munk syndrome may also have some of the following signs and symptoms:

- wasting (atrophy), or thickening, of the nails
- a deformity of the fingers called arachnodactyly— abnormally long, thin, tapered fingers and toes
- lack of normal blood flow to the extremities that results in numbness and tingling in the fingers and/or toes. It also can cause loss of bone tissue at the ends of the fingers and/or toes (acroosteolysis)
- a curve of the bones in the hands causing claw-like features
- flat feet (pes planus)
- recurrent pus-forming (pyogenic) skin infections

Diagnosis

There are no published diagnostic criteria for Haim-Munk syndrome. Researchers use clinical examination of inbred Jewish Cochin descendents to confirm the presence of Haim-Munk. Diagnosis of Papillion-Lefevre syndrome is confirmed by red, thick callused skin on the palms and soles at birth and dental problems that are usually present by age five.

KEY TERMS

Acroosteolysis—Loss of bone tissue at the ends of the fingers and/or toes.

Arachnodactyly—A condition characterized by abnormally long and slender fingers and toes.

Atrophy—Wasting away of normal tissue or an organ due to degeneration of the cells.

Onychogryphosis—Overgrowth of the fingernails and toenails.

Palmoplantar keratoderma—Group of mostly hereditary disorders characterized by thickening of the corneous layer of skin (hyperkeratosis) on the palms and soles as a result of excessive keratin formation (protein in the skin, hair and nails).

Palmoplantar keratosis—A raised thickening of the outer horny layer of the skin on the palms of the hand and the soles of the feet.

Periodontitis—Inflammatory reaction of the tissues surrounding and supporting the teeth that can progress to bone destruction and abscess formation, and eventual tooth loss.

Pes planus—Flat feet.

Pyogenic—Pus forming.

Affected individuals are diagnosed with Haim-Munk syndrome when all of the following features are present:

- palmoplantar keratoderma
- thick, rough, and scaly patches of skin on the forearms and legs
- severe early onset periodontitis
- arachnodactyly
- abnormal changes of the nails

Radiology is used to view the thin and tapering bone deformities in the fingers and dental problems associated with Haim-Munk syndrome.

Genetic testing can confirm the mutation of the cathepsin C gene. Genotyping for polymorphic DNA markers (D11S1887, D11S1367, and D11S1367) are used to identify the presence of the cathepsin C gene mutations associated with Haim-Munk syndrome.

Treatment and management

Treatments include extraction of the teeth and use of dental prosthesis, or dentures. Medications are also used to treat skin lesions associated with this disorder.

Prognosis

A normal life span has been reported for individuals with Haim-Munk syndrome. Loss of the baby teeth may occur by age six and loss of the permanent teeth by age 15; however, general health is not impaired and dentures are well tolerated.

Resources

BOOKS

Winter, Robin M., and Michael Baraitser. *Multiple Congenital Anomalies, A Diagnostic Compendium.* London: Chapman and Hall Medical, 1991.

PERIODICALS

Hart, T. C., et al. "Haim-Munk Syndrome and Papillion-Lefevre Syndrome Are Allelic Mutations in Cathepsin C." *Journal of Medical Genetics* 37 (2000): 88-94.

Hart, T. C., et al. "Localization of a Gene for Prepubertal Periodontitis to Chromosome 11q14 and Identification of a Cathepsin C Gene Mutation." *Journal of Medical Genetics* 37(2000): 95–101.

Stabholz, A., et al. "Partial Expression of the Papillion-Lefevre Syndrome in 2 Unrelated Families." *Journal of Clinical Periodontology* (1996): 764–69.

WEBSITES

GeneClinics <http://www.geneclinics.org>.

Nina B. Sherak, MS, CHES

▌Hair loss syndromes

Definition

Hair loss syndromes are a varied group of disorders and conditions characterized by the gradual or sudden loss of large amounts of hair—most often from the scalp, but sometimes from other areas of the body. Hair loss (or baldness) is sometimes referred to as alopecia. Madarosis is the medical term for the loss of eyelashes (ciliary madarosis) or eyebrows (superciliary madarosis).

Genetic factors are the most common cause of alopecia. Although hair loss, unlike some **genetic disorders**, is not a life-threatening or disabling condition, it often has painful psychological consequences. Good grooming and an attractive appearance are important factors in the contemporary job market as well as interpersonal relationships, and a full head of hair is considered a positive feature. Historically, men have tended to put less weight on their external appearance than women have, but this pattern has changed in the last two decades. Present evidence indicates that men are now as vulnerable to pressures to "look good" as women are, and that hair loss is a frequent focus of men's concerns about their looks. American men spend over two billion dollars each year on hair-replacement products.

Description

Hair loss syndromes can be divided into two major categories, those caused by some type of inflammation, and those caused by genetic factors, aging, or medication side effects. The noninflammatory syndromes are subdivided into two groups according to the pattern of hair loss. The inflammatory syndromes are also subdivided into two groups according to the presence or absence of tissue destruction.

Noninflammatory patterned hair loss

ANDROGENETIC ALOPECIA Androgenetic alopecia is the most common hair loss syndrome, covering about 95% of cases of hair loss. It is also referred to as androgen-dependent or genetic hair loss. In order to understand this form of alopecia, it is useful to begin with some basic facts about the structure and growth cycle of human hair. Hair is composed primarily of keratin, a tough protein that is also found in the fingernails, toenails, and the outermost layer of skin. Each individual hair consists of a hair follicle, which is a small sac that produces the hair shaft, and the hair shaft itself. The average adult scalp contains about 100,000 hair follicles, the number depending on the natural color of the hair. Brunettes have the highest number of scalp follicles (about 155,000), followed by blondes (140,000) and redheads (85,000). The average adult loses between 70 and 100 scalp hairs per day from ordinary combing, brushing, or shampooing. A loss of more than 150 hairs per day is abnormal.

Human hair differs from the hair of other animals in that its growth cycle is not synchronized; an examination of a group of scalp hairs from the same part of the scalp will show that they are in different phases of growth. There are three phases in the human hair growth cycle. Hairs in the anagen, or growth, stage remain in the follicle during an average period of two to eight years, and grow between a quarter-inch and a half-inch per month. About 90% of scalp hairs are in the anagen phase at any one time. At the end of the anagen phase, the hair enters a brief catagen phase lasting between two and four weeks. During this phase the follicle begins to break down. The catagen phase is followed by a telogen, or resting, phase that lasts between two and four months. Hairs in the telogen phase are shed when the growth phase of the next cycle begins and the new hair shaft pushes out the old hair. About 10% of the hairs on the scalp are normally in the telogen phase. These hairs will regrow about six months after they have been shed.

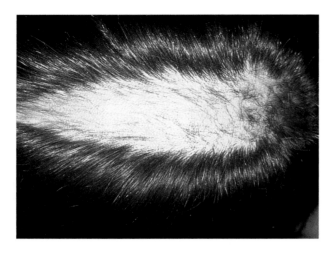

Alopecia, an inherited hair loss syndrome, results in balding.
(*Custom Medical Stock Photo, Inc.*)

What happens in androgenetic baldness is that the hair growth cycle is affected by the rise in the level of androgens (male sex hormones) in the body that occurs at puberty. Women as well as men produce androgens, although in much smaller amounts. The amount of these hormones does not need to be abnormally high for androgenetic hair loss to occur. Males who have a normal level of androgens and a **gene** for baldness will develop male pattern hair loss, or MPHL. There are two androgens that contribute to MPHL, dihydrotestosterone (DHT) and testosterone. Testosterone is converted to DHT by an enzyme called 5-alpha-reductase. In men with genes for baldness, the hair follicles in the scalp remove testosterone from circulation and convert it to DHT. The action of DHT over time shortens the duration of the anagen phase of the hair growth cycle and decreases the proportion of the hairs in the anagen phase. As the anagen phase decreases, the hairs produced are shorter in length and thinner in diameter. As a larger percentage of the hairs are in the resting or telogen phase, more are lost during normal grooming. This process of the shortening and thinning of each hair shaft is called miniaturization. Miniaturization is accompanied by the loss of hair pigment production, so that the miniaturized hairs are also lighter in color. The light-colored fine hairs that are left at the end of the miniaturization process are called vellus hairs.

In MPHL, hair loss tends to occur in certain areas rather than being distributed evenly over the head. One common pattern is recession of the hair at the temples, with the man's hairline moving backward over time in an "M" pattern. The hair at the crown of the head also begins to thin, and may meet the receding hairline so that the remaining hair forms the rough outline of a horseshoe.

In female pattern hair loss, or FPHL, there is an overall thinning of the hair as well as more pronounced hair loss in certain areas of the scalp, usually the crown. Women with FPHL may find that their hairlines recede a little, but rarely to the same extent as happens in men. Androgens play the same role in hair loss in women that they do in men, since the adrenal glands and ovaries secrete small amounts of androgens.

There are other important differences between FPHL and MPHL:

- FPHL generally appears at later ages, in the woman's late twenties or early thirties, whereas MPHL can affect boys as young as 15.

- FPHL is frequently associated with hormonal changes in women, such as those that occur after childbirth; with the use of birth control pills; or after menopause.

- Women very rarely experience complete loss of hair from a specific area of their scalp due to FPHL. The process of miniaturization in FPHL affects the hair follicles at random, so that some hairs are unaffected. These normal thick hairs are interspersed among thinner, miniaturized hairs.

TRACTION ALOPECIA Traction alopecia is a noninflammatory patterned hair loss syndrome in which the pattern of loss is related to pulling or friction on specific areas of the scalp. It is usually caused either by hair styles in which the hair is pulled into tight braids or held too tightly by rubber bands, or by frequent use of electronic headsets (e.g., Walkman radios, hands-free telephones, etc.) for long periods of time. The tension or rubbing damages the hair shafts and hinders the growth of new hair. In some cases the use of tight hair rollers at night or frequent use of blow dryers on high settings contributes to hair loss from traction alopecia.

TRICHOTILLOMANIA Trichotillomania is a psychiatric disorder that results in patterned hair loss. It is characterized by recurrent episodes of pulling or tugging at the hair in order to relieve stress or tension. The most commonly affected areas are the scalp, the eyebrows, and the eyelashes, although some patients with the disorder pull at hair elsewhere on the body. Trichotillomania can usually be differentiated from other hair loss syndromes by laboratory study of a hair sample.

Noninflammatory diffuse hair loss

TELOGEN EFFLUVIUM Telogen effluvium is a common cause of diffuse hair loss, which means that hairs are shed from all parts of the scalp, not just certain patterned areas. Effluvium is a Latin word that means "outflow," and refers to the large amounts of hair that may be lost. Persons affected by telogen effluvium may lose as much as 30%-40% of their hair in a short period of time.

Telogen effluvium results from an abnormal alteration of the hair growth cycle, in which large numbers of hairs in the anagen phase suddenly switch into the telogen phase. Within six weeks to four months after this switch, these hairs begin to shed.

There are number of possible causes for telogen effluvium, including:

• Major surgery.

• Pregnancy and childbirth.

• Crash dieting.

• Nutritional deficiencies, including iron deficiency.

• Malabsorption syndrome.

• Infectious diseases accompanied by high fever, such as scarlet fever, early syphilis, or typhoid.

• Hypothyroidism.

• Medications. A number of medications are known to cause telogen effluvium, including beta blockers; oral contraceptives; retinoids; nonsteroidal anti-inflammatory agents (NSAIDs), such as indomethacin (Indocin) and ibuprofen (Advil); aspirin and other salicylates; lithium; anticoagulants (blood thinners); and anticonvulsants (medications for seizures).

Telogen effluvium usually stops after a few months and new hair grows in. The first regrowth may be finer than usual but the follicles will eventually produce hair of normal thickness.

ANAGEN EFFLUVIUM Anagen effluvium is a type of diffuse hair loss resulting from a sudden interruption of the growth phase. Unlike the time lag that characterizes telogen effluvium, hair loss in anagen effluvium occurs at once. The most common cause of anagen effluvium is chemotherapy, including treatment with methotrexate, bleomycin, vinblastine, vincristine, cyclophosphamide, doxorubicin, daunorubicin, and cytarabine. This form of hair loss, however, can also be caused by poisoning with arsenic, thallium, bismuth, or borax.

Anagen effluvium usually stops as soon as the chemical cause is removed, but it may take several months for hair to regrow completely.

Inflammatory nonscarring hair loss

ALOPECIA AREATA Alopecia areata is a nonscarring recurrent form of hair loss characterized by smooth round or oval patches of bare skin. There may be some mild itching but no visible skin eruptions. Alopecia areata is usually considered an idiopathic disorder, which means its cause is unknown. Some researchers, however, consider it an autoimmune disorder. It is often triggered by stress or anxiety. Alopecia areata usually affects only the scalp, the eyebrows, and (in men) the beard, but may cause hair loss over the entire scalp (alopecia totalis) or even the entire body

(alopecia universalis). The loss of hairs from the eyebrows and eyelashes that may be associated with alopecia totalis is called madarosis.

PSORIASIS Psoriasis is a chronic inflammatory skin disease that frequently affects the elbows and knees as well as the scalp. On the scalp, psoriasis is marked by the appearance of red plaques or patches with silvery scales. These patches may also be found behind the ears. Psoriasis can cause massive but temporary hair loss.

Inflammatory scarring hair loss

In hair loss syndromes marked by tissue scarring, the hair loss is permanent and irreversible. These syndromes should be diagnosed as quickly as possible to minimize the extent of damaged tissue.

LUPUS ERYTHEMATOSUS Lupus erythematosus is an autoimmune disorder than can affect a number of different organ systems. About 85% of lupus patients are women between 20 and 40 years of age. More than 10% of women with lupus develop a form of the disorder known as chronic discoid or chronic cutaneous lupus erythematosus. Chronic discoid lupus can occur on the scalp as well as the face, and is marked by dark red patches or plaques between 0.5 in (1.3 cm) and 0.75 in (1.9 cm) in diameter. The plaques are covered by dry, horny scales that plug the hair follicles and cause permanent hair loss.

LICHEN PLANOPILARIS Lichen planopilaris is a form of lichen planus, an idiopathic recurrent skin disorder that usually affects the wrists, legs, and mucous membranes. It is characterized by itching pinkish-red or purplish patches or pimples on the scalp. Like lupus, lichen planopilaris can cause lasting hair loss.

BACTERIAL OR FUNGAL INFECTIONS Scarring alopecia can be caused by dermatophytes, which are fungi that live on the skin and hair. These fungi include *Trichophyton rubrum*, *Trichophyton tonsurans*, and *Microsporum audouinii*. The dermatophytes infect the skin of the scalp and move down the hair shaft into the follicle, which may be permanently destroyed.

SCLERODERMA **Scleroderma** is a chronic disorder in which the patient's skin and connective tissue become progressively thicker and more rigid. Its cause is not known. As the patient's scalp thickens, the hair is gradually but permanently lost.

INJURIES Scarring alopecia can also result from burns, trauma to the scalp, or radiation treatment.

Genetic profile

Male pattern hair loss (MPHL)

Male pattern hair loss (MPHL) is a polygenic disorder, which means that its appearance is directed by more than one gene. It may be inherited from either the father's or mother's side. The belief that MPHL is inherited only through the mother is a myth. Genes for baldness are, however, dominant, which means that 50% of the children of a balding parent of either sex will inherit the baldness genes. Genetic factors appear to influence the age at onset of MPHL; the extent and speed of hair loss; and the pattern of hair loss. MPHL may begin at any time after the levels of androgens in a boy's blood begin to rise during puberty.

It is important to note that genes for baldness depend on normal levels of androgen in the body to produce androgenetic hair loss. Men who were castrated prior to puberty, or have abnormally low levels of androgen for other reasons, do not go bald even if they have a gene for baldness.

Female pattern hair loss (FPHL)

Female pattern hair loss, or FPHL, is also a dominant disorder. At present, however, there is some disagreement as to whether it runs in families to the same extent as MPHL.

Alopecia areata

About 20% of cases of alopecia areata are thought to have a genetic component.

Demographics

Androgenetic alopecia

Androgenetic alopecia is quite widespread in the general United States population. It is estimated that 35 million American men are affected by this hair loss syndrome. About 25% of Caucasian men begin to show signs of baldness by the time they are thirty, and 67% are either bald or developing a balding pattern by age 60. The first evidence of hair loss, namely a receding hair line at the temples, can be found in 96% of Caucasian males over age 15, including those who will not lose any more hair.

There is less agreement on the incidence of androgenetic alopecia among women in the United States; estimates range from 8% to 87%. A commonly accepted figure is that 21 million women are affected. About 80% of girls begin to show some loss of hair at the hairline during puberty, including some who will not develop FPHL.

Alopecia areata

About 2.5 million people in the United States suffer from alopecia areata. It appears to affect men and women equally.

Trichotillomania

Trichotillomania was once thought to be an uncommon disorder, but more recent research suggests that it occurs fairly frequently among adolescents and young adults. Surveys of college students indicate that 1%-2% are or have been affected by trichotillomania. The male/female ratio is 1:1 in children, but is about 1:4 in college students. The disorder may be underdiagnosed in males because their hair loss is attributed to MPHL.

Signs and symptoms

The signs and symptoms of each hair loss syndrome are included in its description.

Diagnosis

The differential diagnosis of hair loss is usually made on the basis of the patient's history, visual examination of the scalp, and the results of laboratory tests. The more common forms of alopecia can be diagnosed by a family physician, but those that are related to skin disorders may require referral to a dermatologist. There are four key questions that the doctor will ask in evaluating hair loss:

- How long has the patient been losing hair?
- Is there a pattern to the remaining hair?
- Is the hair loss associated with redness, itching, or pain?
- Are there any patches of broken skin, pimples, plaques, or other signs of infection in the affected areas?

Patient history

The patient's medical history may contain information about previous episodes of hair loss; eating and nutritional habits; use of prescription medications; surgery or chemotherapy; occupational exposure to arsenic, thallium, or bismuth; recent illnesses with high fevers; recent periods of severe emotional stress or anxiety; or other factors that may influence hair loss. In addition, the doctor will ask about grooming habits, including the use of dyes, home permanents, hair straighteners, hair sprays, and similar products as well as blow dryers, rollers, and other hair styling equipment.

Laboratory tests

Laboratory tests are performed on samples of the hair itself as part of the differential diagnosis. Microscopic study of a hair sample will indicate, for example, damage to the hair shaft, broken hairs, and changes in the shape of the hair. For example, broken hairs may suggest traction alopecia or trichotillomania. In trichotillomania, there will also be an unusually high number of hairs in the catagen phase. Anagen effluvium produces hairs with tapered or pointed ends, sometimes called "pencil-point" hairs. In telogen effluvium, the hairs have white bulbs at the end and can often be removed from the head by very gentle pulling. In alopecia areata, the area of hair loss is bordered by telltale "exclamation point" hairs.

Hair samples can also be subjected to chemical analysis if heavy metal poisoning is suspected. Arsenic and thallium are absorbed by the hair shaft and can be detected by appropriate tests.

Skin biopsies are most useful in diagnosis when an infection or other inflammatory condition is suspected as the cause of the hair loss. While scarring can often be seen during a visual examination of the scalp, a biopsy may be the only way to tell if the hair follicles have been destroyed, as well as to differentiate among lupus, dermatophyte infection, alopecia areata, and scleroderma. Biopsies may also be useful in determining the presence of traction alopecia or trichotillomania. In these conditions, pieces of hair shaft are sometimes found in the surrounding skin. Some hair follicles may show signs of injury and are interspersed among normal follicles.

Treatment and management

The treatment of hair loss syndromes is determined by their causes.

Medications

TOPICAL APPLICATIONS Topical applications for hair loss syndromes fall into two major categories—those that stimulate the growth of new hair and those that reduce inflammation. The most frequently prescribed topical medication for male pattern hair loss is minoxidil, which was originally developed to lower high blood pressure. It was approved by the FDA for the treatment of androgenetic hair loss in 1988. Minoxidil, sold under the trade name Rogaine, is applied twice a day as a 2% or 5% solution. Rogaine is also sometimes prescribed for female pattern hair loss and alopecia areata. Its chief drawback is its high cost—it costs between $650 and $700 a year to use Rogaine twice a day.

Alopecia areata may be treated with topical corticosteroids, or with injections of triamcinolone acetonide (Kenalog) in the affected areas every three or four weeks. Topical corticosteroids are also used to treat chronic discoid lupus, lichen planopilaris, and psoriasis. Tar shampoos are frequently recommended along with topical steroids to treat psoriasis of the scalp.

ORAL MEDICATIONS One oral medication, finasteride, has been approved by the FDA since 1997 for the treatment of male pattern hair loss. Finasteride, sold under the trade names Propecia or Proscar, works by interfering with the body's production of 5-alpha-reductase, the enzyme that converts testosterone to DHT. It is considered the most effective nonsurgical treatment of MPHL. The usual daily dose of finasteride is 1 mg. Unlike minoxidil, finasteride does not appear to be effective in postmenopausal women. It has not been tested on women of childbearing age because its androgen content could cause birth defects in male children.

Oral antifungal medications are considered better than topical preparations for treating dermatophyte infections of the scalp because topical products do not penetrate around the hair follicle. The mostly commonly prescribed oral antifungal drugs are griseofulvin (Grisactin, Fulvicin), ketoconazole (Nizoral), and fluconazole (Diflucan).

Clomipramine (Anafranil), which is a tricyclic antidepressant, or fluoxetine (Prozac), a selective serotonin reuptake inhibitor (SSRI), have been used in the treatment of trichotillomania.

Surgery

Surgical transplantation is considered the most effective treatment of MPHL, but is not recommended for alopecia areata. Punch grafts or larger skin flaps bearing the patient's own hair are transferred from areas of the head with normal hair growth to the balding areas. Hair transplantation is expensive but is usually permanent. It appears to work best on patients with dark or curly hair.

Scalp reduction is another surgical technique used in treating MPHL, in which bald areas at the top of the scalp are removed. It works best for patients with relatively little hair loss.

Non-surgical hair additions

These devices consist of human hair, synthetic fibers, or combinations of both. They are added to existing hair or attached to the scalp with adhesives to cover areas of hair loss. They include hair weaves, hair pieces, hair extensions, toupees, partial hair prostheses, and similar devices. Non-surgical hair additions are less expensive than surgery but still cost between $750 and $2500, depending on materials and design. They can be used in combination with hair replacement surgery.

KEY TERMS

Alopecia—Loss of hair or baldness.

Alopecia areata—A nonscarring hair loss syndrome characterized by smooth round or oval hairless areas on the scalp.

Anagen—The growth phase of the human hair growth cycle.

Androgens—A group of steroid hormones that stimulate the development of male sex organs and male secondary sexual characteristics.

Catagen—The breakdown phase of the hair growth cycle.

Dihydrotestosterone (DHT)—A male sex hormone formed from testosterone by the enzyme 5-alpha-reductase. DHT causes hair follicles to shut down, shortening the growth phase of the hair growth cycle and leading to miniaturization.

Effluvium—The medical term for massive hair loss or shedding.

Finasteride—An oral medication used to treat male pattern hair loss. Finasteride, sold under the trade names Proscar and Propecia, is an androgen inhibitor.

Keratin—A tough, nonwater-soluble protein found in the nails, hair, and the outermost layer of skin. Human hair is made up largely of keratin.

Madarosis—The medical term for loss of hair from the eyebrows or eyelashes. Madarosis may be associated with a form of alopecia areata called alopecia totalis. It may also result from such diseases as leprosy and syphilis, or from trauma.

Miniaturization—The process of shortening and thinning of the hair shafts that is found in androgenetic alopecia. It is caused by the effects of DHT on the hair follicle.

Minoxidil—A topical medication sold under the trade name Rogaine for the treatment of male pattern hair loss. It is applied to the scalp as a 2% or 5% solution.

Telogen—The resting phase of the hair growth cycle.

Traction alopecia—Hair loss caused by pressure or tension on the scalp related to certain types of hair styles or equipment worn on the head.

Trichotillomania—A psychiatric disorder characterized by hair loss resulting from compulsive pulling or tugging on one's hair.

Vellus hairs—The fine lighter-colored hairs that result from miniaturization.

Psychotherapy

Cognitive-behavioral therapy is considered the most effective form of psychotherapy in treating trichotillomania. Individual psychodynamic psychotherapy is often helpful for persons who are emotionally upset by hair loss, particularly those whose employment depends on their appearance.

Prognosis

The prognoses of hair loss syndromes vary according to their causes. Hair loss caused by inflammatory scarring has the worst prognosis, as syndromes or injuries that form scar tissue destroy the hair follicles, preventing regrowth. The prognosis for alopecia areata is less favorable if the disorder affects large areas of the scalp, begins in adolescence, or has existed for a year or longer before the patient seeks treatment. Alopecia areata that begins in adult life and is limited to a few small areas of the scalp often goes away by itself in a few months, although the condition can recur. Diffuse hair loss related to anagen or telogen effluvium has a good prognosis; although complete regrowth may take some months, the hair does come back once the cause is identified and removed.

The prognosis for androgenetic alopecia varies. Rogaine does not work equally well for all men with MHPL. Those who benefit most from treatment with Rogaine have been bald for less than ten years; have a bald spot on the crown of the head that is smaller than 4 inches across; and still have vellus hairs in their balding areas. In addition, hair that grows in as a result of Rogaine will fall out once the patient stops using it. Finasteride is becoming the first-line nonsurgical treatment for MPHL because it prevents hair loss as well as aiding regrowth; one study indicates that finasteride prevents further loss of hair in 90% of men even five years after they take it, and assists regrowth in 65% of men even two years later.

Resources

BOOKS

"Alopecia." *The Merck Manual of Diagnosis and Therapy.* Edited by Mark H. Beers, MD, and Robert Berkow, MD.

Whitehouse Station, NJ: Merck Research Laboratories, 1999.

American Psychiatric Association. *Diagnostic and Statistical Manual of Mental Disorders.* 4th ed. Washington, DC: American Psychiatric Association, 1994.

Helm, Thomas N., MD. "Hair Disorders." *Conn's Current Therapy.* Edited by Robert E. Rakel, MD. Philadelphia: W. B. Saunders Company, 2000.

ORGANIZATIONS

American Academy of Dermatology. PO Box 4014, 930 N. Meacham Rd., Schaumburg, IL 60168-4014. (847) 330-0230. Fax: (847) 330-0050. <http://www.aad.org>.

American Hair Loss Council. (888) 873-9719. <http://www.ahlc.org>.

American Society for Dermatologic Surgery. 1567 Maple Ave., Evanston, IL 60201. (708) 869-3954.

Dept. of Health and Human Services. Public Health Service, FDA, 5600 Fishers Lane, Rockville, MD 20857.

National Alopecia Areata Foundation (NAAF). PO Box 150760, San Rafael, CA 94915-0760. (415) 456-4644.

WEBSITES

American Hair Loss Council. <http://www.ahlc.org>.

Food and Drug Administration consumer affairs. <http://vm.cfsan.fda.gov/~dms/cos/>.

International Society of Hair Restoration Surgery. <http://www.ishrs.org>.

Rebecca J. Frey, PhD

I Hallermann-Streiff syndrome

Definition

Hallermann-Streiff syndrome is a rare genetic condition which causes characteristic facial features, visual abnormalities, tooth problems, short stature, and occasionally mental impairment.

Description

Hallermann-Streiff syndrome is also known as Francois dyscephaly syndrome, Hallermann-Streiff-Francois syndrome, oculomandibulodyscephaly with hypotrichosis, and oculomandibulofacial syndrome. The distinctive facial features of Hallermann-Streiff syndrome include a very small head that is unusually wide with a prominent forehead, a small underdeveloped jaw, an unusually small mouth, and/or a characteristic beak-shaped nose. Small eyes, clouding of the lens of the eyes (cataracts) and other eye problems often leading to blindness are common. Problems with the teeth, skin, hair, and short stature are also common. Most individuals are of normal intelligence but mental impairment has been reported in some. Most cases of Hallermann-Streiff syndrome occur randomly for unknown reasons and may be the result of mutations, or changes to the genetic material.

Genetic profile

Hallermann-Streiff syndrome is a genetic condition. Genes are units of hereditary material which are passed to a child by his or her parents. The information contained in genes is responsible for the growth and development of all the cells and tissues of the body. Most genes occur in pairs: one copy of each pair is inherited from the mother through the egg cell and one copy of each pair is inherited from the father through the sperm cell. If there is a **gene** alteration (mutation), this may interfere with normal growth and development. The specific gene responsible for Hallermann-Streiff syndrome has not yet been identified.

Most cases of Hallermann-Streiff syndrome occur randomly in families with no other affected individuals. In this situation, the gene alteration is a spontaneous mutation. This means that some unknown event has caused the gene (which functions normally in the parent) to change in either the father's sperm or the mother's egg from which the affected individual was conceived. A person who has Hallermann-Streiff syndrome due to a spontaneous mutation can pass on this mutated gene to offspring who will also be affected. The chance for someone with Hallermann-Streiff syndrome to have a child with the same condition is 50% in each pregnancy. There is also a 50% chance to have a child who is not affected with Hallermann-Streiff syndrome.

There are some reports in the literature which indicate that Hallermann-Streiff syndrome is inherited as a recessive condition. Recessive conditions occur when both copies of a gene pair are changed. The affected individual inherits one mutated gene from each parent. The parents of the affected individual are carriers for one changed copy of the gene pair but are not affected themselves. Carrier couples have a 25% chance in each pregnancy to have a child affected with the condition. Diagnosed individuals are at risk to have an affected child only if their partner is also affected or is a carrier. There is no clear agreement on whether Hallermann-Streiff syndrome can be inherited as a recessive condition. Some have argued that the families reported to have recessive Hallermann-Streiff syndrome in fact do not have this condition but some other condition with features very similar to Hallermann-Streiff syndrome.

Demographics

Hallermann-Streiff syndrome affects both males and females in all ethnic groups. There have been over 150 cases reported in the literature.

Signs and symptoms

Hallermann-Streiff syndrome affects the face, skull, hair, skin, eyes, teeth, and overall growth and development.

Face and skull

The facial features of individuals with Hallermann-Streiff syndrome are distinctive. The face is small with a thin, tapering, pinched nose, and small chin. The head is small and unusually wide with a prominent forehead, a small underdeveloped jaw, and a small mouth. Characteristic changes in the bones of the skull and the long bones of the arms and legs can usually be seen on x ray. The hair is usually sparse, particularly that of the scalp, brows, and lashes. Often there is no hair around the front and sides of the head. The skin of the scalp is thin and taut, and scalp veins are prominent.

Potential complications in Hallermann-Streiff syndrome are related to the narrow upper airway associated with the shape of the skull, particularly the small chin, mouth, and nose. The narrow air passages may result in feeding difficulties and mild aspiration of food. This can lead to severe complications including early lung infection and breathing difficulties. The lung infection can be life-threatening. Some individuals may experience a temporary stop in breathing during sleep because of an obstruction caused by the shape of the skull (obstructive sleep apnea). Individuals with Hallermann-Streiff syndrome are also at increased risk of breathing difficulties when given a general anesthetic before surgery.

Eyes

Individuals with Hallermann-Streiff syndrome may be born with clouding of the lenses of the eyes (congenital cataracts). Congenital cataracts are the most common eye disorder and are usually the reason for a visit to the eye specialist in early life. The cataracts have been reported to spontaneously disappear in some cases. The second most common eye problem is that the eyes are unusually small. Other eye problems may include rapid, involuntary eye movements, crossing of the eyes, and/or decreased visual clarity, and in some cases, blindness.

Teeth

Dental problems are very common. They may include the presence of teeth at birth and the presence of extra teeth. Underdevelopment of tooth enamel and cav-

ities are also common. As well, there may be absence, malformation, and/or improper alignment of certain teeth.

Growth and development

Most individuals with Hallermann-Streiff syndrome are born at term but about one-third are born premature and/or have a low birth weight. Short stature is seen in about half of the individuals with Hallermann-Streiff syndrome. The average final height for females is about 60 in (152 cm) and for males it is about 61 in (155 cm).

Most individuals are of normal intelligence; however, it is estimated that 15-30% of individuals with Hallermann-Streiff syndrome show some degree of mental impairment or slow development. Hyperactivity and seizures have been reported in a small number of individuals.

Other

A small number of individuals with Hallermann-Streiff syndrome have heart defects (such as a hole in the heart). There has also been a report of an individual with a weakened immune system.

Diagnosis

The diagnosis of Hallermann-Streiff syndrome is based on the presence of certain features including the characteristic facial, eye, dental, hair, and skin findings. The main features indicative of Hallermann-Streiff syndrome include a small, wide head with a prominent forehead, the characteristic small jaw and mouth with a pinched nose, cataracts, small eyes, dental abnormalities, sparse or absent hair, thin skin, and short stature. X rays of the bones of the body may be helpful in establishing a diagnosis of Hallermann-Streiff syndrome because there are characteristic changes evident in the bones of individuals with this condition. There is no laboratory test which can be done to confirm the diagnosis. **Genetic testing** to identify the specific genetic alteration causing the condition is not available since the gene for Hallermann-Streiff syndrome has not been identified. Testing for Hallermann-Streiff syndrome in an unborn baby has not been done. It may be possible to detect the abnormal head shape and small chin on ultrasound (sound wave picture) of the developing baby but this has not been documented in the literature.

Treatment and management

There is no cure for Hallermann-Streiff syndrome. In general, an individual with Hallermann-Streiff syndrome requires a team of specialized doctors for treating the various problems which can occur. Assessments by a dentist, dental surgeon, and oral-facial surgeon may also be necessary to evaluate the teeth and difficulties caused by the small chin and mouth. An assessment for possible airway problems is essential. Any individual with Hallermann-Streiff syndrome who shows signs of daytime sleepiness or snoring should be referred to a sleep center for proper diagnosis and treatment of possible obstructive sleep apnea. Treatment for this condition may include surgical procedures such as making a hole in the trachea through the neck to relieve whatever is obstructing the breathing (tracheotomy). Other surgical treatments may include advancing the chin, reducing the size of the tongue, and/or removing the tonsils. Non-surgical treatments may include medications, providing the individual with an oxygen mask, and modifying his or her sleeping position.

An individual with Hallermann-Streiff syndrome should be examined by an eye specialist (ophthalmologist) for signs and symptoms of eye problems. Surgery for some types of eye problems (cataracts, crossed eyes) may be necessary. Individuals who are blind or at risk to lose their eyesight may benefit from being referred to an association for the blind for guidance and counseling.

An examination by a heart specialist (cardiologist) for possible heart problems and by an immune specialist (immunologist) for possible decreased immune function is also recommended. Some types of heart problems may be treated with medications or may require surgical correction.

For individuals with developmental delay or mental impairment, treatment may include special education, speech therapy, occupational therapy, and physical therapy. Drugs may be used to treat hyperactivity, seizures, and other problems.

Some individuals with Hallermann-Streiff syndrome may seek cosmetic surgery for the various effects the syndrome has on the face and skull. Counseling by psychologists may also help individuals with Hallermann-Streiff syndrome cope with the psychological impact of having a facial difference.

Individuals with Hallermann-Streiff syndrome and their families may also benefit from **genetic counseling** for information on the condition and recurrence risks for future pregnancies.

Prognosis

Individuals diagnosed with Hallermann-Streiff syndrome typically have normal intelligence and life-spans when complications of this disorder are properly managed. A major difficulty for individuals with Hallermann-Streiff syndrome is that the visual problems can often lead

> ## KEY TERMS
>
> **Anesthetic**—Drug used to temporarily cause loss of sensation in an area of the body. An anesthetic may either be general, associated with a loss of consciousness, or local, affecting one area only without loss of consciousness. Anesthetics are administered either via inhalation or needle injection.
>
> **Mutation**—A permanent change in the genetic material that may alter a trait or characteristic of an individual, or manifest as disease, and can be transmitted to offspring.
>
> **Trachea**—Long tube connecting from the larynx down into the lungs, responsible for passing air.
>
> **Tracheostomy**—An opening surgically created in the trachea (windpipe) through the neck to improve breathing.
>
> **Ultrasound**—An imaging technique that uses sound waves to help visualize internal structures in the body.

to blindness, despite surgery. Lung infections can be life-threatening to these patients and must be treated immediately. Breathing problems are another serious complication resulting from the abnormal skull formation that narrows the upper airway. Although uncommon, developmental delay and mental impairment have been reported in a minority of individuals affected with Hallermann-Streiff syndrome. These individuals with significant mental impairment may require life-long supervision.

PERIODICALS

Cohen, M. M. "Hallermann-Streiff Syndrome: A Review." *American Journal of Medical Genetics* 41 (1991): 488-499.

David, L. R., et al. "Hallermann-Streiff Syndrome: Experience with 15 Patients and Review of the Literature." *Journal of Craniofacial Surgery* 2 (March 1999): 160-8.

ORGANIZATIONS

FACES: The National Craniofacial Association. PO Box 11082, Chattanooga, TN 37401. (423) 266-1632 or (800) 332-2373. faces@faces-cranio.org. <http://www.faces-cranio.org/>.

National Eye Institute. 31 Center Dr., Bldg. 31, Room 6A32, MSC 2510, Bethesda, MD 20892-2510. <http://www.nei.nih.gov>.

National Organization for Rare Disorders (NORD). PO Box 8923, New Fairfield, CT 06812-8923. (203) 746-6518 or (800) 999-6673. Fax: (203) 746-6481. <http://www.rarediseases.org>.

WEBSITES

"Hallermann-Streiff Syndrome." *Online Mendelian Inheritance in Man.* <http://www.ncbi.nlm.nih.gov/entrez/dispomim.cgi?id=234100> (March 9, 2001).

Nada Quercia, Msc, CGC

Hand-foot-uterus syndrome

Definition

Hand-foot-uterus (HFU) syndrome is characterized by abnormalities of the hand, foot, urinary tract, and reproductive tract.

Description

HFU is a rare genetic condition. Its hallmarks include incurving of the fingers (clinodactyly) and shortened and relocated thumbs. There are also wrist- and ankle-bone fusions, very small feet, short great toes, urinary-tract abnormalities, duplications of the reproductive tract in women, urethral openings on the underside of the penis in men, and curved penis. HFU was first described in 1970. Based on the findings of genital abnormalities in affected males, a 1975 study suggested that the more accurate name of the syndrome would be hand-foot-genital (HFG) syndrome.

Genetic profile

The genetic associations of hand-foot-uterus syndrome are not fully understood. A study in 1997 found mutations (changes) in a **gene** called HOXA13, located on **chromosome** #7, which appears to bring about HFU. It seems that most cases of HFU are caused by a mutation in HOXA13, but other genes may be involved.

Demographics

The ethnic origins of individuals affected by HFU are varied. The syndrome also does not appear to be more common in any specific country.

Signs and symptoms

Signs of HFU syndrome are seen in the hands, feet, urinary tract, and reproductive tract. Individuals in the same family may have different effects of varied severity; this is called intrafamilial variability.

Diagnosis

Diagnosis of HFU is usually made from physical examination by a medical geneticist. Studying x rays of the hands, feet, and reproductive tract also aids in diagnosing the syndrome. Although the HOXA13 gene has clearly been associated with the disease, diagnostic **genetic testing** in affected individuals or in fetuses is not yet available.

Treatment and management

There is no specific therapy that removes, cures, or repairs all effects of hand-foot-uterus syndrome. Management of HFU mainly involves the treatment of specific effects. In people with moderate to severe genital, hand, or urinary-tract abnormalities, surgery may be needed.

Prognosis

Since HFU results in a variety of physical signs and symptoms, the prognosis for each affected individual varies. Most people with mild or moderate hand, genital, or foot abnormalities lead normal lives.

Individuals with severe urinary- and/or reproductive-tract abnormalities may require many surgeries. Their prognoses depend on the severity of the abnormalities and survival of the surgeries. Some people with severe reproductive-tract abnormalities may have difficulty having children.

Resources

BOOKS

Children with Hand Differences: A Guide for Families. Area Child Amputee Center Publications. Center for Limb Differences in Grand Rapids, Michigan. (616) 454-4988.

ORGANIZATIONS

Cherub Association of Families & Friends of Limb Disorder Children. 8401 Powers Rd., Batavia, NY 14020. (716) 762-9997.

WEBSITES

Hensle, Terry W., Steven Y. Tennenbaum, and Elizabeth A. Reiley. *Hypospadias: What Every Parent Should Know.* 1997. <http://207.10.206.114/pediatric/hypospadias.html>

OMIM—Online Mendelian Inheritance of Man. <http://www3.ncbi.nlm.nih.gov/Omim/>

Reach. <http://www.reach.org.uk>

Dawn A. Jacob, MS, CGC

HANE *see* **Heredity angioneurotic edema**

HARD + E, Warburg syndrome *see* **Walker-Warburg syndrome**

▌ Harlequin fetus

Definition

The term harlequin fetus is used to describe an extremely severe form of skin disease in which affected infants have thick, plate-like scales all over their bodies. This abnormality is present from birth. It leads to disfiguration of the facial features and limited movement of the arms, legs, fingers, and toes. Most affected infants die during the first several weeks of life, although longer-term survivors have been reported.

Description

Harlequin fetus represents the most severe presentation of inherited *ichthyosis*. The word **ichthyosis**, which is derived from the Greek word for fish, is a descriptive term used for a group of inherited disorders in which the skin is markedly thickened, ridged, and cracked. The term "harlequin ichthyosis" is therefore used interchangeably with "harlequin fetus." Other synonyms over time have included fetal ichthyosis, ichthyosis intrauterina, keratosis diffusa fetalis, congenital diffuse maligna keratoma, and malignant keratosis.

The ichthyoses as a group are due to a variety of underlying metabolic abnormalities. However, the net effect of each abnormality is the same: keratinization, or differentiation of the cells which make up the skin, does not occur normally. The ichthyoses are separated based on their clinical features and the age at which symptoms appear.

Ichthyosis of the newborn refers to those disorders that present either at birth or shortly thereafter. Each newborn ichthyosis may be due to a different genetic abnormality, even when there is some similarity between clinical features. The harlequin fetus, however, is such a distinct and striking disorder that it is rarely confused with other types of ichthyosis. Affected infants have thick, armor-like skin with deep cracks running in different directions all over their bodies. This gives the appearance of diamond-shaped plaques. The word "harlequin" is often used to describe a variegated pattern, or a combination of patches on a solid background of a contrasting color. The severe skin abnormality leads to an open, fish-mouth appearance as well as a turning outward of the eyelids. Abnormalities of the internal organs are uncommon but have been reported in some individuals. Death often occurs early due to severe skin infection.

Genetic profile

Harlequin fetus (HF) is inherited as an autosomal recessive condition. As such, a child must inherit two copies of the HF **gene** in order to be affected. The presence of one HF gene and one normal gene is consistent with being a gene carrier. Carriers are normal but face a risk of having an affected child with another HF carrier. This risk is 25%, or a one in four chance, that two carriers will each pass on an HF gene to his or her offspring. This risk applies to each pregnancy two carriers have together. Conversely, there is also a 75% chance that two carriers would have an unaffected child.

A gene for harlequin fetus has not yet been identified. It has been speculated that this condition actually represents a varied group of genetic abnormalities, all of which cause a similar clinical picture. This is possible given the number of steps involved in keratinization. If so, it is likely that a different abnormal gene is present in different families.

Demographics

According to the Foundation for Ichthyosis and Related Skin Types (F.I.R.S.T.), harlequin fetus is a very rare form of congenital ichthyosis. There is limited data available to provide a specific incidence figure. However, F.I.R.S.T. provides one estimate as approximately one in every 200,000 individuals. Like other autosomal recessive conditions, HF has been observed more often among the children of consanguineous, or related, couples, such as first cousins, etc. Biologically related individuals are much more likely to carry the same recessive gene and, hence, have offspring with autosomal recessive disorders. Children with HF have, however, also been born to unrelated parents.

Signs and symptoms

Infants affected with harlequin ichthyosis have a striking and unique appearance at birth. Their skin is unusually thick, off-white in color, with deep, moist cracks running in different directions. The facial appearance is distorted with marked ectropion, or turning outward (eversion) of the eyelids. The lips also appear to be

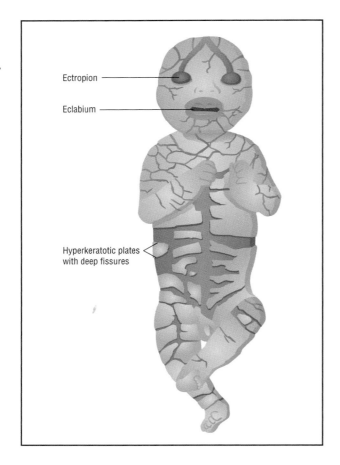

Ectropion

Eclabium

Hyperkeratotic plates
with deep fissures

Harlequin fetus is a severe and usually fatal form of ichthyosis. This rare skin disorder results in thick, scaly skin; turning out of the eyelids (ectropion) and the lips (eclabium); and deep skin fissures. (*Gale Group*)

turned outward. This is referred to as eclabium. The external ears are absent or flattened against the side of the head. The hands and feet are also grayish-white in color. The fingers and toes appear malformed, in part due to the thick scale that surrounds them but probably also due to interference with blood flow to the digits from the constrictions. Nails and body hair may be missing. There is limited mobility of arms and legs.

A consistent pattern of associated internal abnormalities has not been identified in infants with HF. However, abnormalities of the central nervous system, kidneys, and lungs have been described in some affected individuals. Short stature has been observed in those infants who have survived the newborn period.

Diagnosis

A diagnosis of HF is possible based on clinical examination after birth. However, in order to confirm a diagnosis of this particular type of ichthyosis, a skin biopsy is strongly recommended. A sample of skin is submitted for electron microscopy. This specific type of technical examination can identify the characteristic changes within the epidermal cells associated with hyperkeratosis, or overgrowth of the stratum corneum. The cells of the stratum corneum contain protein, keratin, and act as a protective barrier along the surface of the body. The process by which new epidermal cells are formed and gradually changed into the cells of the stratum corneum is referred to as keratinization. It is controlled by a number of different metabolic pathways, and an abnormality at any point can theoretically lead to conditions such as ichthyosis or other serious skin abnormalities.

Prenatal diagnosis of harlequin ichthyosis has been accomplished by biopsy of the fetal skin and microscopic analysis of cells from a sample of amniotic fluid. This is usually accomplished by a combination of fetoscopy and **amniocentesis**. The cellular changes associated with hyperkeratosis begin during the latter part of the second trimester of pregnancy. Prenatal diagnosis of HF has been achieved usually around 21-23 weeks gestation. In 1999, a Japanese group was able to successfully diagnosis HF at the earlier gestational age of 19 weeks in an at-risk family.

Realistically, prenatal diagnosis for HF is available only to those couples that have already had at least one affected child. Based on that family history, the parents will be carriers of a gene for HF and thus at 25% risk of having another affected child. Since a gene for HF has not been identified, carrier testing in the general population is not possible. Also, **prenatal ultrasound** alone will not detect many of the features associated with HF, particularly in a low-risk patient population.

Treatment and management

Infants with HF have a tendency to be born prematurely. Thus, if a prenatal diagnosis of HF has been made, and the family wishes to continue the pregnancy, the woman and her doctor can devise a plan for more intensive monitoring of the remainder of her pregnancy.

Immediate care of a newborn with HF must focus on the following: temperature control, as well as prevention of dehydration, malnutrition, and infection. Infants who are born prematurely may also have breathing problems requiring placement of a breathing tube.

In 1998, guidelines were published for the care of any newborn with a severe form of congenital ichthyosis, including HF:

• The infant should be placed in a humidified incubator immediately after delivery. Antibiotics should be administered via an intravenous (IV) line as a safeguard

KEY TERMS

Amniocentesis—A procedure performed at 16-18 weeks of pregnancy in which a needle is inserted through a woman's abdomen into her uterus to draw out a small sample of the amniotic fluid from around the baby. Either the fluid itself or cells from the fluid can be used for a variety of tests to obtain information about genetic disorders and other medical conditions in the fetus.

Fetoscopy—A technique by which a developing fetus can be viewed directly using a thin, flexible optical device (fetoscope) inserted into the mother's uterus.

Trimester—A three-month period. Human pregnancies are normally divided into three trimesters: first (conception to week 12), second (week 13 to week 24), and third (week 25 until delivery).

against infection. An IV should also be used to provide water and nutrients until the infant can suck sufficiently.

- Medication for pain management should be provided, as needed.

- Sponge baths or tub soaking and the application of skin moisturizers with antibiotics should be performed twice a day to soften the skin and reduce scaliness.

- Creams or ointments containing the drug etretinate should be used to decrease the amount of scale. Etretinate has been a successful mode of treatment for some infants with HF, although treated infants still died at relatively young ages due to complications from their disorder. Careful monitoring for etretinate-related side effects in children, such as bone toxicity, is recommended.

- Artifical tear treatments for infants with severe ectropion.

Prognosis

Most infants with harlequin fetus ichthyosis die within the first few days to weeks of life. Common causes of death include respiratory complications because of prematurity or constriction by the thick scale, dehydration, malnutrition, or severe skin infection. Longer-term survivors have been reported but these children have required intensive, on-going medical care. Etretinate has been an effective form of treatment for some infants but its use has only been for short periods of time since the affected infants have still died. Even with treat-

ment, the ichthyosis does not completely go away. However, over time, the eversion of eyelids and lips gradually resolves. Large, thin scales with reddish edges gradually replace the cracked, thick skin. Variable neurological impairment has been reported among survivors, and, even with attentive medical care, sudden death may still occur.

Resources

BOOKS

Baden, Howard P. "Ichthyosiform Dermatoses." *Emery and Rimoin's Principles and Practice of Medical Genetics.* Edited by David L. Rimoin, J. Micheal Connor, and Reed E. Pyeritz. 3rd ed. St. Louis, MO: Churchill Livingstone, 1997, pp.1205-1214.

"Disorders of Keratinization." *Nelson's Textbook of Pediatrics.* Edited by Richard E. Behrman, Robert M. Kliegman, and Hal B. Jenson. 16th ed. Philadelphia: W. B. Saunders, 2000, p. 2007.

PERIODICALS

Akiyama, Masashi. "Severe Congenital Ichthyosis of the Neonate." *International Journal of Dermatology* 37 (1998): 722-728.

Akiyama, Masashi, Kaoru Suzumori, and Hiroshi Shimizu. "Prenatal Diagnosis of Harlequin Ichthyosis by the Examination of Keratinized Hair Canals and Amniotic Fluid Cells at 19 Weeks Estimated Gestational Age." *Prenatal Diagnosis* 19 (February 1999): 167-171.

Pejaver, Ranjan K., et al. "Etretinate in the Management of Harlequin Siblings." *Indian Journal of Pediatrics* 65 (March-April 1998): 320-323.

ORGANIZATIONS

Foundation for Ichthyosis and Related Skin Types. 650 N. Cannon Ave., Suite 17, Landsdale, PA 19446. (215) 631-1411 or (800) 545-3286. Fax: (215) 631-1413. <http://www.scalyskin.org>.

National Registry for Ichthyosis and Related Disorders. University of Washington Dermatology Department, Box 356524, 1959 N.E. Pacific, Rm. BB1353, Seattle, WA 98195-6524. (800) 595-1265 or (206) 616-3179. <http://www.skinregistry.org>.

WEBSITES

"Ichthyosis Congenita, Harlequin Fetus Type." *Online Mendelian Inheritance in Man.* <http://www.ncbi.nlm.nih.gov/entrez/dispomim.cgi?id=242500>.

Ichthyosis Information. <http://www.ichthyosis.com>.

Terri A. Knutel, MS, CGC

Harlequin ichthyosis *see* **Harlequin fetus**

Haw River syndrome *see* **Dentatorubral-pallidoluysian atrophy**

Hay-Wells syndrome *see* **Ectrodactyly, ecto-dermal dysplasia, clefting syndrome (EEC)**

Heart-hands syndrome *see* **Holt-Oram syndrome**

Hecht syndrome *see* **Trismus-pseudocamptodactyly syndrome**

Hemifacial microsomia

Definition

Hemifacial microsomia is a general diagnosis used to describe facial birth defects of varying severity that may involve certain differences in the eyes, ears, facial bones, mouth, neck, or spine. These defects usually affect only one side of the face, with that side of the face appearing smaller than the other side.

Description

Individuals with hemifacial microsomia have physical differences that are present at birth (congenital). These abnormalities are typically limited to the head and bones of the spinal column (vertebrae) and may be severe or mild. In some cases, the changes are seen on both sides of the face (bilateral). In other cases, they are limited to one side of the face (unilateral).

Different terms may be used for this pattern of differences. Hemifacial microsomia may also be called Goldenhar syndrome, facioauriculovertebral sequence, or oculoauriculovertebral spectrum. This final name describes the common birth defects seen in persons with hemifacial microsomia. The term *oculo* represents the eye, and the term *auriculo* represents the ear. Finally, the term vertebral stands for the physical problems present in the vertebrae.

Genetic profile

Hemifacial microsomia is caused by a disruption of normal facial development. A baby's face forms very early, normally between the eighth and twelfth weeks of pregnancy. Normal facial development depends on many different tissues growing together. When the movement and development of these tissues is disrupted, the face may have abnormal openings, underdevelopment, and/or excess skin. In hemifacial microsomia, some unknown event disrupts normal development of the first and sec-

ond branchial arches, the embryonic structures that later develop into the sides of face, the jaw, and the neck.

The possible causes for the embryonic disruption that leads to hemifacial microsomia are unknown. There are most likely many different factors that may lead to the abnormal development of the facial tissues. In some cases, these factors may be environmental. For example, there are certain medications a woman can take while pregnant that can cause the baby to have the symptoms of hemifacial microsomia. However, in the vast majority of cases, hemifacial microsomia is not caused by something taken during pregnancy.

In other cases, normal development of the facial tissues may be disrupted by genetic factors. The exact genetic factors are unknown. Unlike some other syndromes, there has not been a **gene** identified that, if changed, causes hemifacial microsomia. Studies in a few persons with hemifacial microsomia point to a possible causative genetic difference located on the long arm of **chromosome** 14; however, as of early 2005, this finding requires further study and characterization.

A few families in which hemifacial microsomia occurs show an autosomal recessive **inheritance** pattern, while other families show autosomal dominant pattern of inheritance. However, most cases of hemifacial microsomia are not inherited, meaning that it does not normally run in families.

Hemifacial microsomia typically occurs randomly. Doctors are often unable to explain why it developed. Since it is sporadic in nature, if a child is diagnosed with hemifacial microsomia, the risk for the parents to have another child with hemifacial microsomia is low. In rare cases, one parent may have some of the physical symptoms of hemifacial microsomia. If this is the case, then the risk to have a child with the disorder may be higher.

Demographics

Hemifacial microsomia occurs once in every 3,000–5,000 live births. Males are affected more frequently than females. This syndrome is seen in all ethnic groups and cultures.

Signs and symptoms

The symptoms associated with hemifacial microsomia are highly variable. Some individuals with hemifacial microsomia have many severe abnormalities, while other individuals have few minor birth defects.

The abnormalities seen in hemifacial microsomia are typically limited to the face and vertebrae. Thirty percent of patients have bilateral facial abnormalities. In these patients, the right side is usually affected more

KEY TERMS

Anopthalmia—A medical condition in which an eye is missing.

Anotia—Absence of an ear.

Asymmetry—Without symmetry, as when two halves or parts do not match each other.

Auriculo—Related to the ear.

Bilateral—Relating to or affecting both sides of the body or both of a pair of organs.

Cleft lip—A separation of the upper lip that is present from birth but originates early in fetal development. A cleft lip may appear on one side or both sides and is occasionally accompanied by a cleft palate.

Cleft palate—A congenital malformation in which there is an abnormal opening in the roof of the mouth that allows the nasal passages and the mouth to be improperly connected.

Coloboma—A birth defect in which part of the eye does not form completely and appears to be cleft or notched.

Congenital—Refers to a disorder which is present at birth.

Deoxyribonucleic acid (DNA)—The genetic material in cells that holds the inherited instructions for growth, development, and cellular functioning.

Ear tags—Excess pieces of skin on the outside of the ear.

Epibulbar dermoids—Cysts on the eyeball.

Facial asymmetry—Term used to describe when one side of the face appears different than the other.

Hemivertebra—A defect in which one side or half of a vertebra fails to form.

Hypoplasia—Incomplete or underdevelopment of a tissue or organ.

Macrostomia—A mouth that is larger or wider than normal.

Malar hypoplasia—Small or underdeveloped cheekbones.

Mandible—Lower jaw bone.

Mandibular hypoplasia—Underdevelopment of the lower jaw.

Maxillary hypoplasia—Underdevelopment of the upper jaw.

Maxilla—The main bone forming the upper jaw and the middle of the face.

Microphthalmia—Small or underdeveloped eyes.

Microtia—Small or underdeveloped ears.

Oculo—Related to the eye.

Scoliosis—An abnormal side-to-side curvature of the spine.

Strabismus—An improper muscle balance of the ocular muscles resulting in crossed or divergent eyes.

Unilateral—Refers to one side of the body or only one organ in a pair.

Vertebra—One of the 23 bones that comprises the spine; vertebrae is the plural form.

Vertebral—Related to the vertebrae.

severely. The commonly observed facial asymmetry seen in persons with hemifacial microsomia is caused by hypoplasia (underdevelopment) of the bones of the face. These bones are called the mandible and the maxilla. In addition to the bones of the face, the muscles of the face can also be underdeveloped. Cleft lip and cleft palate are another facial difference associated with hemifacial microsomia. Cleft lip is an abnormal split or opening in the lip that can extend towards the nose or towards the cheek. Cleft palate is an opening in the roof of the mouth. Individuals with hemifacial microsomia can also have wide mouth (macrostomia).

Birth defects of the eye are common in hemifacial microsomia. Cysts on the eyeball (epibulbar dermoids) are common, as is micropthalmia (small eye). Some indi-

viduals with Goldenhar syndrome have a notch of tissue missing from the upper eyelid (*coloboma*). Strabismus (crossing of the eyes) is also prevalent.

Abnormal development of the ears is another characteristic of the hemifacial microsomia spectrum. The ears may be smaller than normal (microtia), or absent (anotia). Ear tags (excess pieces of skin) may be seen on the cheek next to the ear and may extend to the corner of the mouth. The shape of the ears may also be unusual. Hearing loss is common in individuals with hemifacial microsomia.

The vertebral problems seen in many persons with hemifacial microsomia result from improper development of the vertebrae. Vertebrae can be incompletely developed (hemivertebrae), absent, or fused. Ribs can also be abnormal. Approximately 50% of individuals with hemifacial microsomia will have curvature of the spine (**scoliosis**).

Other differences outside of the face and vertebra can occasionally be seen in hemifacial microsomia. Approximately 15% of individuals with hemifacial microsomia have developmental delay or mental retardation. The likelihood for mental retardation increases if the individual has microophthalmia. Heart defects and kidney defects can also occur. Arm defects, though rare, may also occur.

Diagnosis

There is not a genetic test that can diagnose hemifacial microsomia. The diagnosis is made when an individual has the common symptoms associated with the condition. The diagnosis is made by a physician based on the observed physical features.

Treatment and management

Once a child is diagnosed with hemifacial microsomia, additional tests should be performed. A hearing evaluation is necessary to determine if there is hearing loss. If hearing loss is evident, the child should be referred to a hearing specialist. Speech therapy may also be helpful. X rays of the spine are recommended to determine if there are vertebral problems. Individuals with hemifacial microsomia may be followed regularly to check for scoliosis. Renal ultrasounds and ultrasounds of the heart may also be recommended, due to the increased risk for birth defects in these areas. A doctor would make this recommendation. Finally, individuals with hemifacial microsomia should be evaluated by an eye doctor (ophthalmologist).

Surgery may be required to correct the birth defects seen in hemifacial microsomia. Surgery to correct the facial birth defects can improve appearance and function.

Prognosis

The prognosis for individuals with hemifacial microsomia is very good. These individuals typically have a normal lifespan and normal intelligence.

Resources

BOOKS

Gorlin, Robert J., Michael M. Cohen, and Raoul C. M. Hennekam. "Branchial Arch and Oral-Acral Disorders." In *Syndromes of the Head and Neck,* 4th ed. New York: Oxford University Press, 2001.

Jones, Kenneth Lyons. "Oculo-Auriculo-Vertebral Spectrum." In *Smith's Recognizable Patterns of Human Malformation.* Philadelphia: W. B. Sanders, 1997.

PERIODICALS

Schaefer, G. Bradley, Ann Olney, and Peg Kolodziej. "Oculo-auriculo-vertebral Spectrum." *ENT—Ear, Nose & Throat Journal* 77 (1998): 17–18.

ORGANIZATIONS

Alliance of Genetic Support Groups. 4301 Connecticut Ave. NW, Suite 404, Washington, DC 20008. (202) 966-5557. Fax: (202) 966-8553. (April 4, 2005.) <http://www.geneticalliance.org>.

Goldenhar Parent Support Network. 3619 Chicago Ave., Minneapolis, MN 55407-2603. (612) 823-3529.

Goldenhar Syndrome Support Network. 9325 163 St., Edmonton, ALB T5R 2P4. Canada. (April 4, 2005.) <http://www.goldenharsyndrome.org>.

National Organization for Rare Disorders (NORD). PO Box 8923, New Fairfield, CT 06812-8923. (203) 746-6518 or (800) 999-6673. Fax: (203) 746-6481. (April 4, 2005.) <http://www.rarediseases.org>.

WEBSITES

"Hemifacial Microsomia." *Online Mendelian Inheritance in Man.* (April 4, 2005.) <http://www.ncbi.nlm.nih.gov/entrez/dispomim.cgi?id=164210>.

Holly Ann Ishmael, MS, CGC
Judy C. Hawkins, MS, CGC

Hemifacial microsomia with radial defects *see* **Goldenhar syndrome**

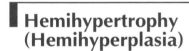

Hemihypertrophy (Hemihyperplasia)

Definition

Hemihypertrophy, more correctly termed hemihyperplasia, is defined as the enlargement of one side of the body or part of the body.

Description

Hemihypertrophy is characterized by unequal (asymmetric) growth of the cranium, face, trunk, limbs, and/or digits. Hemihypertrophy can be an isolated finding, or it can be associated with certain malformation syndromes. Isolated hemihypertrophy refers to hemihypertrophy for which no cause can be found. The degree of asymmetry is variable and very mild cases can go undiagnosed. There are three categories of hemihypertrophy, depending on the body parts involved. The size difference can involve only a specific part of the body

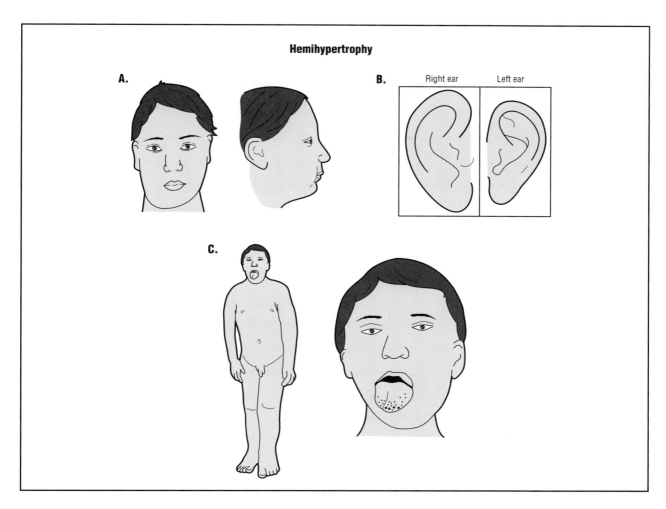

Hemihypertrophy

The enlarged growth of only one side of the body is characteristic of hemihypertrophy. The asymmetric development may be isolated to one organ or limb, or may occur to the entire body. (*Gale Group*)

such as a finger (called simple hemihypertrophy) or an entire half of the body (called total or complex hemihypertrophy). It usually involves only one side of the body, but can involve both sides (called crossed). There is also hemifacial hyperplasia, which involves one side of the face. Usually multiple organ systems are involved, i.e. the skin, vascular system, internal organs, or bones. In complex hemihypertrophy, the right side is more often involved than the left.

Hemihypertrophy may involve not only the part of the body that is visible, but also the underlying internal organs. Enlargement of one kidney, adrenal gland, testis, and ovary has been reported. The enlarged area usually also has thickened skin, more sebaceous (sweat) glands, more hair, may have pigmentary abnormalities, and the bones may be larger or may be deformed. In persons with facial involvement, the asymmetry can include cheek, lip, nose, ear, eye, tongue, jaw, roof of the mouth, or teeth.

The nervous system may also be affected, causing unilateral nerve enlargement or sciatic nerve inflammation. Occasionally a part of the brain is affected causing mental retardation (15% to 20% of cases). Many cases of hemihypertrophy have hamartomatous lesions (birth marks which involve blood vessels) or abnormalities of the genito-urinary system.

As with other overgrowth syndromes, there is an increased risk for childhood cancers in people with isolated hemihypertrophy (about 6%), particularly cancers of the kidney (Wilms tumor, 3% of individuals), adrenals, and liver.

Genetic profile

The cause and exact mechanism of isolated hemihypertrophy is not known. The asymmetry occurs most likely as a result of an increase in the rate of cell growth, or unregulated cell growth. Most cases of hemihypertrophy are not inherited, but there have been seven familial cases reported in which two or more persons were affected. These cases are not well documented and it is possible that the families actually had another genetic syndrome. Males and females are equally affected with this condition.

It is clear that there is not a single **gene** responsible for hemihypertrophy, but the exact number of genes and their locations and functions are not known. It has been suggested that isolated hemihypertrophy may be related to another condition, called **Beckwith-Wiedemann syndrome**, a genetic overgrowth syndrome that can include both hemihypertrophy and Wilms tumor. Beckwith-Wiedemann syndrome has been associated with abnormalities on **chromosome** 11, which contains genes involved with growth, development, and **cancer**.

Good data does not exist for recurrence risk for siblings of patients or for children of affected persons. Case reports suggest a slightly increased risk for siblings and for offspring of affected mothers.

Demographics

Hemihypertrophy occurs in about one in 15,000 live births. Isolated hemihypertrophy occurs in about one in 86,000 live births. There are approximately 200 cases reported. Females and males are affected equally.

Signs and symptoms

Hemihypertrophy is usually recognized at birth by physical examination, but can become more serious over time, especially during puberty. Very mild forms of this condition often go unnoticed and are very common.

Diagnosis

The diagnosis is made by clinical examination of body asymmetry. There are no laboratory tests available for this condition. X ray may show advanced bone age or larger bones in the hypertrophied limbs, supporting a diagnosis of hemihypertrophy, or characteristic bone changes supporting another diagnosis. Other genetic syndromes associated with asymmetry must be excluded, as must other causes of asymmetry, such as atrophy of one side of the body due to neurological disorder or skeletal abnormalities that cause asymmetric hand or limb enlargement.

Prenatal diagnosis is theoretically possible by ultrasound, provided that the difference in size is large enough to be detected or if an embryonic tumor is present, although a confirmed diagnosis is not possible until after birth.

Treatment and management

The treatment for hemihypertrophy is different for each individual and depends on the specific symptoms. If leg-length differences are present, corrective shoes can increase the sole for the unaffected leg to prevent **scoliosis** and walking difficulties. Orthopedic devices such as braces or, more rarely, surgery to lengthen the normal leg may be indicated. Surgery to retard growth of the overgrown leg is controversial and not recommended. Surgery for congenital defects or laser surgery for birth marks may be indicated. Plastic surgery may be considered to correct very discrepant facial features.

A protocol to screen for childhood cancers has been proposed, which includes abdominal ultrasound every three months until age six, every six months until puberty, and careful medical follow-up of patients into adulthood. Surgical intervention is appropriate if cancers are detected. Monitoring of serum alpha fetoprotein levels may also be useful as a marker of hepatic tumors.

Appropriate special education services are necessary for those with mental retardation. Counseling related to social stigmatism may be necessary if severe disfigurement is an issue.

Prognosis

Hemihypertrophy does not alter life span, although complications from associated abnormalities such as childhood cancer and mental retardation can cause problems.

Asymmetry of the limbs can interfere with their proper function and cause pain. Insecurities due to disfigurement are possible and can be addressed through support groups or therapy.

Resources

BOOKS

Buyse, M. L., ed. "Hemihypertrophy." *Birth Defects Encyclopedia.* Boston: Blackwell Scientific Publications, 1990.

Goodman, R. M., and R. J. Gorlin. "Hemihypertrophy." *The Malformed Infant and Child.* New York: Oxford University Press, 1983.

PERIODICALS

Biesecker, L. G., et al. "Clinical Differentiation Between Proteus Syndrome and Hemihyperplasia: Description of a Distinct Form of Hemihyperplasia." *American Journal of Medical Genetics* 79(1998): 311-318.

Hoyme, H. E., et al. "Isolated Hemihyperplasia (Hemihypertrophy): Report of a Prospective Multicenter of the Incidence of Neoplasia and Review." *American Journal of Medical Genetics* 79(1998): 274-278.

ORGANIZATIONS

Klippel-Trenaunay Support Group. 5404 Dundee Rd., Edina, MN 55436. (612) 925-2596.

Proteus Syndrome Foundation. 6235 Whetstone Dr., Colorado Springs, CO 80918. (719)264-8445. abscit@aol.com. <http://www.kumc.edu/gec/support/proteus.html>.

WEBSITES

"Hemihypertrophy." *Online Mendelian Inheritance in Man.* <http://www.ncbi.nlm.nig.gov/entrez/dispomim.cgi?id=235000>.

National Organization of Rare Disorders. <http://www.rarediseases.org>.

Amy Vance, MS, CGC

Hemochromatosis

Definition

Hemochromatosis is an inherited blood disorder that causes the body to retain excessive amounts of iron. This iron overload can lead to serious health consequences, most notably cirrhosis of the liver.

Description

Hemochromatosis is also known as iron overload, bronze **diabetes**, hereditary hemochromatosis, and familial hemochromatosis. The inherited disorder causes increased absorption of intestinal iron, well beyond that needed to replace the body's loss of iron. Iron overload diseases afflict as many as 1.5 million persons in the United States. The most common of these, as well as one of the most common **genetic disorders** in the United States, is hereditary hemochromatosis. Men and women are equally affected by hemochromatosis, but women are diagnosed later in life because of blood loss from menstruation and childbirth. It most commonly appears in patients between the ages of 40–60 years, since it takes many years for the body to accumulate excessive iron. Symptoms appear later in females than in males—usually after menopause.

Hemochromatosis causes excess iron storage in several organs of the body including the liver, pancreas, endocrine glands, heart, skin, joints, and intestinal lining. The buildup of iron in these organs can lead to serious complications, including heart failure, liver **cancer**, and cirrhosis of the liver. It is estimated that about 5% of cirrhosis cases are caused by hereditary hemochromatosis.

Idiopathic pulmonary hemosiderosis, a disorder afflicting children and young adults, is a similar overload disorder characterized by abnormal accumulation of hemosiderin. Hemosiderin is a protein found in most tissues, especially the liver. It is produced by digestion of hematin, an iron-related substance.

Genetic profile

Hereditary hemochromatosis is an autosomal recessive condition. This means that individuals with hemochromatosis have inherited an altered (mutated) **gene** from both of their parents. Affected individuals have two abnormal hemochromatosis genes and no normal hemochromatosis gene.

The gene that causes hemochromatosis has been identified, and the most common abnormalities of the gene have been described. The gene is on **chromosome** 6; it is called HFE. Scientists have not confirmed the function of the normal gene product; they do know that it interacts with the cell receptor for transferrin. Transferrin binds and transports iron in the blood.

Because it is an autosomal recessive condition, siblings of individuals who have hemochromatosis are at a 25% risk to also be affected. However, the likelihood that an individual will develop symptoms depends on which gene mutation he or she has as well as environmental factors. The two most common changes in the HFE gene are C282Y and H63D. The age at which symptoms begin is variable, even within the same family.

Demographics

Hemochromatosis is one of the most common genetic disorders in the United States. Approximately one in nine individuals have one abnormal hemochromatosis gene (11% of the population). Since everyone has two copies of each gene, these individuals have an abnormal HFE gene and a normal gene. They are called carriers. Between one in 200 and one in 400 individuals have two abnormal genes for hemochromatosis and no normal gene.

With most autosomal recessive conditions, an affected person's parents are carriers. If more than one family member has the condition, they are siblings. Hemochromatosis is so common, however, that families are seen in which both parents are affected, or one parent is affected and the other parent is a carrier. More than one generation may be affected, which is not usually seen in rare autosomal recessive conditions.

Signs and symptoms

The symptoms of hemochromatosis include fatigue, weight loss, weakness, shortness of breath, heart palpitations, chronic abdominal pain, and impaired sexual performance. The patient may also show symptoms commonly connected with heart failure, diabetes or cirrhosis of the liver. Changes in the pigment of the skin may appear, such as grayness in certain areas, or a tanned or yellow (jaundice) appearance. The age of onset and initial symptoms vary.

Idiopathic pulmonary hemosiderosis may first, and only, appear as paleness of the skin. Sometimes, the patient will experience spitting of blood from the lungs or bronchial tubes.

Diagnosis

The most common diagnostic methods for hemochromatosis are blood studies of iron, genetic blood studies, magnetic resonance imaging (MRI), and liver biopsy. Blood studies of transferrin-iron saturation and ferritin concentration are often used to screen for iron overload. Ferritin is a protein that transports iron and liver enzymes. Additional studies are performed to confirm the diagnosis.

Blood studies used to confirm the diagnosis include additional iron studies and/or genetic blood studies. Genetic blood studies became available in the late 1990s. **Genetic testing** is a reliable method of diagnosis. However, scientists and physicians studied how accurately having a hemochromatosis mutation predicts whether a person will develop symptoms. Most individuals affected with hemochromatosis (87%) have two iden-

tifiable **gene mutations**, i.e. genetic testing will confirm the diagnosis. Genetic studies are also used to determine whether the affected person's family members are at risk for hemochromatosis. The results of genetic testing are the same whether or not a person has developed symptoms.

MRI scans and/or liver biopsy may be necessary to confirm the diagnosis. MRI studies of the liver (or other iron-absorbing organs), with quantitative assessment of iron concentration, may reveal abnormal iron deposits. For the liver biopsy, a thin needle is inserted into the liver while the patient is under local anesthesia. The needle will extract a small amount of liver tissue, which can be analyzed microscopically to measure its iron content and other signs of hemochromatosis. Diagnosis of idiopathic pulmonary hemosiderosis begins with blood tests and x-ray studies of the chest.

Treatment and management

Patients who show signs of iron overload will often be treated with phlebotomy. Phlebotomy is a procedure that involves drawing blood from the patient, just like blood donation. Its purpose as a treatment is to rid the body of excess iron storage. Patients may need these procedures one or two times a week for a year or more. Less frequent phlebotomy may be continued in subsequent years to keep excess iron from accumulating. Patients who cannot tolerate phlebotomy due to other medical problems can be treated with Desferal (desferrioxamine). Diet restrictions may also be prescribed to limit the amount of iron ingested. Complications from hemochromatosis, such as cirrhosis or diabetes, may also require treatment. Treatment for idiopathic pulmonary hemosiderosis is based on symptoms.

Diet restrictions may help lower the amount of iron in the body, but do not prevent or treat hemochromatosis. Individuals who are affected or who know they have two C282Y and/or H63D genes may reduce iron intake by avoiding iron and mineral supplements, excess vitamin C, and uncooked seafood. If a patient is symptomatic, he/she may be advised to abstain from drinking alcohol.

Prognosis

With early detection and treatment, the prognosis is usually good. All potential symptoms are prevented if iron levels are kept within the normal range, which is possible if the diagnosis is made before an individual is symptomatic. If a patient is symptomatic but treated successfully before he/she develops liver cirrhosis, the patient's life expectancy is near normal. However, if left untreated, complications may arise which can be fatal. These include liver cancer, liver cirrhosis, diabetes

KEY TERMS

Autosomal—Relating to any chromosome besides the X and Y sex chromosomes. Human cells contain 22 pairs of autosomes and one pair of sex chromosomes.

Cirrhosis—A chronic degenerative disease of the liver, in which normal cells are replaced by fibrous tissue. Cirrhosis is a major risk factor for the later development of liver cancer.

Diabetes mellitus—The clinical name for common diabetes. It is a chronic disease characterized by inadequate production or use of insulin.

Phlebotomy—The taking of blood from the body through an incision in the vein, usually in the treatment of disease.

mellitus, congestive heart failure, and difficulty depleting iron overload through phlebotomy. Liver biopsy can be helpful in determining prognosis of more severely affected individuals. Genetic testing may also be helpful, as variable severity has been noted in patients who have two C282Y genes compared to patients with two H63D genes or one of each. Men are two times more likely than women to develop severe complications. The prognosis for patients with idiopathic pulmonary hemosiderosis is fair, depending on detection and complications.

Prevention

Screening for hemochromatosis is cost effective, particularly for certain groups of people. Relatives of patients with hemochromatosis—including children, siblings, and parents—should be tested by the most appropriate method. The best screening method may be iron and ferritin studies or genetic testing. If the affected person's diagnosis has been confirmed by genetic testing, relatives may have genetic testing to determine whether or not they have the genetic changes present in the affected individual. Many medical groups oppose genetic testing of children. Relatives who are affected but do not have symptoms can reduce iron intake and/or begin phlebotomy prior to the onset of symptoms, possibly preventing ever becoming symptomatic.

Population screening for hereditary hemochromatosis is widely debated. Many doctors and scientists want population screening because hemochromatosis is easily and cheaply treated, and quite common. Arguments against treatment include the range of symptoms seen (and not seen) with certain gene mutations, and the risk of discrimination in health and life insurance. Whether or not population screening becomes favored by a majority, the publicity is beneficial. Hemochromatosis is a common, easily and effectively treated condition. However, diagnosis may be difficult because the presenting symptoms are the same as those seen with many other medical problems. The screening debate has the positive effect of increasing awareness and suspicion of hemochromatosis. Increased knowledge leads to earlier diagnosis and treatment of symptomatic individuals, and increased testing of their asymptomatic at–risk relatives.

Resources

BOOKS

Barton, James C., and Corwin Q. Edwards, eds. *Hemochromatosis: Genetics, Pathophysiology, Diagnosis and Treatment.* Cambridge: Cambridge University Press, 2000.

Crawford, Roberta. *The Iron Elephant.* Glyndon, MD: Vida Publishing, 1995.

PERIODICALS

"Iron Overload, Public Health and Genetics." *Annals of Internal Medicine Supplement* 129 (December 1998). <http://www.acponline.org/journals/annals/01dec98/supptoc.htm>.

Motulsky, A.G., and E. Beutler. "Population Screening for Hemochromatosis." *Annual Review of Public Health* 21 (2000): 65-79.

Wolfe, Yun Lee. "Case of the Ceaseless Fatigue." *Prevention Magazine* (July 1997): 88.

ORGANIZATIONS

American Hemochromatosis Society, Inc. 777 E. Atlantic Ave., PMB Z-363, Delray Beach, FL 33483-5352. (561) 266-9037 or (888) 655-IRON (4766). ahs@emi.net. <http://www.americanhs.org>.

American Liver Foundation. 75 Maiden Lane, Suite 603, New York, NY 10038. (800) 465-4837 or (888) 443-7222. <http://www.liverfoundation.org>.

Hemochromatosis Foundation, Inc. PO Box 8569, Albany, NY 12208-0569. (518) 489-0972. s.kleiner@shiva.hunter. cuny.edu. <http://www.hemochromatosis.org>.

Iron Disorders Institute, Inc. PO Box 3021, Greenville, SC 29602. (864) 241-0111. irondis@aol.com. <http://www.irondisorders.org>.

Iron Overload Diseases Association, Inc. 433 Westwind Dr., North Palm Beach, FL 33408. (561) 840-8512. iod@ironoverload.org.

WEBSITES

"Hemochromatosis." *GeneClinics.* <http://www.geneclinics.org/profiles/hemochromatosis/>.

Hemochromatosis Information Sheet. National Institute of Diabetes & Digestive & Kidney Diseases (NIDDK) <http://www.niddk.nih.gov/health/digest/pubs/hemochrom/hemochromatosis.htm>.

Hereditary Hemochromatosis. Lecture by Richard Fass, MD, hematologist, Advanced Oncology Associates, given April 25, 1999. <http://www.advancedoncology.org/listen.htm> in Real Audio.

Michelle Q. Bosworth, MS, CGC

Hemoglobin-beta locus *see* Beta thalassemia

Hemolytic-uremic syndrome

Definition

Hemolytic-uremic syndrome (HUS) is a syndrome defined by the presence of acute hemolytic anemia (low red blood cell count caused by the break up of red cells within the blood stream by a person's own immune system), thrombocytopenia (a low number of platelets), and kidney failure. Having these three symptoms all at once can be caused by a number of problems—some by infections, others by genes, and some are still unknown.

Description

About 90% of HUS cases occur in children less than five years of age. In most cases, there is an early phase of diarrhea, followed by the lowered blood counts and the renal failure. Most patients get better after HUS, a few die during the worst stage of the illness, others go on to have life-long kidney disease, and some will progress to having a form of HUS that comes and goes over the rest of their lives. Which patients will have which outcome is not known during the illness.

Many infectious organisms have been thought to play a role as things that may cause HUS outbreaks, such as one *E. coli* serotype and one *Shigella dysenteriae* serotype. About 40% of patients who ingest *E. coli* 0157:H7 (the implicated serotype) will go on to get some form of diarrhea. Of those that develop diarrhea, about 5% will progress to some form of HUS (ranging in strength from mild to fatal). The bacteria linked to HUS have been shown to produce a toxin that gets released into the bloodstream after the organisms invade the colon's mucosal lining. The toxin, once inside of cells, disrupts protein synthesis. The spreading of organisms that make toxins tends to occur through food products.

Many outbreaks of HUS in the United States have occurred over the last several decades. These outbreaks have been linked to various food sources such as hamburger meat that is not cooked enough, apple juice and apple cider that has not been pasteurized, water, fruits, vegetables, and unpasteurized milk. Hamburger meat is the most common way that *E. coli* spreads. This bacteria is part of the normal flora of cow intestines and it is thought that it gets into the meat during the process of killing and cutting up the cow. When this beef is then not cooked enough to kill the organism, it is able to travel into the human GI (gastro-intestinal) system with ease. The spreading of this disease can also occur with person-to-person contact through a fecal-oral route. Support for this theory includes data from daycare centers that had outbreaks of HUS.

About 10% of cases in children and 50% of cases in adults will be a type of HUS that occurs without diarrhea. Of these cases, some can be linked with other infections, but other cases have no clear cause. Out of these unclear cases, some will be a form of HUS that runs in families. There have been many research studies into families that have many members who have a form of HUS that keeps coming back over the patient's lifetime. Genetic tests of these families have found what may be a **gene** that can cause some cases of HUS.

Patients with HUS all show signs of making thrombi (blood clots) in small vessels. These thrombi form in kidney blood vessels as well as small arteries all over the body. Thus, clots can cause infarcts (starvation and death) of kidney tissue, brain tissue, the bowel, and other organs.

Genetic profile

While most families that have a form of HUS that passes on the disease in an autosomal recessive pathway, there have been some families with signs of autosomal dominant transmission. Genetic tests have found that a region on **chromosome** 1q can play a role in the forms of HUS that run in families. The gene for factor H (a protein regulator of the alternate complement pathway) is the leading gene candidate. Molecular proof linking factor H to cases of HUS that occur without diarrhea was first produced in 1998. Since then, screening of patients and families of patients with HUS not linked to a preceding episode of diarrhea have found a subset of patients who have mutated copies of the factor H gene.

Tests that look at different families with an inherited form of HUS have shown that there are many different point mutations within the factor H gene. All of these mutations led to some reduced level of factor H. With this lower level, many researchers have noticed that patients also have reduced levels of a protein called C3. This protein is part of the complement cascade that is supposed to attack bacteria within the body. Patients with low levels of C3 may be at more risk of having very bad problems arise from infections than patients with normal immune systems. Also, the familial form of HUS is most likely a multifactorial disease (i.e. no one gene mutation causes it by itself) that occurs in certain patients who are predisposed to the disorder.

Demographics

The largest number of cases occur in children between the ages of six months and five years of age. The mean age of children who get HUS is four. Within the United States, this disease most often occurs in epidemics, versus an endemic form that is found in other parts of the world. For example, Argentina has a much higher incidence of HUS than America. Interestingly, the rate of *E. coli* that make the toxins that cause infections is higher in Argentina.

Signs and symptoms

The clinical history most often seen in patients with HUS is of a diarrheal illness that comes before the anemia and renal disease by five to seven days. Some children have symptoms other than diarrhea. These include belly pain, nausea, and throwing up.

When HUS occurs, patients can have many different types of symptoms. Patients tend to have pallor (pale skin), decreased urine output, and fatigue. Even though they tend to have low platelet (the cells that cause blood to clot) counts, they seldom have too much bleeding. About one quarter of patients will have neurologic signs and symptoms that present as seizures, drowsiness, coma, and personality changes. Most of the patients that have HUS with diarrhea will also have hypertension (high blood pressure) that occurs with it. Almost one fifth of patients with HUS will also have some form of pancreatic problems that can lead to the body not making enough insulin and causing **diabetes**. In some cases, the diabetes may last for the rest of the patient's life.

Kidney problems vary from patient to patient in how severe they may be. Some patients only have lower urine output, but others progress to full kidney failure. In some patients who develop HUS *without* diarrhea, the onset of renal failure will be more subtle such that they will present with symptoms of volume overload (too much retained fluid).

Diagnosis

The diagnosis of HUS should be considered in patients who present with symptoms of anemia or renal failure who either give a history of diarrhea before it or have certain problems that show up in their lab tests. Patients will always have low red blood cell counts (anemia) with signs of the ongoing break down of red blood cells. On peripheral smear (blood looked at through a microscope), Burr

cells can be seen. These are red blood cells with bumps sticking out of the surface of the cell. Also schistocytes (pieces of red blood cells that have been destroyed) can be seen under the microscope which provide clues of the ongoing break down of red blood cells (hemolysis).

Diagnosis of familial HUS will depend on the presence of many cases within one family that are not linked to an outside epidemic. Often, the cases will occur over a stretch of many years. As of yet, there is no genetic or lab test that can tell which people will get familial HUS. Prenatal testing is not yet available either.

Treatment and management

There is no certain treatment for patients with HUS other than supportive care. Many types of treatments have been tried in attempts to reduce the amount of clotting that occurs in small vessels, but with little or no success. Antibiotic treatment for children with diarrhea caused by *E. coli* tended to raise, instead of lower, the rate of transformation into HUS. Thus, antibiotics tend to not be used for children with diarrhea. They are of little benefit and may be harmful. Treatment of diarrhea in children should consist of supportive care with ample fluids in order to prevent dehydration.

Careful notice must be paid to fluid intake. It is very easy for kidney failure patients to build up too much volume and have problems with their electrolyte levels. Patients with really low red blood cell counts can be given blood transfusions. Those who get severe renal failure may need dialysis treatment to rid their blood of toxins that would have been cleared by the kidneys. These treatments apply to all forms of HUS including HUS with diarrhea, HUS without diarrhea, and familial HUS. In some patients with recurring familial disease, kidney transplants have been tried, but the disease did recur in many patients.

Prognosis

About 10% of children will die during the acute phase of the illness or will be left with chronic renal or brain damage. Most of the deaths during the acute phase occur in children where organs other than the kidneys are also involved (i.e., brain thrombi formation). Long term effects also include diabetes, rectal stricture (narrowing of the rectum caused by fibrous tissue formation), and neurologic deficits (related to strokes). Of children who have HUS with diarrhea (most of the cases), about 1% will have the illness return.

In adults, the death rate is much higher, at 15 to 30%. Also, 30% of those who do not die from HUS will have chronic kidney damage and 25% may go on to have the disease recur. This difference in age-related recurrence

KEY TERMS

Alternate complement pathway—A cascade of enzymatic reactions that produce antibacterial proteins. This pathway helps to ward off infections.

Idiopathic—Of unknown origin.

Serotype—One form of a bacteria that has unique surface proteins. Each serotype causes a unique antibody response from a person's immune system.

rates and outcomes may be due to the fact that a higher number of adults get the form of HUS that begins without diarrhea.

Resources

BOOKS

Nathan, David, et al. "Schistocytic Hemolytic Anemia with Severe Thrombocytopenia." *Nathan and Oski's Hematology of Infancy and Childhood*. Philadelphia: W.B. Saunders, 1998.

Siegler, Richard. "Hemolytic Uremic Syndrome/Thrombotic Thrombocytopenic Purpura." *Primer on Kidney Diseases*. San Diego, CA: Academic Press, 1998.

PERIODICALS

Landau, Daniel, et al. "Familial Hemolytic Uremic Syndrome Associated with Complement Factor H Deficiency." *Journal of Pediatrics* 138 (March 2001): 412-417.

Wong, Craig, et al. "The Risk of Hemolytic-Uremic Syndrome After Antibiotic Treatment of *Escherichia coli* 0157:H7 Infections." *New England Journal of Medicine* 342, no. 26 (June 2000): 1930-1936.

WEBSITES

"H Factor 1; HF1." *Online Mendelian Inheritance in Man*. <http://www.ncbi.nlm.nih.gov/entrez/dispomim.cgi?id=134370>.

"Hemolytic-Uremic Syndrome; HUS." *Online Mendelian Inheritance in Man*. <http://www.ncbi.nlm.nih.gov/entrez/dispomim.cgi?id=235400>.

Benjamin Morris Greenberg

Hemophilia

Definition

Hemophilia is a genetic disorder—usually inherited—of the mechanism of blood clotting. Depending on the degree of the disorder present in an individual, excess bleeding may occur only after specific, predictable events (such as surgery, dental procedures, or injury), or occur spontaneously, with no known initiating event.

Description

The normal mechanism for blood clotting is a complex series of events involving the interaction of the injured blood vessel, blood cells (called platelets), and over 20 different proteins which also circulate in the blood.

When a blood vessel is injured in a way that causes bleeding, platelets collect over the injured area, and form a temporary plug to prevent further bleeding. This temporary plug, however, is too disorganized to serve as a long-term solution, so a series of chemical events occur, resulting in the formation of a more reliable plug. The final plug involves tightly woven fibers of a material called fibrin. The production of fibrin requires the interaction of several chemicals, in particular a series of proteins called clotting factors. At least thirteen different clotting factors have been identified.

The clotting cascade, as it is usually called, is the series of events required to form the final fibrin clot. The cascade uses a technique called amplification to rapidly produce the proper sized fibrin clot from the small number of molecules initially activated by the injury.

In hemophilia, certain clotting factors are either decreased in quantity, absent, or improperly formed. Because the clotting cascade uses amplification to rapidly plug up a bleeding area, absence or inactivity of just one clotting factor can greatly increase bleeding time.

Hemophilia A is the most common type of bleeding disorder and involves decreased activity of factor VIII. There are three levels of factor VIII deficiency: severe, moderate, and mild. This classification is based on the percentage of normal factor VIII activity present:

- Individuals with less than 1% of normal factor VIII activity level have severe hemophilia. Half of all people with hemophilia A fall into this category. Such individuals frequently experience spontaneous bleeding, most frequently into their joints, skin, and muscles. Surgery or trauma can result in life-threatening hemorrhage, and must be carefully managed.

- Individuals with 1–5% of normal factor VIII activity level have moderate hemophilia, and are at risk for heavy bleeding after seemingly minor traumatic injury.

- Individuals with 5–40% of normal factor VIII activity level have mild hemophilia, and must prepare carefully for any surgery or dental procedures.

Individuals with hemophilia B have symptoms very similar to those of hemophilia A, but the deficient factor is factor IX. This type of hemophilia is also known as Christmas disease.

Hemophilia C is very rare, and much more mild than hemophilia A or B; it involves factor XI.

Genetic profile

Hemophilia A and B are both caused by a genetic defect present on the X **chromosome**. (Hemophilia C is inherited in a different fashion.) About 70% of all people with hemophilia A or B inherited the disease. The other 30% develop from a spontaneous genetic mutation.

The following concepts are important to understanding the **inheritance** of these diseases. All humans have two chromosomes determining their gender: females have XX, males have XY. Because the trait is carried only on the X chromosome, it is called "sex-linked." The chromosome's flawed unit is referred to as the **gene**.

Both factors VIII and IX are produced by a genetic defect of the X chromosome, so hemophilia A and B are both sex-linked diseases. Because a female child always receives two X chromosomes, she nearly always will receive at least one normal X chromosome. Therefore, even if she receives one flawed X chromosome, she will still be capable of producing a sufficient quantity of factors VIII and IX to avoid the symptoms of hemophilia. Such a person who has one flawed chromosome, but does not actually suffer from the disease, is called a carrier. She carries the flaw that causes hemophilia and can pass it on to her offspring. If, however, she has a son who receives her flawed X chromosome, he will be unable to produce the right quantity of factors VIII or IX, and he will suffer some degree of hemophilia. (Males inherit one X and one Y chromosome, and therefore have only one X chromosome.)

In rare cases, a hemophiliac father and a carrier mother can pass on the right combination of parental chromosomes to result in a hemophiliac female child. This situation, however, is rare. The vast majority of people with either hemophilia A or B are male.

About 30% of all people with hemophilia A or B are the first member of their family to ever have the disease. These individuals have had the unfortunate occurrence of a spontaneous mutation; meaning that in their early development, some random genetic accident befell their X chromosome, resulting in the defect causing hemophilia A or B. Once such a spontaneous genetic mutation takes place, offspring of the affected person can inherit the newly-created, flawed chromosome.

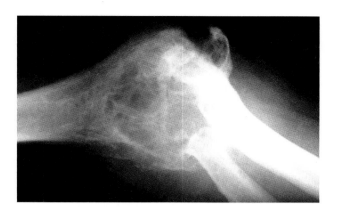

Elbow x ray showing changes to bone structure as a result of hemophilia. (*Custom Medical Stock Photo, Inc.*)

Demographics

Hemophilia A affects between one in 5,000 to one in 10,000 males in most populations.

One recent study estimated the prevalence of hemophilia was 13.4 cases per 100,000 U.S. males (10.5 hemophilia A and 2.9 hemophilia B). By race/ethnicity, the prevalence was 13.2 cases/100,000 among white, 11.0 among African-American, and 11.5 among Hispanic males.

Signs and symptoms

In the case of severe hemophilia, the first bleeding event usually occurs prior to eighteen months of age. In some babies, hemophilia is suspected immediately, when a routine circumcision (removal of the foreskin of the penis) results in unusually heavy bleeding. Toddlers are at particular risk, because they fall frequently, and may bleed into the soft tissue of their arms and legs. These small bleeds result in bruising and noticeable lumps, but don't usually need treatment. As a child becomes more active, bleeding may occur into the muscles; a much more painful and debilitating problem. These muscle bleeds result in pain and pressure on the nerves in the area of the bleed. Damage to nerves can cause numbness and decreased ability to use the injured limb.

Some of the most problematic and frequent bleeds occur into the joints, particularly into the knees and elbows. Repeated bleeding into joints can result in scarring within the joints and permanent deformities. Individuals may develop arthritis in joints that have suffered continued irritation from the presence of blood. Mouth injuries can result in compression of the airway, and, therefore, can be life-threatening. A blow to the head, which might be totally insignificant in a normal individual, can result in bleeding into the skull and brain.

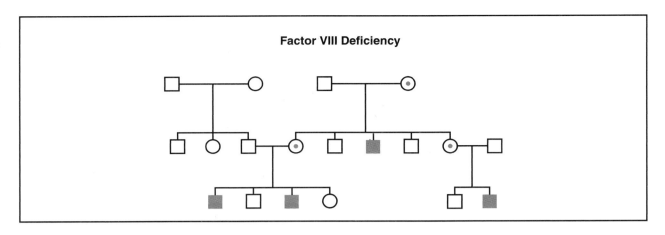

Factor VIII Deficiency

(Gale Group)

Because the skull has no room for expansion, the hemophiliac individual is at risk for brain damage due to blood taking up space and exerting pressure on the delicate brain tissue.

People with hemophilia are at very high risk of hemorrhage (severe, heavy, uncontrollable bleeding) from injuries such as motor vehicle accidents and also from surgery.

Some other rare clotting disorders such as **Von Willebrand disease** present similar symptoms but are not usually called hemophilia.

Diagnosis

Various tests are available to measure, under very carefully controlled conditions, the length of time it takes to produce certain components of the final fibrin clot. Tests called assays can also determine the percentage of factors VIII and IX present compared to normal percentages. This information can help in demonstrating the type of hemophilia present, as well as the severity.

Individuals with a family history of hemophilia may benefit from **genetic counseling** before deciding to have a baby. Families with a positive history of hemophilia can also have tests done during a pregnancy to determine whether the fetus is a hemophiliac. The test called chorionic villius sampling examines proteins for the defects that lead to hemophilia. This test, which is associated with a 1% risk of miscarriage, can be performed at 10–12 weeks. The test called **amniocentesis** examines the **DNA** of fetal cells shed into the amniotic fluid for genetic mutations. Amniocentesis, which is associated with a one in 200 risk of miscarriage, is performed at 16–18 weeks gestation.

Treatment and management

The most important thing that individuals with hemophilia can do to prevent complications of his disease is to avoid injury. Those individuals who require dental work or any surgery may need to be pre-treated

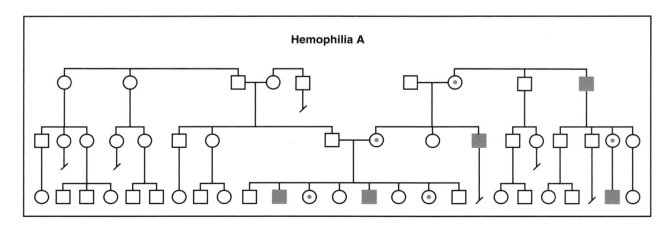

Hemophilia A

(Gale Group)

with an infusion of factor VIII to avoid hemorrhage. Also, hemophiliacs should be vaccinated against hepatitis. Medications or drugs that promote bleeding, such as aspirin, should be avoided.

Various types of factors VIII and IX are available to replace a patient's missing factors. These are administered intravenously (directly into the patient's veins by needle). These factor preparations may be obtained from a single donor, by pooling the donations of as many as thousands of donors, or by laboratory creation through highly advanced genetic techniques.

The frequency of treatment with factors depends on the severity of the individual patient's disease. Patients with relatively mild disease will only require treatment in the event of injury, or to prepare for scheduled surgical or dental procedures. Patients with more severe disease will require regular treatment to avoid spontaneous bleeding.

While appropriate treatment of hemophilia can both decrease suffering and be life-saving, complications associated with treatment can also be quite serious. About 20% of all patients with hemophilia A begin to produce chemicals in their bodies which rapidly destroy infused factor VIII. The presence of such a chemical may greatly hamper efforts to prevent or stop a major hemorrhage.

Individuals who receive factor prepared from pooled donor blood are at risk for serious infections that may be passed through blood. Hepatitis, a severe and potentially fatal viral liver infection, may be contracted from pooled factor preparations. Recently, a good deal of concern has been raised about the possibility of hemophiliacs contracting a fatal slow virus infection of the brain (Creutzfeldt-Jakob disease) from blood products. Unfortunately, pooled factor preparations in the early 1980s were contaminated with human immunodeficiency virus (HIV), the virus which causes AIDS. A large number of hemophiliacs were infected with HIV and some statistics show that HIV is still the leading cause of death among hemophiliacs. Currently, careful methods of donor testing, as well as methods of inactivating viruses present in donated blood, have greatly lowered this risk.

The most exciting new treatments currently being researched involve efforts to transfer new genes to hemophiliacs. These new genes would have the ability to produce the missing factors. As yet, these techniques are not being performed on humans, but there is great hope that eventually this type of **gene therapy** will be available.

Prognosis

Prognosis is very difficult to generalize. Because there are so many variations in the severity of hemo-

KEY TERMS

Amplification—A process by which something is made larger. In clotting, only a very few chemicals are released by the initial injury; they result in a cascade of chemical reactions which produces increasingly larger quantities of different chemicals, resulting in an appropriately-sized, strong fibrin clot.

Factors—Coagulation factors are substances in the blood, such as proteins and minerals, that are necessary for clotting. Each clotting substance is designated with roman numerals I through XIII.

Fibrin—The final substance created through the clotting cascade, which provides a strong, reliable plug to prevent further bleeding from the initial injury.

Hemorrhage—Very severe, massive bleeding that is difficult to control. Hemorrhage can occur in hemophiliacs after what would be a relatively minor injury to a person with normal clotting factors.

Mutation—A permanent change in the genetic material that may alter a trait or characteristic of an individual, or manifest as disease, and can be transmitted to offspring.

Platelets—Small disc-shaped structures that circulate in the blood stream and participate in blood clotting.

Trauma—Injury.

philia, and because much of what befalls a hemophiliac patient will depend on issues such as physical activity level and accidental injuries, statistics on prognosis are not generally available.

Resources

BOOKS

Genetics and Public Health in the 21st Century: Using Genetic Information to Improve Health and Prevent Disease. Edited by Muin J. Khoury, Wylie Burke, and Elizabeth J. Thomson. New York: Oxford University Press, 2000.

Hemophilia. Edited by C.D. Forbes, L.M. Aledort, and R. Madhok. New York: Chapman & Hall, 1997.

Resnick, Susan. *Blood Saga: Hemophilia, AIDS, and the Survival of a Community.* Berkeley: University of California Press, 1999.

PERIODICALS

Soucie, J.M., et al. "Hemophilia Surveillance System Project Investigators: Occurrence of Hemophilia in the United

States." *American Journal of Hematology* 59 (1998): 288+.

Stephenson, J. "New Therapies Show Promise for Patients with Leukemia, Hemophilia, and Heart Disease." *JAMA* 285 (January 1, 2001): 153+.

ORGANIZATIONS

National Hemophilia Foundation. 116 West 32nd St., 11th Floor, New York, NY 10001. (800) 42-HANDI. <http://www.info@hemophilia.org>.

National Organization for Rare Disorders (NORD). PO Box 8923, New Fairfield, CT 06812-8923. (203) 746-6518 or (800) 999-6673. Fax: (203) 746-6481. <http://www.rarediseases.org>.

WEBSITES

March of Dimes. <www.modimes.org>.

National Organization for Rare Disorders. <www.rarediseases.org>.

Jennifer F. Wilson, MS

Hepatocellular carcinoma

Definition

Hepatocellular carcinoma, or liver **cancer**, is a form of cancer with a high mortality rate. Liver cancers can be classified into two types. They are either primary, when the cancer starts in the liver itself; or metastatic, when the cancer has spread to the liver from some other part of the body.

Description

Primary liver cancer

Primary liver cancer is a relatively rare disease in the United States, representing about 2% of all malignancies. It is, however, much more common in other parts of the world, representing from 10–50% of malignancies in Africa and parts of Asia. The American Cancer Society estimated that, in the United States in 2001, at least 16,200 new cases of liver cancer were diagnosed (10,700 in men and 5,500 in women), causing roughly 14,100 deaths.

In adults, most primary liver cancers belong to one of two types: hepatomas, or hepatocellular carcinomas, which start in the liver tissue itself; and cholangiomas, or cholangiocarcinomas, which are cancers that develop in the bile ducts inside the liver. About 75% of primary liver cancers are hepatomas. In the United States, about five persons in every 200,000 will develop a hepatoma;

in Africa and Asia, over 40 persons in 200,000 will develop this form of cancer. Two rare types of primary liver cancer are mixed-cell tumors, or undifferentiated tumors.

There is one type of primary liver cancer that usually occurs in children younger than four years of age and between the ages of 12–15. This type of childhood liver cancer is called a hepatoblastoma. Unlike liver cancers in adults, hepatoblastomas have a good chance of being treated successfully. Approximately 70% of children with hepatoblastomas experience complete cures. If the tumor is detected early, the survival rate is over 90%.

Metastatic liver cancer

The second major category of liver cancer, metastatic liver cancer, is about 20 times as common in the United States as primary liver cancer. Because blood from all parts of the body must pass through the liver for filtration, cancer cells from other organs and tissues easily reach the liver, where they can lodge and grow into secondary tumors. Primary cancers in the colon, stomach, pancreas, rectum, esophagus, breast, lung, or skin are the most likely to spread (metastasize) to the liver. It is not unusual for the metastatic cancer in the liver to be the first noticeable sign of a cancer that started in another organ. After cirrhosis, metastatic liver cancer is the most common cause of fatal liver disease.

Genetic profile

Hepatocellular carcinoma has occasionally been reported to occur in familial clusters. It appears that first-degree relatives (siblings, children, or parents) of people with primary liver cancer are 2.4 times more likely to develop liver cancer themselves. This finding indicates a small overall genetic component, however, specific disease genes have not yet been identified. Certain genetic diseases are associated with a higher risk for liver cancers. These include **Hemochromatosis**, **alpha-1 Antitrypsin** deficiency, glycogen storage disease, tyrosinemia, **Fanconi anemia**, and **Wilson disease**.

Demographics

Hepatocellular carcinoma is the sixth most common cancer of men and eleventh most common cancer of women worldwide, affecting 250,000 to one million individuals annually. Liver cancer is becoming more common in the United States. It is 10 times more common in Africa and Asia where liver cancer is the most common type of cancer. Liver cancer affects men more often than women and, like most cancers, it is more common in older individuals.

Risk factors for primary liver cancer

The exact cause of primary liver cancer is still unknown. In adults, however, certain factors are known to place some individuals at higher risk of developing liver cancer. These factors include:

- Exposure to hepatitis B (HBV) or hepatitis C (HBC) viruses. In Africa and most of Asia, exposure to hepatitis B is an important factor; in Japan and some Western countries, exposure to hepatitis C is connected with a higher risk of developing liver cancer. In the United States, nearly 25% of patients with liver cancer show evidence of HBV infection. Hepatitis is commonly found among intravenous drug abusers.

- Exposure to substances in the environment that tend to cause cancer (carcinogens). These include a substance produced by a mold that grows on rice and peanuts (aflatoxin); thorium dioxide, which was used at one time as a contrast dye for x rays of the liver; and vinyl chloride, a now strictly regulated chemical used in manufacturing plastics.

- Cirrhosis. Hepatomas appear to be a frequent complication of cirrhosis of the liver. Between 30 and 70% of hepatoma patients also have cirrhosis. It is estimated that a patient with cirrhosis has 40 times the chance of developing a hepatoma than a person with a healthy liver.

- Use of oral estrogens for birth control. This association is based on studies of older, stronger birth control pills that are no longer prescribed. It is not clear if newer, lower dose birth control pills increase risk for liver cancer.

- Use of anabolic steroids (male hormones) for medical reasons or strength enhancement. Cortisone-like steroids do not appear to increase risk for liver cancer.

- Hereditary hemochromatosis. Hemochromatosis is a disorder characterized by abnormally high levels of iron storage in the body. It often develops into cirrhosis.

- Geographic location. Liver cancer is 10 times more common in Asia and Africa than in the United States.

- Male sex. The male/female ratio for hepatoma is 4:1.

- Age over 60 years.

Signs and symptoms

The early symptoms of primary, as well as metastatic, liver cancer are often vague and not unique to liver disorders. The long lag time between the beginning of the tumor's growth and signs of illness is the major reason why the disease has such a high mortality rate. At the time of diagnosis, patients are often tired, with fever, abdominal pain, and loss of appetite. They may look emaciated and generally ill. As the tumor grows bigger, it stretches the membrane surrounding the liver (the capsule), causing pain in the upper abdomen on the right side. The pain may extend into the back and shoulder. Some patients develop a collection of fluid, known as ascites, in the abdominal cavity. Others may show signs of bleeding into the digestive tract. In addition, the tumor may block the ducts of the liver or the gall bladder, leading to jaundice. In patients with jaundice, the whites of the eyes and the skin may turn yellow, and the urine becomes dark-colored.

Diagnosis

Physical examination

If the doctor suspects a diagnosis of liver cancer, he or she will check the patient's history for risk factors and pay close attention to the condition of the patient's abdomen during the physical examination. Masses or lumps in the liver and ascites can often be felt while the patient is lying flat on the examination table. The liver is usually swollen and hard in patients with liver cancer; it may be sore when the doctor presses on it. In some cases, the patient's spleen is also enlarged. The doctor may be able to hear an abnormal sound (bruit) or rubbing noise (friction rub) if he or she uses a stethoscope to listen to the blood vessels that lie near the liver. The noises are caused by the pressure of the tumor on the blood vessels.

Laboratory tests

Blood tests may be used to test liver function or to evaluate risk factors in the patient's history. Between 50% and 75% of primary liver cancer patients have abnormally high blood serum levels of a particular protein (alpha-fetoprotein or AFP). The AFP test, however, cannot be used by itself to confirm a diagnosis of liver cancer, because cirrhosis or chronic hepatitis can also produce high alpha-fetoprotein levels. Tests for alkaline phosphatase, bilirubin, lactic dehydrogenase, and other chemicals indicate that the liver is not functioning normally. About 75% of patients with liver cancer show evidence of hepatitis infection. Again, however, abnormal liver function test results are not specific for liver cancer.

Imaging studies

Imaging studies are useful in locating specific areas of abnormal tissue in the liver. Liver tumors as small as an inch across can now be detected by ultrasound or computed tomography scan (CT scan). Imaging studies, however, cannot tell the difference between a hepatoma and other abnormal masses or lumps of tissue (nodules) in the liver. A sample of liver tissue for biopsy is needed

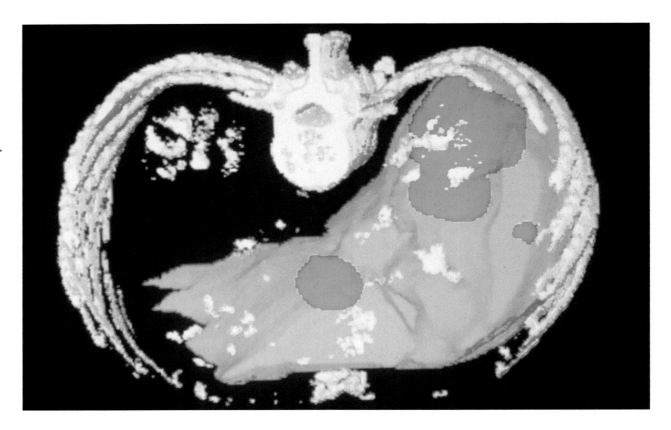

This 3-D CT (computed tomography) scan shows the abdomen of a patient with liver cancer. The metastatic tumors are red and located in the liver (blue). (*Photo Researchers, Inc.*)

to make the definitive diagnosis of a primary liver cancer. CT or ultrasound can be used to guide the doctor in selecting the best location for obtaining the biopsy sample. Chest x rays may be used to see whether the liver tumor is primary or has metastasized from a primary tumor in the lungs.

Liver biopsy

Liver biopsy is considered to provide the definite diagnosis of liver cancer. In about 70% of cases, the biopsy is positive for cancer. In most cases, there is little risk to the patient from the biopsy procedure. In about 0.4% of cases, however, the patient develops a fatal hemorrhage from the biopsy because some tumors are supplied with a large number of blood vessels and bleed very easily.

Laparoscopy

The doctor may also perform a laparoscopy to help in the diagnosis of liver cancer. A laparoscope is a small tube-shaped instrument with a light at one end. The doctor makes a small cut in the patient's abdomen and inserts the laparoscope. A small piece of liver tissue is removed and examined under a microscope for the presence of cancer cells.

Treatment and management

Treatment of liver cancer is based on several factors, including the type of cancer (primary or metastatic); stage (early or advanced); the location of other primary cancers or metastases in the patient's body; the patient's age; and other coexisting diseases, including cirrhosis. Treatment options include surgery, radiation, and chemotherapy. At times, two or all three of these may be used together. For many patients, treatment of liver cancer is primarily intended to relieve the pain caused by the cancer but cannot cure it.

Surgery

The goal of surgery is to remove the entire tumor, curing liver cancer. However, few liver cancers in adults can be cured by surgery because they are usually too advanced by the time they are discovered. If the cancer is contained within one lobe of the liver, and if the patient does not have cirrhosis, jaundice, or ascites, surgery is the best treatment option. Patients who can have their entire tumor removed have the best chance for survival.

If the entire visible tumor can be removed, about 25% of patients will be cured. The operation that is performed is called a partial hepatectomy, or partial removal of the liver. The surgeon will remove either an entire lobe of the liver (a lobectomy) or cut out the area around the tumor (a wedge resection).

Doctors may also offer tumor embolization or ablation. Embolization involves killing a tumor by blocking its blood supply. Ablation is a method of destroying a tumor without removing it. One method of ablation, cryosurgery, involves freezing the tumor, thereby destroying it. In another method of ablation, ethanol ablation, doctors kill the tumor by injecting alcohol into it. A new method of ablation using high-energy radio waves is under development.

Chemotherapy

Chemotherapy involves using very strong drugs, taken by mouth or intravenously, to suppress or kill tumor cells. Chemotherapy also damages normal cells, leading to side effects such as hair loss, vomiting, mouth sores, loss of appetite, and fatigue.

Some patients with incurable metastatic cancer of the liver can have their lives prolonged for a few months by chemotherapy. If the tumor cannot be removed by surgery, a tube (catheter) can be placed in the main artery of the liver and an implantable infusion pump can be installed (hepatic artery infusion). The pump allows much higher concentrations of cancer drugs to be carried directly to the tumor.

Hepatocellular carcinoma is resistant to most drugs. Specific drugs such as doxorubicin and cisplatin have been proven effective against this type of cancer. Systemic chemotherapy can also be used to treat liver cancer. Systemic chemotherapy does not, however, significantly lengthen the patient's survival time.

Radiation therapy

Radiation therapy is the use of high-energy rays or x rays to kill cancer cells or to shrink tumors. In liver cancer, however, radiation is only able to give brief relief from some of the symptoms, including pain. Liver cancers are not sensitive to levels of radiation considered safe for surrounding tissues. Radiation therapy has not been shown to prolong the life of a patient with liver cancer.

Liver transplantation

Removal of the entire liver (total hepatectomy) and liver transplantation are used very rarely in treating liver cancer. This is because very few patients are eligible for this procedure, either because the cancer has spread beyond the liver or because there are no suitable donors. Further research in the field of transplant immunology may make liver transplantation a possible treatment method for more patients in the future.

Future treatments

Gene therapy may be a future treatment for liver cancer. Scientists are still investigating the possible use of **gene** therapy as a treatment for cancer. There is controversy surrounding experimentation with gene therapy on humans. As such, it may be years before science is able to create a clinically available gene therapy treatment.

Prognosis

Liver cancer has a very poor prognosis because it is often not diagnosed until it has metastasized. Fewer than 10% of patients survive three years after the initial diagnosis; the overall five-year survival rate for patients with hepatomas is around 4%. Most patients with primary liver cancer die within several months of diagnosis. Patients with liver cancers that metastasized from cancers in the colon live slightly longer than those whose cancers spread from cancers in the stomach or pancreas.

Prevention

There are no useful strategies at present for preventing metastatic cancers of the liver. Primary liver cancers, however, are 75–80% preventable. Current strategies focus on widespread vaccination for hepatitis B; early treatment of hereditary hemochromatosis; and screening of high-risk patients with alpha-fetoprotein testing and ultrasound examinations.

Lifestyle factors that can be modified in order to prevent liver cancer include avoidance of exposure to toxic chemicals and foods harboring molds that produce aflatoxin. In the United States laws protect workers from exposure to toxic chemicals. Changing grain storage methods in other countries may reduce aflatoxin exposure. Avoidance of alcohol and drug abuse is also very important. Alcohol abuse is responsible for 60–75% of cases of cirrhosis, which is a major risk factor for eventual development of primary liver cancer.

A vaccination for hepatitis B is now available. Widespread immunization prevents infection, reducing a person's risk for liver cancer. Other protective measures against hepatitis include using protection during sex and not sharing needles. Scientists have found that interferon injections may lower the risk for someone with hepatitis C or cirrhosis to develop liver cancer.

Resources

BOOKS

Blumberg, Baruch S. *Hepatitis B and the Prevention of Cancer of the Liver.* River Edge, NJ: World Scientific Publishing Company, Inc., 2000.

Elmore, Lynne W., and Curtis C. Harris. "Hepatocellular Carcinoma." *The Genetic Basis of Human Cancer.* Ed. Bert Vogelstein and Kenneth Kinzler, 681–89. New York: McGraw-Hill, 1998.

Shannon, Joyce Brennfleck. *Liver Disorders Source Book: Basic Consumer Health Information about the Liver, and How It Works.* Detroit: Omnigraphics Inc., 2000.

PERIODICALS

Greenlee, Robert T., et al. "Cancer Statistics, 2001." *CA: A Cancer Journal for Clinicians.* 51 (January/February 2001): 15–36.

Hussain, S. A., et al. "Hepatocellular carcinoma." *Annals of Oncology* 12 (February 2001): 161–72.

Ogunbiyi, J. "Hepatocellular carcinoma in the developing world." *Seminars in Oncology* 28 (April 2001): 179–87.

ORGANIZATIONS

American Cancer Society. 1599 Clifton Rd. NE, Atlanta, GA 30329. (800) 227-2345. <http://www.cancer.org>.

American Liver Foundation. 75 Maiden Lane, Suite 603, New York, NY 10038. (800) 465-4837 or (888) 443-7222. <http://www.liverfoundation.org>.

National Cancer Institute. Office of Communications, 31 Center Dr. MSC 2580, Bldg. 1 Room 10A16, Bethesda, MD 20892-2580. (800) 422-6237. <http://www.nci.nih.gov>.

Rebecca J. Frey, PhD
Judy C. Hawkins, MS

Hepatorenal glycogenosis *see*
Fanconi-Bickel syndrome

Hereditary angioneurotic edema

Definition

Hereditary angioneurotic edema (HANE) is a non-sex linked (autosomal) dominant disease that results from mutations in a **gene** responsible for producing one of the proteins responsible for human immunity. This disease is also known as hereditary angioedema (HAE) or hereditary C1 inhibitor deficiency because it is a deficiency of the protein (C1-INH) that inhibits the action of the enzyme known as C1 which causes this disease.

Description

There are two recognized forms of HANE. Type I represents approximately 80-85% of the cases of hereditary angioneurotic edema. In this type, the protein C1-INH is not produced in sufficient quantities. Type II HANE represents the remaining 15-20% of cases. In this type, C1-INH concentrations are normal, but the C1-INH protein produced is defective.

Related to the two types of hereditary angioneurotic edema are acquired types of this disease (AANE or AAE) that are not based on a defective gene. Type I AAE is caused by a disorder that causes over-growth (proliferation) of the lymph tissues and destroys C1-INH. Type II AAE is caused by the presence of autoantibodies (antibodies that attack the host organism that produced them) that destroy C1-INH. Both of these acquired forms of angioedema can generally be differentiated from the two types of HANE by the age of onset. Symptoms of the acquired diseases usually do not occur until the fourth decade of life, while those of the hereditary forms are generally present prior to puberty.

The human body has two distinct immune systems: the humoral immune system and the cell-mediated immune system. The complement system is a part of the humoral immune system. Humoral means within the humor, or fluids, of the body. Blood, lymph, and bile compose the fluids of the humor. The complement system uses at least 30 different proteins to "mark" any foreign cells in the body that do not have certain protective proteins on their cell membranes which identify them as belonging in the body. These complement proteins are designated C1, C2, C3, et cetera. Once the foreign cells have been "marked," a particular form of white blood cell, called a phagocyte, is dispatched to the area with the marked cells and destroys them.

Phagocytes will eventually destroy any cell that is marked by complement; therefore, it is important to make sure that the complement proteins are not marking non-foreign cells. When cells are improperly marked, these cells will also be destroyed, causing what is called an autoimmune response. In effect, this autoimmune response means that the body is recognizing itself as foreign and attempting to destroy healthy cells. Inhibitors of the various complement proteins are necessary to prevent these proteins from marking the wrong cells or from continuing to mark cells after the foreign cells have been destroyed.

C1 inhibitor (C1-INH) is a chemical that is involved in the regulation of the complement system by inhibiting the action of the first complement protein (C1). C1-INH acts by binding free C1 molecules in the humor, preventing them from being able to function. It also limits the activation of other complement proteins.

Because C1-INH is diminished or defective in people affected with HANE, C1 is not inhibited and this inappropriately initiates the complement reaction which causes the swelling (acute inflammatory response) characteristic of HANE.

C1-INH also binds to the chemicals kallikrein and plasmin that are involved in blood clotting. Kallikrein is necessary for the activation of chemicals that cause dilation of blood vessels to allow increased blood flow to an area that requires more blood than normal. Plasmin is the chemical responsible for dissolving blood clots. A lack of binding of plasmin means that the formation of initial blood clots is difficult, a problem that is exacerbated by high levels of unbound kallikrein, which allows higher than normal blood flow.

With the absence or dysfunction of the C1-INH protein, the functions of blood flow, blood clotting, and immune response are impaired in individuals affected by hereditary angioneurotic edema, leading to swelling of the bodily tissues.

Genetic profile

The central Pyncheon family in Nathaniel Hawthorne's *The House of the Seven Gables* carries an ances-

tral curse of dying from choking on their own blood. Hawthorne describes members of the family who made odd sounds in the throat and chest when agitated, and sometimes died from choking: "This mode of death has been an idiosyncrasy with his family, for generations past....[the] prophecy was probably founded on a knowledge of this physical predisposition in the Pyncheon race." It seems possible that Hawthorne was not only describing the symptoms of HANE but also acknowledging it to be an inherited genetic disorder.

All hereditary forms of HANE are caused by mutations in the gene responsible for the production of C1-INH. This gene is located on the long arm (q) of **chromosome** 11, at the specific location q11.2-q13. There are at least 13 different mutations of the C1-INH gene that cause the symptoms of HANE. Six of these are known to cause type I HANE, while another six are known to cause type II HANE. The final mutation has only been found in one individual. In this case, an acquired form of angioedema was determined to be caused by a mutation in a different region of the C1-INH gene than those mutations causing type I or type II cases of HANE.

Demographics

HANE affects approximately 50,000 people in the United States and Europe. It is estimated to occur in approximately one in every 50,000 to 150,000 live births. HANE appears to affect males and females equally and does not have a racial preference.

As an autosomal dominant trait, only one copy of an abnormal gene needs to be inherited for an individual to be affected. Therefore, if one child is affected with HANE, the likelihood that a second child will be affected with HANE is 50%. In cases of parents related by blood (consanguineous parents) the likelihood of HANE is increased.

Signs and symptoms

Individuals affected with either form of HANE have episodes of swelling of the hands, feet, trunk, face, digestive tract, and airways (angioneurotic edema or angioedema). These attacks of angioedema are often accompanied by attacks of nausea, vomiting, and abdominal pain. The frequency and severity of these attacks is not predictable and varies from individual to individual. These attacks may occur without cause, or they may be triggered by anxiety, stress, or minor traumas, such as dental procedures. If these symptoms are accompanied by hives (urticaria) a diagnosis other than HANE is indicated.

Symptoms of HANE generally first occur prior to puberty and episodes generally increase in severity after puberty.

Diagnosis

A diagnosis of HANE is suspected in individuals who have recurrent attacks of swollen tissues (angioedema). Diagnosis of type I HANE is confirmed by blood tests showing abnormally low levels of C1-INH, C2, and C4. Diagnosis of type II HANE is confirmed by blood tests showing normal levels of C1-INH and C2, but abnormally low levels of C4. Abnormally low levels of C1-INH and C4 without the presence of autoantibodies suggest a diagnosis of type I acquired angioedema, while abnormally low levels of C1-INH and C4 and the presence of autoantibodies suggest a diagnosis of type II acquired angioedema.

Hives (urticaria) are not generally associated with HANE. If hives are present with tissue swelling, this may suggest an allergic reaction, not a case of HANE. Occasionally, individuals affected with HANE also develop hives, but they are usually secondary to the angioedema. In a severe allergic reaction, hives are generally prominent as the major symptom.

Treatment and management

The treatment of both hereditary forms of angioedema is the same. Androgens (male sex hormones) such as winstrol, danazol, and oxandrolone have been shown to be effective in preventing chronic recurrences of swelling. These drugs are seldom used to treat acute attacks. In instances of abdominal attacks, fluid replacement therapy via intravenous injection may be required. Demerol and Compazine suppositories are often prescribed to relieve abdominal pain and vomiting.

Edema (swelling) of the airways is the most life-threatening feature of HANE. Without prompt medical attention, individuals affected with HANE can die from an obstruction of the airway caused by this swelling. Unfortunately, if the attending physician does not recognize HANE, attempts at tracheal intubation (formation of an airway directly in the neck) may aggravate the swelling rather than produce a functioning airway.

Treatment with vapor-heated C1-INH concentrate has proven to be an effective treatment both as a prophylactic (preventative) and a treatment for acute attacks of angioedema in all individuals affected with HANE. The C1-INH concentrate is derived from human blood plasma; therefore it may possibly be contaminated. It is vapor-heated to inactivate possible hepatitis and HIV viruses. However, because HANE is a disease of the immune system, many doctors are reluctant to use C1-INH from other people and many patients are unwilling to accept such a treatment. The use of human recombinant C1-INH should alleviate any concerns arising from possible contamination of the blood supply.

Androgens are still the preventative treatment of choice because they are more cost-effective than treatments with C1-INH. However, androgens should not be given to women who are pregnant, or who might become pregnant. In these cases, C1-INH treatment is required.

In 1999, the U.S. Food and Drug Administration granted Orphan Drug Designations to human recombinant

C1-INH for both preventative and acute treatment of HANE. On March 21, 2000, Baxter Healthcare's Hyland Immuno division and Europe's Pharming Group announced an agreement to jointly develop recombinant human C1-INH. As of the March 2000 press release by these two companies, pre-clinical (animal) studies were expected to be completed in late 2000 and phase I human trials were slated to begin in late 2000 or early 2001. Because of the Orphan Drug Designations from the USFDA, this possible treatment for HANE is automatically "fast-tracked," which means that it could potentially be approved for human use by 2004.

Prognosis

The key to successful management of HANE is a proper medical diagnosis. With proper medical treatment, HANE is completely controllable and individuals affected with HANE suffer no diminishment in quality of life.

Resources

BOOKS

Hawthorne, Nathaniel. *The House of the Seven Gables*. New York, New York: Signet Classics Penguin Books Ltd., 1961.

PERIODICALS

Asghar, S., and M. Pasch. "Therapeutic inhibition of the complement system." *Frontiers in Bioscience* (September 2000): E63-81.

Cicardi, M., et al. "Pathogenetic and clinical aspects of C1 inhibitor deficiency." *Immunobiology* (August 1998): 366-376.

Markovic, S., D. Inwards, A. Evangelos, and R. Phyliky. "Acquired C1 esterase inhibitor deficiency." *Annals of Internal Medicine* (January 2000): 144-150.

Waytes, A., F. Rosen, and M. Frank. "Treatment of hereditary angioedema with a vapor-heated C1 inhibitor concentrate." *New England Journal of Medicine* (June 1996): 1630-1634.

ORGANIZATIONS

Hereditary Angioedema Association. PO Box 492, Live Oak, FL 32064. <http://www.hereditaryangioedema.com>.

National Organization for Rare Disorders (NORD). PO Box 8923, New Fairfield, CT 06812-8923. (203) 746-6518 or (800) 999-6673. Fax: (203) 746-6481. <http://www.rarediseases.org>.

WEBSITES

Angioedema (Hereditary). eMedicine. <http://www.emedicine.com/derm/topic24.htm> (February 23, 2001).

"Angioedema, Hereditary; HAE." *Online Mendelian Inheritance in Man*. <http://www.ncbi.nlm.nih.gov/htbin-post/Omim/dispmim?106100> (February 23, 2001).

The Complement Laboratory at the University of Iowa. <http://ictg.uiowa.edu/clab/what.htm> (February 23, 2001).

OTHER

"Pharming and Baxter to co-develop human C1 inhibitor to treat hereditary angioedema." Pharming Group N.V. Press Release (March 21, 2000).

Paul A. Johnson

Hereditary arthro-opthalmopathy *see* Stickler syndrome

Hereditary colorectal cancer

Definition

Hereditary colorectal **cancer** is cancer of the colon or rectum that develops chiefly as the result of inherited factors.

Description

The colon, or the large intestine, is a long muscular tube that absorbs water from stool and advances the stool towards the rectum. The rectum works in conjunction with the anus to coordinate the process of defecation. The colon and rectum are jointly referred to as the colorectum.

A neoplasm is a portion of abnormal tissue that grows rapidly and out of control. Cancer is the malignant type of neoplasm. Colorectal cancer is a relatively common and dangerous cancer. Tumors originate in the mucosa, or inner lining of the colorectum, and grow inwardly. Eventually, the tumor spreads outwardly until it reaches lymph nodes or other organs in the abdomen. Ultimately, cancer cells may detach from the original tumor and spread to distant parts of the body (such as the liver, lungs, bone, and brain) in a process called metastasis.

The development of colorectal cancer is not a random event, but rather arises in a sequential fashion. The first easily detected step is the appearance of adenomatous polyps. Polyps are grossly defined as elevations of a surface. An adenomatous polyp is derived from the glandular elements of the mucosa. A person may have any number of colorectal adenomatous polyps. Eventually, one or more of these polyps may transform into a cancer. The risk of colorectal cancer increases with the number of polyps. Larger polyps are also more likely to become cancerous than smaller ones. The factors that initiate this adenoma-cancer sequence are inherited and/or acquired from the environment.

Colorectal cancer occurs in certain families much more often than expected by chance alone. In fact, an important and common risk factor for the development of colorectal cancer is the occurrence of colorectal cancer in the family. About 10% of people have a first-degree relative with colorectal cancer. Having a first-degree relative with colorectal cancer increases the chance of developing colorectal cancer by two- to three-fold. The risk becomes even higher when colorectal cancer occurs in a relative at an early age (before 50 years of age) or when more than one relative has the cancer. This suggests that susceptibility of developing colorectal cancer in affected families is due to inherited factors, although shared exposure to environmental stimuli may play a role. Scientists are investigating the genetic factors that may be responsible for the increased risk of colorectal cancer in these cases of common **inheritance**.

The vast majority of cases of colorectal cancer are sporadic; that is, they occur in the absence of a hereditary syndrome, although familial risk may be involved. But rarely, colorectal cancer is inherited as part of a well-defined syndrome. These syndromes altogether account for about 2-5% of all cases of colorectal cancer.

Familial adenomatous polyposis

In the syndrome of **familial adenomatous polyposis** (FAP), adenomas develop in the colon and rectum early in life, at an average age of 15 years. Eventually, hundreds to thousands of adenomas will develop. The presence of such a large number of adenomas ensures that at least one of these adenomas will develop into cancer if the colon is not surgically removed. In people with FAP, the average age of occurrence of colorectal cancer is 39. Some patients will develop cancer in their teens and almost every patient will have cancer by age 45.

Other types of polyps are also common in patients with FAP. Polyps may develop in the stomach or duodenum. Those in the stomach are benign, while those in the duodenum may become malignant. The cancer risk in these other polyps is much less than the risk associated with the colorectal polyps. Patients with FAP may also have abnormalities outside the gastrointestinal tract, such as osteomas, desmoid tumors, extra teeth, and hypertrophy of the retinal pigment epithelium.

Three variants of FAP have been identified. Gardner syndrome is a rare variant of FAP characterized by colorectal polyps and a marked prominence of extraintestinal growths. Examples of the growths include osteomas, epidermoid cysts, and desmoid tumors. Although these growths usually present only cosmetic problems, desmoid tumors can occasionally compress nearby tissue in a harmful way.

Turcot syndrome is another rare type of FAP. Patients with this syndrome have the typical colorectal polyps, as well as malignant tumors of the central nervous system such as medulloblastoma, astrocytoma, ependymoma, and glioblastoma multiforme.

Patients with the attenuated adenomatous polyposis coli form of FAP have many colonic polyps, but not the hundreds or thousands seen in typical FAP. The chance of developing colon cancer approaches but does not reach 100%, and colon cancer usually appears later than in patients with typical FAP.

Hereditary nonpolyposis colorectal cancer

Patients with hereditary nonpolyposis colorectal cancer (HNPCC) have about an 80% risk of developing colorectal cancer if untreated. They may have more polyps than the general population, but not the hundreds or thousands of polyps associated with FAP. The average age for the development of cancer is 45 years old. Frequently, a patient with HNPCC will have multiple cancers at the same time (synchronous) or may develop cancers at different time periods (metachronous).

Extraintestinal cancers sometimes occur in HNPCC. The most common is uterine cancer, but other examples include cancer of the uterus, stomach, small intestine, pancreas, kidney, and ovary.

The Amsterdam criteria are clinical criteria for the diagnosis of HNPCC in a family:

- At least three relatives with colorectal cancer, one of whom must be a first-degree relative of the other two.

- Colorectal cancer involving at least two generations.

- One or more cases of colorectal cancer before the age of 50.

Muir-Torre syndrome is a rare form of HNPCC. In addition to polyps and cancer of the colon and rectum, patients exhibit various types of skin cancer.

Genetic profile

It must be understood that all colorectal cancers stem from genetic mutations. Environmental factors may also contribute to the development of cancer. Sometimes colorectal cancer appears in a patient who has neither affected relatives nor an inherited syndrome. Other cases appear in families that seem genetically susceptible to the development of these cancers. The presence of colorectal cancer in relatives, especially young relatives, increases the risk of developing colorectal cancer. In families affected by the rare syndromes of hereditary colorectal cancer (HNPCC, FAP, and their variants), the genetic mutations are inherited in autosomal dominant fashion.

Whether it appears sporadically or is inherited as part of a syndrome, colorectal cancer is generally linked to mutations in certain categories of genes: proto-oncogenes, tumor suppressor genes, **DNA** mismatch repair genes, or modifier genes. The proto-oncogene category includes the K-ras, src, and c-myc genes. The tumor suppressor genes are the APC (adenomatous polyposis coli) **gene**, the DCC (deleted in colon cancer) gene, the MCC (mutated in colon cancer) gene, the DPC4 gene, and p53. The mismatch repair genes are hMLH1, hMSH2, hPMS1, hPMS2, and hMSH6/GTBP. The modifier genes include the COX2 (cyclooxygenase 2) gene, the CD44v gene, and the phospholipase A2 gene.

The genetic defect in FAP and its three variants (Gardner syndrome, Turcot syndrome, and attenuated adenomatous polyposis coli) reside on the APC gene, which is on the long arm of **chromosome** 5. However, there are a wide variety of mutations within the APC gene that can result in those syndromes. Sometimes Turcot syndrome is associated with the same mutations as those in HNPCC. Mutations of mismatch repair genes, such as hMLH1, hMSH2, hPMS1, hPMS2, and hMSH6/GTBP, are characteristic of the HNPCC syndrome. The transmission of these hereditary colorectal cancer syndromes occurs through mutations of the same genes that are mutated in sporadic cases of colorectal cancer. But it must be emphasized that the hereditary colorectal cancer syndromes are inherited in an autosomal dominant pattern. This means that each child of an affected person has a 50% chance of inheriting the disease.

Families with the inherited syndromes of colorectal cancer can undergo **genetic testing** to determine which individuals have inherited the disease. The tests for the defective genes can detect the mutation in approximately 60 to 80% of FAP families and about 50% of HNPCC families. However, if one person is found to have the mutation, the other family members can be tested with nearly 100% accuracy. Although genetic testing can provide useful information to the patients, it may be associated with psychosocial risks. Thus, genetic testing should be performed only in formal programs. **Genetic counseling** should also be provided.

Demographics

Colorectal cancer is relatively common with approximately 160,000 new cases diagnosed each year. But the syndromes of inherited colorectal cancer are rare. It is estimated that they comprise only two to five percent of all cases of colorectal cancer. FAP occurs in about one in every 10,000 births. The incidence of all colorectal cancer increases with age.

Signs and symptoms

The clinical manifestations of colorectal cancer depend largely on location and tumor size. Tumors in the proximal colon can grow to large sizes before detection. They may cause weight loss, abdominal pain, or bleeding. The bleeding may be readily noticed by the patient as frank blood in the toilet, or smears of blood in the stool. Less extensive bleeding may be detected by the fecal occult blood test, in which a sample of stool obtained during a rectal exam is tested for microscopic amounts of blood. Anemia, or low red blood cell count, detected by a laboratory test may prompt further examination of the colon to determine if a tumor is the source of bleeding. In the smaller, distal colon, tumors are more likely to cause obstruction. This may cause gas pains and decrease in the caliber of the stool. Additionally, these cancers may cause bleeding or a change in bowel habits. In FAP, the first symptom is usually diarrhea.

Diagnosis

The presence of symptoms such as abdominal pain, weight loss, change in bowel habits, or decrease in stool caliber may point to a diagnosis of colorectal cancer. Of course, these symptoms must be interpreted within the context of the patient's age, previous medical history, and family history of colorectal cancer.

Ideally, the diagnosis of colorectal cancer should be made before symptoms develop. A number of screening tests are useful for detecting colorectal cancer. The fecal occult blood test that was discussed earlier is a simple test performed in the office. The normal result is the absence of blood in the stool. If blood is found in the stool, the suspicion for colorectal cancer becomes higher. Standard screening also includes an endoscopic exam—either sigmoidoscopy or colonoscopy. In these exams, a thin, specially lighted tube is inserted directly into the anus and advanced into the colon. The physician can view the inside of the colon and check for polyps or tumors. Sigmoidoscopy allows examination of the lower part of the colon while colonoscopy allows a more extensive view. Sometimes a barium enema is added to the screening procedure. In this test, a dye is injected into the anus and up into the colon. The dye coats the inside of the colon so that tumors can be detected by plain x ray.

New screening tests are currently under investigation. In wireless endoscopy, a tiny pill-sized camera is swallowed. As the camera traverses the gastrointestinal tract, it transmits video footage that can be examined for suspicious abnormalities. Eventually the camera is passed out of the anus with the stool. Virtual colonoscopy generates a three-dimensional image of the colon by applying advanced computer graphics technology to images obtained by computed tomography (CT) scanning. These processes can spare the patient the usual discomfort of traditional endoscopy. However, they are not yet fully developed nor approved for colorectal cancer screening.

If any of the above screening tests identifies an abnormality that appears to be a tumor, the diagnosis must be confirmed by biopsy. This is performed during colonoscopy. A small piece of tissue is removed and examined in the laboratory for cancerous cells.

Most medical organizations recommend that screening should begin in the general population at age 40 to 50. The fecal occult blood test is performed annually and sigmoidoscopy every three to five years. If a first degree relative has colorectal cancer, then screening should begin at 35 to 40 years of age. Alternatively, screening can begin five years earlier than the age of a young relative who has colorectal cancer.

Individuals in families affected by hereditary colorectal cancer syndromes are at high risk for developing cancer early in life. Therefore, screening is initiated at a young age. Screening can be reserved for those family members who have been proven to carry the abnormal gene by genetic testing, or it can be applied to all family members if the specific mutation cannot be identified. Some experts propose that in families with a history of FAP, screening should begin at 10 to 12 years of age and be repeated every one to two years. In families with HNPCC, colorectal screening should begin at 20 to 30 years of age and also be repeated every one to two years.

Since FAP and HNPCC are also associated with other cancers, affected patients should undergo appropriate screening for these malignancies as well. Those with FAP require regular upper endoscopy to detect tumors of the stomach and duodenum. Women with HNPCC should undergo screening for uterine cancer by way of random biopsies of the inner lining of the uterus.

Treatment and management

The treatment of sporadic colorectal cancer requires surgical removal of the tumor and surrounding tissue. Chemotherapy or radiation therapy may also be necessary. But the treatment of colorectal cancer in the hereditary syndromes is more aggressive. In these cases, the entire colon must be removed, since cancer will almost certainly develop in any remaining colon. Sometimes the rectum is also removed; alternatively, the patient may undergo frequent examination of the rectum for polyps or cancers. Experts strongly recommend that individuals with known FAP should consider surgical removal of the colon and/or rectum early in life as a prophylactic measure, before cancer is diagnosed. Although the role of prophylactic surgery in patients with HNPCC is less well-defined, many experts favor it. The patient faces a choice between prophylactic surgery and frequent, lifelong screening.

KEY TERMS

Adenomatous—Derived from glandular structures.

Astrocytoma—Tumor of the central nervous system derived from astrocytes.

Biopsy—The surgical removal and microscopic examination of living tissue for diagnostic purposes.

Central nervous system—In humans, the central nervous system is composed of the brain, the cranial nerves and the spinal cord. It is responsible for the coordination and control of all body activities.

Computed tomography—An imaging procedure that produces a three-dimensional picture of organs or structures inside the body, such as the brain.

Desmoid tumor—Benign, firm mass of scar-like connective tissue.

Distal—Away from the point of origin.

Endoscopy—A slender, tubular optical instrument used as a viewing system for examining an inner part of the body and, with an attached instrument, for biopsy or surgery.

Ependymoma—Tumor of the central nervous system derived from cells that line the central canal of the spinal cord and the ventricles of the brain.

Epidermoid cyst—Benign, cystic tumor derived from epithelial cells.

Glioblastoma multiforme—Tumor of the central nervous system consisting of undifferentiated glial cells.

Medulloblastoma—Tumor of the central nervous system derived from undifferentiated cells of the primitive medullary tube.

Metachronous—Occurring at separate time intervals.

Metastasis—The spreading of cancer from the original site to other locations in the body.

Osteoma—A benign bone tumor.

Polyp—A mass of tissue bulging out from the normal surface of a mucous membrane.

Prophylactic—Preventing disease.

Proximal—Near the point of origin.

Synchronous—Occurring simultaneously.

Some studies have shown that the drug sulindac may reduce the number of adenomatous polyps that develop in FAP and its variants. In addition, certain non-steroidal anti-flammatory drugs such as aspirin may also reduce the incidence of colorectal cancer in general.

Prognosis

Patients with a hereditary colorectal cancer syndrome such as FAP, HNPCC, or its variants, have a much higher likelihood of developing colon cancer than the general population. In the extreme case of typical FAP, essentially 100% of patients will develop colon cancer without surgery. If colon cancer does develop, survival depends on the extent to which the cancer has spread. Cancer that is isolated to the colon is associated with much better survival than cancer that has spread to distant organs such as the liver or lungs.

Resources

BOOKS

"Colon and Rectum." In *Sabiston Textbook of Surgery*, edited by Courtney Townsend Jr., et al. 16th ed. Philadelphia: W. B. Saunders Company, 2001.

"Familial Colon Cancer" and "Predisposition to Colorectal Cancer." In *Sleisenger & Fordtran's Gastrointestinal and Liver Disease*, edited by Mark Feldman, et al. Sixth ed. Philadelphia: W. B. Saunders Company, 1998.

PERIODICALS

Lynch, Henry and Trudy Shaw. "The Genetics of Colorectal Cancer." *Primary Care & Cancer* (June 1999).

Kevin Osbert Hwang, MD

▌Hereditary desmoid disease

Definition

Hereditary desmoid disease (HDD) is a condition that causes people to develop a benign (noncancerous) growth known as a desmoid tumor. Desmoid tumors may also be called fibromatosis.

Description

In HDD, multiple family members from several generations develop desmoid tumors. These tumors are very rare. They account for fewer than 0.1% of all tumors diagnosed. The term "desmoid" comes from the Greek word for "band." That describes these tumors well, as they have a tendon- or ligament-like appearance. They usually occur in the abdomen, but they may also develop in the neck, chest, arms, and legs.

Desmoid tumors may appear due to mutations, or changes, in a **gene** called adenomatous polyposis coli (APC). Most desmoid tumors, though—more than 97%—occur sporadically, meaning that they are not caused by genetic mutations. People who develop sporadic desmoid tumors have no other health problems associated with mutations in the APC gene and have no close family members with the tumors. In the past desmoid tumors were classified as fibrosarcomas (growths associated with **cancer**), but this is no longer the case.

Mutations in the APC gene usually result in **familial adenomatous polyposis** (FAP). This condition causes hundreds to thousands of polyps (tiny growths) to develop in the colon. It is associated with a high risk for developing colon cancer. People who have FAP need to have their health monitored on a regular basis. Colon cancer can be prevented by careful medical screening and removal of the colon.

Some families with FAP develop extra-colonic symptoms (involving organs other than the colon), including desmoid tumors. The combination of colon polyposis and desmoid tumor was once termed "Gardner syndrome," but it is now known that the two conditions are the same. Other extra-colonic features seen in families with FAP are cysts in the jawbone, skin cysts (epidermal cysts), bony bumps on the skull, a specific kind of spot on the retina, and thyroid cancer. About 10% of people with FAP will develop desmoid tumors. However, the risk differs from family to family.

In HDD, multiple family members over two or more generations develop desmoid tumors, but not colon polyposis. Family members in subsequent generations will have an increased risk of developing desmoid tumors.

Genetic profile

Every person diagnosed with HDD has a 50% chance of passing on the condition to each of his/her children. The chances that a child who has the gene mutation associated with HDD will develop a desmoid tumor are thought to be very high, maybe even 100%. It is possible that there may be other genes involved in HDD, but no gene other than APC has been identified. The location of the mutation within the APC gene may predict the symptoms and health problems that a person will experience, but this association is far from perfect.

Demographics

Hereditary desmoid disease is a rare condition. Only four families have been reported in the medical literature.

(It is likely, however, that not all families with HDD have been described in the literature.) Males and females are equally affected.

Signs and symptoms

Desmoid tumors may cause a noticeable lump and/or pain.

Diagnosis

HDD is usually diagnosed solely upon family history. Evaluation for HDD requires filling out a detailed, three-generation family tree. Medical records and/or death certificates should also be examined to confirm or clarify possible diagnoses of desmoid tumors. Medical records for family members developing colon polyps and/or undergoing colon surgery will also be requested in order to evaluate for FAP.

Genetic (or diagnostic) testing for APC **gene mutations** (changes) is another way of making a diagnosis. It may be offered to someone who has developed a desmoid tumor and has a family history of such tumors. If a mutation is identified, the positive test result provides proof of the diagnosis. If no mutation is identified, this negative test result does not necessary remove the diagnosis of HDD.

Diagnostic testing for HDD may be offered to an individual who has no personal history of a desmoid tumor but whose family history is strongly suggestive of HDD. Prenatal diagnosis of HDD is available only if an APC genetic alteration has already been identified in the family. Such "predictive" **genetic testing** is best done with a geneticist (a doctor specializing in genetics) and/or a genetic counselor.

Treatment and management

There is no cure for HDD, nor a method for preventing it. Treatment depends upon the location of the tumor and may include one or more of the following: surgery, chemotherapy, hormonal therapy, and/or radiation. In addition, everyone diagnosed with a desmoid tumor should be evaluated for FAP. This evaluation will include a detailed family history as well as colon screening though sigmoidoscopy or colonoscopy.

Treatment is not required until a tumor develops. Someone who has symptoms, however, must have regular medical check-ups.

There are no proven methods of screening for or preventing desmoid tumors, but it is suggested that people with or at risk for HDD have physical examinations every year. It is very important that an individual's

---

KEY TERMS

Colonoscopy—Procedure for viewing the large intestine (colon) by inserting an illuminated tube into the rectum and guiding it up the large intestine.

Cyst—An abnormal sac or closed cavity filled with liquid or semisolid matter.

Polyp—A mass of tissue bulging out from the normal surface of a mucous membrane.

Polyposis—A descriptive term indicating that hundreds to thousands of polyps have developed in an organ.

Sigmoidoscopy—The visual examination of the inside of the rectum and sigmoid colon, using a lighted, flexible tube connected to an eyepiece or video screen for viewing.

Tumor—An abnormal growth of cells. Tumors may be benign (noncancerous) or malignant (cancerous).

---

physician be aware of the family history and the risk of developing a tumor.

Prognosis

An individual who has a genetic mutation for HDD has a high chance of developing a desmoid tumor. However, the condition is treatable. Prognosis may be affected by a person's overall condition, so being healthy and engaging in healthy behaviors increase the chances of a good outcome.

Resources

ORGANIZATIONS

HCCA. 3601 N. 4th Ave. # 201, Sioux Falls, SD 57104. (800) 264-6783. <http://www.hereditarycc.org/index.html>.

National Organization for Rare Disorders (NORD). PO Box 8923, New Fairfield, CT 06812-8923. (203) 746-6518 or (800) 999-6673. Fax: (203) 746-6481. <http://www.rarediseases.org>.

WEBSITES

Association of Cancer Online Resources. The Desmoid Tumor Online Support Group. <http://listserv.acor.org/archives/desmoid.html>.

OncoLink. <http://www.oncolink.upenn.edu/about_oncolink>.

The University of Texas, MD Anderson Cancer Center. <http://search.mdanderson.org/compass>.

Cindy L. Hunter, CGC

Hereditary hearing loss and deafness

Definition

Hereditary hearing loss and deafness refers to the genetically caused loss or partial impairment of the ability to hear. It is estimated that 50% of congenital and severe early onset deafness occurs due to genetic causes.

Description

Genetic forms of hearing loss may be distinguished as prelingual (beginning before speech develops) or postlingual (beginning after speech develops). These hearing losses can be progressive, in which the hearing impairment increases with time, or, non-progressive, in which the hearing loss is stable over time. Each ear (bilateral) or only one ear (unilateral) may be affected, and the hearing loss may be equal in both ears (symmetric) or different in each ear (asymmetric). Hearing loss may be the only finding the affected person has (nonsyndromic hereditary hearing loss) or the hearing loss may be associated with other physical differences associated with a specific genetic syndrome (syndromic hereditary hearing loss). Hereditary hearing losses cover the entire range from mild hearing loss to total deafness.

Hearing loss can additionally be typed as conductive, sensorineural, or mixed type. Conductive hearing loss results from a blockage of the auditory canal or some other dysfunction of the eardrum or one of the three small bones within the ear (the stapes, the malleus, and the incus) that are responsible for collecting and transmitting sound. In conductive hearing loss, the auditory nerve is normal. Sensorineural hearing loss results from a dysfunction of the auditory nerve. Mixed-type hearing loss involves both conductive and sensorineural types of hearing impairment.

In normal hearing, sound vibrations enter the large fleshy external part of the ear (the pinna) and travel down the auditory canal striking the eardrum (tympanic membrane), which begins to vibrate. As this membrane vibrates, it touches the first of a series of three small bones (the malleus, the incus, and the stapes) that mechanically transfer the vibrations to the cochlea. The cochlea is a fluid-filled tube that bends back on itself such that the two open ends lay one on top of the other. One end is covered by a membrane called the oval window, while the other end is covered by a membrane called the round window. It is the oval window that is struck by the stapes. Since the cochlea is filled with fluid, the oval window cannot vibrate without the assistance of the round window: As the oval window is pushed in by the stapes, the round window bulges out; as

the oval window oscillates out, the round window bulges inward.

The vibrations imparted to the oval window by the stapes striking the round window are picked up by the organ of Corti within the cochlea. It is this structure that is the true receptor, in a nerve sense, of sound waves. The organ of Corti consists of hair cells embedded in a gelatinous membrane (the tectorial membrane) that rests on a basilar membrane. Sensory neurons terminate on the hair cells of the organ of Corti. Vibration of the fluid in the cochlea causes the basilar membrane to move, which causes the hairs to bend, creating an electrical signal. This is picked up by the sensory neurons and then transferred to the auditory nerve (or cochlear nerve), which sends the signal to the brain.

The ear is also involved in maintaining balance. As a result, many individuals affected with hearing loss may also have balance problems. Body position, body movement, and balance are assisted by the vestibular apparatus of the inner ear, which consists of three functional parts. Two of these, the saccule and the utricle, signal what the body position is relative to gravity. The third structure of the vestibular apparatus is the semicircular canal, of which there are three in each ear. These canals contain structures (ampulae) that detect movement of the internal fluid of the canals as the head moves. Most hearing-impaired people with balance problems experience difficulties with the proper functioning of the semicircular canals. Since the function of these canals is partially duplicated by the functioning of the saccule and the utricle, most individuals can "learn" to use these other systems to compensate for the dysfunction in the semicircular canals. Therefore, balance problems associated with hearing loss usually diminish over time.

Syndromic hearing loss

The term syndromic hearing loss is used when a person shows hearing loss in addition to other physical differences such as malformations of the external ear or other medical problems related to the hearing loss. Syndromic hearing loss constitutes approximately 30% of genetic hearing loss. Over 400 different genetic syndromes that include hearing loss have been described. Syndromic hearing loss is generally classified by the overall syndrome that leads to hearing impairment. Some of the more common genetic syndromes associated with hearing loss include **Waardenburg syndrome**, **Usher syndrome**, **Jervell and Lange-Nielsen syndrome**, and Alport syndrome. In these syndromes, hearing loss is associated with various other abnormalities. In Waardenburg syndrome, hearing loss occurs in conjunction with pigment differences in the skin, eyes, and hair. In Usher syndrome, hearing loss is associated with eye abnormalities that progress to blindness. In Jervell and Lange-Nielsen syndrome, hearing loss is associated with heartbeat abnormalities. In Alport syndrome, hearing loss is associated with kidney abnormalities.

Nonsyndromic hearing loss

The term nonsyndromic hearing loss is used when a person shows hearing loss with no other associated physical differences and no associated medical problems. Persons with nonsyndromic hearing loss will not have any visible abnormalities of the external ear; however, they may have abnormalities of the inner and/or middle ear. Nonsyndromic hearing loss constitutes approximately 70% of genetic hearing loss. Nonsyndromic hearing loss is generally classified by the age of onset, the type and degree of audiological impairment, the progressive or nonprogressive nature of the impairment, and the mode of **inheritance**. Nonsyndromic prelingual hearing loss is most frequently of the sensorineural type and most frequently inherited in an autosomal recessive pattern.

Otosclerosis is the most common form of nonsyndromic progressive conductive hearing loss in adults. It is caused by a growth of the spongy bone tissue in the middle ear that prevents the ossicles (malleus, incus, stapes) from being able to move as well as they once did. In certain advanced cases of otosclerosis, there may also be damage to the auditory nerve (sensorineural hearing loss). Otosclerosis may be observed in teenagers, but it is generally first observed in people between the ages of 20 and 50. It is very rare for otosclerosis to occur past the age of 50.

Dominant progressive hearing loss (DPHL) and prebycusis (hearing loss related to aging) are the most common forms of nonsyndromic progressive sensorineural hearing loss. DPHL tends to have an earlier age of onset than prebycusis, but this is highly variable between families. Within families, the age of onset of DPHL is generally fairly constant. The typical age of onset of DPHL is early childhood, but in some families it does not show symptoms until early or middle adulthood. Some individuals affected with DPHL also have problems with balance because of an alteration of the semicircular canal structures within their inner ears. These balance problems are not observed in other individuals with DPHL, suggesting that DPHL is caused by more than one **gene** or gene mutation. Prebycusis is not thought to be due to genetic causes. It is the most common form of hearing loss, and everyone who lives beyond a certain age develops it to some degree. Prebycusis is thought to be caused by the combined effects of aging and the noises from the environment that a person has been exposed to. People who live, work, or entertain themselves in loud environ-

ments generally develop prebycusis to a greater degree than those people who exist in quieter surroundings.

Genetic profile

Hearing loss is genetically heterogeneous. This means that nonrelated persons with genetic hearing loss may have hearing loss due to problems in different genes. Also, persons with genetic hearing loss in one family may show differing symptoms from each other. Additionally, different changes in the same gene may cause syndromic hearing loss in one family and nonsyndromic hearing loss in another family. As of early 2005, more than 100 separate genes associated with hearing loss have been identified. This number is expected to increase markedly as the genetic mutations causing the more than 400 syndromes associated with hearing loss are identified.

Hearing loss can be inherited in different patterns: autosomal dominant inheritance, autosomal recessive inheritance, X-linked inheritance, and mitochondrial inheritance. Approximately 75–80% of nonsyndromic hereditary hearing loss is due to mutations that are autosomal (non-X linked) recessive. Approximately 20% are due to autosomal dominant **gene mutations**. The rare remaining cases of nonsyndromic hereditary hearing loss are attributed to X-linked (about 1%) and mitochondrial disorders (about 1%).

Autosomal dominant hearing loss

Individuals with an autosomal dominant form of hereditary hearing loss have a 50% chance to pass on the gene for the hearing loss in each pregnancy, regardless of the sex of the parent or child. Most persons with this type of hereditary hearing loss have an affected parent; however, this can occur as a new problem in an individual with no family history. In that case, the affected person then has a 50% chance to pass the hearing loss to each of their children.

Otosclerosis is inherited in an autosomal dominant pattern. Otosclerosis shows reduced penetrance. A dominant condition with complete penetrance should show symptoms of the gene mutation in all individuals possessing the mutation (100% penetrance). However, because of the age-related symptoms of otosclerosis, many individuals possessing the genetic mutation known to cause otosclerosis do not have any symptoms of the disease. Similarly, when obtaining a family history, it is very possible that individuals from previous generations died of other causes prior to showing any signs of being affected with otosclerosis. Otosclerosis has been associated with different genetic locations on four chromosomes: 15, 7, 6, and 3. As of early 2005, no genes for otosclerosis have been identified.

The locations of the genes associated with nonsyndromic autosomal dominant deafness are designated as DFNA loci. By early 2005, 21 deafness-causing genes have been isolated at 18 DFNA loci. No single gene accounts for a majority of nonsyndromic autosomal dominant hearing loss.

Waardenburg syndrome is the most common autosomal dominant form of syndromic hereditary hearing loss. Even in a single family, each affected family member may show varying features of the syndrome. Affected persons may show white patches of skin or hair, differently colored eyes, widely spaced eyes, and/or sensorineural hearing loss in varying degrees. Waardenburg syndrome is differentiated into four types according to other abnormal features. Types I and III of Waardenburg syndrome are caused by mutations in the PAX3 gene. Some cases of Waardenburg syndrome Type II are associated with mutations in the MITF gene. Waardenburg syndrome Type IV has been associated with mutations in three genes: EDNRB, EDN3, and SOX10.

The second most common autosomal dominant form of syndromic hereditary hearing loss is **branchiootorenal syndrome** (BOR syndrome). Persons with branchiootorenal syndrome have varying symptoms which that differ between affected family members. Affected persons may have sensorineural, conductive, or mixed-type hearing loss, along with abnormalities of the external ear, cysts on the neck, and/or kidney problems. Mutations in the EYA1 gene located on **chromosome** 8 have been found in about 40% of patients with BOR syndrome. Still other families with BOR syndrome show mutations in the SIX1 gene on chromosome 14. Other genes responsible for BOR syndrome have not yet been characterized.

Autosomal recessive hearing loss

Individuals with an autosomal recessive form of hereditary hearing loss have inherited hearing loss genes from both their mother and their father. Most persons with autosomal recessive hereditary hearing loss do not have parents with hearing loss. In most cases, the parents simply carried silent genes for hearing loss that never caused them problems.

Most of hereditary hearing loss is nonsyndromic and autosomal recessive. The locations of the genes associated with nonsyndromic autosomal recessive deafness are designated as DFNB loci. As of early 2005, 21 deafness-causing genes have been isolated at 19 different DFNB loci. Mutations, or changes, in one gene, the GJB2 gene located at DFNB1 on chromosome 13, account for 50% of all autosomal recessive nonsyndromic hearing loss. GJB2 mutations have been found to account for 30% of hereditary hearing loss where there is

no family history. It is estimated that at least 3% of persons with normal hearing carry a silent mutation in one of their GJB2 genes. If a mother and father each are unaffected carriers of a mutation in GJB2, then they have a 25% chance to have a child with hearing loss in each pregnancy.

The most common type of autosomal recessive syndromic hearing loss is Usher syndrome. Persons with Usher syndrome are born with severe sensorineural hearing loss. They later develop **retinitis pigmentosa**, which is degeneration of the retina, the light sensitive layer of tissue at the back of the inner eye. This leads to visual problems and sometimes total blindness. Usher syndrome is the cause for 50% of cases where people are both deaf and blind. Usher syndrome is estimated to account for 3–6% of all congenital deafness. Usher syndrome has been divided into three types based on the severity of symptoms. The more severe Usher syndrome type I is characterized by vestibular dysfunction and retinal degeneration beginning in childhood. Usher syndrome type I has been localized to seven different chromosomal regions and from these regions five distinct genes have been identified thus far. These genes are designated as USH1B, USH1C, USH1D, USH1F, and USH1G. The moderate Usher syndrome type II is characterized by normal vestibular function and later onset of retinitis pigmentosa. Usher syndrome type II has been localized to three different chromosomal regions; but thus far, from these three regions only one gene, USH2A, has been isolated. The milder Usher syndrome type III is characterized by progressive hearing loss. Usher syndrome type III has been localized to the long arm of chromosome 3, but the gene has not yet been identified.

Pendred syndrome is the second most common type of autosomal recessively inherited hearing loss syndrome. Persons with Pendred syndrome have severe sensorineural hearing loss that is present at birth or it may develop in early childhood. They then develop a goiter, an enlarged thyroid gland, either in puberty or adulthood. In about half of persons with Pendred syndrome, a mutation can be found in the SLC26A4 gene.

X-linked hearing loss

Individuals with X-linked hearing loss have inherited a gene for hearing loss on the X chromosome. Females have two X chromosomes, whereas a male has an X and a Y chromosome. In the case of an X-linked recessive cause for hearing loss, the vast majority of affected persons are male. Females may be carriers, but they will rarely be affected. In the case of an X-linked dominant cause for hearing loss, all of the daughters of an affected father will show the disorder because all must inherit their father's X chromosome to be female.

The chromosomal locations associated with nonsyndromic X-linked deafness are designated as DFN loci. As of early 2005, four chromosomal locations have been associated with X-linked nonsyndromic hearing loss; however, thus far, the only locus that has had a gene identified is DFN3. The identified gene, POU3F4, is located on the long arm of the X chromosome. Persons with mutations at the DFN3 locus show mixed-type hearing loss. The conductive portion of their hearing loss is caused by abnormal attachment of one of the tiny internal ear bones, specifically, the stapes.

Alport syndrome is one example of an X-linked form of syndromic hearing loss. Males with X-linked Alport syndrome always show progressive kidney problems that lead to kidney failure and early death. Many males with X-linked Alport syndrome will develop progressive sensorineural hearing loss beginning after age 10. Additionally, males with X-linked Alport syndrome may have an abnormality in the shape of the lens called anterior lenticonus. Females with X-linked Alport syndrome may also have kidney problems and deafness, but females are expected to have a later onset and less rapid progression of these problems.

Mitochondrial hearing loss

While most genetic data is carried on the chromosomes in the nucleus of the cell, there is also a tiny amount of **DNA** in the mitochondria of cells. The method of inheritance of mitochondrial abnormalities is nearly exclusively maternal (through the mother). The mitochondria that develop in a human are almost all produced by replication of the maternal mitochondria from the egg, or ovum. The sperm contains almost no mitochondria. The percentage of hereditary hearing loss due to abnormalities in mitochondrial DNA is estimated to be around 1%. Hearing loss due to mitochondrial inheritance shows highly variable penetrance and may be either syndromic or nonsyndromic.

Nonsyndromic mitochondrial hearing loss is associated with mutations in either the mitochondrial MTRNR1 gene or the mitochondrial MTTS1 gene. Nonsyndromic mitochondrial hearing loss varies from moderate to profound. One specific mutation in MTRNR1 has been reported in families with nonsyndromic hearing loss and in families with hearing loss induced by exposure to a certain class of antibiotics, the aminoglycosides. If persons with this specific MTRNR1 mutation do not have exposure to an aminoglycoside antibiotic, then they show hearing loss with a median age at onset of 20 years. If persons with this specific mutation are exposed to this class of antibiotics, then they develop hearing loss within a few days to weeks of taking the medication. Persons with hearing loss due to MTTS1

mutations often present with hearing loss beginning in childhood.

Syndromic mitochondrial hearing loss is more common than nonsyndromic mitochondrial hearing loss due to the function of the mitochondria themselves. Because the mitochondria are responsible for energy production, faulty mitochondria result in decreased energy production. This lower level of energy production greatly affects the parts of the body that use most energy, including the brain, heart, and muscles. Therefore people with mitochondrial disorders will generally show a spectrum of physical symptoms, including nervous system problems, visual problems, hearing loss, and muscle weakness. MELAS, MERRF, and Kearns-Sayre syndromes all represent mitochondrial syndromes that include hearing loss.

Demographics

Hearing loss is estimated to affect two to three out of 1,000 babies born in the United States. The incidence of hearing loss increases with age. Approximately 17 out of 1,000 children under age 18 have hearing loss. Of people who are over 65 years old, the incidence of hearing loss is approximately 314 per 1,000. Of people who are 75 years old or older, 40–50% have hearing loss.

Approximately 85–90% of deaf individuals marry another deaf person. Ninety percent of deaf couples have children with normal hearing and 90–95% of deaf children have parents with normal hearing. In general, if a hearing couple has a child with profound childhood deafness of unknown cause, then their risk in each future pregnancy to have another child with hearing loss is approximately one in six.

It is estimated that approximately 10% of the population of the United States has partial hearing loss or deafness. This number is higher worldwide because many nongenetic causes of hearing loss are more prevalent outside of the United States. These nongenetic causes of hearing impairment or loss include rubella, premature birth, meningitis, and incompatibility in the Rh blood factor between mother and fetus.

From studies of pupils at schools for the deaf in the United States, it is estimated that approximately 50% of childhood hearing impairment is genetically based. Another 20–25% of cases are attributed to environmental factors. The remaining 25–30% of cases are classified as of unknown cause.

Otosclerosis is estimated to affect between 10% and 18% of all white and Hispanic women, and between 7% and 9% of all white and Hispanic men. People of Asian descent are affected with otosclerosis at about half the rate seen in whites and Hispanics, with the same observed sex differences. In blacks, only about 1% of the total population is affected with otosclerosis, with minimal differences between males and females. Otosclerosis is exceedingly rare in people of Native American descent.

Signs and symptoms

Syndromic types of hearing loss are generally characterized by the findings and symptoms additional to hearing loss that are associated with the particular syndrome.

Otosclerosis is characterized by an initial loss of hearing in the low frequencies, followed by a loss of the high frequencies, then a loss of the middle frequencies. It may rapidly advance through these stages in some affected individuals, while in other people it may stabilize for a period of years before progressively worsening. Many affected individuals have symptoms only in one ear at first, but otosclerosis almost inevitably will affect both ears. The maximum hearing loss due to otosclerosis without involvement of the auditory nerve is in the moderate range. As an affected person ages and the auditory nerve becomes involved, the hearing loss may progress to severe, or even profound, when this person reaches their 60s and 70s.

There are four main categories of DPHL: early onset, high frequency, mid frequency, and low frequency. Early-onset types of DPHL tend to occur in early childhood and progress at varying rates to deafness. The other three types are categorized by the frequency range in which hearing loss first occurs.

Diagnosis

Hearing is generally tested using earphones. Sounds are sent into the earphones at various decibel and frequency levels. This test allows the observer to determine the amount of hearing loss in decibels and the range of hearing loss in hertz. Since hearing loss is not necessarily the same in both ears, each ear is tested independently. If a hearing loss is found using this simple test, another test is then performed to determine whether the hearing loss is of the conductive or sensorineural type. A device called a bone vibrator is used in place of the earphones. The bone vibrator sends auditory signals through the bones of the ear, bypassing the ear canal and the ossicles of the middle ear. In the case of conductive hearing loss, the affected individual will be able to hear sounds at a lower decibel level using the bone vibrator than using the earphones. In the case of sensorineural hearing loss, the affected individual will generally hear sounds through the bone vibrator at the same decibel level as using the earphones.

Hearing loss is categorized by determining the hearing threshold of the affected person. The hearing threshold is the amount of sound that that individual can just barely hear. The hearing threshold of an individual is the hearing level (HL) of that person. It is measured in decibels (dB). A person with up to a 25 dB HL is categorized as having normal hearing. Mild hearing loss is defined as an HL in the 26–45 dB range. Moderate hearing loss is defined as an HL in the 46–65 dB range. Severe hearing loss is defined as an HL in the 66–85 dB range. Profound hearing loss is defined as an HL greater than 85 dB. The average person speaking English in a conversational tone tends to speak in the 30–60 dB range, depending on the particular sounds being made. Persons with mild hearing loss will generally be able to hear and understand one-on-one conversations if they are close to the speaker. These individuals may have difficulty hearing a speaker who is far away, has a soft voice, or is surrounded by background noise. Persons with moderate hearing loss may have problems hearing conversational speech, even at relatively close range and in the absence of background noises. Persons with severe hearing loss have difficulty hearing in all situations. These people are not usually able to hear speech unless the speaker is talking loudly and is at relatively close range. Persons with profound hearing loss may not hear loud speech or environmental sounds. These people are unlikely to use hearing and speech as primary means of communication.

Hearing loss is also measured in terms of the frequency of the sounds that can or cannot be heard. Frequency is measured in hertz (Hz). The normal hearing range for humans is from approximately 100–8,000 Hz. The normal frequency of the sounds of the English language falls between approximately 240 Hz and 7,500 Hz. In individuals with progressive conductive hearing loss, it is generally the highest frequency range or the lowest frequency range that is lost first; the middle frequency range is generally lost last. In individuals affected with progressive sensorineural hearing loss, it may be any of the three frequency ranges that is lost first. Hearing loss is generally plotted on a graph called an audiogram. This is a graph of frequency (in Hz) versus HL (in dB).

Syndromic hereditary hearing loss is differentially diagnosed by the presence of the nonhearing loss symptoms that the person also possesses. Nonsyndromic hereditary hearing loss is differentially diagnosed from syndromic by the absence of such other symptoms. Types of nonsyndromic hereditary hearing loss are differentially diagnosed by the age of onset of the symptoms; the progressiveness, or nonprogressiveness, of the hearing loss; the degree of symmetry of the hearing loss from one ear to the other; and the type of hearing loss: conductive, sensorineural, or mixed. Occasionally, a

KEY TERMS

Audiogram—A graph of hearing level versus frequency.

Auditory nerve—The nerve responsible for transmitting electrical impulses created within the ear in response to sounds to the brain.

Conductive hearing loss—Hearing loss that is the result of a dysfunction of the parts of the ear responsible for collecting sound. In this type of hearing loss, the auditory nerve is generally not damaged.

Dominant progressive hearing loss—The main type of nonsyndromic progressive sensorineural hearing loss seen in humans.

Hearing threshold—The minimum sound level at which a particular individual can hear; also called the hearing level (HL) of that person.

Mitochondria—Organelles within the cell responsible for energy production.

Mixed-type hearing loss—Hearing loss that involves both conductive and sensorineural losses.

Nonsyndromic hearing loss—Hearing loss that is not accompanied by other symptoms characteristic of a larger genetic syndrome.

Ossicles—Any of the three bones of the middle ear, including the malleus, incus, and stapes.

Otosclerosis—The main type of nonsyndromic progressive conductive hearing loss seen in humans. In very advanced cases, otosclerosis can become of mixed type.

Pedigree analysis—Analysis of a family tree, or pedigree, in an attempt to identify the possible inheritance pattern of a trait seen in this family.

Sensorineural hearing loss (SNHL)—Hearing loss that occurs when parts of the inner ear, such as the cochlea and/or auditory nerve, do not work correctly. It is often defined as mild, moderate, severe, or profound, depending upon how much sound can be heard by the affected individual.

Syndromic hearing loss—Hearing loss accompanied by other symptoms that characterize a larger genetic syndrome of which hearing loss is just one of the characteristics.

Vestibular nerve—The nerve that transmits the electrical signals collected in the inner ear to the brain. These signals, and the responses to them, help maintain balance.

differential diagnosis also includes the inheritance pattern of the nonsyndromic hearing loss. This inheritance pattern is generally determined by obtaining family medical history information on the affected person's family. Tests looking for specific gene changes in specific genes for certain nonsyndromic hearing losses, including prenatal testing, are also beginning to become more available.

Treatment and management

Certain types of conductive hearing loss can be treated by surgery to correct the dysfunctional portion of the ear. Sensorineural hearing loss is generally not able to be repaired by surgery.

Most people with partial hearing loss can benefit from the use of hearing aids and/or sign language. Sign language and writing are often the primary forms of communication used by people suffering from severe, profound, or complete hearing loss.

Prognosis

The prognosis for individuals affected with hereditary hearing loss is largely dependent on the type of hearing loss experienced. In the absence of nonhearing loss-related symptoms, the loss of hearing does not generally present any increased risk of illness and death. Hearing aids and/or the use of sign language can often improve the quality of life of those affected with a hereditary hearing loss.

Resources

BOOKS

Toriello, Helga V., William Reardon, and Robert J. Gorlin, eds. *Hereditary Hearing Loss and Its Syndromes, 2nd ed.* Oxford: Oxford University Press, 2004.

ORGANIZATIONS

American Society for Deaf Children. PO Box 3355 Gettysburg, PA 17325. (800) 942-2732 (parent hotline); (717) 334-7922 (business V/TTY). Fax: (717) 334-8808. Email: asdc@deafchildren.org. (April 4, 2005.) <http://www.deafchildren.org>.

Laurent Clerc National Deaf Education Center at Gallaudet University. 800 Florida Ave. NE, Washington, DC 20002. (April 4, 2005.) <http://clerccenter.gallaudet.edu/>.

League for the Hard of Hearing. 50 Broadway, 6th Floor, New York, NY 10004. Voice: (917) 305-7700. Fax: (917) 305-7888. TTY: (917) 305-7999. (April 4, 2005.) <http://www.lhh.org/index.htm>.

National Association of the Deaf. 814 Thayer, Suite 250, Silver Spring, MD 20910-4500. Voice: (301) 587-1788. TTY: (301) 587-1789. Fax: (301) 587-1791. Email: nadinfo@nad.org. (April 4, 2005.) <http://www.nad.org>.

WEBSITES

"Deafness and Hereditary Hearing Loss Overview." *Gene Reviews*. (April 4, 2005.) <http://www.genereviews.org//profiles/deafnes s-overview/>.

"Hearing, Ear Infections, and Deafness." *National Institute on Deafness and other Communication Disorders*. (April 4, 2005.) <http://www.nidcd.nih.gov/health/hearing/>.

Hereditary Hearing Loss Homepage. (April 4, 2005.) <http://webhost.ua.ac.be/hhh/>.

National Center for Biotechnology Information. (April 4, 2005.) <http://www.ncbi.nlm.nih.gov/>.

Paul A. Johnson
Judy C. Hawkins, MS, CGC

Hereditary hemorrhagic telangiectasia (HHT) *see* Osler-Weber-Rendu syndrome

Hereditary iron-loading anemia *see* Anemia, sideroblastic X-linked

Hereditary multiple exostoses

Definition

Hereditary multiple exostoses (HME) refers to a group of disorders characterized by abnormal bone growth. The major symptom is the development of nodules (bumps) on various bones of the body. Exostoses may produce pain and other complications by pressing on nearby tissue, they may limit movement of joints, and in some cases they must be surgically removed.

Description

An exostosis is a benign (non-cancerous) bony growth. This does not refer to a normally shaped bone that has simply grown larger than normal. Rather, an exostosis is a bump, or nodule, on a bone, usually with overlying cartilage. That is why HME is sometimes referred to as the "bumpy bones" disease. Other names for the disorder include multiple hereditary exostoses (MHE), multiple cartilaginous exostoses, osteochondromatosis, and diaphyseal aclasis.

People with HME typically develop anywhere from several to many exostoses during their life, mostly during childhood and adolescence. Exostoses vary in size, and can develop on most bones in the body. An exostosis may present no problem, or it may cause pain and other complications by pressing on nearby soft tissue (nerves, blood vessels, tendons, internal organs), or on another bone at a joint. Exostoses that do cause problems are often surgically removed. HME can cause differences in the shape of bones, or reduce their growth rate. Thus, people with HME tend to be somewhat shorter than average and may have limited movement in certain joints. People with HME are not at risk for tumor development in other tissues.

HME is an autosomal dominant condition, and most people with the disorder have family members who are affected. A small percentage of people who carry an HME **gene** do not develop any recognizable exostoses. The vast majority of exostoses are benign growths, but a small percentage can become malignant (cancerous).

Genetic profile

Three different types of HME are known to exist—HME type I, HME type II, and HME type III. There appear to be no obvious differences in the presentation and course of the disorder between the three types. Instead, the designations correspond to the three genes—EXT1, EXT2, and EXT3 respectively—that have been linked to HME. The protein produced by the EXT1 gene on **chromosome** number 8 is called exostosin-1, and the EXT2 gene on chromosome number 11 produces exostosin-2. The EXT3 gene is located on chromosome number 19, but its protein product had not been identified.

As noted, HME is an autosomal dominant condition, which means any person who carries an HME gene has a 50% chance of passing it on each time they have a child. Ninety percent of people with HME have a positive family history. In the other 10% of cases, HME occurred in that person for the first time as the result of a new mutation in one of the EXT genes. Regardless of whether someone inherits HME from a parent or it occurs in them for the first time, each of their children is still at 50% risk.

A tumor is the result of cells that undergo uncontrolled replication/division. People often equate the word "tumor" with **cancer**. However, a tumor is simply a growth, and may be malignant (cancerous) or benign (non-cancerous). Technically exostoses are tumors, but they are nearly always benign.

EXT1 and EXT2 belong to a class of genes known as tumor suppressors. In normal circumstances, tumor suppressor genes prevent cells either from replicating at all, or from replicating too quickly. If both copies of a tumor suppressor gene are mutated (inactivated), control of cell replication/division is lost. A person who inherits HME type I or HME type II already has one EXT1 or EXT2 gene inactivated from the moment they are conceived. However, abnormal bone growth does not occur unless the other gene of the pair also becomes inactivated.

This second gene mutation, called loss of heterozygosity (LOH), appears to be an unlikely, random event, which explains why there is not abnormal growth throughout all of the bones. Only the occasional bone cell that undergoes LOH has a chance of becoming an exostosis. Any person without HME can develop a single exostosis, and 2% of all people do. It is simply that exostosis development is much less likely when two random mutations of an EXT gene in a bone cell must occur, rather than just one.

Demographics

The prevalence of HME is estimated at about one in 75,000. There does not appear to be any significant difference in prevalence between the major ethnic groups. Most studies have found that males with an HME gene tend to have more obvious and severe symptoms than females. The reason for this is unknown. This makes it appear as though males are more likely to inherit HME, when in fact they are just more likely to be diagnosed.

Most people with HME have either HME type I or HME type II. Apparently only a small percentage of HME cases are linked to the EXT3 gene. Further study of the HME genes should establish an accurate prevalence for each type.

Signs and symptoms

About half of all people with HME are diagnosed by the time they are three years old. Only 5% of newborns that carry an HME gene show some signs at birth, but 95% of all people with the condition show noticeable signs by the time they are 12 years of age.

Exostoses primarily develop during the period of rapid bone growth—from infancy through late adolescence. As noted, however, a small percentage of newborns already have noticeable exostoses at birth, and rare individuals with HME may develop exostoses as adults. The number of exostoses varies from person to person, even within families. However, the average affected person develops six exostoses during his or her life.

Both the locations and sizes of exostoses vary. The most commonly affected bones are those of the arms (humerus, radius, and ulna), legs (femur, tibia, and fibula), hands (carpals and metacarpals), and feet (tarsals and metatarsals). Exostoses on the arm or leg nearly always develop near the joints (elbow, wrist, knee, or ankle), rather than in the middle of the long bones. About 70% of people with HME have an exostosis or bone deformity around the knee. Flat bones, such as the scapula (shoulder blade) and pelvis, may be affected. The ribs and bones of the shoulder girdle occasionally develop growths, but exostoses are hardly ever seen on the spine or bones of the skull. Some exostoses under the skin may be barely noticeable to the touch (less than 1 cm in height), while others produce a noticeable bump (1-2 cm in height). Growths on the flat bones may be somewhat larger.

The most common problem in HME is exostoses that cause compression and irritation of adjacent soft tissue, such as skin, nerves, and blood vessels. These types of growths can cause chronic pain until they are removed, and accidentally hitting them against something solid can be especially painful. Exostoses that grow near the ends of long bones may interfere with normal movement of a joint. Many children with HME have difficulties with their knees, both in range-of-motion and with angular deformities ("knock-kneed"). An uncommon, but more complicated problem is a large exostosis on the inside of the pelvis that results in compression of the intestine or urinary tract.

HME affects the growth centers of bones (metaphyses and epiphyses), which can result in abnormal modeling (structure) of the affected bones. Reduction in size and bowing of bones are the most frequent structural anomalies seen. Consequently, people with HME tend to be somewhat shorter than average—final height in men averages 170 cm (66 in), while the average height in women is 160 cm (62 in). Differential rates of growth between a child's legs or arms can result in leg- or arm-length discrepancy, sometimes reaching 2 cm (1 in) or more. Leg-length discrepancy can result in hip pain and problems with walking caused by tilting of the pelvis.

The most serious complication in HME is the progression of a benign exostosis to a malignant (cancerous) state, known as a **chondrosarcoma**. This happens in slightly less than 1% of all people with the condition. Chondrosarcomas can develop in children, but those few cases that do occur are usually in adults. An undetected bone malignancy always presents a risk for metastasis—spreading of cancerous cells elsewhere in the body—which is one of the most dangerous complications of any cancer. Most chondrosarcomas should be detected and treated early, however, because they are usually associated with rapid growth of an exostosis accompanied by pain.

Diagnosis

The diagnosis of HME is usually made when noticeable exostoses first appear. Any person who is at risk for the condition because of a family history is more likely to be accurately diagnosed at a younger age. As noted, the occurrence of a single exostosis in an otherwise healthy person is not rare. Therefore, two or more exostoses must be present in order to make the diagnosis of HME (although a single exostosis detected in someone who is known to be at 50% risk for HME is highly suggestive of the diagnosis).

Exostoses are not always detectable by physical examination. Consequently, an x-ray study of the commonly affected bones (skeletal survey) in questionable cases is the best method of confirming or excluding the diagnosis. This is especially true in cases where a child is known to be at risk for HME (positive family history).

Unlike some **genetic disorders** where many people with the condition have the same gene mutation, most individuals/families with HME tested so far have had different mutations in either EXT1 or EXT2. Therefore, while predictive or confirmatory **genetic testing** might be possible within a family (assuming the gene mutation is detectable), direct testing of EXT1/EXT2 in a person with a negative or uncertain family history is not yet reliable enough to use as a diagnostic tool.

Treatment and management

The only treatment for exostoses that present problems is to remove them surgically. In those instances where the exostosis is easily accessible, surgical removal is straightforward and carries very little risk. On the other hand, an exostosis that involves one of the joints or is less accessible—somewhere on the inner surface of the pelvis, for instance—may require involved surgery. A few people with HME will never require surgical intervention, but most have at least one surgery and some will have many. A child who is noted to have uneven or accelerated growth of a long bone in the arm or leg may be offered a procedure to straighten the bone or reduce its growth rate.

No external factors are known to cause or prevent the growth of exostoses. Those persons diagnosed with HME, as well as children at risk, must be taught to monitor themselves for unusual changes in bone growth.

Anyone with HME should have lifelong, periodic examinations by an orthopedic surgeon to look for and address any problematic exostoses, and to screen for chondrosarcoma. Since exostoses and other bone-growth problems occur primarily in childhood, special attention, care, and education about their disorder is often needed for children with HME. A support group especially for children, called MHE and Me, has special materials and a Web site devoted to issues of particular importance to kids (see Resources below).

Prognosis

The majority of people with HME lead active lives, and their life span is not reduced. Surgery to remove problematic exostoses will likely remain the primary

---

KEY TERMS

Chondrosarcoma—A malignant tumor derived from cartilage cells.

Diaphysis—The middle portion, or shaft, of a long bone.

Epiphysis—The end of long bones, usually terminating in a joint.

Exostosis—An abnormal growth (benign tumor) on a bone.

Metaphysis—An area of softer bone and cartilage in long bones between the diaphysis (shaft) and epiphysis (end).

Osteochondromatosis—Another name for hereditary multiple exostoses, meaning a growth of bone and cartilage.

---

method of treatment for some time. The hope is that further analysis of the EXT genes and their protein products will lead at some point to a more targeted approach at reducing or eliminating abnormal bone growths altogether.

Resources

ORGANIZATIONS

MHE and Me—A Support Group for Kids with Multiple Hereditary Exostoses. 14 Stony Brook Dr., Pine Island, NY 10969. (914) 258-6058. <http://www.geocities.com/mheandme>.

Multiple Hereditary Exostoses Coalition. 8838 Holly Lane, Olmstead Falls, OH 44138. (440) 235-6325. <http://www.radix.net/~hogue/mhe.htm>.

Multiple Hereditary Exostoses Family Support Group. 5316 Winter Moss Court, Columbia, MD 21045. (410) 922-5898. <http://www.radix.net/~hogue/mhe.htm>.

Scott J. Polzin, MS

Hereditary nonspherocytic anemia *see*
Pyruvate kinase deficiency

Hereditary pancreatitis

Definition

Hereditary pancreatitis is a rare genetic condition beginning in childhood that is characterized by recurrent episodes of inflammation of the pancreas, causing intense abdominal pain, nausea and vomiting. Most episodes resolve on their own, but serious complications can arise, ranging from **diabetes** and poor digestion, to bleeding, infection, **pancreatic cancer** and death. Medical treatment can help alleviate some of the symptoms, and occasionally surgery may be needed to treat some of the complications.

Description

The pancreas is an organ located in the abdomen that has several functions. First, the pancreas aids in the digestion of food through the production of digestive enzymes. Digestive enzymes are proteins that break down food components, including sugars, fats, and other proteins, so that they can be absorbed and used by the body. Normally, the digestive enzymes are stored within the pancreas in an inactive form. In response to food intake, the enzymes are released from the pancreas and travel through the pancreatic duct into the small intestine where they become activated and begin to digest food.

The second function of the pancreas is to maintain proper sugar balance in the blood. The pancreas produces several hormones, including insulin and glucagon, that are secreted into the bloodstream and act to increase or decrease sugar levels within the blood.

Pancreatitis is a condition in which the pancreas becomes irritated and inflamed. In most cases, the condition is caused by excessive alcohol use, or by the presence of gallstones, but can also be caused by medications, viral infections, injury to the abdomen, abnormal structures of the pancreas, and several metabolic disorders. In some rare instances, pancreatitis is caused by a genetic abnormality that is passed down from parent to child and is called hereditary pancreatitis.

In hereditary pancreatitis, an individual inherits a genetic abnormality in one of the digestive enzymes produced by the pancreas, called trypsin. Normally, trypsin is stored within the pancreas in an inactive state, and only becomes activated when it travels to the small intestine and encounters food to digest. However, in individuals with hereditary pancreatitis, the trypsin becomes activated while still in the pancreas and begins to digest the pancreas itself, causing irritation and inflammation. Damage to the blood vessels in the pancreas can result in bleeding or fluid leaks from the blood vessel into the abdominal cavity. The digestive enzymes also gain access to the bloodstream through the damaged blood vessels, and begin circulating throughout the body, causing further damage.

It is unclear what causes the abnormal trypsin enzyme to become activated and begin digesting the pancreas, but some studies have shown that emotional stress, alcohol, or fatty foods may trigger the process. After time, recurrent episodes of pancreatitis may leave the pancreas permanently irritated and damaged, a condition called chronic pancreatitis.

Genetic profile

Hereditary pancreatitis is a genetic disease and can be inherited or passed on in a family. The genetic abnormality for the disorder is inherited as an autosomal dominant trait, meaning that only one abnormal **gene** is needed to inherit the disease, and that a parent with the disease has a 50% chance of transmitting the abnormal gene and disease to a child.

Changes in the gene for the digestive enzyme trypsin (located on human **chromosome** 7, at 7q35) are responsible for the disease, and more than five different genetic changes in the trypsin gene have been identified. Changes in other genes may also cause hereditary pancreatitis, as recent studies have discovered families with this condition with mutations in other genes, possibly on chromosome 12.

Demographics

The annual incidence of all forms of pancreatitis is about one per 10,000 people. However, hereditary pancreatitis is a rare cause of all pancreatitis and comprises only about 2% of the total cases. While the true prevalence of the condition is difficult to measure, it is estimated that at least 1,000 individuals in the United States are affected by hereditary pancreatitis.

Approximately 100 different families with hereditary pancreatitis have been identified since the condition was first recognized in 1952. The largest concentration of hereditary pancreatitis in the United States is in the central Appalachian region, which extends from southern Ohio to eastern Kentucky and Tennessee, western Virginia and North Carolina, and into northern Georgia.

Signs and symptoms

Hereditary pancreatitis begins with recurrent episodes of pancreatitis during childhood. The age of the first episode of pancreatitis may range from infancy to over 30 years old, but 80% of patients will show the first episode of pancreatitis before 20 years old, and the average individual shows a first episode at approximately 10 to 12 years old.

People who are experiencing an episode of pancreatitis have severe abdominal pain, nausea and vomiting that is greatly worsened by eating. The pain is often described as steady and dull pain that is centered on the

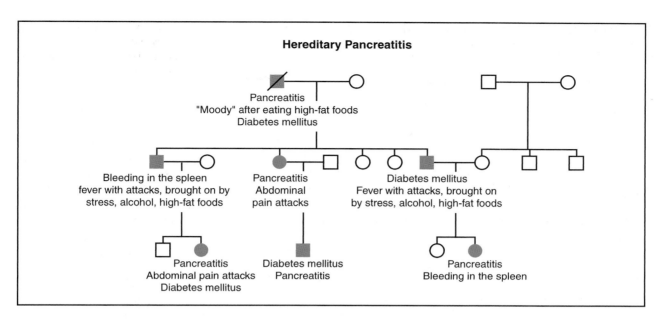

Hereditary Pancreatitis

(Gale Group)

navel and may extend to the back. As a result of fluids that leak from the pancreas and surrounding vessels into the abdomen, the abdomen may swell.

The severity and duration of each episode may range from only occasional abdominal discomfort to prolonged, life-threatening attacks that appear to last for weeks. The number of attacks is also quite variable. For example, severe attacks may occur three or four times in a year followed by a year without attacks.

Most episodes of pancreatitis resolve without problems. However, certain complications can arise which may worsen the condition and threaten the life of the patient. Because of the loss of large amounts of fluid into the abdomen, circulatory shock may occur. Shock occurs when fluid leaks from blood vessels, leaving an insufficient amount of blood volume to provide the body with the oxygen that it needs. Prolonged lack of appropriate levels of oxygen causes damage to many different organs of the body. If not immediately treated, shock can lead to death.

Another complication of pancreatitis is the development of a fluid collection that contains decaying products of an inflamed pancreas and other substances. This fluid collection is called a pseudocyst. A pseudocyst can become life threatening if it becomes infected (abscess) or if the fluid collection ruptures into the abdomen.

Other dangerous and life-threatening complications of pancreatitis include severe bleeding from the pancreas (hemorrhagic pancreatitis), higher risk for the formation of blood clots, and a higher risk of serious infections in the abdomen or damaged pancreas. In addition, people

with hereditary pancreatitis have a much higher risk of developing pancreatic **cancer**, for reasons that are not clear. Studies indicate that people with hereditary pancreatitis are at least 53 times more likely to develop pancreatic cancer than the general population and that 40-75% of people with hereditary pancreatitis will develop pancreatic cancer by the age of 70. Pancreatic cancer is very difficult to treat and is nearly always fatal.

Over time, recurrent episodes of pancreatitis may leave the pancreas permanently damaged and unable to carry out its routine functions. The absence of digestive enzymes normally secreted by the pancreas results in poor digestion, chronic diarrhea, weight loss, and malnutrition (5-45% of people), leaving a person generally weakened. The pancreas may also become unable to secrete insulin in the bloodstream normally, creating imbalances in blood sugar and causing diabetes in 10-25% of people with hereditary pancreatitis.

Diagnosis

Hereditary pancreatitis is diagnosed through a combination of medical history, physical examination, and laboratory testing. The onset of abdominal pain consistent with pancreatitis before the age of 20 in multiple family members without any other risk factor for pancreatitis (drinking large amounts of alcoholic beverages; gallstones) suggests a diagnosis of hereditary pancreatitis. The medical history and physical examination of these individuals during an episode of pancreatitis will show abdominal pain, nausea, vomiting, and abdominal swelling.

KEY TERMS

Abscess—A localized collection of pus or infection that is walled off from the rest of the body.

Amylase—A digestive enzyme found in saliva or pancreatic fluid that breaks down starch and sugars.

Autosomal dominant—A pattern of genetic inheritance where only one abnormal gene is needed to display the trait or disease.

Computed tomography (CT) scan—An imaging procedure that produces a three-dimensional picture of organs or structures inside the body, such as the brain.

Diabetes—An inability to control the levels of sugar in the blood due to an abnormality in the production of, or response to, the hormone insulin.

Digestive enzyme—Proteins secreted by the pancreas that enter the small intestine and break down food so it can be absorbed by the body.

Gastroenterologist—A physician who specializes in disorders of the digestive system.

Hormone—A chemical messenger produced by the body that is involved in regulating specific bodily functions such as growth, development, and reproduction.

Insulin—A hormone produced by the pancreas that is secreted into the bloodstream and regulates blood sugar levels.

Intravenous—A route for administration of fluids, nutrients, blood products, or medications. A small flexible plastic tube is inserted into a vein by way of a needle to establish this route.

Lipase—A digestive enzyme found in pancreatic fluid that breaks down fats.

Nasogastric tube—A long flexible tube inserted through the nasal passageways, down the throat, and into the stomach. Used to drain the contents of the stomach.

Pancreas—An organ located in the abdomen that secretes pancreatic juices for digestion and hormones for maintaining blood sugar levels.

Pseudocyst—A fluid-filled space that may arise in the setting of pancreatitis.

Ranson criteria—A system of measurements, including age and blood testing, that can be used to predict the outcome of a person who has been hospitalized for an episode of pancreatitis.

Shock—An inability to provide the body with the oxygen it requires, sometimes due to large amounts of bleeding or fluid loss.

Trypsin—A digestive enzyme found in pancreatic fluid that breaks down proteins. This enzyme is abnormal in hereditary pancreatitis.

Diagnosis of pancreatitis can be made by noting high levels of pancreatic enzymes (amylase and lipase) circulating in the blood. Further abnormalities in the blood that suggest pancreatitis include: increased white blood cells, changes in the blood substances that occur with dehydration and fluid loss, and decreases in calcium levels.

Other diagnostic methods can be used to track the progress of the disease and monitor for any complications. X rays of the abdomen may show deposits of calcium that occur in 50% of cases of hereditary pancreatitis. Also, the intestines may show signs of inactivity because of the nearby inflammation. Computed tomography scans (CT scans) of the abdomen may reveal the inflammation of the pancreatitis, and are very useful in monitoring for complications such as pseudocyst, infections, and bleeding.

Genetic testing allows for the definitive diagnosis of hereditary pancreatitis by identifying abnormalities in the trypsin gene. However, these tests are currently used only for research purposes and are not generally available.

Treatment and management

There is no cure for hereditary pancreatitis. The goals for treatment consist of pain control, establishing alternate routes of feeding and fluid administration, and prevention or control of complications.

A person experiencing an episode of pancreatitis is nearly always admitted to the hospital for treatment. Since drinking or eating by mouth often worsens the patient's condition, alternative routes are needed. Large amounts of fluid are given by a small tube placed in a vein (intravenous or IV fluids) to replace the fluid that has leaked into the abdomen. This IV route can also be used to administer nutritional products and medications to relieve pain.

Fluids and acid that are produced by the stomach can worsen a patient's condition and increase pain. In order to drain these fluids, a small, flexible tube is inserted through the nose, down the throat and into the stomach (nasogastric tube). The tube is then connected to a weak vacuum to remove the contents of the stomach.

Complications may arise in the setting of pancreatitis. Bleeding may require administration of donor blood products by vein, while infections are treated using antibiotics also given by vein. Abscesses, large pseudocysts or decaying portions of the pancreas may require drainage with a needle or need to be removed surgically. People with a permanently damaged pancreas may require digestive enzyme supplements by mouth to assist with digestion and insulin injections to control diabetes.

People diagnosed with hereditary pancreatitis should be seen regularly by a team of health care professionals, including a primary-care physician, gastroenterologist, and medical geneticist. Individuals with this condition should refrain from drinking alcohol and avoid fatty foods and may benefit from consultation with a licensed nutritionist.

Prognosis

Several systems have been developed to predict the outcome for people who are experiencing an episode of pancreatitis. The most widely used system utilized by health professionals is called "Ranson criteria," which utilizes a list of measurements that are determined during the first two days of the hospital stay.

In general, children who experience an episode of pancreatitis do well and are released from the hospital in three to five days. However, the development of any of the complications of pancreatitis discussed above worsens the prognosis and will likely result in a longer hospital stay. In the extreme, severe complications of pancreatitis can even lead to death.

Most people with hereditary pancreatitis will develop permanent damage to the pancreas as they grow older. Half of people will require surgery, and up to one-fourth will develop diabetes by the age of 70. Of even greater concern, a significant percentage will develop pancreatic cancer, a diagnosis that is nearly always fatal within several years.

Resources

BOOKS

Lankisch, P. G., and P. A. Banks. *Pancreatitis*. Garden City Park, New York: Springer Verlag, 1998.

PERIODICALS

Pietzak, M. M., and D. W. Thomas. "Pancreatitis in childhood." *Pediatric Review* 21 (December 2000): 406-412.

Whitcomb, D. C. "New insights into hereditary pancreatitis." *Current Gastroenterology* 1 (April 1999): 154-160.

ORGANIZATIONS

Pancreatitis Patients' Support Group. PO Box 164, Rochdale, Lancashire, OL11 5GY, United Kingdom. <http://www.zen.co.uk/home/page/ppsg/>.

Pancreatitis Support Network. <http://hometown.aol.com/karynwms/myhomepage/business.html>.

WEBSITES

Applebaum, Suzanne. "Pancreas.org—Information on Pancreatitis and Hereditary Pancreatitis." <http://www.pitt.edu/~sapple/>.

"Hereditary Pancreatitis." National Center for Biotechnology Information. *Online Mendelian Inheritance in Man*. <http://www3.ncbi.nlm.nih.gov/htbin-post/Omim>.

"Pancreatitis." *HealthCyclopedia*. <http://www.healthcyclopedia.com/pancreatitis.html>.

Oren Traub, MD, PhD

Hereditary spastic paraplegia

Definition

Hereditary spastic paraplegia (HSP) is not a single entity, but a group of clinically and genetically diverse hereditary degenerative disorders that have in common degeneration of the corticospinal tracts and posterior column tracts in the spinal cord. The corticospinal tracts are made of nerve fibers that convey motor information from the brain to the limbs. The posterior column carries sensory information regarding position sense from the arms and legs to the brain. The fibers that carry motor information to the legs are more often affected than those of the arms, resulting in progressive stiffness and weakness of leg, thigh, calf, and lumbar spinal muscles. The age of onset, extent of degeneration, and severity of symptoms varies among the affected people, even those among the same family. Some families show a pattern of disease called anticipation, with symptoms developing earlier in each new generation. In most individuals, however, the disease onset occurs between the second and the fourth decades of life.

Description

Dr. Adolf von Strumpell described this disease in 1883. Other names of this disorder are hereditary spastic paraparesis, Strumpell-Lorrain syndrome, Strumpell disease, familial spastic paraparesis, spastic spinal familial paralysis, hereditary Charcot disease, silver syndrome, French settlement disease, and Troyer syndrome. When the only manifested symptom is progressive spasticity, HSP is also known as pure hereditary spastic paraplegia.

Genetic profile

There are at least 20 different types of HSP, and the mode of **inheritance** is known for 11 of them. The risk of an individual inheriting the abnormal **gene** depends on the mode of transmission and whether the mutated gene is present on a sex **chromosome** or an autosome. Mutations in several different genes can result in a similar **phenotype** of HSP and this phenomenon is known as genetic heterogeneity. These genes are generically known as spastic paraplegia gene, or SPG. SPGs are thought to contain genetic information regarding proteins that help in microtubule formation and function. Microtubules form the protein framework of a nerve cell and their dysfunction leads to degeneration of the nerve cells. HSP can be complicated when other neurological impairments are seen in addition to spasticity, or can be uncomplicated. Uncomplicated HSP is inherited as an autosomal dominant mutation in about 70% of cases, but the mutated gene varies from one family to another. Three patterns of inheritance are known for HSP: autosomal dominant HSP, autosomal recessive HSP, and X-linked HSP.

Autosomal dominant HSP

This is the most common form of HSP and the mutated gene is present on an autosome (non-sex chromosome). Only one copy of the abnormal gene is required to produce the disease. There is a 50% chance that an affected person will transmit the gene to an offspring. The disease can be present in both males and females, it can be transmitted from either the mother or the father to a son or a daughter, and there is usually an affected family member in each generation. Exceptions to the latter rule are when the disease has been very mild in earlier generations and has been misdiagnosed as arthritis or walking difficulty due to old age. Also, the person might have been deceased prior to manifesting full-blown symptoms. The SPGs for autosomal dominant HSP are identified in chromosomes 2p, 8q, 12q, 14q, 15q, 19q, and 20. In more than 50% of cases, the two most common **gene mutations** identified are in chromosome 2p and are called spastin and atlastin. In complicated autosomal dominant HSP, the gene is on chromosome 10q. In a rarer form of infantile onset-ascending HSP, there is a deletion mutation in the alsin gene at 2q.

Autosomal recessive HSP

In autosomal recessive HSP, the mutant gene is present on an autosome and two copies of the abnormal gene (one of maternal and one of paternal inheritance) are required for disease expression. Both males and females can express the disease and also transmit the abnormal gene. A mutant HSP gene that is recessive can be passed down silently for generations until someone finally inherits the recessive gene from both parents and develops the disorder. The parents of the affected person

are called carriers, as they carry only one copy of the abnormal gene and do not express the disease. If a mother and father are each carriers for a recessive HSP gene mutation, each of their children has a 25% chance of developing HSP, a 50% chance of being a carrier, and a 25% chance of being normal. It is unlikely for individuals with autosomal recessive HSP to have children with the disorder, because their spouse would have to have the disorder or be a carrier. This is possible only in consanguineous marriages (i.e., marriage between cousins). SPGs identified in this inheritance are located on chromosomes 8, 15q, or 16q. The latter is a mutation of the paraplegin gene. One form of autosomal recessive HSP, the Troyer syndrome, is associated with an SPG on chromosome 13. Two different genes associated with autosomal recessive HSP have also been identified on the X chromosome.

X-linked HSP

This is a rare form in which the mutant gene is located on the X chromosome at Xq28 or Xq22. Transmission is usually by the mother and the risk of inheriting this mutated gene and expressing the disease depends on the patient's gender. Women with an X-linked mutant HSP gene are generally not affected by the disorder, or, if they are affected, usually have less severe symptoms than males. Each son of a woman who is a carrier for X-linked HSP has a 50% chance of developing HSP. Each daughter of a woman who is a carrier for X-linked HSP has a 50% chance of being a carrier (female carriers of X-linked disorders often have no symptoms).

Sporadic HSP

In some instances, a definite mode of inheritance cannot be recognized when there is no other affected family member. This can occur if the inheritance has been autosomal recessive or X linked, where it can skip generations and remain silent and suddenly appear in the present generation. Also, the disease could have been milder (incomplete penetrance) and therefore undiagnosed in prior generations or the affected persons could have passed away prior to full symptom onset. Due to the phenomenon of anticipation, a child may exhibit symptoms even before the parent. Truly sporadic HSP is rare and is due to a new mutation occurring only in the affected individual.

Demographics

As usually happens with other rare neurological diseases, HSP symptoms may overlap or be mistaken with other neurodegenerative disorders. Consequently, HSP incidence is only estimated and is approximately three cases out of 100,000 individuals in the United States and

Europe. About 10,000–20,000 people in the United States are estimated to suffer from this disease, of which about 10% have the complicated form of HSP. Ninety percent of HSP cases are uncomplicated and life expectancy is unaffected.

Signs and symptoms

Previously, HSP was classified into early-onset (type I) HSP and late-onset (type II) HSP. In type I, symptoms of spasticity occurred prior to age 35, but progressed slowly. In type II HSP, symptom onset was after age 35 with weakness, spasticity, mild sensory loss, and bladder problems, and the disease progressed faster. This classification is confusing as both early and late onset disease can occur in the same family due to the phenomenon of anticipation. Therefore categorization into uncomplicated (pure) and complicated HSP is considered a more specific and useful distinction.

Uncomplicated HSP

This is usually the autosomal dominant form and may start at any age, mostly in the second to fourth decades but can also occur in infancy, early childhood, or old age. Atlastin causes childhood onset autosomal dominant HSP and spastin causes the adult onset form. In children, the disease progresses until adolescence and then stabilizes, resulting in partial walking disability. Complete paralysis of the legs is rare in uncomplicated HSP, regardless of age of onset. Progressive difficulty walking is the main problem and occurs due to taut and weak muscles. This manifests initially as stumbling, stubbing the toe, catching of the feet on uneven surfaces and sidewalks, clumsy gait, or difficulty with balance. The muscles that are most commonly affected include those on the inner side, front and back of the thighs and calves, leading to difficulty with hip and ankle flexion. This can lead to uncontrollable shaking (clonus) of the feet and scissoring of the legs while walking. Often the changes are so slowly progressive that patients do not notice subtle symptoms for several years. Arms are affected to a much lesser degree. Spasticity is worsened by cold, high humidity, emotional stress, and infections. Other common symptoms include urinary urgency and frequency, hyperactive tendon reflexes, diminished vibration and position sense in the feet, leg paresthesias, muscle spasms, cramps, and pain. Muscles can atrophy at a late stage. High arched feet (pes cavus) and bunions can occur due to imbalance in the strength and tone of muscles that maintain proper alignment of bones in the feet.

Complicated HSP

This is usually an autosomal recessive form with symptom onset between two and 16 years of age.

Symptoms are progressive and may be associated with other neurological conditions, such as **epilepsy**, mental retardation, peripheral neuropathy, ocular degeneration such as retinopathy, and/or the destruction of optic nerve. Other clinical complications are ataxia (incoordination), dysarthria (difficulty speaking), deafness, nystagmus (involuntary eye movements), decreased functioning of the adrenal glands, and **ichthyosis** (abnormal dryness, scaling, and thickening of the skin). However, these neurological symptoms may be caused by other disorders present at the same time. For instance, a person with uncomplicated HSP may have peripheral neuropathy due to **diabetes**.

Diagnosis

A detailed personal and family history along with physical and neurological examinations are the first tools in HSP diagnosis. The physician will conduct comparative examination of muscle tone and strength between arms and legs and look for signs of weakness in specific muscle groups of the thigh, presence of abnormal increase of deep tendon reflexes in the legs, loss of ankle flexibility, and decrease of sensation in the legs. A thorough clinical examination is vital to avoid misdiagnosing other conditions like vitamin B12 deficiency, vitamin E deficiency, **amyotrophic lateral sclerosis** (ALS), and tropical spastic paraparesis, which mimic HSP. Genetic screening for SPG is the definitive test to avoid misdiagnosis and is commercially available. The University of Michigan Neurogenetic Disorders Clinic is the largest clinical and research program for HSP in the United States, and one of the few that offers comprehensive evaluation, including **genetic testing**. Other ancillary tests like nerve conduction studies, spinal tap, magnetic resonance imaging (MRI), and blood tests will help exclude some of the other mimickers of the disease.

Treatment

There is no curable or preventive treatment for HSP. Symptomatic treatment for muscle spasm and spasticity includes oral medications like baclofen, tizanidine, and benzodiazepines like valium. Major side effects from these include confusion, dry mouth, drowsiness, and sedation. Symptomatic treatment for painful neuropathy includes medications like gabapentin and tricyclic antidepressants. Medications like oxybutynin can help in treating an overactive bladder. Baclofen can also be administered through a mechanical pump implanted in the space around the spinal cord to minimize systemic adverse effects. Newer approaches involve the local injection of botulinum toxin into the spastic muscles and the effect tends to last 3–6 months after an injection. Surgery may be necessary to relieve tendon contractures and

KEY TERMS

Adrenal—A pair of glands located on top of the kidneys that secrete substances or hormones, like steroids and adrenaline, which regulate various functions, such as water balance and stress response.

Amyotrophic lateral sclerosis (ALS)—A neurodegenerative disease that is caused by degeneration of the motor fibers and neurons in the brain, brainstem, and spinal cord, leading to stiffness, weak muscles, and respiratory failure.

Anticipation—The apparent tendency of certain diseases to appear at earlier age and with increasing severity in successive generations.

Ataxia—A condition marked by impaired muscular coordination, most frequently resulting from disorders in the brain or spinal cord.

Atrophy—A wasting away or decrease in size of a cell, tissue, organ, or part of the body caused by lack of nourishment, inactivity, or loss of nerve supply.

Autosomal—Relating to any chromosome besides the X and Y sex chromosomes. Human cells contain 22 pairs of autosomes and one pair of sex chromosomes.

Botulinum toxin—A class of neurotoxins that are produced by a bacteria and that cause paralysis and weakness of muscles.

Bunion—A bulge on the first joint of the big toe, caused by the swelling of a fluid sac under the skin.

Carrier—An individual who possesses an unexpressed abnormal gene of a recessive genetic disorder.

Clonus—A sustained series of involuntary rhythmic jerks following quick stretch of a muscle.

Contractures—An abnormal and usually permanent shortening and contraction of a muscle or tendon that causes a deformity or subnormal range of movement.

Corticospinal tract—A tract of nerve cells that carries motor commands from the brain to the spinal cord.

Dysarthria—Refers to a group of speech disorders caused by disturbances in the strength or coordination of the muscles of the speech mechanism as a result of damage to the brain or nerves.

Epilepsy—Disorders associated with the disturbed electrical discharges in the central nervous system that cause convulsions.

Familial—Tending to occur in more members of a family than expected by chance alone.

Genetic heterogeneity—A condition where the clinical features of a specific disease can be caused by mutations in several different genes.

Icthyosis—A disease condition where the skin becomes rough, thick, and scaly like that of a fish.

Magnetic resonance imaging (MRI)—An imaging technique that utilizes the properties of magnetism to create nondestructive, three-dimensional, internal images of the soft tissues of the body, including the brain, spinal cord, and muscle.

Nerve conduction—A test that measures the speed of conduction of electrical impulses through nerves using a series of electrical shocks delivered through electrodes placed on the skin surface.

Neuropathy—Common term used to denote dysfunction of the nerves in the arms, legs, or face.

Nystagmus—Involuntary, rapid, and repetitive movement of the eyes in either a vertical or horizontal direction.

Paraparesis—Weakness of the legs without complete paralysis.

Paresthesia—Abnormal subjective sensations like numbness, tingling, pain, burning, or prickling that occur due to neuropathy.

Paraplegia—Complete paralysis of the legs.

Penetrance—The extent to which a disease expresses itself in individuals who have the mutation. For example, if all individuals with the abnormal gene exhibit the disease, the disease is said to have complete penetrance.

Phenotype—The externally observable characters of an organism due to genetic and environmental effects on development.

Posterior column—Long fiber tracts that run in the spinal cord, carrying vibratory and position sense from the limbs to the brain.

Retinopathy—Noninflammatory or degenerative condition involving the retina of the eye.

Spasticity—Condition characterized by increased muscle tone and increased resistance to passive stretch.

Spinal tap—A procedure by which a needle is inserted into the space between two lumbar vertebrae to obtain fluid that circulates around the spinal cord.

Tendon reflex—Reflex contraction of the muscle that is observed by tapping on its tendon.

to lengthen spastic muscles. An electrical stimulator device implanted in the nerves near the tailbone can help in stimulating the bladder for complete urinary evacuation.

Supportive care includes physical therapy, which helps to improve muscle strength, range of motion, prevent contractures of joints, and bedsores. Therapies may include stretching, strengthening and aerobic exercises, balance and coordination training, gait training, and appropriate use of assistive devices such as canes, braces, and walkers. They can also include techniques such as massage, ultrasound, electrical stimulation, or whirlpool. Exercise also enhances a sense of well-being, and reduces stress and **depression**.

Prognosis

This varies widely, but most often HSP is compatible with a normal life expectancy. The rate of progression varies considerably and is influenced by the mode of inheritance. Some patients have serious disability not only from the spasticity but also from associated neurological problems. Others however have very mild disability and can lead a very productive and almost normal life. Complications arising from falls and immobility may inadvertently shorten a person's life.

Resources

BOOKS

Bradley, Walter G., R. B. Daroff, G. M. Fenichel, and J. Jankovic. *Neurology in Clinical Practice,* 4th ed. Philadelphia: Butterworth Heinemann, 2004.

PERIODICALS

Fink, John K. "Hereditary Spastic Paraplegia." *Neurologic Clinics of North America* 20 (2002): 711–726.

ORGANIZATIONS

National Institutes of Health/National Institute of Neurological Disorders and Stroke Brain Resources and Information Network. 9000 Rockville Pike, Bethesda, MD 20892. (301) 496 5751. (April 4, 2005.) <http://www.ninds.nih.gov>.

National Organization for Rare Disorders Inc. 55 Kenosia Ave, PO Box 1968, Danbury, CT 06813-1968. (800) 999 6673. (April 4, 2005.) <http://www.rarediseases.org>.

Spastic Paraplegia Foundation. 209 Park Road, Chelmsford, MA 01824. (703) 495 9261. (April 4, 2005.) <http://www.sp-foundation.org>.

Worldwide Education & Awareness for Movement Disorders (WE MOVE). 204 West 84th Street, New York, NY 10024. (April 4, 2005.) <http://www.wemove.org>.

OTHER

Association Strumpell-Lorrain. 7 D rue des Granges, Besancon, Intl 25000, France. (038) 150 2391. (April 4, 2005.) <http://www.perso.wanadoo.fr/asl.spastic>.

Athena Diagnostics Inc. Four Biotech Park, 377 Plantation Street, Worcester, MA 01605. (800) 394 4493. (April 4, 2005.) <http://www.athenadiagnostics.com>.

Chitra Venkatasubramanian, MBBS, MD

Hereditary spherocytosis

Definition

Hereditary spherocytosis (HS) is a relatively common and highly variable inherited disorder of the red blood cells. In HS, red blood cells become sphere-shaped, instead of the usual biconcave (hourglass) shape. The hourglass shape is vital for the blood cells to function—it offers increased surface area so that oxygen and carbon dioxide can diffuse more easily through the cell's tissue, and the shape lets the cells circulate more easily in tight places, like small capillaries. These *spherocytes* are broken down more quickly than normal red blood cells, resulting in anemia and related complications.

Description

Hereditary spherocytosis results from a molecular change in one of the proteins making up the cytoskeleton of the red blood cell. The cytoskeleton consists of the network of proteins that support and maintain the integrity of the red cell membrane. Genetic mutations in membrane proteins lead to loss of these and related membrane components. As the membrane becomes unstable and the surface area of the membrane decreases, spherocytes form. The spleen provides an environment that encourages spherocyte formation. Due to their increased rigidity, spherocytes tend to become trapped in the spleen and then broken down by macrophages, specialized white blood cells. This hemolytic process most often leads to mild, chronic anemia. Depending in part on the particular genetic mutation underlying HS in a given individual, anemia can also be severe and require chronic blood transfusions. Additional complications related to anemia can arise.

Demographics

HS has been seen in individuals of many ethnic backgrounds, but is particularly common among people of northern European background, affecting about one in 5,000 of such individuals.

Genetic profile

About 75% of all cases of HS are due to the presence of an autosomal dominant mutation, one in which the mutated **gene** is passed on from either parent. Most of these cases result from the **inheritance** of a mutation from one parent, but a fourth of these cases are sporadic and due to a new mutation that has occurred in the affected individual. A minority of cases of HS is recessively inherited. HS-causing mutations have been described in four genes, each of which codes for a protein involved in maintaining stability of the red blood cell membrane. The cytoskeleton can be thought of as a "scaffolding" or "frame" that is attached to and maintains the "wall" that is the cell membrane. The red cell membrane is made up of lipids, which are fat and fat-like molecules, and proteins called integral membrane proteins. The cytoskeleton lies just below the cell membrane and is made up of additional proteins, including spectrin, ankyrin, protein 4.1, and others.

Ankyrin

The ankyrin gene is located on the short arm of **chromosome** 8 (8p11.2). As of 1998, a total of 34 mutations in the ankyrin gene have been associated with HS. These account for 35–65% of all HS cases, including both dominant and recessive forms. Dominant-acting mutations tend to be those that result in a shortened ankyrin protein, including so-called frameshift and nonsense mutations. Recessive-acting mutations tend to be those that result in subtler changes to the protein. These include so-called missense mutations that result in the substitution of a single amino acid—the building block of proteins—which can have an effect on protein function. Recessive mutations also include those in the area "upstream" from the gene, in the promoter region that helps determine the quantity of protein made from the gene. Rarely, spherocytosis can be one symptom within a larger syndrome that is due to a deletion of a portion of chromosome 8. Such a microdeletion syndrome can affect several genes including the ankyrin gene, and there can be a range of physical and mental effects.

Spectrin

Spectrin is a cytoskeleton protein made of two components: alpha spectrin and beta spectrin. Two recessive mutations have been identified in the alpha spectrin gene on chromosome 1. This recessive form of the disease tends to have relatively severe hemolytic anemia. 19 mutations have been described in the beta spectrin gene on chromosome 14. These result in dominantly inherited HS.

Band 3 and others

Mutations in the gene for band 3, an integral membrane protein, account for 15–25% of all cases of HS. Five dominant mutations have been described, most of which result in a shortened protein. Disease-causing mutations in other cytoskeleton or red cell membrane proteins are rare but have been described.

Modifying genetic factors

Disease severity is not only affected by the nature of the primary genetic mutation, it is also impacted by other genetic variations. Individuals with HS who also have Gilbert syndrome have an increased risk of gallstones. Gilbert syndrome is caused by a change in the UGT 1A1 gene that results in increased levels of bilirubin. Researchers have also hypothesized that persons with other inherited or acquired forms of hemolytic anemia may also be at increased risk of gallstones if they also have a disease-causing HS mutation. The presence of hereditary **hemochromatosis** in addition to HS increases the propensity toward iron-overload. Hereditary hemochromatosis is a relatively common recessive condition that can lead to organ failure due to iron-overload, if untreated.

Signs and symptoms

Symptoms of HS can be extremely variable. Some individuals may experience onset as early as the neonatal period and require treatment. Others may have only mild anemia that does not require treatment and does not become evident until later in life. Some individuals with few and subtle signs may even go undiagnosed. Variability is largely influenced by the primary underlying genetic mutation, with the recessive forms of the disease tending to be most severe. This does not account for all the variability, however, given that multiple affected individuals within the same family carrying the same genetic mutation may have symptoms of varying severity. The effects of modifying genes or environmental factors may contribute to this additional variability.

Anemia

The red blood cell membrane has increased fragility in HS. Therefore, red cells are more easily broken down, a symptom called hemolytic anemia. This occurs primarily in the spleen. The spleen filters out old and abnormal red blood cells, as well as fights infection from bacteria, particularly the encapsulated type. Anemia can be unnoticeable or mild, or it can be rapid and severe. Rapid, acute breakdown of red blood cells can occur as a result of exposure to chemicals or medications that are known to further increase red cell membrane fragility. It can also occur as a result of infection that increases the hemolytic activity of the spleen or decreases red blood cell production. Acute aplastic anemia events, in which red blood cell production halts, can occur with deficient folate levels or following infection by a specific virus called parvovirus.

Jaundice

Jaundice occurs when the level of bilirubin, a breakdown product of hemoglobin, increases. As red blood cells breakdown rapidly, the liver may not be able to keep up with the increased need to metabolize bilirubin, which can deposit in the skin and eyes causing a yellowish discoloration.

Gallstones

Bilirubin levels can also be increased in the bile. Bile is the fluid secreted by the liver into the intestine. Bile reaches the intestine by passing through the gallbladder and bile duct. Excess bilirubin can form stones in the gallbladder early in life.

Hemochromatosis

Hemochromatosis, or high iron levels, is also characteristic of HS. Iron-overload can lead to dysfunction of organ systems, including the endocrine system, which directs hormone levels.

Other complications

Leg ulcers are also seen in HS, and acute kidney failure due to hemolytic anemia is a rare complication. Rarely, HS can be seen within a syndrome as one symptom in combination with other complications such as neurological problems and other congenital physical differences. Such syndromes may be caused by the deletion of a portion of a chromosome including a gene known to be associated with HS, among other genes.

Diagnosis

HS must be distinguished from other causes of hemolytic anemia that can resemble HS. These include immune hemolytic anemia, G6PD deficiency, unstable hemoglobin traits or diseases, **Wilson disease**, and spherocytosis due to burn injury or toxin exposure (i.e., clostridia—bee, spider, or snake venom). Routine blood tests are typically sufficient to diagnose HS, particularly if an individual is showing symptoms. A peripheral blood smear, which is a slide preparation of a blood sample, will show the presence of a number of spherocytes that are uniform in appearance. Bilirubin levels tend to be elevated. A complete blood count will show several abnormalities. Hemoglobin levels tend to be decreased. Reticulocytes, which are immature red blood cells, tend to be increased. Red blood cells tend to be smaller than normal, which is marked by a decreased mean cell volume (MCV). The mean cell hemoglobin concentration (MCHC) tends to be high, which is a reflection of the overall decrease in the cell volume. Ektacytometry is a specialized test that can demonstrate the fragility of the red blood cell membrane by placing the cells under stress and identifying increased levels and specific patterns of hemolysis. Another specialized test called the rapid flow cytometric test has recently been developed. This test can determine differences in fluorescent staining patterns that distinguish normal red blood cells from those that are characteristic of HS. This test is highly sensitive and specific for HS and should aid in its rapid diagnosis.

Treatment and management

Most individuals with HS do not have symptoms that are severe enough to require treatment. For those with the more severe forms, blood transfusion therapy can effectively improve symptoms until a child is old enough for total or partial removal of the spleen, the organ responsible for most of the red blood cell destruction. Splenectomy most often eliminates HS complications. However, there is some risk remaining for ongoing chronic anemia or acute anemic events, particularly those caused by viruses and other factors that can temporarily halt red blood cell production. Splenectomy can also lead to an increased risk for blood clots, as well as life-threatening bacterial infection given the spleen's role in fighting bacterial infections. Studies have shown that partial, as opposed to total, splenectomy can be effective at ameliorating HS symptoms while also maintaining the bacterial-fighting capacity of the spleen and decreasing the chance for blood clots. Prophylactic antibiotics (e.g., penicillin) and additional vaccinations for common bacterial infections also play a role in decreasing negative side-effects of partial or total splenectomy. Surgery may be needed to remove gallstones that become symptomatic, which usually does not occur until after age 10 years.

Prognosis

Prognosis is very good for all types of HS, particularly the more mild forms. Treatment is very effective for the more severe forms. There is only a small number of affected individuals who still experience anemia and other symptoms following splenectomy.

Resources

BOOKS

Glader, B., and L. Naumovski. "Other Hereditary Red Blood Cell Disorders." In *Emery and Rimoin's Principles and Practice of Medical Genetics.* 3rd ed. New York: Churchill Livingston, 1997.

PERIODICALS

Bader-Meunier, B., et al. "Long-term Evaluation of the Beneficial Effect of Subtotal Splenectomy for Management of Hereditary Spherocytosis." *Blood* 97, no. 2 (January 15, 2001): 399–403.

Campanile, R., et al. "Low Frequency of Ankyrin Mutations in Hereditary Spherocytosis: Identification of Three Novel Mutations." *Human Mutation* 378 (2000).

Gallagher, P.G., et al. "Short Reports: A Recurrent Frameshift Mutation of the Ankyrin Associated with Severe Hereditary Spherocytosis." *British Journal of Haematology* 111, no. 4 (December 2000): 1190–1193.

King, M.J., et al. "Rapid Flow Cytometric Test for the Diagnosis of Membrane Cytoskeleton-association Haemolytic Anaemia." *British Journal of Haematology* 111, no. 3 (December 2000): 924–933.

Miraglia del Giudice, E., et al. "Clinical and Molecular Evaluation of Non-dominant Hereditary Spherocytosis." *British Journal of Haematology* 112, no. 1 (January 2001): 42–47.

WEBSITES

McKusick, V. "Spherocytosis, Hereditary; HS." Entry #182900. *Online Mendelian Inheritance in Man.* (June 2, 2005) <http://www3.ncbi.nlm.nih.gov/entrez/dispomim.cgi?id=182900>.

McKusick, V. "Spherocytosis, Autosomal Recessive." Entry #270970. *Online Mendelian Inheritance in Man.* (June 2, 2005) <http://www3.ncbi.nlm.nih.gov/entrez/dispomim.cgi?id=270970>.

Jennifer D. Bojanowski, MS, CGC

Hermansky-Pudlak syndrome

Definition

Hermansky-Pudlak syndrome (HPS) is a rare inherited disorder of melanin production. Melanin is the pigment that gives color to the skin, hair, and eyes. A lack or decrease of pigment in the skin and eyes is called oculocutaneous **albinism**. HPS is a specific type of oculocutaneous albinism that also includes a bleeding tendency and the storage of ceroid, the byproduct of cell membrane breakdown, in the body's cells.

Description

In 1959, Drs. F. Hermansky and P. Pudlak reported two unrelated people with oculocutaneous albinism who had lifelong bleeding problems. The female died at age 33, and at that time large amounts of pigment were discovered in the walls of her small blood vessels.

Genetic profile

HPS is an autosomal recessive disorder. This means that the disease manifests itself when a person has inherited one nonworking copy of the HPS **gene** from each parent. Parents who carry the gene for HPS are healthy and have typical skin pigmentation. However, each time they have a child, the chance for the child to have HPS is 25%, or one in four. Unless someone in the family has HPS, most couples are unaware of their risk.

Researchers mapped the HPS1 gene to the long arm of **chromosome** 10 in 1995, and later identified its exact location in 1996. The protein produced by the HPS gene helps organelles (specialized parts) of the cell's cytoplasm (portion of the cell between the membrane and nucleus) to develop and function normally.

In 1999, another group of researchers identified a mutation, or gene change, in the AP3B1 gene located on chromosome 5 as another cause of HPS. This gene makes AP3, a molecule that helps to sort proteins within the body's cells.

Demographics

In northwest Puerto Rico, HPS is a common inherited disorder. More than 300 persons are affected. The carrier rate is about one in 21. Intermarriage accounts for the high frequency. Researchers have traced the origin of HPS to southern Spain. Cases have also been reported in the Dutch, Swiss, and Japanese. Both sexes are equally affected. However, females will have more lung symptoms than males.

Signs and symptoms

People with HPS have a broad range of skin color from tan to white, reflecting the partial absence of pigmentation. Hair color ranges from brown to white, also reflecting how much pigmentation is present.

Poor vision and eye abnormalities are common in people with HPS. Visual acuity can approach 20/200. Nystagmus, an irregular rapid back and forth movement of the eyes, is also common. The eyes can have an improper muscle balance called strabismus. Sensitivity to bright light and glare, known as photophobia, is a frequent complaint of people with HPS. These visual problems all result from abnormal development of the eye due to the lack of pigment. Just as skin and hair color vary, so will eye color. Red, brown, hazel, and violet eyes have been reported.

A bleeding tendency distinguishes HPS from other types of albinism. People with HPS will bruise easily and bleed for an extended time after dental extractions and surgical procedures. Platelets are the disc-shaped structures in the blood that cause clotting. In people with HPS, the platelets are missing certain internal components that cause them to clump together during the clotting process.

The third finding of HPS is the accumulation of ceroid in certain cells of the body such as bone marrow and the lung. As ceroid collects in the lungs, it makes the affected individual prone to respiratory infections and progressive lung disease that restricts breathing. Some people also complain of colitis (an inflammation of the colon) and diarrhea (loose, watery stools).

Diagnosis

Diagnosis of HPS can be made by specialized platelet testing and molecular testing for the known **gene mutations**. Very few laboratories are equipped to perform these tests. A person who is suspected to have HPS should consult with a geneticist or genetic counselor to arrange for the appropriate tests. Molecular testing is available for Puerto Rican families who usually have a specific detectable gene alteration, which is a duplication of a small segment of the gene.

Analysis of the person's platelets will determine if they are lacking the critical internal parts, called dense bodies, that help to clot blood. If dense bodies are not present, then HPS is the diagnosis.

For affected people of Puerto Rican ancestry, one unique gene mutation is present. Several other mutations can also be detected, but the lack of a gene mutation does not mean a person does not have HPS, since all mutations have not been identified.

For some families with an affected child, prenatal diagnosis may be possible for future pregnancies. Parents should consult with a genetics specialist when planning a pregnancy.

Treatment and management

For the individual with HPS, vision problems are always present. Many people will meet the legal definition of blindness, but still have enough vision for reading and other activities. Other affected people may be farsighted or nearsighted.

An ophthalmologist, a specialist for the eyes, will help those individuals who have strabismus, a muscle imbalance in the eyes. They can have corrective surgery that will not only improve their physical appearance but also expand their visual field. Surgery, however, cannot restore pigment to the eyes nor correct the optic nerve pathways leading from the brain to the eyes.

Many optical aids can help a person with HPS function better in daily life. Aids like hand-held magnifiers, strong reading glasses, and glasses that have small telescopes fitted in the lens called bioptics can make hobbies, jobs, and other activities easier.

KEY TERMS

Bioptics—Glasses that have small telescopes fitted in the lens.

Ceroid—The byproduct of cell membrane breakdown.

Colitis—Inflammation of the colon.

Cytoplasm—The substance within a cell including the organelles and the fluid surrounding the nucleus.

Diarrhea—Loose, watery stool.

Melanin—Pigments normally produced by the body that give color to the skin and hair.

Mutation—A permanent change in the genetic material that may alter a trait or characteristic of an individual, or manifest as disease, and can be transmitted to offspring.

Nystagmus—Involuntary, rhythmic movement of the eye.

Oculocutaneous albinism—Inherited loss of pigment in the skin, eyes, and hair.

Organelle—Small, sub-cellular structures that carry out different functions necessary for cellular survival and proper cellular functioning.

Photophobia—An extreme sensitivity to light.

Sputum—A mixture of saliva and mucus from the lungs.

Strabismus—An improper muscle balance of the ocular muscles resulting in crossed or divergent eyes.

Protection from excessive sunlight is crucial for people with HPS. Sunscreens of the highest rating should be used to decrease the chance for fatal skin cancers. By wearing clothing that blocks as much sunlight as possible, people with HPS can enjoy outdoor activities. A dermatologist, a specialist in skin disorders, can examine the affected person if any changes in skin color or appearance occur. Annual skin check-ups are important.

As people with HPS reach their 30s, they begin to have lung disease. The first sign is difficulty in breathing, followed by a cough that does not bring up sputum, a mixture of saliva and mucus, from the lungs. Gradually, the lungs develop a tough, fibrous tissue that further limits breathing. The inability to breathe is the most common cause of death for people with HPS.

Prolonged bleeding after tooth extraction, nosebleed, or surgery occurs regularly in people with HPS.

Before any surgery, treatment with desmopressin, a drug that stimulates clotting activity, can be effective. Also, individuals with HPS should avoid aspirin, because it makes blood less likely to clot.

Prognosis

Many people with HPS may have concerns about their physical appearance and decreased vision. Education about the disorder is important to prevent isolation and stigmatization. Once the visual difficulties are addressed, people with albinism can participate in most activities.

Although many preventive efforts can improve the quality of life for a person with HPS, the progressive lung disease cannot be halted. The inability to breathe generally becomes fatal when the affected person is 40–50 years old.

Resources

BOOKS

Kanski, Jack J. *Clinical Ophthalmology: A Systematic Approach.* Woburn, MA: Butterworth-Heinemann Medical, 1999.

Landau, Elaine. *Living with Albinism (First Book).* New York, NY: Franklin Watts, 1998.

PERIODICALS

Dell'Angelica, E. C., et al. "Altered Trafficking of Lysosomal Proteins in Hermansky-Pudlak Syndrome Due to Mutations in the Beta-3A Subunit of the AP-3 Adaptor." *Molecular Cell* 3 (1999): 11-21.

Depinho, R. A., and K. L. Kaplan. "The Hermansky-Pudlak Syndrome, Report of Three Cases and Review of Pathophysiology and Management Considerations." *Medicine* 64 (1985): 192-202.

Gahl, W. A., et al. "Genetic Defects and Clinical Characteristics of Patients with a Form of Oculocutaneous Albinism (Hermansky-Pudlak Syndrome)." *New England Journal of Medicine* 338 (1998): 1258-1264.

Sandberg-Gertzen, H., R. Eid, and G. Jarnerot. "Hermansky-Pudlak Syndrome with Colitis and Pulmonary Fibrosis." *Scan-dinavian Journal of Gastroentology* 34 (1999): 1055-1056.

Wijermans, P. W., and D. B. van Dorp. "Hermansky-Pudlak Syndrome, Correction of Bleeding Time by 1-Desamino-8D-Arginine Vasopressin." *American Journal of Hematology* 30 (1989): 154-157.

Wildenberg, S. C., W. S. Oetting, and C. Almodovar. "Gene Causing Hermansky-Pudlak Syndrome in a Puerto Rican Population Maps to Chromosome 10q2." *Human Genetics* 57 (1995): 755-765.

ORGANIZATIONS

Hermansky-Pudlak Syndrome Network. 39 Riveria Court, Malverne, NY 11565-1602. (800) 789-9477 or (516) 599-2077. <http://www.medhelp.org/web/hpsn.htm>.

National Organization for Albinism and Hypopigmentation. 1530 Locust St. #29, Philadelphia, PA 19102-4415. (215) 545-2322 or (800) 473-2310. <http://www.albinism.org/infobulletins/hermansky-pudlak-syndrome.html>.

WEBSITES

FriendshipCenter.com. <http://www.friendshipcenter.com>.

NORD—National Organization for Rare Disorders. <http://www.rarediseases.org>.

Suzanne M. Carter, MS, CGC

Hermaphroditism

Definition

Hermaphroditism is a rare condition in which ovarian and testicular tissue exist in the same person. The testicular tissue contains seminiferous tubules or spermatozoa. The ovarian tissue contains follicles or corpora albicantia. The condition is the result of a **chromosome** anomaly.

Description

Among human beings, hermaphroditism is an extremely rare anomaly in which gonads for both sexes are present. External genitalia may show traits of both sexes, and in which the chromosomes show male-female mosaicism (where one individual possesses both the male XY and female XX chromosome pairs). There are two different variants of hermaphroditism: true hermaphroditism and pseudohermaphroditism. There are female and male pseudohermaphrodites. True hermaphroditism refers to the presence of both testicular and ovarian tissue in the same individual. The external genitalia in these individuals may range from normal male to normal female. However, most phenotypic males have **hypospadias**. Pseudohermaphroditism refers to gonadal dysgenesis.

Genetic profile

The most common **karyotype** for a true hermaphrodite is 46XX. **DNA** from the Y chromosome is translocated to one of the X-chromosomes. The karyotype for male pseudohermaphrodites is 46XY. Female pseudohermaphroditism is more complicated. The condition is caused by deficiencies in the activity of enzymes. The genetic basis for three enzyme deficiencies have been identified. Deficiency of 3B hydroxysteroid dehydrogenase Type 2 is due to an abnormality on chromosome 1p13.1. Deficiency of 21-Hydroxylase is due to an abnormality on chromosome 6p21.3. Deficiency of 11B-Hydroxylase Type 1 is due to an abnormality on chromosome 8q21.

Demographics

True hermaphrodites are extremely rare. Approximately 500 individuals have been identified in the world to date. Because of the ambiguity of genitalia and difficulties in making an accurate diagnosis, the incidence of pseudohermaphroditism is not well established. The incidence of male pseudohermaphroditism has been estimated at between 3 and 15 per 100,000 people. The incidence of female pseudohermaphroditism has been estimated at between one and eight per 100,000 people.

Signs and symptoms

True hermaphroditism is characterized by ambiguous internal and external genitalia. On internal examination (most often using laparoscopy), there is microscopic evidence of both ovaries and testes. Male pseudohermaphroditism is also characterized by ambiguous internal and external genitalia. However, gonads are often (but not always) recognizable as testes. These are frequently softer than normal. An affected person is often incompletely masculinized. Female pseudohermaphroditism is characterized by female internal genitals. External genitals tend to appear as masculine. This is most commonly characterized by clitoral hypertrophy. Most hermaphrodites are infertile although a small number of pregnancies have been reported.

Diagnosis

True hermaphroditism is often diagnosed after laparoscopic investigation. An initial suspicion of male pseudohermaphroditism is often made by inspection of external genitals. This is confirmed by chromosomal analysis and assays of hormones such as testosterone. Initial suspicion of female pseudohermaphroditism is also made by inspection of external genitals. This is confirmed by analysis of chromosomes and hormonal assay. Laparoscopic examination usually reveals nearly normal female internal genitals.

Treatment and management

Early assignment of gender is important for the emotional well being of any person with **ambiguous genitalia**. A decision to select a gender of rearing is based on the corrective potential of the ambiguous genitalia, rather than using chromosome analysis. Once the decision is made regarding gender, there should be no question in the family's mind regarding the gender of the child from that point on.

KEY TERMS

Corpora albicantia—Plural of corpus albicans. A corpus albicans is the scar tissue that remains on an ovarian follicle after ovulation.

Dysgenesis—Defective or abnormal formation of an organ or part usually occurring during embryonic development.

Follicle—A pouch-like depression.

Mosaicism—A genetic condition resulting from a mutation, crossing over, or nondisjunction of chromosomes during cell division, causing a variation in the number of chromosomes in the cells.

Semineferous tubules—Long, threadlike tubes that are packed in areolar tissue in the lobes of the testes.

Spermatozoa—Mature male germ cells that develop in the seminiferous tubules of the testes.

Corrective surgery is used to reconstruct the external genitalia. In general, it is easier to reconstruct female genitalia than male genitalia, and the ease of reconstruction will play a role in selecting the gender of rearing. Treating professionals must be alert for stress in persons with any form of hermaphroditism and their families.

Prognosis

With appropriate corrective surgery, the appearance of external genitalia may appear normal. However, other problems such as virilization may appear later in life. There is some interest among persons with ambiguous genitalia at birth to reverse their gender of rearing.

Resources

BOOKS

Rappaport, Robert. "Female Pseudohermaphroditism." *Nelson Textbook of Pediatrics.* Edited by Richard E. Behrman et al. 16th ed. Philadelphia, W.B. Saunders, 2000, p. 1760.

Rappaport, Robert. "Male Pseudohermaphroditism." *Nelson Textbook of Pediatrics.* Edited by Richard E. Behrman et al. 16th ed. Philadelphia, W.B. Saunders, 2000, pp. 1761-1764.

Rappaport, Robert. "True Hermaphroditism." *Nelson Textbook of Pediatrics.* Edited by Richard E. Behrman et al. 16th ed. Philadelphia, W.B. Saunders, 2000, pp. 1765-1766.

Wilson, Jean D., and James E. Griffin. "Disorders of Sexual Differentiation." *Harrison's Principles of Internal Medicine.* Edited by Anthony S. Fauci, et al. 14th ed. New York: McGraw-Hill, 1998, pp. 2119-2131.

PERIODICALS

Denes F. T., B. B. Mendonca, and S. Arap. "Laparoscopic Management of Intersexual States." *Urology Clinics of North America* 28, no. 1 (2001): 31-42.

Krstic Z. D., et al. "True Hermaphroditism: 10 Years' Experience." *Pediatric Surgery International* 16, no. 8 (2000): 580-583.

Wiersma, R. "Management of the African Child With True Hermaphroditism." *Journal of Pediatric Surgery* 36, no. 2 (2001): 397-399.

Zuker, K. J. "Intersexuality and Gender Identity Differentiation." *Annual Review of Sexual Research* 10 (1999): 1-69.

ORGANIZATIONS

Genetic Alliance. 4301 Connecticut Ave. NW, #404, Washington, DC 20008-2304. (800) 336-GENE (Helpline) or (202) 966-5557. Fax: (888) 394-3937 info@geneticalliance. <http://www.geneticalliance.org>.

Hermaphrodite Education and Listening Post. PO Box 26292, Jacksonville, NY 32226. help@jaxnet.com. <http://users.southeast.net/~help/>.

Intersex Society of North America. PO Box 301, Petaluma, CA 94953-0301. <http://www.isna.org>.

March of Dimes Birth Defects Foundation. 1275 Mamaroneck Ave., White Plains, NY 10605. (888) 663-4637. resourcecenter@modimes.org. <http://www.modimes.org>.

WEBSITES

Born True Hermaphrodite <http://www.angelfire.com/ca2/BornHermaphrodite/>.

Columbia Electronic Encyclopedia. <http://www.infoplease.com/ce6/sci/A0823491.html>.

Hermaphrodite Education and Listening Post. <http://www.jax-inter.net/~help/>.

Loyola University Strich School of Medicine. <http://matweb.hcuge.ch/matweb/Selected_images/Developmental_genetic_diseases/hermaphroditism.htm>.

National Library of Medicine <http://medlineplus.adam.com/ency/article/001669.htm>.

UK Intersex Association. <http://www.ukia.co.uk/>.

L. Fleming Fallon, Jr., MD, DrPH

High density lipoprotein deficiency *see* Tangier disease

Hirschsprung disease

Definition

Hirschsprung disease, also known as congenital megacolon or aganglionic megacolon, is an abnormality in which certain nerve fibers are absent in segments of the bowel, resulting in severe bowel obstruction.

Description

Hirschsprung disease is caused when certain nerve cells (called parasympathetic ganglion cells) in the wall of the large intestine (colon) do not develop before birth. Without these nerves, the affected segment of the colon lacks the ability to relax and move bowel contents along. This causes a constriction and as a result, the bowel above the constricted area dilates due to stool becoming trapped, producing megacolon (dilation of the colon). The disease can affect varying lengths of bowel segment, most often involving the region around the rectum. In up to 10% of children, however, the entire colon and part of the small intestine are involved.

Genetic profile

Hirschsprung disease occurs early in fetal development when, for unknown reasons, there is either failure of nerve cell development, failure of nerve cell migration, or arrest in nerve cell development in a segment of bowel. The absence of these nerve fibers, which help control the movement of bowel contents, is what results in intestinal obstruction accompanied by other symptoms.

There is a genetic basis to Hirschsprung disease, and it is believed that it may be caused by different genetic factors in different subsets of families. Proof that genetic factors contribute to Hirschsprung disease is that it is known to run in families, and it has been seen in association with some **chromosome** abnormalities. For example, about 10% of children with the disease have **Down syndrome** (the most common chromosome abnormality). Molecular diagnostic techniques have identified many genes that cause susceptibility to Hirschsprung disease. There are a total of six genes: the RET **gene**, the glial cell line-derived neurotrophic factor gene, the endothelin-B receptor gene, endothelin converting enzyme, the endothelin-3 gene, and the Sry-related transcription factor SOX10. Mutations that inactivate the RET gene are the most frequent, occurring in 50% of familial cases (cases which run in families) and 15-20% of sporadic (non-familial) cases. Mutations in these genes do not cause the disease, but they make the chance of developing it more likely. Mutations in other genes or environmental factors are required to develop the disease, and these other factors are not understood.

For persons with a ganglion growth beyond the sigmoid segment of the colon, the **inheritance** pattern is autosomal dominant with reduced penetrance (risk closer to 50%). For persons with smaller segments involved, the inheritance pattern is multifactorial (caused by an interaction of more than one gene and environmental factors, risk lower than 50%) or autosomal recessive (one disease gene inherited from each parent, risk closer to 25%) with low penetrance.

Demographics

Hirschsprung's disease occurs once in every 5,000 live births, and it is about four times more common in males than females. Between 4% and 50% of siblings are also afflicted. The wide range for recurrence is due to the fact that the recurrence risk depends on the gender of the affected individual in the family (i.e., if a female is affected, the recurrence risk is higher) and the length of the aganglionic segment of the colon (i.e., the longer the segment that is affected, the higher the recurrence risk).

Signs and symptoms

The initial symptom is usually severe, continuous constipation. A newborn may fail to pass meconium (the first stool) within 24 hours of birth, may repeatedly vomit yellow or green colored bile and may have a distended (swollen, uncomfortable) abdomen. Occasionally, infants may have only mild or intermittent constipation, often with diarrhea.

While two-thirds of cases are diagnosed in the first three months of life, Hirschsprung disease may also be diagnosed later in infancy or childhood. Occasionally, even adults are diagnosed with a variation of the disease. In older infants, symptoms and signs may include anorexia (lack of appetite or inability to eat), lack of the urge to move the bowels or empty the rectum on physical examination, distended abdomen, and a mass in the colon that can be felt by the physician during examination. It should be suspected in older children with abnormal bowel habits, especially a history of constipation dating back to infancy and ribbon-like stools.

Occasionally, the presenting symptom may be a severe intestinal infection called enterocolitis, which is life threatening. The symptoms are usually explosive, watery stools and fever in a very ill-appearing infant. It is important to diagnose the condition before the intestinal obstruction causes an overgrowth of bacteria that evolves into a medical emergency. Enterocolitis can lead to severe diarrhea and massive fluid loss, which can cause death from dehydration unless surgery is done immediately to relieve the obstruction.

Diagnosis

Hirschsprung disease in the newborn must be distinguished from other causes of intestinal obstruction. The diagnosis is suspected by the child's medical history and

KEY TERMS

Anus—The opening at the end of the intestine that carries waste out of the body.

Barium enema x ray—A procedure that involves the administration of barium into the intestines by a tube inserted into the rectum. Barium is a chalky substance that enhances the visualization of the gastrointestinal tract on x ray.

Colostomy—The creation of an artificial opening into the colon through the skin for the purpose of removing bodily waste. Colostomies are usually required because key portions of the intestine have been removed.

Enterocolitis—Severe inflammation of the intestines that affects the intestinal lining, muscle, nerves and blood vessels.

Manometry—A balloon study of internal anal sphincter pressure and relaxation.

Meconium—The first waste products to be discharged from the body in a newborn infant, usually greenish in color and consisting of mucus, bile and so forth.

Megacolon—Dilation of the colon.

Parasympathetic ganglion cell—Type of nerve cell normally found in the wall of the colon.

physical examination, especially the rectal exam. The diagnosis is confirmed by a barium enema x ray, which shows a picture of the bowel. The x ray will indicate if a segment of bowel is constricted, causing dilation and obstruction. A biopsy of rectal tissue will reveal the absence of the nerve fibers. Adults may also undergo manometry, a balloon study (device used to enlarge the anus for the procedure) of internal anal sphincter pressure and relaxation.

Treatment and management

Hirschsprung disease is treated surgically. The goal is to remove the diseased, nonfunctioning segment of the bowel and restore bowel function. This is often done in two stages. The first stage relieves the intestinal obstruction by performing a colostomy. This is the creation of an opening in the abdomen (stoma) through which bowel contents can be discharged into a waste bag. When the child's weight, age, or condition is deemed appropriate, surgeons close the stoma, remove the diseased portion of bowel, and perform a "pull-through" procedure, which repairs the colon by connecting functional bowel to the

anus. This usually establishes fairly normal bowel function.

Prognosis

Overall, prognosis is very good. Most infants with Hirschsprung disease achieve good bowel control after surgery, but a small percentage of children may have lingering problems with soilage or constipation. These infants are also at higher risk for an overgrowth of bacteria in the intestines, including subsequent episodes of enterocolitis, and should be closely followed by a physician. Mortality from enterocolitis or surgical complications in infancy is 20%.

Prevention

Hirschsprung disease is a congenital abnormality that has no known means of prevention. It is important to diagnose the condition early in order to prevent the development of enterocolitis. **Genetic counseling** can be offered to a couple with a previous child with the disease or to an affected individual considering pregnancy to discuss recurrence risks and treatment options. Prenatal diagnosis is not available.

Resources

BOOKS

Buyse, Mary Louise, MD., ed. "Colon, Aganglionosis." *Birth Defects Encyclopedia*. Oxford: Blackwell Scientific Publications, 1990.

Phillips, Sidney F., and John H. Pemberton. "Megacolon: Congenital and Acquired." *Sleisenger & Fordtran's Gastrointestinal and Liver Disease*. Edited by Mark Feldman, et al. Philadelphia: W. B. Saunders Co., 1998.

PERIODICALS

Kusafuka, T., and P. Puri. "Genetic Aspects of Hirschprung's Disease." *Seminars in Pediatric Surgery* 7 (1998): 148-55.

Martucciello, G., et al. "Pathogenesis of Hirschsprung's Disease." *Journal of Pediatric Surgery* 35 (2000): 1017-25.

Munnes, M., et al. "Familial Form of Hirschsprung Disease: Nucleotide Sequence Studies Reveal Point Mutations in the RET Proto-oncogene in Two of Six Families But Not in Other Candidate Genes." *American Journal of Medical Genetics* 94 (2000): 19-27.

Puri, P., K. Ohshiro, and T. Wester. "Hirschsprung's Disease: A Search for Etiology." *Seminars in Pediatric Surgery* 7 (1998): 140-7.

Salomon, R., et al. "From Monogenic to Polygenic: Model of Hirschsprung Disease." *Pathologie Biologie (Paris)* 46 (1998): 705-7.

ORGANIZATIONS

American Pseudo-Obstruction & Hirschsprung Society. 158 Pleasant St., North Andover, MA 01845. (978) 685-4477.

Pull-thru Network. 316 Thomas St., Bessemer, AL 35020. (205) 428-5953.

Amy Vance, MS, CGC

HLA region *see* **Major histocompatibility complex**

Holoprosencephaly

Definition

Holoprosencephaly is a disorder in which there is a failure of the front part of the brain to properly separate into what is commonly known as the right and left half of the brain. This lack of separation is often accompanied by abnormalities of the face and skull. Holoprosencephaly may occur individually or as a component of a larger disorder.

Description

Types of holoprosencephaly

Holoprosencephaly comes in three different types: alobar, semilobar, and lobar. Each of these classifications is based on the amount of separation between what is commonly known as the left and right halves of the brain. Alobar holoprosencephaly is considered to be the most severe form of the disease, in which the separation between the two halves, or hemispheres, completely fails to develop. Semilobar holoprosencephaly represents holoprosencephaly of the moderate type, where some separation between the hemispheres has occurred. Lobar holoprosencephaly represents the least severe type of holoprosencephaly in which the hemispheres are almost, but not completely, divided.

The severity of the effect of the disease on the brain is often reflected in craniofacial abnormalities (abnormalities of the face and skull). This has led to many health care professionals utilizing the phrase "the face predicts the brain." This phrase is generally but not always accurate. Children may have severe craniofacial abnormalities with mild (lobar) holoprosencephaly, or children may have severe (alobar) holoprosencephaly with mild facial changes. Since the development of the face, skull, and the front of the brain are interconnected, the changes in the face often, but do not always, correspond with changes in the brain. Finally, the designation of these disorders from least severe to most severe can be mildly misleading, since the best predictor of the severity of the disease, according to Barr and Cohen, is how well the brain func-

tions, not its appearance. However, the alobar, semilobar, and lobar categories are universally utilized and give an indication of the severity of the disease, so knowledge of these categories and what they represent is useful.

Other brain abnormalities in holoprosencephaly

All patients with holoprosencephaly lack a sense of smell through the first cranial nerve (the olfactory nerve). Interestingly enough, one has a partial sense of smell through the sense of taste, which is governed by the seventh cranial nerve. The term "smell" and what it means in a conventional and strictly neurological sense differ, so it may be useful to think of persons with holoprosencephaly as lacking a portion of what is in common usage referred to as smell. This deficiency in smell can be detected by testing. One other important structural abnormality should be mentioned. The corpus callosum, which is the part of the brain that connects the right and left hemispheres with each other, is absent or deficient in persons with holoprosencephaly.

Synonyms for holoprosencephaly

Arrhinencephaly and familial alobar holoprosencephaly are synonyms for this disorder.

Genetic profile

Genetic causes of holoprosencephaly

Holoprosencephaly is a feature frequently found in many different syndromes including, but not limited to: **trisomy 13**, **trisomy 18**, tripoloidy, pseudotrisomy 13, **Smith-Lemli-Opitz syndrome**, **Pallister-Hall syndrome**, **Fryns syndrome**, CHARGE association, Goldenhar syndrome, **frontonasal dysplasia**, **Meckel-Gruber syndrome**, velocardiofacial syndrome, Genoa syndrome, Lambotte syndrome, Martin syndrome, and Steinfeld syndrome, as well as several teratogenic syndromes such as diabetic embryopathy, **accutane embryopathy**, and **fetal alcohol syndrome**. Holoprosencephaly has been linked to at least 12 different loci on 11 different chromosomes. Some candidate genes are Sonic hedgehog (abbreviated Shh, and located at 7q36), SIX3 (located at 2p21), and the ZIC2 **gene** (located on **chromosome** 13). The gene causing Smith-Lemli-Opitz syndrome, which affects cholesterol synthesis, also is interesting, since it is also obviously a candidate to cause holoprosencephaly.

Shh, cholesterol, the prechordal plate, and the cause of holoprosencephaly

Holoprosencephaly probably arises in one of two ways (suggested by experiments in animal models).

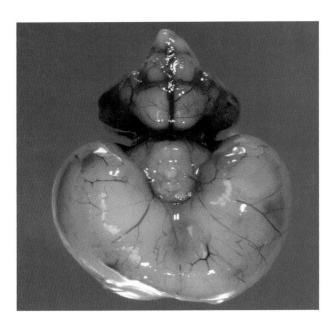

The most severe form of holoprosencephaly, alobar holoprosencephaly, results when the brain fails to separate into the right and left lobes. (*Greenwood Genetic Center*)

Early in the life of an embryo, an area called the prechordal plate forms. The prechordal plate is an area of the embryo which is important for the formation of the brain. The prechordal plate is said to induce brain formation. One can think of the induction process in the following way. If you take a sponge, wet it, and then place a paper towel on top of it, the paper towel will absorb some of the water. In the same way, a signal (the water) goes from the sponge (prechordal plate) to the paper towel (future brain tissue). If the water does not hit the paper towel, brain tissue will not form. This is an extremely simplified version of how the process works, for many reasons. One is that the prechordal plate is not the only "sponge." The notochord is another sponge, which sends out the signal (water) of Shh to form brain and spinal cord and other nervous tissue. Of course, Shh has already been mentioned as a candidate for a gene which causes holoprosencephaly. It turns out it is better than a candidate, because mutations in Shh have been found in some familial forms of holoprosencephaly. Further evidence that Shh plays a role in holoprosencephaly comes from Shh in mice and fish, which both result in holoprosencephaly. Thus, it would be a nice, clear-cut picture if mutations in Shh and Shh alone led to holoprosencephaly, because Shh mutations lead to holoprosencephaly in other animals and Shh is already known to be involved in the formation of neural tissue.

However, Shh is not the only answer. Many persons with holoprosencephaly have perfectly normal Shh genes, and, as previously mentioned, a number of genes have been linked to holoprosencephaly, including genes involved in cholesterol synthesis. So why are so many genes involved?

One possible answer stems from the connection between cholesterol and the Shh signaling pathway. When Shh travels from one tissue to another tissue, there are a number of other genes involved before Shh has its final effect. This process is called signal transduction, and the genes that make it up are part of a signaling pathway. Signal transduction can be compared to a shot in the game of pool. When shooting pool, one must take the cue (Shh), hit the cue ball (another gene; for Shh this would be the gene Patched), and the cue ball goes on to hit the ball that one is interested in sinking (in this case sinking the ball means making a normal brain). Thus, each step depends on the last step and the next step. If one does not have the stick or the cue ball one cannot sink the ball in the pocket. Thus, a number of mutations in genes in the Shh signaling pathway, and not just Shh, could cause holoprosencephaly. Not just that, but other genes involved in cholesterol biosynthesis can have effects on genes in the Shh signaling pathway. Cholesterol appears to affect the function of the gene Patched. In the pool example, a lack of cholesterol would not mean the cue ball is gone, but maybe that the cue ball has a big lump on one side, so the shot is likely to miss.

Another possible answer comes from studies on bone morphogenetic proteins (BMPs) in chickens. Up until now, the problem of holoprosencephaly has been addressed as if it occurs when neural tissue is formed. However, the presence of too much BMP in a chick embryo after the time neural tissue is formed can cause holoprosencephaly. It appears there are two stages that can be interfered with: one that occurs at the time of neural tissue formation involving Shh and another that occurs later involving BMPs. Increased levels of BMPs may cause important neural cells to die. It has been speculated that holoprosencephaly is either a failure to grow neural cells due to failure in Shh pathway, or an excess of neural cells dying possibly due to increased levels of BMPs. Both may end up being true, with some Shh signaling defects early, and BMP mutations later.

Teratogens also cause holoprosencephaly

A **teratogen** is any environmental influence that adversely affects the normal development of the fetus. Teratogens can be skin creams, drugs, or alcohol. Alcohol, when ingested in sufficient amounts during the second week of pregnancy, is thought to lead to some cases of holoprosencephaly. Cytomegalovirus infections in the mother during pregnancy have also been associated with holoprosencephaly. Additionally, in animals, drugs inhibiting cholesterol synthesis have been shown to cause cases of holoprosencephaly. Finally, the drug cyclopamine, which affects the Shh pathway, also causes holoprosencephaly in animals. Cyclopamine was discovered when an abnormally large number of sheep were found to have holoprosencephaly. A local shepherd and scientists determined the drug was found in a fungus called Veratrum californicum.

Demographics

Holoprosencephaly affects males and females at the same rate. Estimates vary on the frequency of the disorder in children with normal chromosomes. The estimates range from one case in every 11,363 births to one case in 53,394 births. It is important to note that this rate of incidence excludes those cases which are caused by **chromosomal abnormalities**, like trisomy 13.

Signs and symptoms

In holoprosencephaly alone, symptoms involve the brain and/or the face and bones of the face and skull. Facial abnormalities exhibit a wide range. In the most severe cases, persons with holoprosencephaly lack eyes and may lack a nose. Less severe is cyclopia, or the presence of a single eye in the middle of the face above the possibly deformed or absent nose. Even less severe are ethmocephaly and cebocephaly, in which the eyes are set close together and the nose is abnormal. In premaxillary agenesis the patient has a midline cleft lip and cleft palate and close-set eyes. If the face is very abnormal, the patient is likely to have alobar holoprosencephaly, the most severe type. In addition to abnormalities of the face, children with alobar holoprosencephaly also have small brains (less than 100g). These children also have small heads unless they have excess cerebrospinal fluid. Excess cerebrospinal fluid can cause the head to be abnormally large.

Persons with holoprosencephaly experience many problems due to brain malformations including in utero or neonatal death. Survivors may experience seizures, problems with muscle control and muscle tone, a delay in growth, problems feeding (choking and gagging or slowness, pauses, and a lack of interest), intestinal gas, constipation, hormone deficiencies from the pituitary, breathing irregularities, and heart rhythm and heart rate abnormalities. These problems are usually least severe in lobar holoprosencephaly and most severe in alobar. Children with holoprosencephaly also experience severe deficiencies in their ability to speak and in their motor skills. An ominous sign that children with holoprosencephaly may exhibit is a sustained (lasting many hours or days) period of irregular breathing and heart rate. This may precede death. However, episodes lasting only minutes are usually followed by a full recovery.

> ## KEY TERMS
>
> **Corpus callosum**—A thick bundle of nerve fibers deep in the center of the forebrain that provides communications between the right and left cerebral hemispheres.
>
> **Craniofacial**—Relating to or involving both the head and the face.
>
> **Induction**—Process where one tissue (the prechordal plate, for example) changes another tissue (for example, changes tissue into neural tissue).
>
> **Neural**—Regarding any tissue with nerves, including the brain, the spinal cord, and other nerves.

Diagnosis

Prenatal ultrasound and computerized tomography can be used to determine whether the fetus has holoprosencephaly and its severity. After birth, physical appearance and/or imaging of the brain can determine a diagnosis of holoprosencephaly. Once a diagnosis of holoprosencephaly has been made, syndromes of which holoprosencephaly is a part must be considered. Forty-one percent of holoprosencephaly cases are thought to have a chromosomal abnormality as the primary cause. Holoprosencephaly is estimated to be found in the context of a larger syndrome in 25% of the remaining patients.

Treatment and management

Although no treatment exists for the underlying disease, symptomatic treatment can reduce the amount of fluid surrounding the brain and assist in feeding. Medical intervention can reduce or eliminate seizures and hormonal deficiencies. However, few treatments exist for the most serious aspects of the disease—breathing and heart arrhythmias (irregular heart rate)—or for the problems associated with developmental delay and poor muscle control. One important aspect of treatment is to help parents understand the effects of the disease and what may be expected from the child. Support groups, like the one listed at the end of this entry, may be important for this purpose. Parents should also be prepared to deal with a large number of health care professionals based on their child's particular needs.

Prognosis

About half of the children born with alobar holoprosencephaly die before the age of four to five months, but a much longer survival time is possible, up to at least 11 years. Children with semilobar and lobar holoprosencephaly may live for any length of time. Depending on the severity of the holoprosencephaly, however, parents should be prepared for differences in their child. For example, children with alobar holoprosencephaly and semilobar holoprosencephaly learn to speak very little, if at all, and children with alobar holoprosencephaly have difficulty even mastering the simple task of reaching and grasping an object. On the other end of the spectrum, children may develop much more normally. It is very important to understand the severity of the disorder to understand the child's abilities and possibilities.

Resources

BOOKS

Sadler, T. W. *Langman's Medical Embryology*. Baltimore: Williams and Williams, 1995, pp. 53-60.

PERIODICALS

Barr, M., and M. Cohen. "Holoprosencephaly survival and performance." *American Journal of Medical Genetics* 89 (1999): 116-120.

ORGANIZATIONS

National Organization for Rare Disorders (NORD). PO Box 8923, New Fairfield, CT 06812-8923. (203) 746-6518 or (800) 999-6673. Fax: (203) 746-6481. <http://www.rarediseases.org>.

Michael V. Zuck, PhD

Holt-Oram syndrome

Definition

Holt-Oram syndrome (HOS) is one of several hereditary conditions characterized by abnormalities of the heart and hands at birth.

Description

HOS involves variable abnormalities of the heart and the hands, or hands and arms. The heart abnormalities may range from disturbances in the electrical conduction pattern of the heart to severe structural defects requiring surgical intervention for survival. The abnormalities of the upper limbs are usually bilateral (occurring on both sides) and asymmetric (not identical from side to side). The severity of the upper limb changes may range from minor signs, such as clinodactyly (inward curvature of the fingers) to disabling defects, such as small or missing bones resulting in very short arms.

Some individuals with HOS are so mildly affected, they do not require any special care or treatment. Other individuals are severely affected and may have significant disability resulting from abnormalities of the arms, or may have limited life spans due to serious heart abnormalities. The signs of HOS are usually limited to the heart and skeleton. HOS does not cause mental retardation.

Some references may use the alternative name of hand-heart syndrome. However, Holt-Oram syndrome is one of many hereditary hand-heart syndromes, so the two names are not truly interchangeable.

Genetic profile

HOS is inherited as an autosomal dominant condition, with variable expressivity (meaning that different individuals with HOS may have very different signs of the condition) and complete penetrance (meaning that every individual that has the genetic change causing the condition has some physical symptoms). An autosomal dominant condition only requires the presence of one abnormal **gene** on a non-sex-linked **chromosome** for the disorder to occur. Some researchers have observed families with incomplete penetrance (meaning that not every individual with the gene abnormality shows symptoms) as well.

In some individuals and families, HOS is caused by mutations in the TBX5 gene located on the long arm of chromosome 12. The TBX5 gene encodes a transcription factor that helps regulate **DNA** expression. Other families with HOS do not show mutations in the TBX5 gene, indicating that mutations in other genes can also cause HOS. HOS families that have TBX5 mutations do not appear to differ significantly from those which do not.

Some patients with HOS have inherited it from an affected parent, whereas others have it as the result of a new change in a gene. The proportion of patients with HOS resulting from new mutations ranges from 8% to 85%. Regardless of where the gene came from, an affected individual has a 50% chance of passing on the gene and the condition to each child. It is difficult to predetermine the severity of symptoms a child may have.

Demographics

Since HOS was first described in 1960, more than 200 cases have been reported in individuals of diverse ethnicity. The incidence of the condition has been estimated as one in 100,000 live births.

Signs and symptoms

All individuals with HOS have some degree of upper limb abnormality, and most (approximately 95%

in familial cases) have defects or dysfunction of the heart. Other body parts and systems are usually not significantly affected by HOS.

Defects of the upper limbs

The limb abnormalities in HOS primarily affect the radial side (the inner or thumb side of the arm/hand). Involvement of the ulnar side (the outer side of the arm/hand, opposite the thumb) may also occur to a lesser degree. In some individuals, the abnormality of the upper limb may be very mild, such as hypoplasia (underdevelopment) of the muscle at the base of the thumb, limited rotation of the arm, or narrow, sloping shoulders. Rarely, severe abnormalities of the upper limbs may be present, resulting in extremely short, "flipper-like" arms. Abnormalities of the upper limb are always bilateral and usually asymmetric. In 90% of patients, the left side is more severely affected.

The thumb is the most commonly affected part of the upper limb in HOS, and is affected in some way in 84% of patients. Some individuals have three phalanges (or bones) in the thumb, resulting in a thumb that can bend in three places, like a finger. In other cases, the thumb may be hypoplastic (underdeveloped). Syndactyly (or skin webbing) may occur between the thumb and index finger.

Abnormalities of the fingers may include hypoplasia, underdevelopment, or absence of one or more fingers. Clinodactyly (inward curvature) of the fifth or "pinky" finger is also common. In some patients, **polydactyly** (extra fingers) has been reported.

The bones of the arms may also be affected by HOS. The radius (the inner bone of the forearm, adjacent to the thumb) may be hypoplastic or even missing. Such patients may have a lesser degree of hypoplasia of the ulna (outer bone of the forearm, opposite the thumb). The upper arm may be short. In rare cases, as noted above, the bones of the arm are dramatically shortened, resulting in a tiny arm.

Individuals with HOS often appear to have narrow, sloping shoulders. This likely results from some degree of hypoplasia of the clavicles (collarbones), as well as decreased musculature which occurs secondarily to bone hypoplasia.

Defects and dysfunction of the heart

The vast majority (95%) of individuals with HOS who have inherited it from an affected parent have heart involvement. Most have a defect in the structure of the heart. In some patients, there is no structural defect in the heart, but abnormalities are present in the pattern of electrical conduction in the heart.

The most common heart abnormalities in people with HOS are septal defects, or holes in the heart. A hole may occur in the wall separating the atria of the heart (atrioseptal defect or ASD), or the wall separating the ventricles of the heart (ventriculoseptal defect or VSD). In rare cases, more severe and complex heart defects may occur, such as hypoplastic left heart (in which the chambers of the left side of the heart are too small to function normally) or tetralogy of fallot (a specific combination of four heart defects). In the case of severe defects, surgical correction is necessary for survival. However, most persons with HOS do not require surgical intervention.

Some individuals with HOS have a cardiac conduction defect, or an abnormal electrical pattern in the heart. The complex motion of the heart requires a system of electrical impulses for coordinated contraction of the muscle fibers. In people with cardiac conduction defects, these electrical impulses may not occur in the normal pattern, resulting in an abnormal heartbeat. In rare cases, this can result in sudden death.

Other defects

Additional skeletal abnormalities occasionally reported in patients with HOS include **scoliosis**, vertebral abnormalities, and minor deformities of the rib cage. Some patients may have abnormalities unrelated to the cardiac or skeletal systems, such as minor eye defects and various birthmarks. It is not clear whether these additional findings are coincidental or part of HOS.

Diagnosis

The diagnosis of HOS is made on the basis of the clinical judgement by a specialist physician, usually a geneticist, following physical examination and review of pertinent tests or studies. Diagnostic criteria may be employed to guide this decision. One commonly used set of criteria for the diagnosis of HOS require that there be 1) defect(s) of the radial side of the hand/arm, as well as 2) septal defect(s) or conduction abnormality of the heart, within one individual or family.

X rays may be necessary to determine involvement of the bones of the upper limb. Diagnosis of structural defects of the heart requires echocardiography, or ultrasound visualization of the heart. Conduction defects of the heart are identified via electrocardiography (EKG). This test involves measuring the electrical activity of the heart and charting the electrical impulses associated with each heartbeat.

Testing to identify changes in the TBX5 gene may be offered, but is not necessary for a diagnosis of HOS. Identification of a change or alteration in the TBX5 gene could provide confirmation of the clinical diagnosis, prenatal diagnosis, or assist in the diagnosis of at risk family members who are minimally affected. Prenatal screening in a pregnancy at-risk for HOS may also be attempted by fetal ultrasonography targeted toward the fetal arms and heart. However, a normal ultrasound examination does not eliminate the possibility of HOS in the unborn baby.

Treatment and management

There is no specific treatment for HOS. Surgery or other treatment may be recommended for cardiac abnormalities. Referral for **genetic counseling** should be considered for families in which HOS has been diagnosed.

Some patients with HOS have life-threatening heart defects that require surgical correction for survival. The most complex heart defects may require multiple surgeries. However, many individuals have asymptomatic or no heart abnormalities. When life-threatening irregularities are present in the heartbeat, a pacemaker device is inserted. These devices correct the abnormal electrical patterns which cause the irregularities and stimulate the heart to beat normally.

Because eye abnormalities have been occasionally reported in HOS, an eye examination may be recommended at the time of diagnosis.

Prognosis

The prognosis for individuals with HOS depends on the severity of associated birth defects, which varies considerably. Positive correlation has been reported between the severity of upper limb and heart defects. In other words, individuals who have more severe hand or arm involvement may be more likely to have a symptomatic heart defect. People who have HOS resulting from new mutations are more likely to have severe defects than those who have inherited it from a parent.

In some cases, HOS may lead to death in early infancy due to multiple septal defects or other complex structural abnormalities of the heart. Severe and unrecognized disturbances of the cardiac conduction system can lead to sudden death. In other cases, heart involvement is limited to asymptomatic irregular heartbeat requiring no treatment.

Several unusual findings have been described with respect to the severity of HOS in families. Affected women have been reported to have a higher chance of having a severely affected child than do affected men. The severity of defects associated with HOS has also been reported to increase with successive generations. The possible explanations for these observations are not known.

KEY TERMS

Atria—The two chambers at the top of the heart, where blood from the lungs or body pools before entering one of the ventricles.

Polydactyly—The presence of extra fingers or toes.

Radius—One of the two bones of the forearm, the one adjacent to the base of the thumb.

Septal defect—A hole in the heart.

Syndactyly—Abnormal webbing of the skin between the fingers or toes.

Ulna—One of the two bones of the forearm, the one opposite the thumb.

Ventricles—One of the chambers (small cavities) of the heart through which blood circulates. The heart is divided into the right and left ventricles.

Resources

BOOKS

Jones, Kenneth L. *Smith's Recognizable Patterns of Human Malformation.* Philadelphia, PA: W.B. Saunders Company, 1997.

PERIODICALS

Newbury, R. A., R. Leanage, J. A. Raeburn, and I. D. Young. "Holt-Oram Syndrome: A clinical genetic study." *Journal of Medical Genetics* (April 1996): 300-307.

Jennifer A. Roggenbuck, MS, CGC

Homocystinuria

Definition

The term homocystinuria is actually a description of a biochemical abnormality, as opposed to the name of a particular disease, although many refer to homocystinuria as a disease. Homocystinuria refers to elevated levels of homocysteine in the urine. This can be caused by different biochemical abnormalities and in fact there are at least eight different **gene** changes that are known to cause excretion of too much homocysteine in the urine. The best known and most common cause of homocystinuria is the lack of cystathionine b-synthase. For the purpose of this entry we will be referring to "classical homocystinuria" that is caused by cystathionine b-synthase deficiency (CBS deficiency).

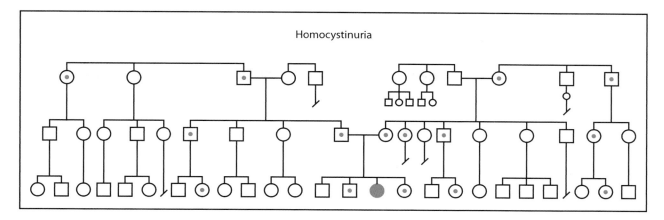

Homocystinuria

(Gale Group)

Description

In Northern Ireland in the early 1960s, homocystinuria was described in individuals who were mentally retarded. Soon after that, it was shown that the cause of the homocystinuria was a deficiency of the enzyme cystathionine b-synthase. This condition is an inborn error of metabolism, meaning that the cause for this condition is present from birth and it affects metabolism.

Metabolism is the sum of all of the chemical processes that take place in the body. Metabolism includes both construction (anabolism) and break down (catabolism) of important components. For example, amino acids are the building blocks for proteins and are converted to proteins through many steps in the process of anabolism. In contrast, proteins can also be broken down into amino acids through many steps in the process of catabolism. These processes require multiple steps that involve different substances called enzymes. These enzymes are proteins that temporarily combine with reactants and in the process, allow these chemical processes to occur quickly. Since practically all of the reactions in the body use enzymes, they are essential for life. At any point along the way, if an enzyme is missing, the particular process that requires that enzyme would not be able to be completed as usual. Such a situation can lead to disease.

Homocysteine is involved with the catabolism of methionine. Methionine is an essential amino acid. Amino acids are the building blocks of proteins. Over 100 amino acids are found in nature, but only 22 are found in humans. Of these 22 amino acids, eight are essential for human life, including methionine. Methionine comes from dietary protein. Generally, the amount of methionine that is consumed is more than the body needs. Excess methionine is converted to homocysteine, which is then metabolized into cystathionine; cystathionine is then converted to cysteine. The cysteine is excreted in the urine. Each step along this pathway is carried out by a specific enzyme and that enzyme may even

require help from vitamin co-factors to be able to complete the job. For example, the conversion of homocysteine to cystathionine by cystathionine b-synthase requires vitamin B6 (pyridoxine). If cystathionine b-synthase is missing, then homocysteine cannot be broken down into cystathionine and cysteine, and instead, homocysteine accumulates and the elevated levels of homocysteine and methionine can be found in the blood. Also, decreased levels of cysteine can be found in the blood. Elevated levels of homocysteine lead to a disease state that, if untreated, affects multiple systems, including the central nervous system, the eyes, the skeleton, and the vascular system.

Genetic profile

Classical homocystinuria or cystathionine b-synthase (CBS) deficiency is an autosomal recessive condition. This means that in order to have the condition, an individual must inherit one copy of the gene for CBS deficiency from each parent. An individual who has only one copy of the gene is called a carrier for the condition. In most cases of autosomal recessive **inheritance** a carrier for a condition does not have any signs, symptoms, or effects of the condition. This is not necessarily the case with CBS deficiency. Individuals who are carriers for CBS deficiency may have levels of homocysteine that are elevated enough to increase the risk for thromboembolic events. So, although carriers may not exhibit obvious physical signs or symptoms of the condition, they may have clinical effects of elevated levels of homocysteine, such as vascular or cardiovascular disease. A carrier for CBS deficiency can have vascular complications, especially if they are also carriers for other clotting disorders such as **factor V Leiden thrombophilia**.

When two parents are carriers for CBS deficiency, there is a one in four or 25% chance, with each pregnancy, for having a child with CBS deficiency. They

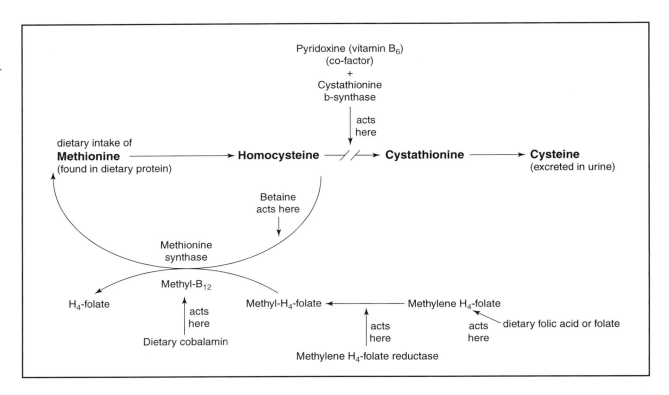

Flow chart for the chemical processes involved in the breakdown of methionine, an essential amino acid found in dietary protein. Homocystinuria results when the enzyme cystathionine b-synthase is missing and does not break down homocystine, a converted form of excess methionine. The elevated levels of methionine and homocystine that result from the failure of homocystine to break down into cystathionine and cystine causes a disease state that affects multiple body systems. (*Gale Group*)

have a one in two or 50% chance for having a child who is a carrier for the condition and a one in four or 25% chance for having a child who is neither affected nor a carrier for CBS deficiency.

The gene for CBS has been mapped to the long arm of **chromosome** 21, specifically at 21q22.3. Approximately 100 different disease-associated gene changes or alterations of the CBS gene have been identified. The two most frequently encountered gene changes are 1278T and G307S. G307S is the most common cause of CBS deficiency in Irish patients and the 1278T gene is the most common cause of CBS deficiency in Italian patients.

Demographics

The worldwide frequency of individuals with CBS deficiency who are identified through newborn screening and clinical detection is approximately one in 350,000; however, newborn screening may be missing half of affected patients and thus the worldwide incidence may be as high as one in 180,000. One study showed that by lowering the cutoff level of methionine from 2 mg per deciliter to 1 mg per deciliter in newborn screening, detection of the deficiency increased from

one in 275,000 to one in 157,000. The incidence of CBS deficiency in the United States population is one in 58,000; in the Irish population it is estimated to be one in 65,000; in the Italian population it is one in 55,000 and in the Japanese population it is one in 889,000. CBS deficiency has been seen in persons of many different ethnic origins living in the United States.

Signs and symptoms

Individuals who have CBS deficiency tend to be tall and thin with thinning and lengthening of the bones. They tend to have a long, narrow face and high arched palate (roof of the mouth). The thinning and lengthening of the long bones causes individuals to be tall and thin by the time they reach late childhood. Their fingers tend to be long and thin as well (referred to as arachnodactyly). They can have curvature of the spine, called **scoliosis**. Their chest can be sunken in (pectus excavatum) or it may protrude out (pectus carinatum). **Osteoporosis** may occur. Also, they tend to have stiff joints. CBS deficiency affects the eyes, causing dislocated lenses and nearsightedness (**myopia**). Untreated individuals or those individuals who do not respond to treatment develop mental retardation or learning disabilities. Affected individuals may also develop psychiatric problems. These psychiatric problems may include **depression**, chronic behavior problems, chronic obsessive-compulsive disorder, and personality disorders. The most frequent cause of death associated with CBS deficiency is blood clots that form in veins and arteries. These are known as thromboembolisms, and include deep vein thrombosis (blood clots that form in the deep veins of the legs, etc.), pulmonary embolus (blood clots that form in the lungs), and strokes. Thromboembolism can occur even in childhood. When thromboembolism does occur in childhood, CBS deficiency should always be considered as a cause for the thromboembolic events. These thromboembolic events can occur in any part of the body. Lastly, another complication of CBS deficiency is severe premature arteriosclerosis (hardening of the arteries).

Diagnosis

Approximately 50% of individuals who have CBS deficiency are diagnosed by newborn screening because they have an elevated level of methionine in their blood. The reason for performing newborn screening is so that infants affected with **genetic disorders** can be identified early enough to be treated. The screening is done by collecting blood from a pin-prick on the baby's heel prior to leaving the hospital, but at least 24 hours after birth. For CBS deficiency, the screening test checks for elevated levels of methionine. If the levels are elevated then follow-up testing to verify the diagnosis is performed. There are other disorders of methionine metabolism, and follow-up testing determines the underlying cause of the positive newborn screen.

If not identified at newborn screening, diagnosis is made by identifying low levels of cysteine in blood and urine. Measurements of the amount of methionine and homocysteine produced by cultured blood cells (lymphoblasts) or cultured skin cells (fibroblasts) also can confirm the diagnosis of CBS deficiency.

DNA testing is available for families in which a gene alteration is identified. Potentially, this makes prenatal diagnosis by chorionic villus sampling (CVS) and **amniocentesis** available for families who have had a previously affected child and in which two identifiable gene alterations for CBS deficiency have been detected. Prenatal diagnosis is also possible by measuring the amount of enzyme activity in cultured cells grown from amniotic fluid.

CBS deficiency has several features in common with **Marfan syndrome**, including the tall, thin build with long limbs and long, thin fingers (arachnodactyly),

a sunken-in chest (pectus excavatum), and dislocated lenses. The dislocated lens in Marfan syndrome tends to be dislocated upward; the tendency for the lens dislocation is to be downward in CBS deficiency. Also, individuals who have Marfan syndrome tend to have lens dislocation from birth (congenital) whereas individuals who have CBS deficiency have not been identified to have lens dislocation before 2 years of age.

Treatment and management

The first choice of therapy for patients with CBS deficiency is administration of pyridoxine (vitamin B6). Vitamin B6 is the cofactor for the cystathionine b-synthase reaction. Potentially, some individuals who have CBS deficiency are not missing the enzyme, but rather have an enzyme that is unable to perform its job. The addition of pyridoxine can help to push the reaction along and thus help to reduce the levels of homocysteine and methionine in the blood. Information suggests that approximately 50% of patients with CBS deficiency respond to high doses of pyridoxine (pyridoxine responsive) and show a significant reduction in levels of homocysteine in the blood. Patients who do not respond to pyridoxine treatment (pyridoxine non-responsive) tend to be more severely affected than the patients who do respond. Those non-responding patients are treated with combinations of folic acid, hydroxycobalamin, and betaine, which stimulate the conversion of homocysteine back to methionine. The reason that the addition of folic acid can help, is because within the methylene H4-folate molecule (MTHFR), there is a molecule known as flavin adenine dinucleotide or FAD. The FAD molecule binds to the MTHFR molecule and helps with the conversion of homocysteine to methionine. Increased levels of folates help bind FAD more tightly to MTHFR, protect the enzyme against heat inactivation, and allow the homocysteine to methionine conversion pathway to proceed. Betaine and cobalamin also help in the conversion of homocysteine to methionine by acting as cofactors. The rationale behind this method of treatment is that although the methionine levels are raised, the net drop in homocysteine is beneficial as it appears that the elevated levels of homocysteine are what cause ectopia lentis, osteoporosis, mental deficiency, and thromboembolic events.

It appears that the addition of dietary betaine in B6-responsive patients is also beneficial. Homocysteine that is not metabolized to cysteine is converted back to methionine in a reaction that uses betaine, so the addition of betaine may help to make this reaction occur and thus reduce the levels of homocysteine.

Other treatments include protein restriction, specifically a low methionine diet with the addition of extra cysteine. Dietary treatment includes avoidance of all high protein foods throughout life, with the use of a nutritional supplement. Special formulas for infants are available. The reasoning behind this is to reduce the methionine and homocysteine levels that accumulate and supplement the low levels of cysteine.

The occurrence of clinically apparent thromboembolism depends upon the age of the affected individual and whether or not he/she responds to pyridoxine treatment. In one study, untreated pyridoxine-responsive patients were at little risk for a thromboembolic event until age 12. After age 12, the risk for thromboembolism increased. By age 20, patients who would have been responsive to pyridoxine had a 25% cumulative risk for a thromboembolic event. In comparison, individuals with CBS deficiency who were untreated and not responsive to pyridoxine treatment had a similar cumulative risk for a thromboembolic event by age 15.

In reference to the two common CBS gene alterations, CBS deficiency caused by the 1278T gene change is pyridoxine responsive. CBS deficiency caused by the G307S gene tends to be pyridoxine non-responsive; however this is not always the case as some individuals with the G307S gene change are pyridoxine responsive.

Very little is known about the risks to an unborn child of a mother with pyridoxine non-responsive CBS deficiency. There have been numerous reports of healthy children born to women and men who have pyridoxine responsive CBS deficiency, however only two reports of children born to pyridoxine non-responsive women have been reported and one had multiple birth defects that may have been related to the mother's condition. Potentially, the mother's elevated levels of homocysteine can cause problems for a developing baby. This could be similar to the process by which infants of mothers who have **phenylketonuria** are affected by the elevated levels of phenylalanine if their mothers are not being treated with dietary restriction during pregnancy.

Prognosis

Untreated CBS deficiency leads to mental retardation, lens dislocation, and a decreased life expectancy because of complications associated with blood clots. If untreated from early infancy, approximately 20% of affected patients will have seizures. If treated from birth, prevention or long term delay of the complications of CBS deficiency can be expected.

Resources

BOOKS

Scriver, C. R., A. L. Beaudet, W. S. Sly, and D. Valle, eds. *The Metabolic Basis of Inherited Disease.* 6th ed. New York: McGraw-Hill Medical Publishing Division, 1989.

ORGANIZATIONS

National Organization for Rare Disorders (NORD). PO Box 8923, New Fairfield, CT 06812-8923. (203) 746-6518 or (800) 999-6673. Fax: (203) 746-6481. <http://www.rarediseases.org>.

WEBSITES

Climb: Children Living with Inherited Metabolic Diseases Support Group. <http://www.climb.org.uk>.

Renee A. Laux, MS

Homogentisic acid oxidose deficiency *see* Alkaptonuria

Human Genome Project

Definition

The Human Genome Project (HGP) was an international project to sequence the **DNA** of the human genome. The sequencing work was conducted in many laboratories around the world, but the majority of the work was done by five institutions: the Whitehead Institute for Medical Research in Massachusetts (WIMR), the Baylor College of Medicine in Texas, the University of Washington, the Joint Genome Institute in California, and the Sanger Centre near Cambridge in the United Kingdom. Most of the funding for these centers was provided by the United States National Institutes of Health and Department of Energy, and the Wellcome Trust, a charitable foundation in the United Kingdom.

Description

Completely sequencing the human genome was first suggested at a conference in Alta, Utah, in 1984. The conference was convened by the U.S. Department of Energy, which was concerned with measuring the mutation rate of human DNA when exposed to low-level radiation, similar to conditions after an attack by nuclear weapons. The technology to make such measurements did not exist at the time, and the sequence of the genome was one step required for this aim to become possible. The genome was estimated to be 3000Mb long, however, and sequencing it seemed an arduous task, especially using the sequencing technology of the time. If most of the DNA was "junk" (not coding for genes), scientists assumed that they could speed the process along by targeting specific genes for sequencing. This could be done by sequencing complementary DNAs (cDNA), which are derived from mRNAs used to code for proteins in the cell. Despite several advocates for this method, it was decided that the whole genome would be sequenced, with a 2005 target completion date. Goals for the Human Genome Project included identifying all of the approximately 20,000–25,000 genes in human DNA; determine the sequence of the three billion base pairs that make up human DNA; store this information in retrievable databases; and address the ethical, legal, and social issues that would inevitably arise from the project. The Human Genome Project quickly became the world's premier science project for biology, involving large factory-like laboratories rather than small laboratories of independent geneticists.

The strategy employed by the HGP involved three stages, and is termed hierarchical shotgun sequencing. The first stage involved generating physical and genetic maps of the human genome. The second stage was placing clones from a genomic library onto these maps. The third stage was fragmenting these genomic clones into smaller overlapping clones (shotgun cloning), which were a more suitable size for sequencing. Then, the complete sequence of each **chromosome** could be reconstructed by assembling the fragments of sequence that overlapped with each other to generate the sequence of the genomic clone. The sequence of each genomic clone could then be fitted together using the assembly (contig) of genomic clones on the genetic and physical map.

Although the ultimate aim was high-quality sequence of the human genome, it was recognized that the genetic and physical maps generated by the first stage of the HGP would be by themselves very useful for genetic research. The first generation physical map was constructed by screening a yeast artificial chromosome (YAC) genomic library to isolate YACs, and overlaps were identified by restriction enzyme digest "fingerprints" and STS content

mapping. These STSs were sequenced around the highly polymorphic CA-repeat markers (microsatellites) that were used to generate the genetic map. Genetic maps were also constructed. These use recombination between markers in families to deduce the distance separating and order of these markers. The first human genetic map used restriction fragment length polymorphisms (RFLPs) as markers, which only have two alleles per marker, but common microsatellites were used to create a high-resolution genetic map.

The second stage of human genome sequencing was made simpler by the development of bacterial artificial chromosomes (BACs), cloning vectors that could carry up to 150kb of DNA. Before then, it was assumed that a contig of YACs and cosmids, carrying up to 2Mb and 40kb of DNA, respectively, would be assembled. These two types of genomic clone were found to be liable to rearrangement; the DNA in the vector could be in chunks that were not necessarily in the same order as in the genome. The BAC vector did not rearrange DNA, and could carry more DNA than many other types of genomic clone.

The third stage was made easier by development of high-throughput DNA sequencing and affordable computing power to enable reassembly of the sequence fragments. It was these developments that led to the idea of whole genome shotgun sequencing of the human genome. In contrast to the HGP plan involving the use of genetic contigs and physical maps as a framework for genomic clones and sequence, scientists suggested that the whole genome could be fragmented into small chunks for sequencing, and then reassembled using overlap between fragment sequences (whole-genome shotgun sequencing). This required large amounts of computing power to generate the correct assembly, but was considerably faster than the HGP approach. Many scientists did not believe that this method would assemble the genome properly, and suggested that overlap between small fragments could not be the only guide to assembly, because the genome contained many repeated DNA sequences. However, American biochemist J. Craig Venter believed the method could work, and formed Celera, a private company that would sequence the human genome before the HGP.

Celera demonstrated that the whole-genome shotgun method would work by sequencing the genome of a model organism, the fruit fly *Drosophila melanogaster*. Despite the successful sequencing of the fly, many people were still skeptical that the method would be successful for the bigger human genome. The publicly funded HGP, in light of Celera's competition, decided to concentrate, like Celera, on a draft of the human genome sequence (3× coverage—that is, each nucleotide has been sequenced an average of three times), before generating a more accurate map of 8× coverage. Celera had an advantage, because the HGP had agreed to release all its data as it was generated on to a freely accessible database, as part of the Bermuda rules (named after the location of a series of meetings during the early stages of the HGP). This allowed Celera to use HGP data to link its sequence fragments with the BAC contigs and genetic/physical maps.

The human genome draft sequence of both groups were published in February 2001 by Celera and the HGP consortium in the journals *Science* and *Nature*, respectively. Celera had imposed restrictions on access to its genomic data, and this was a source of disagreement between the private company and the HGP. Celera scientists argue that their methods are cheaper and quicker than the HGP framework method, but HGP scientists, in turn, argue that Celera's assembly would not have been possible without the HGP data. No matter who eventually takes credit, the finalized complete sequence was completed in 2003.

For human geneticists in general, and medical researchers in particular, the genome sequence is abundantly useful. The ability to identify genes, single nucleotide polymorphisms, from a database search speeds up research. Previously, mapping and finding (positional cloning) a **gene** would take several years of research, a task which now takes several minutes. The investment in the sequencing centers will continue to be of use, with a mouse sequencing project underway, and many genomes of pathogenic bacteria sequenced.

This study of genomes and parts of genomes has been called genomics. The medical benefits of genomics were emphasized throughout the project partly to ensure continuing government support. These benefits are not likely to be immediate or direct, but the genome sequence will have a significant effect on pharmacogenomics, which studies how genetic variants affect how well a drug can treat a disease. In addition, through pharmacogenomics it is hoped that there will be a substantial increase in the design of more effective drugs with lower toxicity by tailoring drug treatment to a patient's individual genetically determined drug metabolism.

The HGP has also given scientists more powerful tools in elucidating the determinants of **cancer** susceptibility. In many ways, cancer can be considered as a complex genetic trait, where the interaction between a person's genes and environment interact in such a way to confer a variable degree of risk of developing cancer. Through information gained from the HGP, a significant amount of information has been gleaned about high-penetrance genes that are responsible for some familial aggregations of cancer, such as the BRCA mutations and their association with **breast cancer**.

The impact on nonscientists has been substantial, with the HGP suggested to be the ultimate in self knowledge.

Resources

PERIODICALS

Taramelli, R., and F. Acquati. "The Human Genome Project and the Discovery of Genetic Determinants of Cancer Susceptibility." *European Journal of Cancer* 40 (2004): 2537–2543.

Van Omen, G. J. B. "The Human Genome Project and the Future of Diagnostics, Treatment, and Prevention." *Journal of Inherited Metabolic Disease* 25 (2002): 183–188.

Edward J. Hollox, PhD
Edward R. Rosick, DO, MPH, MS

Hunter syndrome *see*
Mucopolysaccharidosis type II

Huntington chorea *see*
Huntington disease

Huntington disease

Definition

Huntington disease is a progressive, neurodegenerative disease causing uncontrolled physical movements and mental deterioration. The disease was discovered by George Huntington of Pomeroy, Ohio, who first described a hereditary movement disorder.

Description

Huntington disease is also called Huntington chorea, from the Greek word for "dance," referring to the involuntary movements that develop as the disease progresses. It is occasionally referred to as "Woody Guthrie disease" for the American folk singer who died from it. Huntington disease (HD) causes progressive loss of cells in areas of the brain responsible for some aspects of movement control and mental abilities. A person with HD gradually develops abnormal movements and changes in cognition (thinking), behavior and personality.

Demographics

The onset of symptoms of HD is usually between the ages of 30 and 50; although in 10% of cases, onset is in late childhood or early adolescence. Approximately

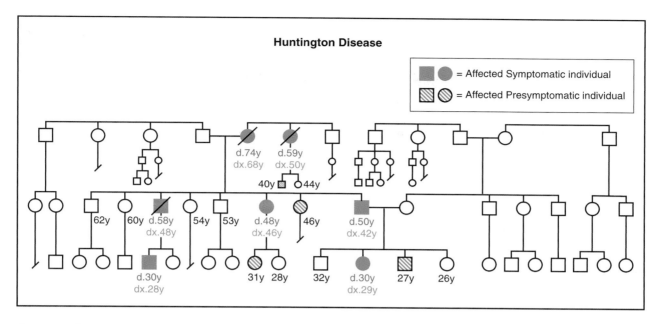

Huntington Disease

◼ ● = Affected Symptomatic individual

▨ ◒ = Affected Presymptomatic individual

(Gale Group)

30,000 people in the United States are affected by HD, with another 150,000 at risk for developing this disorder. The frequency of HD is four to seven per 100,000 persons.

Genetic profile

Huntington disease is caused by a change in the **gene** (an inherited unit which contains a code for a protein) of unknown function called huntingtin. The nucleotide codes (building blocks of genes arranged in a specific code that chemically form proteins), contain CAG repeats (40 or more of these repeat sequences). The extra building blocks in the huntingtin gene cause the protein that is made from it to contain an extra section as well. It is currently thought that this extra protein section, or portion, interacts with other proteins in brain cells where it occurs, and that this interaction ultimately leads to cell death.

The HD gene is a dominant gene, meaning that only one copy of it is needed to develop the disease. HD affects both males and females. The gene may be inherited from either parent, who will also be affected by the disease. A parent with the HD gene has a 50% chance of passing it on to each offspring. The chances of passing on the HD gene are not affected by the results of previous pregnancies.

Signs and symptoms

The symptoms of HD fall into three categories: motor or movement symptoms, personality and behavioral changes, and cognitive decline. The severity and rate of progression of each type of symptom can vary from person to person.

Early motor symptoms include restlessness, twitching and a desire to move about. Handwriting may become less controlled, and coordination may decline. Later symptoms include:

- Dystonia, or sustained abnormal postures, including facial grimaces, a twisted neck, or an arched back.

- Chorea, in which involuntary jerking, twisting or writhing motions become pronounced.

- Slowness of voluntary movements, inability to regulate the speed or force of movements, inability to initiate movement, and slowed reactions.

- Difficulty speaking and swallowing due to involvement of the throat muscles.

- Localized or generalized weakness and impaired balance ability.

- Rigidity, especially in late-stage disease.

Personality and behavioral changes include **depression**, irritability, anxiety and apathy. The person with HD may become impulsive, aggressive, or socially withdrawn.

Cognitive changes include loss of ability to plan and execute routine tasks, slowed thought, and impaired or inappropriate judgment. Short-term memory loss usually occurs, although long-term memory is usually not affected. The person with late-stage HD usually retains knowledge of his environment and recognizes family members or other loved ones, despite severe cognitive decline.

Diagnosis

Diagnosis of HD begins with a detailed medical history, and a thorough physical and neurological exam. Family medical history is very important. Magnetic resonance imaging (MRI) or computed tomography scan (CT scan) imaging may be performed to look for degeneration in the basal ganglia and cortex, the brain regions most affected in HD.

A genetic test is available for confirmation of the clinical diagnosis. In this test, a small blood sample is taken, and **DNA** from it is analyzed to determine the CAG repeat number. A person with a repeat number of 30 or below will not develop HD. A person with a repeat number between 35 and 40 may not develop the disease within their normal life span. A person with a very high number of repeats (70 or above) is likely to develop the juvenile-onset form. An important part of **genetic testing** is extensive **genetic counseling**.

Prenatal testing is available. A person at risk for HD (a child of an affected person) may obtain fetal testing without determining whether she herself carries the gene. This test, also called a linkage test, examines the pattern of DNA near the gene in both parent and fetus, but does not analyze for the triple nucleotide repeat (CAG). If the DNA patterns do not match, the fetus can be assumed not to have inherited the HD gene, even if present in the parent. A pattern match indicates the fetus probably has the same genetic makeup of the at-risk parent.

Treatment and management

There is no cure for HD, nor any treatment that can slow the rate of progression. Treatment is aimed at reducing the disability caused by the motor impairments, and treating behavioral and emotional symptoms.

Physical therapy is used to maintain strength and compensate for lost strength and balance. Stretching and range of motion exercises help minimize contracture, or muscle shortening, a result of weakness and disuse. The physical therapist also advises on the use of mobility aids such as walkers or wheelchairs.

Motor symptoms may be treated with drugs, although some studies suggest that anti-chorea treatment rarely improves function. Chorea (movements caused by abnormal muscle contractions) can be suppressed with drugs that deplete dopamine, an important brain chemical regulating movement. As HD progresses, nat-ural dopamine levels fall, leading to loss of chorea and an increase in rigidity and movement slowness. Treatment with L-dopa (which resupplies dopamine) may be of some value. Frequent reassessment of the effectiveness and appropriateness of any drug therapy is necessary.

Occupational therapy is used to design compensatory strategies for lost abilities in the activities of daily living, such as eating, dressing, and grooming. The occupational therapist advises on modifications to the home that improve safety, accessibility, and comfort.

Difficulty swallowing may be lessened by preparation of softer foods, blending food in an electric blender, and taking care to eat slowly and carefully. Use of a straw for all liquids can help. The potential for choking on food is a concern, especially late in the disease progression. Caregivers should learn the use of the Heimlich maneuver. In addition, passage of food into the airways increases the risk for pneumonia. A gastric feeding tube may be needed, if swallowing becomes too difficult or dangerous.

Speech difficulties may be partially compensated by using picture boards or other augmentative communication devices. Loss of cognitive ability affects both speech production and understanding. A speech-language pathologist can work with the family to develop simplified and more directed communication strategies, including speaking slowly, using simple words, and repeating sentences exactly.

Early behavioral changes, including depression and anxiety, may respond to drug therapy. Maintaining a calm, familiar, and secure environment is useful as the disease progresses. Support groups for both patients and caregivers form an important part of treatment.

Experimental transplant of fetal brain tissue has been attempted in a few HD patients. Early results show some promise, but further trials are needed to establish the effectiveness of this treatment.

Prognosis

The person with Huntington disease may be able to maintain a job for several years after diagnosis, despite the increase in disability. Loss of cognitive functions and increase in motor and behavioral symptoms eventually prevent the person with HD from continuing employment. Ultimately, severe motor symptoms prevent mobility. Death usually occurs 15–20 years after disease onset. Progressive weakness of respiratory and swallowing muscles leads to increased risk of respiratory infection and choking, the most common causes of death. Future research in this area is currently focusing on nerve cell transplantation.

KEY TERMS

Cognition—The mental activities associated with thinking, learning, and memory.

Computed tomography (CT) scan—An imaging procedure that produces a three-dimensional picture of organs or structures inside the body, such as the brain.

Deoxyribonucleic acid (DNA)—The genetic material in cells that holds the inherited instructions for growth, development, and cellular functioning.

Heimlich maneuver—An action designed to expel an obstructing piece of food from the throat. It is performed by placing the fist on the abdomen, underneath the breastbone, grasping the fist with the other hand (from behind), and thrusting it inward and upward.

Neurodegenerative—Relating to degeneration of nerve tissues.

Resources

BOOK

Watts R. L., and W. C. Koller, eds. *Movement Disorders*. New York: McGraw-Hill, 1997.

ORGANIZATION

Huntington Disease Society of America. 140 W. 22nd St. New York, NY 10011. (800) 345-HDSA.

Laith Gulli, MD

Hurler syndrome *see*
  Mucopolysaccharidosis type I

Hutchinson-Gilford progeria syndrome
  see **Progeria**

Hydrocephalus

Definition

Hydrocephalus is an abnormal expansion of cavities (ventricles) within the brain that is caused by the accumulation of cerebrospinal fluid. Hydrocephalus comes from two Greek words: *hydros* means water and *cephalus* means head.

There are two main varieties of hydrocephalus: congenital and acquired. An obstruction of the cerebral aqueduct (aqueductal stenosis) is the most frequent cause of congenital hydrocephalus. Acquired hydrocephalus may result from **spina bifida**, intraventricular hemorrhage, meningitis, head trauma, tumors, and cysts.

Description

Hydrocephalus is the result of an imbalance between the formation and drainage of cerebrospinal fluid (CSF). Approximately 500 milliliters (about a pint) of CSF is formed within the brain each day, by epidermal cells in structures collectively called the choroid plexus. These cells line chambers called ventricles that are located within the brain. There are four ventricles in a human brain. Once formed, CSF usually circulates among all the ventricles before it is absorbed and returned to the circulatory system. The normal adult volume of circulating CSF is 150 ml. The CSF turn over rate is more than three times per day. Because production is independent of absorption, reduced absorption causes CSF to accumulate within the ventricles.

There are three different types of hydrocephalus. In the most common variety, reduced absorption occurs when one or more passages connecting the ventricles become blocked. This prevents the movement of CSF to its drainage sites in the subarachnoid space just inside the skull. This type of hydrocephalus is called "noncommunicating." In a second type, a reduction in the absorption rate is caused by damage to the absorptive tissue. This variety is called "communicating hydrocephalus."

Both of these types lead to an elevation of the CSF pressure within the brain. This increased pressure pushes aside the soft tissues of the brain. This squeezes and distorts them. This process also results in damage to these tissues. In infants whose skull bones have not yet fused, the intracranial pressure is partly relieved by expansion of the skull, so that symptoms may not be as dramatic. Both types of elevated-pressure hydrocephalus may occur from infancy to adulthood.

A third type of hydrocephalus, called "normal pressure hydrocephalus," is marked by ventricle enlargement without an apparent increase in CSF pressure. This type affects mainly the elderly.

Hydrocephalus has a variety of causes including:

- congenital brain defects
- hemorrhage, either into the ventricles or the subarachnoid space
- infection of the central nervous system (syphilis, herpes, meningitis, encephalitis, or mumps)
- tumor

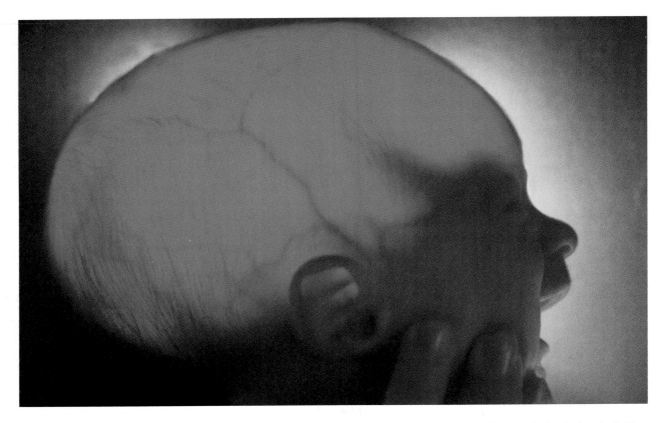

Shining a bright light behind an infant with hydrocephalus, one can observe the excessive fluid accumulation in the skull. (*Corbis Corporation, Bellevue*)

Genetic profile

Hydrocephalus that is congenital (present at birth) is thought to be caused by a complex interaction of genetic and environmental factors. Aqueductal stenosis, an obstruction of the cerebral aqueduct, is the most frequent cause of congenital hydrocephalus. The genetic factors are not well understood. According to the British Association for Spina Bifida and Hydrocephalus, in very rare circumstances, hydrocephalus is due to hereditary factors, which might affect future generations.

Demographics

Hydrocephalus is believed to occur in approximately 1–2 of every 1,000 live births. The incidence of adult onset hydrocephalus is not known. There is no known way to prevent hydrocephalus.

Signs and symptoms

Signs and symptoms of elevated-pressure hydrocephalus include:

• headache

• nausea and vomiting, especially in the morning

• lethargy

• disturbances in walking (gait)

• double vision

• subtle difficulties in learning and memory

• delay in children achieving developmental milestones

Irritability is the most common sign of hydrocephalus in infants. If this is not treated, it may lead to lethargy. Bulging of the fontanelles, or the soft spots between the skull bones, may also be an early sign. When hydrocephalus occurs in infants, fusion of the skull bones is prevented. This leads to abnormal expansion of the skull.

Symptoms of normal pressure hydrocephalus include **dementia**, gait abnormalities, and incontinence (involuntary urination or bowel movements).

Diagnosis

Imaging studies—x ray, computed tomography scan (CT scan), ultrasound, and especially magnetic resonance imaging (MRI)—are used to assess the presence and location of obstructions, as well as changes in brain tissue that have occurred as a result of the hydrocephalus.

KEY TERMS

Cerebral ventricles—Spaces in the brain that are located between portions of the brain and filled with cerebrospinal fluid.

Cerebrospinal fluid—Fluid that circulates throughout the cerebral ventricles and around the spinal cord within the spinal canal.

Choroid plexus—Specialized cells located in the ventricles of the brain that produce cerebrospinal fluid.

Fontanelle—One of several "soft spots" on the skull where the developing bones of the skull have yet to fuse.

Shunt—A small tube placed in a ventricle of the brain to direct cerebrospinal fluid away from the blockage into another part of the body.

Stenosis—The constricting or narrowing of an opening or passageway.

Subarachnoid space—The space between two membranes surrounding the brain, the arachnoid and pia mater.

Lumbar puncture (spinal tap) may be performed to aid in determining the cause when infection is suspected.

Treatment and management

The primary method of treatment for both elevated and normal pressure hydrocephalus is surgical installation of a shunt. A shunt is a tube connecting the ventricles of the brain to an alternative drainage site, usually the abdominal cavity. A shunt contains a one-way valve to prevent reverse flow of fluid. In some cases of noncommunicating hydrocephalus, a direct connection can be made between one of the ventricles and the subarachnoid space, allowing drainage without a shunt.

Installation of a shunt requires lifelong monitoring by the recipient or family members for signs of recurring hydrocephalus due to obstruction or failure of the shunt. Other than monitoring, no other management activity is usually required.

Some drugs may postpone the need for surgery by inhibiting the production of CSF. These include acetazolamide and furosemide. Other drugs that are used to delay surgery include glycerol, digoxin, and isosorbide.

Some cases of elevated pressure hydrocephalus may be avoided by preventing or treating the infectious diseases which precede them. Prenatal diagnosis of congenital brain malformation is often possible.

Prognosis

The prognosis for elevated-pressure hydrocephalus depends on a wide variety of factors, including the cause, age of onset, and the timing of surgery. Studies indicate that about half of all children who receive appropriate treatment and follow-up will develop IQs greater than 85. Those with hydrocephalus at birth do better than those with later onset due to meningitis. For individuals with normal pressure hydrocephalus, approximately half will benefit by the installation of a shunt.

Resources

BOOKS

Drake, James M., and Christian Sainte-Rose. *Shunt Book.* Boston: Blackwell Science Inc., 1995.

Toporek, Chuck, and Kellie Robinson. *Hydrocephalus: A Guide for Patients, Families & Friends.* Cambridge, Mass.: O'Reilly & Associates, 1999.

PERIODICALS

Grant, Beth. "Hydrocephalus: diagnosis and treatment." *Radiologic Technology* 69, no. 2 (Nov–Dec 1997): 17–35.

"Hydrocephalus." *Review of Optometry* 137, no. 8 (August 15, 2000): 56A.

ORGANIZATIONS

Association for Spina Bifida and Hydrocephalus. 42 Park Rd., Peterborough, PE1 2UQ United Kingdom. 01 73 355 5988. Fax: 017 3355 5985. postmaster@asbah.org. <http://www.asbah.demon.co.uk>.

Columbia Presbyterian Medical Center. Dept. of Neurological Surgery, 710 West 168 St., New York, NY 10032. (212) 305-0378. Fax: (212) 305-3629. <http://cpmcnet. columbia.edu/dept/nsg/PNS/Hydrocephalus.html>.

Hydrocephalus Association. 870 Market St., Suite 705, San Francisco, CA 94102. (415) 732-7040 or (888) 598-3789. (415) 732-7044. hydroassoc@aol.com. <http:// neurosurgery.mgh.harvard.edu/ha>.

Hydrocephalus Foundation, Inc. (HyFI), 910 Rear Broadway, Saugus, MA 01906. (781) 942-1161. HyFI1@netscape.net. <http://www.hydrocephalus.org>.

WEBSITES

"Hydrocephalus." *American Association of Neurological Surgeons/Congress of Neurological Surgeons* <http:// www.neurosurgery.org/pubpages/patres/ hydrobroch.html>.

"Hydrocephalus." Beth Israel Medical Center, New York, NY. *Institute for Neurology and Neurosurgery.* <http:// nyneurosurgery.org/child/hydrocephalus/ hydrocephalus.htm>.

"Hydrocephalus." National Library of Medicine. *MEDLINEplus.* <http://www.nlm.nih.gov/medlineplus/ hydrocephalus.html>.

L. Fleming Fallon, Jr., MD, PhD, DrPH

Hydrolethalus syndrome

Definition

Hydrolethalus syndrome is a rare disorder that results in severe birth defects and often, stillbirth.

Description

Hydrolethalus syndrome is a condition that causes improper fetal development. Multiple malformations along the body's midline, such as heart and brain defects, a cleft lip or palate, an abnormally shaped nose or jaw, and incomplete lung development result from this syndrome. The birth defects are typically extreme enough to cause stillbirth or death within a few days of birth. A less common name for hydrolethalus syndrome is Salonen-Herva-Norio syndrome, after the Finnish researchers who first described it in 1981.

Genetic profile

Hydrolethalus syndrome is passed on through an autosomal recessive pattern of **inheritance**. Autosomal means that the syndrome is not carried on a sex **chromosome**, while recessive means that both parents must carry the **gene** mutation in order for their child to have the disorder. Some cases of hydrolethalus syndrome have been observed in cases where the parents are related by blood (consanguineous). Parents with one child affected by hydrolethalus syndrome have a 25% chance that their next child will also be affected with the disease.

Each parent passes 23 chromosomes, or units of genetic information, to the infant. Structurally, each chromosome has a short segment or "arm," called the p arm, and a long arm, called the q arm, extending from a central region called the centromere. Along each arm the chromosome is further divided by numbering the bands down the arm according to their appearance under a microscope. Each band corresponds to specific genes. Based on studies of genetic material from affected and non-affected families, studies in 1999 assigned the gene location for hydrolethalus syndrome to 11q23-25, or somewhere between the 23rd and 25th band of the q arm of chromosome 11.

Demographics

The majority of cases of hydrolethalus syndrome have been reported in people of Finnish ancestry. In Finland the incidence of hydrolethalus syndrome is estimated at one in every 20,000. Less than twenty cases have been reported outside of Finland.

Hydrolethalus syndrome affects fetal development in the womb and is a syndrome of infants only, due to the extremely serious birth defects caused by the disorder. No cases of survival into childhood or adulthood have been reported. The syndrome appears to affect both males and females with equal probability.

Signs and symptoms

Prenatal symptoms include an excess of amniotic fluid in the womb (hydramnios). Babies with hydrolethalus syndrome are often delivered pre-term and may be stillborn.

After birth, the following conditions may be observed as a result of hydrolethalus syndrome:

- fluid in the skull and swelling leading to an abnormally large head (hydrocephalus)
- defects in the structure of the heart
- incomplete development of the lungs
- the presence of extra fingers and toes (**polydactyly**), especially an extra big toe or little finger
- clubfoot
- a cleft lip or palate
- a small lower jaw (micrognathia)
- abnormal eye and nose formation
- a keyhole-shaped defect at the back of the head
- abnormal genitalia

Diagnosis

Hydrolethalus syndrome can be diagnosed prenatally by ultrasound scanning in as early as the eleventh week of gestation. After birth, the presence of multiple malformations, especially the extreme swelling of the skull and other brain and spinal cord defects, can confirm the diagnosis. A family history and **genetic testing** may be useful in making the diagnosis certain.

Treatment and management

There is no treatment for hydrolethalus syndrome other than management of the specific medical conditions of the infant. **Genetic counseling** is particularly important in the prenatal treatment and management of hydrolethalus syndrome. This is because the severity of symptoms almost always causes death of the infant within a few days of birth, even if the fetus survives to full term.

Prognosis

The prognosis for infants with hydrolethalus syndrome is extremely poor. Most affected infants are stillborn or die within the first day of life. Only a handful of

KEY TERMS

Hydramnios—A condition in which there is too much amniotic fluid in the womb during pregnancy.

Hydrocephalus—The excess accumulation of cerebrospinal fluid around the brain, often causing enlargement of the head.

Micrognathy—Having a very small and receding jaw.

Polydactyly—The presence of extra fingers or toes.

cases of survival past the neonatal period have been reported and the longest survival period was 44 days.

Resources

PERIODICALS

Visapaa, Ilona, et al. "Assignment of the locus for hydrolethalus syndrome to a highly restricted region on 11q23-25." *American Journal of Human Genetics* (September 1999): 1086-95.

ORGANIZATIONS

March of Dimes Birth Defects Foundation. 1275 Mamaroneck Ave., White Plains, NY 10605. (888) 663-4637. resourcecenter@modimes.org. <http://www.modimes. org>.

National Organization for Rare Disorders (NORD). PO Box 8923, New Fairfield, CT 06812-8923. (203) 746-6518 or (800) 999-6673. Fax: (203) 746-6481. <http:// www.rarediseases.org>.

WEBSITES

"Entry 236680: Hydrolethalus syndrome." *OMIM—Online Mendelian Inheritance in Man.* <http:// www.ncbi.nlm.nih.gov/htbin-post/Omim/ dispmim?236680>. (April 20, 2001).

Jeanty, Philippe, and Sandra Silva. "Hydrolethalus syndrome." *TheFetus.Net.* <http://www.thefetus.net> (April 20, 2001).

Paul A. Johnson

Hydrometrocolpos syndrome *see* McKusick-Kaufman syndrome

▋ Hydrops fetalis

Definition

Refers to the abnormal accumulation of fluid in the skin, body cavities, umbilical cord, and placenta of an unborn baby. Hydrops fetalis (HF) can result from many different diseases and structural defects. HF is traditionally divided into two major categories: immune HF and nonimmune HF. Immune hydrops fetalis is caused by Rh incompatibility, and was the most common cause of HF until the advent of anti-Rh antibody treatment (Rho-GAM®) during pregnancy. All other causes of HF are termed nonimmune HF. Nonimmune hydrops fetalis may be caused by chromosomal aberrations, other **genetic disorders**, infections, anemias, structural birth defects such as **congenital heart disease**, and many other conditions. Currently in the United States nonimmune HF consists of about 90% and immune HF consists of about 10% of cases.

Description

HF occurs when a baby has a condition or birth defect that causes accumulation of excess fluid, known as edema, in the skin and other body cavities. Immune HF occurs when a mother's blood group is Rh negative (this means that she does not have the Rh protein on the surface of her blood cells) and her baby's blood group is Rh positive (the baby has the Rh protein on its blood cells). During the pregnancy a small amount of the baby's blood crosses into the mother's circulatory system. When this happens, the mother's immune system recognizes the Rh protein on the baby's blood cells as foreign and makes antibodies to the Rh protein. The antibodies can then cross back over to the baby and attack its blood cells, destroying them and causing anemia. The anemia causes heart failure, subsequent edema, and, ultimately, HF. The mother's immune response becomes greater with each subsequent pregnancy in which the baby has Rh-positive blood and thus the HF becomes worse. Administration of anti-Rh antibodies during all of an Rh-negative mother's pregnancies will prevent her from ever developing an immune response to Rh-positive blood and thus will prevent HF.

The most common causes of nonimmune HF include heart disease (congenital malformations and arrhythmia), **chromosome** aberrations (**Turner syndrome** and **Down syndrome**), and anemia (alpha-thalassemia, fetomaternal transfusion, and twin-twin transfusion). Other causes include infections, metabolic disorders, and tumors. In all there are over 100 separate causes of nonimmune HF.

All disorders that cause HF do so by three common mechanisms that include heart failure, hypoproteinemia (low levels of protein in the blood stream), and vascular or lymphatic obstruction. Some disorders combine two or more of these mechanisms to cause HF. Most disorders cause some degree of heart failure. Anemia causes heart failure by increasing the work of the heart so much that it fails (this is termed high output heart failure).

Isolated congenital heart disease or conditions that have congenital heart disease as a feature often will develop heart failure due to a poorly functioning heart (this is termed low output heart failure). Conditions that block the flow of blood or lymph can cause edema and HF. Examples include tumors and congenital malformations of the blood and lymphatic vessels. Conditions that lower that amount of protein in the blood can cause edema and HF by allowing fluid to easily leak out of the vessels and collect in the soft tissues and body cavities. Examples include metabolic conditions that damage the liver and prevent it from producing enough protein such as **Gaucher disease** and Sly disease.

Genetic profile

Many causes of hydrops fetalis do not have a genetic etiology. Because the recurrence risk can range from 0–100% depending on the underlying cause, an accurate diagnosis is important. Infectious causes are not genetic and should not recur in subsequent pregnancies. Other causes of HF have a specific genetic profile. Immune causes are due to a difference in the antigens on the mother and baby's blood cells. This can recur in subsequent pregnancies if anti-Rh antibodies are not given to the mother. Recurrence can either be 50% or 100% depending on the father's Rh-antigen status.

If hydrops fetalis is caused by a chromosome aberration, the risk of recurrence is about 1%, as most of these conditions occur sporadically and are not inherited. Malformations causing HF, such as congenital heart disease, are most commonly inherited as multifactorial traits. This type of **inheritance** pattern is caused by multiple genes and environmental factors working in combination. The recurrence risk for a multifactorial trait is about 3–5% with each subsequent pregnancy.

Higher risk for recurrence occurs when a single **gene** condition is the cause of HF. Autosomal recessive conditions such as alpha-thalassemia, Gaucher disease, and Sly disease have a recurrence risk of 25% with each subsequent pregnancy. The X-linked recessive disorder G-6-P-deficiency has a recurrence risk of 50% with each additional male child and 0% for each additional female child.

Some dominant conditions can cause HF; these are often lethal and usually represent a new mutation in that child. In these cases the recurrence risk is about 1%. Other dominant conditions such as **myotonic dystrophy** and lymphedema distichiasis are variable and recurrence may be 50% with each child.

Demographics

The incidence of HF in the United States is one in 3,000 pregnancies in all populations. In developing countries where Rh antibodies are not used, the rate can be much higher, due to a higher rate of immune HF cases. In Southeast Asia the most common cause is alpha-thalassemia. Alpha-thalassemia is so common in Southeast Asia that it remains as the most common cause of HF in the world today.

Signs and symptoms

All babies with HF have edema of the skin, soft tissues, and placenta. Often the body cavities will show fluid collections including the abdominal cavity (ascites), pleural cavity, and pericardial cavity. The back of the neck is particularly prone to fluid collections and can sometimes contain so much fluid that it appears as a large cystic mass called a cystic hygroma. Internal organs such as the liver, spleen, and heart can become enlarged with accumulated fluid. All of these signs may be seen in the newborn or before birth using ultrasonography.

Other signs of hydrops fetalis are variable and often depend on the underlying cause. Common to most causes of HF are decreased movements during the pregnancy, respiratory distress from poor lung development due to compression of the lungs by accumulated fluid, and heart failure.

Diagnosis

HF is easily diagnosed at birth by the swollen appearance of an affected baby, but the diagnosis is often made during the pregnancy by ultrasonography. Determining the cause of the HF is more challenging, but necessary for possible treatment and recurrence risk assessment. Testing the mother for infections such as toxoplasmosis, rubella, cytomegalovirus (CMV), herpes, syphilis, and parvovirus B19 can rule out most infectious causes of HF. A high-resolution ultrasound will help determine if a baby has any major structural malformations or tumors that could cause HF. At the same time as the ultrasound a percutaneous umbilical artery blood sampling (PUBS) procedure can be done. This procedure consists of passing a needle through the mother's abdomen into the uterine cavity and then into the baby's umbilical cord to withdraw a small amount of blood. This blood is then used to test for Rh antibodies, anemia, chromosome aberrations, and other suspected conditions. These diagnostic steps will determine the cause for the HF in many cases, but sometimes the cause remains unknown.

Treatment and management

As discussed in the description section, immune HF is easily prevented by administration of anti-Rh

KEY TERMS

Alpha-thalassemia—Autosomal recessive disorder where no functional hemoglobin is produced. Leads to severe untreatable anemia.

Arrhythmia—Abnormal heart rhythm, examples are a slow, fast, or irregular heart rate.

Congenital heart disease—Structural abnormality of the heart at birth. Examples include a ventricular septal defect and atrial septal defect.

Down syndrome—A genetic condition characterized by moderate to severe mental retardation, a characteristic facial appearance, and, in some individuals, abnormalities of some internal organs. Down syndrome is always caused by an extra copy of chromosome 21, or three rather than the normal two. For this reason, Down syndrome is also known as *trisomy 21*.

Gaucher disease—Autosomal recessive metabolic disorder caused by dysfunction of the lysosomal enzyme beta-glucosidase.

Lymphedema distichiasis—Autosomal dominant condition with abnormal or absent lymph vessels. Common signs include a double row of eyelashes (distichiasis) and edema of the limbs beginning around puberty.

Myotonic dystrophy—A form of muscular dystrophy, also known as Steinert's condition, characterized by delay in the ability to relax muscles after forceful contraction, wasting of muscles, as well as other abnormalities.

Pericardial cavity—Space occupied by the heart.

Pleural cavity—Area of the chest occupied by the lungs.

Sly disease—Autosomal recessive metabolic disorder caused by dysfunction of the lysosomal enzyme beta-glucuronidase.

Turner syndrome—Chromosome abnormality characterized by short stature and ovarian failure, caused by an absent X chromosome. Occurs only in females.

coccygeal teratomas (tumor seen in newborns) and some other structural malformations.

Prognosis

The prognosis is poor. A baby who is diagnosed by ultrasonography before birth has a less than 30% chance of survival. Babies who are born alive have a 50% chance of survival. The specific cause of HF influences the chances of survival with chromosome aberrations having a higher mortality rate and infectious etiologies having a lower mortality rate.

Resources

BOOKS

Machin, Geoffrey A. "Hydrops, Cystic Hygroma, Hydrothorax, Pericardial Effusion, and Fetal Ascites." *Potter's Pathology of the Fetus and Infant.* Edited by Enid Gilbert-Barness. St. Louis: Mosby, 1997, pp. 163–77.

PERIODICALS

Norton, Mary E. "Nonimmune Hydrops Fetalis." *Seminars in Perinatology* 18 (August 1994): 321–332.

Steiner, Robert D. "Hydrops Fetalis: Role of the Geneticist." *Seminars in Perinatology* 18 (August 1994): 516–524.

WEBSITES

"Hydrops Fetalis." (2000). Lucile Packard Children's Hospital. Stanford University Medical Center. <http://www.packardchildrenshospital.org/health/hrnewborn/hydrops_lh.htm>.

Premer, Danna, M.D. "Hydrops Fetalis." (2000). <http://www.peds.umn.edu/divisions/neonatology/hydrops.html>.

Randall Stuart Colby, MD

Hyperactivity of childhood *see* **Attention deficit hyperactivity disorder (ADHD)**

Hyperglycinemia with ketoacidosis and lactic acidosis (propionic type) *see* **Propionic acidemia**

antibodies to Rh negative pregnant women. Most nonimmune HF causes have no specific treatment other than early delivery and supportive care. HF caused by some types of anemia can be treated by a blood transfusion via a PUBS procedure. Fetal arrhythmia can often be treated by antiarrhythmia medications taken by the mother. Fetal operations are indicated for HF caused by sacro-

Hyperlipoproteinemia

Definition

Hyperlipoproteinemia refers to a group of acquired and inherited disorders whose common denominator is excessive levels of lipids (fats) in the blood, caused by a metabolic disorder. It is also referred to as hyperlipidemia. The condition is a major cause of coronary heart disease (CHD).

Description

The acquired form of hyperlipoproteinemia occurs as a condition secondary to another disease, such as **diabetes** mellitus, hypothyroidism, or nephrosis. The hereditary, or inherited, form of hyperlipoproteinemia is classified into five major types.

Lipids are an essential part of human metabolism and are a primary source of energy for the body. Lipids are produced by cells in the body and along with carbohydrates and proteins, are components of all life. But lipids are essentially oil-based and as such do not mix with a water-based liquid such as blood. Yet both must be carried through the body's circulatory system. So to get around this obstacle, lipids attach themselves to proteins. This combination of lipids and proteins is called lipoproteins, which are water-soluble particles that can be carried through the blood stream.

Some of the chemicals in the lipoproteins are fatty nutrients that are absorbed by the intestines for use in other parts of the body. Cholesterol is carried by lipoproteins through the blood stream to the liver and ultimately to the bowel for excretion. If the substances in the lipoproteins are not properly balanced, cholesterol will stay in the tissues instead of being excreted. It can also build up in blood vessels, eventually restricting and even blocking blood flow.

There are five different densities of lipoproteins, each containing triglycerides, cholesterol, phospholipids (lipids with phosphorus attached), and special proteins. The lipoproteins are high-density lipoproteins (HDL), low-density lipoproteins (LDL), intermediate-density lipoproteins, very low-density lipoproteins (VLDL), and chylomicrons. HDL is commonly called "good" cholesterol and LDL "bad" cholesterol. The two major lipoprotein groups are HDL and LDL.

HDL helps prevent fat buildup throughout the body by carrying cholesterol from the arteries to the liver, where it is disposed of. Abnormally low levels of HDL, fewer than 30 milligrams per deciliter (mg/dL) of blood, are associated with a greater risk for coronary heart disease and stroke. LDL carries most of the cholesterol in the body, so an excess of LDL, usually 160 mg/dL of blood, can clog the arteries with cholesterol buildup. This can lead to atherosclerosis, commonly referred to as hardening of the arteries, or acute myocardial infarction (heart attack).

The five types of inherited hyperlipoproteinemia are:

- Type I, characterized by high levels of chylomicrons and triglycerides and a deficiency of lipoprotein lipase, an enzyme that accelerates the breakdown of lipoproteins. Disease onset is usually in infancy.

- Type II, broken into two subtypes, type II-a and type II-b. Both subtypes display high levels of blood cholesterol. People with type II-b also have high levels of triglycerides in their blood. Disease onset is usually after age 20.

- Type III, also called broad beta disease, is characterized by high blood levels of cholesterol and triglycerides, and the presence of a lipoprotein called apolipoprotein E (apo E) **genotype** E2/E2. Disease onset is usually in adults.

- Type IV, characterized only by high triglyceride levels in the blood. Disease onset is usually during puberty or early adulthood.

- Type V, characterized by increased blood levels of chylomicrons and triglycerides and low levels of LDL and HDL. Disease onset is usually in children or adults.

Genetic profile

Type III hyperlipoproteinemia is an autosomal recessive disorder that affects males and females. Autosomal means that the **gene** does not reside on the sex **chromosome**. People with only one abnormal gene are carriers but since the gene is recessive, they do not have the disorder. Their children could be carriers of the disorder but not show symptoms of the disease. Both parents must have one of the abnormal genes for a child to have symptoms of type III hyperlipoproteinemia. When both parents have the abnormal gene, there is a 25% chance each child will inherit both abnormal genes and have the disease. There is a 50% chance each child will inherit one abnormal gene and become a carrier of the disorder but not have the disease itself. There is a 25% chance each child will inherit neither abnormal gene and not have the disease nor be a carrier.

The other types of hyperlipoproteinemia are autosomal dominant. This means they occur when an abnormal gene from one parent is capable of causing the disease even though the matching gene from the other parent is normal. The abnormal gene dominates the outcome of the gene pair. This means that there is a 50% chance that each child of the couple will have the disease. Consequently, there is a 50% chance each child will not inherit the defective gene and will not have the disease.

Demographics

Hyperlipoproteinemia can affect people regardless of age, gender, race, or ethnicity. All adults, starting at age 20, should be tested for hyperlipoproteinemia at least once every five years, recommends the National Cholesterol Education Program (NCEP) of the National Institutes of Health (NIH). People considered at high risk for hyperlipoproteinemia should be tested more often and include those with a diet high in fat and cholesterol, have a family history of the disorder, use oral contraceptive or take estrogen, or who have diabetes mellitus, hypothyroidism, nephrosis, or **alcoholism**. Ethnic groups that have a higher risk of developing hyperlipoproteinemia include Latinos, Native Americans, African-Americans, and Pacific Islanders.

Signs and symptoms

It is very common for people with hyperlipoproteinemia to show no outward signs of the disorder. But there are several general signs that may indicate a person has the disorder, including obesity, yellowish skin, fatty yellow patches or nodules on the skin, especially the eyelids, neck, and back, inflamed tendons, an enlarged spleen, inflamed pancreas, nausea and vomiting, or abdominal pain. However, these are also symptoms of a variety of other conditions so for hyperlipoproteinemia to be diagnosed, blood tests are needed.

Diagnosis

Diagnosis involves a series of blood tests to measure lipid levels and determine the type of hyperlipoproteinemia. Blood tests, usually taken after a 12-hour fast, include measurement of total serum cholesterol, HDL, LDL, VLDL, triglycerides, and for the presence of apolipoprotein E. When hyperlipoproteinemia secondary to another disorder has been excluded and inherited hyperlipoproteinemia seems likely, first-degree relatives should be tested. These include parents, children, and siblings.

Treatment and management

Hyperlipoproteinemia treatment is usually based on a three-fold attack: diet, exercise and lipid-lowering medications. People who are overweight should begin a program to slowly but consistently lose weight until they are at or near the recommended weight for their height and body frame. It is essential to eat a diet low in fat. Exercise also plays a vital role. A minimum of 20 minutes of aerobic exercise three times a week is beneficial and 30 minutes or more daily is ideal. The exercise can take the form of running, jogging, cycling, swimming, cardiovascular machines, or even walking briskly.

Eating healthy and exercising regularly, while extremely beneficial, are not always enough to bring lipid levels to the desired range. Prescription medications are often required. There is a wide range of medications available to manage lipid levels. The most prescribed are HMG-CoA-reductase inhibitors, commonly called "statins," which hinder the body's production of cholesterol. Statins include cerivstatin (Baycol), fluvastatin (Lescol),

lovastatin (Mevacor), pravastatin (Pravacol), atorvastatin (Lipitor), and simvastatin (Zocor). Other first-line medications include bile acid sequestrants, cholestyramine (Questran), colesevelan (Welchol), and colestipol (Colestid). Also, probucol (Lorelco) is sometimes used.

The type of drug prescribed may vary, depending on the lipid test results and the type of hyperlipoproteinemia that is diagnosed. For example, people with type III of the disorder respond better when prescribed fibric acid derivatives such as gemfibrozil (Lopid), clofibrate (Atromid-S), and fenofibrate (Tricor) or nicotinic acid (niacin).

Other factors which have a negative effect on hyperlipoproteinemia include smoking, excessive alcohol consumption, and stress. It is also important to treat underlying conditions, such as diabetes, heart disease, pancreatitis (inflamed pancreas), and thyroid problems.

Prognosis

The prognosis is good for type I hyperlipoproteinemia with treatment. For type II, the prognosis is good for II-b and fair for II-a with early diagnosis and treatment. The prognosis for type III is good when the prescribed diet is strictly followed. The prognosis is uncertain for types IV and V, due to the risk of developing premature coronary artery disease in type IV and pancreatitis in type V.

Resources

BOOKS

Carlson, Lars., et al. *Treatment of Hyperlipoproteinemia.* New York: Lippincott-Raven Publishers, 1984.

Rifkind, Basil M., ed. *Drug Treatment of Hyperlipidemia.* New York: Marcel Dekker, 1991.

PERIODICALS

Abel, Allen. "The Tumblebrutus Solution." *Saturday Night* (February 1997): 26-29.

Baer, Daniel. "Lipid Tests." *Medical Laboratory Observer* (May 1992): 11-14.

Gotto, Antonio M. Jr., et al. "Hyperlipidemia: A Complete Approach." *Patient Care* (February 15, 1989): 34-48.

ORGANIZATIONS

Inherited High Cholesterol Foundation. University of Utah School of Medicine, 410 Chipeta Way, Room 167, Salt Lake City, UT 84104. (888) 244-2465.

National Cholesterol Education Program. National Heart, Lung and Blood Institute. PO Box 30105, Bethesda, MD 20824. (301) 592-8573. <http://www.nhlbi.nih.gov>.

National Organization for Rare Disorders (NORD). PO Box 8923, New Fairfield, CT 06812-8923. (203) 746-6518 or (800) 999-6673. Fax: (203) 746-6481. <http://www.rarediseases.org>.

WEBSITES

"Hyperlipidemia Types I, II, III, IV, V (Hyperlipoproteinemia)." *HealthGate.* <http://www.healthgate.com/ped/sym204.html>.

Ken R. Wells

Hypermobility syndrome *see* Larsen syndrome

Hypochondrogenesis

Definition

Hypochondrogenesis is a lethal genetic **skeletal dysplasia** caused by a mutation in the COL2A1 **gene**. This condition is characterized by a severe limb and trunk shortening with a disproportionately large head.

Infants with this disorder usually die soon after birth of respiratory failure.

Description

Hypochondrogenesis is a rare form of skeletal **dysplasia** (or dwarfing syndrome) caused by mutations in the COL2A1 gene. The COL2A1 gene provides the instruction for the formation of collagen II, which is a major building block of cartilage, a major component of bone. Because of these mutations, infants with hypochondrogenesis have defects in their bone formation that cause them to have severely shortened limbs (arms and legs) and a small chest with short ribs. As infants with hypochondrogenesis have small chests and abnormal ribs, their lungs are underdeveloped, which leads to respiratory (breathing) difficulties at birth. In addition, the vertebrae or spinal bones in the neck and part of the sacrum (pelvis) do not harden, or ossify, properly. The face of an infant with hypochondrogenesis is flat and oval-shaped, with widely spaced eyes, a small chin, and, in some cases, an opening in the roof of the mouth called a cleft palate. Rarely, fetuses with hypochondrogenesis can develop a condition called **hydrops fetalis** in which excess fluid builds up in the abdomen and body before birth. One report has suggested that some infants with hypochondrogenesis may also have heart defects.

There are many causes for impaired growth or dwarfism, including hormone imbalances, metabolic problems, and problems with bone growth. Hypochondrogenesis belongs to a class of dwarfism referred to as a chrondrodystrophy or skeletal dysplasia and results from a problem with bone growth. All skeletal dysplasias are the result of a problem with bone formation or growth. There are more than 100 different types of skeletal dysplasias. Hypochondrogenesis is also sometimes referred to as a collagenopathy because the specific abnormality in hypochondrogenesis is a problem in the formation of collagen.

The collagenopathies are a group of disorders that affect connective tissue, the tissue that supports the body's joints and organs. Collagenopathies, as a group, are caused by defects in either type II or type IX collagen. Hypochondrogenesis is caused by a defect in the formation of type II collagen. Collagen is a complex molecule that provides structure, strength, and elasticity to connective tissue.

There are other skeletal dysplasias that have features very similar to hypochondrogenesis. Consequently, hypochondrogenesis is considered to belong to a spectrum, or continuum, of skeletal dysplasias that vary in severity. This spectrum includes anchondrogenesis type II at the severe end and **spondyloepiphyseal dysplasia** congenita (SEDc) at the milder end. Infants with achondrogenesis type II also have the same spinal changes as seen in hypochondrogenesis, but the condition is generally more severe and is invariably lethal. Infants with spondyloepiphyseal dysplasia congenita have the same findings as an infant with hypochondrogenesis, but their condition tends to be milder. Infants with SEDc can survive, but generally have many complications due to their severe skeletal problems.

Genetic profile

Hypochondrogenesis is caused by a mutation, or change, in the COL2A1 gene located on the long arm of **chromosome** 12 (12q13.11-q13.2). Hypochondrogenesis has autosomal dominant **inheritance**; however, there is usually no prior history of the condition in the family. In an autosomal dominant disorder, only one gene has to have a mutation for the person to have the disorder. Every individual has two COL2A1 genes: one from their father and one from their mother. However, all infants with hypochondrogenesis are born to average-stature parents. The infant's hypochondrogenesis is the result of a *de novo*, or new, mutation. The occurrence of hypochondrogenesis is almost always due to a *de novo* mutation. This *de novo* mutation typically occurs in one of the type II collagen gene from an average-sized parent. No one knows the cause of *de novo* mutations. Because infants with hypochondrogenesis do not survive to reproductive age, there is no risk of their passing on this mutated gene. Because most *de novo* mutations occur sporadically, the recurrence risk is small.

Several different types of mutations in the COL2A1 gene are responsible for hypochondrogenesis. These mutations may include small deletions, or missing pieces, of the COL2A1 gene, missense mutations that lead to the substitution of one amino acid for another, and other changes that leave out important parts of the protein. All of these changes interfere with the formation of mature triple-stranded type II collagen molecules, which results in hypochondrogenesis by affecting tissues that are rich in type II collagen.

Demographics

Hypochondrogenesis occurs equally in males and females. There is no exact prevalence data for hypochondrogenesis, but collectively, collagenopathies are found in about one in 10,000 people. Because achondrogenesis and hypochondrogenesis can be difficult to tell apart, the incidence data reflect the incidence of both disorders. Hypochondrogenesis and achondrogenesis type II together occur in approximately one in 40,000–60,000 births. With the advent of **DNA** testing and the ability to make a more definitive diagnosis, it should soon be possible to have an incidence figure for hypochondrogenesis alone.

Signs and symptoms

Physical findings

Type II collagen is a major building block of the spine, cartilage, and the vitreous protein in the eye. Defects in this collagen and the cartilage that it forms cause infants with hypochondrogenesis to have micromelia (extremely short limbs), a short trunk (or body) with shortened ribs, and a head that appears large. Their faces have a characteristic appearance with a flat oval-shaped face, wide-set eyes (hypertelorism), small chin, and, occasionally, an infant with hypochondrogenesis will also have a cleft palate or opening on the roof of the mouth. They may also have heart defects.

X-ray findings

Infants with hypochondrogenesis also have very characteristic or unique x-ray findings. In order to understand what these findings are, it is important to know a little bit about how x rays work. X rays are a form of energy that is able to pass through some objects and not others. When x rays pass through a body, more x rays are absorbed by the denser parts (such as teeth and bone) than by softer tissues (such as muscles and digestive organs). X rays create a negative image on the x-ray film. Soft tissues, such as blood, muscles, and digestive organs, appear darker or do not appear at all because the x rays pass directly through the tissues onto the film. Bones and teeth appear brighter because fewer x rays penetrate these structures and reach the film during exposure.

When looking at the x ray of an infant with hypochondrogenesis, it is easy to see abnormalities with their bones. Because their vertebra are underdeveloped and have not hardened, they are quite difficult to see on an x ray; they should be easy to see. Those vertebrae that can be seen are usually abnormally shaped. The ribs appear very thin. In addition to vertebral and rib abnormalities, the bones of the pelvis and in particular the hip socket are abnormally shaped. Hip sockets are usually curved, but in hypochondrogenesis these bones are flattened and smaller than usual.

While the findings in hypochondrogenesis are distinctly abnormal, it is important to distinguish these findings from those seen in achondrogenesis type II and those seen in spondyloepiphyseal dysplasia congenita. The x-ray findings of achondrogenesis type II are more severe than those of hypochondrogenesis, and the findings of SEDc are generally milder than those seen in hypochondrogenesis.

Diagnosis

The diagnosis of hypochondrogenesis can be made prenatally by ultrasound, or shortly after birth. A number of different tests, including x rays, biopsies, and DNA testing, is used to confirm the diagnosis. Consultation with experts in the field of skeletal dysplasias may also be helpful.

The diagnosis of hypochondrogenesis can also be made prenatally (during pregnancy), either by ultrasound (sonogram) or by prenatal DNA testing. Sonograms use sound waves to provide an image of a fetus. The structural abnormalities of hypochondrogenesis, including severely shortened limbs, shortened truck with abnormal ribs, and unossified vertebral bones, can be observed during the second trimester of pregnancy. Because of overlapping features with other skeletal dysplasias, it can be very difficult to definitively diagnose hypochondrogenesis by sonogram. DNA testing can have a role in clarifying ambiguous ultrasound findings.

The neonatal diagnosis in infants is made by physical examination shortly after birth. Severe shortening of the limbs, a small trunk, abnormal facial features, and a cleft palate are often seen and raise the suspicion of the diagnosis of hypochondrogenesis. The diagnosis cannot be made by physical examination alone as hypochondrogenesis and numerous other skeletal dysplasias look very similar.

X rays are often helpful in establishing the diagnosis of hypochondrogenesis. X-ray findings include under-ossified vertebra, abnormally thin ribs, and abnormally shaped hip bones. The x-ray findings of achondrogenesis type II are generally more severe, and the findings of SEDc are less severe.

Biopsies are the collection of tissue that can then be examined under a microscope. In hypochondrogenesis, a skin biopsy may be done to obtain skin cells for DNA analysis. Biopsies of the connective tissue may also be collected so that the collagen and other connective tissues can be examined microscopically.

DNA testing can also be performed on a blood or skin sample. The presence of a mutation in the COL2A1 gene would confirm the diagnosis of hypochondrogenesis. As of 2005, it is estimated that DNA testing will detect greater that 90% of mutations in the COL2A1 gene. Because scientists have not yet found all of the mutations in this gene, the absence of a detectable mutation does not completely rule out the diagnosis. The COL2A1 gene is a large gene with many possible mutations. Because of this, the results of DNA testing may take 4–6 weeks.

Prenatal testing can also be done using DNA technology. A sample of tissue from a fetus is obtained by either chorionic villi sampling (CVS) or by **amniocentesis**. Chorionic villi sampling is generally done between 10 and 12 weeks of pregnancy, and amniocentesis is done between 14 and 18 weeks of pregnancy. Chorionic villi sampling involves removing a small amount of tissue from the developing placenta. The tissue in the placenta contains the same DNA as the fetus. Amniocentesis involves removing a small amount of fluid from around the fetus. This fluid contains some fetal skin cells from which DNA can be isolated. The fetal DNA is then tested to determine whether there are any mutations in the COL2A1 gene. This test is not done in low-risk couples and may only be available if a specific mutation has already been characterized in a family.

Because hypochondrogenesis is such a rare disorder and has a great deal of overlap with other skeletal dysplasia, it can be very difficult to diagnose definitively. It can be helpful to consult with skeletal dysplasia experts who may suggest further specialized testing to help clarify the diagnosis.

Treatment and management

There is no cure or treatment for hypochondrogenesis. If the diagnosis is made prior to birth, the parents may wish to meet with a neonatalogist to discuss management of the birth.

If hypochondrogenesis is detected during a pregnancy, patients have the option to terminate the pregnancy based upon the lethality of this condition. This is a very personal decision and should be made following serious counseling about the nature and outcome of this diagnosis.

Once the diagnosis has been firmly established, there is no need for resuscitation and ventilatory support for the infant given the established lethality of the conditions. Infants should be provided with basic supportive care, including warmth, nourishment and comfort.

If the diagnosis has not been confirmed prior to birth, resuscitation and ventilatory (breathing) support are appropriate to allow time for a thorough diagnostic evaluation. X rays should be performed, and skin and connective and blood tissue should be collected.

The diagnosis of hypochondrogenesis is shocking for families. The bleak prognosis and lack of treatment can be devastating. Families should be reassured that there is nothing that they did or did not do that could have prevented the outcome. The family needs time to process the information about the diagnosis. The family should also be provided emotional support. The neonatal staff can aid in collecting reminders of the baby, including footprints, photographs, and locks of hair, that can help the family as they deal with the crisis. In addition to providing emotional support, it is equally important to make sure that the parents understand the genetic diagnosis and its implications for future pregnancies. They need to understand the sporadic nature of this diagnosis and that it is unlikely to recur in a future pregnancy. Because the interpretation of some of the test results are complicated, it is best that the family be referred to a genetics center for counseling following the diagnosis of hypochondrogenesis.

Prognosis

The prognosis for an infant with hypochondrogenesis is bleak. Some infants are stillborn, and those that are live born die shortly after birth due to respiratory failure. Survival can range from a few days to a few weeks. If an infant with suspected hypochondrogenesis does survive the newborn period, it is assumed that they actually have spondyloepiphyseal dysplasia congenita. In cases where the diagnosis is ambiguous, DNA testing can help to confirm the diagnosis and may allow for a more accurate prognosis.

Resources

BOOKS

Ilse, Sherokee. *Empty Arms: Coping After Miscarriage, Stillbirth and Infant Death.* Maple Plain, MN: Wintergreen Press, 2000.

ORGANIZATIONS

The Cedar-Sinai Skeletal Dysplasia Registry. (April 10, 2005.) <http://www.csmc.edu/3805.html>.

Compassionate Friends. P. O. Box 3696, Oak Brook, IL 60522-3696. (877) 969-0010. E-mail: nationaloffice@compassionatefriends.org. Web sites

The Genetic Home Reference. (April 10, 2005.) <http://ghr.nlm.nih.gov/condition=hypochondrogenesis>.

The Greenberg Center for Skeletal Dysplasias. (April 10, 2005.) <http://www.hopkinsmedicine.org/greenbergcenter/SED.htm>.

Help After Neonatal Death. (April 10, 2005.) <http://www.handonline.org/resources/groups/index.html>.

Kathleen A. Fergus, MS, CGC

Hypochondroplasia

Definition

Hypochondroplasia is an autosomal dominant mutation that results in short stature with disproportionately short arms and legs, but normal head size.

Description

Hypochondroplasia is a genetic form of short stature (dwarfism) due to a problem of bone growth and development. There are many causes for short stature including hormone imbalances, metabolic problems, and problems with bone growth. Hypochondroplasia is a common form of short stature and belongs to a class of dwarfism referred to as a chrondrodystrophy or **skeletal dysplasia**. All skeletal dysplasias are the result of a problem with bone formation or growth. There are over 100 different types of skeletal **dysplasia**.

Because the features of hypochondroplasia are so mild, the disorder may go undiagnosed. Although infants with hypochondroplasia may have low birth weight, hypochondroplasia is often not evident until between two and six years of age. In general, individuals with hypochondroplasia have disproportionate short stature with an average height of 51-57 in (130-145 cm). The degree of disproportion of the limbs to the body is variable.

Most individuals with hypochondroplasia have a normal IQ although some studies suggest that up to 10% of individuals with hypochondroplasia may have mild mental retardation or learning disabilities. This finding is controversial and more studies are currently underway to verify it. The motor development of infants with hypochondroplasia is normal. In rare cases, individuals with hypochondroplasia may experience neurologic problems due to spinal cord compression. The spinal canal (which holds the spinal cord) can be smaller than normal in patients with hypochondroplasia.

Genetic profile

Hypochondroplasia is caused by a mutation, or change, in the fibroblast growth factor receptor 3 **gene** (FGFR3) located on the short arm of **chromosome** 4.

FGFR (fibroblast growth factor receptor) genes provide the instruction for the formation of a cell receptor. Every cell in the body has an outer layer called a cell membrane that serves as a filter. Substances are transported into and out of the cells by receptors located on the surface of the cell membrane. Every cell has hundreds of different types of receptors. The fibroblast growth factor receptors transport fibroblast growth factor into a cell. Fibroblast growth factors play a role in the normal growth and development of bones. When the receptors for fibroblast growth factor do not work properly, the cells do not receive enough fibroblast growth factor and the result is abnormal growth and development of bones.

Approximately 70% of hypochondroplasia is caused by mutations in the FGFR3 gene. The genes (or gene) responsible for the other 30% of cases are not known. The FGFR3 gene is comprised of 2,520 bases. In a normal (non-mutated) gene, base number 1620 codes for the amino acid asparagine. In most individuals with hypochondroplasia, a mutation changes the asparagine to the amino acid lysine. Two specific mutations account for approximately 70% of hypochondroplasia. These small substitutions change the amino acid that affects the protein structure. Both of these small substitutions cause a change in the fibroblast growth factor receptor (FGFR) that affects the function of this receptor.

The remaining 30% of patients diagnosed with hypochondroplasia do not show FGFR3 **gene mutations**. It has not yet been made clear if these patients have a different gene abnormality, an unrecognized FGFR3 gene mutation, or are normal variants. Another possibility is that these individuals actually have another disorder in which short stature results.

Mutations in the FGFR3 gene are inherited in an autosomal dominant manner. Every individual has two FGFR3 genes—one from their father and one from their mother. In an autosomal dominant disorder, only one gene has to have a mutation for a person to have the disorder. An individual with hypochondroplasia has a 50% chance of passing on his or her changed (mutated) gene to offspring. An individual can inherit a mutated gene from one parent or the mutation can occur for the first time in the individual. Mutations that arise for the first time in affected individuals are called *de novo* mutations. The causes of mutations are not known.

Demographics

Because hypochondroplasia has such a wide range of variability, many people mildly affected with hypochondroplasia may never be diagnosed. Thus, the true incidence of hypochondroplasia is unknown. No studies have been done to determine the incidence of hypochondroplasia but it is assumed to be a relatively common disorder with an incidence equal to achondroplasia—one in 15,000 to one in 40,000.

Signs and symptoms

Individuals with hypochondroplasia have disproportionate short stature, limb abnormalities, and rhizomelic

shortening of the limbs. Rhizomelic shortening of the limbs means that those segments of a limb closest to the body (the root of the limb) are more severely affected. In individuals with hypochondroplasia, the upper arms are shorter than the forearms and the upper leg (thigh) is shorter than the lower leg. In general, the upper limbs are more affected than the lower limbs in individuals with hypochondroplasia.

In addition to shortened limbs, individuals with hypochondroplasia have other characteristic limb differences such as a limited ability to rotate and extend their elbows. They can develop bowed legs, a finding that usually improves as they get older. Their hands and feet are short and broad, as are their fingers and toes. Their final adult height is usually 51-57 inches (130-145 cm). Their body habitus or shape is described as thick and stocky with a relatively long trunk. They may have lumbar lordosis (curved back) giving them a swayed back appearance.

Diagnosis

The diagnosis of hypochondroplasia can be extremely difficult to make for a number of reasons. There is no one physical feature or x ray finding specific to hypochondroplasia and there is a great deal of overlap between individuals with hypochondroplasia and individuals in the general population. Many of the physical findings of hypochondroplasia (short stature, bowed legs and a stocky build) are seen in individuals without hypochondroplasia. The same is true for the "typical" x ray findings. All of the possible x ray findings associated with hypochondroplasia can also be seen in unaffected individuals. There is no consensus on specific criteria necessary for diagnosis; however, it is usually made based on a combination of physical and x ray findings and is rarely made in infants.

DNA testing for hypochondroplasia is also complicated because testing will only detect 70% of the mutations that cause hypochondroplasia. DNA testing can be performed on blood samples from children or adults. If an individual is suspected of having hypochondroplasia and a mutation is detected, then the diagnosis is confirmed. If a mutation is not detected, then the diagnosis of hypochondroplasia has neither been confirmed nor ruled out. This individual could be one of the 30% of individuals with hypochondroplasia due to unknown mutations or they could have short stature due to another disorder.

Prenatal testing for hypochondroplasia can be performed using DNA technology. A sample of tissue from a fetus is obtained by either chorionic villus sampling (CVS) or by **amniocentesis**. Chorionic villus sampling is generally done between 10 and 12 weeks of pregnancy and amniocentesis is done between 16 and 18 weeks of pregnancy. Chorionic villus sampling involves removing a small amount of tissue from the developing placenta. The tissue in the placenta contains the same DNA as the fetus. Amniocentesis involves removing a small amount of fluid from around the fetus. This fluid contains some fetal skin cells. DNA can be isolated from these skin cells. The fetal DNA is then tested to determine if it contains either of the two mutations responsible for **achondroplasia**.

Prenatal DNA testing for hypochondroplasia is not routinely performed in low-risk pregnancies. This type of testing is generally limited to high-risk pregnancies, such as when one parent has hypochondroplasia. This testing can also only be performed if the mutation causing hypochondroplasia in the parent has been identified.

Treatment and management

There is no cure for hypochondroplasia. Because of the wide range of variability of this condition there is no consensus on the medical management of individuals with hypochondroplasia either. Individuals with more severe cases are the only individuals likely to need medical management. The recommendations for the medical management of individuals with achondroplasia have been outlined by the American Academy of Pediatrics' Committee on Genetics and should be used as a guide for the management of individuals with severe hypochondroplasia. The potential medical complications of hypochondroplasia range from mild to moderate. Early intervention may avert some of the long-term consequences of these complications.

As children with hypochondroplasia develop, certain conditions and behaviors should be monitored. Their height, weight, and head circumference should be measured regularly and plotted on growth curves developed for children with achondroplasia as a guide. Neurologic problems such as lethargy, abnormal reflexes, or loss of muscle control should be seen by a neurologist to make sure that they are not experiencing compression of their spinal cord. Compression of the spinal cord is rare in individuals with hypochondroplasia but can occur because of the abnormal size of their spinal canal.

Children with hypochondroplasia should also be monitored for sleep apnea. Sleep apnea occurs when an individual stops breathing during sleep. This can occur for several reasons including obstruction of the throat by the tonsils and adenoids, spinal cord compression and obesity. Individuals with hypochondroplasia are more prone to sleep apnea due to the changes in their spinal canal and foramen magnum. Treatment for sleep apnea depends on the cause of the sleep apnea. Obstructive

sleep apnea is treated by surgically removing the tonsils and adenoids. Weight management may also play a role in the treatment of sleep apnea.

The bowed legs of children with hypochondroplasia usually improve as they get older and rarely require surgical intervention. Children with hypochondroplasia can often have an increased risk for middle ear infections which can be treated with oral antibiotics and the surgical placement of ear tubes.

Children with visible physical differences can have difficulties in school and socially. Support groups such as Little People of America can be a source of guidance on how to deal with these issues. It is important that children with hypochondroplasia not be limited in activities that pose no danger.

Two treatments have been used to try to increase the final adult height of individuals with hypochondroplasia–limb-lengthening and growth hormone therapy. There are risks and benefits to both treatments and they are still considered experimental.

Limb-lengthening involves surgically attaching external rods to the long bones in the arms and legs. These rods run parallel to the bone on the outside of the body. Over a period of 18-24 months, the tension on these rods is increased which results in the lengthening of the underlying bone. This procedure is long, costly, and has potential complications such as pain, infections and nerve problems. Limb-lengthening can increase overall height by 12-14 in (30.5-35.6 cm). This is an elective surgery and individuals must decide for themselves if it would be of benefit to them. The optimal age to perform this surgery is not known.

Growth hormone therapy has been used to treat some children with hypochondroplasia. Originally there was doubt about the effectiveness of this treatment because children with hypochondroplasia are not growth hormone deficient. Studies have shown mixed results. Some children with hypochondroplasia show improvement in their growth rate and others do not. It is too early to say how effective this treatment is because the children involved in this study are still growing and have not reached their final adult height.

Prognosis

The prognosis for most people with hypochondroplasia is very good. In general, they have minimal medical problems, normal IQ, and most achieve success and have a long life regardless of their stature. The most serious medical barriers to an excellent prognosis are the neurologic complications that very rarely arise in hypochondroplasia, including mild mental retardation and spinal cord compression.

Successful social adaptation plays an important role in the ultimate success and happiness of an individual with hypochondroplasia. It is very important that the career and life choices of individuals with achondroplasia not be limited by preconceived ideas about their abilities.

Resources

ORGANIZATIONS

Human Growth Foundation. 997 Glen Cove Ave., Glen Head, NY 11545. (800) 451-6434. Fax: (516) 671-4055. <http://www. hgf1@hgfound.org>.

Little People of America, Inc. National Headquarters, PO Box 745, Lubbock, TX 79408. (806) 737-8186 or (888) LPA-2001. lpadatabase@juno.com. <http://www.lpaonline.org>.

MAGIC Foundation for Children's Growth. 1327 N. Harlem Ave., Oak Park, IL 60302. (708) 383-0808 or (800) 362-4423. Fax: (708) 383-0899. mary@magicfoundation.org. <http://www.magicfoundation.org/ghd.html>.

WEBSITES

Human Growth Foundation. <http://www.hgfound.org/>.

Little People of America: An Organization for People of Short Stature. <http://www.lpaonline.org/lpa.html>.

MAGIC Foundation for Children's Growth. <http://www.magicfoundation.org>.

Kathleen Fergus, MS

Hypophosphatasia

Definition

Hypophosphatasia is an inherited bone disease whose clinical symptoms are highly variable, ranging from a profound lack of mineralization of bone with death occurring prior to delivery up to early loss of teeth in adulthood as the only sign. Still other affected individuals may have the characteristic biochemical abnormality but no outward clinical signs of the disorder. Hypophosphatasia is due to consistently low levels of an important enzyme in the body, alkaline phosphatase.

Description

The term hypophosphatasia was first coined in 1948 by a Canadian pediatrician, Dr. J.C. Rathbun. He used it to describe a male infant who developed and then died from severe rickets, weight loss, and seizures. Levels of the enzyme alkaline phosphatase were below normal in samples of blood and bone from this child.

Rickets is a condition resulting from a deficiency of vitamin D in children, causing inadequate strengthening of developing cartilage and newly formed bone. While this disorder shares many clinical characteristics with hypophosphatasia, the two conditions are separate and distinct. A major difference is that rickets are typically not lethal.

In 1953, the clinical features of hypophosphatasia were expanded to include not only abnormal mineralization of bone but also premature loss of the permanent teeth in adulthood. Since then, hypophosphatasia has been further divided into six different clinical forms. Each form is defined by the severity of the disease and the age at which symptoms first appear.

Alkaline phosphatase (ALP) is present in nearly all plants and animals. There are at least four different genes known to encode different forms of ALP in humans. Hypophosphatasia is due to a deficiency of the form of ALP that is particularly abundant in the liver, bones, and kidneys. This is often referred to as the tissue non-specific form of ALP, or TNSALP. This form of alkaline phosphatase is important in the mineralization, or hardening, of the bones of the skeleton as well as the teeth. Thus, abnormalities in either the production or function of this enzyme have a direct effect on the formation and strength of these parts of the body. In general, the more severe forms of hypophosphatasia are associated with lower serum TNSALP activity for that individual's age.

Genetic profile

The first report of siblings affected with hypophosphatasia was published in 1950, providing supportive evidence that it is an inherited abnormality as opposed to one that is acquired. This is an important distinction, particularly since rickets alone is often due to a lack of vitamin D in a person's diet. Good sources of vitamin D include fortified milk and sunlight. Rickets can therefore be an acquired medical problem.

Nearly all forms of hypophosphatasia are inherited as an autosomal recessive condition. In order to be affected, an individual must inherit two copies of a hypophosphatasia **gene**, or one copy from each carrier parent. Carriers have one normal gene and one hypophosphatasia gene and are typically asymptomatic. In some families, hypophosphatasia carriers have been found to have low to low-normal levels of TNSALP in their blood. As a general rule, however, it is difficult to detect carriers with biochemical tests due to the wide range of enzyme levels found among both carriers and non-carriers.

Two hypophosphatasia carriers face a risk of 25%, or a one in four chance, of both passing on the disease gene and having an affected child. On the other hand, there is a 75% chance that they will have an unaffected, normal child. These risks apply to each pregnancy.

In contrast, evidence suggests that some of the more mild adult forms of hypophosphatasia may be inherited as an autosomal dominant trait. In this mode of **inheritance**, a single copy of a hypophosphatasia gene can cause clinical abnormalities. An affected individual would consequently have a 50% risk of passing on the abnormal gene to each of his or her children.

The gene for TNSALP is located near the tip of the short arm of **chromosome** 1 at band 1p36.1-p34. Mutations in this gene are responsible for both the autosomal recessive and autosomal dominant forms of hypophosphatasia. Although it is not yet entirely clear how mutations in this gene cause impaired mineralization of bone, more recent work has shown that the type of mutation and its location within the gene each have an effect on the severity of disease. A wide range of mutations have been described to date. A common mutation for any form of hypophosphatasia has not yet been identified in most populations. Consequently, genetic analysis of TNSALP in most families requires extensive study of the entire gene.

Demographics

Hypophosphatasia has been described worldwide and is believed to occur in all races. The most severe form of the disease is estimated to occur in approximately one in every 100,000 live births. This corresponds to a carrier frequency of roughly one in every 200–300 individuals. The milder childhood and adult forms of hypophosphatasia are probably more common than the severe perinatal form.

Of note, hypophosphatasia is especially common among Mennonite families from Manitoba, Canada, where mating between blood relatives is not unusual. The frequency of severe disease in this population is approximately one in every 2,500 newborns with a corresponding carrier frequency of one in every 25. The number of mutations identified in this group is smaller than the general population.

Signs and symptoms

Each individual who has hypophosphatasia has clinical features derived from generalized impairment of skeletal mineralization. Six different clinical forms have been recognized. The prognosis associated with each form is dependent upon the severity of the disease and the age at which the condition is first recognized. Although affected individuals within a family tend to have similar abnormalities, it is possible to see clinical variability even between relatives.

Perinatal (lethal) hypophosphatasia

This is the most severe form of hypophosphatasia. Affected fetuses are often diagnosed during pregnancy with profound undermineralization of their bones. The limbs are typically shortened and abnormal. Bone fractures may be present. An excessive amount of amniotic fluid (polyhydramnios) during pregnancy is common. Many affected infants die prior to delivery, or are stillborn. Those who survive delivery are often irritable, have a high-pitched cry, and fail to gain weight. Respiratory failure is a common cause of death. This is usually due to deformities of the chest and associated underdevelopment of the lungs.

Infantile hypophosphatasia

Many infants with this form of the disease appear normal at birth and initially begin to develop normally. However, difficulties such as poor feeding and poor weight gain along with early clinical signs of rickets often begin before six months of age. Bony abnormalities of the chest as well as an increased susceptibility to fractures make affected infants more prone to developing pneumonia. Over 50% of affected children die during infancy, usually from severe respiratory failure. Those infants who do survive often suffer from episodes of recurrent vomiting and from abnormal kidney function due to excess loss of calcium from bone. Additionally, they may develop a misshapen head due to early closure of specific bones of the skull. Spontaneous overall improvement in health has, however, also been reported.

Childhood hypophosphatasia

The most common clinical feature in this form of hypophosphatasia is loss of the primary (deciduous) teeth before the age of five. This premature loss is directly related to abnormal dental cementum. It is this structure that normally establishes the appropriate connection of the teeth to the jaw. In hypophosphatasia, it is frequently completely missing or present but either underdeveloped or abnormally developed.

Rickets is another feature commonly seen in this later onset form. Rickets frequently lead to delayed walking as a toddler, short stature, and a characteristic waddling gait. Other rachitic deformities may also be present such as bowed legs or enlargement of the wrists, knees, and ankles.

Adult hypophosphatasia

Most affected individuals are formally diagnosed in adulthood. However, a careful review of an individual's health often reveals a childhood history of rickets and early loss of the primary teeth. This is typically followed by relatively good health during adolescence and young adulthood.

Dental and skeletal abnormalities, however, gradually recur. The age at their onset as well as their severity varies between individuals. Early loss or even extraction of the permanent teeth is common. Other skeletal abnormalities, however, are of greater concern. Osteomalacia is a common complaint. Osteomalacia is the adult form of rickets. It is characterized by increasing softness of the bones. This, in turn, leads to increased flexibility and fragility and causes deformities. Clinically, osteomalacia is typified by chronic pain in the feet due to recurrent, poorly healing stress fractures. Affected adults may also experience discomfort in their thighs and hips from painful thin zones of decalcification (pseudofractures) in the bones of the thigh.

Odontohypophosphatasia

The only clinical abnormality associated with this form of hypophosphatasia is dental disease. It may occur in children or adults. Neither rickets nor osteomalacia has been found to occur.

Pseudo-, or false, hypophosphatasia

This is an especially rare clinical form documented in only a few infants. The physical features all resemble those seen in the infantile form of the disease. However, in contrast to all of the other forms of hypophosphatasia, the total alkaline phosphatase activity has been consistently normal or even increased in blood samples from the affected children. It is unclear what the exact biochemical or molecular abnormality is in these children.

Diagnosis

After birth, a diagnosis of hypophosphatasia is based on a combination of physical examination, x ray, and biochemical studies. X ray can be particularly helpful in differentiating between the more severe forms of hypophosphatasia (perinatal, infantile) and other inher-

ited bone diseases. In the perinatal form, the skeleton generally appears completely undermineralized, occasionally absent. Bone fractures may be observed. The x-ray findings in the infantile form are similar to those seen in the perinatal form, but are usually much less severe.

Biochemical analysis may be performed on a routine blood sample. The serum may be used to determine the level of alkaline phosphatase activity. This usually represents TNSALP, and, in affected individuals, is generally low. However, it is important that the sample be obtained and handled correctly in the laboratory so as not to interfere with the enzyme activity and raise the likelihood of an incorrect result. Also, the values from each individual should be interpreted carefully as variation normally occurs based on a person's sex and his or her age.

The genetic abnormality that causes hypophosphatasia leads to an inactive form of TNSALP in most cases. As a result, the chemicals on which the enzyme would normally act begin to accumulate, or increase, in the blood and urine. This accumulation is what hastens the defective calcification of bone. In theory, these substances could be measured to establish a diagnosis of hypophosphatasia. Although none have yet been proven to alone be reliable in all situations, a few appear more promising than others. These include pyridoxal-5-phosphate (PLP), phosphoethanolamine, or inorganic pyrophosphate. Abnormal (high) results lend further support to a diagnosis of hypophosphatasia when other clinical signs have also been recognized.

Prenatal diagnosis of hypophosphatasia has been successfully reported, although prior to the advent of molecular testing, it wasn't always completely reliable. Prenatal testing has been most widely used for the detection of the perinatal lethal form of hypophosphatasia. In some cases, the severe bone abnormalities of this type have been missed with a standard mid-pregnancy ultrasound but subsequently identified at an ultrasound performed much later. While this may be due, in part, to inexperience of the person performing the ultrasound, the highly variable clinical nature of hypophosphatasia is also to blame. A fetal x ray may be performed as a follow-up to any suspicious **prenatal ultrasound** evaluation.

Both chorionic villus sampling (CVS) and **amniocentesis** have been performed but have also on occasion been complicated by technical factors. For example, cultured cells from either a villus or amniotic fluid sample may be used to determine ALP activity. Because there are four forms of ALP in humans, the TNSALP form, which is abnormal in hypophosphatasia, may not be directly analyzed. An accurate interpretation of test results may therefore not be possible.

Direct analysis of the TNSALP gene thus holds the greatest promise for accurate prenatal diagnosis. Many different TNSALP mutations have been identified; many have been found in individual families only. It is also not unusual for two carrier parents to each have a different mutation. Direct analysis is therefore only currently possible for those families who have had at least one affected child and whose mutations have already been determined. Either CVS or amniocentesis may be used in these families for mutation studies. Rapid prenatal diagnosis of hypophosphatasia in the context of a negative family history is difficult.

Treatment and management

For those families in whom the underlying mutations are unknown, the most reliable method of prenatal diagnosis for perinatal lethal hypophosphatasia includes a combination of either CVS or amniocentesis for biochemical studies as well as serial ultrasound evaluations during pregnancy. If a diagnosis is made with certainty relatively early in pregnancy, the expectant parents should be offered the option of pregnancy termination.

There is no established, effective medical therapy for any form of hypophosphatasia. Care is mainly directed toward the prevention or correction of disease-related complications. Expert dental care is highly recommended for those individuals with dental abnormalities. Physical therapy and orthopedic management are important in the care and treatment of bone complications such as fractures. Young children with the infantile form should also be monitored carefully for increasing pressure within the head from early fusion of the bones of the skull. Traditional treatments for rickets or osteomalacia, such as vitamin D or other mineral supplements, should be avoided as these bone symptoms represent only one component of an inherited, rather than acquired, complex medical problem.

Prognosis

The prognosis associated with hypophosphatasia is directly related to the severity of the disease. In general, those individuals with the most severe skeletal abnormalities tend to do much worse than those with only mild clinical symptoms. Hence, infants who are diagnosed either during pregnancy or who have significant bone deformities at birth generally die within the first few days or weeks of life. These infants may also be stillborn. The prognosis associated with the infantile form of hypophosphatasia is variable: while over half of affected infants die during their first year due to serious breathing abnormalities, others spontaneously improve and may do well. Childhood disease is associated with skeletal

KEY TERMS

Amniocentesis—A procedure performed at 16-18 weeks of pregnancy in which a needle is inserted through a woman's abdomen into her uterus to draw out a small sample of the amniotic fluid from around the baby. Either the fluid itself or cells from the fluid can be used for a variety of tests to obtain information about genetic disorders and other medical conditions in the fetus.

Chorionic villus sampling (CVS)—A procedure used for prenatal diagnosis at 10-12 weeks gestation. Under ultrasound guidance a needle is inserted either through the mother's vagina or abdominal wall and a sample of cells is collected from around the fetus. These cells are then tested for chromosome abnormalities or other genetic diseases.

Enzyme—A protein that catalyzes a biochemical reaction or change without changing its own structure or function.

Rachitic—Pertaining to, or affected by, rickets. Examples of rachitic deformities include curved long bones with prominent ends, a prominent middle chest wall, or bony nodules at the inner ends of the ribs.

deformities in some cases. Symptoms may improve, however, during adolescence only to occasionally reappear in adulthood. Finally, adult-onset hypophosphatasia is associated with ongoing, orthopedic problems once skeletal symptoms begin. Women, in particular, may notice increased bone loss and fractures after menopause.

Resources

BOOKS

Whyte, Michael P. "Hypophosphatasia." *The Metabolic and Molecular Bases of Inherited Disease.* 7th Edition. Edited by Charles R. Scriver, Arthur L. Beaudet, William S. Sly, and David Valle. New York: McGraw-Hill, Inc., 1995, pp. 4095-4110.

PERIODICALS

Deeb, A. A., S. N. Bruce, A. A. M. Morris, and T. D. Cheetham. "Infantile hypophosphatasia: Disappointing results of treatment." *Acta Pediatrica* 89, no. 6 (June 2000): 730-33.

Gehring, B., E. Mornet, H. Plath, M. Hansmann, P. Bartmann, and R. E. Brenner. "Perinatal hypophosphatasia: Diagnosis and detection of heterozygote carriers within the family." *Clinical Genetics* 56, no. 4 (October 1999): 313-17.

ORGANIZATIONS

MAGIC Foundation for Children's Growth. 1327 N. Harlem Ave., Oak Park, IL 60302. (708) 383-0808 or (800) 362-4423. Fax: (708) 383-0899. mary@magicfoundation.org. <http://www.magicfoundation.org/ghd.html>.

National Institutes of Health, Osteoporosis and Related Bone Diseases. National Resource Center, 1232 22nd Street NW, Washington, DC 20037-1292. Fax: (202) 223-0344. <http://www.osteo.org/hypoph.html>.

WEBSITES

OMIM—Online Mendelian Inheritance in Man. <http://www.ncbi.nlm.nih.gov/omim>.

Terri A. Knutel, MS, CGC

Hypophosphatemia

Definition

Hypophosphatemia is a group of inherited disorders in which there is abnormally low levels of the substance phosphate in the blood, leading to softening of the bones. This condition can result in rickets, a childhood disease in which soft and weak bones can lead to the development of bone deformities. While there is no cure, treatment can prevent the bone changes and allow proper growth of bones.

Description

Bone is one of the strongest tissues of the human body. As the main component of the adult skeleton, it provides support for movement, protects the brain and organs of the chest from injury, and contains the bone marrow, where blood cells are formed. Bone is made up of several components, including a substance called hydroxyapatite. Hydroxyapatite is made of calcium and phosphate and is partially responsible for the strength of bone.

Because of the importance of hydroxyapatite, the strength of bone is dependent on the proper levels of calcium and phosphate within the body. A lack of calcium or phosphate in the diet or a failure in maintaining proper levels of calcium or phosphate in the blood can lead to abnormalities of bone growth. Another factor required for proper development of bone is vitamin D. Vitamin D is either obtained through foods in the diet, or is made by the body in response to sunlight exposure. Vitamin D is converted to another substance within the body called calcitriol. Calcitriol promotes bone development by helping to absorb calcium and phosphate from the diet and by preventing the loss of calcium and phosphate in the urine.

Hypophosphatemia is a group of inherited disorders in which there is abnormally low phosphate levels in the blood because large amounts of phosphate exit the body through the urine. In some forms of the disease there may also be problems in the conversion of vitamin D to calcitriol. Research suggests that inherited hypophosphatemia syndromes result from an abnormality in the way the kidney handles phosphate. Normally, the kidney prevents phosphate from leaving the body in the urine, but in hypophosphatemia, an abnormality in the way the kidney handles phosphate leads to large losses of phosphate in the urine. This results in abnormally low levels of phosphate in the blood, leading to poor hydroxyapatite formation and soft bones. Insufficient levels of phosphate for bone formation results in rickets, a childhood condition in which there is abnormal bone development, growth, and repair (when this occurs in adults, it is called osteomalacia). Inherited hypophosphatemia was first described by R. W. Winters in 1958 and has been referred to in the past as vitamin D-resistant rickets or familial hypophosphatemic rickets.

Genetic profile

Hypophosphatemia is a group of conditions that can be inherited or passed on in a family. The different types of hypophosphatemia have different causes, patterns of **inheritance**, and symptoms.

The most common and widely studied form of hypophosphatemia is hereditary hypophosphatemia type I, also known as X-linked hypophosphatemia (XLH). The abnormality in XLH is in a **gene** called PHEX. It is not known precisely how this gene affects phosphate handling by the kidney. Changes in other genes have been shown to cause hypophosphatemia, but the mechanism is similarly unclear. While most occurrences of hypophosphatemia are passed from parent to child, there are several examples of new genetic changes arising in a child with no relatives with hypophosphatemia.

There are different patterns of inheritance in different forms of hypophosphatemia, including autosomal dominant inheritance and X-linked dominant inheritance. In autosomal dominant inheritance, only one abnormal gene is needed to display the disease, and the chance of passing the gene to offspring is 50%.

X-linked dominant inheritance is similar to autosomal dominant inheritance in that only one abnormal gene is needed to display the disease. However, in X-linked dominant inheritance, the genetic abnormality is located on the X **chromosome**. Females have two X chromosomes, whereas males only have one X chromosome. Females have a 50% chance of passing the abnormal gene on to either a son or a daughter, as the mother always contributes one X chromosome to a child. On the other hand, males with the abnormal X chromosome will always pass the abnormal gene to a daughter (the father will contribute the abnormal X chromosome), but never to a son (the father will contribute a normal Y chromosome, and not the abnormal X chromosome)

Demographics

Hypophosphatemia has been estimated to be present in between one in 10,000 and one in 100,000 people, but one in 20,000 people is the most widely quoted figure. It is not known whether this disease is present equally among different geographical areas and ethnic groups. The first reports of the condition found hypophosphatemia in a Bedouin (nomadic Arab) tribe.

Signs and symptoms

Major symptoms of hypophosphatemia include poor growth, bone pain, abnormally bowed legs, weakness, tooth abscesses and sometimes listlessness and irritability in infants and young children. Although the disease affects all bones, the legs are more severely affected than the arms, ribs, or pelvis. The bowed legs are often noted by 12 months of age, and the altered growth increases in severity as the child grows older. Because of poor hydroxyapatite formation, people may experience fractures, and abnormal healing follows, further contributing to growth abnormalities. As a result of poor bone development and poor healing, people with hypophosphatemia often have short stature and may have a waddling walk. Other, less common manifestations of hypophosphatemia include high blood pressure and hearing loss or deafness.

While most symptoms are the same in the different types of hypophosphatemia, there may be small changes in the severity and age at which the person will experience the symptoms.

Diagnosis

If there is no family history of hypophosphatemia, diagnosis is usually guided by physical exam. Obvious bow leg deformities will lead to x rays of the legs and knees, which will show characteristic bone abnormalities. Other studies of bone strength using radioactive tracer materials can be used, or a bone biopsy (surgical excision of a small portion of bone for inspection with a microscope) can be performed to confirm that there is less hydroxyapatite than normal.

Laboratory tests aid in determining the cause of poor bone growth and rickets. In XLH, the serum phosphorus is low and the levels of serum calcium and calcitriol are low or sometimes normal. However, urine levels of phosphate are high, indicating that phosphate is being lost in the urine and that the kidney is not reabsorbing the phosphate properly. Another laboratory finding in XLH is the presence of increased alkaline phosphatase, a enzyme that breaks down bone. However, alkaline phosphatase is often elevated in growing children compared to normal adult values. Other forms of hypophosphatemia may have other variations in laboratory findings, including normal calcitriol levels or high levels of calcium in the urine and can be used to distinguish between the different types of hypophosphatemia.

Treatment and management

There is no cure, but medical and surgical treatment can greatly improve the outcome of people with hypophosphatemia. Goals of treatment include improvement in growth, reduction in severity of bone disease, bowed legs, and activity limitations, and minimizing the complications that may develop from the treatment itself.

Medical treatment is directed toward increasing the blood phosphate levels by using phosphate salts and calcitriol, both given by mouth. However, phosphate may have to be given five times a day because it is rapidly lost in the urine, and phosphate often causes diarrhea. Despite these drawbacks, the response to the medications is very good, and bowed legs may straighten over several years of growth. Scientific studies are also being performed to determine if growth hormone can help in achieving normal growth and height development.

Health care providers are able to monitor the person's ability to take the medication by checking the phosphate levels in the urine and the blood. It is recommended that these tests be performed in small children every three months to determine if they are receiving adequate amounts of phosphate. Later, the monitoring can be decreased to every four to six months. It is also recommended that childhood x rays of the knee be performed every one to two years to see whether medication changes are needed.

Some problems may result from the medications used to treat hypophosphatemia. High levels of calcium can build up in the bloodstream causing problems with the kidneys and the parathyroid (a gland in the neck). Because of these problems, routine calcium measurements and kidney ultrasound studies should be performed to determine if additional medications should be added or changes in medications should be made.

Treatment with medication is sometimes not enough to reverse the bone abnormalities. In cases such as these, surgery can be performed to reshape or even lengthen the bones.

Prognosis

With early diagnosis and treatment, the prognosis for people with hypophosphatemia is excellent. Adult heights of 170 cm may be achievable, compared to

KEY TERMS

Biopsy—The surgical removal and microscopic examination of living tissue for diagnostic purposes.

Calcitriol—A substance that assists in bone growth by helping to maintain calcium and phosphate levels in the blood. Vitamin D is converted into this substance by the body.

Calcium—One of the elements that make up the hydroxyapatite crystals found in bone.

Hydroxyapatite—A mineral that gives bone its rigid structure and strength. It is primarily composed of calcium and phosphate.

Hypophosphatemia—The state of having abnormally low levels of phosphate in the bloodstream.

Osteomalacia—The adult form of rickets, a lack of proper mineralization of bone.

Parathyroid glands—A pair of glands adjacent to the thyroid gland that primarily regulate blood calcium levels.

Phosphate—A substance composed of the elements phosphorus and oxygen that contributes to the hydroxyapatite crystals found in normal bones.

Rickets—A childhood disease caused by vitamin D deficiency, resulting in soft and malformed bones.

130-165 cm without treatment. While some degree of abnormal bone growth may always be detectable, people with hypophosphatemia will generally live normal life spans.

Resources

BOOKS

Brenner, B. M., ed. *Brenner and Rector's The Kidney.* Philadelphia: W.B. Saunders, 2000.

Behrman, R. E., ed. "Familial Hypophosphatemia." *Nelson Textbook of Pediatrics.* Philadelphia: W.B. Saunders, 2000, pp. 2136-2137.

Goldman, L., ed. "Osteomalacia and Rickets." *Cecil Textbook of Medicine.* Philadelphia: W.B. Saunders, 2000, pp. 1391-1398.

Wilson, J. D., ed. "Rickets and Osteomalacia." In *Williams Textbook of Endocrinology.* Philadelphia: W.B. Saunders, 1998, pp. 1228-1230.

PERIODICALS

Carpenter, T. O. "New perspectives on the biology and treatment of X-linked hypophosphatemic rickets." *Pediatric Clinics of North America* 44 (April 1997): 443-466.

Subramanian R., and R. Khardori. "Severe hypophosphatemia. Pathophysiologic implications, clinical presentations, and treatment." *Medicine* 79 (January 2000): 1-8.

WEBSITES

OMIM—Online Mendelian Inheritance in Man. National Center for Biotechnology Information, National Center for Biotechnology Information, National Library of Medicine. <http://www3.ncbi.nlm.nih.gov/htbin- post/ Omim>.

XLH Network. <http://georgia.ncl.ac.uk/VitaminD/ vitamind.html>.

Oren Traub, MD, PhD

Hypophosphatemic rickets
see **Hypophosphatemia**

Hypospadias and epispadias

Definition

Hypospadias is a congenital defect, primarily of males, in which the urethra opens on the underside (ventrum) of the penis. The corresponding defect in females is an opening of the urethra into the vagina and is rare.

Epispadias (also called bladder exstrophy) is a congenital defect of males in which the urethra opens on the upper surface (dorsum) of the penis. The corresponding defect in females is a fissure in the upper wall of the urethra and is quite rare.

Description

In a male, the external opening of the urinary tract (external meatus) is normally located at the tip of the penis. In a female, it is normally located between the clitoris and the vagina.

In males with hypospadias, the urethra opens on the inferior surface or underside of the penis. In females with hypospadias, the urethra opens into the cavity of the vagina.

In males with epispadias, the urethra opens on the superior surface or upper side of the penis. In females with epispadias, there is a crack or fissure in the wall of the urethra and out of the body through an opening in the skin above the clitoris.

During the embryological development of males, a groove of tissue folds inward and then fuses to form a tube that becomes the urethra. Hypospadias occurs when the tube does not form or does not fuse completely.

Epispadias is due to a defect in the tissue that folds inward to form the urethra.

During the development of a female, similar processes occur to form the urethra. The problem is usually insufficient length of the tube that becomes the urethra. As a result, the urethra opens in an abnormal location, resulting in a hypospadias. Occasionally, fissures form in the bladder. These may extend to the surface of the abdomen and fuse with the adjacent skin. This is most often identified as a defect in the bladder although it is technically an epispadias.

Hypospadias in males generally occur alone. Female hypospadias may be associated with abnormalities of the genital tract, since the urinary and genital tracts are formed in the same embryonic process.

Because it represents incomplete development of the penis, some experts think that insufficient male hormone may be responsible for hypospadias.

Genetic profile

Hypospadias and epispadias are congenital defects of the urinary tract. This means that they occur during intrauterine development. There is no genetic basis for the defects. Specific causes for hypospadias are not known. This means that blood relatives do not have increased chances of developing them.

Demographics

In males, the incidence of hypospadias is approximately one per 250 to 300 live births. Epispadias is much less common, having an incidence of about one per 100,000 live male births.

In females, hypospadias is much less common than in males. It appears about once in every 500,000 live female births. Epispadias is even rarer. Reliable estimates of the prevalence of epispadias in females are not available. Epispadias in females is often diagnosed and recorded as a bladder anomaly.

Signs and symptoms

Hypospadias is usually not associated with other defects of the penis or urethra. In males, it can occur at any site along the underside of the penis. In females, the urethra exits the body in an abnormal location. This is usually due to inadequate length of the urethra.

Epispadias is associated with bladder abnormalities. In females, the front wall of the bladder does not fuse or close. The bladder fissure may extend to the external abdominal wall. In such a rare case, the front of the pelvis is also widely separated. In males, the bladder fissure extends into the urethra and simply becomes an opening somewhere along the upper surface of the penis.

Hypospadias is associated with difficulty in assigning gender to babies. This occurs when gender is not obvious at birth because of deformities in the sex organs.

Diagnosis

Male external urinary tract defects are discovered at birth during the first detailed examination of the newborn. Female urethral defects may not be discovered for some time due to the difficulty in viewing the infant vagina.

Treatment and management

Surgery is the treatment of choice for both hypospadias and epispadias. All surgical repairs should be undertaken early and completed without delay. This minimizes psychological trauma.

In males with hypospadias, one surgery is usually sufficient to repair the defect. With more complicated hypospadias (more than one abnormally situated urethral opening), multiple surgeries may be required. In females with hypospadias, surgical repair is technically more complicated but can usually be completed in a brief interval of time.

Repairing an epispadias is more difficult. In males, this may involve other structures in the penis. Males should not be circumcised since the foreskin is often needed for the repair. Unfortunately, choices may be required that affect the ability to inseminate a female partner. Reproduction requires that the urethral meatus be close to the tip of the penis. Cosmetic appearance and urinary continence are usually the primary goals. Surgery for these defects is successful 70 to 80% of the time. Modern treatment of complete male epispadias allows for an excellent genital appearance and achievement of urinary continence.

In females, repair of epispadias may require multiple surgical procedures. Urinary continence and cosmetic appearance are the usual primary considerations. Urinary continence is usually achieved although cosmetic appearance may be somewhat compromised. Fertility is not usually affected. Repair rates that are similar or better than those for males can usually be achieved for females.

Hypospadias in both males and females is more of a nuisance and hindrance to reproduction than a threat to health. If surgery is not an option, the condition may be allowed to persist. This usually leads to an increased risk of infections in the lower urinary tract.

Prognosis

With adequate surgical repair, most males with simple hypospadias can lead normal lives with a penis that appears and functions in a normal manner. This includes fathering

KEY TERMS

Bladder—This is the organ that stores urine after it flows out of the kidneys and through the ureters.

Circumcision—The surgical removal of the foreskin of the penis.

Continence—Normal function of the urinary bladder and urethra, allowing fluid flow during urination and completely stopping flow at other times.

External meatus—The external opening through which urine and seminal fluid (in males only) leave the body.

Genital tract—The organs involved in reproduction. In a male, they include the penis, testicles, prostate and various tubular structures to transport seminal fluid and sperm. In a female, they include the clitoris, vagina, cervix, uterus, fallopian tubes and ovaries.

Urethra—The tubular portion of the urinary tract connecting the bladder and external meatus through which urine passes. In males, seminal fluid and sperm also pass through the urethra.

children. Females with simple hypospadias also have normal lives, including conceiving and bearing children.

The prognosis for epispadias depends on the extent of the defect. Most males with relatively minor epispadias lead normal lives, including fathering children. As the extent of the defect increases, surgical reconstruction is generally acceptable. However, many of these men are unable to conceive children. Most epispadias in females can be surgically repaired. The chances of residual disfigurement increase as the extent of the epispadias increases. Fertility in females is not generally affected by epispadias.

Resources

BOOKS

Duckett, John W. "Hypospadias." *Campbell's Urology.* Edited by Patrick C. Walsh, et al. Philadelphia: W. B. Saunders, 1998, pp. 2093-2116.

Gearhart, John P., and Robert D. Jeffs. "Exstrophy-epispadias complex and bladder anomalies." *Campbell's Urology.* Edited by Patrick C. Walsh, et al. Philadelphia: W. B. Saunders, 1998, pp. 1977-1982.

Nelson, Waldo E., et al., ed. "Anomalies of the bladder." *Nelson Textbook of Pediatrics.* Philadelphia: W. B. Saunders, 2000, pp. 1639-1642.

Nelson, Waldo E., et al., ed. "Anomalies of the penis and urethra." *Nelson Textbook of Pediatrics.* Philadelphia: W. B. Saunders, 2000, pp. 1645-1650.

PERIODICALS

Kajbafzadeh, A. M., P. G. Duffy, and P. G. Ransley. "The evolution of penile reconstruction in epispadias repair: A report of 180 cases." *Journal of Urology* 154, 2 pt 2 (1995): 858-61.

Shapiro, E., H. Lepor, and R. D. Jeffs. "The inheritance of the exstrophy-epispadias complex." *Journal of Urology* 132, no. 2 (1984): 308-10.

ORGANIZATIONS

Association for the Bladder Exstrophy Community. PO Box 1472, Wake Forest, NC 27588-1472. (919) 624-9447. <http://www.bladderexstrophy.com/support.htm>.

Hypospadias Association of America. 4950 S. Yosemite Street, Box F2-156, Greenwood Village, CO 80111. hypospadiasassn@yahoo.com. <http://www.hypospadias.net>.

Support for Parents with Hypospadias Boys. <http://clubs.yahoo.com/clubs/mumswithhypospadiaskids>.

University of California–San Francisco. <http://itsa.ucsf.edu/~uroweb/Uro/hypospadias/index.html>.

WEBSITES

Hatch, David A., MD. "Abnormal Development of the Penis and Male Urethra." *Genitourinary Development.* <http://www.meddean.luc.edu/lumen/MedEd/urology/abnpendv.htm>.

"Hypospadias." *Atlas of Congenital Deformities of the External Genitalia.* <http://www.atlasperovic.com/contents/9.htm>.

"Hypospadias." *Columbia Presbyterian Hospital.* <http://cpmcnet.cpmc.columbia.edu/dept/urology/pediatric/hypospadias.html>.

"Hypospadias." *University of Michigan.* <http://www.urology.med.umich.edu/clinic/pediatric/hypospadias.html>.

Johns Hopkins University Pediatric Urology Center. "Epispadias." *Johns Hopkins Exstrophy Database.* <http://www.med.jhu.edu/pediurol/pediatric/exstrophy/database/web4d.html>.

Society for Pediatric Urology. <http://www.spu.org/>.

The Penis.com. <http://www.the-penis.com/hypospadias.html>.

L. Fleming Fallon, Jr., MD, PhD, DrPH

Hypothalamic hamartobastoma *see* **Pallister-Hall syndrome**

Hypotonia-obesity-prominent incisors syndrome *see* **Cohen syndrome**

Hypoxanthine guanine phosphoribosyl-transferase 1 (HPRT1) *see* **Lesch-Nyhan syndrome**

I

I-cell disease *see* **Mucolipidosis**

Ichthyosis

Definition

Derived from the Greek word meaning fish disease, ichthyosis is a congenital (meaning present at birth) dermatological (skin) disease that is represented by thick, scaly skin.

Description

The ichthyoses are a group of genetic skin diseases caused by an abnormality in skin growth that results in drying and scaling. There are at least 20 types of ichthyosis. Ichthyosis can be more or less severe, sometimes accumulating thick scales and cracks that are painful and bleed. Ichthyosis is not contagious because it is inherited.

Genetic profile

Depending on the specific type of ichthyosis, the **inheritance** can be autosomal recessive, autosomal dominant, X-linked recessive, X-linked dominant, or sporadic. Autosomal recessive means that the altered **gene** for the disease or trait is located on one of the first 22 pairs of chromosomes, which are also called "autosomes." Males and females are equally likely to have an autosomal recessive disease or trait. Recessive means that two copies of the altered gene are necessary to express the condition. Therefore, a child inherits one copy of the altered gene from each parent, who are called carriers (because they have only one copy of the altered gene). Since carriers do not express the altered gene, parents usually do not know they carry the altered gene that causes ichthyosis until they have an affected child. Carrier parents have a 1-in-4 chance (or 25%) with each pregnancy, to have a child with ichthyosis.

Autosomal dominant inheritance also means that both males and females are equally likely to have the disease but only one copy of the altered gene is necessary to have the condition. An individual with ichthyosis has a 50/50 chance to pass the condition to his or her child.

The last pair of human chromosomes, either two X (female) or one X and one Y (male) determines gender. X-linked means the altered gene causing the disease or trait is located on the X **chromosome**. Females have two X chromosomes while males have one X chromosome. The term "recessive" usually infers that two copies of a gene—one on each of the chromosome pair—are necessary to cause a disease or express a particular trait. X-linked recessive diseases are most often seen in males, however, because they have a single X chromosome, and no "back-up." So, if a male inherits a particular gene on the X, he expresses the altered gene, even though he has only a single copy of it. Females, on the other hand, have two X chromosomes, and therefore can carry a gene on one of their X chromosomes yet not express any symptoms. (Their second X, or "back-up," functions normally). Usually a mother carries the altered gene for X-linked recessive ichthyosis unknowingly, and has a 50/50 chance with each pregnancy to transmit the altered gene. If the child is a male, he will have ichthyosis, while if the child is a female, she will be a carrier for ichthyosis like her mother.

X-linked dominant inheritance means that only one gene from the X chromosome is necessary to produce the condition. Mothers with the altered gene are affected, and have a 50/50 chance to pass the condition to any child, who will also have ichthyosis. In some cases, X-linked dominant inheritance is lethal in males, which means that male fetuses with X-linked dominant ichthyosis are miscarried. This is true for a rare disorder called Conradi-Hunerman, in which ichthyosis is just one feature.

New mutations—alterations in the **DNA** of a gene—can cause disease. In these cases, neither parent has the disease-causing mutation. This may occur because the mutation in the gene happened for the first time only in the egg or sperm for that particular pregnancy. New mutations are thought to happen by chance and are therefore referred to as "sporadic," meaning that they occur occasionally and are not predictable.

Demographics

The most common form of ichthyosis is called ichthyosis vulgaris (*vulgar* is Latin for common), and occurs in approximately one person in every 250 and is inherited in an autosomal dominant manner. The most rare types of ichthyosis occur in fewer than one person in one million and are inherited in an autosomal recessive manner. Ichthyosis occurs regardless of the part of the world the child is from, or the ethnic background of the parents.

Signs and symptoms

The skin is made up of several layers, supported underneath by a layer of fat that is thicker or thinner depending on location. The lower layers contain blood vessels, the middle layers contain actively growing cells, and the upper layer consists of dead cells that serve as a barrier to the outside world. This barrier is nearly waterproof and highly resistant to infection. Scattered throughout the middle layers are hair follicles, oil and sweat glands, and nerve endings. The upper layer is constantly flaking off and being replaced from beneath by new tissue. In ichthyosis, the skin's natural shedding process is slowed or inhibited, and in some types, skin cells are produced too rapidly.

The abnormality in skin growth and hydration called ichthyosis may present with symptoms at birth or in early childhood. Ichthyosis can itch relentlessly, leading to such complications of scratching as lichen simplex (dermatitis characterized by raw patches of skin). Either the cracking or the scratching can introduce infection, bringing with it discomfort and complications.

Diagnosis

A dermatologist will often make the diagnosis of ichthyosis, based on a clinical exam. However, a skin biopsy, or DNA study (from a small blood sample) is necessary to confirm the diagnosis. Evaluation for associated problems is done by a complete physical medical examination.

For some types of ichthyosis, the abnormal gene has been identified and prenatal testing is available. At present this is true for the autosomal recessive congenital ichthyoses, which includes: lamellar ichthyosis (LI), autosomal recessive lamellar ichthyosis

(ARLI), congenital ichthyosiform erythroderm (CIE), and non-bullous congenital ichthyosiform erythroderma (NBCIE).

There are four different genes that have been located for the autosomal recessive congenital ichthyoses, however, testing is available for only one gene called transglutaminase-1 (TGM1) located on chromosome 14. Once a couple has had a child with ichthyosis, and they have had the genetic cause identified by DNA studies (performed from a small blood sample), prenatal testing for future pregnancies may be considered. (Note that prenatal testing may not be possible if both mutations cannot be identified.) Prenatal diagnosis is available via either chorionic villus sampling (CVS) or **amniocentesis**. CVS is a biopsy of the placenta performed in the first trimester of pregnancy under ultrasound guidance. Ultrasound is the use of sound waves to visualize the developing fetus. The genetic makeup of the placenta is identical to the fetus and therefore the TGM1 gene can be studied from this tissue. There is approximately a one in 100 chance for miscarriage with CVS. Amniocentesis is a procedure done under ultrasound guidance in which a long thin needle is inserted through the mother's abdomen into the uterus, to withdraw a couple of tablespoons of amniotic fluid (fluid surrounding the developing baby) to study. The TGM1 gene can be studied using cells from the amniotic fluid. Other genetic tests, such as a chromosome analysis, may also be performed through either CVS or amniocentesis.

Treatment and management

Most treatments for ichthyosis are topical, which means they are applied directly to the skin, not taken internally. Some forms of ichthyosis requires two forms of treatment—a reduction in the amount of scale buildup and moisturizing of the underlying skin. Several agents are available for each purpose. Reduction in the amount of scale is achieved by keratolytics. Among this class of drugs are urea, lactic acid, and salicylic acid. Petrolatum, 60% propylene glycol, and glycerin are successful moisturizing agents, as are many commercially-available products. Increased humidity of the ambient air is also helpful in preventing skin dryness.

Because the skin acts as a barrier to the outside environment, medicines have a hard time penetrating, especially through the thick skin of the palms of the hands and the soles of the feet. This resistance is diminished greatly by maceration (softening the skin). Soaking hands in water macerates skin so that it looks like prune skin. Occlusion (covering) with rubber gloves or plastic wrap will also macerate skin. Applying medicines and then covering the skin with an occlusive dressing will facilitate entrance of the medicine and greatly magnify its effect.

KEY TERMS

Amniocentesis—A procedure performed at 16-18 weeks of pregnancy in which a needle is inserted through a woman's abdomen into her uterus to draw out a small sample of the amniotic fluid from around the baby. Either the fluid itself or cells from the fluid can be used for a variety of tests to obtain information about genetic disorders and other medical conditions in the fetus.

Amniotic fluid—The fluid which surrounds a developing baby during pregnancy.

Autosomal dominant—A pattern of genetic inheritance where only one abnormal gene is needed to display the trait or disease.

Autosomal recessive—A pattern of genetic inheritance where two abnormal genes are needed to display the trait or disease.

Dermatologist—A physician that specializes in disorders of the skin.

Emollient—Petroleum or lanolin based skin lubricants.

Keratin—A tough, nonwater-soluble protein found in the nails, hair, and the outermost layer of skin. Human hair is made up largely of keratin.

Keratinocytes—Skin cells.

Keratolytic—An agent that dissolves or breaks down the outer layer of skin (keratins).

Retinoids—A derivative of synthetic vitamin A.

Sporadic—Isolated or appearing occasionally with no apparent pattern.

X-linked dominant inheritance—The inheritance of a trait by the presence of a single gene on the X chromosome in a male or female, passed from an affected female who has the gene on one of her X chromosomes.

X-linked recessive inheritance—The inheritance of a trait by the presence of a single gene on the X chromosome in a male, passed from a female who has the gene on one of her X chromosomes. She is referred to as an unaffected carrier.

Secondary treatments are necessary to control pruritus (itching) and infection. Commercial products containing camphor, menthol, eucalyptus oil, aloe, and similar substances are very effective as antipruritics. If the skin cracks deeply enough, a pathway for infection is created. Topical antibiotics like bacitracin are effective

in prevention and in the early stages of these skin infections. Cleansing with hydrogen peroxide inhibits infection as well.

Finally, there are topical and internal derivatives of vitamin A called retinoids that improve skin growth and are used for severe cases of acne, ichthyosis, and other skin conditions.

Prognosis

This condition requires continuous care throughout a lifetime. Properly treated, in most cases it is a cosmetic problem. There are a small number of lethal forms, such as **harlequin fetus**.

Resources

BOOKS

Baden, Howard P. "Ichthyosiform Dermatoses." *Dermatology in General Medicine*. Edited by Thomas B. Fitzpatrick, et al. New York: McGraw-Hill, 1993, 531-544.

Parker, Frank. "Skin Diseases of General Importance." *Cecil Textbook of Medicine.* Edited by J. Claude Bennett and Fred Plum. Philadelphia: W. B. Saunders, 1996, 2204.

Sybert, Virginia P. *Genetic Skin Disorders*. Oxford Monographs on Medical Genetics. No. 33. New York: Oxford University Press, 1997.

ORGANIZATIONS

Alliance of Genetic Support Groups. 4301 Connecticut Ave. NW, Suite 404, Washington, DC 20008. (202) 966-5557. Fax: (202) 966-8553. <http://www.geneticalliance.org>.

Foundation for Ichthyosis and Related Skin Types. 650 N. Cannon Ave., Suite 17, Landsdale, PA 19446. (215) 631-1411 or (800) 545-3286. Fax: (215) 631-1413. <http://www.scalyskin.org>.

National Organization for Rare Disorders (NORD). PO Box 8923, New Fairfield, CT 06812-8923. (203) 746-6518 or (800) 999-6673. Fax: (203) 746-6481. <http://www.rarediseases.org>.

National Registry for Ichthyosis and Related Disorders. University of Washington Dermatology Department, Box 356524, 1959 N.E. Pacific, Rm. BB1353, Seattle, WA 98195-6524. (800) 595-1265 or (206) 616-3179. <http://www.skinregistry.org>.

WEBSITES

Immune Deficiency Foundation. <www.primaryimmune.org>.

The National Registry for Ichthyosis and Related Skin Types. <http://depts.washington.edu/ichreg/ichthyosis.registry>.

Catherine L. Tesla, MS, CGC

Ichthyosis bullosa of siemens *see* **Ichthyosis**

Ichthyosis congenita *see* **Ichthyosis**

Ichthyosis-spastic neurologic disorder-oligo-
phrenia syndrome *see* **Sjögren Larsson
syndrome**

Idiopathic basal ganglia calcification (IBGC)
see **Fahr disease**

Imprinting

Definition

Genetic imprinting is the differential expression of a **gene** depending on whether it was maternally or paternally inherited. It is a method by which the gene expression can be silenced, and made nonfunctional. Imprinting is believed to play a critical role in fetal growth and development, but the exact purpose for imprinting has not been determined.

Description

Normal genetic imprinting process

A gene is made up of long sequences of **DNA**. When DNA is changed into **RNA** and then into protein, the processes involved are known as transcription and translation. For a gene to exert an effect on the individual's system, it has to be transcribed and translated. Some genes are constitutively (consistently) transcribed. Others are only transcribed when their products are needed.

Genetic imprinting is a natural phenomenon that does not follow the pattern of traditional Mendelian genetics. Mendelian genetics demonstrate that an individual inherits two functional copies (alleles) of every non-sex linked gene. One copy is paternally inherited, and the other is maternally inherited. When genes follow the Mendelian **inheritance** pattern, both the paternal and maternal copies are functionally expressed, regardless of which parent it came from. Imprinting, however, demonstrates that the expression of some genes is affected by which parent they originated from. A gene is imprinted when the expression of its activity depends on the sex of the parent that transmitted the copy of the gene. The activity of these genes is specifically regulated based on whether it is maternally or paternally marked with a signal sequence. Usually, one allele is silenced so that only one parental copy is active. The silenced copy is the imprinted copy. An imprinted gene is temporarily silenced. Genes that are silenced are not transcribed and translated, and so exert no effect on the system. There are no expression products from an imprinted gene. An individual with a maternally imprinted gene will only have expression products from the paternal allele. An individual with a paternally imprinted gene will only have expression products from the maternal allele. The result is only one functional copy of the gene that came from the parent with the normal, non-imprinted **chromosome**.

The imprinted chromosome was silenced during the formation of parental egg or sperm, before the offspring ever inherited it. Imprinting occurs in each generation when new egg and sperm cells are produced. A female that inherits a paternally imprinted gene will maintain the paternal imprint during the embryonic stage. However, the female will eventually form her own egg cells that may be used to reproduce. In her new egg cells (gametes), the original paternal imprint will be erased, and replaced with her own imprinted patterns. The same is true for males that inherit maternally imprinted genes. The imprinting is not permanent in that it will be erased when gametes, or sperm, are formed. This germline conversion process is regulated by the imprinting center, a piece of DNA located within the imprinted chromosome. Relatively few human genes are imprinted. Imprinted genes tend to cluster together in the same genomic regions. A maternally imprinted gene has a signal on it, often a chemical methyl group, which causes it to be silenced. Imprinted genes are referred to as "epigenetic," because the alterations that silence them do not involve actual mutations to the DNA sequence.

Genetic imprinting is a normal process that occurs in several dozen mammalian genes. It is thought to play a role in the transmission of nutrients from the mother to the fetus and to the newborn. Imprinted genes tend to impact fetal growth and the behavior of the newborn infant. Abnormalities involving imprinting patterns may result in many different diseases.

Complications in the genetic imprinting process

Multiple types of complications may arise involving imprinted genes. Normally, if there is a mutation in one of a pair of chromosomes that deletes its function, the other copy still functions and expresses a gene product. With an imprinted gene, if the one normal, functional gene is deleted or mutated, there is no back-up functionality on the imprinted chromosome. In this manner, the mutation of the normal, active copy of an imprinted gene may result in disease. Another complication may occur if, as a result of an error, cells receive all or part of a pair of chromosomes from a single parent. This is known as uniparental disomy. With imprinted genes, the cell receives either two imprinted copies or two active copies. If both copies are imprinted, there are no functional genes present.

Loss of activity and gain of inappropriate activity can both be harmful. A mutation in a gene that is imprinted may also activate the gene. This loss of imprinting leads to two active copies of a gene where neither copy is silenced. Too many active copies of a gene may result in overexpression, which can result in disease. Some types of **cancer** are associated with failure to imprint genes that encode for growth factors. Overexpression of these growth factors contributes to uncontrolled cell growth and the development of cancer. Environmental factors such as exposure to toxins may sometimes cause changes in DNA that alter imprinted gene expression, resulting in genetic diseases such as cancer and behavioral disorders.

Two of the best-studied diseases caused by genomic imprinting are **Prader-Willi syndrome** (PWS) and **Angelman syndrome** (AS). Both syndromes are caused by alterations in chromosome 15. Many different genes within this chromosomal region express different products based on whether they were inherited maternally or paternally. A paternally imprinted chromosome 15 with a deletion causes approximately 70% of cases of PWS. Approximately 29% of cases are caused by inheriting both maternal copies of chromosome 15, with a rare 1% involving a mutation in the imprinting center itself. All of these alterations lead to PWS, a neurobehavioral disorder characterized by excessive eating habits, obesity, short stature, mental retardation, and small hands and feet. Approximately 70% of cases of AS are caused by a deletion within the same region of chromosome 15, but on the maternal copy. Various other types of alterations cause the remaining 30%. Although AS involves the same chromosomal region, the impact of a functional paternal chromosome as opposed to a maternal chromosome, is profoundly different. Angelman syndrome is characterized by hyperactivity, an unusual facial appearance, short stature, mental retardation, spasticity, inappropriate laughter, and seizures. While PWS affects approximately one in every 10,000–15,000 live births, AS is relatively rare.

As of 2005, the National Institutes of Health (NIH) is in the process of assessing preliminary evidence that suggests assisted reproduction techniques such as *in vitro* fertilization (IVF) may be interfering with the imprinting process and lead to increased risk for related congenital abnormalities in offspring. These techniques may interfere with genetic processing that takes place during early embryogenesis. An increased incidence in **genetic disorders** involving imprinting has been found in children conceived by IVF. There may be an increased incidence of Beckwith Wiedemann syndrome (BWS), a

disorder associated with overgrowth and malformations due to an imprinting defect in chromosome 11. An increase in BWS has also been reported in monozygotic twin gestations, increasing the evidence that disturbances occurring during the preimplantation stage may affect imprinting.

KEY TERMS

Allele—One of two or more different genes encoding specific and inheritable characteristics that occupy corresponding locations on a pair of chromosomes.

Chemical methyl group—One carbon and three hydrogen molecules that can be attached as a signal to DNA in the regulation of gene expression.

Embryogenesis—The formation and growth of the embryo.

Epigenetic—Implying a modification outside of actual mutation of the DNA sequence, such as the addition of a methyl group.

Gamete—A reproductive cell; an ovum or sperm

Germline—The cell line from which gametes arise.

Mendelian genetics—A set of parameters describing the traditional method of the transmission of genes from one generation to the next.

Spasticity—Increased muscular tone or contractions that cause stiff or awkward movements.

Uniparental disomy—The inheritance of both copies of a chromosome from one parent, with none from the other parent.

Resources

BOOKS

Lewin, Benjamin. *Genes, Fifth Edition.* Oxford: Oxford University Press, 1994.

Moore, Keith L., and T. V. N. Persaud. *The Developing Human, Clinically Oriented Embryology, Seventh Edition.* St. Louis, MO: Elsevier Science, 2003.

Thompson & Thompson Genetics in Medicine, Sixth Edition. St. Louis, MO: Elsevier Science, 2004.

PERIODICALS

Reik, W., and J. Walter. "Genomic Imprinting: Parental Influence on the Genome." *Nature Reviews Genetics* 2 2001: 21–32.

WEBSITES

Genomic Imprinting and Assisted Reproduction: Is There a Cause for Concern? NIH. (April 5, 2005.) <http://www.nichd.nih.gov/cdbpm/pp/fetalGrowth/wilkins_haug1.htm>.

Maria Basile, PhD

Incontinentia pigmenti

Definition

Incontinentia pigmenti (IP) is an X-linked dominant disorder affecting primarily the skin, hair, teeth and nails (all components of the epidermis). This disease may have been initially described by Garrod in 1906. It was completely characterized by Bloch and Sulzberger in 1928. For this reason, incontinentia pigmenti has also been referred to as Bloch-Sulzberger syndrome.

Description

Incontinentia pigmenti has been traditionally classified into two types: type I and type II. Much debate has occurred over whether or not type I or sporadic, incontinentia pigmenti is actually the same disease as type II or familial, male-lethal type incontinentia pigmenti. The debate on this issue continues in the medical literature. The growing consensus is that sporadic (type I) incontinentia pigmenti is not, in fact, the same disease as familial, male-lethal (type II) incontinentia pigmenti. Type II (familial, male-lethal) incontinentia pigmenti is considered to be the "classic" case of incontinentia pigmenti that matches the disease characterized by Bloch and Sulzberger in 1928.

Genetic profile

The locus of the **gene** mutation responsible for incontinentia pigmenti type II has been mapped to the long end of the X **chromosome** at gene location Xq28. The affected gene is known as the NEMO gene.

A chromosome is a long chain of **deoxyribonucleic acid (DNA)**, a double-stranded molecule composed of individual units called nucleotides. The two strands that make up a single DNA molecule are held together by a matching (base pairing) of the nucleotides on one strand with the nucleotides on the other strand. Each set of a nucleotide on one strand paired with its nucleotide on the other strand is called a base pair.

A gene is a particular segment of a particular chromosome. Within the segment containing a particular gene there are two types of areas: introns and exons. Introns are sections of the particular chromosomal segment that do not actively participate in the functioning of the gene. Exons are those sections that do actively participate in gene function. A typical gene consists of several areas of exons divided by several areas of introns.

The NEMO gene was completely sequenced by the International Incontinentia Pigmenti Consortium in 2000. The NEMO gene consists of approximately 23,000 base pairs that compose 10 exons. The first exon of this gene, which is the exon that tells this gene to "turn on," has been found to have three variants; these are designated: 1a, 1b, and 1c.

The NEMO gene is known to partially overlap with the gene responsible for the production of glucose-6-phosphate dehydrogenase (G6PD). Mutations in the G6PD gene cause an under-production of red blood cells (anemia) that results in an insufficient amount of oxygen being delivered to the tissues and organs. Anemia resulting from mutations in the G6PD gene is observed with higher frequencies in Africans, Mediterraneans, and Asians.

The locus of the gene mutation responsible for type I incontinentia pigmenti has been mapped to band Xp11, on the short arm of the X chromosome. Individuals affected with this disorder show many of the signs of incontinentia pigmenti type II, but it is not an inherited condition. Type I incontinentia pigmenti is only exhibited as a sporadic and *de novo* trait. This means that when an affected individual has the symptoms of type I IP, that individual did not inherit this condition from his or her parents; rather the condition was caused by a mutation that occurred after conception.

Demographics

Incontinentia pigmenti is observed with higher frequencies in Africans, Mediterraneans, and Asians than in other portions of the population. This was originally thought to be due to the greater ability to observe the skin-related symptoms in these individuals. But, with the additional evidence that the NEMO gene and the G6PD gene overlap and that anemia resulting from mutations in the G6PD gene also disproportionately affects these populations, this anecdotal explanation has to be discarded.

More than 95% of all patients diagnosed with IP are female. The occurrence in males is probably due to a spontaneous (de novo) mutation in the NEMO gene that is not as severe as the typical mutation leading to IP or the misdiagnosis of type I IP. Approximately 70% of all IP affected individuals have been found to have the same mutation in the NEMO gene. In these families, 100% lethality prior to birth is observed in males.

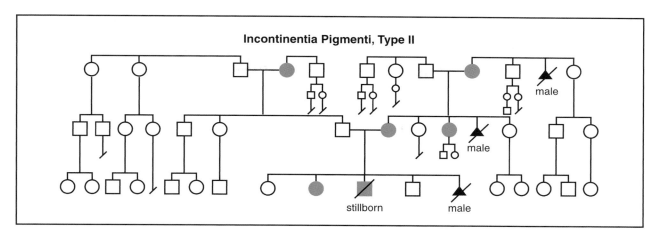

Incontinentia Pigmenti, Type II

(Gale Group)

Signs and symptoms

Familial, male-lethal (type II) IP is characterized by progressive rashes of the skin. These have been classified into four stages: the red (erythematic) and blister-like (vesicular) stage; the wart-like (verrucous) stage; the darkened skin (hyperpigmented) stage; and the scarred (atrophic) stage.

The first, or erythematic vesicular, stage consists of patches of red skin containing blisters and/or boils. This condition usually appears in affected individuals at or near birth and is generally localized to the scalp, the arms, and the legs. This stage generally lasts from a few weeks to a few months and may recur within the first few months of life. It rarely recurs after the age of 6 months. This condition is often misdiagnosed as chicken pox, herpes, impetigo, or scabies. Each of these alternative diseases is potentially life-threatening in an infant, so most IP affected infants are treated for one of these diseases before the appropriate diagnosis of incontinentia pigmenti can be made.

The second, or verrucous, stage of IP is characterized by skin lesions that look like adolescent acne (pustules). Upon healing, these pustules generally leave darkened skin. This stage almost exclusively affects the arms and legs, but it may be observed elsewhere. The verrucous stage may occur at birth, which may indicate that the erythematic vesicular stage occurred prior to birth. But, more generally, the second stage of IP skin disorder is observed after the first stage has completed. The verrucous stage tends to persist for months. Rarely it may last for an entire year.

The third, or hyperpigmented, stage is characterized by "marbled skin," in which darkened areas of skin seem to make swirling patterns across the normal and less pig-mented skin. This third stage generally occurs between six and 12 months of life. In 5-10% of affected individuals, this third stage is present at birth. These areas of hyperpigmentation tend to fade with age such that they are barely visible in adults affected with type II IP.

Areas of scarred skin caused by the first two stages characterize the fourth, or atrophic, stage. These scars are often noticeable before the third stage has begun to fade. Adolescents and adults affected with type II IP will generally have pale, hairless patches or streaks, most visibly on the scalp or calves, that are associated with this fourth stage. In many adults affected with IP, the skin abnormalities may have faded to such a significant degree that they are no longer noticeable to the casual observer. Many type II IP affected individuals have a loss or lack of hair on the crown of the head (alopecia). This is suspected to be caused by the underlying skin atrophies of IP.

More than 80% of individuals affected with type II IP have abnormalities of the teeth including missing teeth, late eruption of both the baby teeth and the adult teeth, unusually pegged or cone-shaped teeth, and deficiencies in the enamel. A smaller percentage (approximately 40%) of affected individuals have irregular formations of the finger and toe nails including missing nails, thickened nails, and ridged or pitted nails. In a small number of cases, the skin lesions associated with the first two stages of skin abnormalities may be present underneath a nail. In these cases, it is possible for this lesion to develop into a benign tumor that may cause abnormal bone development in the affected finger or toe.

Approximately 30% of all individuals affected with IP experience visual problems. Less than ten percent of type II IP affected individuals have vision problems related to an abnormal growth of blood vessels in the retina which may, if untreated, lead to a detachment of the retina possibly resulting in blindness. These symptoms generally are seen before the affected individual reaches the age of five. Other vision problems that have been observed in type II IP affected individuals include crossed eyes or "wall eyes" resulting from an improper alignment of the eyes (strabismus); partial or complete opaqueness in one or both lens (cataract); and, occasionally abnormally small eyes (microphthalmia). Because of these vision problems, some individuals affected with IP are blind at birth or will go blind if corrective treatment is not sought.

The incidence of breast development anomalies in type II IP affected girls is quite common. It is estimated to be more than ten times that of the general population. These anomalies range from the presence of an extra nipple to the complete absence of breasts.

Approximately 25% of all IP affected individuals have disorders of the central nervous system. These include mental retardation, slow motor development, **epilepsy**, an abnormally small brain (microcephaly) and increased muscle tone in both legs (spastic diplegia) or in all four limbs (spastic tetraplegia) similar to that seen in the classic case of **cerebral palsy**.

Diagnosis

The genetic mutation responsible for type I incontinentia pigmenti has been fully mapped and sequenced; therefore, it is possible to perform a genetic test for the existence of this disease. However, most cases are still diagnosed on a clinical basis.

Clinical diagnosis of type I IP is based primarily on the skin abnormalities seen at birth. These skin problems may still be misdiagnosed as chicken pox or herpes. This misdiagnosis is easily corrected when the affected individual begins to develop the later stages of the skin anomalies. All suspected male infants should have a chromosome test performed to confirm diagnosis.

In older patients with scarred skin, a skin biopsy that shows "loose" melanin (the pigment that produces color in the skin) confirms a diagnosis of IP.

When the skin appears normal, a diagnosis of IP is indicated when an individual shows one or more of the physical symptoms characteristic of IP: teeth abnormalities, missing patches of hair (alopecia), and/or overgrowth and scarring of the retinal blood vessels; and, that individual is female, has two or more IP affected daughters, is the daughter or sister of an affected woman, or has experienced the miscarriage of two or more male fetuses.

The presence of seizures within the first weeks of life indicate central nervous system involvement in the IP affected individual and indicate an extremely high likelihood of subsequent developmental delay.

Treatment and management

Usually no treatment for the skin conditions associated with IP is necessary other than the control of secondary infection that may occur.

In a female newborn where IP is suspected, an eye exam to look for retinal abnormalities, or any of the other possible eye disorders associated with IP, should be conducted within the first few days after birth. Older affected individuals should have regular eye exams to ensure that retinal abnormalities do not develop. Laser treatments and freezing treatments (cryopexie) are often required to prevent retinal detachment.

Dental treatment is often necessary to repair damaged enamel or for cosmetic reasons in the cases of missing teeth or abnormally shaped teeth.

In cases where there is involvement of the central nervous system, the necessary treatments are on a symptomatic basis. These may include early and continuing intervention programs for developmental delays, anticonvulsants to control seizures, muscle relaxants to control spasticity, and/or surgery to release the permanent muscle, tendon, and ligament tightening (contracture) at the joints that is characteristic of longer term spasticity.

Prognosis

Incontinentia pigmenti is generally fatal in males prior to birth. Females, and the few surviving males, who are affected with IP can expect a normal life span if treatment is undertaken to repair or manage any of the associated symptoms.

Resources

PERIODICALS

"Gene discovery should help diagnose incontinentia pigmenti." *Baylor College of Medicine Press Release* (May 24, 2000).

Smahl, A., et al. "Genomic rearrangement in NEMO impairs NF-kB activation and is a cause of incontinentia pigmenti." *Nature* (May 25, 2000): 466-72.

ORGANIZATIONS

National Incontinentia Pigmenti Foundation. 30 East 72nd St., New York, NY 10021. (212) 452-1231. Fax: (212) 452-1406. <http://imgen.bcm.tmc.edu/NIPF>.

National Organization for Rare Disorders (NORD). PO Box 8923, New Fairfield, CT 06812-8923. (203) 746-6518 or (800) 999-6673. Fax: (203) 746-6481. <http://www.rarediseases.org>.

WEBSITES

McKusick, Victor A. "#308300 Incontinentia Pigmenti; IP." [September 16, 1998]. *OMIM—Online Mendelian Inheritance in Man.* <http://www.ncbi.nlm.nih.gov/htbin-post/Omim/dispmim?308300>. (February 15, 2001).

"Nutrition: Incontinentia Pigmenti." [June 16, 1998]. *Vanderbilt Medical Center Pediatric Digital Interactive Library.* <http://www.mc.vanderbilt.edu/peds/pidl/nutrit/incont.htm>. (February 15, 2001).

Paul A. Johnson

Infantile autism *see* Autism

Infantile refsum disease
Definition

Infantile **refsum disease** (IRD) is an inherited disorder characterized by the reduction or absence of cellular peroxisomes and by the accumulation of various unmetabolized substances in the blood and bodily tissues. The disorder arises in infancy and results in visual and hearing impairments, decreased muscle tone, poor growth, mental retardation, decreased coordination, liver damage, and abnormal development of facial structures. There is no cure for the disorder, and treatment is limited to the relief of symptoms.

Description

Living bodies are built up of millions of individual cells specifically adapted to carry out particular functions. Within cells are even smaller structures, called organelles, which perform different jobs and enable the cell to serve its ultimate purpose. One type of organelle is the peroxisome, whose function is to break down waste materials or to process materials that, if allowed to accumulate, would prove toxic to the cells.

Peroxisomes break down various materials through the use of enzymes (proteins that assist in biochemical reactions), and 80 different peroxisomal enzymes have been identified. These enzymes are made by the cell and transported into the peroxisome by a complex process, requiring at least 15 other proteins. In some cases, an absence or deficiency of these proteins results in a failure to transport enzymes into peroxisomes, leaving the cell unable to metabolize various substances. These substances build up in the blood stream and deposit in various tissues, causing damage.

Infantile refsum disease (IRD) results from an abnormality in the transport of enzymes into the peroxisome, manifesting as absent or reduced functioning peroxisomes. As a consequence of peroxisome deficiency, various substances accumulate in the bloodstream, including phytanic acid, pipecolic acid, hydroxycholestanoic acids, glyoxylate, and substances called very-long-chain fatty acids (VLCFA). Mutations in at least two different genes that encode proteins that participate in the transport of enzymes to the peroxisome have been identified in IRD.

IRD is thought to be the mildest form of **leukodystrophy**, a group of **genetic disorders** including **Zellweger syndrome** and neonatal **adrenoleukodystrophy**, that damage the fatty sheaths surrounding nerves. In the past, IRD was thought to be a variant of adult refsum disease (also called classical refsum disease) because both disorders demonstrate high levels of phytanic acid due to a peroxisomal abnormality. However, later studies demonstrated that the peroxisomal abnormality in IRD is global, affecting many different enzymes, as opposed to the abnormality in adult refsum disease, where only one specific peroxisomal enzyme is abnormal. Indeed, people with IRD show the accumulation of many substances in their bloodstream in addition to phytanic acid and experience different and more severe symptoms than those experienced by people with adult refsum disease. Currently, the two diseases are regarded as separate and distinct entities with different genetic, biochemical, and clinical profiles.

Genetic profile

IRD is a genetic condition and is inherited or passed on in a family. The genetic abnormality for the disorder is inherited as an autosomal recessive trait, meaning that two mutant genes are needed to display the disease. A person who carries one mutant **gene** does not display the disease and is called a carrier. A carrier has a 50% chance of transmitting the gene to their children. A child must inherit the same abnormal gene from each parent to display the disease.

IRD is caused by an abnormality in proteins that assist in the transport of enzymes into the peroxisome. Mutations in the genes for at least two different peroxisomal transport proteins have been identified. The first gene is designated PEX1 (mapped to human **chromosome** 7, locus 7q21-q22) and encodes for a protein called peroxisome biogenesis factor-1. The second gene is designated PEX2 (mapped to human chromosome 8, locus 8q21.1) and encodes for a protein called peroxisomal membrane protein-3.

Demographics

The combined incidence of all leukodystrophy disorders is estimated to be between 1 in 25,000 and 1 in 50,000. It is unclear whether these disorders are distributed equally among different geographical areas and ethnic groups. Because of some overlap with other leukodystrophy disorders, the incidence and prevalence of IRD in the general population is not clear.

Signs and symptoms

Symptoms associated with IRD arise at birth or very early infancy and affect many different organ systems and tissues, resulting in severe disease. Babies with IRD show decreased muscle tone and a failure to grow at appropriate rates. Characteristic facial features are often present, including prominent forehead and folds at the

inner aspect of the eye, flat face and bridge of the nose, and low-set ears. While affected children are able to walk, the gait may be irregular due to abnormalities in muscle coordination.

High levels of unmetabolized substances can deposit in the fatty sheaths surrounding nerves, causing damage and resulting in peripheral neuropathy. Peripheral neuropathy is the term for dysfunction of the nerves outside of the spinal cord, causing loss of sensation, muscle weakness, pain, and loss of reflexes. Nerves leading to the ears can be affected, resulting in hearing loss or deafness. IRD also results in cerebellar ataxia, an abnormality in a specific part of the brain (the cerebellum), resulting in loss of coordination and unsteadiness. In contrast to adult refsum disease, people with IRD have extensive impairments in cognitive function resulting in severe mental retardation.

IRD often affects the eyes, causing **retinitis pigmentosa**, a degeneration of the retina resulting in poor nighttime vision, followed by loss of peripheral vision and eventually loss of central vision late in the course of the disease. Nystagmus (uncontrollable movements of the eye) may also be present due to related nervous system damage. Other manifestations of IRD include enlargement of the liver, poor digestion, and abnormally low blood cholesterol. Early **osteoporosis** (decalcifications of the bone) may also develop, leading to bone fractures or compression of the spinal bones.

Diagnosis

IRD is diagnosed though a combination of consistent medical history, physical exam findings, and laboratory and **genetic testing**. Typically, parents bring newborns to their physicians because of the signs of low muscle tone. Other times, the characteristic facial abnormalities or a failure to grow at appropriate rates is noted. These findings raise suspicion for a genetic syndrome or metabolic disorder, and further tests are conducted.

Laboratory tests reveal several abnormalities. Blood samples from patients with IRD show accumulation of various substances including phytanic acid, pipecolic acid, hydroxycholestanoic acids, glyoxylate, and VLCFA. Other measurements demonstrate low levels of plasmalogen, a substance normally produced by action of the peroxisomal enzymes. Immunoblot tests that measure levels of specific proteins will show deficiencies in many peroxisomal enzymes. Additional studies will reveal abnormal electrical responses from the retina and various nerve groups.

Finally, genetic testing can be preformed. When a diagnosis of IRD is made in a child, genetic testing of the

KEY TERMS

Autosomal recessive—A pattern of genetic inheritance where two abnormal genes are needed to display the trait or disease.

Carrier—A person who possesses a gene for an abnormal trait without showing signs of the disorder. The person may pass the abnormal gene on to offspring.

Cerebellar ataxia—Unsteadiness and lack of coordination caused by a progressive degeneration of the part of the brain known as the cerebellum.

Enzyme—A protein that catalyzes a biochemical reaction or change without changing its own structure or function.

Mutant—A change in the genetic material that may alter a trait or characteristic of an individual or manifest as disease.

Organelle—Small, sub-cellular structures that carry out different functions necessary for cellular survival and proper cellular functioning.

Peripheral neuropathy—Any disease of the nerves outside of the spinal cord, usually resulting in weakness and/or numbness.

Peroxisome—A cellular organelle containing different enzymes responsible for the breakdown of waste or other products.

Retinitis pigmentosa—Progressive deterioration of the retina, often leading to vision loss and blindness.

PEX1 and PEX2 genes can be offered to determine if a specific gene change can be identified. If a specific change is identified, carrier testing can be offered to relatives. In families where the parents have been identified to be carriers of the abnormal gene, diagnosis of IRD before birth is possible. Prenatal diagnosis is performed on cells obtained by **amniocentesis** (withdrawal of the fluid surrounding a fetus in the womb using a needle) at about 16-18 weeks of pregnancy or by chorionic villus sampling (CVS) where cells are obtained from the chorionic villi (a part of the placenta) at 10-12 weeks of pregnancy.

Treatment and management

There is no cure or standard course of treatment for IRD. Currently, treatment of patients has generally involved only supportive care and symptomatic therapy. Several studies suggest that a diet that is free of phytanic acid can limit symptoms of IRD, but this is not nearly as effective as in adult refsum disease. A useful adjunct to dietary treatment is plasmapheresis. Plasmapheresis is a procedure by which determined amounts of plasma (the fluid component of blood that contains the unmetabolized substances) is removed from the blood and replaced with fluids or plasma that are free of accumulated substances. While treatment strategies may mitigate some of the symptoms experienced by the patient with IRD, they do not slow the progression of the disorder.

Experimental studies are underway to investigate whether several different agents can be of additional use. Patients with IRD have reduced levels of docosahexaenoic acid and arachidonic acid that can be corrected with the administration of oral supplements. There are some reports of improvement in symptoms with these therapies, and trials to formally investigate these claims are now in progress. Other scientific laboratories are investigating the usefulness of agents that stabilize peroxisomes in the treatment of IRD, but the experiments are still in their early stages.

Patients with IRD should be seen regularly by a multidisciplinary team of health care providers, including a pediatrician, neurologist, ophthalmologist, cardiologist, medical geneticist specializing in metabolic disease, nutritionist, and physical/occupational therapist. **Genetic counseling** can help people with IRD, those who are carriers of the abnormal gene, or those who have a relative with the disorder, learn more about the disease, **inheritance**, testing, and options available to them so they can make informed decisions appropriate to their families.

Prognosis

For patients with IRD, some success has been achieved with multidisciplinary early intervention, including physical and occupational therapy, hearing aids, alternative communication, nutrition, and support for the parents. Although most patients continue to function in the profoundly or severely retarded range, some make significant gains in self-help skills, and a small percentage may reach stable condition in their teens. Despite these few successes, the prognosis for individuals with IRD is poor; death generally occurs in the second decade of life.

Resources

BOOKS

"Peroxisomal Disorders." *Nelson Textbook of Pediatrics*, edited by R. E. Behrman. Philadelphia: W. B. Saunders, 2000, pp. 318-384.

PERIODICALS

Bader, P. I., et al. "Infantile refsum disease in four Amish sibs." *American Journal of Medical Genetics* 90 (January 2000): 110-114.

Naidu, S., H. Moser. "Infantile refsum disease." *American Journal of Neuroradiology.* 12 (November 1991):1161-1163

Torvik, A., et al. "Infantile refsum's disease: A generalized peroxisomal disorder." *Journal of Neurological Science* 85 (May 1988): 39-53.

ORGANIZATIONS

Infantile refsum disease support and information. 6004 NE 108th Avenue, Vancouver, WA, 98662. (360) 891-5878. <http://home.pacifier.com/~mstephe/>.

WEBSITES

Infantile Refsum Disease Webring. <http://www.angelfire.com/nc/homefireplace/IRDring.html>.

National Center for Biotechnology Information. *OMIM—Online Mendelian Inheritance in Man.* <http://www3.ncbi.nlm.nih.gov/htbin-post/Omim>.

NINDS Infantile refsum Disease Information Page. <http://www.ninds.nih.gov/health_and_medical/disorders/refsum_infantile_doc.htm>.

Oren Traub, MD, PhD

Inheritance

Definition

Inheritance (generally) and heredity (scientifically) both refer to the transmission of genes from parent to offspring, along with the physical, behavioral, and biochemical traits/characteristics they produce.

Description

Throughout history, people have puzzled over heredity. While it is obvious that physical traits and behavioral traits are passed from parent to offspring, both in plants and animals, the puzzling aspects of heredity are the exceptions and quirks in what should be a very basic process. For instance, apparently hereditary characteristics sometimes skip a generation or two, disappear altogether, or appear in an individual or generation for the first time, seemingly from nowhere. A further mystery, the finer points of which are still being unraveled, lay in the mechanism of exactly how traits get from parent to offspring. Even more perplexing to those in the past was the occurrence/recurrence of congenital anomalies and disorders, resulting in physical and/or behavioral disability.

Answers to many of the questions about heredity were deduced in the mid-nineteenth century by a scientist, Gregor Mendel, at a monastery in what is now Czechoslovakia. The deductions he made from the results of his experiments came to be known as Mendel's laws of heredity, since shortened to just Mendelian inheritance. These are the patterns of inheritance, dominant and recessive, with which most people are familiar. However, geneticists have learned in recent years that even Mendel's laws are not immutable, and that other non-Mendelian types of inheritance also exist.

A common misconception is that genetic is synonymous with hereditary, and that the terms can be used interchangeably. In fact, while something that is hereditary is always genetic, something that is genetic is not necessarily hereditary. For example, all **cancer** at the most basic level is genetic, caused by errors in the genetic control of cell division and proliferation. However, only a small proportion of individuals with cancer inherited the causative **gene** mutation from a parent. In most cases, an external agent (carcinogen) induces a genetic mutation in a cell somewhere in the body (e.g., tobacco smoke in a lung cell, or ultraviolet radiation in a skin cell), an error in **DNA** replication results in a mutation, or both. **Gene mutations** that occur anywhere in the body other than sperms, eggs, or their precursor cells (germline) are called somatic mutations, and are not hereditary. As noted, a small percentage of cases of any particular type of cancer (usually about 5–10% for the most common types) exhibit a hereditary pattern. Most often, it is a predisposition to developing cancer that is inherited, placing someone at increased risk for cancer. In fact, most common diseases, such as **diabetes**, hypertension, heart disease, etc., are thought to follow the same general pattern as cancer, with a small percentage of cases due to heredity, most due to environmental effects acting on normal, but susceptible, variants of genes, and the remaining proportion caused by purely environmental or purely somatic genetic events.

Classifying the different types of heredity can be done in various ways. However, most people are only familiar with traditional types of Mendelian inheritance, and know little or nothing about other types of heredity. Accordingly, inheritance can be classified as either Mendelian or non-Mendelian, and then further divided and subdivided on that basis.

Mendelian inheritance

All somatic cells in humans (except mature red blood cells) normally contain 46 chromosomes, in 23 pairs. Sperms and eggs carry 23 chromosomes, one of each pair. The process of sperm development is spermatogenesis, egg development is oogenesis, and the general term for both is gametogenesis. The process that is the basis for Mendelian inheritance is meiosis, which takes place only during gametogenesis (**chromosome** duplication and cell division in somatic cells is mitosis). During meiosis, the 46 chromosomes in precursor cells in testes and ovaries duplicate to produce a total of 92. Two cell divisions then take place, reducing the number of chromosomes per cell to 23. During spermatogenesis, the process results in four sperm, but oogenesis produces only one egg (along with two nonfunctional polar bodies with 46 and 23 chromosomes each). All eggs normally carry a single X chromosome, whereas half of all sperm carry an X, and the other half carry a Y chromosome.

Humans have 24 different chromosomes, the first 22 numbered sequentially, with the twenty-third and twenty-fourth designated as X and Y. Chromosomes 1 through 22 are called autosomes. The X and Y are the sex chromosomes, although only the Y chromosome has any effect in determining sex (gender). Although it is commonly believed that female gender is determined by an XX chromosome constitution, and likewise males are XY, this is misleading. Male and female genders are determined by specific genes and hormonal influences. Certain genetic conditions result in males that are 46,XX, and others in females that are 46,XY. Therefore, it is appropriate and technically more accurate to state that females and males typically or usually have 46,XX and 46,XY chromosome constitutions, respectively.

Mendelian inheritance is either autosomal or sex linked, and dominant or recessive. Given the small number of genes on the Y chromosome and their relative unimportance in producing genetic disease, for all practical purposes, sex-linked inheritance is equivalent to X-linked inheritance. Sex-linked inheritance should also not be confused with sex-influenced inheritance, which involves autosomal inheritance with different phenotypic results in males and females due to hormonal differences. For the purposes of the criteria and terminology that follow, **genetic disorders** will be assumed, rather than normal characteristics (e.g., blue eyes, brown eyes, etc.) that might follow dominant or recessive inheritance patterns.

Genetic conditions that display Mendelian inheritance are often referred to as single-gene disorders. However, this is somewhat of a misnomer, since these conditions nearly always involve two genes, one on each chromosome of a particular pair. To clarify, the word gene is typically used in a broad context, and includes all the variations of that gene, known as alleles.

For instance, there may be a single gene for eye color, with different alleles for brown, blue, green, etc. Some changes in genes result in alleles with no functional difference, or in neutral variations, such as the eye color example. Other genetic changes (mutations) result in alleles associated with disease. If an individual has two identical alleles of a gene, they are considered homozygous; if the alleles are different, that person is said to be heterozygous. Hemizygous refers to the presence of only one allele of a gene, instead of the expected two. Males are normally hemizygous for all the genes on the X and Y chromosomes, since they have only one copy of each. Hemizygosity for an autosomal gene may cause disease, and the symptoms may be different based on whether it is the maternal or paternal allele (gene) that is missing.

Autosomal dominant

The hallmarks of autosomal dominant inheritance include:

- A disorder that is caused by an anomaly in an autosomal gene, requiring only one disease-causing allele to produce symptoms (i.e., heterozygotes affected).

- The condition affects and can be transmitted by both sexes equally.

- A carrier of the gene, whether affected or not, has a 50% chance of transmitting it to each child.

- A later age of onset, with milder symptoms and greater variability, as compared to recessive disorders (on average).

- Sporadic (isolated) cases are not uncommon, and are usually the result of new mutations (no previous family history).

Some conditions (e.g., **Huntington disease**) display what has been referred to as true dominance, which means that individuals with one-disease allele (heterozygotes) exhibit the same signs and symptoms as individuals with two-disease alleles (homozygotes). In other conditions, the effects of the gene are additive. For example, it is not unusual for two heterozygous individuals with **achondroplasia** (a common dwarfing condition) to meet and have children. With each conception, there is a 25% chance the child will receive a normal gene from each parent (homozygous unaffected), a 50% chance of receiving one normal gene and one achondroplasia gene (heterozygous, affected-like parents), and a 25% chance of receiving the achondroplasia gene from each parent, which results in severe limb shortening and other skeletal problems that result in death before or shortly after birth. It could be argued that this type of situation more closely resembles autosomal recessive inheritance, with heterozygotes simply showing more pronounced symptoms than most other recessive disorders.

Other important issues complicating autosomal dominant inheritance include reduced penetrance, variable expression, and possible gonadal mosaicism in the parent of an isolated case. If each person who carries the gene for a particular disorder exhibits symptoms, the gene is said to have 100% penetrance. Therefore, reduced penetrance means that some proportion less than 100% of heterozygotes will develop detectable signs of the condition. For some disorders that have been well studied, penetrance figures at specific ages have been calculated (e.g., a disorder is 50% penetrant at age 30, 70% penetrant at age 50, and so on). Variable expression simply means that two individuals with the same disease allele, even within the same family, may show markedly different ages of onset and/or severity of symptoms.

Autosomal recessive

The hallmarks of autosomal recessive inheritance include:

- The genetic disorder is fully expressed only in individuals homozygous for the disease-causing gene.

- The disorder is usually found only in siblings, with males and females at equal risk.

- When both parents are carriers (unaffected heterozygotes), the risk in each pregnancy of having an affected child is 25%.

- An unaffected sibling of an affected individual has a 66% (two-thirds) chance of being a carrier.

- The incidence of consanguinity in general is increased in autosomal recessive disorders, with a higher likelihood the more rare the condition. Conversely, consanguinity noted in the parents of a child with an unidentified disorder suggests autosomal recessive inheritance as a possible cause.

Many sporadic cases of recessive disorders are noted, because modern families tend to be small and geographically dispersed. Unfortunately, in some cases, the only way that autosomal recessive inheritance is proved is when a second or third affected child is born.

If an affected person has children with a carrier of the same disorder, each child has a 50% risk of being affected, and a 50% risk of being a carrier. If two individuals are affected by the same genetic disorder and have children (rare, but more likely for recessive disorders involving deafness, blindness, or other symptoms that tend to bring people together), all of their children will be affected.

X-linked recessive

The hallmarks of X-linked recessive inheritance include:

- The genetic disorder in which females are carriers, and usually only males are affected.

- There is no male-to-male transmission, since males transmit an X chromosome only to daughters.

- All sons of an affected male will be unaffected, but all daughters will be carriers.

- Typically, carrier females have a 25% chance in each pregnancy of having an affected child (50% chance of transmitting the X chromosome with the disease gene, but only half of those will be passed to boys).

Unlike carriers of autosomal recessive disorders, who, at most, usually show only clinically insignificant biochemical or physical changes, female carriers of X-linked recessive disorders often show mild to moderate effects of the disorder. In rare cases, they may even be as severely affected as their affected male relatives. While it is true that females normally have two X chromosomes and males have only one, it is also true that most of one of the X chromosomes in each cell are randomly inactivated in females shortly after conception. If, by chance, most cells in the body have an active X chromosome that carries the disease gene, a female carrier can show marked symptoms of the disorder. If the reverse is true, she will likely appear completely unaffected.

Women are considered obligate carriers if they have more than one affected son, or an affected male relative and a proven carrier daughter, or an affected son and an affected brother or maternal uncle. Women are at risk for being carriers if they have one affected son, or one affected brother, or one affected maternal uncle, or a sister with an affected son (since any of them may have a new mutation).

An isolated case of a diagnosed X-linked disorder may be the result of a new mutation in the affected individual or in the mother, or may be the result of carrier status transmitted to the mother by her mother. Clarification of this point can make the difference between 50% (mother is a carrier) and negligible (new mutation) in the recurrence risk for the next male pregnancy, and in the risk for daughters or sisters to be carriers. Unfortunately, carrier status of the mother may be very difficult to determine unless reliable carrier testing is available. Molecular **genetic testing** is making this possible for an increasing number of diseases (e.g., **Duchenne muscular dystrophy** and **fragile X syndrome**). An isolated case of an X-linked disorder may also be the result of germline mosaicism in the mother in which some of her eggs carry the mutation and others do not.

X-linked dominant

X-linked dominant disorders are rare. Females are usually affected more mildly than males. However, since both males and females can show symptoms, the inheritance pattern may resemble autosomal dominant inheritance, with the critical difference being no male-to-male transmission in X-linked inheritance. A few X-linked dominant disorders are lethal in males (e.g., **incontinentia pigmenti**).

Non-Mendelian inheritance

Chromosomal heredity

For purposes of broad classification, chromosome anomaly syndromes are considered either numerical or structural. As the term implies, numerical chromosome anomalies involve a change in the total number of chromosomes in each cell, most often presenting as a trisomy, such as the most common type of **Down syndrome** (trisomy 21). Numerical chromosomal syndromes are not considered to be hereditary. Structural chromosome anomalies can take various forms, but most often involve a translocation of some type, either an exchange of chromosomal material between two chromosomes (reciprocal translocation), or two chromosomes attached to each other to form a single chromosome (Robertsonian translocation). Either type of translocation can be balanced (no extra or missing chromosomal material, just rearranged) or unbalanced (missing and/or extra chromosomal material). Individuals who carry a balanced translocation have no ill health effects from it, but when they produce sperms or eggs, the translocation can be passed on in an unbalanced form, which can produce a syndrome of some type in a child, or very often results in repeated pregnancy loss. There is also an equally likely chance that a sperm or egg will receive the translocation in the balanced state as the parent carries it, or receive a normal chromosome complement. Other types of structural chromosome anomalies include ring chromosomes, and different types of inversions of material within a single chromosome, each of which can be hereditary, and present reproductive risks.

Mitochondrial inheritance

Mitochondria are tiny structures (organelles) in the cytoplasm of cells that are the primary site of energy production. They are also the only location outside of the nucleus that contains DNA. The DNA exists in a ring structure, with about 2–10 rings per mitochondrion. Additionally, depending on cell type, there may be anywhere from several dozen to more than a hundred

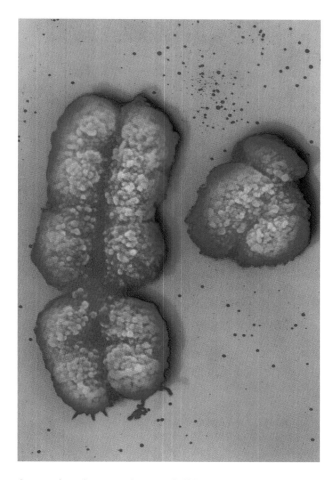

A scanning electron micrograph (SEM) of the female X chromosome (left) and male Y chromosome (right). *(Photo Researchers, Inc.)*

mitochondria per cell. Approximately 70 mitochondrial genes have been identified, many of which are associated with specific genetic disorders.

Mitochondrial inheritance is unusual in that, with rare exceptions, a person inherits all their mitochondria through the egg from their mother. Again, with few exceptions, a typical mitochondrial inheritance pattern involves an affected female who transmits the condition to all of her children, but none of her affected sons will pass on the disorder. However, this straightforward pattern is usually complicated by the fact that each mitochondrion may be mosaic for the gene mutation (e.g., five rings with the mutation and five rings with normal DNA), any particular cell is likely to be mosaic for mitochondria that are themselves mosaic, and this complicated mosaic pattern can apply to any egg that results in conception. All of which makes it nearly impossible to predict specific recurrence risks or the degree of severity if a child is affected.

KEY TERMS

Allele—One of two or more alternate forms of a gene.

Autosomal—Relating to any chromosome besides the X and Y sex chromosomes; human cells contain 22 pairs of autosomes and one pair of sex chromosomes.

Hemizygous—Having only one copy of a gene or chromosome.

Heterozygous—Having two different versions of the same gene.

Homozygous—Having two identical copies of a gene or chromosome.

Mitochondrial inheritance—Inheritance associated with the mitochondrial genome, which is inherited almost exclusively from the mother.

Penetrance—The proportion of individuals with a dominant gene mutation, expressed as a percentage, who actually exhibit recognizable signs or symptoms of the disorder.

Phenotype—The physical expression of an individual's genes.

Sex-linked—A gene located on, and thus a trait linked to, the X or Y chromosomes.

Uniparental disomy (UPD)—An unusual genetic status in an individual in which one parent is the source of both chromosomes of a pair.

Uniparental disomy

Uniparental disomy (UPD) refers to an unusual genetic status in an individual in which one parent is the source of both chromosomes of a pair. Again, before it was possible to analyze chromosomes at the microscopic (DNA) level, the logical assumption was that one chromosome of each pair is always maternal in origin, and the other one paternal in origin. Through various means, this supposed rule of heredity was found to have exceptions.

There are two possible mechanisms for the occurrence of UPD. The first involves a conception in which the embryo is trisomic for a particular chromosome and, at some early stage one of the extra chromosomes is "lost" during mitotic cell division. The result is a normal, diploid cell, and every cell produced from it from that point on will also be diploid. The remaining trisomic cell(s) may produce only a small percentage of the total cells in the body (mosaicism), or they may die off completely. In any case, if the disomic (diploid) cells contain

the two chromosomes contributed by either the sperm or the egg, the result is UPD. This process is sometimes referred to as trisomy rescue. The other, less likely possibility is that one gamete at conception carries an extra chromosome (24 total, which is common), but the other gamete is coincidentally missing that same chromosome. If UPD involves two identical chromosomes (the first stage of meiosis produces two pairs of identical chromosomes at each position/number), the situation is further distinguished as uniparental isodisomy. On the other hand, if the chromosome constitution at that position is the same as the parent's, it is termed uniparental heterodisomy. Uniparental isodisomy presents a much greater risk of transmitting an autosomal recessive disorder than does the alternative.

Gonadal mosaicism

Just as individuals may be mosaic for chromosome anomalies, such as mosaic Down syndrome, so also can mosaicism for single-gene anomalies exist. Mosaicism can have both medical (the individual's health) and reproductive (the individual's children's health) implications. Medical significance is determined by the degree of somatic mosaicism, while reproductive risks depend on the presence or absence of gonadal (germline) mosaicism. A person may have either type of mosaicism, but most cases probably involve both. While the presence of mosaicism in a particular tissue can be proved, the actual level (percentage of abnormal cells) can never be determined, since doing so would require genetic testing of every cell. Likewise, without testing every cell, the absence of mosaicism cannot be confirmed.

Epigenetic effects (imprinting)

Epigenetics is the study of heritable changes in gene expression that occur without a change in DNA sequence. **Imprinting**, the selective deactivation of certain genes in sperm, and others in eggs, is the best-known and most dramatic epigenetic effect. There is also mounting evidence that certain maternal biochemical or physical influences on the embryo/fetus may alter the function of some genes. As a general rule, imprinting is removed and then reapplied during gametogenesis. It remains to be seen whether other types of epigenetic effects are similarly reversible. However, the discovery of new exceptions to old rules continues, with no evidence of slowing down.

Resources

BOOKS

Connor, Michael, and Malcolm Ferguson-Smith. *Essential Medical Genetics*, 5th edition. Oxford: Blackwell Science, Ltd., 1997.

Harper, Peter S. *Practical Genetic Counselling*, 5th edition. Oxford: Butterworth-Heinemann, 1998.

ORGANIZATIONS

Alliance of Genetic Support Groups. 4301 Connecticut Ave. NW, Suite 404, Washington, DC 20008. (202) 966-5557.

March of Dimes Birth Defects Foundation. 1275 Mamaroneck Ave., White Plains, NY 10605. (888) 663-4637. (April 20, 2005.) <http://www.marchofdimes.com/>.

National Society of Genetic Counselors. 233 Canterbury Dr., Wallingford, PA 19086-6617. (610) 872-1192. (April 20, 2005.) <http://www.nsgc.org/>.

WEBSITES

National Library of Medicine: Genetics Home Reference. (April 20, 2005.) <http://ghr.nlm.nih.gov>.

Scott J. Polzin, MS

Ivemark syndrome *see* **Asplenia**

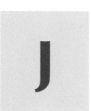

J

Jackson-Weiss syndrome

Definition

Jackson-Weiss syndrome (JWS) is a hereditary disease of varying severity affecting the skull, the face, and the feet. JWS is inherited in an autosomal dominant manner.

Description

Jackson-Weiss syndrome is characterized by a small midface, unusual skull shape, and foot abnormalities. The feet display very wide big toes and webbing of the skin between the second and third toes. Additionally, the toes are angled inward. Bony foot defects apparent on x ray include short, wide foot bones and fusion of some of the foot and ankle bones.

The hallmark skull differences associated with JWS are caused by the premature closure of skull sutures, or skull plates. Other features include a small jaw, flattening of the nasal bridge and the middle third of the face, and a beaked nose. The eyes may be crossed and are widely set and slanting downward with droopy eyelids. High arching of the roof of the mouth or cleft palate, an incomplete closure of the roof of the mouth, may also be present. Mental retardation has been reported in some individuals with JWS.

Genetic profile

Jackson-Weiss syndrome is inherited in an autosomal dominant manner. This means that possession of only one copy of the defective **gene** is enough to cause disease. When a parent has Jackson-Weiss syndrome each of his or her children have a 50% chance to inherit the disease-causing mutation. JWS is believed to have a high rate of penetrance. This means that almost all people who inherit the altered gene will manifest symptoms. JWS has also occurred spontaneously in babies with no family history of it or any similar disorder. This is known as a sporadic occurrence.

JWS has been associated with changes in two different fibroblast growth factor receptor genes, the FGFR1 and FGFR2 genes. The fibroblast growth factor receptor genes serve as a blueprint for proteins important in inhibiting growth during and after embryonic development. FGFR1 is located on human **chromosome** 8 in an area designated as 8p11.2-p11.1. FGFR2 is located on human chromosome 10 in an area designated as 10q26.

FGFR1 has been associated with JWS in only one reported patient who had an unusual presentation of the disorder. This patient displayed JWS's characteristic toes, foot bone fusion, and short fingers, but only very mild skull and facial differences. The genetic change seen in this patient had been seen before in a patient with symptoms much like **Pfeiffer syndrome**, another inherited disorder that affects the skull, face, and hands.

Most commonly, JWS is associated with changes in FGFR2. Mutations in FGFR2 are also associated with the more common **Crouzon syndrome**, a similar inherited disease that affects the skull and face. It appears that the same mutations can be associated with different diseases. Some families, like the original Amish family diagnosed with Jackson-Weiss syndrome, have members who may appear to have Crouzon syndrome or Pfeiffer syndrome. The family as a whole, however, was diagnosed as having Jackson-Weiss syndrome. In 1996, two scientists proposed that the name Jackson-Weiss syndrome should strictly be used in families like the original JWS family where different family members display features of more than one of these similar disorders (Crouzon, Pfeiffer, and Apert syndromes). There is controversy regarding this suggestion.

Demographics

JWS has been described in different races and geographic regions. The original Jackson-Weiss family was a large Amish family with at least 138 affected members. JWS affects both sexes equally. The strongest risk factor for JWS is a family history of the disorder. No precise estimates on the frequency of JWS are available.

Signs and symptoms

Jackson-Weiss syndrome's hallmarks are variable skull differences, flattened mid-face, and wide big toes that angle inward toward each other. The hands are usually not involved. Rarely, deafness or mental retardation can be seen in people with JWS.

Skull abnormalities vary between individuals. Abnormalities in skull shape happen when the sutures, or open seams between the bony plates that form the skull, fuse before they normally would. Premature closure of the skull sutures is known as **craniosynostosis**. Growth of the brain pushes outward on skull plates that have not yet fused. In JWS different sutures may be involved leading to different head shapes. The face may be lopsided due to skull deformity.

Facial differences also vary between individuals with Jackson-Weiss syndrome. Some individuals have no obvious facial differences. The hallmark face of Jackson-Weiss syndrome has very prominent, bulging, down slanting, sometimes crossed, eyes that are slightly further apart than normal with droopy eyelids. The middle third of the face is underdeveloped and somewhat flattened with a beaked nose. The forehead is rounded prominently and the hairline may be slightly lower on the forehead than usual. The chin may be small and the lower jaw may come forward more than normal. Some people with JWS may have cleft palate or a steeply arched palate (roof of the mouth). These changes may cause unusually nasal sounding speech or more serious speech difficulties.

The feet display unusually wide big toes that curve inward toward each other. The large bones of the foot may be fused or abnormally shaped. Smaller bones of the feet and toes may be abnormally shaped or absent. These bony abnormalities may be obvious only on x ray. The fingers and toes may be abnormally short with webbing of the skin between the second and third toes. Extra toes may be present at birth.

Diagnosis

Characteristic facial features and unusual toes may be obvious to an untrained eye, but a thorough physical exam by a physician is necessary to check for less obvious differences. Bony differences may not be obvious, appearing only on x ray. Bony differences in the feet were found consistently, even in seemingly unaffected individuals, in the original Jackson-Weiss syndrome family. X ray is considered to be a very important element in diagnosing

---

KEY TERMS

Amniocentesis—A procedure performed at 16-18 weeks of pregnancy in which a needle is inserted through a woman's abdomen into her uterus to draw out a small sample of the amniotic fluid from around the baby. Either the fluid itself or cells from the fluid can be used for a variety of tests to obtain information about genetic disorders and other medical conditions in the fetus.

Autosomal—Relating to any chromosome besides the X and Y sex chromosomes. Human cells contain 22 pairs of autosomes and one pair of sex chromosomes.

Chorionic villus sampling (CVS)—A procedure used for prenatal diagnosis at 10-12 weeks gestation. Under ultrasound guidance a needle is inserted either through the mother's vagina or abdominal wall and a sample of cells is collected from around the fetus. These cells are then tested for chromosome abnormalities or other genetic diseases.

Sporadic—Isolated or appearing occasionally with no apparent pattern.

JWS. X rays are also important in determining what specific type of abnormal skull plate fusion is present.

DNA testing is available for Jackson-Weiss syndrome. This testing is performed on a blood sample in children and adults to confirm a diagnosis made on physical features. Prenatal **genetic testing** is also available. An unborn baby can be tested for JWS with DNA extracted from cells obtained via chorionic villus sampling or **amniocentesis**.

Treatment and management

There is no medication or cure for Jackson-Weiss syndrome. Treatment, if necessary, depends on an individual's symptoms. Surgery is always offered to correct the most severe physical complications, like cleft palate. Foot and facial abnormalities can also be treated with surgery if they are bothersome to an affected individual. Cosmetic surgery on the face can yield excellent results. In many cases facial differences are so mild that surgical intervention is not recommended. Counseling and support groups may be helpful to patients experiencing emotional difficulty due to physical differences.

Genetic counseling is offered to persons who have this inheritable disorder. Parents with this disease have a 50% chance of passing it to each of their children.

Prenatal diagnosis for JWS is available. This prenatal genetic testing cannot, however, predict the severity or scope of an individual's symptoms. In the future, parents with genetic diseases like Jackson-Weiss syndrome may be able to opt for disease diagnosis from a cell of an embryo before the embryo is introduced to the mother's womb. This testing is called preimplantation genetic diagnosis and is already available in some centers in the United States.

Prognosis

The life span of individuals with JWS is normal. Intelligence is often normal, though borderline intelligence and mental retardation have been described in some patients with JWS.

Resources

PERIODICALS

Roscioli, T., et al. "Clinical Findings in a Patient with FGFR1 P252R Mutation and Comparison with the Literature." *American Journal of Medical Genetics* 93 (2000): 22-28.

Tartaglia, Marco, et al. "Jackson-Weiss syndrome: identification of two novel FGFR2 missense mutations shared with Crouzon and Pfeiffer craniosynostotic disorders." *Human Genetics* 101 (1997): 47-50.

ORGANIZATIONS

Children's Craniofacial Association. PO Box 280297, Dallas, TX 75243-4522. (972) 994-9902 or (800) 535-3643. contactcca@ccakids.com. <http://www.ccakids.com>.

FACES. The National Craniofacial Association. PO Box 11082, Chattanooga, TN 37401. (423) 266-1632 or (800) 332-2373. faces@faces-cranio.org. <http://www.faces-cranio.org/>.

WEBSITES

Online Mendelian Inheritance in Man. <http://www3.ncbi.nlm.nih.gov/Omim>.

Robin, Nathaniel, MD. "Craniosynostosis Syndromes (FGFR-Related)." [October 12, 1998]. *Gene Clinics: Clinical Genetic Information Resource.* University of Washington, Seattle. <http://www.geneclinics.org/profiles/craniosynostosis/index.html>.

Judy C. Hawkins, MS

Jacobsen syndrome

Definition

Jacobsen syndrome is a rare **chromosome** disorder that affects multiple aspects of physical and mental development.

Description

Jacobsen syndrome is characterized by a distinctive facial appearance, some degree of mental impairment, and certain types of birth defects, especially of the heart. Other common medical complications include recurrent infections, decreased platelet count, failure to thrive, and slow growth. The syndrome derives its name from a Danish physician, Dr. Petra Jacobsen, who first described an affected child in 1973. It is also known as 11q deletion syndrome or partial 11q monosomy syndrome because a specific region of one copy of chromosome 11 is missing and thus an affected person has one out of a possible two copies of the genes in that region. It is the loss of these genes that leads to the multiple problems found in Jacobsen syndrome.

Genetic profile

The loss of genetic material from a specific segment of chromosome 11q, which at least includes the critical region at band 11q24.1, leads to the manifestations of Jacobsen syndrome. There are several ways in which this portion of chromosome 11 can be deleted. In at least two-thirds of Jacobsen syndrome cases there is a partial chromosome 11q deletion (a terminal deletion) that begins at band q23 and extends through the end of the chromosome. The remainder of cases are attributed to the loss of this chromosome 11q genetic material due a deletion within, but not including, the end of the chromosome (an interstitial deletion), or due to a chromosome rearrangement such as an unbalanced chromosome translocation or a ring chromosome.

Most deletions and chromosome rearrangements responsible for Jacobsen syndrome are not familial; they are the result of a new or *de novo* genetic change that occurred only in the gamete (the egg or sperm) contributed by the mother or father of that individual. Less often, the origin of chromosome deletion or rearrangement is familial. In a minority of cases a parent of an affected child has a folate-sensitive fragile site at chromosome band 11q23.3 that can cause chromosomal breakage and subsequent deletion of chromosome 11q when inherited. Also, there are children who have inherited an unbalanced chromosome translocation from a parent who is a balanced translocation carrier.

Demographics

Although it is not known how many people have Jacobsen syndrome, estimates are that one person in every 100,000 is affected by the disorder. More females than males have the disorder with 70–75% of cases being females.

Signs and symptoms

Symptoms of Jacobsen syndrome are variable and the prognosis for an affected child depends on the presence of life-threatening birth defects or medical problems. Individuals with Jacobsen syndrome have a distinctive physical appearance. The face is characterized by wide-spaced eyes (hypertelorism), droopy eyelids (ptosis), redundant skin covering the inner eye (epicanthal folds), a broad or flat nasal bridge, a short nose with upturned nostrils, a small chin (micrognathia), low-set ears, and a thin upper lip. As many as 90–95% of affected individuals have a malformation of the skull, trigonocephaly, a defect that results from premature closure of one of the cranial sutures. A small head size (microcephaly) is found in over one-third of cases. Overall, individuals with Jacobsen syndrome are smaller than their peers or siblings. Prenatal growth retardation occurs about 75% of the time. A newborn with Jacobsen syndrome is usually small at birth and continues to have delayed growth and subsequent short stature. Feeding problems that can result in failure to thrive are also common.

Children with Jacobsen syndrome usually have some degree of developmental delay or mental retardation, ranging from mild to severe. Nearly all affected individuals also have decreased muscle tone (hypotonia) or increased muscle tone (hypertonia) as well as fine and gross motor delays. Occasionally, brain abnormalities are present.

Multiple types of physical abnormalities are known to occur in individuals with Jacobsen syndrome. **Congenital heart disease** is present in about half of affected children and, if severe, can pose a significant health problem. Other common internal abnormalities include **pyloric stenosis**, undescended testes, inguinal hernia, kidney defects, and urinary tract abnormalities. Craniofacial abnormalities such as strabismus, ptosis, colobomas, a high-arched palate, and external ear anomalies are frequent. Orthopedic problems, mainly joint contractures and abnormalities of the digits (the fingers and toes), have been described in some cases.

In addition to congenital defects, there are a variety of other health problems found in individuals with Jacobsen syndrome. Illnesses including recurrent respiratory infections, sinusitis, and otitis media occur more frequently in children with Jacobsen syndrome. Gastrointestinal problems such as gastroesophageal reflux and chronic constipation may occur. Blood disorders such as thrombocytopenia and pancytopenia are often seen in childhood and may improve with time.

Diagnosis

Most individuals with Jacobsen syndrome are diagnosed after birth. The diagnosis is usually made through a blood test called chromosome analysis in an infant or child who has mental retardation and a typical facial appearance. The **karyotype** will show a deletion or rearrangement of the longer segment, known as the q arm, of one copy of chromosome 11. Jacobsen syndrome can be diagnosed before birth. There have been reports of prenatal diagnosis through **amniocentesis** after an ultrasound demonstrated one or more fetal abnormalities. Another technique, known as FISH (fluorescent in-situ hybridization), may be used to further define the chromosome 11q deletion breakpoints; this laboratory test is being done on a research basis to identify the disease-causing genes in the Jacobsen syndrome critical region.

Treatment and management

There is no cure for Jacobsen syndrome nor is there a therapy that can replace the missing genes from the deleted segment of chromosome 11. In addition to routine pediatric exams, there are management strategies and treatments that aim to prevent or minimize some of the serious health consequences associated with Jacobsen syndrome.

At the time of diagnosis a series of evaluations should be undertaken in order to appropriately guide medical management. Pediatric specialists in genetics, cardiology, orthopedics, ophthalmology, and neurology should be consulted, especially since some problems can be treated if caught early. Important tests may include a karyotype, a cardiac echocardiogram, a renal sonogram, a platelet count, a blood count, a brain imaging study, hearing and vision screenings, and a dental exam.

A neurodevelopmental evaluation should be initiated in infancy or at the time of diagnosis with implementation of age-appropriate early intervention services such as speech therapy, occupational therapy, and physical therapy. An ear, nose, and throat specialist (ENT) may be needed to treat problems such as otitis media. Craniofacial and neurosurgery consults may be indicated if trigonocephaly or other forms of **craniosynostosis** are present.

Some children may require a gastroenterology specialist to evaluate problems such as failure to thrive, chronic constipation, and/or severe gastroesophageal reflux, some or all of which may require surgical intervention. Boys with Jacobsen syndrome should be examined for undescended testes, a problem found in half of males and one that often requires surgery.

Prognosis

Approximately 25% of affected children die before two years of age mainly from cardiac defects, a tendency to bleed, or infection. Except for respiratory infections,

Band—A specific region of a chromosome that is identified by its characteristic staining pattern and location within a chromosome, as seen in a karyotype. A band is either part of the short arm (p arm) or the long arm (q arm) of a chromosome and is further defined by a numeric location, such as chromosome band 11q24.1.

Chromosome—A microscopic thread-like structure found within each cell of the body and consists of a complex of proteins and DNA. Humans have 46 chromosomes arranged into 23 pairs. Changes in either the total number of chromosomes or their shape and size (structure) may lead to physical or mental abnormalities.

Coloboma—A birth defect in which part of the eye does not form completely.

Congenital—Refers to a disorder which is present at birth.

Cranial suture—Any one of the seven fibrous joints between the bones of the skull.

Craniosynostosis—Premature, delayed, or otherwise abnormal closure of the sutures of the skull.

Deletion—The absence of genetic material that is normally found in a chromosome. Often, the genetic material is missing due to an error in replication of an egg or sperm cell.

Echocardiogram—A non-invasive technique, using ultrasonic waves, used to look at the various structures and function of the heart.

Failure to thrive—Significantly reduced or delayed physical growth.

Folate-sensitive fragile site—A chromosome location which, under folate-deficient conditions, appears as a gap in the chromosome and is susceptible to breakage.

Gastroesphageal reflux—The return of the contents of the stomach back up into the esophagus.

Gene—A building block of inheritance, which contains the instructions for the production of a particular protein, and is made up of a molecular sequence found on a section of DNA. Each gene is found on a precise location on a chromosome.

Inguinal hernia—A condition in which part of the intestines protrudes through a tear in the muscles of the abdomen.

Karyotype—A standard arrangement of photographic or computer-generated images of chromosome pairs from a cell in ascending numerical order, from largest to smallest.

Monosomy—Missing an entire copy of a chromosome or a piece of one copy of a chromosome.

Otitis media—Inflammation of the middle ear, often due to fluid accumulation secondary to an infection.

Pancytopenia—An abnormal reduction in the number of erythrocytes (red blood cells), leukocytes (a type of white or colorless blood cell), and blood platelets (a type of cell that aids in blood clotting) in the blood.

Pyloric stenosis—Narrowing of the stomach due to thickening of the pyloris muscle at the end of the stomach.

Ring chromosome—An abnormal chromosome in which the terminal ends of the short (p) and long (q) arms have been lost and the remaining p and q arms subsequently join to form a ring.

Strabismus—An improper muscle balance of the ocular musles resulting in crossed or divergent eyes.

Thrombocytopenia—A persistent decrease in the number of blood platelets usually associated with hemorrhaging.

Translocation—The transfer of one part of a chromosome to another chromosome during cell division. A balanced translocation occurs when pieces from two different chromosomes exchange places without loss or gain of any chromosome material. An unbalanced translocation involves the unequal loss or gain of genetic information between two chromosomes.

Trigonocephaly—An abnormal development of the skull characterized by a triangular shaped forehead.

the remainder of children are generally healthy. Most individuals described here are children or adolescents. Little is known about the course of this syndrome in adulthood, and the life expectancy for those who live beyond age two is unknown.

Resources

BOOKS

Jones, Kenneth Lyons. *Smith's Recognizable Patterns of Human Malformation*. Philadelphia: W.B. Saunders Company, 1997.

PERIODICALS

Jones, Christopher, et al. "Co-localisation of CCG repeats and chromosome deletion breakpoints in Jacobsen syndrome: evidence for a common mechanism of chromosome breakage." *Human Molecular Genetics* 9, no. 8: 1201–08.

McClelland, S. M., et al. "Nuchal thickening in Jacobsen syndrome." *Ultrasound in Obstetrics and Gynecology* 12 (1998): 280–82.

Ono, J., et al. "Partial deletion of the long arm of chromosome 11: ten Japanese children." *Clinical Genetics* 50 (1996): 474–78.

Penny, Laura A., et al. "Clinical and Molecular Characterization of Patients with Distal 11q Deletions." *American Journal of Human Genetics* 56 (1995): 676–83.

Pivnick, E. K., et al. "Jacobsen syndrome: report of a patient with severe eye anomalies, growth hormone deficiency, and hypothyroidism associated with deletion 11(q23q25) and review of 52 cases." *Journal of Medical Genetics* 33 (1996): 772–78.

Tunnacliffe, Alan, et al. "Localization of Jacobsen syndrome breakpoints on a 40-Mb physical map of distal chromosome 11q." *Genome Research* 9 (1999): 44–52.

ORGANIZATIONS

European Chromosome 11q Network. <http://www.11q.org>.

OTHER

11q Research and Resource Home Page. <http://www.11q.net>.

The Fragile WEB Site. <http://web.ukonline.co.uk>.

Dawn Cardeiro, MS, CGC

Jervell and Lange-Nielsen syndrome

Definition

Jervell and Lange-Nielsen syndrome (JLNS) is a rare inherited disorder characterized by congenital deafness and cardiac arrhythmias (irregularities in the electrical activity of the heart that can lead to cardiac arrest and sudden death).

Description

JLNS results from mutations, or changes, in either one of two genes that encode proteins that combine to form potassium ion channels. One of the potassium channels is important for proper heart function. It is also critical in the functioning of the cochlea of the inner ear. People with JLNS lack this channel and, thus, are born with profound deafness in both ears, as well as with cardiac abnormalities.

JLNS was first described in 1957 by A. Jervell and F. Lange-Nielsen. It is also known by the names cardio-auditory syndrome of Jervell and Lange-Nielsen; cardo-cardiac syndrome; surdocardiac syndrome; deafness-functional heart disease; and deafness, congenital, and functional heart disease. The cardiac (heart) symptoms of JLNS are very similar to those of long-QT syndrome (LQTS), including a longer-than-normal "QT interval" on an electrocardiogram (ECG or EKG) test. Thus, JLNS is sometimes called QT prolonged with congenital deafness.

Genetic profile

JLNS is caused by mutations in either the KVLQT1 (KCNQ1) **gene** or the KCNE1 (MinK or IsK) gene. It is an autosomal recessive disorder, which means it occurs only in people with two copies of the mutant gene, one from each parent. The mutations in the two copies do not have to be identical. Someone who inherits one copy of the mutant gene and one copy of the normal gene has LQTS types 1 or 5.

Demographics

Although it is the third most common type of autosomal recessive hearing loss, JLNS is a very rare disorder. Worldwide, there are an estimated two to six cases per one million people. Norway, however, has a much higher incidence of JLNS, estimated at one in 200,000.

Because JLNS requires two copies of the abnormal gene, one from each parent, it most often is found in the offspring of related parents, such as cousins (termed a "consanguineous" marriage). Individuals who carry one copy of the abnormal gene and one normal gene copy will have LQTS, but will have normal hearing or only partial hearing loss. However, a child of two such individuals has a 25% chance of having JLNS. Thus, although JLNS occurs across racial and ethnic groups, it is more common in small isolated groups where marriage between relatives is frequent.

Signs and symptoms

The deafness associated with JLNS usually is apparent in infancy or early childhood. Although the severity of JLNS varies, children with acute JLNS are profoundly deaf in both ears.

Depending on the severity of the disorder, the cardiac symptoms of JLNS may be overlooked. Thus, people with JLNS can be at serious risk for sudden death. In addition to a prolonged QT interval on an ECG/EKG, cardiac arrhythmias, dizziness, periods of unconsciousness (syncopic episodes), and seizures are common symptoms of JLNS. These symptoms most often occur

Action potential—The wave-like change in the electrical properties of a cell membrane, resulting from the difference in electrical charge between the inside and outside of the membrane.

Arrhythmia—Abnormal heart rhythm, examples are a slow, fast, or irregular heart rate.

Autosomal recessive—A pattern of genetic inheritance where two abnormal genes are needed to display the trait or disease.

Beta-adrenergic blocker—A drug that works by controlling the nerve impulses along specific nerve pathways.

Cochlea—A bony structure shaped like a snail shell located in the inner ear. It is responsible for changing sound waves from the environment into electrical messages that the brain can understand, so people can hear.

Congenital—Refers to a disorder which is present at birth.

Depolarization—The dissipation of an electrical charge through a membrane.

Electrocardiogram (ECG, EKG)—A test used to measure electrical impulses coming from the heart in order to gain information about its structure or function.

Endolymph—The fluid in the inner ear.

Fibrillation—A rapid, irregular heartbeat.

Heterozygous—Having two different versions of the same gene.

Homeostasis—A state of physiological balance.

Homozygous—Having two identical copies of a gene or chromosome.

Ion channel—Cell membrane proteins which control the movement of ions into and out of a cell.

QT interval—The section on an electrocardiogram between the start of the QRS complex and the end of the T wave, representing the firing or depolarization of the ventricles and the period of recovery prior to repolarization or recharging for the next contraction.

Repolarization—Period when the heart cells are at rest, preparing for the next wave of electrical current (depolarization).

Syncope—A brief loss of consciousness caused by insufficient blood flow to the brain.

Tachycardia—An excessively rapid heartbeat; a heart rate above 100 beats per minute.

Torsade de pointes—A type of tachycardia of the ventricles characteristic of Jervell and Lange-Nielsen syndrome.

---

upon awakening, during strenuous physical activity, or during moments of excitement or stress.

Diagnosis

Deaf children, particularly those with a family history of sudden death, syncopic episodes, or LQTS should be screened for JLNS, using an ECG to detect a prolonged QT interval. **Genetic testing** for JLNS is possible for high-risk individuals.

Individuals with JLNS sometimes have normal or borderline-normal QT intervals on an ECG/EKG. Additional ECGs/EKGs performed during exercise may reveal an abnormal QT interval. ECGs/EKGs of the parents may also reveal a prolonged QT interval.

Treatment and management

Since JLNS can result in sudden death, including sudden infant death syndrome (SIDS), treatment is essential. Beta-blockers are the most common treatment for the ventricular arrhythmia of JLNS. Treatment with these drugs usually continues for life. Beta-blockers such as propranolol are considered to be safe medications. Any side effects from propranolol are usually mild and disappear once the body has adjusted to the drug. However, beta-blockers can interact dangerously with many other medications.

Surgery may reduce cardiac arrhythmias in people with JLNS. A mechanical device called a pacemaker or an automatic implanted cardioverter defibrillator (AICD) may be used to regulate the heartbeat or to detect and correct abnormal heart rhythms. Sometimes a pacemaker or AICD is used in combination with beta-blockers.

In 2000, the first cochlear implant in the inner ear of a child with JLNS was reported. The child gained limited hearing and improved speech.

Preventative measures

All individuals who have been diagnosed with JLNS must avoid reductions in blood potassium levels, such as those that occur with the use of diuretics (drugs that reduce fluids in the body). People with JLNS must also avoid a very long list of drugs and medications that can increase the QT interval or otherwise exacerbate the syndrome.

People with JLNS usually are advised to refrain from competitive sports and to practice a "buddy system" during moderate exercise. Family members are advised to learn cardiopulmonary resuscitation (CPR) in case of cardiac arrest.

Prognosis

Cochlear implants may improve the hearing of people with JLNS. The cardiac abnormalities of JLNS usually can be controlled with beta-blockers. However, without treatment, there is a high incidence of sudden death due to cardiac events.

Family members of a JLNS individual should be screened with ECGs/EKGs for a prolonged QT interval, since they are at risk of having LQTS. **Genetic counseling** is recommended for people with JLNS, since their children will inherit a gene causing LQTS.

Resources

PERIODICALS

Chen, Q., et al. "Homozygous Deletion in KVLQT1 Associated with Jervell and Lange-Nielsen Syndrome." *Circulation* 99 (1999): 1344-47.

Schmitt, N., et al. "A Recessive C-terminal Jervell and Lange-Nielsen Mutation of the KCNQ1 Channel Impairs Subunit Assembly." *The EMBO Journal* 19 (2000): 332-40.

Steel, Karen P. "The Benefits of Recycling." *Science* 285 (August 27, 1999): 1363-1364.

ORGANIZATIONS

American Heart Association. 7272 Greenville Ave., Dallas, TX 75231-4596. (214) 373-6300 or (800) 242-8721. inquire@heart.org. <http://www.americanheart.org>.

American Society for Deaf Children. PO Box 3355, Gettysburg, PA 17325. (800) 942-ASDC or (717) 334-7922 v/tty. <http://www.deafchildren.org/asdc2k/home/home.shtml>.

Deafness Research Foundation. 575 Fifth Ave., 11th Floor, New York, NY 10017. (800) 535-3323. drf@drf.org.

EAR (Education and Auditory Research) Foundation. 1817 Patterson St., Nashville, TN 37203. (800) 545-HEAR. earfound@earfoundation.org. <http://www.theearfound.org>.

European Long QT Syndrome Information Center. Ronnerweg 2, Nidau, 2560. Switzerland 04(132) 331-5835. jmettler@bielnews.ch. <http://www.bielnews.ch/cyberhouse/qt/qt.html>.

Sudden Arrhythmia Death Syndrome Foundation. PO Box 58767, 508 East South Temple, Suite 20, Salt Lake City, UT 84102. (800) 786-7723. sads@sads.org. <http://www.sads.org>.

WEBSITES

Contie, Victoria L. "Genetic Findings Help Tame the Runaway Heart." *NCAA Reporter,* [November-December 1997]. <http://www.ncrr.nih.gov/newspub/nov97rpt/heart.htm>

"Genetics of Long QT Syndrome/Cardiac Arrest." *DNA Sciences.* 2001. <http://my.webmd.com/content/article/3204.676>

Long QT Syndrome European Information Center. <http://www.qtsyndrome.ch/lqts.html>

Narchi, Hassib, and Walter W. Tunnessen Jr. "Denouement and Discussion: Jervell and Lange-Nielsen Syndrome (Long QT Syndrome)." *Archives of Pediatrics and Adolescent Medicine,* 153, no. 4 (April 1999). <http://archpedi.ama-assn.org/issues/v153n4/ffull/ppm8451-1b.html>

Margaret Alic, PhD

Joubert syndrome

Definition

Joubert syndrome is a well documented but rare autosomal recessive disorder. The syndrome is characterized by partial or complete absence of the cerebellar vermis (the connective tissue between the two brain hemispheres), causing irregular breathing and severe muscle weakness. Other features of the syndrome include jerky eye movements, abnormal balance and walking, and mental handicap. There may be minor birth defects of the face, hands and feet.

Description

Marie Joubert (whose name is given to the condition) gave a detailed description of the syndrome in 1969. She wrote about four siblings (three brothers, one sister) in one family with abnormal breathing, jerky eye movements (nystagmus), poor mental development, and ataxia (staggering gait and imbalance). X ray examination showed that a particular section of the brain, called the cerebellar vermis, was absent or not fully formed. This specific brain defect was confirmed on autopsy in one of these individuals. Her initial report also described a sporadic (non-inherited) patient with similar findings, in addition to **polydactyly**. Another name for Joubert syndrome is Joubert-Bolthauser syndrome.

Genetic profile

There have been numerous instances of siblings (brothers and sisters), each with Joubert syndrome. The parents were normal. A few families have also been seen where the parents were said to be closely related (i.e. may have shared the same altered **gene** within the family). For these reasons, Joubert syndrome is an autosomal recessive disorder. Autosomal means that both males and females can have the condition. Recessive means that both parents would be carriers of a single copy of the responsible gene. Autosomal recessive disorders occur when a person inherits a particular pair of genes that do not work correctly. The chance that this would happen to children of carrier parents is 25% (one in four) for each pregnancy.

It is known that the cerebellum and brain stem begin to form between the sixth and twelfth week of pregnancy. The birth defects seen in Joubert syndrome must occur during this crucial period of development. As of 2001, the genetic cause remains unknown.

Demographics

Joubert syndrome affects both males and females, although more males (ratio of 2:1) have been reported with the condition. The reason why more males have the condition remains unknown.

Joubert syndrome is found worldwide, with reports of individuals of French Canadian, Swedish, German, Swiss, Spanish, Dutch, Italian, Indian, Belgian, Laotian, Moroccan, Algerian, Turkish, Japanese, and Portuguese origin. In all, more than 200 individuals have been described with Joubert syndrome.

Signs and symptoms

The cerebellum is the second largest part of the brain. It is located just below the cerebrum, and partially covered by it. The cerebellum consists of two hemispheres, separated by a central section called the vermis. The cerebellum is connected to the spinal cord, through the brain stem.

The cerebellum (and vermis) normally works to monitor and control movement of the limbs, trunk, head, and eyes. Signals are constantly received from the eyes, ears, muscle, joints, and tendons. Using these signals, the cerebellum is able to compare what movement is actually happening in the body, with what is intended to happen. Then, it sends an appropriate signal back. The effect is to either increase or decrease the function of different muscle groups, to make movement both accurate and smooth.

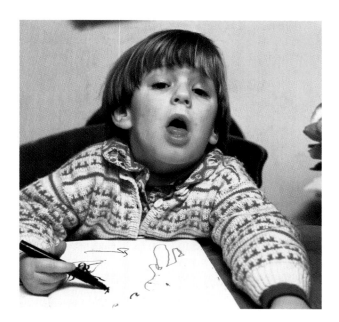

This child is diagnosed with Joubert syndrome. Common symptoms of this disorder include mental retardation, poor coordination, pendular eye movement, and abnormal breathing patterns. *(Photo Researchers, Inc.)*

In Joubert syndrome, the cerebellar vermis is either absent or incompletely formed. The brain stem is sometimes quite small. The absence or abnormal function of these brain tissues causes problems in breathing and vision, and severe delays in development.

One characteristic feature of Joubert syndrome is the pattern of irregular breathing. Their breathing alternates between deep rapid breathing (almost like panting) with periods of severe apnea (loss of breathing). This is usually noticeable at birth. The rate of respiration may increase more than three times that of normal (up to 200 breaths per minute) and the apnea may last up to 90 seconds. The rapid breathing occurs most often when the infant is awake, especially when they are aroused or excited. The apnea happens when the infants are awake or asleep. Such abnormal breathing can cause sudden death or coma, and requires that these infants be under intensive care. For unknown reasons, the breathing tends to improve with age, usually within the first year of life.

Muscle movement of the eye is also affected in Joubert syndrome. It is common for the eyes to have a quick, jerky motion of the pupil, known as nystagmus. The retina (the tissue in the back of the eye that receives and transmits visual signals to the brain) may be abnormal. Some individuals (most often the males) may have a split in the tissue in the iris of the eye. Each of these problems will affect their vision, and eye surgery may not be beneficial.

The central nervous system problem affects the larger muscles of the body as well, such as those for the arms and legs. Many of the infants will have severe muscle weakness and delays in development. They reach normal developmental milestones, such as sitting or walking, much later than normal. For example, some may learn to sit without support around 19–20 months of age (normal is six to eight months). Most individuals are not able to take their first steps until age four or older. Their balance and coordination are also affected, which makes walking difficult. Many will have an unsteady gait, and find it difficult to climb stairs or run, even as they get older.

Cognitive (mental) delays are also a part of the syndrome, although this can be variable. Most individuals with Joubert syndrome will have fairly significant learning impairment. Some individuals will have little or no speech. Others are able to learn words, and can talk with the aid of speech therapy. They do tend to have pleasant and sociable personalities, but problems in behavior can occur. These problems most often are in temperament, hyperactivity, and aggressiveness.

Careful examination of the face, especially in infancy, shows a characteristic appearance. They tend to have a large head, and a prominent forehead. The eyebrows look high, and rounded, and the upper eyelids may be droopy (ptosis). Their mouth many times remains open, and looks oval shaped in appearance. The tongue may protrude out of the mouth, and rest on the lower lip. The tongue may also quiver slightly. These are all signs of the underlying brain abnormality and muscle weakness. Occasionally, the ears look low set on the face. As they get older, the features of the face become less noticeable.

Less common features of the syndrome include minor birth defects of the hands and feet. Some individuals with Joubert syndrome have extra fingers on each hand. The extra finger is usually on the pinky finger side (polydactyly). It may or may not include bone, and could just be a skin tag. A few of these patients will also have extra toes on their feet.

Diagnosis

The diagnosis of Joubert syndrome is made on the following features. First, there must be evidence of the cerebellar vermis either being absent or incompletely formed. This can be seen with a CT scan or MRI of the brain. Second, the physician should recognize the infant has both muscle weakness and delays in development. In addition, there may be irregular breathing and abnormal eye movements. Having four of these five criteria is enough to make the diagnosis of Joubert syndrome. Most individuals are diagnosed by one to three years of age.

Treatment and management

During the first year of life, many of these infants require a respiratory monitor for the irregular breathing. For the physical and mental delays, it becomes necessary to provide special assistance and anticipatory guidance. Speech, physical and occupational therapy are needed throughout life.

Prognosis

The unusual pattern of breathing as newborns, especially the episodes of apnea, can lead to sudden death or coma. A number of individuals with Joubert syndrome have died in the first three years of life. For most individuals, the irregular breathing becomes more normal after the first year. However, many continue to have apnea, and require medical care throughout their life. Although the true life span remains unknown, there are some individuals with Joubert syndrome who are in their 30s.

Resources

ORGANIZATIONS

Joubert Syndrome Foundation Corporation. c/o Stephanie Frazer, 384 Devon Drive, Mandeville, LA 70448.

OTHER

Alliance of Genetic Support Groups. <http://www.geneticalliance.org.htm>.

Joubert Syndrome Foundation Corporation. <http://www.joubertfoundation.com>.

Kevin M. Sweet, MS, CGC

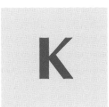

K

Kabuki syndrome

Definition

Kabuki syndrome is a rare disorder characterized by unusual facial features, skeletal abnormalities, and intellectual impairment. Abnormalities in different organ systems can also be present, but vary from individual to individual. There is no cure for Kabuki syndrome, and treatment centers on the specific abnormalities, as well as on strategies to improve the overall functioning and quality of life of the affected person.

Description

Kabuki syndrome is a rare disorder characterized by mental retardation, short stature, unusual facial features, abnormalities of the skeleton and unusual skin ridge patterns on the fingers, toes, palms of the hands and soles of the feet. Many other organ systems can be involved in the syndrome, displaying a wide variety of abnormalities. Thus, the manifestations of Kabuki syndrome can vary widely among different individuals.

Kabuki syndrome (also known as Niikawa-Kuroki syndrome) was first described in 1980 by Dr. N. Niikawa and Dr. Y. Kuroki of Japan. The disorder gets its name from the characteristic long eyelid fissures with eversion of the lower eyelids that is similar to the make-up of actors of Kabuki, a traditional Japanese theatrical form. Kabuki syndrome was originally known as Kabuki Make-up syndrome, but the term "make-up" is now often dropped as it is considered offensive to some families.

Scientific research conducted over the past two decades suggests that Kabuki syndrome may be associated with a change in the genetic material. However, it is still not known precisely what this genetic change may be and how this change in the genetic material alters growth and development in the womb to cause Kabuki syndrome.

Genetic profile

As stated above, the etiology of Kabuki syndrome is not completely understood. While Kabuki syndrome is thought to be a genetic syndrome, little or no genetic abnormality has been identified as of yet. **Chromosome** abnormalities of the X and Y chromosome or chromosome 4 have occurred in only a small number of individuals with Kabuki syndrome, but in most cases, chromosomes are normal.

In almost all cases of Kabuki syndrome, there is no family history of the disease. These cases are thought to represent new genetic changes that occur randomly and with no apparent cause and are termed sporadic. However, in several cases the syndrome appears to be inherited from a parent, supporting a role for genetics in the cause of Kabuki syndrome. Scientists hypothesize that an unidentified genetic abnormality that causes Kabuki syndrome is transmitted as an autosomal dominant trait. With an autosomal dominant trait, only one abnormal **gene** in a gene pair is necessary to display the disease, and an affected individual has a 50% chance of transmitting the gene and the disease to a child.

Demographics

Kabuki syndrome is a rare disorder with less than 200 known cases worldwide, but the prevalence of the disease may be underestimated as only a handful of physicians have first-hand experience diagnosing children with Kabuki syndrome. Kabuki syndrome appears to be found equally in males and females. Earlier cases were reported in Japanese children but the syndrome is now known to affect other racial and ethnic groups.

Theoretical mathematical models predict that the incidence of Kabuki syndrome in the Japanese population may be as high as one in 32,000.

Signs and symptoms

The signs and symptoms associated with Kabuki syndrome are divided into cardinal symptoms (i.e. those that are almost always present) and variable symptoms (those that may or may not be present). The cardinal and variable signs and symptoms of Kabuki syndrome are summarized in the table below.

Diagnosis

The diagnosis of Kabuki syndrome relies on physical exam by a physician familiar with the condition and by radiographic evaluation, such as the use of x rays or ultrasound to define abnormal or missing structures that are consistent with the criteria for the condition (as described above). A person can be diagnosed with Kabuki syndrome if they possess characteristics consistent with the five different groups of cardinal symptoms: typical face, skin-surface abnormalities, skeletal abnormalities, mild to moderate mental retardation, and short stature.

Although a diagnosis may be made as a newborn, most often the features do not become fully evident until early childhood. There is no laboratory blood or genetic test that can be used to identify people with Kabuki syndrome.

Treatment and management

There is no cure for Kabuki syndrome. Treatment of the syndrome is variable and centers on correcting the different manifestations of the condition and on strategies to improve the overall functioning and quality of life of the affected individual.

For children with heart defects, surgical repair is often necessary. This may take place shortly after birth if the heart abnormality is life threatening, but often physicians will prefer to attempt a repair once the child has grown older and the heart is more mature. For children who experience seizures, lifelong treatment with anti-seizure medications is often necessary.

Children with Kabuki syndrome often have difficulties feeding, either because of mouth abnormalities or because of poor digestion. In some cases, a tube that enters into the stomach is surgically placed in the abdomen, and specially designed nutritional liquids are administered through the tube directly into the stomach.

People with Kabuki syndrome are at higher risk for a variety of infections, most often involving the ears and the lungs. In cases such as these, antibiotics are given to treat the infection, and occasionally brief hospital stays are necessary. Most children recover from these infections with proper treatment.

Nearly half of people affected by Kabuki syndrome have some degree of hearing loss. In these individuals, formal hearing testing is recommended to determine if they might benefit from a hearing-aid device. A hearing aid is a small mechanical device that sits behind the ear and amplifies sound into the ear of the affected individual. Occasionally, hearing loss in individuals with Kabuki syndrome is severe, approaching total hearing loss. In these cases, early and formal education using American Sign Language as well as involvement with the hearing-impaired community, schools, and enrichment programs is appropriate.

Children with Kabuki syndrome should be seen regularly by a team of health care professionals, including a primary care provider, medical geneticist familiar with the condition, gastroenterologist, and neurologist. After growth development is advanced enough (usually late adolescence or early adulthood), consultation with a reconstructive surgeon may be of use to repair physical abnormalities that are particularly debilitating.

During early development and progressing into young adulthood, children with Kabuki syndrome should be educated and trained in behavioral and mechanical methods to adapt to any disabilities. This program is usually initiated and overseen by a team of health care professionals including a pediatrician, physical therapist, and occupational therapist. A counselor specially trained to deal with issues of disabilities in children is often helpful is assessing problem areas and encouraging healthy development of self-esteem. Support groups and community organizations for people with disabilities often prove useful to the affected individuals and their families, and specially equipped enrichment programs should be sought. Further, because many children with Kabuki syndrome have poor speech development, a consultation and regular session with a speech therapist is appropriate.

Prognosis

The abilities of children with Kabuki syndrome vary greatly. Most children with the condition have a mild to moderate intellectual impairment. Some children will be able to follow a regular education curriculum, while others will require adaptations or modifications to their schoolwork. Many older children may learn to read at a functional level.

The prognosis of children with Kabuki syndrome depends on the severity of the symptoms and the extent to which the appropriate treatments are available. Most of the medical issues regarding heart, kidney or intestinal abnormalities arise early in the child's life and are improved with medical treatment. Since Kabuki syndrome was discovered relatively recently, very little is known regarding the average life span of individuals affected with the condition, however, present data on Kabuki syndrome does not point to a shortened life span.

KEY TERMS

Autosomal dominant—A pattern of genetic inheritance where only one abnormal gene is needed to display the trait or disease.

Cardinal symptoms—A group of symptoms that define a disorder or disease.

Gastric tube—A tube that is surgically placed though the skin of the abdomen to the stomach so that feeding with nutritional liquid mixtures can be accomplished.

Gastroenterologist—A physician who specializes in disorders of the digestive system.

Kabuki—Traditional Japanese popular drama performed with highly stylized singing, dancing, makeup, and clothing.

Neurologist—A physician who specializes in disorders of the nervous system, including the brain, spine, and nerves.

Resources

BOOKS

Behrman, R.E., ed. *Nelson Textbook of Pediatrics.* Philadelphia: W.B. Saunders, 2000.

PERIODICALS

Kawame, H. "Phenotypic Spectrum and Management Issues in Kabuki Syndrome." *Journal of Pediatrics* 134 (April 1999): 480-485.

Mhanni, A.A., and A.E. Chudley. "Genetic Landmarks Through Philately—Kabuki Theater and Kabuki Syndrome." *Clinical Genetics* 56 (August 1999): 116-117.

ORGANIZATIONS

CardioFacioCutaneous Support Network. 157 Alder Ave., McKee City, NJ 08232. (609) 646-5606.

Kabuki Syndrome Network. 168 Newshaw Lane, Hadfield, Glossop, SK13 2AY. UK 01457 860110. <http://www.ksn-support.org.uk>.

National Organization for Rare Disorders (NORD). PO Box 8923, New Fairfield, CT 06812-8923. (203) 746-6518 or (800) 999-6673. Fax: (203) 746-6481. <http://www.rarediseases.org>.

WEBSITES

"Entry 147920: Kabuki Syndrome." *OMIM—Online Mendelian Inheritance in Man.* <http://www.ncbi.nlm.nih.gov/entrez/dispomim.cgi?id=147920>.

Oren Traub, MD, PhD

▌Kallmann syndrome

Definition

Kallmann syndrome is a disorder of hypogonadotropic hypogonadism, delayed puberty and anosmia.

Description

Hypogonadotropic hypogonadism (HH) occurs when the body does not produce enough of two important hormones, luteinizing hormone (LH) and follicle stimulating hormone (FSH). This results in underdeveloped gonads and often infertility. Anosmia, the inability to smell, was first described with hypogonadotropic hypogonadism in 1856, but it was not until 1944 that Kallmann reported the **inheritance** of the two symptoms together in three separate families. Hence, the syndrome of hypogonadotropic hypogonadism and anosmia was named Kallmann syndrome (KS).

Kallmann syndrome (KS) is occasionally called **dysplasia** olfactogenitalis of DeMorsier. Affected people usually are detected in adolescence when they do not undergo puberty. The most common features are HH and anosmia, though a wide range of features can present in an affected person. Other features of KS may include a small penis or undescended testicles in males, kidney abnormalities, cleft lip and/or palate, **clubfoot**, hearing problems, and central nervous system problems such as synkinesia, eye movement abnormalities, and visual and hearing defects.

Genetic profile

Most cases of Kallmann syndrome are sporadic. However, some cases are inherited in an autosomal dominant pattern, an autosomal recessive pattern, or an X-linked recessive pattern. In most cells that make up a person there are structures called chromosomes. Chromosomes contain genes, which are instructions for how a person will grow and develop. There are 46 chromosomes, or 23 pairs of chromosomes, in each cell. The first 22 chromosomes are the same in men and women and are called the autosomes. The last pair, the sex chromosomes, are different in men and women. Men have an X and a Y **chromosome** (XY). Women have two X-chromosomes (XX). All the genes of the autosomes and the X-chromosomes in women come in pairs.

Autosomal dominant inheritance occurs when only one copy of a **gene** pair is altered or mutated to cause the condition. In autosomal dominant inheritance, the second normal gene copy cannot compensate, or make up for, the altered gene. People with autosomal dominant inheritance have a 50% chance of passing the gene and the condition onto each of their children.

Autosomal recessive inheritance occurs when both copies of a gene are altered or mutated to cause the condition. In autosomal recessive inheritance, the affected person has inherited one altered gene from their mother and the other altered gene from their father. Couples who both have one copy of an altered autosomal recessive gene have a 25% risk with each pregnancy to have an affected child.

X-linked recessive inheritance is thought to be the least common form of inheritance in KS, but is the most well understood at the genetic level. With X-linked recessive inheritance, the altered gene that causes the condition is on their X chromosome. Since men have only one copy of the X chromosome, they have only one copy of the genes on the X chromosome. If that one copy is altered, they will have the condition because they do not have a second copy of the gene to compensate. Women, however, can have one altered copy of the gene and not be affected as they have a second copy to compensate. In X-linked recessive conditions, women are generally not affected with the condition. Women who are carriers for an X-linked recessive condition have a 25% chance of having an affected son with each pregnancy.

Though all three patterns of inheritance have been suggested for Kallmann syndrome, only one gene has been found that causes Kallmann syndrome. The gene, KAL, is located on the X chromosome and is responsible for most cases of X-linked recessive Kallmann syndrome. The gene instructs the body to make a protein called anosmin-1. When this gene is altered in a male, Kallmann syndrome occurs. Of those families who have an X-linked recessive form of KS, approximately one-half to one-third has identifiable alterations in their KAL gene.

Demographics

Kallmann syndrome is the most frequent cause of hypogonadotropic hypogonadism and affects approximately one in 10,000 males and one in 50,000 females. Kallmann syndrome is found in all ethnic backgrounds. Because the incidence of KS in males is about five times greater than KS in females, the original belief was that the X-linked form of Kallmann syndrome was the most common. However, it is now assumed that the X-linked recessive form is the least common of all KS. The reason for Kallmann syndrome being more frequent in males is not known.

Signs and symptoms

Embryology

Normally, a structure in the brain called the hypothalamus makes a hormone called gonadotrophin releas-ing hormone (GnRH). This hormone acts on the pituitary gland, another structure in the brain, to produce the two hormones: follicle stimulating hormone (FSH) and luteinizing hormone (LH). Both of these hormones travel to the gonads where they stimulate the development of sperm in men and eggs in women. FSH is also involved in the release of a single egg from the ovary once a month. Hypogonadotropic hypogonadism results when there is an alteration in this pathway that results in inadequate production of LH or FSH. In Kallmann syndrome, the alteration is that the hypothalamus is unable to produce GnRH.

How hypogonadotropic hypogonadism and the inability to smell are related can be explained during the development of an embryo. The cells that eventually make the GnRH in the hypothalamus are first found in the nasal placode, part of the developing olfactory system (for sense of smell). The GnRH cells must migrate, or move, from the nasal placode up into the brain to the hypothalamus. These GnRH cells migrate by following the path of another type of cell called the olfactory neurons. Neurons are specialized cells that are found in the nervous system and have long tail-like structures called axons. The axons of the olfactory neurons grow from the nasal placode up into the developing front of the brain. Once they reach their final destination in the brain, they form the olfactory bulb, the structure in the brain that helps process odors allowing the sense of smell. The GnRH cells follow the pathway of the olfactory neurons up into the brain to reach the hypothalamus.

In Kallmann syndrome, the olfactory neurons are unable to grow into the brain. Hence, the GnRH cells can not follow their pathway. As a result, the olfactory bulb does not form, resulting in the inability to smell. The GnRH cells can not follow the pathway of the axons and do not reach their final destination in the hypothalamus. Hence, no GnRH is made to stimulate the pituitary to make FSH and LH, resulting in hypogonadotropic hypogonadism.

In X-linked recessive KS, the KAL gene instructs the body to make the protein anosmin-1. This protein is involved in providing the pathway in the brain for which the olfactory axons grow. If it is altered in any way, the axons will not know where to grow in the brain and the GnRH cells will be unable to follow. The protein anosmin-1 is also found in other parts of the body, possibly explaining some of the other symptoms sometimes seen in Kallmann syndrome.

Other features

The features of Kallmann syndrome can vary among affected individuals even within the same family. The two features most often associated with Kallmann syndrome are HH and the inability to smell. Males can also have a small penis and undescended testicles at birth (testicles are still in body and have not dropped down into the scrotal sac). Clubfoot, cleft lip and/or cleft palate can also be present at birth. Clubfoot occurs when one or both feet are not properly placed onto the legs and can appear turned. Cleft lip and/or cleft palate occur when the upper lip and/or the roof of the mouth fail to come together during development. Kidney abnormalities, most often unilateral **renal agenesis** (one kidney did not form) are especially common in those males with X-linked recessive KS. Choanal atresia (pathway from the nose is blocked at birth) and structural heart defects have also been seen in KS.

Central nervous system problems can also occur in Kallmann syndrome. These can include nystagmus (involuntary eye movement), ataxia (involuntary body movement), hearing loss and problems with vision. Synkinesia is especially common in men with the X-linked recessive form of KS. Some people with KS are also mentally retarded. **Holoprosencephaly**, when the brain fails to develop in two halves, can also be seen in some individuals with KS.

Diagnosis

Individuals with Kallmann syndrome are usually diagnosed when they do not undergo puberty. Hormone testing shows that both LH and FSH are decreased. Affected individuals often do not realize they cannot smell. MRI can often detect the absence of the olfactory bulb in the brain. Renal ultrasound can determine if a kidney is missing.

Genetic testing for alterations in the KAL gene is the only genetic testing available. Even with families with clear X-linked recessive inheritance, genetic testing does not always detect an alteration in the KAL gene. Hence, diagnosis is still very dependent upon clinical features.

Treatment and management

When a child with KS is born with structural abnormalities such as cleft lip and/or palate, clubfoot or heart defects, surgery is often required to fix the defect. Taking sex hormones treats delayed puberty; women take estrogen and men take testosterone. Once puberty is completed, taking GnRH or both LH and FSH can treat hypogonadism. For most affected individuals, treatment is successful and infertility is reversed. However, a small portion of people will not respond to treatment.

When an isolated case of Kallmann syndrome is diagnosed, evaluation of first-degree family members, such as parents and siblings, should be completed. This

KEY TERMS

Hormone—A chemical messenger produced by the body that is involved in regulating specific bodily functions such as growth, development, and reproduction.

Hypothalamus—A part of the forebrain that controls heartbeat, body temperature, thirst, hunger, body temperature and pressure, blood sugar levels, and other functions.

Neuron—The fundamental nerve cell that conducts impulses across the cell membrane.

Pituitary gland—A small gland at the base of the brain responsible for releasing many hormones, including luteinizing hormone (LH) and follicle-stimulating hormone (FSH).

Puberty—Point in development when the gonads begin to function and secondary sexual characteristics begin to appear.

Synkinesia—Occurs when part of the body will move involuntarily when another part of the body moves.

should include a detailed family history, measuring hormone levels, assessing sense of smell, and renal ultrasound to look for kidney abnormalities. This information may help to diagnosis previously unrecognized cases of Kallmann syndrome. Furthermore, this information may be important for **genetic counseling** and determining whom in the family is at risk for also having Kallmann syndrome.

Prognosis

For individuals with the most common features of Kallmann syndrome, hypogonadism and the inability to smell, prognosis is excellent. In most cases, hormone treatment is able to reverse the delayed puberty and hypogonadism. For those individuals with other symptoms of Kallmann syndrome, prognosis can depend on how severe the defect is. For example, structural heart defects can be quite complex and sometimes surgery can not fix them. Furthermore, no treatment is available for the mental retardation in the portion of affected individuals with this symptom.

Resources

PERIODICALS

Rugarli, Elena, and Andrea Ballabio. "Kallmann Syndrome: From Genetics to Neurobiology." *JAMA* 270, no. 22 (December 8, 1993): 2713–2716.

ORGANIZATIONS

American Society for Reproductive Medicine. 1209 Montgomery Highway, Birmingham, AL 35216-2809. (205) 978-5000. <http://www.asrm.com>.

RESOLVE, The National Infertility Association. 1310 Broadway, Somerville, MA 02144-1779. (617) 623-0744. resolveinc@aol.com. <http://www.resolve.org>.

WEBSITES

Pediatric Database (PEDBASE) <www.icondata.com/health/pedbase/files/KALLMANN.HTM>.

Carin Lea Beltz, MS

Kartagener syndrome

Definition

Kartagener (pronounced KART-agayner) syndrome refers to a condition that involves difficulty with clearing mucus secretions from the respiratory tract, male infertility, and situs inversus. The defining characteristic of this syndrome is the situs inversus, which is a reversal of abdominal and thoracic organs.

Description

This syndrome is named after Kartagener, a physician from Switzerland. In the 1930s, Kartagener and a colleague described a familial form of bronchiectasis with situs inversus and nasal polyps. This came to be known as Kartagener syndrome. Kartagener syndrome is also known as the Siewert syndrome, after another physician, Siewert, who described the syndrome in the early 1900s.

Individuals who have Kartagener syndrome form a subset of the disorder called primary ciliary dyskinesia. Originally, primary ciliary dyskinesia was known as immotile cilia syndrome. The name, immotile cilia syndrome, is no longer used since the discovery that the cilia are actually not immotile, but rather, abnormal in movement. Individuals who have Kartagener syndrome, basically have primary ciliary dyskinesia, plus partial or complete situs inversus. The situs inversus is what sets Kartagener syndrome apart from primary ciliary dyskinesia.

Kartagener syndrome is caused by abnormalities of the cilia that line the respiratory tract and also form the flagella of sperm. Cilia are tiny hair-like structures that contain a bundle of small parallel tubes that form a central core. This core is called the axoneme. Ciliary move-ment is accomplished by the bending of the axoneme. One of the most important associated structures that enable ciliary movement to occur are sets of tiny arms that project from each tubule. These tiny arms are called dynein arms.

Cilia line the cells of the lungs, nose and sinuses. Before reaching the lungs, air travels through the airway where it is moistened and filtered. The nasal passages and airway are lined with mucus membranes. The mucus covering the mucus membrane traps dirt and other foreign particles that have been breathed in. The cilia, lining the membranes, beat in a wavelike manner moving the layer of mucus and carrying away the dirt and debris that has been trapped. This mucus can then be coughed out or swallowed into the stomach.

In Kartagener syndrome, the cilia do not move, move very little, or move abnormally. Because the cilia do not function properly, the mucus is not cleared from the respiratory tract, which leads to sinus infection (sinusitis) and chronic changes of the lung (bronchiectasis), which make it difficult to exhale. Mucus clearance from the middle ear can also be affected and over time can lead to hearing loss.

The male infertility in Kartagener syndrome is also caused by abnormal cilia movement. One spermatozoon consists of a head, midpiece, and a tail or flagellum. The tail of a spermatozoon is a long flagellum consisting of a central axoneme. This axoneme enables the movement of the flagellum so that the spermatozoon can propel its way to the fallopian tube and burrow through the egg coat to fertilize the egg. In Kartagener syndrome, these cilia are either immotile, or are not able to move normally to complete the journey to the fallopian tubes, nor may they be able to burrow through the egg coat. This results in male infertility.

As stated above, situs inversus is what sets Kartagener syndrome apart from primary ciliary dyskinesia. Complete situs inversus involves reversal of both the abdominal and thoracic organs so that they form a mirror image of normal. In partial situs inversus, the thoracic organs may be reversed, while the abdominal organs are normally positioned, or vice versa. Approximately one in 10,000 adults have situs inversus. Only about 20% of individuals who have complete situs inversus are diagnosed to have Kartagener syndrome. Of those with complete situs inversus who are diagnosed to have Kartagener syndrome, there is only a small risk for associated cardiac defects. Partial situs inversus may occur in individuals who have Kartagener syndrome as well. Partial situs inversus has a higher association with other abnormalities, including polysplenia or **asplenia** (extra or absent spleen) and cardiac defects.

One theory behind the association of situs inversus with the underlying cause of Kartagener syndrome is that the lack of ciliary movement in the developing embryo may result in incorrect organ rotation in approximately 50% of affected individuals. In fact, 50% of patients with PCD will have situs inversus and thus be diagnosed to have Kartagener syndrome. However, this is a theory supported only by some researchers.

Genetic profile

Kartagener syndrome is an autosomal recessive condition. This means that in order to have the condition, an individual needs to inherit two copies of the **gene** for the condition, one from each parent. Individuals who carry only one gene for an autosomal recessive syndrome are called heterozygotes. Heterozygotes for Kartagener syndrome have normal ciliary function and do not have any clinical features of the condition. If two carriers of Kartagener syndrome have children, there is a 25% chance, with each pregnancy, for having a child with Kartagener syndrome.

The components that form the cilium contain several hundred different proteins. Each is coded for by different **DNA** sequences, potentially on different chromosomes. A defect in any of these codes could produce an abnormal or missing protein that is a building block for the cilium and thus could cause abnormal ciliary structure and movement, resulting in Kartagener syndrome.

When the same condition can be caused by different genetic abnormalities, this is known as genetic heterogeneity. In fact, several different defects in cilia have been seen in association with Kartagener syndrome, including; overly long cilia, overly short cilia, absent cilia and randomly oriented cilia, suggesting genetic heterogeneity. Studies have suggested that the most common defect of cilia in Kartagener syndrome is the lack of dynein arms. There have been rare cases in which individuals have Kartagener syndrome, yet have no detectable abnormality of the cilia, even though the ciliary function is abnormal. Results of one study involving a genome-wide linkage search performed on 31 families, with multiple individuals affected with either PCD or Kartagener syndrome, strongly suggested extensive heterogeneity. Potential regions involving genes responsible for PCD or Kartagener syndrome were localized on chromosomes 3, 4, 5, 7, 8, 10, 11, 13, 15, 16, 17 and 19.

Demographics

Kartagener syndrome occurs in approximately one in 32,000 live births, which is half the incidence of primary ciliary dyskinesia (one in 16,000 live births). Kartagener syndrome is not found more commonly in any particular sex, ethnic background or geographic region. Males, however, may be diagnosed more often than females because of infertility investigation.

Signs and symptoms

Newborns who have Kartagener syndrome may present with neonatal respiratory distress. Often when individuals are diagnosed to have Kartagener syndrome in later childhood, problems such as neonatal respiratory distress may be identified in their history. Symptoms that may present in childhood include; recurrent ear infections (otitis media) that can lead to hearing loss, chronic productive cough, reactive airway disease, pneumonia, chronic bronchitis, runny nose (rhinitis) with a thin discharge, and sinus infection (sinusitis). Situs inversus usually does not present symptomatically, unless it is associated with a congenital heart defect.

The most common clinical expression of Kartagener syndrome in adults includes chronic upper and lower airway disease presenting as sinusitis and bronchiectasis. Clubbing of the digits (fingers) may occur as the result of chronic hypoxia (lack of oxygen) from bronchiectasis. In males of reproductive age, male infertility is almost universal. In females who have Kartagener syndrome, infertility is not usually a characteristic. This suggests that the egg transport down the fallopian tube is associated more with muscle contractions than with ciliary movement.

Several other conditions should be considered when the aforementioned symptoms present, including; **Cystic fibrosis** (CF), immune deficiencies and severe allergies. Although the causes of Kartagener syndrome and CF are completely different, the symptoms of these two diseases are very similar. Often when the symptoms present, children with Kartagener syndrome are tested for CF first because the incidence of CF is much higher (one in 2,400) than the incidence of Kartagener syndrome. CF is also associated with male infertility.

Diagnosis

Diagnosis of Kartagener syndrome is confirmed by identifying the ciliary abnormalities of structure and movement. This is accomplished by biopsy of the mucus membranes of the respiratory tract and/or by examination of sperm, looking for ciliary dyskinesia. Situs inversus can be identified by x ray or ultrasound examination. Infertility investigation may elicit the possibility of Kartagener syndrome in a patient previously undiagnosed. After a diagnosis is made, **genetic counseling** should be provided to discuss the **inheritance** pattern, to help identify other possible affected family members and to discuss reproductive options.

KEY TERMS

Bronchiectasis—An abnormal condition of the bronchial tree, characterized by irreversible widening and destruction of the bronchial walls of the lungs.

Cystic fibrosis—A respiratory disease characterized by chronic lung disease, pancreatic insufficiency and an average age of survival of 20 years. Cystic fibrosis is caused by mutations in a gene on chromosome 7 that encodes a transmembrane receptor.

Dyskinesia—Impaired ability to make voluntary movements.

Tympanoplasty—Any of several operations on the eardrum or small bones of the middle ear, to restore or improve hearing in patients with conductive hearing loss.

As Kartagener syndrome is an autosomal recessive disorder, individuals who have had a child with Kartagener syndrome have a 25% chance, with each future pregnancy, of having another child with Kartagener syndrome. Prenatal diagnosis may be possible for a couple with a previously affected child, by performing ultrasound examination to identify a fetus who has situs inversus. Although, if the fetus does not exhibit situs inversus, it is still possible for the fetus to have PCD. Also, it is important to remember that identifying a fetus who has situs inversus in a family not known to be at an increased risk for Kartagener syndrome, does not mean that the fetus has Kartagener syndrome as only 20% of individuals who have situs inversus have Kartagener syndrome. DNA testing for Kartagener syndrome is not possible.

Treatment and management

Treatment for Kartagener syndrome involves treatment of the symptoms. Treatment for sinusitis includes the use of antibiotics to treat and prevent recurrent infection. Occasionally, surgery to relieve the sinusitis and remove nasal polyps that may be present is necessary. Daily chest physiotherapy to loosen mucus secretions is a common therapy as well, and if started early in life can help to prevent or delay development of bronchiectasis. Tympanoplasty in children with recurrent ear infections is often necessary.

Advances in reproductive technology allow for men who have Kartagener syndrome to have the opportunity to have children. A procedure called intracytoplasmic sperm injection or ICSI, now allow immotile or dysmotile sperm to fertilize an egg. ICSI involves injection of a single sperm into single eggs in order for fertilization to occur. This procedure first involves ovulation induction and egg retrieval to obtain eggs for attempt at fertilization by ICSI. In Vitro Fertilization (ICSI) pregnancy rates vary from center to center. Overall pregnancy rates of 10%–40% have been quoted worldwide, utilizing these procedures.

The chance for an affected male and his unaffected partner to have a child who has Kartagener syndrome is small. If the disease incidence is one in 32,000, then the chance for the unaffected woman to be a carrier of Kartagener syndrome is approximately one in 100 and the chance for having an affected child would be expected to be approximately one in 200 (0.5%). However, all children of affected males or females will be carriers for Kartagener syndrome.

Prognosis

The severity of Kartagener syndrome is variable. With the advent of antibiotic use for infection control, the life expectancy of a patient with Kartagener syndrome is close to or within the normal range, if there are no immediate problems in the newborn period.

Resources

BOOKS

Jones, Kenneth Lyons. *Smith's Recognizable Patterns of Human Malformation.* Philadelphia: W. B. Saunders Company, 1997.

PERIODICALS

Guichard, Cècile, et al. "Axonemal Dynein Intermediate-Chain Gene (DNAI1) Mutations Result in Situs Inversus and Primary Ciliary Dyskinesia (Kartagener Syndrome)." *American Journal of Human Genetics* (April 2001): 1030.

ORGANIZATIONS

American Lung Association. 1740 Broadway, New York, NY 10019-4374. (212) 315-8700 or (800) 586-4872. <http://www.lungusa.org>.

National Organization for Rare Disorders (NORD). PO Box 8923, New Fairfield, CT 06812-8923. (203) 746-6518 or (800) 999-6673. Fax: (203) 746-6481. <http://www.rarediseases.org>.

WEBSITES

OMIM Online Mendelian Inheritance in Man. Entries 244400 and 242650. <http://www.ncbi.nlm.nih.gov/entrez/query.fcgi?db=OMIM>.

Tucker, Michael. "Clinical In Vitro Fertilization and Culture." *IVF.com.* <http://www.ivf.com/insem.html>.

Renee A. Laux, MS

Karyotype

Definition

Karyotype refers to the arrangement of chromosomes in their matched (homologous) pairs. For the purposes of this definition, we will be referring to human chromosomes, although there is a karyotype characteristic for each species. The human chromosomes are arranged and numbered according to the International System for Human Cytogenetic Nomenclature (ISCN). The most recent recommendations of the ISCN are from 1995. Karyotype either refers to the actual composition of the chromosomes in a body cell of an individual or species, or to the actual diagram or photograph of those chromosomes, arranged in their pairs.

Description

The normal human karyotype consists of 23 pairs of chromosomes. There are 22 pair of autosomes, which are the chromosomes that are not the sex chromosomes. The genes on these chromosomes instruct our bodies as to how they look and function. The 23rd pair of chromosomes are the sex chromosomes. Typically, females have two X sex chromosomes and males have one X sex **chromosome** and one Y sex chromosome.

Karyotype construction

In the construction of the karyotype, the chromosomes are numbered 1 to 22 from longest to shortest. The last pair are the sex chromosomes and are placed on the karyotype after the 22nd pair. The chromosomes can be separated into groups, based on their length and the position of the centromere. Group A consists of chromosome pairs 1, 2 and 3. They are the longest chromosomes and their centromeres are in the center of the chromosomes (metacentric). Group B consists of chromosome pairs 4 and 5. They are long; however, their centromeres lie toward the top of the chromosomes (submetacentric). Group C consists of chromosome pairs 6, 7, 8, 9, 10, 11 and 12 and also includes the X chromosome. They are medium-sized and their centromeres either lie in the middle or toward the top of the chromosomes. Group D consists of chromosome pairs 13,14 and 15. They are medium-sized and their centromeres lie at the top of the chromosomes (acrocentric). Additionally, the D group chromosomes have satellites. Group E consists of chromosome pairs 16, 17 and 18. They are relatively short chromosomes and their centromeres lie in the center or towards the top of the chromosomes. Group F consists of chromosomes 19 and 20. They are short chromosomes with centromeres that lie in the center of the chromosome. Lastly, group G consists of chromosome pairs 21,

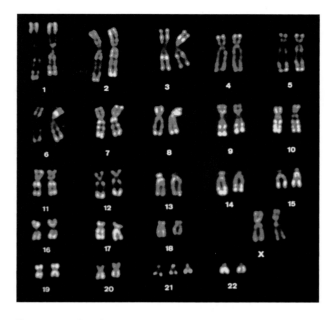

Karyotype showing three copies of chromosome 21. This indicates Down syndrome. *(Custom Medical Stock Photo, Inc.)*

22 and the Y chromosome. These are short chromosomes with their centromeres at the top. Chromosome pairs 21 and 22 have satellites. The Y chromosome does not have satellites.

The actual chromosomes are only individually distinguishable during a certain stage of cell division. This stage is called the metaphase stage. Chromosome preparations are made from pictures of the chromosomes during the metaphase stage of division. The metaphase spread is what the technician sees in one cell under the microscope and what the photograph of that one cell is referred to. Usually, the chromosomes in a metaphase preparation are banded by special staining techniques used in the laboratory. Each numbered chromosome is unique in its banding pattern so that all number 1s look the same and all number 2s look the same, etc. Although, there can be small normal familial variations in chromosomes. Because of banding, the chromosomes are more easily distinguishable from each other and the banding makes it is easier to see differences or abnormalities. For example, if a chromosome is missing a piece, or two chromosomes are attached to each other (translocation), it is much easier to see with banded chromosomes than with unbanded chromosomes.

Chromosome preparations can be made from any potentially dividing cells, including; blood cells, skin cells, amniotic fluid cells (the fluid surrounding an unborn baby), placental tissue or chorionic villi (tissue that forms the placenta and can be used in prenatal diagnosis).

KEY TERMS

Acrocentric—A chromosome with the centromere positioned at the top end.

Centromere—The centromere is the constricted region of a chromosome. It performs certain functions during cell division.

Homologous chromosomes—Homologous chromosomes are two chromosomes of a doublet set that are identical, particularly for the genes that are on them.

Metacentric—When a chromosome has the centromere in the middle of the chromosome it is called a metacentric chromosome.

Satellites of chromosomes—Small segments of genetic material at the tips of the short arms of chromosomes 13, 14, 15, 21, and 22.

Submetacentric—Positioning of the centromere between the center and the top of the chromosome.

ISCN formulas exist to describe any chromosome complement. The basic formula for writing a karyotype is as follows. The first item written is the total number of chromosomes, followed by a comma. The second item written is the sex chromosome complement. The typical female karyotype is written as 46,XX and the typical male karyotype is written as 46,XY.

Formulas for abnormal karyotypes

Many formulas for writing abnormal karyotypes have been determined. Some common examples follow. A plus or a minus sign before a chromosome number is used to show that the entire chromosome is extra or missing. Also, the total number of chromosomes will be different than 46. For example, the condition **Down syndrome** occurs when an individual has an extra number 21 chromosome. For a male, this karyotype is written as 47,XY,+21. An individual may also have extra or missing parts of chromosomes. The short arm of a chromosome is called the p arm and the long arm is called the q arm. For example, the condition **Wolf-Hirschhorn syndrome** is caused by a missing part of the top arm of chromosome 4. For a female, this karyotype would be written as 46,XX,del(4)(p16). The chromosome that is involved in the change is specified within the first set of parentheses and the breakpoint for the missing material is defined in the second set of parentheses. A final example is a balanced translocation karyotype. A balanced translocation means that there is no missing or extra genetic material

as the result of the translocation. There are many types of translocations. One type is called a robertsonian translocation. A robertsonian translocation occurs when two acrocentric chromosomes are attached together. One common example is a translocation involving chromosomes 13 and 14. If a male has a balanced robertsonian translocation of chromosomes 13 and 14, this is written as 45,XY,der(13;14). The "der" stands for derivative, as the new 13;14 chromosome is considered a derivative. There are only 45 separate chromosomes now, which is why 45 is the number written in the karyotype. There are many more formulas for the abundant abnormal chromosome findings in individuals. For further detailed information, please refer to the resource listed below.

Resources

BOOKS

Mitelman, Felix, ed. *An International System for Human Cytogenetic Nomenclature (1995)*. Farmington, CT: S. Karger AG, 1995.

Renee A. Laux, MS

Karyotype analysis *see* **Karyotype**

Keller syndrome *see* **FG syndrome**

Kennedy disease

Definition

Kennedy disease (KD) is a disorder characterized by degradation of the anterior horn cells of the spinal cord resulting in slow progressive muscle weakness and atrophy. Men with Kennedy disease often have breast enlargement (gynecomastia), testicular atrophy, and may have infertility.

Description

Kennedy disease, also referred to as spinobulbar muscular atrophy (SBMA), arises primarily from degradation of the anterior horn cells of the spinal cord, resulting in proximal weakness and atrophy of voluntary skeletal muscle. Anterior horn cells control the voluntary muscle contractions from large muscle groups such as the arms and legs. For example, if an individual wants to move his/her arm, electrical impulses are sent from the brain to the anterior horn cells to the muscles of the arm, which then stimulate the arm muscles to contract, allowing the arm to move. Degradation is a rapid loss of functional motor neurons. Loss of motor neurons results in progressive symmetrical atrophy of the voluntary muscles. Progressive symmetrical atrophy refers to the loss of function of muscle groups from both sides of the body. For example, both arms and both legs are equally affected by similar degrees of muscle loss and the inability to be controlled and used properly. Progressive loss indicates that muscle loss is not instantaneous, rather muscle loss occurs consistently over a period of time. These muscle groups include those skeletal muscles that control large muscle groups such as the arms, legs and torso. The weakness in the legs is generally greater than the weakness in the arms.

Proximal weakness is in contrast to distal weakness, and indicates that muscles such as the arms and the legs are affected rather than the muscles of the hands, feet, fingers, and toes. However, the motor neuron of the brainstem and sensory neurons of the dorsal root ganglia are also affected in KD. Motor neurons are the neurons that control large muscle groups (arms, legs, torso) of which anterior horn cells are a subgroup. Sensory neurons are a distinct class of neurons that control an individual's senses. An example would be pain receptors that cause an involuntary reaction to a stimuli such as when a person accidentally grasps a boiling hot kettle and immediately releases the kettle. Dorsal root ganglia are analogous to a headquarters for neurons, through which essentially all neuronal stimuli are processed.

Diagnosis

Kennedy disease is suspected clinically in a male with an early adulthood onset of proximal muscle weakness of the limbs, fasticulations (small local contractions of the musculature that is visible through the skin) of the tongue, lips or area around the mouth, absence of hyperactive reflexes and spasticity, and often evidence of enlarged breasts and/or small testes with few or no sperm.

The diagnosis is made by a specific molecular genetic test that measures the number of "repeats" in a particular part of the androgen receptor (AR) **gene**. The alteration of the AR gene that causes Kennedy disease is an expansion of a CAG trinucleotide repeat in the first PART of the gene. In unaffected individuals, between 11 to 33 copies OF the CAG trinucleotide are present. In patients with Kennedy disease, this number rises to 40 to 62. The greater the number of expanded repeats, the earlier the age of onset.

Genetic profile

Kennedy disease is an X-linked recessive disease, meaning the abnormal gene is found on the X **chromo-**some and two copies of the abnormal gene must be present for the disorder to occur. Since males only inherit one X chromosome (the other is the Y chromosome) they will always express an X-linked disorder if the abnormal gene is on the X chromosome they receive. Females on the other hand inherit two X chromosomes. Even if one X chromosome contains the abnormal gene, the second X chromosome with a normal functioning gene can usually compensate for the other. Males lack the second X chromosome that may be able to mask the effect of the abnormal gene.

The disease was first characterized in 1968. The KD-determining gene, androgen receptor (AR), maps to the proximal long arm of the X-chromosome.

The AR protein is a member of the steroid-thyroid hormone receptor family and is involved in transcription regulation. Transcription regulation is the molecular process that controls the "reading" of the genetic **DNA** information and turning it into **RNA** which is the material which generates proteins.

Demographics

Because of the X-linked **inheritance** pattern of Kennedy disease, only males are affected by this disorder. Females may be carriers of the disease if they possess an abnormal gene on one of her X chromosomes. Due to the rare nature of this disease, and the fact that it may frequently be misdiagnosed as another form of neuromuscular disease, no particular race or ethnicity appears to be at greater risk than another.

Kennedy disease is primarily an adult disease, with an onset between the third and fifth decade of life. Once symptoms present, the disease is slowly progressive. In addition to neuronal cell loss, breast enlargement (gynecomatia), reduced fertility and testicular atrophy have also been reported in affected males.

Treatment and management

To date, there is not treatment for SBMA. However, there are possible mechanisms through which treatment could be developed. **Gene therapy** could be used for SBMA to replace the abnormal gene associated with SBMA with a copy carrying fewer CAG repeats. Currently this is not possible or available.

As the bulbar muscles of the face are affected, eating and swallowing can become difficult. Due to the weakening of the respiratory muscles breathing can also be labored. It is therefore essential for patients to undergo chest physiotherapy (CPT). CPT is a standard set of procedures designed to trigger and aid coughing in patients. Coughing is important as it clears the patient's lungs and

KEY TERMS

Anterior horn cells—Subset of motor neurons within the spinal cord.

Atrophy—Wasting away of normal tissue or an organ due to degeneration of the cells.

Degradation—Loss or diminishing.

Dorsal root ganglia—The subset of neuronal cells controlling impulses in and out of the brain.

Intragenic—Occuring within a single gene.

Motor neurons—Class of neurons that specifically control and stimulate voluntary muscles.

Motor units—Functional connection with a single motor neuron and muscle.

Sensory neurons—Class of neurons that specifically regulate and control external stimuli (senses: sight, sound).

Transcription—The process by which genetic information on a strand of DNA is used to synthesize a strand of complementary RNA.

Voluntary muscle—A muscle under conscious control, such as arm and leg muscles.

throat of moisture and prevents secondary problems, such as pneumonia.

As symptoms progress, patients may require a ventilator to aid breathing.

Prognosis

The majority of patients with SBMA have a normal life span. About 10% of older, severely affected patients with SBMA may die from pneumonia or asphyxiation secondary to weakness of the bulbar muscles.

Resources

BOOKS

Zajac, J. D., and H. E. MacLean. "Kennedy's Disease: Clinical Aspects." *Genetic Instabilities and Hereditary Neurological Diseases,* edited by R. D. Wells and S. T. Warren. New York: Academic Press, 1998, pp. 87-100.

PERIODICALS

Crawford, T. O., and C. A. Pardo. "The Neurobiology of Childhood Spinal Muscular Atrophy." *Neurobiology of Disease* 3 (1996): 97-110.

Ferlini, A., et al. "Androgen Receptor CAG Repeat Analysis in the Differential Between Kennedy's Disease and Other Motoneuron Disorders." *American Journal of Human Genetics* 55 (1995): 105-111.

ORGANIZATIONS

Kennedy Disease (SBMA) Support Group. 1804 Quivira Road, Washington, KS 66968. (785) 325-2629. gryphon@grapevine.net. <http://www.geocities.com/HotSprings/Villa/1989>.

National Ataxia Foundation. 2600 Fernbrook Lane, Suite 119, Minneapolis, MN 55447. (763) 553-0020. Fax: (763) 553-0167. naf@mr.net. <http://www.ataxia.org/>.

WEBSITES

The Andrew's Buddies web site. *FightSMA.com* <http://www.andrewsbuddies.com/news.html>.

Families of Spinal Muscular Atrophy. <http://www.fsma.org>.

Muscular Dystrophy Association. <http://www.mdausa.org>.

Philip J. Young
Christian L. Lorson, PhD

Ketotoic hyperglycinemia
see **Propionic acidemia**

Killian-Teschler-Nicola syndrome
see **Tetrasomy 12p**

Kinky hair disease
see **Menkes syndrome**

Klein-Waardenburg syndrome,
see **Waardenburg syndrome**

Klinefelter syndrome

Definition

Klinefelter syndrome is a **chromosome** disorder in males. People with this condition are born with at least one extra X chromosome.

Description

Klinefelter syndrome is a condition where one or more extra X-chromosomes are present in a male. Boys with this condition appear normal at birth. They enter puberty normally, but by mid-puberty have low levels of testosterone causing small testicles and the inability to make sperm. Affected males may also have learning disabilities and behavior problems such as shyness and immaturity and are at an increased risk for certain health problems.

Genetic profile

Chromosomes are found in the cells in the body. Chromosomes contain genes, structures that tell the body

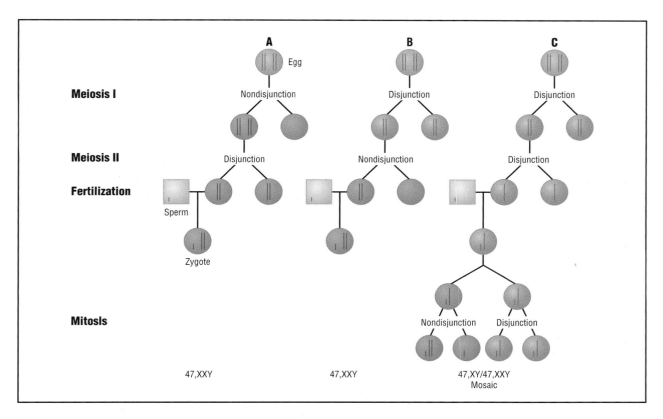

	A	B	C
Meiosis I	Egg		
	Nondisjunction	Disjunction	Disjunction
Meiosis II	Disjunction	Nondisjunction	Disjunction
Fertilization	Sperm		
	Zygote		
Mitosis			Nondisjunction Disjunction
	47,XXY	47,XXY	47,XY/47,XXY Mosaic

Nondisjunction, failure of paired chromosomes to separate, can result at different stages of meiosis or mitosis. When nondisjunction occurs in the first (A) or second (B) phase of meiosis the resulting karyotype will be 47,XXY. If the chromosomes fail to separate during mitosis (C) a mosaic karyotype (46,XY/47,XXY) will result. *(Gale Group)*

how to grow and develop. Chromosomes are responsible for passing on hereditary traits from parents to child. Chromosomes also determine whether the child will be male or female. Normally, a person has a total of 46 chromosomes in each cell, two of which are responsible for determining that individual's sex. These two sex chromosomes are called X and Y. The combination of these two types of chromosomes determines the sex of a child. Females have two X chromosomes (the XX combination); males have one X and one Y chromosome (the XY combination).

In Klinefelter syndrome, a problem very early in development results in an abnormal number of chromosomes. Most commonly, a male with Klinefelter syndrome will be born with 47 chromosomes in each cell, rather than the normal number of 46. The extra chromosome is an X chromosome. This means that rather than having the normal XY combination, the male has an XXY combination. Because people with Klinefelter syndrome have a Y chromosome, they are all male.

Approximately one-third of all males with Klinefelter syndrome have other chromosome changes involving an extra X chromosome. Mosaic Klinefelter syndrome

occurs when some of the cells in the body have an extra X chromosome and the other have normal male chromosomes. These males can have the same or milder symptoms than non-mosaic Klinefelter syndrome. Males with more than one additional extra X chromosome, such as 48,XXXY, are usually more severely affected than males with 47,XXY.

Klinefelter syndrome is not considered an inherited condition. The risk of Klinefelter syndrome reoccurring in another pregnancy is not increased above the general population risk.

Demographics

Klinefelter syndrome is one of the most common **chromosomal abnormalities**. About one in every 500 to 800 males is born with this disorder. Approximately 3% of the infertile male population have Klinefelter syndrome.

Signs and symptoms

The symptoms of Klinefelter syndrome are variable and not every affected person will have all of the features of the condition. Males with Klinefelter syndrome appear normal at birth and have normal male genitalia. From childhood, males with Klinefelter syndrome are taller than average with long limbs. Approximately 20–50% have a mild intention tremor, an uncontrolled shaking. Many males with Klinefelter syndrome have poor upper body strength and can be clumsy. Klinefelter syndrome does not cause homosexuality. Approximately one-third of males with Klinefelter syndrome have breast growth, some requiring breast reduction surgery.

Most boys enter puberty normally, though some can be delayed. The Leydig cells in the testicles usually produce testosterone. With Klinefelter syndrome, the Leydig cells fail to work properly causing the testosterone production to slow. By mid-puberty, testosterone production is decreased to approximately half of normal. This can lead to decreased facial and pubic hair growth. The decreased testosterone also causes an increase in two other hormones, follicle stimulating hormone (FSH) and luteinizing hormone (LH). Normally, FSH and LH help the immature sperm cells grow and develop. In Klinefelter syndrome, there are few or no sperm cells. The increased amount of FSH and LH cause hyalinization and fibrosis, the growth of excess fibrous tissue, in the seminiferous tubules, where the sperm are normally located. As a result, the testicles appear smaller and firmer than normal. With rare exception, men with Klinefelter syndrome are infertile because they can not make sperm.

While it was once believed that all boys with Klinefelter syndrome were mentally retarded, doctors now know that the disorder can exist without retardation. However, children with Klinefelter syndrome frequently have difficulty with language, including learning to speak, read, and write. Approximately 50% of males with Klinefelter syndrome are dyslexic.

Some people with Klinefelter syndrome have difficulty with social skills and tend to be more shy, anxious, or immature than their peers. They can also have poor judgement and do not handle stressful situations well. As a result, they often do not feel comfortable in large social gatherings. Some people with Klinefelter syndrome can also have anxiety, nervousness and/or **depression**.

The greater the number of X-chromosomes present, the greater the disability. Boys with several extra X-chromosomes have distinctive facial features, more severe retardation, deformities of bony structures, and even more disordered development of male features.

Diagnosis

Diagnosis of Klinefelter syndrome is made by examining chromosomes for evidence of more than one X chromosome present in a male. This can be done in preg-

---

---

nancy with prenatal testing such as a chorionic villus sampling or **amniocentesis**. Chorionic villus sampling is a procedure done early in pregnancy (approximately 10–12 weeks) to obtain a small sample of the placenta for testing. An amniocentesis is done further along in pregnancy (from approximately 16–18 weeks) to obtain a sample of fluid surrounding the baby for testing. Both procedures have a risk of miscarriage. Usually these procedures are done for a reason other than diagnosing Klinefelter syndrome. For example, a prenatal diagnostic procedure may be done on an older woman to determine if her baby has **Down syndrome**. If the diagnosis of Klinefelter syndrome is suspected in a young boy or adult male, chromosome testing can also be on a small blood or skin sample after birth.

Treatment and management

There is no treatment available to change chromosomal makeup. Children with Klinefelter syndrome may benefit from a speech therapist for speech problems or other educational intervention for learning disabilities. Testosterone injections started around the time of puberty may help to produce more normal development including more muscle mass, hair growth and increased sex drive. Testosterone supplementation will not increase testicular size, decrease breast growth or correct infertility.

Prognosis

While many men with Klinefelter syndrome go on to live normal lives, nearly 100% of these men will be sterile (unable to produce a child). However, a few men with Klinefelter syndrome have been reported who have fathered a child through the use of assisted fertility services. Males with Klinefelter syndrome have an increased

---

risk of several conditions such as **osteoporosis**, autoimmune disorders such as lupus and arthritis, **diabetes**, and both breast and germ cell tumors.

Resources

BOOKS

Bock, R. *Understanding Klinefelter's Syndrome: A Guide for XXY Males and Their Families.* National Institutes of Health, USA, 1993.

Probasco, Teri, and Gretchen A. Gibbs. *Klinefelter Syndrome.* Richmond, IN: Prinit Press, 1999.

PERIODICALS

Smyth, Cynthia M., and W. J. Bremner. "Klinefelter Syndrome." *Archives of Internal Medicine* 158 (1998): 1309–1314.

Smyth, Cynthia M. "Diagnosis and Treatment of Klinefelter Syndrome." *Hospital Practice* (September 15, 1999): 111–120.

Staessen, C., et al. "Preimplantation Diagnosis for X and Y Normality in Embryos from Three Klinefelter Patients." *Human Reproduction* 11, no. 8. (1996): 1650–1653.

ORGANIZATIONS

American Association for Klinefelter Syndrome Information and Support (AAKSIS) 2945 W. Farwell Ave., Chicago, IL 60645-2925. (773) 761-5298 or (888) 466-5747. Fax: (773) 761-5298. <http://www.aaksis.org aaksis@aaksis.org>.

Klinefelter Syndrome and Associates, Inc. PO Box 119, Roseville, CA 95678-0119. (916) 773-2999 or (888) 999-9428. Fax: (916) 773-1449. ksinfo@genetic.org. <http://www.genetic.org/ks>.

Klinefelter's Organization. PO Box 60, Orpington, BR68ZQ. UK <http://hometown.aol.com/KSCUK/index.htm>.

WEBSITES

Klinefelter Syndrome Support Group Home Page. <http://klinefeltersyndrome.org/index.html>.

Carin Lea Beltz, MS

▌Klippel-Feil sequence

Definition

Individuals with Klippel-Feil sequence (KFS) were originally described as having a classic triad of webbed neck (very short neck), low hairline, and decreased flexibility of the neck. More commonly, abnormal joining or fusion of two or more vertebrae (bones) of the cervical spine (neck bones) characterizes Klippel-Feil sequence.

Description

Klippel-Feil sequence is extensive fusion of multiple cervical vertebrae (the uppermost bones of the spine). There may be complete fusion or multiple irregular bony segments in the bones of the upper back (cervical and often upper thoracic spine). Premature and extensive arthritis and osseous (bony) spurring affecting the joints of the spine (facet joints) are common in individuals with Klippel-Feil sequence.

There are three classifications of Klippel-Feil sequence.

- Group 1 exhibits fusion of the lower skull (head) and the first bone of the spine (the first cervical vertebrae (C1)). The second and third spinal bones (cervical vertebrae C2 and C3) are also usually fused together in Group 1. The normal cervical spine has seven bones or vertebrae. Normally half of the ability of humans to bend their heads forward (flexion) and backwards (extension) occurs in the joints between the base of the skull and the uppermost spinal bone. The other half of the motions of flexion and extension occur in the rest of the upper spine. Therefore, the danger is due to the excessive motion of the neck between the joints that are fused.

- Group 2 has fusion of bones (vertebrae) below the second cervical bone (C2). Group 2 also has an abnormal skull and upper spinal bone connection.

- Group 3 has an open space between two fused segments of spinal bones.

Genetic profile

Although this is usually a sporadic occurrence, an abnormal **gene** responsible for Klippel-Feil sequence has been found on the q (long) arm of **chromosome** 8. The human cell contains 46 chromosomes arranged in 23 pairs. Most of the genes in the two chromosomes of each pair are identical or almost identical with each other. However, with KFS individuals, there appears to be a reversal or inversion on part of chromosome 8.

Demographics

Approximately one out of every 42,000 people has Klippel-Feil sequence. The classic triad is seen in 52% of individuals with the syndrome. Men and women are affected equally, however, some studies have shown slightly higher numbers for women. There have been some reports of Klippel-Feil sequence being more common among infants born with **fetal alcohol syndrome** (FAS) because FAS affects bone development of the fetus. However, there is a genetic component that passes the syndrome on through the generations in a dominant **inheritance** pattern.

Signs and symptoms

The first clinical signs are the classic triad of webbed neck, low hairline, and decreased flexibility of the neck. However, the presence of abnormalities of the cervical spine found with x rays is the hallmark diagnosis. Other signs and symptoms may be found, but vary from person to person.

Some patients may exhibit wryneck or Torticollis, which is a twisting of the neck to one side that results in abnormal carriage of the head. The individual may have differences between the two sides of his face, known as facial asymmetry. Patients may also have **scoliosis** (abnormal curves of the spine).

A variety of miscellaneous abnormalities may clinically manifest themselves in Klippel-Feil sequence. Deafness occurs in about 30% of the cases. Ear abnormalities such as very small ear lobes (microtia), or deformed bones within the ear (ossicles) may be present. They may even have a small or absent internal ear.

Abnormalities of the blood vessels such as a missing radial artery in the forearm may decrease the size of the thumbs (thenar hypoplasia). Anomalies of the right subclavian artery (artery under the clavicle or collar bone) have been reported as well as higher incidences of artery anomalies of the upper neck (cervical vertebrae). Anomalies of the genital areas and urinary system are also common.

Individuals diagnosed with Klippel-Feil sequence frequently have problems with cervical nerves and nerves that go from the neck to the arms and hands. Individuals can have pain that starts in their neck and travels into the arms if the nerve roots coming off of the spinal cord are irritated or pinched.

Diagnosis

Klippel-Feil syndrome is usually diagnosed in early childhood or adolescence. Observing the clinical signs of having the classic triad of webbed neck, low hairline, and limited cervical ranges of motion initiates the diagnosis. When further testing is done such as x ray, the diagnosis is confirmed by the fusion of multiple cervical vertebrae.

Treatment and management

If the individual has a very mild case of Klippel-Feil sequence, then the person can lead a normal life with only minor restrictions. These restrictions, such as avoiding contact sports that would place the neck at risk, are necessary because of the instability of the cervical spine. This is due to the increased motion between the fused cervical vertebrae.

Symptoms, such as pain, that occur with the arthritis and degeneration of the joints may also result. The individuals should be treated with pain medication and possible cervical traction. If neurological symptoms occur, the treatment of choice is fusion of the symptomatic area. However, due to the severe consequences of not having the preventive surgery, surgery is still the treatment most performed.

Prognosis

There have been reports of death following minor trauma because of injuries to the spinal cord in the cervical spine. Most commonly, individuals with Klippel-Feil will develop pain. Some diseases are acquired or occur because of the increased motion of the vertebrae. Degenerative disc disease, or destruction of the cushion like disc between the vertebrae, is also very common and affects the entire lower cervical spine. Spondylotic osteophytes, or bone spurs in the spine, form as a result of this degeneration. This laying down of new bone may lead to narrowing of the canal through which the spinal cord travels (spinal stenosis).

Because of the instability of the spinal cord, surgery may prevent a dangerous and fatal accident. Pain that originates in the neck and travels into the arms (radiculopathy) is common near the sites of the surgical fusion of vertebrae. One study found that 25% of the individuals who had surgery would have had neurological problems within ten years, therefore requiring additional surgery.

Resources

BOOKS

Guebert, Gary M., et al. "Congenital Anomalies and Normal Skeletal Variants." In *Essentials of Skeletal Radiology,* edited by Terry Yochum and Lindsay Rowe. 2nd ed. Baltimore: Williams & Wilkins, 1996.

Juhl J. H., A. B. Crummy, and J. E. Kuhlman, eds. *Paul and Juhl's Essentials of Radiologic Imaging.* 7th ed. Philadelphia: Lippencot-Raven, 1998.

PERIODICALS

Clarke, Raymond A., et al. "Familial Klippel-Feil Syndrome and Paracentric Inversion inv(8)(q22.2q23.3)." *American Journal of Human Genetics* 57 (1995): 1364–1370.

Clarke, Raymond A, et al. "Heterogenectiy in Klippel-Feil Syndrome: A New Classification." *Pediatric Radiology* 28 (1998): 967–974.

Hilibrand, A. S., et al. "Radiculopathy and Myelopathy at Segments Adjacent to the Site of a Previous Anterior Cervical Arthrodesis." *Journal of Bone and Joint Surgery* 81-A, no. 4 (1999): 519–528.

Nagashima, Hideki. "No Neurological Involvement for More Than 40 Years in Klippel-Feil Syndrome with Hypermobility of the Upper Cervical Spine." *Archives of Orthopedic Trauma and Surgery* 121 (2001): 99–101.

Thomsen, M. N., et al. "Scoliosis and Congenital Anomalies Associated with Klippel-Feil Syndrome Types I-Ill." *Spine* 22, no. 4 (1997): 396–401.

ORGANIZATIONS

National Institutes of Health (NIH). PO Box 5801, Bethesda, MD 20824. (800) 352-9424. nihinfo@Ood.nih.gov. <http://www.ninds.nih.gov/health>.

National Organization for Rare Disorders (NORD). PO Box 8923, New Fairfield, CT 06812-8923. (203) 746-6518 or (800) 999-6673. Fax: (203) 746-6481. <http://www.rarediseases.org>.

WEBSITES

KFS Circle of Friends support group. <http://www.fortunecity.com/millenium/bigears/99/kfs.html>.

KFS Connection Online, An online Klippel-Feil Support group. <http://members.aol.com/kfsconxpgs/links.htm>.

Jason S. Schliesser, D.C.

Klippel-Trenaunay-Weber syndrome

Definition

Klippel-Trenaunay-Weber syndrome (KTWS) is most often defined by the presence of three classic characteristics: vascular abnormalities, prominent varicose veins or darkened skin patches, and limb enlargement.

Description

KTWS was first described by Drs. Klippel and Trenaunay in 1900. The condition is also known by the names Klippel-Trenaunay syndrome (KTS) and Angioosteohypertrophy syndrome.

Vascular abnormalities in KTWS may involve the capillary, venous, arterial, and lymphatic systems. Limb enlargement resulting in asymmetry of the limbs is quite common. This usually affects the lower limbs, but occasionally the upper limbs as well. Vein enlargement and varicose veins are also typically a part of KTWS. Other occasional abnormalities in KTWS may involve the fingers and toes, other skin changes, **glaucoma**, mental delays, seizures, and blood platelet problems.

Genetic profile

In most cases, KTWS occurs by chance alone. There is usually no family history and very little chance of the condition occurring again, even to the same parents. In 2004, researchers reported that abnormalities in the **VG5Q gene** on **chromosome** 5 were found to cause a susceptibility to KTWS. VG5Q is a gene known to be important for blood vessel development, so abnormalities within it might naturally lead to some symptoms of KTWS.

A few families with multiple people who may have KTWS have been noted. Ceballos-Quintal, et al., described a family with three people who were suspected to have KTWS, in three separate generations. Each person had different symptoms seen in KTWS. This family history suggests autosomal dominant **inheritance** in rare cases of KTWS. In dominant inheritance, an affected individual has a 50% chance of having an affected child with KTWS, regardless of that child's gender. It is also common to see families with histories of the condition in this type of inheritance pattern.

Demographics

KTWS is a relatively uncommon condition that is found worldwide, affecting males and females equally. Additionally, it appears to affect people of all ages, though the average age that children may come for medical care is four years.

Signs and symptoms

Vascular abnormalities

Problems may occur as a result of an abnormal communication between a group of blood vessels and the skin. An abnormal grouping of blood vessels may reach the skin, causing the appearance of a large hemangioma on the skin. Additionally, the blood vessel walls may enlarge or swell, causing large, blood-filled spaces within the body. Internal bleeding can be a serious complication in some cases. There may also be swelling or masses of tissue from problems in the lymphatic system. These may disturb neighboring tissues and internal organs.

Veins and arteries may join abnormally, which can cause an improper flow of blood between the body's vein and artery systems. The deep veins can be incorrectly developed, sometimes being smaller than usual or even duplicated. Ultimately, this can disrupt the proper circulation of blood between various parts of the body.

Varicose veins are common in KTWS. People may have prominent veins that involve their feet or entire legs.

The lymphatic system, meant to help blood and fluid circulate, can be problematic in those with KTWS. Lymphatic fluid can collect abnormally, causing an enlargement and swelling of surrounding tissues. Smaller swellings can occur in various parts of the body like the neck, armpits, or other locations where the lymph nodes are naturally located.

Skin abnormalities

Abnormal capillary formations can cause dark patches on the skin, which look similar to a hemangioma. These are usually reddish in color and can be large. They are most often seen on the lower limbs, but in 17–21% of people with KTWS the entire limb or one side of the body is affected. The dark skin patches usually have an irregular and linear border to them. When seen on the torso of someone's body, they do not usually cross from the left to right sides. Other skin abnormalities can include smaller streaks and patches of dark skin.

Limb abnormalities

Limb enlargement is a very common sign of KTWS. In the vast majority of people, one leg is larger than the other. In others, an arm or a combination of both the arm and leg are affected. About 70% of people with KTWS have lengthening of an extremity, and an increase in thickness occurs in at least 50%.

Enlargement and vascular abnormalities usually occur together in the same limb. The enlargement of the limbs is presumed to be due to a combination of factors: underlying bone overgrowth, lymphatic swelling, muscle overgrowth, and thickened skin.

Other limb abnormalities can include enlargement of the fingers or toes, webbing between these digits, extra digits, or missing digits.

Other signs of KTWS

Glaucoma can be seen in KTWS, either first appearing at birth or in early childhood. Seizures can be part of the condition and, rarely, mental retardation as well.

Individuals with extensive vein or lymphatic abnormalities can develop a blood-clotting problem in which their platelet count is lower than usual. This is sometimes incorrectly referred to as the Kasabach-Merritt syndrome, which actually occurs when the blood platelet count is extremely low.

Diagnosis

As of early 2005, there is no clinical **genetic testing** available for KTWS. Research taking place in the United States and Belgium offers screening of genes that may be implicated in the condition, but it is only offered as part of a research study. Most people with KTWS are diagnosed because of signs and symptoms they have.

Children may first come to medical attention for KTWS at birth or shortly afterward because they are born with dark patches on their skin or a limb that is larger than the other. A careful evaluation by a team of physicians, including a pediatrician, medical geneticist, and a dermatologist, can help to identify whether the diagnosis is KTWS.

KTWS has occasionally been suspected during a pregnancy in cases where significant limb enlargement was seen on a **prenatal ultrasound**. Roberts, et al., reported a case from 1999 where a prenatal ultrasound showed that the developing baby had limb and digit enlargement with increased blood flow and fluid-filled sacs.

In this case, suspecting KTWS helped to determine the best type of delivery for the baby and the mother. The baby was born by a Caesarean section, which helped reduce the complications to him and his mother from his limb enlargement and fluid collections. When the baby was born, he was found to have large red skin patches on the affected limb, and KTWS was highly suspected.

There are symptoms of KTWS that overlap with other conditions. **Sturge-Weber syndrome** usually has dark skin patches and vascular abnormalities, glaucoma, seizures, and mental delays. However, significant limb enlargement is not usually a part of Sturge-Weber syndrome.

Parkes-Weber syndrome involves vascular abnormalities, but these differ from those seen in KTWS. For example, Parkes-Weber syndrome does not usually involve the lymphatic system. Additionally, Parkes-Weber syndrome can have symptoms that affect the heart, which are not typically seen in KTWS.

Treatment and management

There is no known cure for KTWS. However, treatments are available to help with some symptoms of the condition. These typically involve a large team of specialists that may include a pediatrician, vascular surgeon, orthopedist, orthopedic surgeon, hematologist, medical geneticist, genetic counselor, ophthalmologist, neurologist, social worker, and therapist.

Custom-made compression stockings can be worn to reduce swelling, create a barrier for minor trauma, and help blood drain from an enlarged body part. Parents can find it a challenge to encourage a young child to wear such stockings, but they may work well for older children and adults. Compression stockings do not usually permanently reduce the size of the enlarged limb.

Swelling can also be reduced with manual drainage, a gentle massage of the affected area. A physical therapist, occupational therapist, or massage therapist typically performs this. Air-driven pumps can also help reduce swelling. The affected limb is covered in an air-filled plastic sleeve, which places gentle pressure to stimulate fluid movement from the swollen limb.

Some people have seen reduction in the redness of their skin patches through laser treatments using pulses of light. It may require a series of these treatments, and skin changes may still be noticeable or even unchanged after the treatment is finished.

If there is increased bleeding or a low amount of platelets is suspected, blood testing can check the platelet level. This can be carefully monitored through a series of blood tests, and in some cases a blood transfusion may be required. If a patient has internal bleeding that causes damage to some internal organs or tissues, surgery to control this bleeding or remove affected tissues may be needed.

In some cases, bacterial infections can warrant the use of antibiotics to stop the infection.

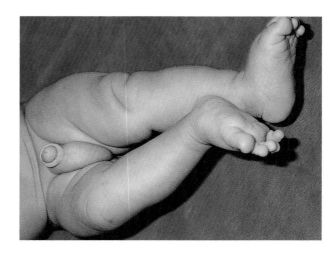

Limb enlargement is a very common sign of Klippel-Trenaunay-Weber syndrome. In the vast majority of people, as depicted here, one leg is larger than the other. (© L. I., Inc. / Custom Medical Stock Photo.)

Ultrasounds, x rays, magnetic resonance imaging (MRI) scans, lymphoscintigraphy, and angiography can help obtain details about limb enlargement. These all attempt to gain information about the specific tissues or organs affected by limb enlargement and abnormal blood flow.

Surgical treatments may be needed for some with KTWS, though the goal is often to avoid this whenever possible. Abnormal blood vessels may need to be repaired by removing them or rejoining them. Varicose veins may need to be removed, but these can sometimes return even after treatment. Women with KTWS who are pregnant may have bleeding complications depending on the location of any vascular abnormalities, and should be monitored closely during their pregnancies.

Minor leg length differences can sometimes be treated with a shoe insert that is worn on the foot of the shorter leg. If a leg causes a significant asymmetry, a procedure called epiphysiodesis may be necessary. This surgical treatment can stop bone growth in an affected leg, but requires destroying a portion of the underlying bone to do it. It must be timed well to coordinate with the normal bone growth that occurs in childhood and adolescence.

In rare cases, limb or digit amputation may be needed to improve function for a person with KTWS. This is typically done when other helpful options have not been successful.

Seizures can occur in KTWS, and these may be treated with anti-seizure medications. Glaucoma may be

KEY TERMS

Angiography—Procedure that shows the system of blood vessels and the blood flow in a portion of the body. Requires an injection of dye to help see the vessels.

Arterial—Term used to describe an artery or the entire system of arteries.

Caesarean section—Surgical method to deliver a baby that requires making an incision in the mother's abdomen to remove the infant.

Capillary—Very narrow tube that carries liquid like blood or lymphatic fluid.

Glaucoma—An eye disease that usually involves high pressure in the eye, which can lead to vision problems or blindness if left untreated.

Hemangioma—Abnormality resulting from a collection of vascular tissue like blood vessels, which can cause a dark reddish patch on the skin.

Lymphoscintigraphy—Procedure that helps to look at the lymph nodes in the body. Requires an injection of radioactive material to help see the lymph nodes and lymphatic system.

Magnetic resonance imaging (MRI) scan—Procedure that shows internal organs and tissues of the body using magnetic fields and signals.

Platelet—Cell in the blood that helps with clotting.

Ultrasound—Procedure that shows internal organs and tissues of the body using sound waves.

Venous— Term used to describe a vein or the entire system of veins.

X ray—Procedure that shows internal organs and tissues of the body using radiation.

identified from a careful eye examination and treated with eye drops, pills, ointments, or laser therapy to reduce the pressure in the eye and maintain vision.

Mental retardation is rare in KTWS, but may be assessed by a child development team or early childhood program. Extra assistance is sometimes available through early intervention programs and special education in schools. Social workers are useful to connect families to helpful resources.

A psychologist, genetic counselor, or therapist can be helpful for some with KTWS. Living with visible skin changes can be difficult, and some may find it easier to talk to an objective person or to talk with other affected families in a support group.

Prognosis

Prognosis can vary widely in KTWS. Complications, especially the vascular abnormalities, can be serious and cause death if symptoms are severe enough and treatment is not successful. The exact expected lifespan for the average person with KTWS is not known, but is highly dependent on the symptoms experienced.

The best way to increase one's prognosis is to utilize a team of specialists that is familiar with KTWS. Through early identification and monitoring of symptoms, treatments can be started sooner and appropriate medical decisions can be made to help the individual and the family.

Resources

PERIODICALS

Jacob, A. G., et al. "Klippel-Trenaunay Syndrome: Spectrum and Management." *Mayo Clinic Proceedings* 73, no. 1 (January 1998): 28–36.

WEBSITES

Genetic Alliance–Advocacy, Education and Empowerment. 2005 (March 15, 2005). <http://www.geneticalliance.org>.

Online Mendelian Inheritance in Man. (March 15, 2005.) <http://www.ncbi.nlm.nih.gov/entrez/query.fcgi?db=OMIM>.

ORGANIZATIONS

The Klippel-Trenaunay Syndrome Support Group. Phone: (952) 925-2596. Email: ktnewmembers@yahoo.com. <http://www.k-t.org>.

Deepti Babu, MS, CGC

Knobloch syndrome
see **Encephalocele**

Konigsmark syndrome
see **Hereditary hearing loss and deafness**

Kowarski syndrome
see **Pituitary dwarfism syndrome**

Krabbe disease

Definition

Krabbe disease is an inherited enzyme deficiency that leads to the loss of myelin, the substance that wraps nerve cells and speeds cell communication. Most affected individuals start to show symptoms before six months of age and have progressive loss of mental and motor function. Death occurs at an average age of 13 months. Other less common forms exist with onset in later childhood or adulthood.

Description

Myelin insulates and protects the nerves in the central and peripheral nervous system. It is essential for efficient nerve cell communication (signals) and body functions such as walking, talking, coordination, and thinking. As nerves grow, myelin is constantly being built, broken down, recycled, and rebuilt. Enzymes break down, or metabolize, fats, carbohydrates, and proteins in the body including the components of myelin.

Individuals with Krabbe disease are lacking the enzyme galactosylceramidase (GALC), which metabolizes a myelin fat component called galactosylceramide and its by-product, psychosine. Without GALC, these substances are not metabolized and accumulate in large globoid cells. For this reason, Krabbe disease is also called globoid cell **leukodystrophy**. Accumulation of galactosylceramide and psychosine is toxic and leads to the loss of myelin-producing cells and myelin itself. This results in impaired nerve function and the gradual loss of developmental skills such as walking and talking.

Genetic profile

Krabbe disease is an autosomal recessive disorder. Affected individuals have two nonfunctional copies of the GALC **gene**. Parents of an affected child are healthy carriers and therefore have one normal GALC gene and one nonfunctional GALC gene. When both parents are carriers, each child has a 25% chance to inherit Krabbe disease, a 50% chance to be a carrier, and a 25% chance to have two normal GALC genes. The risk is the same for males and females. Brothers and sisters of an affected child with Krabbe disease have a 66% chance of being a carrier.

The GALC gene is located on **chromosome** 14. Over 70 mutations (gene alterations) known to cause Krabbe disease have been identified. One specific GALC gene deletion accounts for 45% of disease-causing mutations in those with European ancestry and 35% of disease-causing mutations in those with Mexican ancestry.

Demographics

Approximately one in every 100,000 infants born in the United States and Europe will develop Krabbe disease. A person with no family history of the condition has a one in 150 chance of being a carrier. Krabbe disease occurs in all countries and ethnic groups but no cases have been reported in the Ashkenazi Jewish population. A Druze community in Northern Israel and two Moslem Arab villages near Jerusalem have an unusually high incidence of Krabbe disease. In these areas, about one person in every six is a carrier.

Signs and symptoms

Ninety percent of individuals with Krabbe disease have the infantile type. These infants usually have normal development in the first few months of life. Before six months of age, they become irritable, stiff, and rigid. They may have trouble eating and may have seizures. Development regresses leading to loss of mental and muscle function. They also lose the ability to see and hear. In the end stages, these children usually cannot move, talk, or eat without a feeding tube.

Ten percent of individuals with Krabbe disease have juvenile or adult type. Children with juvenile type begin having symptoms between three and ten years of age. They gradually lose the ability to walk and think. They may also have paralysis and vision loss. Their symptoms usually progress slower than in the infantile type. Adult Krabbe disease has onset at any time after age 10. Symptoms are more general including weakness, difficulty walking, vision loss, and diminished mental abilities.

Diagnosis

There are many tests that can be performed on an individual with symptoms of Krabbe disease. The most specific test is done by measuring the level of GALC enzyme activity in blood cells or skin cells. A person with Krabbe disease has GALC activity levels that are zero to five percent of the normal amount. Individuals with later onset Krabbe disease may have more variable GALC activity levels. This testing is done in specialized laboratories that have experience with this disease.

The fluid of the brain and spinal cord (cerebrospinal fluid) can also be tested to measure the amount of protein. This fluid usually contains very little protein but the protein level is elevated in infantile Krabbe disease. Nerve-conduction velocity tests can be performed to measure the speed at which the nerve cells transmit their signals. Individuals with Krabbe disease will have slowed nerve conduction. Brain imaging studies such as computerized tomography (CT scan) and magnetic resonance imaging (MRI) are used to get pictures from inside the brain. These pictures will show loss of myelin in individuals with Krabbe disease.

DNA testing for GALC mutations is not generally used to make a diagnosis in someone with symptoms but it can be performed after diagnosis. If an affected person has identifiable known mutations, other family members can be offered DNA testing to find out if they are carriers. This is helpful since the GALC enzyme test is not always accurate in identifying healthy carriers of Krabbe disease.

If an unborn baby is at risk to inherit Krabbe disease, prenatal diagnosis is available. Fetal tissue can be obtained through chorionic villus sampling (CVS) or **amniocentesis**. Cells obtained from either procedure can be used to measure GALC enzyme activity levels. If both parents have identified known GALC **gene mutations**, DNA testing can also be performed on the fetal cells to determine if the fetus inherited one, two, or no GALC gene mutations.

Some centers offer preimplantation diagnosis if both parents have known GALC gene mutations. In-vitro fertilization (IVF) is used to create embryos in the laboratory. DNA testing is performed on one or two cells taken from the early embryo. Only embryos that did not inherit Krabbe disease are implanted into the mother's womb. This is an option for parents who want a biological child but do not wish to face the possibility of terminating an affected pregnancy.

Treatment and management

Once a child with infantile Krabbe disease starts to show symptoms, there is little effective treatment. Supportive care can be given to keep the child as comfortable as possible and to counteract the rigid muscle tone. Medications can be given to control seizures. When a child can no longer eat normally, feeding tubes can be placed to provide nourishment.

Affected children who are diagnosed before developing symptoms (such as through prenatal diagnosis) can undergo bone marrow transplant or stem cell transplant. The goal of these procedures is to destroy the bone marrow which produces the blood and immune system cells. After the destruction of the bone marrow, cells from a healthy donor are injected. If successful, the healthy cells travel to the bone marrow and reproduce. Some children have received these transplants and had a slowing of their symptom's progression or even improvement of their symptoms. However, these procedures are not always successful and research is being done in order to reduce complications.

Scientists are also researching **gene therapy** for Krabbe disease. This involves introducing a normal GALC gene into the cells of the affected child. The goal

is for the cells to integrate the new GALC gene into its DNA and copy it, producing functional GALC enzyme. This is still in research stages and is not being performed clinically.

Prognosis

Prognosis for infantile and juvenile Krabbe disease is very poor. Individuals with infantile type usually die at an average age of 13 months. Death usually occurs within a year after the child shows symptoms and is diagnosed. Children with juvenile type may survive longer after diagnosis but death usually occurs within a few years. Adult Krabbe disease is more variable and difficult to predict but death usually occurs two to seven years after diagnosis.

Resources

BOOKS

Wenger, D. A., et al. "Krabbe Disease: Genetic Aspects and Progress Toward Therapy." *Molecular Genetics and Metabolism* 70 (2000): 1-9.

ORGANIZATIONS

Hunter's Hope Foundation. PO Box 643, Orchard Park, NY 14127. (877) 984-HOPE. Fax: (716) 667-1212. <http://www.huntershope.org>.

United Leukodystrophy Foundation. 2304 Highland Dr., Sycamore, IL 60178. (815) 895-3211 or (800) 728-5483. Fax: (815) 895-2432. <http://www. ulf.org>.

WEBSITES

Wenger, David A. "Krabbe Disease." *GeneClinics*. <http://www.geneclinics.org/profiles/krabbe/details.html>.

Amie Stanley, MS

KEY TERMS

Globoid cells—Large cells containing excess toxic metabolic "waste" of galactosylceramide and psychosine.

Motor function—The ability to produce body movement by complex interaction of the brain, nerves and muscles.

Mutation—A permanent change in the genetic material that may alter a trait or characteristic of an individual, or manifest as disease, and can be transmitted to offspring.

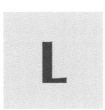

Lamellar ichthyosis *see* **Ichthyosis**

Langer-Giedion syndrome *see*
Trichorhinophalangeal syndrome

Langer mesomelic dysplasia *see*
Dyschondrosteosis

Langer-Saldino syndrome *see*
Achondrogenesis

Larsen syndrome

Definition

Larsen syndrome is an inherited condition characterized by congenital dislocation of multiple body joints along with other unusual features of the face, hands, and bones.

Description

This condition was first described in 1950 by Larsen, Schottstaedt, and Bost, who compiled information on six people with sporadic cases of Larsen syndrome.

Larsen syndrome has been called both a **skeletal dysplasia** (a condition caused by abnormalities of bone structure), and a hypermobility syndrome (a condition involving abnormally loose joints). It is most likely caused by inherited abnormalities of connective tissue that affect both bone and joint structure.

Present at birth are multiple dislocations of the elbows, hips, and most commonly the knees. Persons with Larsen syndrome have other distinctive physical features that can include a prominent forehead, widely spaced eyes, long cylindrical fingers, and short bones of the hand. Sometimes present are other birth defects such as structural heart defects, cleft palate, cataracts, extra bones of the wrist, and abnormalities of the vertebrae.

Most people have moderate symptoms that can be treated, allowing for a relatively normal life span. However, a small number of babies have a severe form of the condition and die at birth.

Genetic profile

There are likely to be multiple different causes for Larsen syndrome. Both recessive and dominant patterns of **inheritance** have been described thus far.

Some cases are sporadic, meaning the affected person is the first in the family to have the condition. Many sporadic cases are thought to be caused by new dominant mutations (spontaneous changes in the genetic material). A person with sporadic Larsen syndrome has a change in the genetic material that is not present in either parent but can be passed on, with 50/50 odds in each child, to his or her offspring.

Patients have been reported who have affected brothers or sisters but unaffected parents. Most of these cases probably represent a recessive form of Larsen syndrome in which a person must have two copies of a genetic change in order to be affected. The parents of a person with a recessive condition must each have one copy of the genetic change in order to have an affected child.

There are rare instances in which a person with Larsen appears to have the recessive form but then gives birth to an affected child. These cases are most likely dominant rather than recessive. It can be difficult to be certain of the inheritance pattern in some families and genetic counselors must be careful to address both forms of inheritance when discussing chances of recurrence.

The autosomal dominant form of Larsen syndrome is thought to be due to mutations in a **gene** called LAR1, on the short arm of **chromosome** 3. The exact structure and function of this gene is not yet known. There may be other genes responsible for a proportion of cases of dominant Larsen syndrome; however, no other candidate genes have been located.

Another dominantly inherited condition called Atelosteogenesis Type III (AOIII) has features which overlap with Larsen syndrome, and may, in fact, be a variant of Larsen caused by mutations in the same gene.

Demographics

Larsen syndrome is an extremely rare genetic condition that occurs in about one in every 100,000 births.

A variant of Larsen syndrome is found in high frequency on La Reunion island near East Africa. Over 40 affected children have been reported, with an incidence of one in 1,500 births. This variant is thought to be recessive but the responsible gene has not yet been located.

Signs and symptoms

The symptoms of Larsen syndrome are widely variable from person to person and can range from lethal to very mild, even among members of the same family.

Typical characteristics at birth are multiple joint dislocations that can include hips, elbows, wrists, and knees. Babies can be born with their knees in hyperextension with their ankles and feet up by their ears, a deformation called genu recurvatum. **Clubfoot** is common and persistent flexion, or contractures, of other joints, such as the wrist and fingers, can also occur.

Persons with Larsen syndrome often have distinctive facial features. Common findings, in addition to a large forehead and wide spaced eyes, are flat cheekbones and a flat bridge of the nose, which is sometimes indented and called "saddle nose." The hands are often short but the fingers are long and lack the normal tapered ends.

Other birth defects can occur but are not present in all people. Cleft palate, cataracts, and heart defects of the valves or between the upper or lower chambers occur occasionally.

Often, babies have floppy muscle tone giving them a "rag doll" appearance. Respiratory problems are frequently seen at birth because of laxity of the trachea. Feeding and swallowing difficulties are common.

Abnormalities of the bones are frequent. Underdevelopment and abnormal shape of some of the vertebral bones can lead to problems such as **scoliosis** or kyphosis. Abnormalities of the epiphyses (centers of bone growth) can develop in childhood. Height is often reduced, and an adult height of four to five feet is not uncommon. The joints between the bones of the ear may be abnormal and may cause conductive hearing loss.

Hypermobility of joints lasts throughout life and may lead to early-onset arthritis, recurrent dislocations, and may necessitate joint replacement at an early age. Cervical spine instability is a very serious complication of Larsen syndrome as it can cause compression of the spinal cord and lead to paralysis or death.

The condition does not affect intelligence and children can expect to have normal school experiences, with the exception of physical education, which will need to be adapted to each child's needs.

Diagnosis

Larsen syndrome should be suspected in any baby having multiple joint dislocations at birth. As of 2001, there is no genetic test to confirm the diagnosis and, thus, diagnosis must be based on clinical and x ray findings. Babies suspected to have the condition warrant a complete evaluation by a medical geneticist (a physician specializing in genetic syndromes).

Larsen syndrome is sometimes misdiagnosed as another condition called arthrogryposis, which involves multiple joint contractions. Larsen syndrome can be distinguished from this and other syndromes involving joint dislocations or contractions because of the unusual constellation of features found in the face and hands. Extra bones of the wrist, often seen in Larsen syndrome, are extremely rare in other syndromes.

Some people have very mild symptoms and may not have joint dislocations or other problems at birth. The diagnosis can be missed in these people unless they are carefully evaluated.

A person with dominantly inherited Larsen syndrome has a 50% chance with each pregnancy of having a child with the same disorder. **Genetic counseling** can help couples sort out their options for parenthood. Some couples would choose to adopt rather than take the chance of an affected child, others would go ahead with a pregnancy, and others would choose to have prenatal diagnosis. The only form of prenatal diagnosis available to date is ultrasound.

Fetal ultrasound performed by a specialist at 18-20 weeks of pregnancy can sometimes reveal signs of Larsen syndrome. Knee dislocations and hyperextension, club feet, fixed flexion of elbows, wrists, and fingers, and some of the characteristic facial features can sometimes be noted by ultrasound in affected fetuses. Physical findings from ultrasound can suggest but do not confirm the diagnosis of Larsen syndrome in a fetus.

Treatment and management

Treatment will vary according to the symptoms of a particular child. Joint problems require long-term

KEY TERMS

Arthrogryposis—Abnormal joint contracture.

Carrier—A person who possesses a gene for an abnormal trait without showing signs of the disorder. The person may pass the abnormal gene on to offspring.

Clubfoot—Abnormal permanent bending of the ankle and foot. Also called *talipes equinovarus*.

Congenital—Refers to a disorder that is present at birth.

Connective tissue—A group of tissues responsible for support throughout the body; includes cartilage, bone, fat, tissue underlying skin, and tissues that support organs, blood vessels, and nerves throughout the body.

Contrature—A tightening of muscles that prevents normal movement of the associated limb or other body part.

Deformation—An abnormal form or position of a part of the body caused by extrinsic pressure or mechanical forces.

Epiphysis—The end of long bones, usually terminating in a joint.

Hypermobility—Unusual flexibility of the joints, allowing them to be bent or moved beyond their normal range of motion.

Joint dislocation—The displacement of a bone from its socket or normal position.

Kyphosis—An abnormal outward curvature of the spine, with a hump at the upper back.

Magnetic resonance imaging (MRI)—A technique that employs magnetic fields and radio waves to create detailed images of internal body structures and organs, including the brain.

Scoliosis—An abnormal, side-to-side curvature of the spine.

Skeletal dysplasia—A group of syndromes consisting of abnormal prenatal bone development and growth.

orthopedic care. Dislocations, clubfeet, and joint contractures are treated with intensive physical therapy, splints, casting, and/or surgery. Physical therapy is also important after joint surgery to build up muscles around the joint and preserve joint stability. Occupational therapy may be helpful for children with wrist and finger contractures.

Respiratory problems at birth may necessitate oxygen or assistive breathing devices. If not alleviated by medication or special feeding techniques, eating and swallowing problems may require tube feeding. Heart problems, cleft palate, and cataracts often warrant surgical correction. Special care is needed if laxity of the trachea is present because of an increased risk for respiratory problems during and after surgery.

People with chronic pain associated with hypermobile joints often can be helped by techniques taught in a pain management clinic.

Magnetic resonance imaging (MRI) of the neck is recommended in childhood to screen for cervical vertebral problems. Early diagnosis and surgical stabilization of the spine can help patients avoid paralysis and death from spinal cord compression. Scoliosis is usually treated by bracing, or by a surgically placed metal rod. Artificial hip and knee replacements may be needed in early-to-mid adulthood because of degeneration of unstable joints.

Regular medical examinations are crucial to assess the condition of the bones, joints, spine, heart, and eyes. Hearing should be evaluated on a periodic basis, especially in children, because of the potential for conductive hearing loss. Ophthalmologic examinations are recommended periodically to screen for cataracts.

Prognosis

The effects of the syndrome vary markedly from person to person. Therefore, prognosis is based on the findings in a given individual. The usual causes of early death are either severe respiratory problems or compression of the cervical spine from vertebral instability.

If careful and consistent orthopedic treatment is initiated early, prognosis can be good, with a normal life span. Weak and unstable joints and limited range of motion from contractures may cause walking difficulties and restrict other physical activities. Contact sports and heavy lifting should be avoided as anything that puts extra strain or pressure on the joints can cause harm. Swimming is a good activity because it helps strengthen muscles without joint strain.

Resources

PERIODICALS

Becker, R., et al. "Clinical Variability of Larsen Syndrome: Diagnosis in a Father after Sonographic Detection of a Severely Affected Fetus." *Clinical Genetics* 57 (2000): 148-150.

Tongsong, T., et al. "Prenatal Sonographic Diagnosis of Larsen Syndrome." *Journal of Ultrasound Medicine* 19 (2000): 419-421.

ORGANIZATIONS

Arthritis Foundation. 1330 West Peachtree St., Atlanta, GA 30309. (800) 283-7800 or (404)965-7537. <http://www.arthritis.org>.

Scoliosis Research Society. 6300 N. River Rd., Ste 727, Rosemont, IL 60018-4226. (847)698-1627. Fax: (847) 823-0536. Goulding@aaos.org. <http://www.srs.org/>.

WEBSITES

Hypermobility Syndrome Association. <http://www.hypermobility.org/>.

Larsen Syndrome Resource Page. <http://www.stormloader.com/nita/ls.html>.

Barbara J. Pettersen

Late onset multiple carboxylase deficiency *see* **Biotinidase deficiency**

Laterality sequence

Definition

Laterality sequence refers to a variable group of developmental anomalies in which some or all of an affected individual's internal organs form on the opposite side of the body than is standard. The heart, stomach, and spleen may form on the right side of the body, instead of the left. The liver and gallbladder may form on the left side of the body, instead of the right. Laterality refers to a side of the body. A sequence is a chain of events that occurs as a result of a single abnormality or problem.

Description

All humans display a characteristic placement of internal organs with the heart, stomach, and spleen towards the left, and the liver and gallbladder on the right. This placement of organs is called situs solitus. Very early in fetal development, the embryo forms a left-right axis that determines which side is left and which side is right. The axis can then instruct the body to form organs towards one side or the other. When the left-right axis does not form correctly, all or some of the organs form in the wrong location and result in a laterality sequence defect.

The first documented cases of laterality sequence occurred in the 1600s with Fabricus' description of an individual's symptoms of reversed liver and spleen, and

Marco Severino's recognition of dextrocardia. Laterality sequence defects range in features and descriptions. Features of laterality sequence anomalies include abnormal placement of all or some organs, dextrocardia (heart on the right side of the body), **asplenia** (no spleen), polysplenia (multiple spleens), complex congenital heart defects, intestinal malrotation, abnormal lung formation, symmetrical liver, midline abnormalities, and **neural tube defects**. Other terms for laterality sequence defects include situs inversus, situs inversus viscerum, situs transverses, heterotaxy, situs ambiguous, isomerism sequence, asplenia syndrome, Ivemark syndrome, polysplenia syndrome, partial situs inversus, and dextrocardia.

Genetic profile

Laterality sequence defects can occur due to genetic or multifactorial causes. Most cases of laterality sequence defects are sporadic and multifactorial. Multifactorial conditions result from the combination of environmental and genetic factors that contribute to the development of laterality sequence defects. First-degree relatives of an individual affected by a multifactorial condition have an increased risk that is based on family studies. A family who has one child with an isolated case of a laterality sequence, with no other affected children, runs a 3–5% risk of having a future child being affected by a laterality sequence defect.

Although all of the genes that are known to be involved in laterality sequence defects encode proteins that help determine the laterality of an individual, the **inheritance** pattern of inherited laterality sequence defects depends on the specific **gene** defect. New genetic mutations that cause laterality defects are still being discovered. Current genes associated with laterality defects include ZIC3 (also known as HTX1, zinc finger protein ZIC 3, Xq26.2), CRELD1 (Cysteine-rich with EGF-like domains located at 3p25.3), DNAH11, LEFTB (formerly LEFTY2), CRC (CRYPTIC located on **chromosome** 2), EBAF (transforming growth factor beta 1q42.1), NKX2 (homeobox protein Nkx-2.55 5q34), and ACVR2B (encoding activin receptor IIB located at 3p22-p21.3).

Most cases of inherited laterality defects travel through the family in an autosomal recessive manner. In an autosomal recessive condition, two copies of the mutant, or nonworking, gene are needed to develop the symptoms of laterality sequence. In these cases, both parents each carry one copy of a mutant gene. Individuals with only one copy of a nonworking gene for a recessive condition are known as carriers, and have no problems related to the condition. In fact, each person carries between five and 10 nonworking genes for harmful, recessive conditions. However, when two people with the same mutant recessive gene have children together, there is a 25% chance, with each pregnancy, for the child to inherit two mutant copies, one from each parent. That child then has no working copies of the gene and, therefore, has the signs and symptoms associated with genetic defects. **Gene mutations** that result in autosomal recessive forms of laterality defects include DNAH11. DNAH11, located on the short arm of chromosome 7 (7p21), is expressed in the node of the embryo at day 7.5, and is involved in left-right axis determination of the organs. Mutations in the coding region of DNAH11 account for situs inversus totalis.

Additional autosomal recessive laterality defects can also be a feature of other inherited conditions, such as **Kartagener syndrome** and Ivemark syndrome. Kartagener syndrome is an autosomal recessive disorder characterized by bronchiectasis, sinusitis, dextrocardia, and infertility that can be caused by several different genetic locations and mutations. Approximately 25% of individuals affected by situs inversus have Kartagener syndrome. Ivemark syndrome refers to the congenital absence of the spleen, usually accompanied by complex cardiac malformations, malposition and maldevelopment of the abdominal organs, and abnormal lobation of the lungs.

Some cases of laterality sequence defects are inherited in an autosomal dominant pattern. In an autosomal dominant inheritance pattern, the genes that cause laterality sequence are carried on one of the 22 pairs of numbered autosomal chromosomes, rather than on the X or Y sex chromosomes. Furthermore, in autosomal dominant conditions, only one copy of the mutant, or nonworking, gene is necessary for the development of laterality sequence. An individual who inherits a normal gene copy from one parent and an abnormal gene copy from the other parent is likely to have a lateral sequence anomaly. The children of an individual with one normal gene copy and one mutated copy have a 50% chance of inheriting laterality sequence. One known form of laterality sequence that is found inherited in an autosomal dominant manner occurs in patients with a nonworking copy of CFC1. CFC1 is located on chromosome 2 and is involved in the formation of the left-to-right axis in human development. Accordingly, individuals who have one nonworking copy of CFC1 have randomized organ positioning (heterotaxia).

Some cases of laterality sequence defects are inherited in an X-linked recessive pattern. As opposed to genes that are carried on one of the 22 pairs of numbered autosomal chromosomes, X-linked genes are found on the sex chromosomes called X. Females have two X chromosomes, while males have a single X chromosome and a single Y chromosome. When a female inherits a mutated gene on the X chromosome, she is known as a carrier. She often has no problems related to that condition, because the gene on her other chromosome continues to function properly. However, males only inherit one copy of the information stored on the X chromosome. When a male inherits a mutated copy of the gene that causes an X-linked recessive condition, he will experience the symptoms associated with the disease. The chance for a carrier female to have an affected son is 50%, while the chance to have an unaffected son is 50%. The chance for a carrier female to have a daughter who is also a carrier for the condition is 50%, while the chance for her to have a daughter who is not a carrier is 50%. An affected male has a 100% chance of having carrier daughters and a 0% chance of having affected sons. In 1997, an X-linked recessive form of laterality sequence caused by mutations in HTX1 located on the long arm of the X chromosome (Xq26.2) was described. In the same year, it was determined that the gene is a zinc finger protein, and was named ZIC3. Currently, the gene is known as both ZIC3 and HTX1. ZIC3 is involved in the development of the left-right axis, and mutations account for approximately 1% of individuals affected by heterotaxy. Accordingly, mutations in ZIC3 cause inability of the embryo to establish normal left-right asymmetry.

Demographics

Laterality sequence defects occur in about one in 8,500–25,000 live births. It occurs in individuals of all ethnic backgrounds. An equal number of males and females are affected by laterality sequence defects.

Signs and symptoms

Different laterality sequence defects can be described by the positioning of the various organs and associated malformations.

Complete situs inversus or situs transversus is a laterality defect resulting in a mirror image of the normal organ formation with heart, spleen, and stomach on the right, and the liver and gallbladder on the left side, respectively. The normal pulmonary anatomy is reversed so that the left lung has three lobes and the right lung has two lobes. The remaining internal structures also are a mirror image of the normal.

Heterotaxy or situs ambiguous refers to random positioning of individual organs that can result in multiple malformations with severe heart defects, livers found in the middle of the body, spleen abnormalities, and intestines turned in the opposite direction than is standard (gastrointestinal malrotation). Often, structures normally found on one side of the body are duplicated or absent. Two primary subtypes of heterotaxy are based on the presence or absence of certain organs. In classic right isomerism, or asplenia, patients have a right atrium on both sides of the body, a centrally located liver, no spleen, and both lungs have three lobes. In left isomerism, or polysplenia, patients have left atria on both sides, multiple spleens, and both lungs have two lobes.

Dextrocardia refers to right-sided positioning of the heart. There are various forms of dextrocardia, ranging from a normally configured heart that is positioned further to the right than normal to mirror-image dextrocardia in which the positions of the heart chambers and major vessels are exactly the reverse of the standard arrangement.

Laterality sequence defects caused by mutations in DNAH11 are characterized by situs inversus viscerum, intrauterine growth retardation, congenital heart defects, such as transposition of the great vessels, ventricular septal defect, atrial septal defect, truncuscommunis, and dextrocardia, right pulmonary isomerism, and right spleen. Mutations in DNAH11 may also be associated with Kartagener syndrome that includes bronchiectasis, sinusitis, dextrocardia, and infertility.

Laterality sequence defects caused by mutations in CFC1 result in visceral heterotaxy including a variable group of congenital anomalies that include complex cardiac malformations and situs inversus or situs ambiguous.

Laterality sequence defects caused by mutations in ZIC3 include a variable group of congenital anomalies that include complex cardiac malformations (corrected transposition of great arteries, ventricular septal defect, and **patent ductus arteriosus**), dextrocardia, situs inversus, asplenia, polysplenia, situs inversus viscerum, pulmonic stenosis, and poor growth (intrauterine growth retardation). Some individuals with mutations in ZIC3 have been found to have isolated heart defects only. Female carriers have been described with uterine septums and hypertelorism (wide-spaced eyes).

Diagnosis

Laterality defects may be discovered before birth and in infancy because of associated heart defects or other health problems. Laterality defects also may remain asymptomatic in childhood and are discovered by chance in adult life as affected individuals seek medical attention for an unrelated condition. Clinical testing for several genes associated with laterality defects (ACVR2B, CFC1, CRELD1, EBAF, NKX2-5, and ZIC3) is available; however, diagnosis is still primarily based on imaging through means such as ultrasound, magnetic resonance imaging (MRI), and computed tomography (CT) scan.

Some symptoms of laterality sequence defects such as heart defects, poor growth (intrauterine growth retardation), and possibly organ reversal may be identified through a screening ultrasound around 18 weeks gestation of pregnancy. Accuracy of diagnosis of laterality sequence defects depends on the position, size, and maturity of the fetus, as well as an adequate volume of amniotic fluid and mother's size. A fetal echocardiogram can also help characterize a heart defect or placement before birth. If there is a known gene mutation present in an affected family member, prenatal diagnosis may be available through tests, such as **amniocentesis**.

Diagnosis of a laterality sequence defect in infancy is most often made as a result of a heart defect or other serious medical issue related to the organ positioning and/or number of organs. Laterality sequence defects can be verified through use of x rays, ultrasound, or CT scan. The location and relationships of the abdominal organs, veins of the liver, heart arteries and veins, heart chambers, and heart valves should be reviewed carefully.

Diagnosis in adulthood is based on clinical manifestations and exams such as abdominal and thoracic radiography and electrocardiogram. CT is the preferred examination for definitive diagnosis of situs inversus with dextrocardia because it provides good detail for confirming visceral organ position, cardiac position, and great vessel branching. MRI is usually reserved for difficult cases or for patients with associated cardiac anomalies. The features of laterality sequence defects are variable and require thorough evaluation of the internal organs for full diagnosis.

Treatment and management

The treatment and management of laterality sequence defects depend on the type of defect. Infants and children with laterality defects can have congenital heart defect and other associated birth defects that require surgery. Many adults with incidental detection of their laterality sequence anomalies will not need special treatment or management unless they are ill or need surgery. The recognition of situs inversus is important for preventing surgical mishaps that result from the failure to recognize reversed anatomy or an atypical history. The reversal of the organs may lead to some confusion, as many signs and symptoms will be opposite from the standard side. Laterality sequence defects can also complicate organ transplantation operations as donor organs will most likely come from normal individuals whose organs and vessels are a mirror image of the transplanted patients. Accordingly, in the event of a medical problem, the knowledge that the individual has a laterality defect can increase the time and accuracy of diagnosis and increase the safety of surgery.

KEY TERMS

Complete situs inversus—A laterality defect resulting in a mirror image of the normal organ formation with heart, spleen, and stomach on the right, and the liver and gallbladder on the left side.

Dextrocardia—Right-sided positioning of the heart.

Heterotaxy—Random organ positioning in an individual that can result in multiple malformations with severe heart defects, livers found in the middle of the body, spleen abnormalities, and intestines turned in the opposite direction from normal (gastrointestinal malrotation).

Left-right axis—The developmental feature in a fetus that determines which side of the body is left and which side is right; it conducts the location and positioning of the fetus' internal organs.

Situs solitus—Normal organ placement in the body with the heart, stomach, and spleen placed towards the left, and the liver and gallbladder on the right.

Prognosis

Many patients with laterality sequence defects such as total situs inversus present with no significant medical problems and have normal life expectancy. Total organ reversal results in normal relationships between the left-right positions of the organs and their blood supplies. In other forms of laterality sequence defects, such as those associated with Kartagener's syndrome, issues such as chronic respiratory problems and infertility can occur. Infants affected by complex cardiac defects may die as a result of their congenital heart defects. Prognosis in isolated dextrocardia depends on the congenital cardiac defects present. Women have been described with a uterine septum that can result in difficulties maintaining a pregnancy.

Resources

BOOKS

McManus, Chris. *Right Hand, Left Hand: The Origins of Asymmetry in Brains, Bodies, Atoms, and Cultures.* London: Weidenfeld and Nicolson, 2002.

PERIODICALS

Strong, Eric. "Abnormalities in the Determination of Lateral Symmetry." New York Times. November 1998. (April 10, 2005.) <http://endeavor.med.nyu.edu/~strone01/anatomy.html>.

Walmsley, R., et al. "Diagnosis and Outcome of Dextrocardia Diagnosed in the Fetus." *Am J Cardiol.* 2004 Jul 1;94(1): 141–3.

ORGANIZATIONS

Congenital Heart Information Network (C.H.I.N.). 1561 Clark Drive, Yardley, PA 19067. (215) 493-3068. E-mail: mb@tchin.org. (April 10, 2005.) <http://tchin.org/>.

WEB SITES

Biology Daily: Situs inversus. (April 10, 2005.)<http://www.biologydaily.com/biology/Situs_inversus>.

Dextrocardia with Situs Inversus. (April 10, 2005.) <http://www.laughs.com.au/sid/>.

OMIM-Online Mendelian Inheritance of Man. (April 10, 2005.) <http://www.ncbi.nlm.nih.gov/Omim>.

"Situs Inversus." Emedicine. (April 10, 2005.) <http://www.emedicine.com/radio/topic639.htm>.

Virtual Hospital. (April 10, 2005.) <http://www.vh.org/adult/provider/anatomy/AnatomicVariants/OrganSystem/Text/Stomach.html>.

Laurence-Moon-Bardet-Biedel syndrome *see* **Bardet-Biedel syndrome**

Leber congenital amaurosis

Definition

Leber congenital amaurosis (LCA) is a group of autosomal recessive-inherited eye disorders which lead to blindness at birth or within the first few years of life. Other manifestations of the disease may include hearing loss, mental retardation and decreased physical coordination.

Description

Vision is an important and complex sense by which the qualities of an object, such as color, shape, and size, are perceived through the detection of light. For proper vision, a critical series of biological steps must occur; if any of the steps in the process is abnormal, visual impairment or blindness may occur.

The process of vision begins with light that bounces off an object and passes through the outer coverings and lens of the eye and projects onto a layer of cells at the back of the eye called the retina. The retina contains two kinds of specialized cells types, called the rods and cones, that are responsible for sensing visual stimuli. When rods and cones are stimulated by light, impulses

Location of genetic abnormality for specific types of Leber congenital amaurosis

Type	Abnormal	Mutant gene	Gene location
LCA1	Retinal-specific guanylate cyclase	RETGC/GUC2D	17p13.1
LCA2	Retinal pigment epithelium-specific protein	RPE65	1p31
LCA3	Unknown	Unknown	14q24
LCA4	Arlhydrocarbon-interacting protein-like1	AIPL1	17p13.1
LCA5	Unknown	Unknown	6q11–q16
LCA due to CRX defect	Cone-rod homeobox protein	CRX	19q13.3

are conducted through the optic nerve to a region in the back of the brain known as the occipital lobe. The occipital lobe contains the visual cortex, the area of the brain that processes visual stimuli and integrates signals sent by the retina to obtain a composite image of an object.

Leber congenital amaurosis (LCA) is a term for a group of inherited conditions in which the rod and cone receptors in the retina are defective or missing. Without the proper function of these specialized cells, light cannot be sensed normally.

LCA is often referred to by other names, such as: congenital absence of the rods and cones, congenital retinal blindness, congenital **retinitis pigmentosa**, Leber congenital tapetoretinal degeneration, or Leber congenital tapetoretinal **dysplasia**. The disorder was first described by the German ophthalmologist, Theodor Leber, in 1869, who subsequently showed that it was an inherited defect. Although similarly named, LCA should not be confused with another disorder of sight, Leber optic atrophy, that was also discovered by Theodor Leber.

Genetic profile

Mutations in any one of at least six different **gene** groups may result in LCA. Each of the known genes produce proteins, which are located within the retinal rod and cone cells. These proteins participate in the detection of an incoming stimulus of light and the subsequent transmission of signals out of the retinal cells to the visual cortex of the brain. The different types of LCA and the corresponding genetic abnormality is described in the table below. These six identified mutations likely account for less than half of all diagnosed cases of LCA, and thus, there are additional mutations resulting in LCA that remain to be discovered.

LCA is a genetic condition and can be inherited or passed on in a family. The genetic defects for the disorder are all inherited as autosomal recessive traits, meaning that two mutant genes of the same group are needed to display the disease. A person who carries one mutant

gene does not display the disease and is called a carrier. A carrier has a 50% chance of transmitting the gene to their children, who must inherit the same defective gene from each parent to display the disease. Since there are different genes that are responsible for causing LCA, two individuals with different types of LCA will have an unaffected child, as it is impossible for the child to inherit two of the same type of defective genes from the parents.

Demographics

LCA has been reported to account for at least 5% of all cases of inborn blindness, but several reports suggest that is an underestimation. In 1957, scientific investigators reported that one form of LCA was responsible for 10% of blindness in Sweden. Several years later, similar rates of LCA were found in people living in the Netherlands. While this suggests that the geographical distribution of LCA is not uniform and may be higher in certain ethnic groups, a comprehensive study has never been performed.

Signs and symptoms

Because there are different types of LCA, there is considerable variation in the symptoms experienced by an affected infant. Most infants with LCA are often blind at birth or lose their sight within the first few years of life, however some people with LCA may have residual vision. In these patients, visual acuity is usually limited to the level of counting fingers or detecting hand motions or bright lights, and patients are extremely farsighted. There may be some small improvement in vision during the first decade of life as the visual system reaches maturity, but it is uncommon for children to be able to navigate without assistance or to be able to read print.

Other symptoms of LCA may include crossed eyes, sluggish pupils, rapid involuntary eye movements, unusual sensitivity to light, and the clouding of the lenses of the eyes. Many children with LCA habitually press on their eyes with their fists or fingers. This habitual pressing on the eyes is known as an oculo-digital reflex and may represent an instinctual attempt to provide the eveloping visual cortex of the brain with a stimulus to replace the loss of normal visual stimuli. As a result of this behavior, the eyes may become thin and conical in shape and appear sunken or deep. In some cases, LCA is associated with hearing loss, **epilepsy**, decreased coordination, kidney problems, or heart abnormalities. Mental retardation may be present in approximately 20% of individuals affected with LCA.

Diagnosis

Infants are usually brought to medical attention within the first six months of life when parents note a lack of visual responsiveness and the unusual roving eye movements characteristic of the disease. As with any evidence of loss of vision, a prompt and thorough evaluation is initiated to determine the cause of the visual defect, and steps may include physical tests designed to measure brain and eye function, CT scans (a method using x rays controlled by a sophisticated computer) of the brain and eye, and even tests to look for genetic and metabolic causes of blindness.

Eye examinations of infants with LCA usually reveal a normal appearing retina. By early adolescence, however, various changes in the retinas of patients with LCA become readily apparent; blood vessels often become narrow and constricted, and a variety of color changes can also occur in the retina and its supportive tissue.

One of the most important tests in diagnosing LCA is called electroretinography (ERG). This test measures electrical impulses which are produced in the retina when light is sensed by the rod and cone cells. It is useful in distinguishing whether blindness is due to a problem in the retina versus a problem in the visual cortex of the brain. When ERG tests are performed on people with LCA, there is no recordable electrical activity arising from the eye, indicating the problem is based in the retina rather than in the brain.

Thus, an absence of activity on ERG, combined with the absence of diagnostic signs of other conditions which result in blindness, point to a diagnosis of LCA. Although several abnormal genes have been identified which are responsible for LCA, genetic analysis and prenatal diagnosis is rarely performed outside of research studies.

Treatment and management

Currently, there is no treatment for LCA, and thus, patient and family education and adaptive assistance is critical. Some people with remaining vision may benefit from vision-assistance technology such as electronic, computer-based, and optical aids, but severely visually-impaired individuals often utilize traditional resources such as canes and companion-guide dogs. Orientation and mobility training, adaptive training skills, job placement and income assistance are available through hospital physical and occupation therapy programs and various community resources. It should be noted that up to 20% of patients with LCA may have associated mental retardation and will require additional adaptive and vocational assistance.

Most people with LCA are unable to read print and instead utilize Braille, an alphabet represented by raised dots that can be felt with the fingertips. People with LCA often attend schools specially designed to meet the needs of visually-impaired students and may require modifica-

tions to their home and work environments in order to accommodate their low or absent vision. As almost all patients with LCA are legally blind, they will not be able to drive or operate heavy machinery. **Genetic counseling** may assist affected individuals with family planning.

Scientists have isolated several mutant genes that can each cause LCA. Ongoing scientific research is directed toward understanding how these genes function in the retina and toward locating the remaining genes that cause LCA. With this information, scientists can better develop a means of prevention and treatment. A dramatic example of this principle was provided in 2000, when researchers were able to restore vision in mice with LCA2. By giving oral doses of a chemical compound derived from vitamin A, the scientists were able to restore the animals' visual functions to almost normal levels after just two days. The researchers report that they will attempt the same experiments in dogs with LCA2 before trying the treatment in humans. It should be noted that LCA2 causes only 10% of the known cases of LCA, and the treatment in this experimental study does not work for other types of LCA.

Prognosis

While children born with LCA may have variable symptoms and differing levels of visual acuity, they can lead productive and healthy lives with adaptive training and assistance. In those patients who do not have associated problems with their brain, heart, or kidney, life span is approximately the same as the general population, otherwise the prognosis is variable and depends on the extent of the complication.

Resources

BOOKS

"Disorders of Vision" In *Nelson Textbook of Pediatrics,* edited by R. E. Behrman. Philadelphia: W. B. Saunders, 2000, pp. 1900-1928.

PERIODICALS

Dharmaraj, S. R., et al. "Mutational Analysis and Clinical Correlation in Leber Congenital Amaurosis." *Ophthalmic Genetics* 21 (September 2000): 135-150.

Gamm, D. M., and A.T. Thliveris. "Implications of Genetic Analysis in Leber Congenital Amaurosis." *Archives of Ophthalmology* 119 (March 2001): 426-427.

Lambert, S. R., A. Kriss, and D. Taylor. "Vision in Patients with Leber Congenital Amaurosis." *Archives of Ophthalmology* 11 (February 1997): 293- 294.

Perrault, I. "Leber Congenital Amaurosis." *Molecular Genetics and Metabolism* 68 (October 1999): 200-208.

ORGANIZATIONS

Foundation Fighting Blindness. Executive Plaza 1, Suite 800, 11350 McCormick Rd., Hunt Valley, MD 21031-1014. (888) 394-3937. <http://www.blindness.org>.

WEBSITES

"Entry 20400: Leber Congenital Amaurosis, Type 1." *OMIM—Online Mendelian Inheritance in Man.* <http://www.ncbi.nlm.nih.gov/entrez/dispomim.cgi?id=20400>.

Leber's Links: Leber's Congenital Amaurosis. <http://www.freeyellow.com/members4/leberslinks/index.html>.

Oren Traub, MD, PhD

Lebers hereditary optic neuropathy
see **Lebers hereditary optic atrophy**

Lebers hereditary optic atrophy

Definition

Lebers hereditary optic atrophy is a painless loss of central vision (blurring of objects and colors appearing less vivid) that usually begins between the ages of 25 and 35 (but can occur at any age) and leads to legal blindness. Other minor problems may be present such as tremors, numbness or weakness in arms and legs, or loss of ankle reflexes. It was first described in 1871 by Theodore Leber and is the most common cause of optic atrophy.

Description

Lebers hereditary optic atrophy is also called Lebers hereditary optic neuropathy or LHON. The beginning of visual blurring in both eyes is called the acute phase of LHON. In about half the patients, both eyes are affected at the same time. In the remainder of patients, central vision is lost in one eye over a period of a few weeks, then a month or two later, the second eye is affected. Once both eyes are affected, a few weeks usually pass before the eyesight stops getting worse. Other less common patterns of central vision loss in LHON can be very sudden loss in both eyes, or very gradual loss occurring over several years. After the acute phase, there is rarely any significant change in eyesight during the remainder of the person's life. People with LHON are usually left with some peripheral vision, which is seeing around the edges, or out of the corner of the eye. This final phase is called the atrophic phase because the optic discs are atrophic (cells have wasted away) and rarely change.

The optic disc is the center part of the retina (back of the eye) and is where the clearest vision—both in detail and color—comes from. The retina is what interprets what a person sees and sends this message to their brain, along the pathway known as the optic nerve. In LHON, both the retina and the optic nerve stop working properly. The rest of the eye works normally, so that light enters the eye through the pupil (black circle in the center of the iris, the colored part of the eye) as it should. However, even though the light is focused on the retina properly, in LHON, this information isn't converted into signals for the brain to process. When a person wears prescription glasses, the purpose is to help focus light properly on the retina. In LHON, light is already focused as it should be, so glasses will not improve vision. Magnifying glasses and telescopes do help, however, because they make things look bigger. When a person looks through a magnifier or telescope they use more of their retina to see, and some undamaged cells of the retina may be able to provide some information to the brain.

Suddenly losing vision is a shock. Patients diagnosed with LHON may feel they have no useful sight left, and often, their family and friends treat them as the stereotypic blind person. In reality, LHON usually leaves an affected person with some useable vision. A variety of visual aids are available to enhance this.

Genetic profile

In 60% of patients with LHON, there is a positive family history of LHON, while the remaining cases are considered sporadic (occur by chance), where only one person in the family has LHON. In 1988 it was discovered that LHON is caused by a mutation in a mitochondrial **gene**. Mitochondria are the energy producing organelles (structures) of cells. They have their own genetic material called mitochondrial **DNA**, which is separate from the usual genetic material contained in the center of the cell (or nucleus). Each mitochondria has several copies of its' circular DNA. DNA is the chemical that makes up genes. Genes code for certain traits, and in some cases, can code for disease. Mutations in the DNA of a mitochondria may be present in all copies (called homoplasmy), or may be present in a portion of the mitochondria's DNA (called heteroplasmy). About 15% of individuals with LHON are heteroplasmic, which means some of their mitochondrial DNA has a mutation, and some does not. This may have a bearing on the chance to develop symptoms, and on the risk of transmission.

There are three specific DNA changes or mutations that are found in the majority (90-95%) of LHON cases. The remaining LHON patients have other various mitochondrial mutations. In genetics, mutations are designated in such a way as to tell a scientist where they are located in the mitochondrial DNA and what the DNA alteration is:

- G11778A (i.e., mutation is located at position 11778; DNA change is G [guanine] to A [adenine]—a change in the base pairs that make up DNA)

- T14484C

- G3460A

Not all persons who have one of these mutations will develop LHON, since it is thought that additional genetic or environmental factors are necessary to develop central vision loss. In general, males with one of these mutations have a 40% lifetime risk to develop symptoms of LHON, while females have a 10% risk, although the actual risk varies slightly from mutation to mutation. In addition, the older a person in whom a mutation has been identified becomes without symptoms, the less likely they will lose their vision at all. If a person is going to experience vision loss from LHON, the majority of people with a mutation will express symptoms by the age of 50 years.

Environmental factors that can reduce the blood supply to the retina and optic nerve, and "trigger" the vision loss in LHON to begin include heavy drinking or smoking, exposure to poisonous fumes such as carbon monoxide, high levels of stress, and certain medications. A person in whom a mutation has been identified is considered more susceptible to some of these exposures and are advised not to smoke and to moderate their alcohol intake if they are asymptomatic.

The other important concept to understand in relation to mitochondrial disease is that mitochondria are only inherited from the mother. Therefore, a woman with a mitochondrial mutation (whether she has symptoms or not) will pass it to all of her offspring. Sons who inherit the mutation will not pass it to any of their children, while daughters who inherit the mutation will pass it to all of their children. This is in contrast to nuclear DNA, where half the genetic material is inherited from each parent.

Demographics

Males have LHON more often than females, however, females may develop LHON at a slightly older age and may have more severe symptoms, including a multiple sclerosis-like illness. **Multiple sclerosis** is a progressive degeneration of nerve cells that causes episodes of muscle weakness, dizziness, and visual disturbances, followed by remission. The onset of LHON usually occurs by 50 years if a mitochondrial DNA mutation is present, although it can present as late as the sixth or seventh decade of life.

Signs and symptoms

Symptoms of LHON include a painless sudden loss of central vision, both in visual detail and color, in both eyes over a period of weeks to months. Peripheral vision (seeing out of the corner of the eye) remains. Additional symptoms involving the neurological system may be present such as tremors, numbness or weakness in arms or legs, or loss of ankle reflexes. Symptoms vary by gender and type of mutation present. The following mutations are frequently identified and well understood:

- G11778A—the most common mutation and usually the most severe vision loss

- T14484C—usually has the best long term prognosis or outcome

- G3460A—has an intermediate presentation

Persons who have a multiple sclerosis-like illness can have any of the three mutations. This phenomena—

Lebers hereditary optic atrophy

Acute phase—The initial phase of LHON where visual blurring begins in both eyes, and central vision is lost.

Atrophic phase—The final phase of LHON where cells in the optic disc and optic nerve have atrophied, resulting in legal blindness. Peripheral vision remains.

Central vision—The ability to see objects located directly in front of the eye. Central vision is necessary for reading and other activities that require people to focus on objects directly in front of them.

Heteroplasmy—When all copies of mitochondrial DNA are not the same, and a mix of normal and mutated mitochondrial DNA is present.

Homoplasmy—When all copies of mitochondrial DNA are the same, or have the same mutation.

Lebers hereditary optic atrophy or Lebers hereditary optic neuropathy (LHON)—Discovered in 1871 by Theodore Leber, the painless loss of central vision in both eyes, usually occurring in the second or third decade of life, caused by a mutation in mitochondrial DNA. Other neurological problems such as tremors or loss of ankle reflexes, may also be present.

Lifetime risk—A risk which exists over a person's lifetime; a lifetime risk to develop disease means that the chance is present until the time of death.

Mitochondria—Organelles within the cell responsible for energy production.

Mitochondrial inheritance—Inheritance associated with the mitochondrial genome which is inherited exclusively from the mother.

Multiple sclerosis (MS)—A progressive degeneration of nerve cells that causes episodes of muscle weakness, dizziness, and visual disturbances, followed by periods of remission.

Mutation—A permanent change in the genetic material that may alter a trait or characteristic of an individual, or manifest as disease, and can be transmitted to offspring.

Ophthalmologist—A physician specializing in the medical and surgical treatment of eye disorders.

Optic disc—The region where the optic nerve joins the eye, also referred to as the blind spot.

Optic nerve—A bundle of nerve fibers that carries visual messages from the retina in the form of electrical signals to the brain.

Peripheral vision—The ability to see objects that are not located directly in front of the eye. Peripheral vision allows people to see objects located on the side or edge of their field of vision.

Pupil—The opening in the iris through which light enters the eye.

Retina—The light-sensitive layer of tissue in the back of the eye that receives and transmits visual signals to the brain through the optic nerve.

Sporadic—Isolated or appearing occasionally with no apparent pattern.

where different mutations give different clinical outcomes—is called a genotype-phenotype correlation. The word **genotype** describes the specific findings in DNA, while the word **phenotype** is used to describe the clinical presentation.

Diagnosis

Suspicion of LHON is usually made by an ophthalmologist after a complete eye examination. **Genetic testing** for the presence/absence of mitochondrial mutations can then be performed from a small blood sample. After a symptomatic person with LHON in a family has been identified to have a mitochondrial mutation, other asymptomatic at-risk relatives can also be tested. At-risk relatives would include the affected persons' mother, siblings, and the offspring of any females found to have the mutation. Testing for asymptomatic children who are

at-risk is not currently offered since no treatment is available for LHON; these individuals could opt for testing upon becoming a legal adult (i.e. reaching 18 years of age). Prenatal diagnosis for LHON is presently not available in the United States, but may be offered elsewhere. With genetic testing for LHON, it is important to remember that the presence of a mitochondrial mutation does not predict whether the condition will occur at all, the age at which it will begin, the severity, or rate of progression.

Treatment and management

There is no proven treatment available for LHON, although some studies report benefit from various vitamin therapies or other medications. Management of LHON is supportive, utilizing visual aids such as magnifiers.

Prognosis

The loss of central vision tends to remain the same (legally blind) over a lifetime once a person with LHON has reached the atrophic phase.

Resources

ORGANIZATIONS

International Foundation for Optic Nerve Disease. PO Box 777, Cornwall, NY 12518. <http://www.ifond.org>.

United Mitochondrial Diseases Foundation. PO Box 1151, Monroeville, PA 15146-1151. <http://www.umdf.org>.

WEBSITES

Leber's Optic Neuropathy. <http://www.leeder.demon.co.uk/pages/lhonhome.htm>.

Catherine L. Tesla, MS, CGC

Leigh syndrome

Definition

Leigh syndrome is a rare inherited neurometabolic disorder characterized by degeneration of the central nervous system (brain, spinal cord, and optic nerve), meaning that it gradually loses its ability to function properly.

Description

First described in 1951, Leigh syndrome usually occurs between the ages of three months and two years. The disorder worsens rapidly; the first signs may be loss of head control, poor sucking ability and loss of previously acquired motor skills, meaning the control of particular groups of muscles. Loss of appetite, vomiting, seizures, irritability, and/or continuous crying may accompany these symptoms. As the disorder becomes worse, other symptoms such as heart problems, lack of muscle tone (hypotonia), and generalized weakness may develop, as well as lactic acidosis, a condition by which the body produces too much lactic acid. In rare cases, Leigh syndrome may begin late in adolescence or early adulthood, and in these cases, the progression of the disease is slower than the classical form.

The disorder usually occurs in three stages, the first between eight and 12 months involving vomiting and failure to thrive, the second in infancy, characterized by loss of motor ability, eye problems and respiratory irregularity. The third stage occurs between two and 10 years of age and is characterized by hypotonia and feeding difficulties.

In most cases, Leigh syndrome is inherited as an autosomal recessive genetic trait. However, X-linked recessive, autosomal dominant, and mitochondrial **inheritance** can also occur. Several different types of genetic enzyme defects are thought to cause Leigh syndrome, meaning that the disorder may be caused by defective enzymes, the proteins made by the body to speed up the biochemical reactions required to sustain life.

Commonly known as Leigh's disease, Leigh syndrome is also known as Leigh necrotizing encephalopathy, necrotizing encephalomyelopathy of Leigh's and subacute necrotizing encephalopathy (SNE). When it occurs in adolescence and adulthood, it may be called adult-onset subacute necrotizing encephalomyelopathy.

Genetic profile

Several different types of genetic metabolic defects are thought to lead to Leigh syndrome. A deficiency of one or a number of different enzymes may be the cause.

Classic Leigh syndrome

The usual form of Leigh syndrome is inherited as an autosomal recessive genetic trait. It has been linked to a genetic defect in one of two genes known as E2 and E3, which cause either a deficiency of the enzyme pyruvate dehydrogenase, or an abnormality in other enzymes that make pyruvate dehydrogenase work. Other cases of autosomal recessive Leigh syndrome are associated with other genetic enzyme deficiencies (i.e., NADH-CoQ and Cytochrome C oxidase), although the **gene** or genes responsible for these deficiencies are not known. All of these different genetic defects seem to have a common effect on the central nervous system.

In autosomal recessive inheritance, a single abnormal gene on one of the autosomal chromosomes (one of the first 22 "non-sex" chromosomes) from both parents can cause the disease. Both of the parents must be carriers in order for the child to inherit the disease and neither of the parents has the disease (since it is recessive).

A child whose parents are carriers of the disease has a 25% chance of having the disease; a 50% chance of being a carrier of the disease, meaning that he is not affected by the disease, and a 25% chance of receiving both normal genes, one from each parent, and being genetically normal for that particular trait.

X-linked Leigh syndrome

Evidence also exists for an X-linked recessive form of Leigh syndrome, which has been linked to a specific defect in a gene called E1-alpha, a part of the enzyme pyruvate dehydrogenase.

X-linked recessive disorders are conditions that are coded on the X **chromosome**. All humans have two chromosomes that determine their gender: females have XX, males have XY. X-linked recessive, also called sex-linked, inheritance affects the genes located on the X chromosome. It occurs when an unaffected mother carries a disease-causing gene on at least one of her X chromosomes. Because females have two X chromosomes, they are usually unaffected carriers. The X chromosome that does not have the disease-causing gene compensates for the X chromosome that does. Generally for a woman to have symptoms of the disorder, both X chromosomes would have the disease-causing gene. That is why women are less likely to show such symptoms than males.

If a mother has a female child, the child has a 50% chance of inheriting the disease gene and being a carrier who can pass the disease gene on to her sons. On the other hand, if a mother has a male child, he has a 50% chance of inheriting the disease-causing gene because he has only one X chromosome. If a male inherits an X-linked recessive disorder, he is affected. All of his daughters will also be carriers.

Mitochondrial Leigh syndrome

Evidence also exists that Leigh syndrome may be inherited in some cases from the mother as a **DNA** mutation inside mitochondria. Hundreds of tiny mitochondria are contained in every human cell. They control the production of cellular energy and carry the genetic code for this process inside their own special DNA, called mtDNA. The mtDNA instructions from the father are carried by sperm cells, and during fertilization, these instructions break off from the sperm cell and are lost. All human mtDNA, therefore comes from the mother. The specific mtDNA defect that is thought to be responsible for some cases of Leigh syndrome, mtDNA nt 8993, is associated with the ATPase 6 gene. An affected mother passes it along to all of her children, but only the daughters will pass the mutation onto the next generation.

When mutations occur on mtDNA, the resulting genes may outnumber the normal ones. And until mutations are present in a significant percentage of the mitochondria, symptoms may not occur. Uneven distribution of normal and mutant mtDNA in different tissues of the body means that different organ systems in individuals from the same family may be affected, and a variety of symptoms may result in affected family members.

Adult–onset Leigh syndrome

In cases of adult-onset Leigh syndrome, the disorder may be inherited in yet another way, as an autosomal dominant genetic trait. In autosomal dominant inheritance, a single abnormal gene on one of the autosomal chromosomes (one of the first 22 "non-sex" chromosomes) from either parent can cause the disease. One of the parents will have the disease (since it is dominant) and will be the carrier. Only one parent needs to be a carrier in order for the child to inherit the disease. A child who has one parent with the disease has a 50% chance of also having the disease.

Demographics

Leigh syndrome is very rare. It is thought that the classic form of the disorder accounts for approximately 80% of cases and affects males and females in equal numbers. In both X-linked Leigh syndrome and adult-onset Leigh syndrome, almost twice as many males as females are affected. In adult-onset cases, progression of the disease is slower than the classical form.

Signs and symptoms

The symptoms of developmental delay, hypotonia, and lactic acidosis are present in almost all cases of Leigh syndrome. Other symptoms that may occur with the disorder are:

- Respiratory: Hyperventilation, breathing arrest (apnea), shortness of breath (dyspnea), respiratory failure. Respiratory disturbance may occur in as many as 70% of cases.

- Neurological: Muscle weakness, clumsiness, shaking, failure of muscular coordination (ataxia).

- Ocular: Abnormal eye movements, sluggish pupils, blindness.

- Cardiovascular: heart disease and malformation.

- Seizures may also occur.

Diagnosis

The diagnosis of Leigh syndrome is usually made by clinical evaluation and a variety of tests.

Advanced imaging techniques

The main body part affected is the nerve cells (gray matter) of the brain with areas of dead nerve cells (necrosis) and cell multiplication (capillary proliferation) in the lowest part of the brain (brain stem). A CT scan or magnetic resonance imaging MRI of the brain may reveal these abnormalities. Also, cysts may be present in the outer portion of the brain (cerebral cortex).

Laboratory testing

Biochemical findings are high levels of pyruvate and lactate in the blood and slightly low sugar (glucose)

KEY TERMS

Apnea—An irregular breathing pattern characterized by abnormally long periods of the complete cessation of breathing.

Asymmetric septal hypertrophy—A condition in which the septum (the wall that separates the atria of the heart) is abnormally excessively thickened. In microscopic examination, normal alignment of muscle cells is absent (myocardial disarray).

Ataxia—A deficiency of muscular coordination, especially when voluntary movements are attempted, such as grasping or walking.

Central nervous system (CNS)—In humans, the central nervous system is composed of the brain, the cranial nerves and the spinal cord. It is responsible for the coordination and control of all body activities.

Degenerative disorder—A disorder by which the body or a part of the body gradually loses its ability to function.

Enzyme—A protein that catalyzes a biochemical reaction or change without changing its own structure or function.

Hypertrophic cardiomyopathy—A condition in which the muscle of the heart is abnormally excessively thickened. In microscopic examination, normal alignment of muscle cells is absent (myocardial disarray).

Hypotonia—Reduced or diminished muscle tone.

Lactic acidosis—A condition characterized by the accumulation of lactic acid in bodily tissues. The cells of the body make lactic acid when they use sugar as energy. If too much of this acid is produced, the person starts feeling ill with symptoms such as stomach pain, vomiting, and rapid breathing.

Metabolism—The total combination of all of the chemical processes that occur within cells and tissues of a living body.

Mitochondria—Organelles within the cell responsible for energy production.

Motor skills disorder—A disorder that affects motor coordination or its development, and the control of particular groups of muscles that perform activities.

Necrosis—Death of a portion of tissue differentially affected by disease or injury.

Neurometabolic disorder—Any disorder or condition that affects both the central nervous system (CNS) and the metabolism of the body.

---

levels in the blood and cerebrospinal fluid (CSF), a clear fluid that bathes the brain and spinal cord. Laboratory tests may reveal high levels of acidic waste products in the blood, indicative of lactic acidosis as well as high levels of pyruvate and alanine. The enzyme pyruvate carboxylase may be absent from the liver. An inhibitor of thiamine triphosphate (TTP) production may be present in the blood and urine of affected individuals. Blood glucose may be somewhat lower than normal. Some children with the disorder may have detectable deficiencies of the enzymes pyruvate dehydrogenase complex or cytochrome C oxidase.

Related disorders

Symptoms of other disorders are very similar to those of Leigh syndrome, and comparisons may be useful to distinguish between them. These disorders are:

- Wernicke encephalopathy
- Kufs disease
- Batten disease
- Tay-Sachs disease
- Sandhoff disease
- Niemann-Pick disease
- Alpers disease

Prenatal testing

Genetic counseling may be of benefit for families with a history of Leigh syndrome. Prenatal testing is available to assist in prenatal diagnosis. Prior testing of family members is usually necessary for prenatal testing.

Either chorionic villus sampling (CVS) or **amniocentesis** may be performed for prenatal testing. CVS is a procedure to obtain chorionic villi tissue for testing. Examination of fetal tissue can reveal information about the changes that lead to Leigh syndrome. Chorionic villus sampling can be performed at 10–12 weeks pregnancy.

Amniocentesis is a procedure that involves inserting a thin needle into the uterus, into the amniotic sac, and withdrawing a small amount of amniotic fluid. DNA can be extracted from the fetal cells contained in the amniotic fluid and tested. Amniocentesis is performed at 15–18 weeks pregnancy.

Tissue obtained from CVS or in amniotic fluid that shows evidence of the genetic abnormalities responsible for Leigh syndrome confirms the diagnostic. Other forms of prenatal testing may be available for Leigh syndrome.

Treatment and management

The most common treatment for the disorder is the prescription of thiamine or vitamin B1. This may result in a temporary improvement of the symptoms and slightly slow the progress of the disease.

Patients lacking the pyruvate dehydrogenase enzyme complex may benefit from a high-fat, low-carbohydrate diet.

To treat lactic acidosis, oral sodium bicarbonate or sodium citrate may also be prescribed. To control severe lactic acidosis, intravenous infusion of tris-hydroxy-methyl aminomethane (THAM) may be beneficial. Both treatments help reduce abnormally high acid levels in the blood and the accumulation of lactic acid in the brain.

If eye problems occur, the individual with Leigh syndrome may benefit from treatment from an ophthalmologist.

Treatment should also include assistance with locating support resources for the family and the individual with Leigh syndrome.

Prognosis

Prognosis for individuals with classical Leigh syndrome is poor. Death usually occurs within a few years, although patients may live to be 6 or 7 years of age. Some patients have survived to the mid-teenage years. Children who survive the first episode of the disease may not fully recover physically and neurologically. In addition, they are likely to face successive bouts of devastating illness that ultimately cause death.

Resources

BOOKS

Jorde, L. B., et al., eds. *Medical Genetics*. 2nd ed. St. Louis: Mosby, 1999.

ORGANIZATIONS

Arc (a National Organization on Mental Retardation). 1010 Wayne Ave., Suite 650, Silver Spring, MD 20910. (800) 433-5255. <http://www.thearclink.org>.

Association for Neuro-Metabolic Disorders. 5223 Brookfield Lane, Sylvania, OH 43560-1809. (419) 885-1497.

Children Living with Inherited Metabolic Diseases. The Quadrangle, Crewe Hall, Weston Rd., Crewe, Cheshire, CW1-6UR. UK 127 025 0221. Fax: 0870-7700-327. <http://www.climb.org.uk>.

Children's Brain Disease Foundation. 350 Parnassus Ave., Suite 900, San Francisco, CA 94117. (415) 566-5402.

Epilepsy Foundation of America. 4351 Garden City Dr., Suite 406, Landover, MD 20785-2267. (301) 459-3700 or (800) 332-1000. <http://www.epilepsyfoundation.org>.

Lactic Acidosis Support Trust. 1A Whitley Close, Middlewich, Cheshire, CW10 0NQ. UK (016) 068-37198.

March of Dimes Birth Defects Foundation. 1275 Mamaroneck Ave., White Plains, NY 10605. (888) 663-4637. resourcecenter@modimes.org. <http://www.modimes.org>.

National Institute of Neurological Disorders and Stroke. 31 Center Drive, MSC 2540, Bldg. 31, Room 8806, Bethesda, MD 20814. (301) 496-5751 or (800) 352-9424. <http://www.ninds.nih.gov>.

National Organization for Rare Disorders (NORD). PO Box 8923, New Fairfield, CT 06812-8923. (203) 746-6518 or (800) 999-6673. Fax: (203) 746-6481. <http://www.rarediseases.org>.

United Mitochondrial Disease Foundation. PO Box 1151, Monroeville, PA 15146-1151. (412) 793-8077. Fax: (412) 793-6477. <http://www.umdf.org>.

WEBSITES

Online Mendelian Inheritance in Man. <http://www.ncbi.nlm.nih.gov:80/entrez/query.fcgi?db=OMIM>.

Jennifer F. Wilson, MS

LEOPARD syndrome *see* Multiple lentigines syndrome

Leprechaunism *see* Donohue syndrome

▌Lesch-Nyhan syndrome

Definition

Lesch-Nyhan syndrome is a rare genetic disorder that affects males. Males with this syndrome develop physical handicaps, mental retardation, and kidney problems. It is caused by a total absence of an enzyme. Self injury is a classic feature of this genetic disease.

Description

Lesch-Nyhan syndrome was first described in 1964 by Dr. Michael Lesch and Dr. William Nyhan. The syndrome is caused by a severe change (mutation) in the

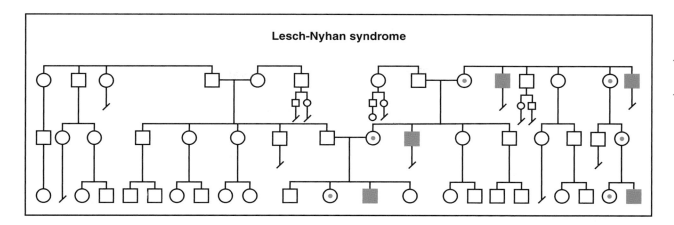

Lesch-Nyhan syndrome

(Gale Group)

HPRT gene. This gene is responsible for the production of the enzyme called hypoxanthine-guanine phosphoribosyltransferase (HPRT). HPRT catalyzes a reaction that is necessary to prevent the buildup of uric acid. A severe mutation in the HPRT gene leads to an absence of HPRT enzyme activity which, in turn, leads to markedly elevated uric acid levels in the blood (hyperuricemia). This buildup of uric acid is toxic to the body and is related to the symptoms associated with the disease. Absence of the HPRT enzyme activity is also thought to alter the chemistry of certain parts of the brain, such as the basal ganglia, affecting neurotransmitters (chemicals used for communication between nerve cells), acids, and other chemicals. This change in the nervous system is also related to the symptoms associated with Lesch-Nyhan syndrome.

Males with Lesch-Nyhan syndrome develop neurological problems during infancy. Infants with Lesch-Nyhan syndrome have weak muscle tone (hypotonia) and are unable to develop normally. Affected males develop uncontrollable writhing movements (athetosis) and muscle stiffness (spasticity) over time. Lack of speech is also a common feature of Lesch-Nyhan syndrome. The most dramatic symptom of Lesch-Nyhan syndrome is the compulsive self-injury seen in 85% of affected males. This self injury involves the biting of their own lips, tongue, and finger tips, as well as head banging. This behavior leads to serious injury and scarring.

Genetic profile

Severe changes (mutations) in the HPRT gene completely halt the activity of the enzyme HPRT. There have been many different severe mutations identified in the HPRT gene. These mutations may be different within families. Since the HPRT gene is located on the X **chromosome**, Lesch-Nyhan syndrome is considered an X-linked disorder and therefore only affects males.

A person's sex is determined by their chromosomes. Males have one X chromosome and one Y chromosome. Females, on the other hand, have two X chromosomes. Males who possess a severe mutation in their HPRT gene will develop Lesch-Nyhan syndrome. Females who possess a severe mutation in their HPRT gene will not; instead they are carriers. This is because females have another X chromosome without the mutation that prevents them from getting this disease. If a woman is a carrier, she has a 50% risk with each pregnancy to pass on her X chromosome with the mutation. Therefore, with every male pregnancy she has a 50% risk to have an affected son, and with every female pregnancy she has a 50% risk to have a daughter who is a carrier.

Demographics

Lesch-Nyhan syndrome affects approximately one in 380,000 live births. It occurs evenly among races. Almost always, only male children are affected. Women carriers usually do not have any symptoms. Women carriers can occasionally develop inflammation of the joints (gout)as they get older.

Signs and symptoms

At birth, males with Lesch-Nyhan syndrome appear completely normal. Development is usually normal for the first few months. Symptoms develop between three to six months of age. Sand-like crystals of uric acid in the diapers may be one of the first symptoms of the disease. The baby may be unusually irritable. Typically, the first sign of nervous system impairment is the inability to lift their head or sit up at an appropriate age. Many patients with Lesch-Nyhan will never learn to walk. By the end of the first year, writhing motions (athetosis), and spasmodic movements of the limbs and facial muscles (chorea) are clear evidence of defective motor development.

The compulsive self-injury associated with Lesch-Nyhan syndrome begins, on average, at three years. The self-injury begins with biting of the lips and tongue. As the disease progresses, affected individuals frequently develop finger biting and head banging. The self-injury can increase during times of stress.

Males with Lesch-Nyhan disease may also develop kidney damage due to kidney stones. Swollen and tender joints (gout) is another common problem.

Diagnosis

The diagnosis of Lesch-Nyhan syndrome is based initially on the distinctive pattern of symptoms. Measuring the amount of uric acid in a person's blood or urine can not definitively diagnose Lesch-Nyhan syndrome. It is diagnosed by measuring the activity of the HPRT enzyme through a blood test. When the activity of the enzyme is very low it is diagnostic of Lesch-Nyhan syndrome. It can also be diagnosed by **DNA** testing. This is also a blood test. DNA testing checks for changes (mutations) in the HPRT gene. Results from DNA testing are helpful in making the diagnosis and also if the family is interested in prenatal testing for future pregnancies.

Prenatal diagnosis is possible by DNA testing of fetal tissue drawn by **amniocentesis** or chorionic villus sampling (CVS). Fetuses should be tested if the mother is a carrier of a change (mutation) in her HPRT gene. A woman is at risk of being a carrier if she has a son with Lesch-Nyhan syndrome or someone in her family has Lesch-Nyhan syndrome. Any woman at risk of being a carrier should have DNA testing through a blood test.

Treatment and management

There are no known treatments for the neurological defects of Lesch-Nyhan. The medication Allopurinol can lower blood uric acid levels. This medication does not correct many of the symptoms. Some patients with Lesch-Nyhan syndrome have their teeth removed to prevent self-injury. Restraints are recommended to reduce self-destructive behaviors.

Prognosis

With strong supportive care, infants born with Lesch-Nyhan can live into adulthood with symptoms continuing throughout life.

KEY TERMS

Amniocentesis—A procedure performed at 16-18 weeks of pregnancy in which a needle is inserted through a woman's abdomen into her uterus to draw out a small sample of the amniotic fluid from around the baby. Either the fluid itself or cells from the fluid can be used for a variety of tests to obtain information about genetic disorders and other medical conditions in the fetus.

Athetosis—A condition marked by slow, writhing, involuntary muscle movements.

Basal ganglia—A section of the brain responsible for smooth muscle movement.

Chorea—Involuntary, rapid, jerky movements.

Chorionic villus sampling (CVS)—A procedure used for prenatal diagnosis at 10-12 weeks gestation. Under ultrasound guidance a needle is inserted either through the mother's vagina or abdominal wall and a sample of cells is collected from around the fetus. These cells are then tested for chromosome abnormalities or other genetic diseases.

Enzyme—A protein that catalyzes a biochemical reaction or change without changing its own structure or function.

Mutation—A permanent change in the genetic material that may alter a trait or characteristic of an individual, or manifest as disease, and can be transmitted to offspring.

Neurotransmitter—Chemical in the brain that transmits information from one nerve cell to another.

Palsy—Uncontrollable tremors.

Spasticity—Increased muscle tone, or stiffness, which leads to uncontrolled, awkward movements.

At present, there are no preventive measures for Lesch-Nyhan syndrome. However, recent studies have indicated that this genetic disorder may be a good candidate for treatment with gene replacement therapy. Unfortunately, the technology necessary to implement this therapy has not yet been perfected.

Resources

BOOKS

Jinnah, H. A., and Theodore Friedmann. "Lesch-Nyhan Disease and Its Variants." *The Metabolic and Molecular*

Bases of Inherited Disease. New York: McGraw-Hill, 2001.

PERIODICALS

Lesch, M., and W. L. Nyhan. "A Familial Disorder of Uric Acid Metabolism and Central Nervous System Function." *American Journal of Medicine* 36 (1964): 561–570.

Mak, B. S., et al. "New Mutations of the HPRT Gene in Lesch-Nyhan Syndrome." *Pediatric Neurology* (October 2000): 332–335.

Visser, J. E., et al. "Lesch-Nyhan Disease and the Basal Ganglia." *Brain Research Reviews* (November 1999): 450–469.

ORGANIZATIONS

Alliance of Genetic Support Groups. 4301 Connecticut Ave. NW, Suite 404, Washington, DC 20008. (202) 966-5557. Fax: (202) 966-8553. <http://www.geneticalliance.org>.

International Lesch-Nyhan Disease Association. 114 Winchester Way, Shamong, NJ 08088-9398. (215) 677-4206.

Lesch-Nyhan Syndrome Registry. New York University School of Medicine, Department of Psychiatry, 550 First Ave., New York, NY 10012. (212) 263-6458.

National Organization for Rare Disorders (NORD). PO Box 8923, New Fairfield, CT 06812-8923. (203) 746-6518 or (800) 999-6673. Fax: (203) 746-6481. <http://www.rarediseases.org>.

WEBSITES

GeneClinics <http://www.geneclinics.org/profiles/lns/details.html>.

Pediatric Database (PEDBASE) <http://www.icondata.com/health/pedbase/files/LESCH-NY.HTM>.

Holly Ann Ishmael, MS, CGC

Leukodystrophy

Definition

Leukodystrophy describes a collection of about 15 rare **genetic disorders** that effect the brain, spinal cord and peripheral nerves. It is characterized by imperfect growth or development of the white matter covering nerve fibers in the brain.

Description

Leukodystrophy comes from the Greek words *leuko* meaning white (referring to the white matter of the nervous system) and *dystrophy* meaning imperfect growth or development. The white matter is called the myelin sheath and is an extremely complex substance composed of at least 10, and probably more, chemicals. The myelin sheath protects the axon (a long and single-nerve cell process that acts as a wire to conduct impulses away from the cell body), much the way insulation does to an electric wire.

Each type of leukodystrophy affects one of these chemicals. Leukodystrophies covered in this essay are Alexander's disease, childhood ataxia with central nervous system hypomyelination (CACH), also known as vanishing white matter disease, cerebralautosomal dominant arteriopathy with subcortical infarcts and leukoencephalopathy (**CADASIL**), cerebrotendinous xanthomatosis (CTX), metachromatic leukodystrophy, ovarioleukodystrophy syndrome, and Van der Knapp syndrome, also called vacuolating leukodystrophy with subcortical cysts.

Leukodystrophies covered as separate entries in this encyclopedia are **adrenoleukodystrophy** (ALD)/adrenomyeloneuropathy (AMN), Aicardi-Goutieres syndrome, **canavan disease** (spongy degeneration), **Krabbe disease** (globoid cell leukodystrophy), neonatal adrenoleukodystrophy, **Pelizaeus-Merzbacher disease** (X-linked spastic paraplegia), **Refsum disease**, and **Zellweger syndrome**.

Genetic profile

Genes are the blueprint for the human body that directs the development of cells and tissue. Mutations in some genes can cause genetic disorders such as leukodystrophy. Every cell in the body has 23 pairs of chromosomes, 22 pairs of which are called autosomes and contain two copies of individual genes. The 23rd pair of chromosomes is called the sex **chromosome** because it determines a person's sex. Males have an X and a Y chromosome while females have two X chromosomes.

All of the leukodystrophies discussed in this article have an autosomal recessive pattern of **inheritance** that affects males and females. People with only one abnormal **gene** are carriers but since the gene is recessive, they do not have the disorder. Their children will be carriers of the disorder but not show symptoms of the disease. Both parents must have one of the abnormal genes for a child to have symptoms of an autosomal recessive leukodystrophy. When both parents have the abnormal gene, there is a 25% chance each child will inherit both abnormal genes and have the disease. There is a 50% chance each child will inherit one abnormal gene and become a carrier of the disorder but not have the disease itself. There is a 25% chance each child will inherit neither abnormal gene and not have the disease nor be a carrier.

Demographics

All of the leukodystrophies discussed here appear to affect all racial and ethnic groups and all geographic populations. However, metachromatic leukodystrophy has been found in a higher frequency in highly inbred groups, such as the Habbanite Jewish population. Van der Knapp syndrome has a high prevalence among Turkish and Asian-Indian people.

Signs and symptoms

The most common signs seen in most leukodystrophies include gradual changes in an infant or child who previously appeared healthy. These changes may appear in body tone, movements, gait, speech, the ability to eat, hearing, vision, behavior, and memory. Specific signs and symptoms for individual leukodystrophies include:

- Metachromatic, with the most common and most severe form occurring between the ages of six months and two years with symptoms such as irritability, decreased muscle tone, muscle wasting, and difficulty learning to walk and talk. Onset symptoms in older children and adults include deterioration of intellectual performance, and behavioral or psychiatric problems. Blindness, seizures, and paralysis occur as the disease progresses.

- Alexander's disease, which usually begins in infancy (six to 24 months of age) and affects mostly males. Initial signs are physical and mental retardation and as the disease progresses, enlargement of the brain and head, spasticity, and seizures. In children and adults, symptoms are the same but occur less frequently and progress more slowly.

- CACH is usually diagnosed in infancy and initial symptoms include motor and speech difficulties that progressively worsen. Later symptoms include difficulty swallowing, seizures, and coma.

- CADASIL can be diagnosed in children and adults but usually shows up at around age 45. The initial symptom is usually migraine headaches, followed in about 10 years by ischemic attacks and small strokes followed by mood disturbances and **dementia. Epilepsy** sometimes occurs.

- CTX may present initial symptoms of cataracts, mild mental retardation, fatty tumors (called xanthomas) in tendons, especially the Achilles tendon or heel cord. Later symptoms include seizures, emotional or psychiatric disturbances, and impaired motion or muscle movement.

- Ovarioleukodystrophy syndrome usually has onset symptoms of walking difficulties and/or mental retardation.

- Van der Knapp syndrome can have onset at or shortly after birth with the symptom of an extremely enlarged head. But onset usually occurs between ages four and five with initial symptoms of cerebella ataxia followed by spasticity. Later symptoms include mental slowing and learning problems and sometimes epileptic seizures and severe walking impairment.

Diagnosis

Leukodystrophies are occasionally misdiagnosed as **muscular dystrophy**, since they all are neurological disorders involving white matter. **Genetic testing** is usually in order for all leukodystrophies except Alexander's disease and Van der Knapp syndrome for which the specific genetic abnormalities are unknown. A nerve conduction velocity (NCV) test is sometimes used to evaluate nerve damage in people with metachromatic leukodystrophy. The NCV test sends small electrical shocks through one end of a nerve. The time it takes to travel to the other end of the nerve is measured to help determine the severity of nerve damage. Diagnosis of CTX is made by measuring the levels of bile alcohol in the blood or urine, or of cholestanol in the blood. Cholestanol is similar chemically to cholesterol but can be distinguished from it by special chemical tests. MLD and Van der Knapp syndrome diagnosis are usually made by a brain imaging scan called magnetic resonance imaging (MRI). A series of biochemical tests is sometimes used to diagnose MLD.

Treatment and management

With the exception of CTX, none of the leukodystrophies covered here are treatable. In some of the disorders, specific symptoms can be treated. For example some infections associated with MLD, such as pneumonia, can be treated with antibiotics. In ovarioleukodystrophy syndrome, ovarian insufficiency can be treated with hormone replacement therapy. But there are no treatments available for most of the conditions associated with leukodystrophies, such as mental retardation, dementia, deterioration of speech, vision, and mobility, and degeneration of myelin (white matter). In CTX, administration of certain bile acids, especially chenododeoxycholic acid, can prevent further progression of the disorder and in some cases may bring improvement.

Prognosis

The prognosis varies between leukodystrophy types but overall, most people with leukodystrophy can expect a shortened life span. Infants with Alexander's disease generally do not live past the age of five or six. Infants with metachromatic leukodystrophy (MLD) usually do not live past age 10. In children and adults, Alexander's

KEY TERMS

Arteriopathy—Damage to blood vessels.

Ataxia—A deficiency of muscular coordination, especially when voluntary movements are attempted, such as grasping or walking.

Bile acids—Steroid acids such as cholic acid that occur in bile, an alkaline fluid secreted by the liver and passed into a part of the small intestine where it aids in absorption of fats.

Bile alcohol—A steroid acid with an alcohol group attached.

Cataract—A clouding of the eye lens or its surrounding membrane that obstructs the passage of light resulting in blurry vision. Surgery may be performed to remove the cataract.

Dementia—A condition of deteriorated mental ability characterized by a marked decline of intellect and often by emotional apathy.

Hypomyelination—The death of myelin on a nerve or nerves.

Ischemic attack—A period of decreased or no blood flow.

Leukoencephalopathy—Any of various diseases, including leukodystrophies, affecting the brain's white matter.

Spasticity—Increased muscle tone, or stiffness, which leads to uncontrolled, awkward movements.

Subcortical infarcts—Obstruction of nerve centers below the cerebral cortex of the brain.

disease and MLD progress more slowly but life expectancy is still shortened. Life expectancy with CACH is also shortened, with few people living beyond age 40 years. CADASIL progresses slowly but death occurs on average about 21–22 years after onset of symptoms. Life expectancy is closer to normal with CTX provided it is diagnosed and treated early. Ovarioleukodystrophy is a relatively newly identified disorder and there is not enough information available to make a prognosis of life expectancy, other than to say it is probably reduced. The average life expectancy is also unknown for Van der Knapp syndrome; several patients have died in their 20s but others are still alive in their 40s.

A number of government agencies and private foundations are currently funding research into many of the leukodystrophies, including identifying the cause of individual disorders, developing therapies to prevent disease progression, and to prevent onset of disease. However, little research is being done on therapies to repair damage already done by the disorders, or of restoring functions lost because of the disorders, according to The Myelin Project, a private research foundation.

Resources

BOOKS

Scheltens, P. *White Matter Disease.* Basel, Switzerland: S. Karger Publishing AG, 1999.

ORGANIZATIONS

National Organization for Rare Disorders (NORD). PO Box 8923, New Fairfield, CT 06812-8923. (203) 746-6518 or (800) 999-6673. Fax: (203) 746-6481. <http://www.rarediseases.org>.

United Leukodystrophy Foundation. 2304 Highland Dr., Sycamore, IL 60178. (815) 895-3211 or (800) 728-5483. Fax: (815) 895-2432. <http://www. ulf.org>.

WEBSITES

Delayed Myelin. Myelin Associated Infant-Childhood Development Disorders. <http://www.delayedmyelin.homestead.com>.

The Myelin Project. <http://www.myelin.org>.

Ken R. Wells

Li-Fraumeni syndrome

Definition

Li-Fraumeni syndrome (LFS) is a hereditary condition in which individuals have an increased risk for developing certain kinds of tumors. The characteristic tumors of LFS are adrenocortical carcinoma, **breast cancer**, brain **cancer**, leukemia, and sarcoma. Li-Fraumeni syndrome has previously been known as the Sarcoma, Breast, Leukemia and Adrenal gland (SBLA) syndrome.

Description

Li-Fraumeni syndrome is an inherited condition that is associated with a significantly increased risk for developing certain kinds of cancer. It is classified as a hereditary cancer syndrome and was first described in 1969. Hereditary cancer syndromes typically result in multiple family members developing cancer, in family members developing the same kind(s) of cancer, in family members developing cancer at a young age, and in family members developing more than one primary cancer. In contrast, most people who develop cancer are diagnosed later in life and do not have multiple close family members who develop the same kind of cancer.

Five cancers are characteristic of LFS: adrenocortical carcinoma, breast cancer, brain cancer, leukemia, and sarcoma. Other types of cancer such as melanoma, colon cancer, and stomach cancer have been seen in families with LFS, but it is not certain whether these tumors are truly a part of LFS.

Adrenocortical carcinoma is a rare cancer affecting a specific part of the adrenal gland called the adrenal cortex. There are two adrenal glands and each one sits on the upper part of a kidney. Adrenal glands produce hormones and if a cancer is present, more hormones may be produced. In LFS, adrenocortical carcinomas typically develop in childhood.

Brain cancer refers to a tumor developing in the brain. The brain tumors that occur in LFS tend to develop in young adulthood, although they may develop at any age.

Breast cancer is a cancer affecting the breast and in LFS women are often diagnosed in their twenties, thirties, and forties. Although breast cancer in men is rare, it does occur both within families with LFS and in the general population.

Leukemia refers to cancer of the blood. There is more than one type of leukemia; the type depends upon the kind of blood cell involved and whether the cancer is fast (acute) or slow (chronic) growing. Overall, acute lymphocytic leukemia (ALL) is the most common leukemia in children, and acute myelogenous leukemia (AML) is common in young adults. Chronic myelogenous leukemia (CML) is a common leukemia in older individuals. Li-Fraumeni syndrome is typically associated with acute leukemias and are most often diagnosed in children, adolescents, and young adults.

Sarcoma refers to a soft-tissue tumor, meaning that the tumor has developed in bone, muscle, or connective tissue. Osteosarcoma refers to a sarcoma that has developed in the bone. Rhabdomyosarcoma is a sarcoma that has developed in the muscle. Both of these sarcomas are associated with LFS and typically are diagnosed in children and in adults before the age of 35 years. A third type of sarcoma, Ewing's sarcoma, occurs in bone but is not associated with LFS.

An individual inheriting the familial LFS **gene** alteration has a significantly increased risk for developing one of the five characteristic cancers in his/her lifetime. This risk is about 85–90% by age 60. Much of this risk occurs in childhood through middle adulthood with the majority of individuals developing cancer by the time they reach 30 years of age.

Age of onset for cancers associated with Li-Fraumeni syndrome	
Age of onset	**Type of cancer**
Infancy	Development of adrenocortical carcinoma
Under 5 years of age	Development of soft-tissue sarcomas
Childhood and young adulthood	Acute leukemias and brain tumors
Adolescence	Osteosarcomas
Twenties to thirties	Premenopausal breast cancer is common

Genetic profile

Li-Fraumeni syndrome follows autosomal dominant **inheritance**, meaning that every individual diagnosed with LFS has a 50% chance of passing on the condition to each of his/her children. Nearly every individual inheriting the LFS gene alteration will develop at least one of the characteristic tumors. However, not every family member inheriting the LFS gene alteration will develop the same kind of tumor. Additionally, some family members may develop more than one tumor whereas other family members may develop one tumor. For example, a family history may include a father who was diagnosed with a brain tumor at age 50, a daughter who was diagnosed with an adrenocortical carcinoma at age three and breast cancer at age 43 years, and a granddaughter who was diagnosed with sarcoma at age seven.

The majority of families with LFS have an alteration in a gene located on the short arm of **chromosome** 17 at location p53. There may be another gene(s) involved in LFS, but no other gene has been identified yet.

Demographics

Li-Fraumeni syndrome is a rare condition. About 300 families worldwide have been reported in the medical literature. Males and females are equally affected.

Signs and symptoms

General symptoms of cancer include unexplained weight loss, weakness, fatigue, and pain. Symptoms specific to each characteristic tumor are listed below. It should be noted that the same kind of cancer may cause different symptoms in different people as well as that individuals with LFS may develop other kinds of cancer; consequently, any new and/or unusual symptom should be evaluated by a physician.

Adrenocortical carcinomas may cause abdominal pain. In some cases, the tumor causes extra hormones to be produced, and if so, the individual may experience high blood pressure, **diabetes**, deepening of the voice, swelling of the sexual organs and/or breasts, or growth of hair on the face.

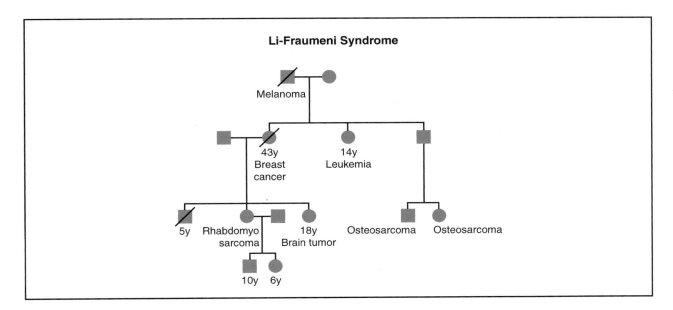

Li-Fraumeni Syndrome

Melanoma

43y
Breast
cancer

14y
Leukemia

5y

Rhabdomyo
sarcoma

18y
Brain tumor

Osteosarcoma   Osteosarcoma

10y 6y

(Gale Group)

Brain cancer may result in a number of symptoms including vomiting, seizures, headaches, behavioral changes, changes in eating or sleeping patterns, fatigue, or clumsiness.

Breast cancer typically results in a lump. Occasionally, the nipple may invert or the skin over the lump may dimple. In rare cases, the breast may suddenly become red and swollen. Breast cancer can be identified before symptoms develop by the use of mammography.

Leukemia may result in unusual bruising, a pale appearance, and/or recurrent infections. Little red or purple spots, called petechiae, may develop on the skin.

Sarcomas result in different symptoms depending upon the type of sarcoma. Osteosarcomas often lead to swelling and pain, symptoms that may be confused with an injury. Rhabdomyosarcomas cause a lump to develop and swelling.

Diagnosis

Evaluation of a family history for LFS requires a detailed three-generation family tree as well as medical records and/or death certificates to confirm or clarify the tissues involved as well as the age of the individual at the time of his/her diagnosis. Diagnosis of LFS depends upon the types of tumors family members have developed and the ages at which the tumors were diagnosed. A set of criteria for diagnosing LFS has been established.

A family may not meet the criteria for diagnosis of LFS but may have features that suggest LFS. Families such as these may be said to be "Li-Fraumeni-like"

(LFL). Two sets of criteria have been developed for LFL, which, like the diagnostic criteria, are based upon the high incidence of tumors in these families and the earlier ages of diagnosis.

Caution needs to be used when evaluating a family history of early-onset breast cancer because several other genes besides p53 are known to increase the risk for developing breast cancer at young ages. The clinical features of these other genes need to be taken into account and evaluated.

Genetic testing for p53 **gene mutations** is available and provides an additional method for making a diagnosis. It may be offered to an individual who has developed one of the tumors characteristic of LFS and who has a family history that meets the diagnostic criteria. If a mutation is identified, the positive test result provides proof of the diagnosis. If no mutation is identified, this negative test result does not necessary remove the diagnosis of LFS. Genetic testing may not identify a mutation for two reasons. First, laboratory techniques are not perfect and not every mutation in the p53 gene has been or can be identified; about 70 to 80% of mutations are identifiable. Second, there may be another gene(s) involved in LFS.

Genetic testing for LFS may also be offered to an individual who has no personal history of cancer but whose family history meets the diagnostic criteria for LFS or is strongly suggestive of LFS. It is usually offered in order to determine this individual's risk for developing cancer and to help with decisions regarding medical screening. Genetic testing in this case is referred to as predictive or presymptomatic genetic testing. Predictive

KEY TERMS

Chemotherapy—Treatment of cancer with synthetic drugs that destroy the tumor either by inhibiting the growth of the cancerous cells or by killing the cancer cells.

Mammography—X rays of the breasts; used to screen for breast cancer.

Metastasis—The spreading of cancer from the original site to other locations in the body.

Primary tumor—The organ or tissue where the tumor began.

Radiation therapy—Treatment using high-energy radiation from x-ray machines, cobalt, radium, or other sources.

Stage—The extent of the tumor. Tests will be done to determine if the tumor is localized to the organ or if it has spread to the lymph nodes and/or other organs. Treatment depends upon the stage of the cancer.

Tumor—An abnormal growth of cells. Tumors may be benign (noncancerous) or malignant (cancerous).

genetic testing should not be done unless a p53 genetic alteration has already been identified in an affected family member.

Genetic testing for diagnostic and predictive purposes is associated with significant risks and limitations, uncertain benefits, and is best done with a geneticist or genetic counselor knowledgeable about LFS and the implications of genetic testing. Predictive genetic testing for LFS does not clearly provide a benefit for all family members at risk for inheriting a familial p53 gene alteration because medical screening and prevention methods are not available for the tumors associated with LFS.

Prenatal diagnosis of LFS is available only if a p53 genetic alteration has already been identified in the family. Prenatal diagnosis of LFS is considered to be predictive genetic testing and therefore, the issues surrounding predictive genetic testing exist in this situation. An additional issue is how the test result will be used with regard to continuation of the pregnancy. Individuals considering prenatal diagnosis of LFS should confirm its availability prior to conception.

Treatment and management

There is no cure or method for preventing LFS. Treatment depends upon the tumor(s) an individual develops. An individual does not require treatment until a tumor develops, and then the treatment will be specific to the type of tumor. An individual without symptoms should undergo regular medical check-ups.

In general, tumors are treated by surgery, chemotherapy, and/or radiation therapy. Adrenocortical carcinomas and breast cancers, depending upon the stage of the tumor, use one or more of these treatments. Brain cancer is treated by surgery and/or radiation. In some cases, chemotherapy is also used. Leukemia is primarily treated by chemotherapy. In some cases, bone marrow transplantation is used. Osteosarcoma is treated by surgery. Rhabdomyosarcoma is treated by surgery, chemotherapy, and radiation therapy.

There are no proven methods of screening for or preventing cancer in individuals with LFS, other than perhaps breast cancer. It is very important that an individual's physician is aware of the family history and the cancer risk. It has been suggested that children of a parent with LFS be followed by having a complete physical examination, urinalysis, complete blood count (CBC), and abdominal ultrasound examination once each year. For adults at risk for having inherited a familial p53 gene alteration, it has been suggested that they undergo a complete physical examination with skin, nervous system, and rectal examinations once a year, and that women undergo a clinical breast examination every six months and mammography once a year. There is controversy concerning the use of mammography in women with LFS because of some suggestion that p53 gene alterations are sensitive to radiation. In general, an individual may decrease his/her chance of developing cancer by not smoking, exercising on a regular basis, eating a healthy diet, limiting sun exposure, and limiting his/her alcohol intake. Lastly, an individual with or at risk for LFS should not delay seeing his/her physician if he/she notices a new or unusual symptom.

Prognosis

An individual who has LFS has a very high chance of developing a cancerous tumor by the time he/she is 60 years old. In contrast, individuals in the general population have about a 2% risk for developing cancer. The cancers associated with LFS each have a different prognosis, so an individual's prognosis is highly dependent upon the type of cancer he/she has developed. In some cases, prognosis is associated with how early the cancer has been found. For example, breast cancer found early has a better prognosis than breast cancer found later. In general, the cancers typically seen in LFS are curable if caught early. For this reason, regular medical screening is important. Prognosis may also be affected by the individual's overall health; consequently, being healthy and engaging in healthy behaviors may increase the chances of a good outcome.

Resources

BOOKS

Buckman, Robert. *What You Really Need to Know about Cancer: A Comprehensive Guide for Patients and Their Families*. Baltimore: The Johns Hopkins University Press, 1995.

Offit, Kenneth. "Li-Fraumeni Syndrome." In *Clinical Cancer Genetics: Risk Counseling and Management*. New York: Wiley-Liss, 1998, pp.157-162.

PERIODICALS

National Institute of Health: National Cancer Institute. *When someone in your family has cancer*. (December 1995).

National Institute of Health: National Cancer Institute. *Taking time: Support for people with cancer and the people who care about them*. (January 1997).

National Institute of Health: National Cancer Institute. *Understanding gene testing*. (December 1995).

ORGANIZATIONS

National Cancer Institute. Office of Communications, 31 Center Dr. MSC 2580, Bldg. 1 Room 10A16, Bethesda, MD 20892-2580. (800) 422-6237. <http://www.nci.nih.gov>.

National Organization for Rare Disorders (NORD). PO Box 8923, New Fairfield, CT 06812-8923. (203) 746-6518 or (800) 999-6673. Fax: (203) 746-6481. <http://www.rarediseases.org>.

WEBSITES

National Cancer Institute. "Kids Home." *CancerNet*. <http://cancernet.nci.nih.gov/occdocs/KidsHome.html>.

National Cancer Institute. "Young people with cancer: Handbook for parents." *CancerNet*. <http://cancernet.nci.nih.gov/Young_People/yngconts.html>.

OncoLink. University of Pennsylvania. <http://www.oncolink.upenn.edu/>.

Schneider, K. A., and F. P. Li. "Li-Fraumeni Syndrome." *GeneClinics*. Univeristy of Washington, Seattle. <http://www.geneclinics.org/>.

Cindy L. Hunter, MS, CGC

▌Limb-girdle muscular dystrophy

Definition

Limb-girdle muscular dystrophy (LGMD) encompasses a diverse group of hereditary degenerative muscle disorders characterized by weakness and deterioration of the proximal skeletal muscles.

Description

The term limb-girdle **muscular dystrophy** is used to describe a group of muscular dystrophies that cause a muscle deterioration that primarily affects the voluntary muscles around the limb girdle. The muscles of the limb girdle include those around the shoulders and hips. As the disease develops, the distal muscles of the limbs can become affected. Most individuals' muscles of the heart are not affected, but exceptions can occur. There are at least 15 different LGMDs, each having a different range of symptoms. Each of the muscular dystrophies results in an absent, deficient, or abnormal protein that is required for normal structure and function of the muscles. It can be difficult to differentiate LGMD from other muscular dystrophies and muscle disorders that can also result in a weakness in the limb girdle.

Genetic profile

Each type of limb-girdle muscular dystrophy is caused by changes in a different type of **gene** that produces a protein normally involved in the functioning of the skeletal muscles. Each gene is found at a specific location on a **chromosome**. Every person inherits two copies of gene, one from their mother and one from their father. Each type of gene produces a specific type of protein. A change (mutation) in a gene can cause it to produce an abnormal protein, an increased or decreased amount of normal protein, or to stop producing protein altogether. Abnormal or decreased amounts of skeletal muscle proteins can affect the development or functioning of the muscle cells, causing the symptoms of LGMD. Most forms of LGMD are autosomal recessive, although some rare forms are autosomal dominant.

An autosomal recessive form of LGMD is caused by a change in both genes of a pair. One of the changed genes is inherited from the egg cell of the mother and one is inherited from the sperm cell of the father. Parents who have a child with an autosomal recessive form of LGMD are called carriers, since they each possess one changed LGMD gene and one unchanged LGMD gene. Carriers do not have any symptoms as they have only one unchanged gene, which produces enough normal protein to prevent the symptoms of LGMD. Each child born to parents who are both carriers for the same type of LGMD has a 25% chance of having LGMD, a 50% chance of being a carrier, and a 25% chance of being neither a carrier nor affected with LGMD. Parents who are each a carrier for a different type of LGMD are not at increased risk for having children affected with LGMD.

The autosomal dominant forms of LGMD are caused by a change in only one gene of a pair. This changed

TABLE 1

Genetic causes of the limb-girdle muscular dystrophies

Type	Mode of Inheritance	Gene Involved	Chromosomal Location
*Alpha- sarcoglycanopathy	Recessive	LGMD2D (SGCA)	17q12-q21.3
*Beta- sarcoglycanopathy	Recessive	LGMD2E (SGCB)	4q12
*Gamma- sarcoglycanopathy	Recessive	LGMD2C (SGCG)	13q12
*Delta- sarcoglycanopathy	Recessive	LGMD2F (SGCD)	5q33
Calpainopathy	Recessive	LGMD2A (CAPN3)	15q15.1-q21.1
Dysferlinopathy/Miyoshi distal myopathy	Recessive	LGMD2B (DYSF)	2p13.3-p13.1
Telethoninopathy	Recessive	LGMD2G(TCAP)	17q12
LGMD2H	Recessive	LGMD2H(TRIM32)	9q31-34.1
LGMD2I	Recessive	LGMD2I(FKRP)	19q13.3
LGMD1A	Dominant	LGMD1A(TTID)	5q31
LGMD1B	Dominant	LGMD1B(LMNA)	1q21.2
Caveolinopathy	Dominant	LGMD1C (CAV3)	3p25
LGMD1D	Dominant	LGMDID	7q
LGMD1E	Dominant	unknown	unknown
Bethlem myopathy	Dominant	COL6A1	21q22.3
	Dominant	COL6A2	21q22.3
	Dominant	COL6A3	2q37

*Each tupe of sarcoglycanopathy can result from a gene change that results in complete absence sarcoglycan protein or decreased amounts of sarcoglycan protein

gene is inherited from either the mother or the father. If the changed gene is inherited, each child born to a carrier of LGMD has a 50% chance of inheriting the condition. Sometimes the change occurs spontaneously when the egg and sperm come together to form the first cell of the baby. In this case, other relatives, such as siblings, are probably not at increased risk for inheriting LGMD. People with an autosomal dominant form of LGMD have a 50% chance of passing the condition on to their children. Some people who possess an autosomal dominant LGMD gene change do not have any symptoms.

Demographics

The incidence of LGMD is difficult to estimate as it can have a wide variety of symptoms. The rate of incidence of LGMD is one in 14,500–123,000 people, and is found equally in men and women. LGMD is also difficult to differentiate from other muscular disorders. Some forms of LGMD are found more commonly in people of a certain ethnic background.

Signs and symptoms

Each type of LGMD has a different range of symptoms. The symptoms can even vary between individuals with the same type of LGMD. The age of onset of symptoms can occur from infancy to adulthood. The most common symptom of LGMD is muscle weakness and deterioration and involves the muscles around the hips and shoulders. The disorder progresses at a different rate in each person. Although individuals with an onset of the disorder in adulthood may have a slower progression and

milder symptoms, the exact progression and extent of muscle deterioration cannot be predicted,.

The first noticeable symptom of LGMD is often a waddling gait due to weakness of the hip and leg muscles. Difficulties in rising from a chair or toilet seat and difficulties in climbing stairs are common. Eventually, walking may become impossible and lead to resorting to a wheelchair or scooter for locomotion. Enlargement or a decrease in size of the calf muscles can also be seen. Some individuals with LGMD also experience contractures and muscle cramps. The limited mobility associated with LGMD can result in muscle soreness and joint pain.

Lifting heavy objects, holding the arms outstretched, and reaching over the head can become impossible for people affected with LGMD because of weaknesses in the shoulder muscles. Some individuals with LGMD may eventually have difficulties swallowing and feeding themselves. Sometimes the back muscles can become weakened and result in **scoliosis** (curvature of the spine).

LGMD can occasionally result in a weakening of the heart muscles and/or the respiratory muscles. Some people may experience a weakening of the heart muscles (cardiomyopathy). Others may develop a conduction defect, an abnormality in the electrical system of the heart that regulates the heartbeat. A weakening of the muscles necessary for respiration can cause breathing difficulties. LGMD does not affect the brain and the ability to reason and think. Individuals with LGMD also do maintain normal bladder and bowel control and sexual functioning.

TABLE 2

Frequency of limb-girdle muscular dystrophy

Type	Frequency	Most Common In:
Alpha-sarcoglycanopathy		None
Beta-sarcoglycanopathy	Majority with severe disease—	Amish
Gamma-sarcoglycanopathy	10% of those with mild disease	North Africans; Gypsies
Delta-sarcoglycanopathy		Brazilian
Calpainopathy	Approximately 10%- 30%	Amish; La Reunion Isle.; Basque (Spain);Turkish
Dysferlinopathy	Approximately 10%	Libyan Jewish
Telethoninopathy	Rare	Italian
LGMD2H	Unknown	Unknown
LGMD2I	Unknown	Unknown
LGMD1A	Rare	Unknown
LGMD1B	Rare	Unknown
Caveolinopathy	Rare	Unknown
LGMD1D	Rare	Unknown
LGMD1E	Rare	Unknown
Bethlem myopathy	Rare	Unknown

Diagnosis

No single test can diagnose LGMD. A diagnosis is based on clinical symptoms, physical examinations, and a variety of tests. The physician will first take a medical history to establish the type of symptoms experienced and the pattern of muscle weakness. Questions will usually be asked about the family history to see whether other relatives have similar symptoms.

It is necessary for the doctor to establish whether the weakness is due to problems with the muscles or due to a problem with the nerves that control the muscles. Sometimes this can be accomplished through a physical examination. Electromyography testing is often performed to establish whether the weakness is in the nerves or the muscles. During electromyography, a needle electrode is inserted into the muscle and measurements are taken of the electrical activity of the muscle in response to stimulation by the nerves.

A blood test that measures the amount of creatine kinase is often performed. Creatine kinase is an enzyme that is produced by damaged muscles. High levels of creatine kinase suggest that the muscle is being destroyed, but the high levels cannot indicate the cause of the damage. The most common causes of increased creatine kinase levels are muscular dystrophy and muscle inflammation.

A muscle biopsy will often be performed if LGMD is suspected. During the muscle biopsy, a small amount of muscle is surgically removed. The muscle sample is examined to check for changes that are characteristic of muscular dystrophies. The amount and type of muscle proteins present in the sample can sometimes help to confirm a diagnosis of LGMD and can sometimes indicate the type of LGMD.

Ultimately, a diagnosis can be difficult to make as there are many types of LGMD and a wide range of symptoms. It can also be difficult to differentiate LGMD from other muscular dystrophies that have similar symptoms, such as Becker and Duchenne muscular dystrophies. Anyone suspected of having LGMD should, therefore, consider undergoing testing for other types of muscular dystrophies.

DNA testing for some forms of LGMD is now available through clinical and commercial laboratories. DNA testing is complicated by the many genes and the types of **gene mutations** (changes) that can cause LGMD. Some research laboratories are looking for the gene mutations that cause LGMD and may detect the gene mutation or mutations responsible for LGMD in a particular individual. DNA testing may be performed on a sample of blood cells or a sample of muscle cells. If an autosomal dominant gene mutation is detected in someone with LGMD, then both of the individual's parents can be tested to see if the gene mutation was inherited. If the gene mutation was inherited, siblings can be tested to see if they have inherited the mutated gene. If autosomal recessive gene mutations are detected, relatives, such as siblings, can be tested to see if they are carriers.

Prenatal testing for LGMD is only available if DNA testing has detected an autosomal dominant LGMD gene

TABLE 3

Symptoms of the limb-girdle muscular dystrophies

Type	Age of Onset	Early Symptoms	Late Symptoms
*Sarcoglycanopathy (complete deficiency)	3–15 years (8.5 average)	Proximal weakness; Difficulty walk/run; Enlarged calf muscle	Contractures; Curvature in the spine; Wheelchair dependence; Possible Cardiac conduction defect; Dilated cardiomyopathy
**Sarcoglycanopathy (partial deficiency	Adolescence/Young adulthood	Muscle cramps; Intolerance to exercise	
Calpainopathy	2–40 years (8–15 average)	Proximal weakness; Jutting backwards of shoulder blades (scapular winging); Decreased size of calf muscles; Contractures; Curvature in the spine	Wheelchair dependence
Dysferlinopathy	17–23 years	Some patients have distal weakness and some have proximal weakness; Inability to tip-toe; Difficulties walk/run	
Telethoninopathy	Early teens		Wheelchair dependence
LGMD2H	8–27 years		Wheelchair dependence
LGMD2I	1.5–27 years		Wheelchair dependence
LGMD1A	18–35 years	Proximal leg and arm weakness; Tight Achilles tendon; Problems with articulation of speech; Nasal sounding speech	Distal weakness
LGMD1B	4–38 years (50% onset childhood)	Proximal lower limb weakness;	Contractures; Irregular heart beat; Sudden death due to cardiac problems (if untreated)
LGMD1D	<25 years	Proximal muscle weakness; Cardiac conduction defect; Dilated cardiomyopathy	All patients remain able to walk
LGMD1E	9–49 years (30 average)	Proximal lower and upper limb muscle weakness	Contractures; Difficulties swallowing
Caveolinopathy	Approx. 5 years	Mild to moderate proximal weakness; Muscle cramping; Enlargement of the calf muscles; Some have no symptoms	
Bethlem myopathy	<2 years	Floppy muscles in infancy; Proximal muscle weakness; Contractures	2/3 of patents are wheelchair dependent by age 50

*Includes alpha, beta, gamma and delta sarcoglycanopathies that result in complete absence of a sarcoglycan protein
**Includes alpha, beta, gamma and delta sarcoglycanopathies that result in decreased amounts of a sarcoglycan protein

mutation in one parent or an autosomal recessive gene mutation in both parents. Cells for prenatal testing are obtained through an **amniocentesis** or chorionic villus sampling (CVS). These cells are analyzed for the LGMD gene mutation or mutations that were found in one or both parents.

Treatment and management

Physical therapy and exercises can often help keep the muscles and joints mobile and prevent contractures. Muscle and joint pain can be treated through exercise, warm baths, and pain medications. Surgical treatment of complications, such as a curved spine, may be necessary. Breathing exercises can sometimes help if breathing becomes difficult. If breathing independently becomes impossible, a portable mechanical ventilator can be used. A wheelchair or scooter can help when a person can no longer walk. Medications are often prescribed for cardiomyopathies and heart conduction defects. A device such as a pacemaker that creates normal contractions of the heart muscle may be necessary for some people with heart muscle abnormalities.

Gene therapy may one day cure or improve LGMD. Gene therapy introduces unchanged copies of a LGMD gene into the muscle cells. The goal of therapy is for the normal LGMD gene to produce normal protein that will allow the muscle cells to function normally. Gene therapy clinical trials are still in their infancy. It will take quite a few years, however, for gene therapy to become a viable way to treat LGMD.

Prognosis

The prognosis of LGMD varies tremendously. Most people with LGMD, however, do not have severe symptoms and most experience a normal life expectancy. Cardiac and respiratory difficulties can, however, decrease the lifespan.

Resources

PERIODICALS

Bushby, K. "Making Sense of the Limb-girdle Muscular Dystrophies." *Brain* 122 (1999): 1403–1420.

Kirschner, J, and C. G. Bonnemann. "The Congenital and Limb-girdle Muscular Dystrophies: Sharpening the Focus, Blurring the Boundaries." *Arch Neurol* 61, no. 2 (2004): 189–199.

KEY TERMS

Amniocentesis—A procedure performed between 16 and 18 weeks of pregnancy in which a needle is inserted through a woman's abdomen into the uterus to draw out a small sample of the amniotic fluid from around the fetus; either the fluid itself or cells from the fluid can be used for a variety of tests to obtain information about genetic disorders and other medical conditions in the fetus.

Amniotic sac—Contains the fetus that is surrounded by amniotic fluid.

Autosomal dominant—A pattern of genetic inheritance where only one abnormal gene is needed to display the trait or disease.

Autosomal recessive—A pattern of genetic inheritance where two abnormal genes are needed to display the trait or disease.

Cardiac conduction defect—Abnormality of the electrical system of the heart that regulates the heartbeat.

Carrier—A person who possesses a gene for a trait without showing signs of the disorder; the person may pass the mutated gene on to offspring.

Chromosome—A microscopic thread-like structure found within each cell of the body and consists of a complex of proteins and DNA; humans have 46 chromosomes arranged into 23 pairs.

Contracture—A tightening of muscles that prevents normal movement of the associated limb or other body part.

Dilated cardiomyopathy—A diseased and weakened heart muscle that is unable to pump blood efficiently.

Distal muscles—Muscles that are furthest away from the center of the body.

DNA testing—Analysis of DNA (the genetic component of cells) in order to determine mutations in genes that may indicate a specific disorder.

Gene—A building block of inheritance, which contains the instructions for the production of a particular protein, and is made up of a molecular sequence found on a section of DNA. Each gene is found on a precise location on a chromosome.

Limb girdles—Areas around the shoulders and hips.

Prenatal testing—Testing for a disease, such as a genetic condition, in an unborn baby.

Protein—Important building blocks of the body, composed of amino acids, involved in the formation of body structures and controlling the basic functions of the human body.

Proximal muscles—The muscles closest to the center of the body.

Scapular winging—The jutting back of the shoulder blades that can be caused by muscle weakness.

Skeletal muscle—Muscle under voluntary control that attaches to bone and control movement.

Laval, S. H., and K. M. Bushby. "Limb-girdle Muscular Dystrophies—From Genetics to Molecular Pathology." *Neuropathology and Applied Neurobiology* 30 (2004): 91–105.

Zatz, M., M. Vainzof, and M. R. Passos-Bueno. "Limb-girdle Muscular Dystrophy: One Gene with Different Phenotypes, One Phenotype with Different Genes." *Current Opinion in Neurology* 13, no. 5 (October 2000): 511–517.

ORGANIZATIONS

Muscular Dystrophy Association. 3300 East Sunrise Dr., Tucson, AZ 85718. (520) 529-2000 or (800) 572-1717. <http://www.mdausa.org/>.

Muscular Dystrophy Association Canada. 2345 Yonge St., Suite 900, Toronto, ONT M4P 2E5, Canada. (416) 488-2699. E-mail: info@mdac.ca. (April 21, 2005.) <http://www.mdac.ca/>.

Muscular Dystrophy Campaign. 7-11 Prescott Place, London, SW4 6BS, United Kingdom. +44(0) 7720 8055. E-mail: info@muscular-dystrophy.org. (April 21, 2005.) <http://www.muscular-dystrophy.org/>.

WEB SITES

Gordon, Erynn, Elena Pegoraro, and Eric Hoffman. "Limb-girdle Muscular Dystrophy Overview." Gene Clinics. (April 21, 2005.) <http://www.geneclinics.org/profiles/lgmd-overview/index.html>.

Suzanne M. Carter, MS, CGC

Lipoprotien-lipase deficiency
see Hyperlipoproteinemia Type I

Lissencephaly

Definition

Lissencephaly, literally meaning smooth brain, is a rare birth abnormality of the brain that results in profound mental retardation and severe seizures.

Lissencephaly is caused by an arrest in development of the fetal brain during early pregnancy. The cerebral cortex, the top layer of the brain controlling higher thought processes, does not develop the normal sulci, the indentations or valleys in the cortex, and gyri, the ridges or convolutions seen on the surface of the cortex. Instead, the cortex in a person with lissencephaly is thickened and smooth with disorganized neurons that have not migrated to their proper places. The typical cortex has six layers of neurons, but brains with lissencephaly usually have only four.

Description

The condition was first reported in 1914 by pathologists Culp and Erhardt, who described a human brain with a smooth surface, lacking the normal gyri. They called it lissencephaly.

Lissencephaly is one of a number of conditions called "neural migration disorders" that occur because the developing neurons do not proceed correctly to their normal place in the brain's cortex during fetal development. In fact, the brain of a person with lissencephaly, with its smooth and immature cortex, resembles a typical human fetal brain at about 10 to 14 weeks of development.

Children with lissencephaly are almost always severely to profoundly mentally retarded, and the vast majority develop seizures that are difficult to treat. Life expectancy is reduced, and survivors need constant care.

Lissencephaly can occur as an isolated birth abnormality or can be one of many birth abnormalities occurring together in a specific inherited syndrome. There are at least 10 inherited syndromes that include lissencephaly and many more that include variants of this brain malformation. Lissencephaly can also occur by itself without other characteristics.

Some cases of lissencephaly are caused by new changes in the genetic material of that particular baby—these cases are caused by sporadic, or random, **gene mutations** (also called *de novo*). This means that the genetic change is not present in the parents or anyone else in the family. Some cases of lissencephaly are caused by rearrangements of **chromosome** material that can be inherited from a healthy parent. Other types of lissencephaly are inherited in an autosomal recessive pattern. This means that a couple who has a child with an autosomal recessive lissencephaly syndrome has a 25% chance in any future pregnancy to have another affected child. There are also types of lissencephaly caused by changes in a **gene** or genes on the X chromosome. X-linked lissencephaly affects mainly males, who have only one X chromosome. Females who carry an X-linked gene change on one of their two X chromosomes often have mild brain changes.

Other known causes of lissencephaly include viral infections of the fetus or insufficient blood supply to the brain during the first trimester of pregnancy.

Genetic profile

There are a number of subtypes of lissencephaly that are distinguished by differences in the physical structure of the brain. Classical, or type 1, lissencephaly and cobblestone **dysplasia**, or type 2, lissencephaly are the most common subtypes.

Classical, or type 1, lissencephaly consists of a brain surface that is completely smooth except for a few shallow valleys (sulci). The cortex is thicker than normal and there are clumps of neurons found in areas outside the cortex (heterotopia). The corpus callosum, the band of tissue between the hemispheres of the brain, is often small and is sometimes absent. The posterior ventricles, the fluid-filled spaces in the center of the brain, are often larger than normal.

Type 1 lissencephaly can be seen in a number of genetic syndromes and can also occur by itself in a condition called Isolated Lissencephaly Sequence (ILS). The vast majority of cases of ILS is a result of mutations or deletions (missing sections) in one of two different genes involved in brain development.

The gene causing the majority of cases of ILS is called the LIS1 and is located on the short arm of chromosome 17. Between 40% and 64% of persons with ILS have a deletion of a portion of the LIS1 gene, and about 24% have a mutation that disrupts the normal function of the gene. Most deletions and mutations in the LIS1 gene are sporadic and are not present in other family members.

Another 12% of persons with ILS have a mutation in a gene called XLIS (or DCX), located on the long arm of the X chromosome. Mutations in XLIS cause X-linked lissencephaly in males and may or may not cause symptoms in the mothers who carry the mutation.

There are also a few cases of ILS that appear to be inherited in an autosomal recessive pattern. The mutated genes for this and other types of ILS have not been discovered.

An example of a genetic syndrome involving type 1 lissencephaly is **Miller-Dieker syndrome** (MDS). This disorder is caused by a deletion of part of the short arm of chromosome 17 (17p13) that includes the LIS1 gene. In addition to lissencephaly, children with MDS have distinctive facial features including a high forehead, short upturned nose, and thin lips. They also have narrowing at the temples and a small jaw, although these traits can also be seen in ILS and other lissencephaly syndromes. Children with MDS occasionally have other birth abnormalities of the heart, kidneys, or palate. Calcium deposits in the midline of the brain are common in MDS, but not in ILS or other syndromes.

Disorder	Inheritance	Gene location	Proportion of patients	Gene name	Protein product	Clinical test
MDS (Miller-Dieker syndrome)	AD	17p13.3	100%	LIS1	Platelet activating factor Acetylhydrolase 45K	Yes
ILS1 (Isolated lissencephaly sequence 1)	AD	17p13.3	>40%	LIS1	Platelet activating factor acetylhydrolase 45K	Yes
X-linked lissencephaly and subcortical band heterotropia	X-linked	Xq22.3–q23	Unknown	XLIS	Unknown	No
Cobblestone lissencephaly (lissencephaly type 2)	AR	Unknown	Unknown	Unknown	Unknown	No

Type 2 lissencephaly is also called cobblestone dysplasia because of the pebbled appearance to the surface of the cerebral cortex. Brains with cobblestone dysplasia often show abnormalities of the white matter, enlarged ventricles, underdeveloped brainstem and cerebellum, and absence of the corpus callosum. There are four known syndromes that include cobblestone dysplasia: cobblestone lissencephaly without other birth defects (CLO); Fukuyama congenital **muscular dystrophy** (FCMD); muscle-eye-brain disease (MEB); and **Walker-Warburg syndrome** (WWS). These disorders are quite rare and all are inherited in an autosomal recessive pattern. Diagnosis depends on MRI studies and clinical evaluations. There are no specific genetic tests available for clinical use for these conditions.

There are other rare syndromes involving lissencephaly and variants of lissencephaly, some of which are autosomal recessive and some X-linked. None of the genes responsible for these other conditions has been identified.

Demographics

Lissencephaly affects fewer than one in 100,000 individuals and occurs in all parts of the world. The sporadic and autosomal recessive types of lissencephaly occur equally in males and females. X-linked syndromes that include lissencephaly occur mainly in boys, although carrier mothers sometimes have milder signs.

Signs and symptoms

Many babies with lissencephaly appear normal at birth, although some have immediate respiratory problems. After the first few months at home, parents typically notice feeding problems, inability to visually track objects, and lessened activity in their child. Breath-holding spells (apnea) and muscle weakness are also common. Seizures frequently begin within the first year of life, are usually severe, and are difficult to treat with medication. Muscle weakness changes to spasticity (a condition of excessive muscle tension) over time. Repeated pneumonias from swallowing food down the airway and into the lungs are common.

Head size is usually within normal limits at birth; however, as the baby's body grows, head growth lags and a small head (microcephaly) results. Babies with isolated lissencephaly often have hollowing at the temples and small jaws, both thought to be a result of the abnormal brain shape. Genetic syndromes involving lissencephaly will include other symptoms and signs.

Diagnosis

The diagnosis of lissencephaly is initially based on tests using magnetic resonance imaging (MRI) and CT testing. MRI findings in type 1 lissencephaly include a lack of, or very shallow, convolutions on the surface of an unusually thick cerebral cortex. Enlargement of the ventricles is sometimes present.

On average, persons with Miller-Dieker syndrome have more severe MRI findings than persons with ILS. It is sometimes possible to distinguish between chromosome 17-related lissencephaly (ILS and MDS) and X-linked ILS based on MRI findings. The smooth brain appearance is more striking in the back portion of the brain in persons with chromosome 17 LIS1 deletions and mutations. In contrast, it is more conspicuous in the front part of the brain in persons with XLIS mutations. In addition, underdevelopment of part of the cerebellum is more commonly seen in persons with XLIS mutations.

Individuals with subcortical band heterotopia (SBH), a milder form of lissencephaly often seen in female carriers of XLIS, often have minor changes in the gyri, shallow sulci, and ribbons of white and gray matter beneath the cortex that show up on MRIs.

MRI findings in type 2 lissencephaly can include a cobblestone appearance of the cortex, enlarged ventricles, abnormalities of the white matter, and changes in the cerebellum, corpus callosum and brain stem.

A CT scan can be done to look for calcium deposits in the midline of the brain. Calcium deposits are common in MDS but not found in other lissencephaly syndromes.

In addition to MRI and CT testing, a careful clinical evaluation and examination by a medical geneticist is necessary to confirm the diagnosis and evaluate the child for the presence of a syndrome. It is essential for a child to have a precise diagnosis in order for genetic counselors to be able to give the family complete and accurate information about the inheritance pattern and chances for the condition to recur in future children.

To confirm the diagnosis of MDS or ILS, chromosome testing and other specialized genetic tests are often helpful. A test called fluorescence in situ hybridization (FISH) is used to detect LIS1 gene deletions. High resolution chromosome testing can often determine whether a deletion is sporadic or due to an inherited chromosome rearrangement. If necessary, mutation analysis, looking for specific errors in the sequence of the LIS1 or XLIS gene, can be performed.

Parents of a child with ILS who has a confirmed deletion or mutation in LIS1, and who have normal genetic studies themselves, have a less than 1% chance of having another child with ILS. Similarly, MDS with a confirmed sporadic deletion in LIS1 has a low chance of recurring. MDS caused by a chromosome rearrangement carries a higher chance of happening again. Actual risks depend on the specific rearrangement.

XLIS mutations are often inherited from a carrier mother. If a woman has **genetic testing** and is confirmed to have an XLIS mutation, she will have a 25% chance with each pregnancy to have an affected male and a 25% chance to have a carrier female who may have SBH.

If a detectable mutation, deletion, or chromosome rearrangement has been confirmed in the affected family member, prenatal diagnosis is available during future pregnancies. Ultrasound of the fetal anatomy during pregnancy cannot diagnose lissencephaly. However, ultrasound performed by a specialist at 18 to 22 weeks of pregnancy can sometimes detect other birth abnormalities that occur in some of the syndromes involving lissencephaly.

Treatment and management

There is no treatment or cure for lissencephaly. Seizures occur in almost all children with lissencephaly and are often difficult to control, even with the strongest anti-seizure medications. A severe type of seizure called infantile spasms can occur and may need to be treated with injections of adrenocorticotropic hormone (ACTH), although this treatment is not always effective.

Feeding difficulties can include choking, gagging, or regurgitating food or liquid. Aspiration, swallowing food down the trachea and into the lungs, is a serious problem that can lead to pneumonia. Liquids and thin foods can be thickened to make swallowing easier. There are medications available to help with reflux. Children who continue to have serious problems may need a permanent feeding tube placed into the stomach to ensure adequate nutrition.

Physical and occupational therapy can help prevent or reduce tightening of the joints and help to normalize

muscle tone. However, the improvements are often limited and temporary.

Prognosis

Persons with classical lissencephaly usually need lifelong care for all basic needs. Many babies will not live past infancy, but the average age of survival depends on the particular syndrome involved, the type of lissencephaly, and the severity of the brain abnormalities in a given child. Babies with MDS usually die by two years of age, but the majority of persons with ILS live into childhood, although often not into adulthood. Many babies with cobblestone dysplasia die in infancy; however, some affected people have lived into their 20s. In contrast, persons with SBH have very variable signs and symptoms, may be asymptomatic, mildly affected or severely retarded, and may have near-normal or normal life spans.

Resources

PERIODICALS

Berg, M. J., et al. "X-linked Female Band Heterotopia-Male Lissencephaly Syndrome." *Neurology* 50 (1998): 1143-1146.

Dobyns, W. B., et al. "Differences in the Gyral Pattern Distinguish Chromosome 17-linked and X-linked Lissencephaly." *Neurology* 53 (1999): 270-277.

Dobyns, W. B., et al. "Lissencephaly and Other Malformation Syndromes of Cortical Development: 1995 Update." *Neuropediatrics* 26 (1995): 132-147.

Matsumoto, N., et al. "Mutation Analysis of the DCX Gene and Genotype/Phenotype Correlation in Subcortical Band Heterotopia." *European Journal of Human Genetics* 9 (January 2001): 5-12.

ORGANIZATIONS

American Epilepsy Society. 342 North Main St., West Hartford, CT 06117. (860) 586-7505. Fax: (860 586-7550. info@aesnet.org. <http://www.aesnet.org>.

Epilepsy Foundation of America. 4351 Garden City Dr., Suite 406, Landover, MD 20785-2267. (301) 459-3700 or (800) 332-1000. <http://www.epilepsyfoundation.org>.

Lissencephaly Network, Inc. 716 Autumn Ridge Lane, Fort Wayne, IN 46804-6402. (219) 432-4310. Fax: (219) 432-4310. lissennet@lissencephaly.org. <http://www.lissencephaly.org>.

WEBSITES

Dobyns, William B. [1999]. "Lissencephaly Overview." *GeneClinics: Lissencephaly Overview.* University of Washington, Seattle. <http://www.geneclinics.org/profiles/lis-overview/>.

Lissencephaly Contact Group (UK). <http://www.lissencephaly.org.uk/index.htm>.

*The Lissencephaly Research Project (University of Chicago)*http://www.genes.uchicago.edu/ucgs/lissproj.html

NINDS Lissencephaly Information Page. <http://www.ninds.nih.gov/health_and_medical/disorders/lissencephaly.htm?format=printable>.

Barbara J. Pettersen

Liver cancer *see* **Hepatocellular carcinoma**

Long bone deficiencies associated with cleft lip/palate
see **Roberts SC phocomelia**

Long QT syndrome

Definition

Long QT syndrome (LQTS) is the overarching term used to describe a family of genetic or acquired disorders that are characterized by irregular heartbeats caused by problems in the heart's electrical activity (cardiac arrhythmias). The cardiac arrhythmias of Long QT syndrome can lead to cardiac arrest and sudden death. The syndrome is characterized by a longer-than-normal QT interval on an electrocardiogram.

Description

Long QT syndrome (LQTS) is one of the sudden arrhythmia death syndromes (SADS). It is a major cause of sudden, unexplained death in children and young adults, resulting in as many as 3,000–4,000 deaths per year in the United States. Its characteristic symptoms include seizures or fainting, often in response to stress, and long QT intervals found on an electrocardiogram.

LQTS was first described by C. Romano and coworkers in 1963, and by O. C. Ward in 1964 as a syndrome that was almost identical to **Jervell and Lange-Nielsen syndrome**, but without congenital deafness. Therefore, LQTS also is known as Romano-Ward syndrome or Ward-Romano syndrome.

LQTS involves irregularities in the recharging of the heart's electrical system that occurs after each heartbeat or contraction. The QT interval is the period of relaxation or recovery that is required for the repolarization, or recharging, of the electrical system following each heart contraction. Depolarization, or electrical activity that causes heart contraction, and repolarization are orchestrated by the flow of potassium, sodium, and calcium through the heart cell's ion channels. As sodium channels in the heart open, positively charged sodium ions flow into the cells, making the inner surfaces of the cell membranes more positive than the outside and creating the action potential, or electrical charge. During depolarization, the sodium channels shut and, after a delay, potassium channels open and allow positively charged potassium ions to move out of the cells, returning the cell membranes to their resting state in preparation for the next heart contraction.

Individuals with LQTS have an unusually long period of relaxation or recovery called the QT interval after each heart contraction. If the electrical impulse for the next contraction arrives before the end of the QT recovery period, a specific arrhythmia arises in the ventricles, or lower chambers, of the heart. This arrhythmia is called polymorphous ventricular tachycardia, meaning fast heart (above 100 beats per second), or *torsade de pointes*, which means turning of the points. A normal heartbeat begins in the right atrium of the heart and progresses down to the ventricles. In ventricular tachycardia or *torsade de pointes*, the heartbeat may originate in the ventricle. Usually this very fast and abnormal heartbeat reverts to normal. If it does not, it leads to ventricular fibrillation, in which the heart beats too quickly, irregularly, and ineffectively. This can result in cardiac arrest and death. Variations in the QT interval from one heart cell to another also can cause arrhythmias and ventricular fibrillation in LQTS.

LQTS usually results from changes, or mutations, in one of seven or more genes. These genes encode proteins that form the ion channels in the heart. Depending on the other functions of the **gene** that is mutated, features beyond irregular heartbeats may occur in individuals affected by the different forms of LQTS. Although some mutations causing LQTS can arise spontaneously in an individual, they are most often passed on from parent to offspring. Thus, LQTS usually runs in families.

Acquired LQTS is caused by factors other than genetic **inheritance** or mutation. Many different medications, including heart medicines, antibiotics, digestive medicines, psychiatric drugs, and antihistamines, as well as certain poisons, can result in LQTS. Some of these drugs block potassium ion channels in the heart. Diuretic medications can cause LQTS by lowering levels of potassium, magnesium, and calcium in the blood. Mineral imbalances, resulting from chronic vomiting, diarrhea, anorexia, or starvation can also result in LQTS. Additional medical issues, such as strokes, some neurological problems, or **alcoholism**, also can cause LQTS. However, since only certain individuals develop LQTS under these circumstances, multiple genetic factors also play a role in the acquired disorder.

Genetic profile

Although all of the genes that are known to be involved in LQTS encode proteins that form sections or subunits of ion channels through cellular membranes, the type of LQTS depends on the specific gene defect. Although new genetic mutations that cause LQTS are still being discovered, the majority of inherited LQTS

cases result from mutations in KVLQT1 or KCNE1, causing LQT1, or mutations in HERG or KCNE2, causing LQT2.

Most types of LQTS are autosomal dominant **genetic disorders**: the genes that cause LQTS are carried on one of the 22 pairs of numbered autosomal chromosomes, rather than on the X or Y sex chromosomes. Furthermore, in autosomal dominant conditions, only one copy of the mutant, or nonworking, gene is necessary for the development of LQTS. An individual who inherits a normal gene copy from one parent and an abnormal gene copy from the other parent is likely to have LQTS. The children of an individual with one normal gene copy and one mutated copy have a 50% chance of inheriting LQTS.

Some types of LQTS are inherited in an autosomal recessive pattern. In an autosomal recessive pattern, two copies of the mutant, or nonworking, gene are needed to develop the symptoms of LQTS. In these cases, both parents each carry one copy of a mutant gene. Individuals with only one copy of a nonworking gene for a recessive condition are known as carriers and have no problems related to the condition. In fact, each person carries between five and 10 nonworking genes for harmful, recessive conditions. However, when two people with the same nonworking recessive gene have children together, there is a 25% chance, with each pregnancy, for the child to inherit two nonworking copies, one from each parent. That child then has no working copies of the gene and has the signs and symptoms associated with a recessive condition.

Long QT syndrome 1 and long QT syndrome 5

Long QT syndrome 1 (LQT1) is the most common form of LQTS. It is caused by any of a number of **gene mutations** in the KVLQT1 (KvLQT1) gene located on the short arm of **chromosome** 11 (11p15.5); KVLQT1 also is known as KCNQ1. The KVLQT1 gene codes a critical part of a voltage-gated potassium ion channel that helps the heart beat. Even if the KVLQT1 creates an abnormal potassium ion channel part, it can still join with the other parts of the channel. A potassium ion channel that is constructed with an abnormal part or subunit does not work as well as a channel formed of all normal parts. Most mutations in KVLQT1 causing LQT1 are passed down in an autosomal dominant pattern through the family; however, some mutations in this gene may be passed down in an autosomal recessive pattern. In these cases, LQTS is present only in individuals with two abnormal KVLQT1 genes, one inherited from each parent. The pattern of inheritance depends on which type of LQTS-causing mutation is present in the family because some mutations cause a potassium ion channel part that works better than other mutations. Mutation analysis of the KVLQT1 gene and/or a detailed medical family history can determine the inheritance pattern of LQT1 in a specific family.

The KCNE1 (MinK or IsK) gene on chromosome 21 codes for another critical part of the voltage-gated potassium ion channel that combines with the part encoded by KVLQT1. Together, they form the ion channel that is responsible for the heart's potassium current. The channel encoded in KCNE1 and KVLQT1 is a slow ion channel that starts working when the heart is in depolarization. Depolarization of the heart causes the channel to open and potassium ions to move freely out of the cells during repolarization. Mutations in KCNE1 also can cause a defective potassium channel protein, resulting in a LQT1 form of LQTS; however, LQTS resulting from mutations in KCNE1 may also be referred to as long QT syndrome 5 (LQT5). Mutations in potassium channel genes reduce the number of functional potassium channels in the heart and lengthen the QT interval by delaying depolarization.

Jervell and Lange-Nielsen syndrome

Jervell and Lange-Nielsen syndrome (JLNS) is a specific autosomal recessive form of LQTS. In JLNS, an individual has inherited two copies of an abnormal KVLQT1 or KCNE1 gene: one inherited from the mother and the other from the father. The syndrome is characterized by congenital deafness as well as a prolonged QT interval.

Long QT syndrome 2 and long QT syndrome 6

Long QT syndrome 2 (LQT2) is the second most common form of LQTS. Mutations in the HERG gene (so named because it is the human equivalent of a fruit fly gene called ether-a-go-go) can result in LQT2. HERG, located on chromosome 7 (7q35-q36), encodes a protein part of another potassium ion channel found in the heart. Mutations in HERG result in loss of the potassium current called IKr.

Long QT syndrome 6 (LQT6) is caused by mutations in the KCNE2 gene. The KCNE2 or MiRP1 (for MinK-related) gene is located on chromosome 21 (21q22.1). The gene encodes a protein part that combines with the protein encoded by HERG to form a potassium ion channel used in the heart. Mutations in potassium channel genes reduce the number of functional potassium channels in the heart and lengthen the QT interval by delaying depolarization.

Long QT syndrome 3

Mutations in the SCN5A gene can result in an uncommon form of LQTS known as long QT syndrome

3 (LQT3). SCN5A, on the short arm of chromosome 3 (3p21), encodes a part of a cardiac sodium ion channel. Some mutations in this gene prevent the channel from being turned off or inactivated. Thus, although the channel opens normally and sodium ions flow into the cells with each contraction, the channel does not close properly. Sodium ions continue to leak into the cells, which prolongs the action potential.

Brugada syndrome

Brugada syndrome is caused by a mutation in SCN5A, located on the short arm of chromosome 3 (3p21). The type of mutation that causes Brugada decreases the flow of sodium ions into the cells and shortens the time of action potential. The symptoms of Brugada syndrome, which includes ventricular arrhythmia, cardiac arrest, and sudden death, are caused by the shortened action potential.

Long QT syndrome 4

Long QT syndrome 4 (LQT4) is most often referred to as sick sinus syndrome with bradycardia. LQT4 is associated with mutation in the ankyrin-B gene called ANK2, which is located on the long arm of chromosome 4 (4q25-q27). ANK2 plays a vital role in the organization of a sodium pump that exchanges sodium and calcium in and out of the heart. A mutation in the ANK2 gene reduces ability to get necessary proteins and calcium to the heart cells. Individuals with LQT4 have the typical cardiac dysfunction seen in LQTS. However, a long QT interval is not always seen in individuals with LQT4, so it is considered a condition distinct from classical long QT syndromes.

Long QT syndrome 7

Long QT syndrome 7 (LQT7) is also known as Andersen cardiodysrhythmic periodic paralysis, Andersen syndrome, periodic paralysis, potassium-sensitive cardiodysrhythmic type, and Andersen-Tawil syndrome. LQT7 is associated with mutations in the KCNJ2 gene located on the long arm of chromosome 17 (17q23.1-q24.2). Mutations in KCNJ2 decrease the ability of a potassium channel in the heart to react to a specific important protein, called phosphatidylinositol 4,5-bisphosphate (PIP2), and move potassium in and out of the body's muscles. The movement of potassium in and out of the body's muscles allows movement of the arms, legs, and other muscles.

Long QT syndrome with syndactyly

Long QT syndrome with syndactyly is also known as Timothy syndrome. Long QT syndrome with syndactyly is caused by new mutations in the CACNA1C gene located on the short arm of chromosome 12 (12p13.3). Mutations in CACNA1C keep calcium ion channels open and pulling in calcium ions. By constantly pulling in calcium ions, repolarization is delayed and the chance for an irregular heart beat, or arrhythmia, is increased.

Other forms of LQTS

A small number of individuals with LQTS have mutations in more than one of the known genes and may have symptoms of multiple LQTS types. Other families with inherited LQTS lack mutations in any of these known genes, suggesting the existence of other genes that can cause LQTS. Furthermore, individuals with identical LQTS genes may differ significantly in the severity of their symptoms, again suggesting the existence of other genes that can cause or modify LQTS. Between 2000 and 2005, several large studies characterized the presence of gene variants or alleles in genes, including KCNA5, KCNQ1, KCNH2, KCNE1, and KCNE2, that help control the length of the QT interval.

Demographics

Large-scale studies of LQTS, such as the International Registry for LQTS established in 1979, have revealed that the disorder is much more prevalent than was originally thought. Inherited LQTS is estimated to occur in one out of every 5,000–10,000 individuals and it occurs in all racial and ethnic groups. LQTS may result in fetal death, may account for some cases of sudden infant death syndrome (SIDS), and has been implicated in many instances of sudden death and unexplained drowning among individuals who were previously without symptoms.

As an autosomal, non-sex-linked genetic disorder, LQTS should affect males and females in equal numbers. However, it appears to be more prevalent among women. Nearly 70% of the time, a female is the first member of a family recognized as having LQTS. Females are two to three times more likely than males to exhibit symptoms of LQTS. However, in general, males manifest symptoms of LQTS at an earlier age than females. At puberty, the QT interval shortens in males, whereas in females it stays the same or shortens only slightly. Therefore, unaffected women have slightly longer QT intervals than unaffected men. Men with LQT1 or LQT2 have shorter QT intervals than either women or children with these two forms of the disorder. Women also are more likely than men to develop drug-induced or acquired LQTS. These gender-related differences may be due to the effects of the female hormone estrogen on the regulation of cardiac ion channels, particularly potassium channels.

Signs and symptoms

Tragically for many individuals with LQTS, sudden death by cardiac arrest is the first symptom. For this reason, LQTS sometimes is referred to as a "silent" killer. Approximately one-third of deaths from LQTS are not preceded by showing any symptoms of the disease. At least one-third of the individuals carrying a gene variant that causes LQTS do not exhibit any symptoms. Sudden infant death syndrome (SIDS) claims the lives of one or two out of every 1,000 infants. In 1998, the results of the Multicenter Italian Study of Neonatal Electrocardiography and a SIDS study found that a large number of SIDS victims had prolonged QT intervals.

Common symptoms of LQTS include dizziness, sudden loss of consciousness or fainting spells (syncopes), or convulsive seizures. These occur because the heart is unable to pump sufficient blood to the brain. Following a loss of consciousness or syncope, the *torsade de pointes* rhythm (fast heart beat of the lower heart chambers) usually reverts spontaneously to a normal rhythm within one minute or less, and the individual regains consciousness. These symptoms may first appear during infancy or early childhood, although sometimes no symptoms are evident until adulthood. Some individuals may experience syncopal episodes from childhood on, whereas others may experience one or two episodes as children, with no recurrence throughout adulthood. On average, males with LQTS first exhibit symptoms at about age eight and females at about age 14. These symptoms usually occur upon awakening, during strenuous physical activity, a fast change in posture, or during moments of excitement or stress.

Affected newborn infants and children under the age of three may exhibit slower than normal resting heart rates. Individuals with LQTS may experience irregular heartbeats accompanied by chest pain.

Symptoms of LQTS can vary depending on the specific gene mutation. Certain mutations in the KVLQT1 gene that cause LQT1 may result in arrhythmias when an individual is under stress. Exercise is a major trigger for cardiac events in LQT1. Swimming can trigger syncopic episodes and appears to be a gene-specific trigger in individuals with KVLQT1 mutations. Sudden loud noises, such as telephones or alarm clocks, are more likely to trigger arrhythmias and syncopic episodes in individuals with LQT2. Cardiac events, including syncope, aborted cardiac arrest, and sudden death, are more common among individuals with LQT1 or LQT2 than among those with LQT3. However, cardiac events are more likely to be lethal in individuals with LQT3. Certain variants of the SCN5A gene that cause LQT3 result in abnormal heart rhythms during sleep.

Individuals with LQT4 have the typical cardiac dysfunction seen in LQTS: slow heart beat (sinus node bradycardia) leading to the abnormal function of the body's natural pacemaker (sinus node dysfunction), severely abnormal heartbeat of the lower heart chambers (ventricular fibrillation), rapid heartbeat (ventricular tachycardia), and episodes of severely abnormal heartbeat in the heart's upper chambers (atrial fibrillation) in adulthood (though not childhood), and risk of sudden death. However, a long QT interval is not always seen in individuals with LQT4, so it is considered a condition distinct from classical long QT syndromes. Individuals with some of the variants of the KCNE2 gene that cause LQT6 may be adversely affected by exercise and some medications.

Individuals with LQT7 are affected by episodes in which they cannot move (potassium-sensitive periodic paralysis), heart problems, and unusual face and body features. The symptoms of LQT7 can include short stature, wide-spaced eyes (hypertelorism), low-set ears, small chin (hypoplastic mandible), palate abnormalities, curved fingers and toes (clinodactyly), fused fingers and toes (syndactyly), curved back (**scoliosis**), periodic paralysis, long QT interval, abnormal heart beat in the upper and lower chambers of the heart, rapid heart beat, and sudden death.

Long QT syndrome with syndactyly is characterized by symptoms in multiple parts of the body that include lethal heart arrhythmias, webbing of fingers and toes, heart defects present at birth, immune deficiency, severe low blood sugar that comes and goes, developmental delays, and **autism**.

Diagnosis

A diagnosis of LQTS most often comes from an electrocardiogram (ECG or EKG). An ECG records the electrical activity of the heart, using electrical leads placed at specific sites on the body. The electrical activity due to the depolarization and repolarization of the heart is recorded by each lead and added together. The recordings, on paper or on a monitor, show a series of peaks, valleys, and plateaus.

The QRS complex is a sharp peak and dip on the ECG that occurs as the electrical impulses fire the cells of the ventricles, causing contraction and depolarization of the action potential. The *torsade de pointes* (turning of the points) refers to these spikes in the QRS complex. Sometimes it is possible to diagnose *torsade de pointes* from an ECG. The T wave on the ECG occurs as the cells recover and prepare to fire again with the next heartbeat. Thus, the T-wave represents the repolarization of the ventricles. The QT interval on the ECG is the period from the start of the depolarization of the ventricles (Q), as the electrical current traverses the ventricles from the

inside to the outside, through the repolarization of the ventricles (T), as the current passes from the outside to the inside. The QT interval represents the firing and recovery cycle of the ventricles. In LQTS, the QT interval on the ECG may be a few one-hundredths of a second longer than normal. A QT interval that is longer than 440 milliseconds is considered to be prolonged. There also may be abnormalities in the T-wave of the ECG.

ECGs may vary depending on the specific mutation that is the cause of the LQTS. Furthermore, up to 12% of individuals with LQTS may show normal-appearing or borderline-normal QT intervals. An individual's ECGs can vary, and additional ECGs or ECGs performed during exercise may reveal an abnormal QT interval. ECGs of parents or siblings also may contribute to a diagnosis, since one parent, and possibly siblings, may carry a gene variation that causes LQTS and, therefore, may exhibit a prolonged QT interval on an ECG.

Children with LQTS may exhibit a low heart rate; specifically, a resting heart rate that is below the second percentile for their age. A fast heart rate of 140–200 beats per minute may indicate tachycardia resulting from LQTS. Convulsive seizures due to LQTS sometimes are misdiagnosed as **epilepsy**, particularly in children. Some individuals with LQTS may have low levels of potassium in their blood.

Some individuals with LQTS may be identified by the combination of the standard diagnostic measurement with ECG and physical examination. Long QT syndrome with syndactyly, LQT7, and Jervell and Lange-Nielsen syndrome have features, such as a hearing impairment, fused fingers, or facial features, that may lead to a diagnosis.

Currently, there is not a specific diagnostic test that can identify all cases of LQTS. The difficulty in developing a comprehensive test is due to the fact that more than 200 specific changes in many different genes have been found to be responsible for LQTS. Additionally, approximately half of the individuals diagnosed with LQTS do not carry any of the known genetic variations. However, when family members are known to carry a specific LQTS gene mutation, **genetic testing** may be used to diagnose LQTS in other family members.

Treatment and management

Beta-adrenergic blockers, or beta-blockers, are the most common treatment for the ventricular arrhythmia resulting from LQTS. Propranolol is the most frequently prescribed drug. It lowers the heart rate and the strength of the heart muscle contractions, thereby reducing the oxygen requirement of the heart. Propranolol also regulates abnormal heart rates and reduces blood pressure.

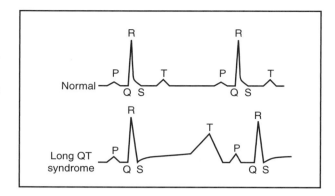

Normal

Long QT syndrome

A comparison of the "QT" interval found in a normal patient versus one diagnosed with long QT syndrome obtained from an electrocardiogram. The typical QT interval is 400-440 milliseconds, but for patients with long QT syndrome the interval exceeds 460 milliseconds. This lengthened interval is obvious in the comparison above. *(Gale Group)*

Approximately 90% of individuals with LQTS can be treated successfully with these drugs. However, since the prophylactic effects disappear within one or two days of stopping the beta-blocker, treatment with these drugs usually lasts for life. Since the first symptom of LQTS may be sudden death, younger individuals with prolonged QT intervals or with family histories of LQTS commonly are treated with beta-blockers, even in the absence of symptoms.

Beta-blockers such as propranolol are considered to be safe medications. Any side effects from propranolol are usually mild and disappear once the body has adjusted to the drug. However, propranolol and other beta-blockers can interact dangerously with many other medications.

As knowledge of the causes of LQTS increases, other drugs may prove to be more effective for treating some forms of LQTS. For example, mexiletine, a sodium-channel blocker, is used to shorten the QT interval in individuals with LQT3 that results from mutations in the SCN5A gene.

Elevating the levels of blood potassium may relieve symptoms of LQTS in individuals with mutations in potassium channel genes. For example, increased blood potassium raises the outward potassium current in the HERG-encoded channel. Thus, treatment with potassium can compensate to some extent for the shortage of functional potassium ion channels in individuals with LQT2, thereby shortening the QT interval.

Left cardiac sympathetic denervation, the surgical cutting of a group of nerves connecting the brain and the heart, may reduce cardiac arrhythmias in individuals with LQTS. Pacemakers or automatic implanted cardioverter defibrillators (AICDs) are also used to regulate the heartbeat or to detect and correct abnormal heart rhythms. Sometimes, a pacemaker or AICD is used in combination with beta-blockers.

Since the likelihood of developing symptoms of LQTS after about age 45 is quite low, individuals who are at least middle-aged when first diagnosed may not be treated. However, all individuals that have been diagnosed with LQTS must avoid reductions in blood potassium levels, such as those that occur with the use of diuretic drugs. Additionally, individuals with LQTS must avoid a very long list of drugs and medications that can increase the QT interval or otherwise exacerbate the syndrome.

Infants in LQTS families should be screened with ECGs and monitored closely, due to the 41-fold increase in the risk of SIDS.

Individuals with LQTS usually are advised to refrain from competitive sports and to have someone around them during moderate exercise. Family members may be advised to learn cardiopulmonary resuscitation (CPR) in case of cardiac arrest.

Individuals with LQTS require special attention and careful management before, during, and after surgery. In 2005, recommendations before surgery where developed, and include: monitoring baseline QT interval; using adequate amounts of beta-blocker medications, maintaining a quiet and calm environment; preparing a defibrillator to be available for immediate use; using premedications as needed; ensuring patient is adequately anesthetized before laryngoscopy and tracheal intubation to avoid sympathetic stimulation; and using of topical anesthesia before intubation. During the operation, recommendations include: monitoring the QT interval, keeping a quiet and calm environment, and avoiding patient hypothermia. Specific agents are recommended to be used for general anesthesia, including propofol for induction or as continuous infusion throughout, isoflurane as volatile agent of choice, vecuronium for muscle relaxation (dose appropriately to avoid pharmacologic reversal), and fentanyl for analgesia. After surgery, careful monitoring of the patient and their QT interval is recommended until the patient has recovered from anesthesia and the monitored QT interval has returned to baseline. It is also recommended to ensure adequate pain control after surgery.

Prognosis

The prognosis usually is quite good for LQTS patients who receive treatment. Symptoms may disappear completely and, often, at least some of the ECG abnormalities revert to normal. In contrast, the death rate for LQTS can be very high among untreated individuals.

Women with LQTS usually do not experience an increase in cardiac events during pregnancy or delivery. However, they may experience an increase in serious

KEY TERMS

Action potential—The wave-like change in the electrical properties of a cell membrane, resulting from the difference in electrical charge between the inside and outside of the membrane. The action potential acts as a signal for certain activities and processes in the body.

Arrhythmia—Abnormal heart rhythm; examples are a slow, fast, or irregular heart rate.

Beta-adrenergic blocker—A drug that works by controlling the nerve impulses along specific nerve pathways.

Depolarization—The dissipation of an electrical charge through a membrane. In the heart, depolarization causes the heart muscle to contract.

Electrocardiogram (ECG, EKG) —A test used to measure electrical impulses coming from the heart in order to gain information about its structure or function.

Fibrillation—A rapid, irregular heartbeat.

Ion channel—Cell membrane proteins that control the movement of ions into and out of the cell.

QT interval—The section on an electrocardiogram between the start of the QRS complex and the end of the T wave, representing the firing or depolarization of the ventricles and the period of recovery prior to repolarization, or recharging, for the next contraction.

Repolarization—Period when the heart cells are at rest, preparing for the next wave of electrical current (depolarization).

Syncope—A brief loss of consciousness caused by insufficient blood flow to the brain.

Tachycardia—An excessively rapid heartbeat; a heart rate above 100 beats per minute.

Torsade de pointes—Term that means turning of the points; a type of fast heart beat or tachycardia of the ventricles that is characteristic of long QT syndrome.

Resources

PERIODICALS

Ackerman, M. J., D. J. Tester, and C. J. Porter. "Swimming, a Gene-Specific Arrhythmogenic Trigger for Inherited Long QT Syndrome." *Mayo Clin Proc.* 74 (November 1999): 1088–94.

Fahje, C. J. "An Overview of Congenital Long QT Syndrome." *J Contin Educ Nurs* 36(Jan–Feb 2005): 14–15.

Kies, S. J., C. M. Pabelick, H. A. Hurley, R. D. White, and M. J. Ackerman. "Anesthesia for Patients with Congenital Long QT Syndrome." *Anesthesiology* 2005 Jan;102(1): 204–10.

Li, H., J. Fuentes-Garcia, and J. A. Towbin. "Current Concepts in Long QT Syndrome." *Pediatr Cardiol.* 21 (November 2000): 542–50.

Wang, Q., Q. Chen, and J. A. Towbin. "Genetics, Molecular Mechanisms and Management of Long QT Syndrome." *Ann. Med.* 30, no. 1 (February 1998): 58–65.

ORGANIZATIONS

Cardiac Arrhythmias Research and Education Foundation, Inc. 2082 Michelson Dr., #301, Irvine, CA 92612-1212. (949) 752-2273 or (800) 404-9500. E-mail: care@longqt.org. (April 11, 2005.) <http://www.longqt.org>.

SADS Foundation. PO Box 58767, 508 East South Temple, Suite 20, Salt Lake City, UT 84102. (800) 786-7723. (April 11, 2005.)<http://www.sads.org>.

WEB SITES

Cardiac Arrhythmias Research and Education Foundation (CARE). "Gender Differences in Long QT—What Are They?" (April 11, 2005.) <http://www.longqt.org/genderdiff.html>.

Cardiac Arrhythmias Research and Education Foundation (CARE). "The Long QT Syndrome and Pregnancy." (April 11, 2005.) <http://www.longqt.org/longqtpreg.html>.

First International Symposium on Long QT syndrome on Internet. (April 11, 2005.)<http://lqts-symposium.org/ing_home.shtml>.

Health on the Net Foundation. "Heart Misfiring May Cause Some Cases of SIDS." (2002) (April 11, 2005.)<http://www.hon.ch/News/HSN/510372.html>.

Mayo Clinic. "Long QT Syndrome." (April 11, 2005.) <http://www.mayoclinic.com/invoke.cfm?objectid=47C52B5C-DA54-4EF4-864C9B4F3F60A5CB>.

episodes of irregular heartbeat in the months following delivery. This is especially true for women who have experienced syncopic episodes prior to pregnancy. This increase in symptoms may be due to the physical and emotional stress of the postpartum period. Women who receive beta-blocker therapy during pregnancy and following delivery experience far fewer cardiac events. Beta-blockers do not appear to adversely affect a pregnancy, nor do they appear to harm the fetus.

Dawn Jacob Laney, MS
Margaret Alic, PhD

Lou Gehrig disease
see **Amyotrophic lateral sclerosis**

Lowe oculocerbrorenal syndrome
see **Lowe syndrome**

Lowe oculocerebrorenal syndrome

Definition

Lowe oculocerebrorenal syndrome is a rare genetic condition that affects males. It is caused by an enzyme deficiency. It affects many body systems including the eyes, the kidneys, and the brain.

Description

Lowe oculocerebrorenal syndrome was first described by Dr. Charles Lowe in 1952. The syndrome is caused by a change (mutation) in the OCRL1 **gene**. This gene is responsible for the production of the enzyme phosphatidylinositol 4,5-bisphosphate 5-phosphatase. A mutation in the OCRL1 gene leads to a decrease in enzyme activity. This decrease in the activity of phosphatidylinositol 4,5-bisphosphate 5-phosphatase is responsible for the physical and mental problems associated with Lowe oculocerebrorenal syndrome. The reason why a deficiency of this enzyme causes Lowe oculocerebrorenal syndrome is still unknown. Phosphatidylinositol 4,5-bisphosphate 5-phosphate phosphatase is thought to be limited to a specific part of the cell called the "Golgi apparatus." The relationship between the function of the Golgi apparatus, the enzyme deficiency, and the features of Lowe oculocerebrorenal syndrome is unclear.

The name Lowe oculocerebrorenal syndrome describes the body systems most commonly affected by this genetic disease. The term "oculo" refers to the eye problems commonly seen in individuals with the disease. Cataracts (cloudiness of the lens of the eye) are a classic feature and are usually present at birth (congenital). Other eye problems are also common. The term "cerebro" refers to the brain dysfunction commonly seen in the disease. The majority of affected males have mental retardation and behavior disturbances. The term "renal" represents the associated kidney problems, which can interfere with normal bone development and eventually lead to kidney failure.

Genetic profile

Changes (mutations) in the OCRL1 gene decrease the activity of the enzyme phosphatidylinositol 4,5-bisphosphate 5-phosphatase. There have been many different mutations identified in the OCRL1 gene. These mutations may be different between families. The OCRL1 gene is located on the X **chromosome**. Since the OCRL1 gene is located on the X chromosome, Lowe oculocerebrorenal syndrome is considered to be X-linked. This means that it only affects males.

A person's sex is determined by his or her chromosomes. Males have one X chromosome and one Y chromosome, while females have two X chromosomes. Males who possess a mutation in their OCRL1 gene will develop Lowe oculocerebrorenal syndrome. Females who possess a mutation in their OCRL1 gene will not; they are considered to be carriers. This is because females have another X chromosome without the mutation that allows normal function, and prevents them from getting this disease. If a woman is a carrier, she has a 50% risk with any pregnancy to pass on her X chromosome with the mutation. Therefore, with every male pregnancy she has a 50% risk of having an affected son, and with every female pregnancy she has a 50% risk of having a daughter who is a carrier.

Demographics

Lowe oculocerebrorenal syndrome affects approximately one in 100,000 live births. It occurs evenly among ethnic groups. Almost always, only male children are affected. Women carriers usually do not have physical or mental problems related to the disease.

Signs and symptoms

The signs and symptoms of Lowe oculocerebrorenal syndrome are variable. Some individuals with Lowe oculocerebrorenal syndrome have many severe symptoms, while other affected individuals have fewer, more mild symptoms.

Eye problems are a common feature of Lowe oculocerebrorenal syndrome. Congenital cataracts are a classic feature of the disorder. These cataracts may be one of the first symptoms noticed during infancy. Approximately 50% of males with Lowe oculocerebrorenal syndrome will develop increased pressure behind the eye (**glaucoma**). This pressure can damage the eye. Other eye problems include strabismus (crossed or divergent eyes), nystagmus (uncontrollable rhythmic eye movements), and microphthalmia (small eyes).

The nervous system (brain and nerves) is also typically affected by Lowe oculocerebrorenal syndrome. Mental retardation is a common feature of Lowe oculocerebrorenal syndrome. It can vary between mild and severe. Some males with Lowe oculocerebrorenal syndrome have normal intelligence. Seizures and behavior disturbances can also be seen in individuals with Lowe oculocerebrorenal syndrome. Behavior disturbances can include temper tantrums, aggression, obsessions, and repetitive hand movements. One of the first signs of brain dysfunction caused by Lowe oculocerebrorenal syndrome is muscle weakness (hypotonia) during infancy.

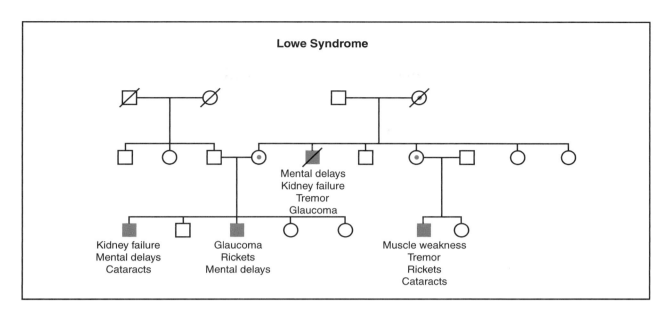

Lowe Syndrome

Mental delays
Kidney failure
Tremor
Glaucoma

Kidney failure
Mental delays
Cataracts

Glaucoma
Rickets
Mental delays

Muscle weakness
Tremor
Rickets
Cataracts

(Gale Group)

Kidney problems are another common finding in individuals with Lowe oculocerebrorenal syndrome. The kidneys normally filter chemicals and acids from the body. The kidneys allow the body to keep needed substances and to remove unneeded substances through the urine. Individuals with Lowe oculocerebrorenal syndrome cannot do this properly, allowing needed substances (calcium, phosphate, etc.) to be excreted in the urine. This kidney disturbance can ultimately lead to kidney failure.

Individuals with Lowe oculocerebrorenal syndrome frequently have slow growth and have short stature. Problems with bones can also develop due to the loss of certain substances through the kidneys. Rickets and easily breakable bones are common features. Joints may also become inflamed in individuals with Lowe oculocerebrorenal syndrome.

Diagnosis

The diagnosis of Lowe oculocerebrorenal syndrome is based initially on the presence of the symptoms of the disorder. Lowe oculocerebrorenal syndrome is definitively diagnosed by measuring the activity of the enzyme phosphatidylinositol 4,5-bisphosphate 5-phosphatase. When the activity of this enzyme is very low it is diagnostic of Lowe oculocerebrorenal syndrome. In order to perform this test a small piece of skin must be removed from the patient's body (skin biopsy). The enzyme is then measured from cells in this skin sample. In some cases it is also possible to look for a mutation in the OCRL1 gene. The presence of mutation confirms the diagnosis of Lowe oculocerebrorenal syndrome in males.

Determining if a woman is a carrier of Lowe oculocerebrorenal syndrome can be done several different ways. Females who carry a mutation in their OCRL1 gene commonly have changes in the lens of the eye. These changes can only be detected by an ophthalmologist with a special eye examination. These changes do not cause vision problems. The eye difference seen in carriers of Lowe oculocerebrorenal syndrome is best observed once females reach adulthood. Recent reports suggest that a detailed eye exam can detect 90% of carriers. In addition to eye examinations, carrier detection can also be performed with **DNA** testing. If the OCRL1 mutation has been identified in an affected male in the family, the females in the family can undergo DNA testing.

Prenatal diagnosis is possible by measuring the activity of phosphatidylinositol 4,5-bisphosphate 5-phosphatase in fetal tissue drawn by **amniocentesis** or chorionic villus sampling (CVS). In cases where the mutation is known, DNA testing can be used in prenatal diagnosis. Fetuses should be tested if the mother is a carrier of a Lowe oculocerebrorenal syndrome. A woman is at risk of being a carrier if she has a son with Lowe oculocerebrorenal syndrome or someone in her family with Lowe oculocerebrorenal syndrome. Any woman at risk of being a carrier can undergo testing to determine if she is at risk to have a son with Lowe oculocerebrorenal syndrome.

Treatment and management

There is currently no cure for Lowe oculocerebrorenal syndrome. Individuals with Lowe oculocerebrorenal syndrome benefit from therapies and regular medical care.

KEY TERMS

Amniocentesis—A procedure performed at 16-18 weeks of pregnancy in which a needle is inserted through a woman's abdomen into her uterus to draw out a small sample of the amniotic fluid from around the baby. Either the fluid itself or cells from the fluid can be used for a variety of tests to obtain information about genetic disorders and other medical conditions in the fetus.

Cataract—A clouding of the eye lens or its surrounding membrane that obstructs the passage of light resulting in blurry vision. Surgery may be performed to remove the cataract.

Cerebro—Related to the head or brain.

Chorionic villus sampling (CVS)—A procedure used for prenatal diagnosis at 10-12 weeks gestation. Under ultrasound guidance a needle is inserted either through the mother's vagina or abdominal wall and a sample of cells is collected from around the fetus. These cells are then tested for chromosome abnormalities or other genetic diseases.

Congenital—Refers to a disorder which is present at birth.

Germ line mosaicism—A rare event that occurs when one parent carries an altered gene mutation that affects his or her germ line cells (either the egg or sperm cells) but is not found in the somatic (body) cells.

Glaucoma—An increase in the fluid eye pressure, eventually leading to damage of the optic nerve and ongoing visual loss.

Mutation—A permanent change in the genetic material that may alter a trait or characteristic of an individual, or manifest as disease, and can be transmitted to offspring.

Nystagmus—Involuntary, rhythmic movement of the eye.

Oculo—Related to the eye.

Renal—Related to the kidneys.

Rickets—A childhood disease caused by vitamin D deficiency, resulting in soft and malformed bones.

Strabismus—An improper muscle balance of the ocular musles resulting in crossed or divergent eyes.

Physical therapy, occupational therapy, and speech therapy may be recommended due to developmental delays. Regular eye exams by an ophthalmologist are also recommended. Patients with Lowe oculocerebrorenal syndrome should be followed by a nephrologist (kidney doctor). Dialysis may ultimately be recommended for kidney failure.

Prognosis

The life span of males with Lowe oculocerebrorenal syndrome is limited by their multiple medical problems. Death by middle age is common. However, medical advances are improving the quality of life for individuals with this genetic condition.

Resources

BOOKS

Nussbaum, Robert L., and Sharon Suchy. "The Oculocerebrorenal Syndrome of Lowe (Lowe Syndrome)." *The Metabolic and Molecular Bases of Inherited Disease*. New York: McGraw Hill, 2001.

PERIODICALS

Monnier, Nicole, V. Satre, E. Lerouge, F. Berthoin, and J. Lunardi. "OCRL1 Mutation Analysis in French Lowe Syndrome Patients: Implications for Molecular Diagnosis Strategy and Genetic Counseling." *Human Mutation* 16 (2000) :157–65.

Roschinger, Wulf, A. Muntau, G. Rudolph, A. Roscher, and S. Kammerer. "Carrier Assessment in Families with Lowe Oculocerebrorenal Syndrome: Novel Mutations in the OCRL1 Gene and Correlation of Direct DNA Diagnosis with Ocular Examination." *Molecular Genetics and Metabolism* 69 (2000): 213–22.

ORGANIZATIONS

Alliance of Genetic Support Groups. 4301 Connecticut Ave. NW, Suite 404, Washington, DC 20008. (202) 966-5557. Fax: (202) 966-8553. <http://www.geneticalliance.org>.

Lowe Syndrome Association. 222 Lincoln St., West Lafayette, IN 47906-2732. (765) 743-3634. <http://www.lowesyndrome.org>.

National Organization for Rare Disorders (NORD). PO Box 8923, New Fairfield, CT 06812-8923. (203) 746-6518 or (800) 999-6673. Fax: (203) 746-6481. <http://www.rarediseases.org>.

WEBSITES

On-line Mendelian Inheritance (OMIM). <www.ncbi.nlm.nih.gov/htbin-post/Omim/dispmim?309000>.

Holly Ann Ishmael, MS

Lynch cancer family syndrome
see **Hereditary colorectal cancer**

Lynch syndrome
see **Muir-Torre syndrome**

Lysosomal trafficking regulator
see **Chediak-Higashi syndrome**